Solved Papers

Radiodiagnosis

for PG Students

A must for MD, DNB and DMRD Radiodiagnosis Students

Solved Papers
Radiodiagnosis
for PG Students

A must for MD, DNB and DMRD Radiodiagnosis Students

Soumik Das
DM (Neuroimaging and Interventional Radiology)
MD (Radiodiagnosis) DNB (Radiodiagnosis) MNAMS
Assistant Professor
Department of Radiodiagnosis
IPGME&R and SSKM Hospital
Kolkata, West Bengal, India

Foreword

Barindranath Mallick
MD (Radiodiagnosis)
President
IRIA-West Bengal State Chapter
Professor and Head of the Department
Calcutta National Medical College and Hospital
Kolkata, West Bengal, India

JAYPEE

JAYPEE BROTHERS MEDICAL PUBLISHERS
The Health Sciences Publisher
New Delhi | London

Jaypee Brothers Medical Publishers (P) Ltd

Headquarters
Jaypee Brothers Medical Publishers (P) Ltd
EMCA House, 23/23-B
Ansari Road, Daryaganj
New Delhi 110 002, India
Landline: +91-11-23272143, +91-11-23272703
+91-11-23282021, +91-11-23245672
Email: jaypee@jaypeebrothers.com

Corporate Office
Jaypee Brothers Medical Publishers (P) Ltd
4838/24, Ansari Road, Daryaganj
New Delhi 110 002, India
Phone: +91-11-43574357
Fax: +91-11-43574314
Email: jaypee@jaypeebrothers.com

Overseas Office
J.P. Medical Ltd
83 Victoria Street, London
SW1H 0HW (UK)
Phone: +44 20 3170 8910
Fax: +44 (0)20 3008 6180
Email: info@jpmedpub.com

Website: www.jaypeebrothers.com
Website: www.jaypeedigital.com

Inquiries for bulk sales may be solicited at: jaypee@jaypeebrothers.com

Solved Papers Radiodiagnosis for PG Students

First Edition: **2025**

ISBN: 978-93-6616-431-1

Printed at: Samrat Offset Pvt. Ltd.

Dedicated to

My dearest whose sincere thoughts and silent prayers are always with me.

Contributors

Soumik Das DM (Neuroimaging and Interventional Radiology) MD (Radiodiagnosis) DNB (Radiodiagnosis) MNAMS
Assistant Professor
Department of Radiodiagnosis
IPGME&R and SSKM Hospital
Kolkata, West Bengal, India

Shis Mahammad Pail MD (Radiodiagnosis)
Associate Consultant
Department of Radiodiagnosis
Institute of Neurosciences Kolkata
Kolkata, West Bengal, India

Kasturi Rakshit
Junior Resident
Department of Radiodiagnosis
IPGME&R and SSKM Hospital
Kolkata, West Bengal, India

Lipika Afroz
Junior Resident
Department of Radiodiagnosis
IPGME&R and SSKM Hospital
Kolkata, West Bengal, India

Mehtaab Alam
Junior Resident
Department of Radiodiagnosis
IPGME&R and SSKM Hospital
Kolkata, West Bengal, India

Anisha Sharma
Junior Resident
Department of Radiodiagnosis
IPGME&R and SSKM Hospital
Kolkata, West Bengal, India

Hasibur Rahaman
Junior Resident
Department of Radiodiagnosis
IPGME&R and SSKM Hospital
Kolkata, West Bengal, India

Suparna Sahu MD (Radiodiagnosis) DNB (Radiodiagnosis) EDiR
Senior Resident
Department of Radiodiagnosis
NRS Medical College and Hospital
Kolkata, West Bengal, India

Priyanka Rathore MD (Radiodiagnosis) DNB (Radiodiagnosis)
PDCC Interventional Radiology Resident
Department of Radiodiagnosis
IPGME&R and SSKM Hospital
Kolkata, West Bengal, India

Manideepa Maiti
Junior Resident
Department of Radiodiagnosis
IPGME&R and SSKM Hospital
Kolkata, West Bengal, India

Sayeka Khatun
Junior Resident
Department of Radiodiagnosis
Murshidabad Medical College and Hospital
Berhampore, West Bengal, India

Himadri Shee
Junior Resident
Department of Radiodiagnosis
IPGME&R and SSKM Hospital
Kolkata, West Bengal, India

Rohan Dey
Junior Resident
Department of Radiodiagnosis
IPGME&R and SSKM Hospital
Kolkata, West Bengal, India

Arghya Chattopadhyay
Junior Resident
Department of Radiodiagnosis
IPGME&R and SSKM Hospital
Kolkata, West Bengal, India

Omkar Oraon
Junior Resident
Department of Radiodiagnosis
IPGME&R and SSKM Hospital
Kolkata, West Bengal, India

Sayanwita Majumder
Junior Resident
Department of Radiodiagnosis
IPGME&R and SSKM Hospital
Kolkata, West Bengal, India

Azhar Molla
Junior Resident
Department of Radiodiagnosis
IPGME&R and SSKM Hospital
Kolkata, West Bengal, India

Saikat Sen
Junior Resident
Department of Radiodiagnosis
IPGME&R and SSKM Hospital
Kolkata, West Bengal, India

Foreword

This book, *Solved Papers Radiodiagnosis for PG Students* is a unique comprehensive text for students of Radiodiagnosis appearing for their final MD and DNB examination. The questions over the last 5 years have been classified topic wise at the beginning of each chapter which will give the student an overview of the important questions to be prepared for their final theory examination. The answers are concise and in line with the standard textbooks of "Radiodiagnosis" which will help them to revise the relevant topics prior to the examinations.

Dr Soumik Das is presently attached as an Assistant Professor in the Department of Radiodiagnosis, Institute of Postgraduate Medical Education and Research, Kolkata, West Bengal, India. He has excelled in academics all throughout his career. He is skilled in diagnostic as well as interventional radiology. He is an excellent teacher and is favored by all his students. He is liked by all his colleagues, seniors, and juniors alike for his kind, sensitive, and down-to-earth personality. He is a member of Indian Radiological and Imaging Association (IRIA), Indian Society of Vascular and Interventional Radiology (ISVIR), Indian Society of Neuroradiology (ISNR), Society of Therapeutic Neurointervention (STNI) and National Academy of Medical Sciences (MNAMS). He has several publications in many national and international journals.

I hope that his book will be helpful for all exam-going residents in the subject of "Radiodiagnosis".

I wish him every success in his academic journey and peace and happiness in his life.

Barindranath Mallick
MD (Radiodiagnosis)
President
IRIA-West Bengal State Chapter,
Professor and Head of the Department,
Calcutta National Medical College and Hospital, Kolkata, West Bengal, India

Preface

It gives me immense pleasure and satisfaction to present this book, *Solved Papers Radiodiagnosis for PG Students* before you. The entire book is designed to facilitate preparation of MD and DNB candidates for their final theory examination. You must revise thoroughly covering all important aspects before the final theory examination. It is therefore necessary to know the important topics to emphasize for the examination. Also, it is practically difficult to revise all the topics from standard textbooks before the examination. So, in this book, I have tried to cover the last five years' questions along with their relevant answers in a lucid point-wise manner with schematic diagrams and flowcharts as necessary that can be easily understood, remembered, revised prior to the examinations, and represented in the answer within the time constraints of the examination. I hope that all exam-going residents in the subject of "Radiodiagnosis" will find this review question-answer book comprehensive and useful for theory examination preparation.

I have tried to minimize errors in the book. Inconvenience from any inadvertent errors is deeply regretted.

Any constructive criticism and suggestions from readers are welcome. I will try to incorporate their valuable opinions in the subsequent editions.

Soumik Das

Acknowledgments

I would like to convey my sincere regards and gratitude to Almighty for providing me the opportunity to be a part of the team which created this book.

Firstly, I wish to express my gratitude to my parents, my grandmother, and other family members who continuously encouraged me in all possible ways to carry on this monumentous task. I believe that their blessings are always with me.

I am greatly indebted to my teachers in school. They had a profound influence on my life and character. Their continuous support and motivation helped me to realize my dreams. I would like to pay my tribute to all my outstanding teachers of Ramakrishna Mission Residential College, Narendrapur, Kolkata, West Bengal, India, for their constant encouragement. I would also like to thank all my friends from school and college who have always stood by me in times of need.

I would like to express my gratitude and regards to our respected MBBS teachers of Medical College Kolkata, Kolkata, West Bengal, India. I am also grateful to our faculty, staff, and other teachers for sharing their knowledge and experience during MD (Radiodiagnosis) course in Medical College Kolkata.

I was extremely fortunate to meet Dr. Arun Kumar Gupta Sir at NIMHANS during my DM in Neuroimaging and Interventional Radiology course. His enthusiastic teaching and sharing of experience on the modern-day practice of radiology in various clinical situations motivated me immensely.

I would also like to acknowledge my loving friend, Dr. Sourav Talukder, who has always supported me in every sphere of my life.

It was a God-sent opportunity that Mr. Bikram Sardar, Commissioning Editor of M/s Jaypee Brothers Medical Publishers Pvt. Ltd., New Delhi, India approached me for a book for exam-going students of Radiodiagnosis. I would like to thank him for always guiding me properly in every step of this journey.

I sincerely thank Mr. Sabyasachi Hazra, Associate Director (Publishing) of M/s Jaypee Brothers Medical Publishers Pvt. Ltd., for his prompt support and guidance in making this title a reality in such a short span of time.

I would like to convey my regards to our Director Sir who has always been very encouraging in all academic pursuits. I feel greatly indebted to the Head of the Department of Radiodiagnosis, Prof. Sukharanjan Howlader, other faculty members and colleagues of this institution, who have always stood by me providing moral support and enthusiasm for compilation of this book.

I would like to acknowledge all those residents who have contributed chapters for this book. Without their active support, it was practically impossible to assemble this book in time.

Last but not least, I wish to acknowledge the authors of various textbooks of radiology which I have used for compilation and framing of answers of this book.

I am deeply grateful to Shri Jitendar P Vij (Group Chairman), Mr. Ankit Vij (Managing Director), Mr. MS Mani (Group President), Ms. Pooja Bhandari [Director—Production (Books and Journals)], and Mr. Akhilesh Saxena (Development Editor) of M/s Jaypee Brothers Medical Publishers (P) Ltd., New Delhi, India, for their professional support and dedication to bringing this book to life. Their team has been phenomenal for being there for me round the clock. Without their active help and kind cooperation, compilation of this book would not have been possible.

Soumik Das

Contents

Scan the QR code for detailed Index

CHAPTER

1 Applied Physics in Imaging

Suparna Sahu, Anisha Sharma, Himadri Shee

QUESTIONS

Radiophysics

1. Discuss the biological effects of radiation. What are the AERB guidelines for radiation safety? [6+4] [MD (WBUHS) 24, MD (WBUHS) 23, MD (WBUHS) 21, MD (WBUHS) 20, MD (WBUHS) 18, DNB Dec 21, DNB June 21, AIIMS Dec 23]
2. What is grid? Describe different types of grids and its applications. [2+4+4] [MD (WBUHS) 23, DNB June 21]
3. Write short note on ALARA principle. [5] [MD (WBUHS) 20]
4. Write short note on stationary grid. [5] [MD (WBUHS) 20]
5. Write short note on Autotransformer. [5] [MD (WBUHS) 20]
6. Discuss "AERB Guidelines for X-ray layout". [10] [MD (WBUHS) 20, AIIMS May 23]
7. Describe in detail the various components of X-ray tube with a schematic diagram. What is X-ray and how it is produced? [6+4] [MD (WBUHS) 21]
8. Write short note on wedge filter. [5] [MD (WBUHS) 21]
9. Write in detail the radiographic techniques of the following with a schematic diagram. (a) Towne's view, (b) Skyline view of patella. [5+5] [MD (WBUHS) 21]
10. Write short notes on radiographic intensifying screen and TLD. [10] [MD (WBUHS) 24, MD (WBUHS) 22, MD (WBUHS) 19, AIIMS May 23, DNB Dec 20, DNB June 20]
11. Define scatter radiation. Discuss briefly the parameter which influence scatter radiation and method to reduce scatter radiation. [2+4+4] [MD (WBUHS) 22, AIIMS Dec 24, DNB June 22]
12. What is digital radiography? Discuss its advantages and disadvantages. [3+7] [MD (WBUHS) 22, AIIMS May 24]
13. Handheld digital radiography system. [5]
14. Write short note on zero lead apron. [5] [DNB June 22]
15. Write short note on breast tomosynthesis. [5] [DNB June 22]
16. Write short note on artificial intelligence. [5] [DNB June 22, DNB June 20]
17. Any 5 chest radiographic views. Technique and indications. [10] [DNB Dec 21]
18. Labeled diagram of X-ray tube. Functioning of X-ray tube. Causes of tube failure. [10] [DNB Dec 21]
19. X-ray film. [5] [DNB Dec 21]
20. Computed radiography. [5] [DNB Dec 21]
21. ALARA and eLORA. [5] [DNB Dec 21]
22. (a) Rotating anode tube. (b) Photoelectric effect. [5+5] [DNB Dec 20, DNB June 20]

Ultrasound Imaging

1. What is sonoelastography? Describe the role of sonoelastography in breast and liver diseases. [2+4+4] [MD (WBUHS) 24, MD (WBUHS) 20]
2. Write short note on tissue harmonic imaging. [5] [MD (WBUHS) 20, MD (WBUHS) 21, DNB Dec 20]
3. Define Doppler principle. How Doppler principle application is utilized in medical imaging? [10] [MD (WBUHS) 20]
4. Write short note on ultrasound contrast agent. [5] [DNB Dec 21]
5. Discuss the role of sonoelastography and MR elastography in evaluation of diffuse liver disease. Discuss the role of sonoelastography in evaluation of breast lesion. [6+4] [MD (WBUHS) 22, MD (WBUHS) 20, MD (WBUHS) 17, AIIMS Dec 23, DNB June 22, DNB June 21]
6. Role of sonoelastography in obstetrics and gynecology. [5]
7. Color Doppler artifacts and how to prevent it. [10] [DNB June 22]
8. Ultrasound contrast agents. [5] [MD (WBUHS) 19, AIIMS Dec 24]
9. HIFU—principle and clinical uses. [5] [DNB Dec 21]
10. Principle of color Doppler imaging. [5] [DNB Dec 21]
11. First and second generation of ultrasound contrast agent and its application. [10] [DNB June 21]
12. Ultrasound artifacts. [5] [DNB June 20, AIIMS May 23, AIIMS May 24]
13. PC-PNDT Act and its applications. [5] [DNB June 20, AIIMS May 23, AIIMS May 24, MD (WBUHS) 24]

Computed Tomography

1. Discuss the principle and utility of dual energy CT. [6+4] [MD (WBUHS) 23, MD (WBUHS) 20, MD (WBUHS) 17, AIIMS Dec 23, DNB Dec 20, DNB June 20]
2. Describe the principles of MDCT and various reconstruction methods. What are the techniques of radiation dose reduction? [4+3+3] [RG 18, MD (WBUHS) 22, MD (WBUHS) 21]
3. Briefly outline the evolution of present day CT scanners citing the key specific change through different generations. [10] [MD (WBUHS) 24, MD (WBUHS) 19]
4. Mobile CT scan and its applications. [5]
5. What are the limitations of standard coronary CT scan with a retrospective ECG-gated acquisition? Describe the current and novel imaging strategies to overcome these limitations. [5+5]
6. CT enterography. [5]
7. CT enteric contrast agents. [5] [DNB Dec 21]
8. Cone beam CT. [5] [DNB June 21]

Magnetic Resonance Imaging

1. Discuss the principle of MR spectroscopy in brief and its utility in differentiation of brain lesions. [3 + 7] [MD (WBUHS) 23, MD (WBUHS) 19, DNB June 20]
2. Write short note on DTI. [5] [MD (WBUHS) 24, MD (WBUHS) 20]
3. Write short note on MR perfusion. [5]
4. Discuss the principle of MR perfusion. Elaborate the role of MR perfusion in neuroimaging. [4+6] [MD (WBUHS) 21, MD (WBUHS) 20]
5. Write in brief the basic principle and application of various MRI sequence. [10] [MD (WBUHS) 19]
6. Discuss the principle of diffusion weighted imaging and its utility in differentiation of brain lesions. [3+7] [MD (WBUHS) 22, DNB Dec 21, DNB June 21]
7. Briefly describe the techniques of MR neurography and black blood imaging of brain. [5+5]
8. What are the advantages and limitations of 3T over 1.5T MRI? Briefly discuss MRI safety. [6+4] [DNB June 21]
9. Pulmonary MRI. [5]

10. Hepatobiliary MRI contrast agents. [5] [MD (WBUHS) 24]
11. What is K-space and various techniques using it?
12. Chemical shift imaging in MRI—technique, advantages, and disadvantages. [10] [DNB June 22]
13. Various fat suppressed sequence—describe them. [10] [DNB June 22]
14. MR perfusion techniques. [10] [DNB June 22, MD (WBUHS) 24]
15. Parallel imaging and its use. [10] [DNB June 22]
16. Principle and pitfalls of TOF-MRA. [5] [DNB Dec 21]
17. (a) What is nephrogenic systemic fibrosis, (b) risk factors for NSF, and (c) method of prevention? [10] [DNB June 21]
18. MR artifacts. [5] [DNB June 21, DNB Dec 20]
19. (a) Describe the principle and technique of phase contrast MR angiography. (b) Discuss its advantages, limitations and clinical applications. [2+2+2+2+2] [DNB June 20]

Digital Subtraction Angiography

1. DSA—basic principles and role in radiological interventions. [5+5] [MD (WBUHS) 23]
2. Write short note on Seldinger technique. [5] [MD (WBUHS) 24, MD (WBUHS) 21]
3. Write short note on pulse fluoroscopy. [5] [DNB June 22]
4. Describe image intensifier with the help of a diagram and briefly discuss its properties and limitations. [5+2+3] [MD (WBUHS) 24, DNB Dec 20]

Contrast Media

1. Discuss about the radiographic contrast media. [10] [MD (WBUHS) 22, MD (WBUHS) 21, DNB Dec 18, AIIMS May 24, AIIMS May 23]
2. How will you manage a patient with acute radiographic contrast media reaction? [10] [DNB Dec 21, DNB Dec 20, DNB June 20, MD (WBUHS) 19, RG 18, AIIMS Dec 24]

Miscellaneous

1. Write short note on PACS. [5] [MD (WBUHS) 20]
2. Write in brief about problem of storage requirements in PACS. Describe its solutions. [5+5] [MD (WBUHS) 22]
3. Discuss postmortem imaging and its applications. [10] [AIIMS May 24]
4. Technique, indications, contraindications and complications of HSG. [10] [DNB June 21]

Recent Advances

1. Discuss the principle and clinical application of PET-CT. [3+7] [MD (WBUHS) 23, MD (WBUHS) 21, MD (WBUHS) 20, MD (WBUHS) 18, DNB Dec 21, DNB Dec 18]
2. Write short note on fusion imaging. [5] [MD (WBUHS) 20, AIIMS Dec 24]
3. High-intensity focused ultrasound (HIFU): principle, instrumentation, and its applications. [3+3+4] [MD (WBUHS) 21]
4. (a) Principle of RFA, (b) application in benign and malignant lesions. [10] [DNB June 21, MD (WBUHS) 18]
5. Recent developments in noninvasive lymphatic imaging techniques for visualizing the central lymphatic anatomy and flow dynamics. [10] [DNB Dec 20]
6. PET-MRI. [5] [DNB June 20, DNB Dec 18]

ANSWERS

Radiophysics

1. Discuss the biological effects of radiation. What are the AERB guidelines for radiation safety? [6+4] [MD (WBUHS) 24, MD (WBUHS) 23, MD (WBUHS) 21, MD (WBUHS) 20, MD (WBUHS) 18, DNB Dec 21, DNB June 21, AIIMS Dec 23]

Radiation interacts with cell (basic unit of life) and produces various biological effects.
The knowledge about biological effects will help us to minimize the exposure and its effects while working in the field of radiation.

Types of Ionizing Radiation

- **Indirectly ionizing radiations:**
  - X- and gamma rays—electromagnetic radiations
  - Neutrons—uncharged particles
- **Directly ionizing radiations:**
  - Electrons, protons—charged particles
  - Both types of radiation transfer part or all of their energy when they interact with matter.

The smallest unit of body is called a cell.
The most sensitive organelle of the cell is the nucleus.
- Nucleus contains 46 thread like structures which are called chromosomes
- Each chromosome contains one very complex sensitive molecule called deoxyribonucleic acid (DNA)

DNA is the ultimate sensitive target molecule
- When DNA is damaged by radiation, its coded language is also damaged resulting in death of cell or abnormal modification of cell.

Mechanisms of Induction of Radiation Damage

- **Direct effect**: Due to direct deposition of energy in the Target Molecule—Deoxyribonucleic Acid-DNA. Proportion of Direct Effect ≈30%
- **Indirect effect**: Due to deposition of energy in the surrounding water and reaction of free radical formed in the water with the Target Molecule—DNA Proportion of Indirect Effect ≈70%

Effects also depend on Radiation Quality

- Charged particles like α and protons are more harmful
- Uncharged particles like X and γ are relatively less harmful

Damage due to exposure may lead to the following **(Fig. 1)**
- Inhibition of cell division

Delay or inhibit the process of cell division, which may impair the functions of tissues or organs
- Chromosome aberrations lead to rearrangement of genetic information. Serve as biological dosimeter (detectable above 100 mSv)
- Gene mutation—alteration in the information content of genes
  - Cell death

Some Tissues are More Sensitive than Others [Radiosensitivity (RS)]

- High RS—Bone marrow, spleen, thymus, lymphatic nodes, gonads, lymphocytes (exception to the RS laws)
- Medium RS—Skin, mesoderm organs (liver, heart, and lungs)
- Low RS—Muscle, bones, nervous system

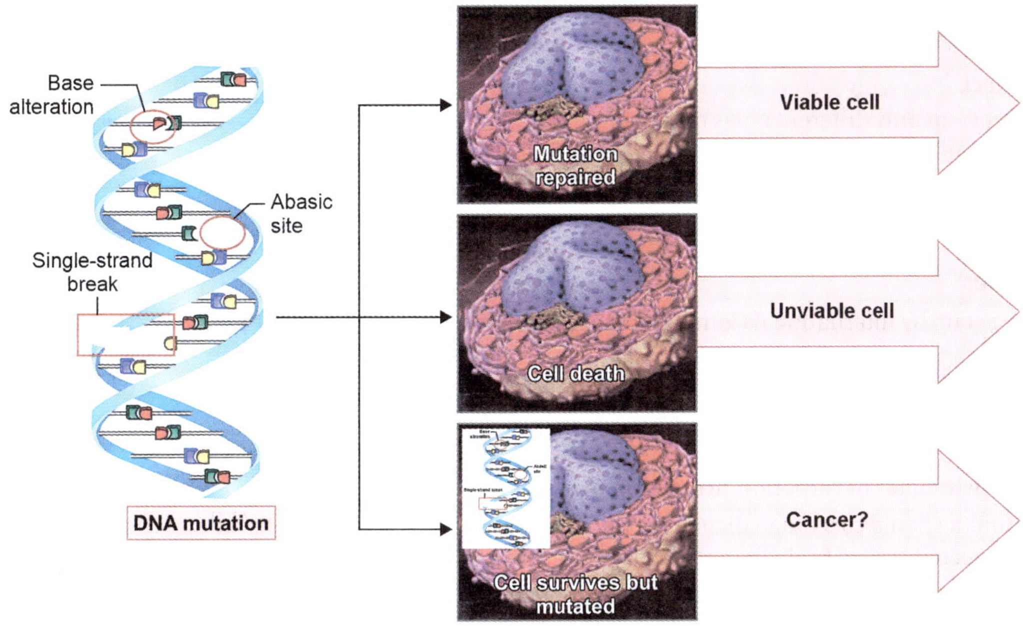

FIG. 1: Outcomes after cell exposure to radiation.

Biological Effects of Ionizing Radiation (Table 1)

TABLE 1: Biological effects of ionizing radiation.

Deterministic (Threshold/non-stochastic) 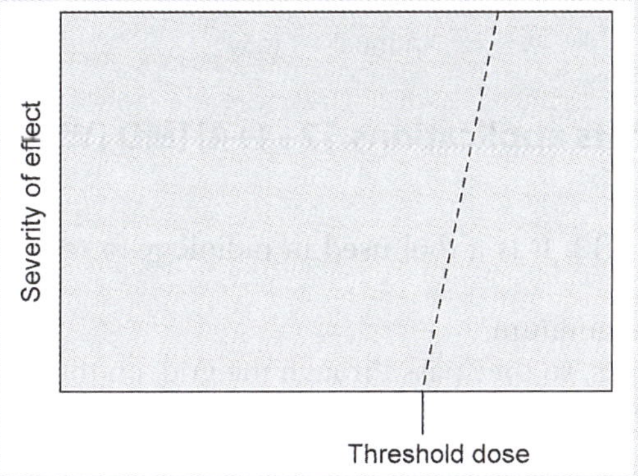 	Existence of a dose threshold value (below this dose, the effect is not observable) • Severity of the effect increases with dose • A large number of cells are involved, e.g., lens opacities, skin injuries, infertility, epilation, etc. Due to cell killing • Have a dose threshold typically several Gy • Specific to particular tissues • Severity of harm is dose dependent Cataracts of the lens of the eye 2–10 Gy Permanent sterility in males 3.5–6 Gy and in females 2.5–6 Gy Temporary sterility in males 0.15 Gy and in females 0.6 Gy
Stochastic (non-threshold) 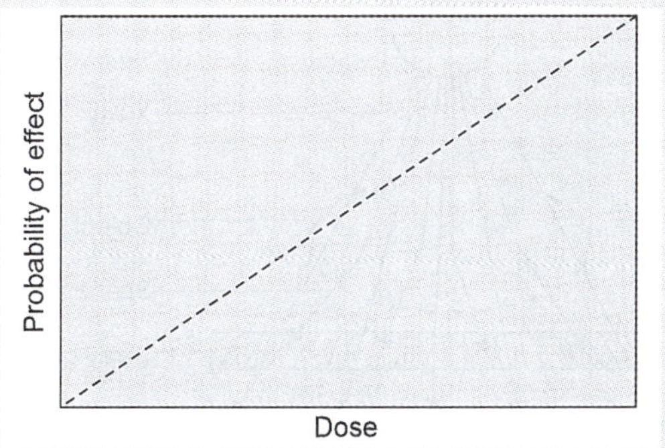 	No threshold dose for occurrence • Probability of the effect increases with dose • Generally occurs with a single cell, e.g., cancer, genetic effects • Due to cell changes (DNA) and proliferation towards a malignant disease • Severity (example cancer) independent of the dose • No dose threshold—applicable also to very small doses • Probability of effect increases with dose

Stochastic effects: Categorized as per the cell affected

- **Somatic effect**
  - Early effect
  - Late effect—mainly different types of cancer
- **Hereditary (genetic) effect**
  - Late effect—chromosomal aberrations
  - 3-5 Gy Lethal Dose (LD 50/60)

AERB Guidelines

Guidelines are set up by International Commission of Radiological Protection (ICRP)

Aims of radiological protection

- To prevent deterministic effects
- To limit the occurrence of stochastic effects to acceptable limits

Three cardinal principles of radiation protection are

1. **Justification**: It should carry high diagnostic information so that the risk benefit ratio becomes high, e.g., role of CT brain in suspected case of brain hemorrhage.

   Levels of justification are there—first-doing more good than no harm to society, second-justification of the procedure in improving diagnosis or treatment, thirdly-application of the procedure to individual
2. **Optimization**: As low as reasonably achievable—ALARA, appropriate selection of methods, design, construction in day-to-day practice
3. **Dose limitation**: To set the maximum permissible dose **(Table 2)**.

AERB Dose Limits

TABLE 2: AERB dose limits for occupational worker and public.

Occupational worker	100 mSv for 5-year period	Annual—30 mSv
Public	1 mSv/yr for 5 years	Annual—1 mSv

2. What is grid? Describe different types of grids and its applications. [2+4+4] [MD (WBUHS) 23, DNB June 21]

Grid—radiographic grid was invented by Dr Gustave Bucky in 1913. It is a tool used in radiology to reduce scatter radiation.[1]

These are made of lead stripes with the interspace is made by aluminum.

Primary radiation is oriented in the same axis of the lead stripes, so they pass through the grid, on the other hand scatter radiation arises from patient in multiple direction, these are mostly absorbed by lead **(Fig. 2)**.

Types of grids with its applications:

Parallel Grids

In these types of grids, the lead strips are all oriented parallel to one another. When such a grid is used at excessively short focus-film distances, the more slanting rays towards the periphery of beam strike the sides of the more peripheral lead strips called peripheral cut off.

To counter this problem focused grids are used.

Focused Grid

The focused grid is designed to minimize the problem of peripheral grid cut off as in case of parallel grid. The focused grid is composed of strips of lead angled towards the edge so that they lie on imaging lines of the divergent X-ray beam.

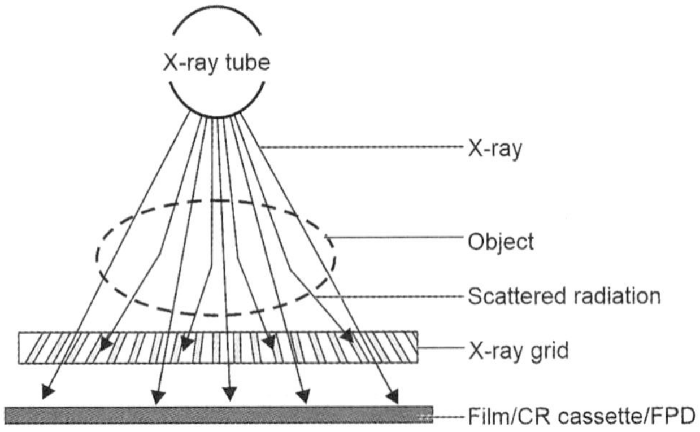

FIG. 2: X-ray grid and its relative position with respect to the X-ray tube, object (patient) and cassette.

X-ray focused grid is marked with its intended focal distance and the side of the grid that should face the X-ray tube. If radiographs are made at distances other than those specified by the manufacturer of the grid, cut off will occur.

Crossed Grids

Linear grids clean up scattered radiation in only one direction, which is along the axis of grid. Crossed grids are made to overcome this problem. These grids consist of two parallel or focused grids placed at right angle to one another. Positioning of the grid is critical; the central ray of the X-ray beam must coincide with the center of grid.

Moving Grids

- Hollis S Potter suggested the idea of moving the grid while the X-ray exposure is being made.
- A shortcoming of the stationary grids is that they produce grid lines on the radiograph.
- Grid lines are the images made when primary X-rays are absorbed in the grid strips.
- A device that moves grid during exposure is called moving grid/Potter bucky diaphragm/bucky diaphragm.
- To be effective the grid must move side to side, perpendicular to the level strips. Moving grids are usually focused grids.

Three basic types of moving grid mechanisms:

1. **Single stroke grid**: A single stroke mechanism causes the grid to move continuously across the film while the X-ray exposure is being made. Usually, it is spring loaded and requires a manual cocking of the mechanism before each exposure. They are not used in modern radiographic equipment.
2. **Reciprocating grid**: A reciprocating grid is a moving grid that is motor driven. It does not require resetting after each exposure. This is the most commonly used grid in modern radiographic equipment.
3. **Oscillating grid**: The main difference between reciprocating and oscillating grids is their pattern of motion. The motion of a reciprocating grid is to and fro whereas that of an oscillating grid is circular.

3. Write short note on ALARA Principle. [5] [MD (WBUHS) 20]

ALARA principle—full form—as low as reasonably achievable.

This principle was established in 1954 by NCRP (National Council on Radiation Protection).

Now-a-days it is considered as the main guideline for radiation protection.

Cardinal Factors Comprise ALARA

1. Time
2. Distance
3. Shielding

1. **Time**: Exposure time should be kept minimum.
   Exposure = Exposure rate X time
   So, it is proportional in relation.
2. **Distance**: Exposure is inversely proportional to the square of distance, so distance should be large
   exposure ∞ $1/D^2$
3. **Shielding**: The concept is to put a barrier between the radiation source and exposed person.
   Commonly used materials are lead, concrete, and barium plaster.

Types of shielding:

1. Shielding of X-ray source/tube
2. Shielding of control room
3. Shielding of the personnel (example, lead apron, thyroid shield, and glove)
4. Shielding of patient

In USA, the concept of ALARA has modified as ALARP—as low as reasonably practicable.

AERB Dose Limit (Table 3)

TABLE 3: AERB Dose limits for occupational worker and public.

Dose limit	*Occupational workers*	*Public*
5 years	100 mSV	1 mSV/year
Annual	30 mSV	1 mSV

4. Write short note on stationary grid. [5] [MD (WBUHS) 20]

Stationary Grid

- In 1913, Gustav Bucky introduced fixed or stationary grid.
- It is made of strips of lead arranged in two parallel series that intersected at right angles. The modern stationary grid is made of closely spaced extremely thin lead stripes separated by radiolucent material, usually plastic or aluminum.
- The grid may be a parallel grid, in which the lead strips are parallel to each other, or a focused grid, in which the lead strips are angled toward the center.
- Disadvantage of the stationary grid is that the lead strips leave "blank" or white lines on the film. Known as "grid lines."
- Solution of these problem is moving grid, conceptualized Dr Hollis Potter in 1920.

Attachment: A moving grid is attached to the table while a stationary grid is placed on a radiographic cassette.

Grid type: Low-frequency grids are used with moving grids, while medium and high-frequency grids are used with stationary grids.

Use: Mainly used in portable radiography, mammography.

5. Write short note on autotransformer. [5] [MD (WBUHS) 20]

Transformer **(Fig. 3)** is one of the major components of X-ray generator. The main role of the generator is to provide electrical power to the X-ray tube by which selection of X-ray energy, quantity, etc., are done.[2]

Transformer "transforms" an input voltage to output voltage.

It follows the principle of electromagnetic induction.

Generic transformer is composed of two electrically insulated wires wrapped around iron core.

Autotransformer is composed of an iron core wrapped by a single coil which is attached to a power source.

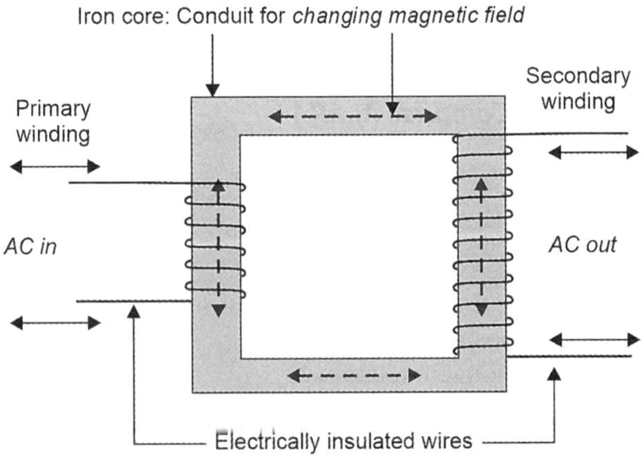

FIG. 3: Transformer.

Simple autotransformer has fixed number of input turns and several output taps to provide variable output of lower voltage.

Switching transformer **(Fig. 4)** has several taps on both input and output sides, making it more flexible. It is also possible to change the output voltage either down or up in relation to input in small increments.

6. Discuss "AERB guidelines for X-ray layout". [10] [MD (WBUHS) 20, AIIMS May 23]

From radiation protection view every imaging unit should be planned and functioned according to the guidelines of AERB **(Fig. 5)**.

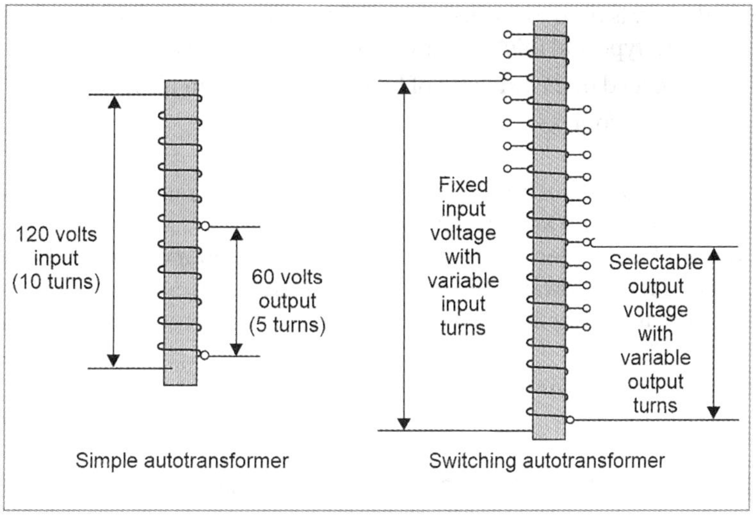

FIG. 4: Switching transformer.

Area should be divided into three regions:

1. Public area
2. Staff area
3. Work area

Radiation safety is important in diagnostic radiology, not only because of regulatory requirements but also because of radiation workers, members of public and patient safety considerations.

In radiation protection, the guiding philosophy is ALARA (as low as reasonably achievable).

In diagnostic radiology, the main source of occupational exposure is scattered radiation from the patient—particularly in fluoroscopically guided procedures.

The objective of radiation shielding in diagnostic X-ray facilities is to protect:

- Workers of X-ray department
- Members of the public
- Persons working adjacent to or near the X-ray facility

The purpose of layout planning of medical X-ray facility is to ensure that radiation exposure to radiation workers and members of the public does not exceed the dose limits prescribed by competent authority (i.e., Chairman, AERB).

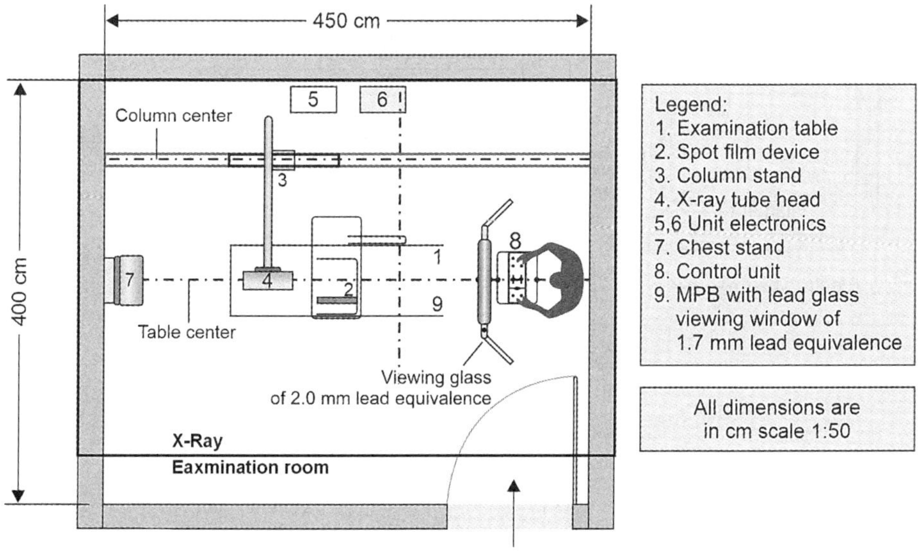

FIG. 5: AERB guidelines for X-ray installation layout.

Shielding in diagnostic radiology is used to reduce exposure to radiation workers and the members of general public. The decision to utilize shielding, its type and thickness are functions of photon energy and intensity of ionizing radiation.

- Room shielding done by 2 mm lead or 25 mm later of high-quality barium plaster
- 225 mm of solid brick/150 mm of concrete
- ½ brick and ½ inch plaster

The room housing an X-ray unit shall not be <18 m^2 for general-purpose radiography and conventional fluoroscopy equipment and no single dimension of the X-ray room shall be <4.0 m.

There shall be no windows and ventilation shall be above 2 m from the floor outside. Table shall be oriented such that the primary (chest stand) is not directed towards the main door or darkroom.

The users should procure and use protective accessories such as mobile protective barriers, lead rubber aprons, lead rubber flaps, gloves, thyroid shields, etc.

All walls of the examination room are 23 cm (9 inch) thick—made of bricks.

Single leaf door lined with 2.0 mm lead.

7. Describe in detail the various components of X-ray tube with a schematic diagram. What is X-ray and how it is produced? [6+4] [MD (WBUHS) 21]

X-ray tube is a device in which X-rays are produced on the principle of energy conversion.

X-rays are produced when a fast-moving stream of electrons is suddenly decelerated in the "target" anode of an X-ray tube.

In this process, only 1% energy converted into X-rays; remaining 99% energy converted into heat.

Structure of X-ray Tube (Fig. 6)

External structure: Consists of three parts:

1. Support structure
2. Protective housing
3. Glass or metal envelope

Internal structure:

- **Cathode assembly***:* Electrically negative

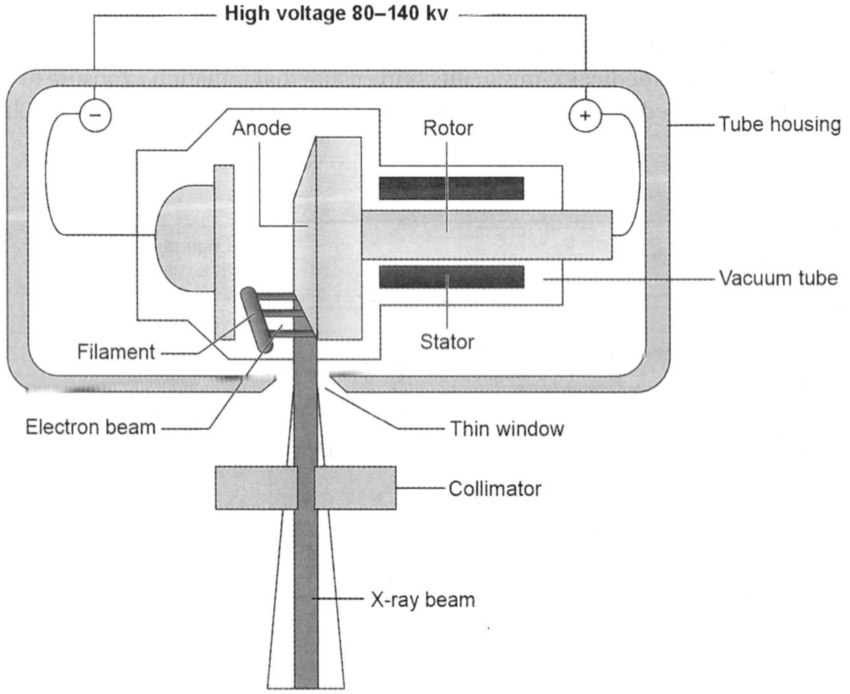

FIG. 6: Schematic diagram of X-ray tube.

- **Filament**:
  - Filament is made of tungsten wire 10–20 mm in length and 2–5 mm in width.
  - Tungsten is used because of:
    - High-melting point = 3370°C
    - Ductile-can be drawn into thin but strong wires
    - Little tendency to vaporize
    - Trace of thorium in the tungsten filament increases the efficiency of electron emission and prolongs life.

A low-voltage circuit (also provided by the generator) produces a current (filament current) through a wire filament at the cathode of the tube. The current in the wire filament causes it to heat up and emit electrons, a process called thermionic emission.

Modern tubes are dual filament and dual focal spot tubes

Only one filament is activated for a given exposure.

- **Larger filament**: To accommodate imaging applications that require high X-ray tube output in a short exposure time
- **Smaller filament**: For use in applications in which resolving capability is crucial or in which motion blurring is not a concern.
- **Connecting wires**: Filament current (low voltage, high ampere) supply 10 V voltage and 3–5 A current to heat the filament up to 2200°C.
- **Focusing cup**: It is negatively charged concave metal (Ni) cup behind the filament light weight, poor thermal conductivity and high melting point. Confines the electrons to a narrow beam and focuses them on a small focal spot on the target.
- **Anode**: It has positive electrical charge and attract electrons.

Purpose of Anode

1. Serves as a target surface for the high-voltage electrons
2. Conducts the high-voltage from the cathode back into the X-ray generator circuit
3. Serves as the primary thermal conductor

Focal spots—large or small.

Tungsten is chosen as the target material for general radiography because of its high atomic number and high melting point.

Tungsten is typically alloyed with 10% rhenium to improve its resistance to thermal damage.

Tungsten is not a good conductor and is usually used as a thin overlay on a molybdenum substrate (for a rotating anode) or as a thin inlay within a copper substrate (for a fixed anode).

Stationary Anode

- Limited heat capacity
- Low energy applications
  - Dental—Tungsten target as a thin inlay in a copper substrate.

Rotating Anode

- Tungsten target
- Mo disc and stem—make anode light, high melting point and poor heat conductor
- Length of stem—short as possible, decrease inertia
- Backed by graphite—improves heat loading

Rotating assembly (stator and rotor) with Ag as lubricant and ball bearings at both ends.

Heat loss by radiation to glass envelope and then by conduction to oil bath.

X-ray: It is a type of electromagnetic radiation having smaller wavelengths.

It has sinusoidally varying electric field and magnetic field travelling at right angles to each other and perpendicular to the direction of propagation.

TABLE 4: Mechanism of X-ray production.

<table>
<tr><td>
Bremsstrahlung radiation

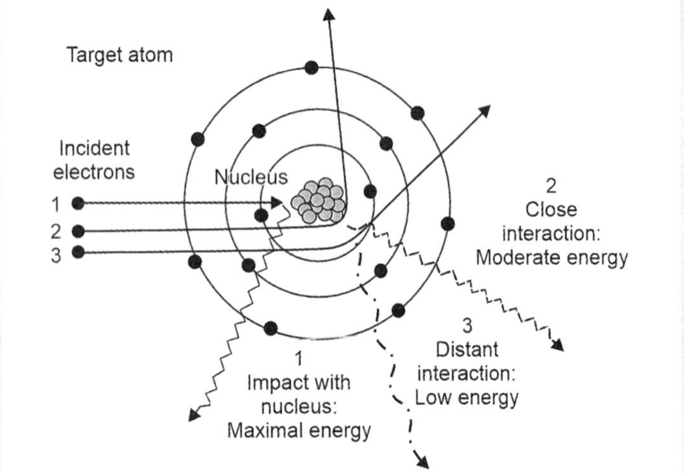

</td><td>

- In the Bremsstrahlung (brake radiation or general radiation), moving electron is deflected by the attractive force of the nucleus of an atom
- This causes the electron to lose energy in the form of radiation
- Contributes maximum to the X-rays produced
- This radiation is polyenergetic and heterogenous
- The energy of this X-ray is determined by the proximity of the electron to the nucleus
- Maximum energy of X-ray beam = energy of incoming electron, these determined by the tube potential
- The deceleration also depends upon atomic number of Target
- Tungsten is a common target material, chosen both for its high atomic number (Z = 74) and its high melting point
</td></tr>
<tr><td>
Characteristic radiation

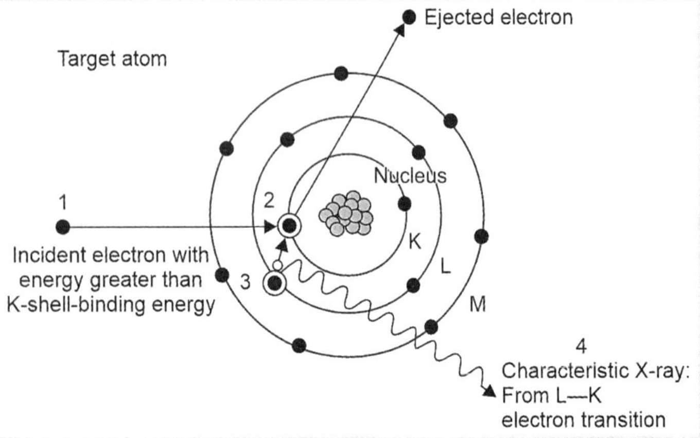

</td><td>

- Electron beam strikes an inner shell electron of an atom to eject it out
- The void filled by another electron from an outer orbit
- Difference in the energy is emitted as radiation
- This term is used because the energy of resulting X-ray is the characteristic of the atom from which it is originated
- The energy of X-ray = binding energy of the destination shell-binding energy of the origination shell
- For characteristic X-rays to be produced, the energy of the accelerated electrons must exceed the K-shell binding energy of the target material (69.4 keV for tungsten, 20 keV for molybdenum)
- When an electron from an outer shell falls toward the nucleus to fill an inner vacancy, the excess energy can also be released to an orbital electron. When this occurs, and the electron is ejected from the atom, it is called Auger electron
</td></tr>
</table>

- It is an indirectly ionizing EM radiation.
- Wilhelm Conrad Roentgen discovered X-rays on November 8, 1895.
- He called them X-rays, because the letter x represents unknown in mathematics.
- X-rays are produced when a fast-moving stream of electrons is suddenly decelerated in the "target" anode of an X-ray tube.
- In this process, only 1% energy converted into X-rays; remaining 99% energy converted into heat.

X-rays may be produced by two mechanisms **(Table 4)**:

1. Bremsstrahlung radiation
2. Characteristic radiation

8. Write short note on Wedge filter. [5] [MD (WBUHS) 21]

Filters are used to absorb low energy X-ray so that high energy X-rays are used to produce the image, the process by which mean energy of the X-ray beam is increased is called beam hardening.

Usually, aluminum is used as material for filter.

Wedge filter **(Fig. 7)** is most commonly used compensating filter, used in specific regions or body parts having variable tissue thickness.

- It is to ensure uniform exposure along the body part.
- Shape-wedge
- Less radiation is absorbed by the thinner part of the filter so more amount of X-ray is transmitted through the thicker part.

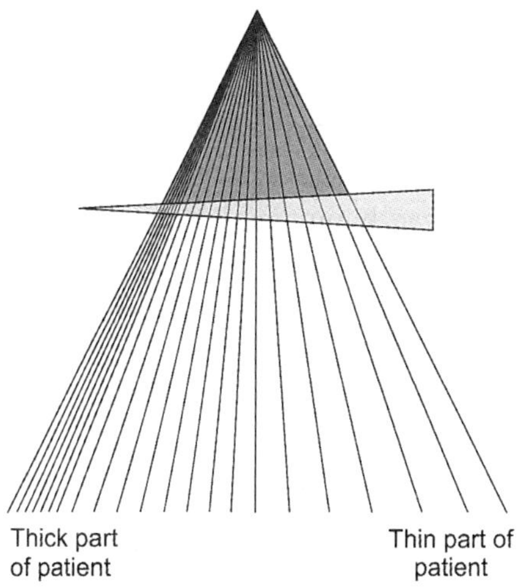

FIG. 7: Wedge filter.

Uses

1. Fluoroscopy
2. Imaging of upper and lower thorax
3. Foot and ankle
4. Lower limb angiography

9. Write in detail the radiographic techniques of the following with a schematic diagram. a) Towne's View, b) Skyline view of patella. [5+5] [MD (WBUHS) 21]

Towne's View

This is an angled anteroposterior view of skull **(Figs. 8 and 9)**

Indication

- Posterior fossa is well visualized in this view, lambdoid suture
- Used to see medial or lateral displacement in cases of skull fracture
- Any displacement of sutures in case of neoplastic cause or Paget disease

Structures Seen

1. Petrous part of pyramids
2. Posterior clinoid process
3. Dorsum sellae

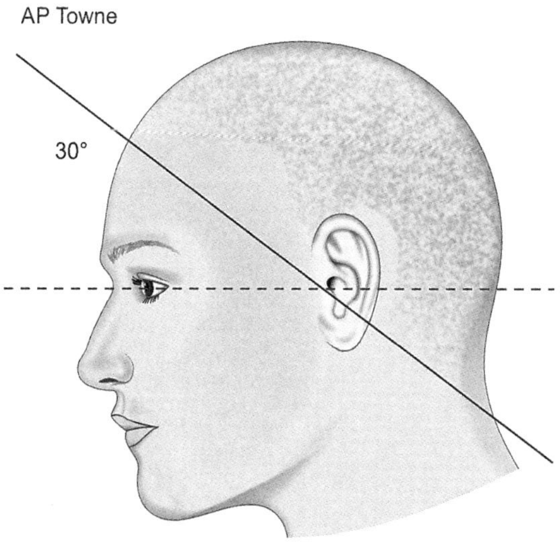

FIG. 8: Schematic diagram of Towne's view.

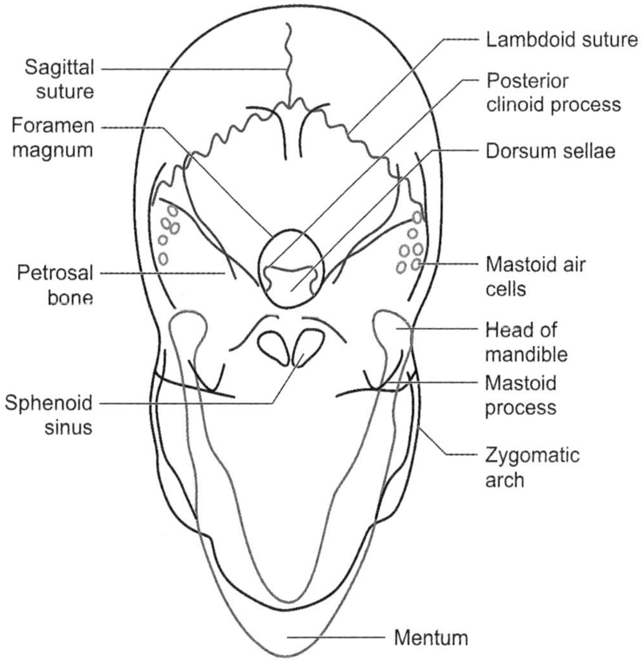

FIG. 9: Main structures seen in Towne's view.

Technique

Patient Position

- Patient supine or sitting erect
- Nuchal ridge is placed against the image detector
- Infraorbitomeatal line perpendicular to the receptor
- Beam 30 degree caudal to orbitomeatal line or 37 degrees caudal to infraorbitomeatal line.

Technical Aspects

- **Centering point**: Equidistance from external auditory meatus through foramen magnum
- **Collimation**:
  - Upper—skull vertex
  - Inferior—foramen magnum
- **Detector**: 24 × 30 cm
- **Grid**: Used

Skyline View

The skyline or axial view of the patella-femoral joint shows valuable information about its shape and anatomy. It gets a piece of the patella's axial projection (kneecap). It works well for patients who can stay in a semi-reclined (half-lying down) position on the examination table **(Figs. 10A and B)**.

- **Tube tilt**: 10° cephalad
- **Patient position**: Prone. The knee is fully flexed. If the patient is unable to fully flex the knee, angle the CR cephalad so that a 45° angle exists between the lower leg and the CR.
- **CR**: Set the CR between the patella and the femoral condyles. Center film to the CR.

Indication

- This view is used in trauma and orthopedics to check for patellar fractures or subluxations and patellofemoral joint disease.
- To identify infections, osteoporosis, bone abnormalities, or abnormal bone development.
- To diagnose dislocation of the knee.

Technical Factors

- **Superior-inferior axial projection**
- **Centering point**: The central ray will be angled 160° from the vertical axis (or 30° from horizontal) superior-inferior toward the base of the patella.

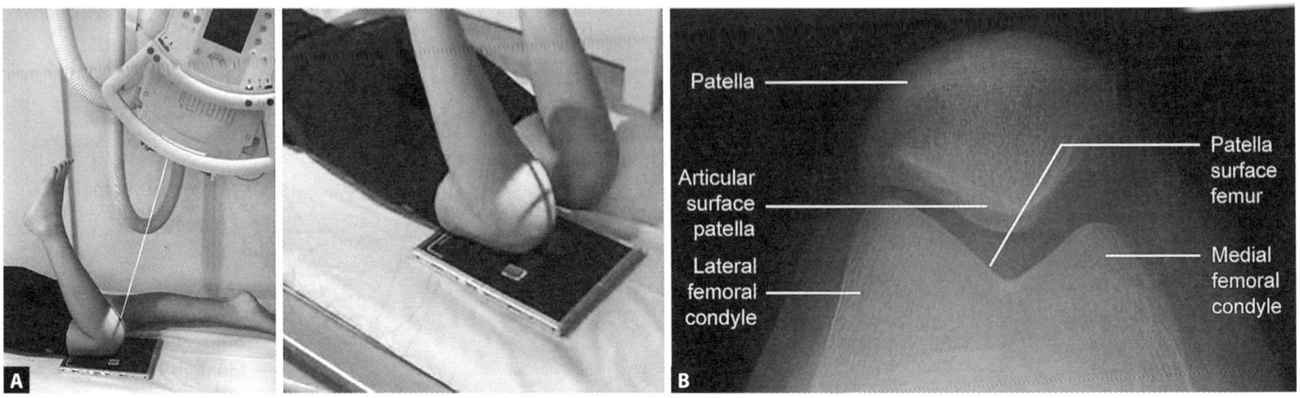

FIGS. 10A and B: (A) Skyline view of patella; (B) Main structures seen in skyline view of patella.

- **Collimation**
  - Laterally to include the skin margins of the knee
  - Inferior to include the femoropatellar joint space
  - Superior to include skin margin
- **Orientation**: Landscape
- **Detector size**: 18 cm × 24 cm
- **Exposure**
- **SID**
  - 100–120 cm
- **Grid**: Not used

10. Write short notes on radiographic intensifying screen and TLD. [10] [MD (WBUHS) 24, MD (WBUHS) 22, MD (WBUHS) 19, AIIMS May 23, DNB Dec 20, DNB June 20]

Radiographic Intensifying Screen

Radiographic Screens—Crucial Component of Radiography

Problem of low sensitivity of X-ray films was overcome with the help of intensifying screen which not only improve the image quality but also significantly reduced the radiation exposure

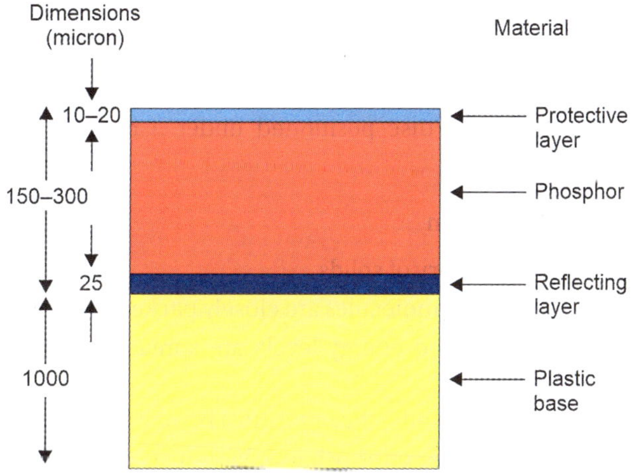

FIG. 11: Layers of intensifying screen.

Basic components of screen **(Fig. 11)**:

1. **Base or support**: Made of polyester or cardboard provides structural support, withstand handling or mechanical stress
2. **Reflecting coat**: Made of titanium oxide or barium sulphate, about 1 mL thick, interaction of X-ray with phosphor produce light, this layer helps in reflecting the light to the front of the screen
3. **Phosphor layer**: Central layer, made of phosphor which convert X-ray to light, when X-rays interact with phosphor crystal—fluorescence—emits light

   Original phosphor-calcium tungstate, recently rare earth phosphor-gadolinium oxysulfide, thallium activated lanthanum oxybromide used, these are high speed screen. X-ray to light conversion efficiency of rare earth screens is significantly high.
4. **Protective layer**:
   - Layer over phosphor to provide protection from static electricity, physical damage.
   - Largely made of cellulose mixed with another polymer.
   - Because of this layer, screens can be cleaned without damaging the phosphor layer.

It is important to note that the color of the light emitted (wavelength) must match the light sensitivity of the film used. This is known as spectral matching:

- **Conventional films**: Sensitive to ultraviolet and blue lights
- **Orthochromatic films**: Sensitive to ultraviolet, blue and green light

  Intensification factor: Measure of reduction of dose reduction with use of screen

  Intrinsic conversion efficiency ratio of light energy emitted by crystals to X-ray absorbed, as for example—calcium tungstate—5%

  Screen efficiency: Ability of the light to escape screen and expose film

To check adequacy of screen—film contact—simply a piece of wire can be kept over cassette and radiograph taken-sharpness of image denoted the contact.

Thermoluminescent Dosimeters

Thermoluminescence: The property of certain materials to emit light when they are stimulated by heat.

Materials

- Lithium fluoride (LiF),
- Lithium borate ($Li_2B_4O_7$),
- Calcium fluoride (CaF_2), and
- Calcium sulfate ($CaSO_4$)
  Known as phosphors

General Features of TLD Badge

- Consists of a TLD card loaded in a cassette
- **TLD card**: Teflon discs mechanically clipped over three symmetrical circular holes on a nickel plated aluminum plate.
- **TLD cassette**: Made of high impact plastic **(Fig. 12)**
  - The first disc sandwiched between a pair of filter combination of 1 mm Al and 0.9 mm Cu
  - The second disc sandwiched between a pair of 1.5 mm thick plastic filters
  - The third disc positioned under a circular open window

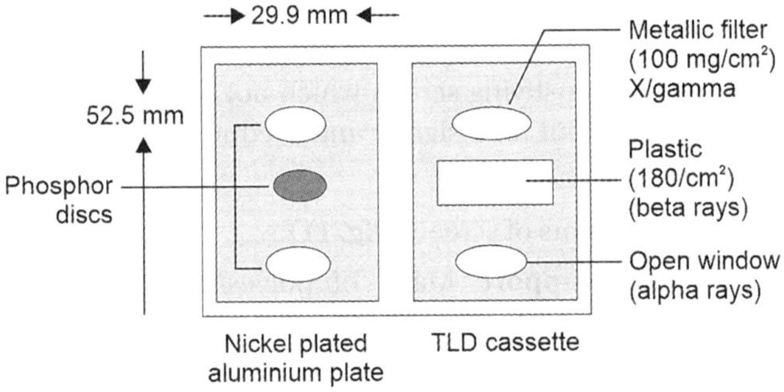

FIG. 12: TLD cassette.

TLD—Mechanism

- Band theory of solids
- In a solid, molecules are closely packed together
- The allowed energy levels are spread into energy bands
- Valence band—the outermost band which is occupied by electrons is completely filled
- **Next higher energy band**: Vacant and is referred into as conduction band
- **Between the two energy bands**: Forbidden zone—electrons are forbidden to stay here
- Impurities are added deliberately which introduce discrete energy shells within the forbidden zone that were previously unoccupied → electron traps
- Irradiation → excitation → electrons are raised from the valence band → conduction band
- If electron comes in the vicinity of an impure atom, it is trapped
- By application of heat → a hole is created in the vicinity of the electron trap → electron falls back into the valence band → energy given in the form of light

Measurement

- Intensity of light is plotted as a function of the temperature **(Fig. 13)** → **Glow curve**
- Highest peak, area under the curve ∞ the energy of the radiation.

Annealing Effects

400 C for 1 hour

- Resets trap structure
- Eliminates any electrons in residual traps

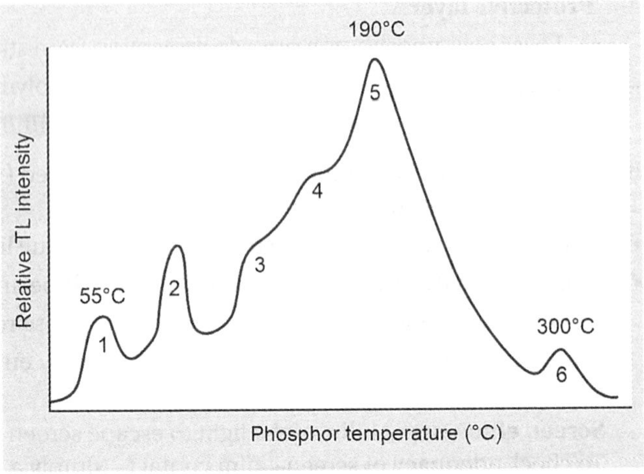

FIG. 13: Measurement of radiation absorbed by TLD badge.

Reused

How to Use

Whenever working in the radiation field, TLD badge should be always worn by the person TLD badge should not be shared

Control: Each institution should keep apart one TLD card loaded in a TLD holder as **CONTROL** which is required for correct dose evaluation

- **The control badge**: Stored in a radiation free area—no likelihood of any radiation exposure

Where to wear

During radiography

- TLD is worn anteriorly
    - At the level of upper chest below the lead apron

During fluoroscopy

- A protective apron should always be worn
- Ideally two dosimeters should be used
- At the collar level outside the lead apron
- At the level of trunk underneath the lead apron
- **Collar level badge**: dose reading to the unprotected regions of head and neck
- **Trunk level badge**: dose reading to the protected organs
- If only one dosimeter is worn it must be worn inside the lead apron.

11. Define scatter radiation. Discuss briefly the parameter which influence scatter radiation and method to reduce scatter radiation. [2+4+4] [MD (WBUHS) 22, AIIMS Dec 24, DNB June 22]

Scatter Radiation

Definition: In the diagnostic energy range (10–100 kev), the interactions are always with orbital electrons. It can be-transmitted, absorbed, scattered.

X-ray image formed by transmitted photons, scatter radiation is produced by the electrons which are deflected from their original path and loose some energy.

This secondary radiation makes no contribution to the formation of images but they reduce overall image contrast and produce fog.

Characteristics

1. Isotropic in energy in all direction
2. Can not be removed by grid or filters
3. They are result of Compton scattering (diagnostic energy X-ray) or coherent scattering (low energy X-ray)
4. Compton scatter travels in all direction, most of it travels in a forward direction
5. More oblique in nature
6. With increase in energies energy of primary radiation more scatter in forward direction
7. Amount of scatter depends on:
    - Volume of tissue
    - Thickness of patient
    - kVp used

Effects of Scatter Radiation

- Increase overall density of the film which is not useful in production of image thus produces of fog
- Reduces contrast

- Reduce light transmitting ability of film
- Result in the formation of noise

Sources of Scatter Radiation

- Patient himself
- Glass walls of X-ray tube
- Tabletop
- Cassette
- Back scatter from floor
- Back scatter from wall

Causes of increased scatter radiation:

1. Increase field size
2. Patient thickness
3. Increase kVp

Measures to Reduce Scatter Radiation

A. **Air gap technique**: It uses an increased OID to reduce scatter reaching the receptor, used in chest X-ray and X-ray cervical spine in lateral view.
   - Disadvantage—reduce the sharpness of the image, mAs of the study needs to be increased.

B. **Compression**: Reduces scatter by diminishing the volume of tissue through which X-ray will travel, improves—spatial resolution and contrast

C. **Beam restricting device (Fig. 14)**
   a. Apertures—piece of lead with a hole in it, easy to use, directly placed below the X-ray tube
   b. Cones and cylinders—similar to apertures
   c. Collimators—made of two sets of lead shutter, located below the tube window—consists of longitudinal and lateral blades with its own control which makes it useful to produce field in different size, field shape is always rectangular or square, it is attached with a light source

D. Filtration—used to increase the amount of useful electrons and decrease low energy photons. Two types—
   - Inherent filtration—by tube itself-Aluminum
   - Added filtration—separate from tube

E. Radiographic grid—Dr Gustave Bucky invented grid, it is made up of lead strips with interspace material being Aluminum, it allows passage of primary beam and reduces the scatter radiation.

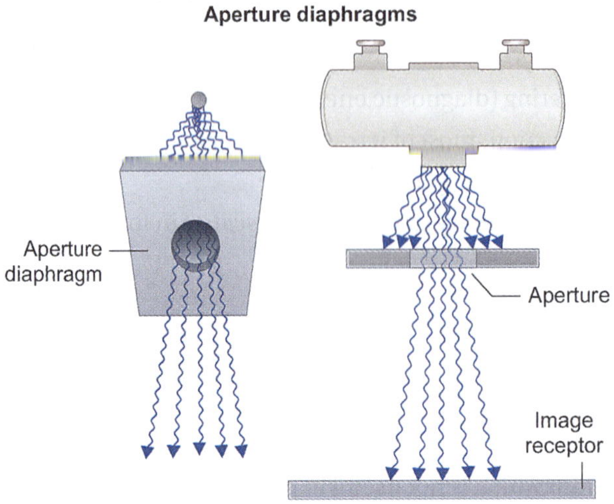

FIG. 14: Beam restricting devices to reduce scatter radiation.

12. What is digital radiography? Discuss its advantages and disadvantages. [3+7] [MD (WBUHS) 22, AIIMS May 24]

- Radiography is an art and science of recording images produced by X-rays on film
- Digital radiography replacing film screen radiography (FSR) in most of the centers
- The main difference between digital radiography and FSR is the detector we use to capture the image
- Hardware is essentially same (X-ray tube, stand, etc.)
- Receptor receives X-rays and exposes a digital plate that transformed to an electrical image
- Screen and cassette replaced by reusable image receptor or detector

Physical Principles of Digital Radiography

- SFR—film serves as both detector and storage medium
- Digital radiography—digital detectors are used only to generate the digital image
- Digital image then stored on a digital medium
- Postprocessing software used to convert the raw digital data into clinically meaningful image

Steps in Digital Radiography (Fig. 15)

Digital imaging comprises four separate steps:

1. Generation
2. Processing
3. Archiving
4. Presentation of the image

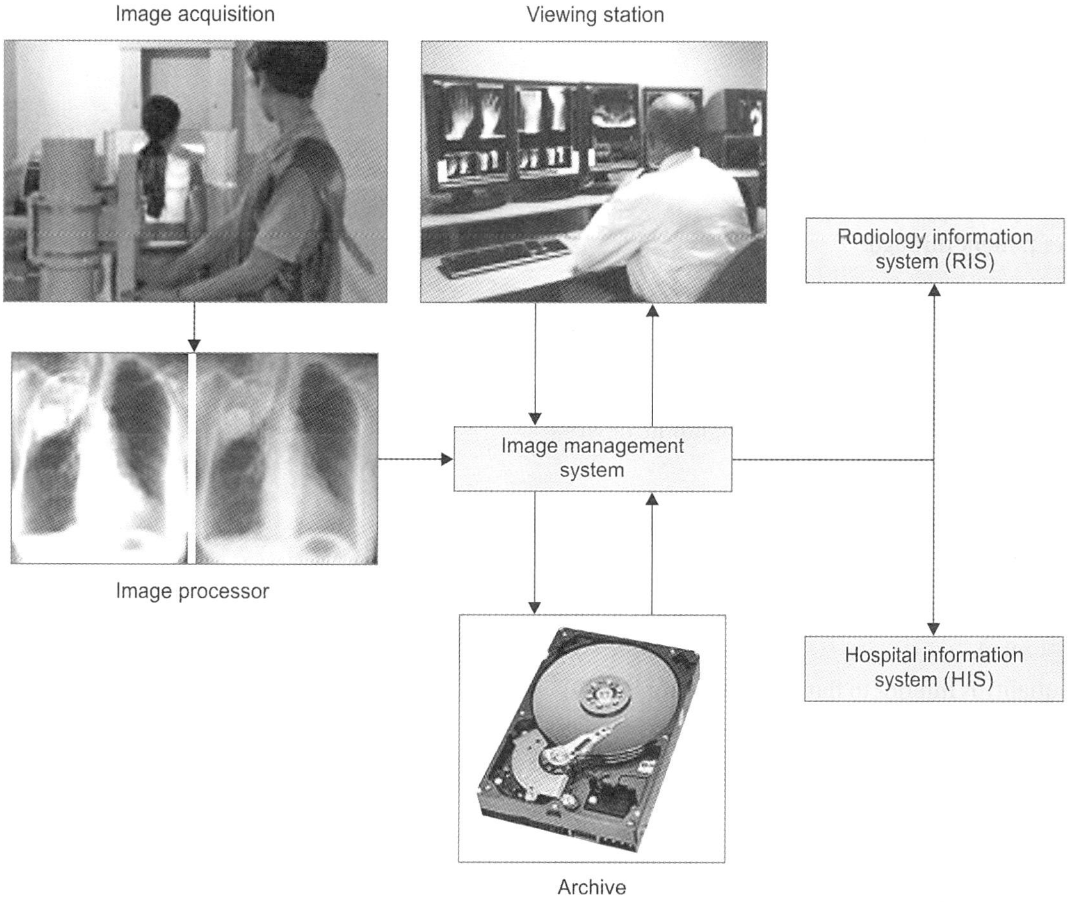

FIG. 15: Digital radiography workflow.

Limitations of FSR

1. Intolerant to exposure errors
2. Defined latitude
3. Cannot be transmitted or duplicated without loss of quality
4. Acquisition, display and storage of the images are not separable
5. Cannot be manipulated
6. Storage
7. Quality deteriorates with time

Types of Digital Radiography (Flowchart 1)

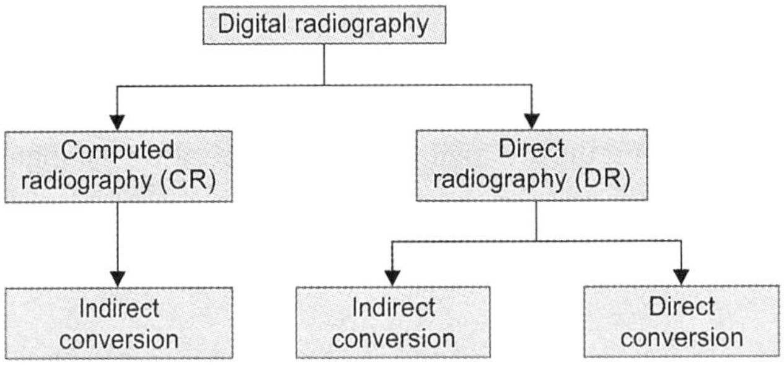

FLOWCHART 1: Types of digital radiography.

Advantages of Digital Radiography

1. Images do not deteriorate with time
2. True reproduction of image copy
3. Manipulation possible
4. Allow implementation of PACS
5. Distribution of images electronically
6. Wide dynamic range
7. A higher patient through

Computed Radiography (CR)

Advantages

1. Wide dynamic range—reduced rates of failed X-ray exposure
2. Easily be integrated into existing radiographic devices
3. Easy to use for bedside examinations
4. Multiple cassette sizes available

Disadvantages

1. Technique is time and labor consuming like SFR-removing cassette from X-ray set and put into scanner to scan the plate (~1 min)
2. Image quality is inferior to flat panel detectors (FPD)
3. Spatial resolution usually lower than SFR
4. CR DICOM reader usually carries less information

Direct Radiography (DR)

Advantages

1. Superior image quality compared to other methods
2. Image generation with flat-panel detectors is almost a real-time process (<10 sec)

13. Handheld Digital Radiography System. [5]

- In the era of analogue to digital conversion and miniaturization of device handheld radiography is a new choice.
- It is mainly used in dental radiography
- The first handheld portable dental X-ray devices came in 90s
- Intended to be used in the military field

Types of handheld X-ray devices

1. NOMAD
2. Non-FDA-cleared device
3. Tube-based X-ray fluorescence (XRF).

Handheld X-ray units are held by the operator. The distance from the body is variable and depends on how the device is held.

The devices replace wall-mounted or semi-mobile X-ray equipment (on a tripod or mobile support) and are distinguished from those in two keyways:

Since the operator is unable to stand back from radiation protection shields while holding the handheld portable X-ray machines, special methods of (scatter) radiation protection must be offered.

Compared to the conventional wall-mounted direct current units, the output dosage rate of the more recent handheld devices is usually lower (determined by current, waveform, filtering, and cone length).

Some uses permitted with the handheld unit would be:

1. Home healthcare
2. Special needs patients (individuals who require assistance for disabilities such as medical, mental, or psychological)
3. Sedated patients
4. Forensic work
5. In outreach programs

The current handheld portable X-ray devices resemble a photographic camera or have a "shotgun" design **(Fig. 16)**. The devices are used as a replacement for wall-mounted or semi mobile X-ray devices.

The handheld X-ray device uses direct current, operates at a fixed 60 kV, 2.3 mA, and has a 0.4 mm focal spot with a 20 cm source-to-skin distance.

It has been clinically shown that handheld device produces diagnostic-quality X-rays and will work equally well with both film and digital imaging media.

Handheld device provides all the benefits of DC performance: highest quality images and lowest patient dosage.

Handheld X-ray devices as high-frequency, 60 kV DC X-ray generator provides constant radiation output.

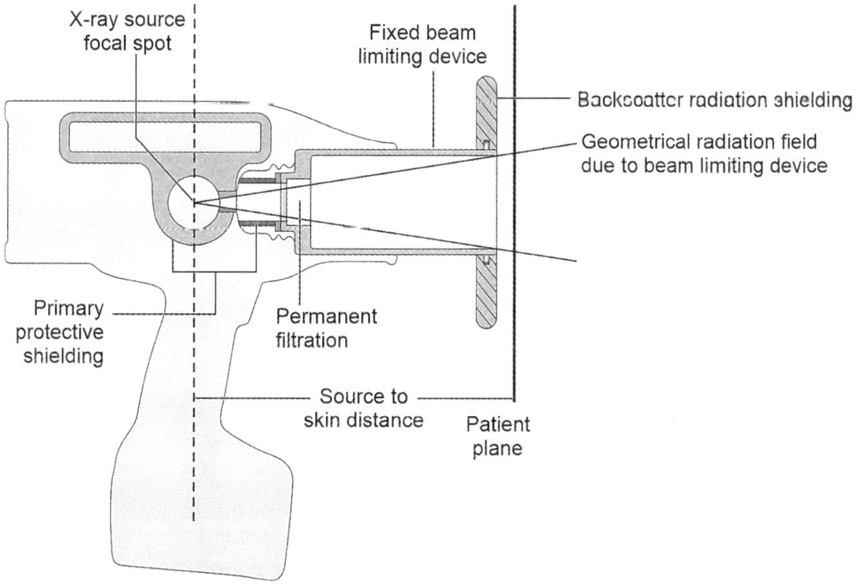

FIG. 16: Handheld digital radiography system.

Advantages of handheld radiography for dental professionals

- Twice as fast as with conventional X-ray systems
- Reduce number of retakes by up to 50%
- Movable, no need of multiple units
- Flexible to take X-ray in any preferred position
- There are less chances of cone-cut and other errors in taking X-rays
- No need to follow accurate angulations. usually, 90° or perpendicular to the film or sensor is maintained
- Light weight, cordless, easily transportable
- No need for special stands, cables, remotes
- Hundreds of diagnostic quality images from a single battery charge
- Works with sensors, film, phosphor plates
- Exceptionally valuable in dental surgery suites
- Perfect for use with sedated patients, children, geriatric or special needs
- Ideal for general dentistry, humanitarian work, clinics, mobile, home health, hospitals
- It is rechargeable one so there is no need of current to operate the device.

Disadvantages of handheld radiography for dental professionals

- The main drawback is that ALARA principal is not followed
- The device must be angled and the operator cannot be completely within the protection zone
- Compulsory lead apron is necessarily should be worn by the operator
- Sometime the radiofrequency which is used to produce X-ray leads disturbs other operating machines
- An experienced operator is needed.

14. Write short note on zero lead apron. [5] [DNB June 22]

Occupational exposure is a serious concern. In this era of interventional radiology where many procedures are done by minimally invasive techniques, but that comes with the cost of prolonged exposure. Because of its high atomic number and high attenuation coefficient, Lead is primarily used as shielding material.

Disadvantages of Lead

- Toxic material
- Difficult to dispose
- Heavy weight
- Difficult to wear for prolonged period.
- **Lead apron**: 0.25 mm—wt 1-5 kg.
- **Lead**: 0.5 mm—wt 3-7 kg.

Because of the abovementioned difficulties, concept of zero lead apron has come, which consists of material like bismuth, antimony, tin, strontium—these components also have high atomic number.

Advantages

- Lightweight (20% to 40% lighter than lead)
- Composite material
- Easy to handle.

Efficiency: It is found that performance of non-lead and lead protective apron (0.25 mm and 0.35 mm Pb equivalent) is similar to scattered X-ray also in clinical setting.

15. Write short note on breast tomosynthesis. [5] [DNB June 22]

Breast Tomosynthesis

- **Breast cancer**: Leading cause of mortality and morbidity in women around the world.
- **Screening modality**: Digital mammography

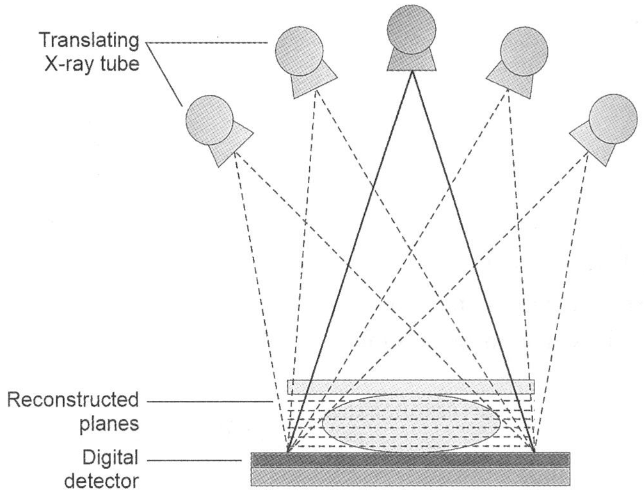

FIG. 17: Digital breast tomosynthesis (DBT).

- **Disadvantages**: 2D/Two Dimensional
  - Less accurate characteristics
  - Many times, lesions are obscured/overlapped.
  - To overcome this situation DBT has been conceptualized. It gives 3D volumetric data by adding 3rd dimension - depth along the Z-axis.

Technique: Using X-ray source which will move in a fashion of arc, multiple projections are taken **(Fig. 17)**.

Reconstruction algorithms are applied to produce series of tomographic images, which can be interpret like CT or MR Stack as thin as 1 mm section can be made. Different manufacturers have developed different techniques with varying arc angles to perform DBT.

Radiation dose: Radiation dose with DBT is significantly higher than full field digital mammography although most of the DBT images are below the FDA limit, i.e., 300 millirad per exposure.

Potential Benefits of DBT

- Small lesion characterization detection.
- Reduction in recall rates.
- Improved sensitivity off screening.
- Primary benefit is expected to be more for masses asymmetric and distortion.

16. Write short note on artificial intelligence. [5] [DNB June 22, DNB June 20]

- Currently, in every aspect of our lives, we are upgraded with the help of AI.
- Introduction of AI in medical imaging came in late 90's.
- Introduction of PACS has led to collection of large amount of data which make the implementation faster and easier.
- **Imaging**: The main role of AI is seen in neuroimaging followed by breast, lung, musculoskeletal abdominal and so on.

AI Characteristics (Flowchart 2)

1. By automation of repetitive tasks it can discover new paradigms.
2. Adding intelligence to existing products
3. Deep accuracy through deep network.

Deep learning: It is a type of supervised learning, it basically resembles neural network of brain known as artificial network having three—input, hidden and output layers. Strength of connection between these layers depicts the accuracy of the AI.

Application of AI in Radiology

1. Collecting requisition
2. Schedule an exam
3. Image acquisition
4. Detection of finding and features
5. Interpretation of finding
    - CNS—detection of bleed, microbleed
    - Diffusion perfusion mismatch instroke patient
    - Pulmonary—detection, classification of pulmonary nodules
    - Breast-CAD—to find mass lesion, architectural distortion
    - Orthopedic—bone age estimation
    - Detection of calcium score
6. Postprocessing, fusion, archival, storage, etc.
7. Image quality check
8. Comparison with previous report
9. Automated dose estimation
10. Scheduling for follow-up/integration of other investigations

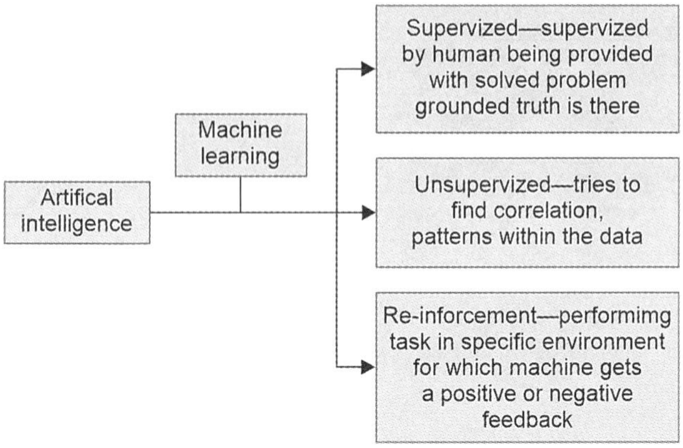

FLOWCHART 2: Characteristics of artificial intelligence.

Challenges of AI

1. Chance of ethical issue
2. AI algorithms by private sector may lead to biased result with a favor to specific drug or intervention
3. AI device failure—question comes of reliability
4. Loss of human control—may lead to leakage of personal data
5. Sympathy or practical—lack of emotional intelligence

17. Any 5 chest radiographic views. Technique and indications. [10] [DNB Dec 21]

Postero-Anterior

- Central ray at T5
- FFD-180 cm
- After second full inspiration
- 50 to 60 kvP
- 10 to 15 mAs
- Dose-0.3 mGy

AP

- Supine
- Erect
- Semi-erect
- Central ray at T7
- FFD-100 cm

Lateral View

- FFD- 72 inches (180 cm)
- 60 to 70 kVp

- 10 to 15 mAs
- Dose 1.5 mGy
- CR-right angles to middle of film in mid-axillary line (T7 or inferior aspect of scapula)

Lordotic Views

- Lindblom method/AP Lordotic
  - AP axial or AP oblique projection
  - Patient reclines against IR in lordosis
  - Tube angulation- 30 degree cephalad.
  - Demonstrate the apices and such conditions as interlobar effusion.
- PA-Lordotic/Fleischner method
  - Patient stands as for PA projection, clasps the sides of the vertical bucky and bends backwards 30-40 degree at the waist.
  - Central ray is directed at right angle towards the middle of the film.
  - RML collapse or an interlobar pleural effusion and apices.

Decubitus

- Lateral positions (ventral or dorsal decubitus)—cross table views
- Affected side against vertical grid device
- Central ray—mid-axillary line at T6.
- Change in level of fluid
- Pulmonary areas hidden in standard projection

18. Labeled diagram of X-ray tube. Functioning of X-ray tube. Causes of tube failure. [10] [DNB Dec 21]

X-ray tube is a device in which X-rays are produced on the principle of energy conversion.

X-rays are produced when a fast-moving stream of electrons is suddenly decelerated in the "target" anode of an X-ray tube.

In this process, only 1% energy converted into X-rays; remaining 99% energy converted into heat.

Structure of X-ray Tube (Fig. 18)

- **External structure**: Consists of three parts:
  1. Support structure
  2. Protective housing
  3. Glass or metal envelope
- **Internal structure**:
  - *Cathode assembly:* Electrically negative
  - *Filament:*
  - Filament is made of tungsten wire 10-20 mm in length and 2-5 mm in width.
  - Tungsten is used because of:
    - High melting point = 3370°C
    - Ductile-can be drawn into thin but strong wires
    - Little tendency to vaporize
    - Trace of thorium in the tungsten filament increases the efficiency of electron emission and prolongs life.

A low-voltage circuit (also provided by the generator) produces a current (filament current) through a wire filament at the cathode of the tube. The current in the wire filament causes it to heat up and emit electrons, a process called thermionic emission.

Modern tubes are dual filament and dual focal spot tubes

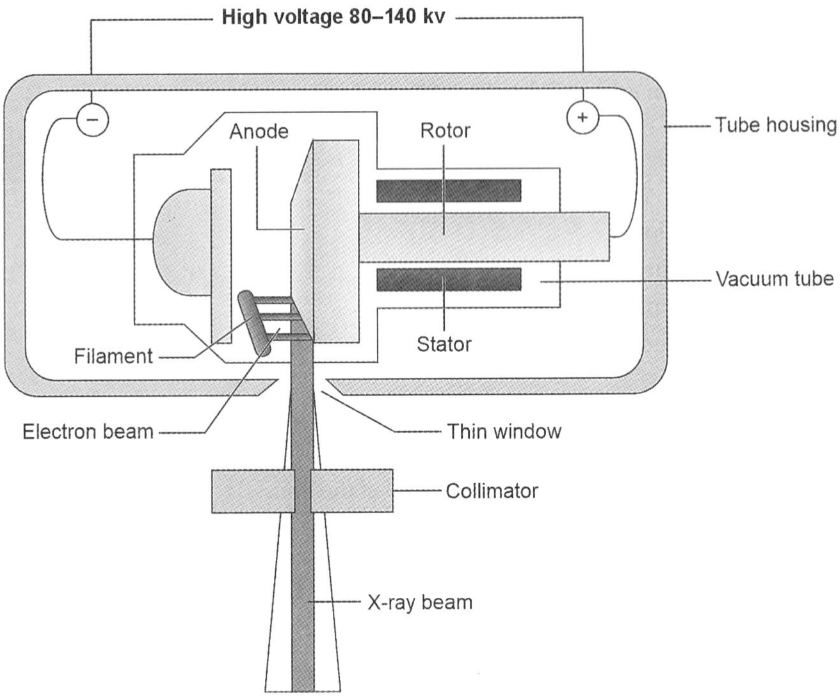

FIG. 18: Schematic diagram of X-ray tube.

Only one filament is activated for a given exposure.

- **Larger filament**: To accommodate imaging applications that require high X-ray tube output in a short exposure time
- **Smaller filament**: For use in applications in which resolving capability is crucial or in which motion blurring is not a concern.
- **Connecting wires**: Filament current (low voltage, high ampere) supply 10V voltage and 3–5 A current to heat the filament up to 2200°C.
- **Focusing cup**: It is negatively charged concave metal (Ni) cup behind the filament light weight, poor thermal conductivity and high melting point. Confines the electrons to a narrow beam and focuses them on a small focal spot on the target.
- **Anode**: Has positive electrical charge and attract electrons

Purpose of Anode

1. Serves as a target surface for the high-voltage electrons
2. Conducts the high-voltage from the cathode back into the X-ray generator circuit
3. Serves as the primary thermal conductor.

Focal spots—large or small.

Tungsten is chosen as the target material for general radiography because of its high atomic number and high melting point.

The tungsten is typically alloyed with 10% rhenium to improve its resistance to thermal damage.

Tungsten is not a good conductor and is usually used as a thin overlay on a molybdenum substrate (for a rotating anode) or as a thin inlay within a copper substrate (for a fixed anode).

Stationary Anode

- Limited heat capacity
- Low energy applications
- Dental—Tungsten target as a thin inlay in a copper substrate.

Rotating Anode

- Tungsten target
- Mo disc and stem—make anode light, high melting point and poor heat conductor
- Length of stem—short as possible, decrease inertia
- Backed by graphite—improves heat loading

Rotating assembly (stator and rotor) with Ag as lubricant and ball bearings at both ends.

Heat loss by radiation to glass envelope and then by conduction to oil bath.

Causes of Tube Failure

Common Causes of Tube Failure

- Extremely high voltage.
- Burnt out filament.
- Anode melting.
- Puncturing of glass tube
- Damage to bearings

Practical Steps in Extending the Useful Tube Life

- Filament life is shortened by application of large filament currents. Therefore, the boost or preparation time (booster circuit) should be kept as short as possible.
- Maximum tube rating should never be exceeded.
- The anode should be warmed up before subjective to a large load. Heat produced by a large power load on cold anode causes uneven expansion that may crack the anode disc. The anode should not be run unnecessarily as the life of the bearings is reduced as total rotation time increases.
- Adequate cooling of the tube housing must be provided.

Factors Governing Tube Life

- **Filament factor**: Undue heating of the filament causes it to vaporize leading to reduction in its diameter and deposition on the glass envelope.
- **Anode factors**: The three anode factors are—radiographic tube rating chart, anode thermal capacity and anode cooling curve

Radiographic Tube Rating Chart

- When the rate of temperature rise, exceeds a limiting value, localized melting or cracking occurs as a result of thermal stresses.
- Melting of the metal causes it to vaporize and coats the glass.
- Roughening of the target leads to reduced X-ray output.
- The safe limits of exposure factors can easily be found referring to the appropriate tube rating chart provided by the manufacturer. A chart indicates the maximum "safe" exposure time for any selected combination of kV and mA for a single exposure.

Factors Affecting the Tube Rating

- Rectification—maximum tube rating is less for half wave than for full wave rectification
- Size of the tube focus—maximum rating is less for smaller focal spot or track
- Tube design—tube with speed disc rotation and smaller anode angle have more tube rating
- Cold versus hot tubes—the chart applies to a relatively cool tube which has not been subjected to heavy loading before use.

Cooling Mechanisms

- **Anode thermal capacity and anode cooling curve**: Excessive heat accumulation may reach the anode stem and the induction motor which may become deformed to slow down or stop the rotor. Thus, starting with a known amount of heat already present in the anode, we must allow enough time to elapse for it to cool down sufficiently to permit the additional heat load.

- The thermal capacity of an anode is measured in heat units
- HU = kVp × mA × sec (for single phase generators)
- HU = kVp × mA × sec × 1.4 (for three phase and constant potential generators)
- A typical anode has a heat loading of 25,000 HU
- If the anode has been heated to its full storage capacity by a large number of exposures, additional exposures are limited by the cooling rate of the anode.
- The cooling rate is determined from the cooling curves. The anode cooling curve gives the rate at which anode cooling starts at any particular value.
- Housing factors—excessive heat may bring the oil to the boiling point and even cause the housing to explode, hence special cooling curves are available for the housing as well.

19. X-ray film. [5] [DNB Dec 21]

X-ray film also known as photographic film which carries the information of attenuated X-ray beam.

It consists of photosensitive material coated on a thin sheet like material.

Consists of 4 layers **(Fig. 19)**:

1. Base—made of polyester, mechanical support
2. Adhesive layer—made of gelatin
3. Emulsion—silver halide crystal
4. Super-coat—gelatin

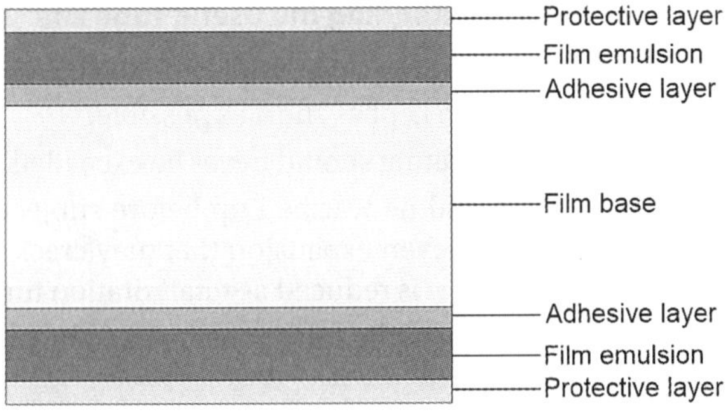

FIG. 19: Layers of X-ray film.

Base

Skeleton of the film with the property of being transparent, chemically nonreactive, non-inflammable and waterproof.

Previously, cellulose nitrate was used as base, now a days polyester is being used.

Adhesive Layer

Sticks emulsion to base, made of pure gelatin, sometimes dyes are added to this to prevent crossover.

Emulsion

- Made of photo-sensitive material-silver halide crystals dispersed in gelatin.
- 90-99% bromide and 1-10% iodide.
- Large grains are generally used—because of their increased sensitivity
- Although too much large grains can cause image unsharpness

Super-coat

- Thin layer of gelation
- Protects emulsion from abrasion

Types of Films

1. Double emulsion—emulsion layer on both side
   - Used in general radiography
   - Increased sensitivity
   - Increased contrast
   - But chance of cross over is there

2. Single emulsion:
    - Emulsion layer on one side, other side—nonemulsion side has anti-curl layer of gelation with dye
    - Used in mammography

Film can be of:

a. Screen type—with the intensifying screen-general radiography
b. Non-screen type—with no intensifying screen-increased radiation dosedental radiography, duplication film.

20. Computed radiography. [5] [DNB Dec 21]

Types of Digital Radiography (Flowchart 3)

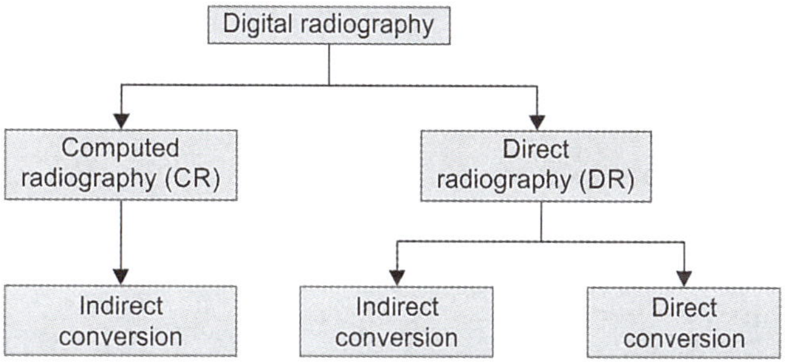

FLOWCHART 3: Types of digital radiography.

Computed Radiography (CR)

- Principles of photostimulated luminescence
- Use photostimulable phosphor plates for image capture with a separate image readout process
- **Commonly used material BaFBr**: Eu
- Surface coat protects phosphor from physical damage

Imaging Plates (Fig. 20)

Generation of Image

- X-rays → electrons to higher energy levels (in crystals)
- X-ray energy can be stored for several hours
- The readout process should start immediately after exposure
- Amount of stored energy decreases over time

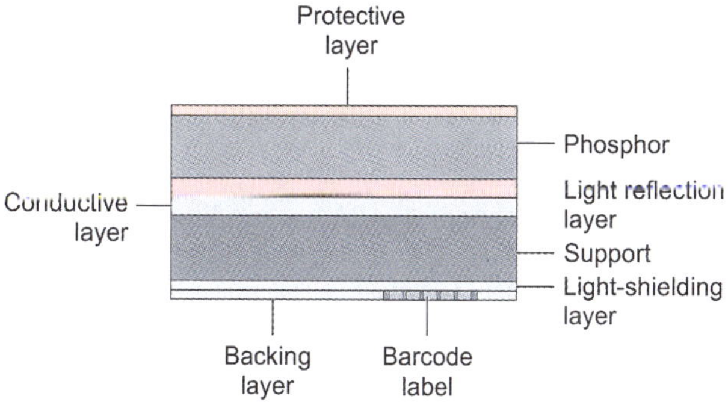

FIG. 20: Cross-section of CR imaging plate.

Readout Process

- Detective layer is scanned with a high-energy laser beam
- Stored energy is set free as emitted light (different wavelength from laser beam)
- This light is collected by photodiodes and converted digitally into an image.

Advantages

1. Wide dynamic range -reduced rates of failed X-ray exposure
2. Easily be integrated into existing radiographic devices
3. Easy to use for bedside examinations
4. Multiple cassette sizes available

Disadvantages

1. Technique is time and labor consuming like SFR-removing cassette from X-ray set and put into scanner to scan the plate (~1 min)

2. Image quality is inferior to flat panel detectors (FPD)
3. Spatial resolution usually lower than SFR
4. CR DICOM reader usually carries less information

21. ALARA and eLORA. [5] [DNB Dec 21]

ALARA

Principle—full form - As low as reasonably achievable

- This principle was established in 1954 by NCRP (National Council on Radiation Protection).
- Now-a-days, it is considered as the main guideline for radiation protection.

Three cardinal factors comprise ALARA.

1. Time
2. Distance
3. Shielding

1. **Time**: Exposure time should be kept minimum.
   Exposure = Exposure rate X time
   So, it is proportional in relation.
2. **Distance**: Exposure is inversely proportional to the square of distance, so distance should be large
   Exposure ∞ $1/D^2$
3. **Shielding**

- The concept is to put a barrier between the radiation source and exposed person.
- Commonly used material are lead, concrete, barium plaster.

Types of shielding

1. Shielding of X-ray source/tube
2. Shielding of control room
3. Shielding of the personnel (example, lead apron, thyroid shield, and glove)
4. Shielding of patient

In USA, the concept of ALARA has modified as ALARP—as low as reasonably practicable

AERB Dose Limit (Table 5)

TABLE 5: AERB dose limits for occupational worker and public.

Dose limit	*Occupational workers*	*Public*
5 years	100 mSV	1 mSV/yr
Annual	30 mSV	1 mSV

eLORA

With the limited resources, the AERB faces a significant task in effectively and efficiently regulating all of these facilities to ensure the safety and security of radiation facilities due to the growing use of ionizing radiation technologies.

AERB took the initiative to automate the regulatory procedures related to the use of ionizing radiation in India in order to tackle the challenge by deploying eLORA (e-Licensing of Radiation Applications), a state-of-the-art e-Government system.

eLORA is a web-based I and CT (Information and Communication Technology) application establishing direct communication channel between AERB and its stakeholders for exchange of information and communication transaction for delivering its regulatory services as well as for achieving higher efficiency, reliability and transparency in dealings.

The eLORA system is designed to automate the comprehensive business processes of radiological application regulations targeted to large number of facilities involved in use of ionizing radiation as well as radiation workers working with them for safe service.

The components of eLORA are chosen to achieve Business Solution with Security, Performance, Availability, Scalability, Manageability and Maintainability. The infrastructure of eLORA system is based on virtualization technology which has helped in achieving cost effectiveness at the investment level and further during operations at the data center.

The processed developed in eLORA system is as per statutory requirements given by Government of India [e.g. Atomic Energy (Radiation Protection) Rules, 2004] and technical documents developed by AERB (viz., regulatory codes, manuals, and standards)

AERB regulates spectrum of facilities and activities ranging from nuclear power plants, nuclear fuel cycle, particle accelerator, etc., to medical X-rays, nucleonic gauges, etc. The facilities and activities vary in numbers as well as their spread across the country.

AERB makes use of various regulatory processes to discharge its responsibilities in an effective manner. These processes ensure use of graded approach for efficient regulation. The major processes are:

1. Development of safety requirements and guidance for utilities and users
2. Licensing process for various facilities and activities based on safety requirements and guidance
3. Regulatory inspections for checking compliance with license conditions as well as safety requirements
4. Development of Regulatory Safety Documents
5. AERB develops and lays down safety requirements and guidance for utilities and users in form of Regulatory Safety Documents. Regulatory safety documents are issued under provisions of Atomic Energy (Radiation Protection) Rules, 2004. The regulatory safety documents are developed with a view to cover the entire spectrum of regulated nuclear and radiation facilities and activities, as applicable, with graded approach.

Licensing/Consenting

Regulatory "Consent" includes "Licence", "Authorisation", "Approval", "Registration" and "Certification".

The consenting process involves safety review and assessment to check the compliance to the regulatory requirements and consequent to the satisfactory compliance, stagewise issuance of consents for stages namely, Siting, Construction, Commissioning, Operation and De-Commissioning.

22. (a) Rotating anode tube. (b) Photoelectric effect. [5+5] [DNB Dec 20, DNB June 20]

Anode is of two types—stationary and rotating

Rotating Anode (Fig. 21)

The purpose of rotating anode is to spread the heat during an exposure over a large area of anode. Use of rotating anode helps in increasing the effective surface area, thereby improving the tube heat capacity. The rotor and stator are elements of electric induction motor used to rotate anode during X-ray exposure. Anode rotation speeds range from 3,000 rpm (revolutions per minute) to 10,000 rpm for a high-speed anode. The rotor is connected to the anode disk by the anode stem, which is typically made of molybdenum or stainless steel. The stem is designed to protect the bearings from heat damage, a common cause of X-ray tube failure.

By rotating the target rapidly during the exposure time, the effective surface area of target is substantially increased, allowing instantaneous heat load on target to be increased. In turn higher heat load allows higher X-ray output. A particular challenge to designer of rotating anode was how to achieve rotation of anode while maintaining vacuum in the tube.it was solved by using electric induction motor. An alternating current in stator (outside the envelope) windings induces a changing magnetic field within the envelope. The rotor (within the envelope) rotates in response to change in magnetic field, causing the attached target disk to rotate.

Spiral groove bearing is the most advanced design today. It uses a liquid metal lubricant (usually metallic silver or barium), which as a metal provides excellent heat conduction.

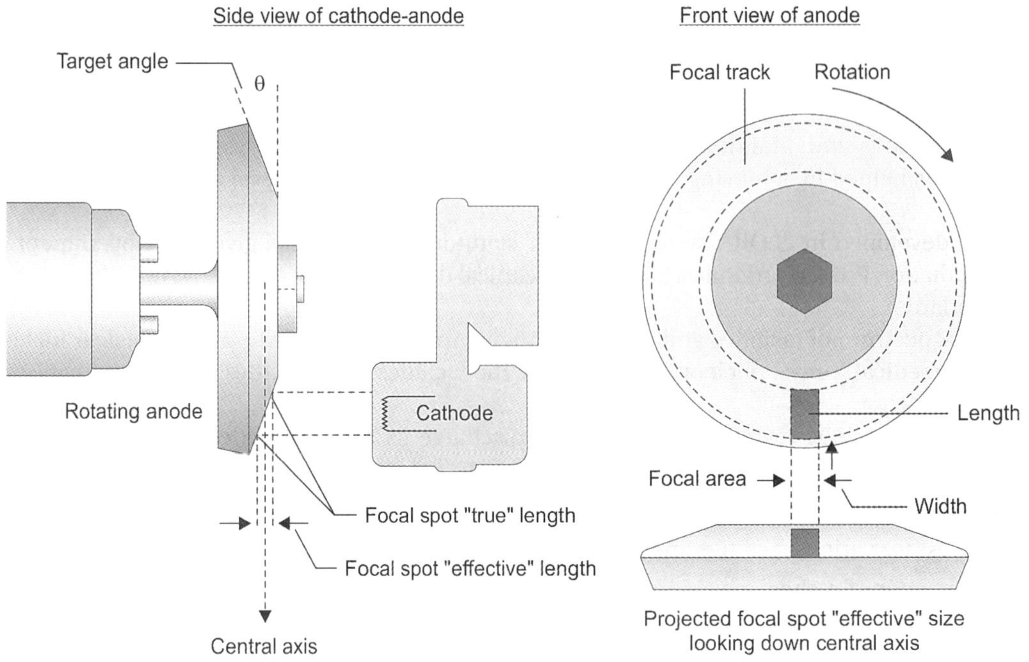

FIG. 21: Rotating anode tube.

Interaction of Radiation and Matter

1. Photoelectric effect
2. Compton effect
3. Coherent scattering
4. Pair production
5. Photo disintegration

Photoelectric Effect (Fig. 22)

PE effect is directly proportional to Z^3/E^3

Z-magnifies the difference in tissue composed of different elements such as bone and soft tissue, and the difference in contrast media and soft tissue like in barium and IVP studies

Most likely to occur when photon energy and electron binding energy are nearly same. A 34 Kev electron is most likely to interact with K shell of iodine (binding energy 33.2Kev) than a 100 Kev photon.

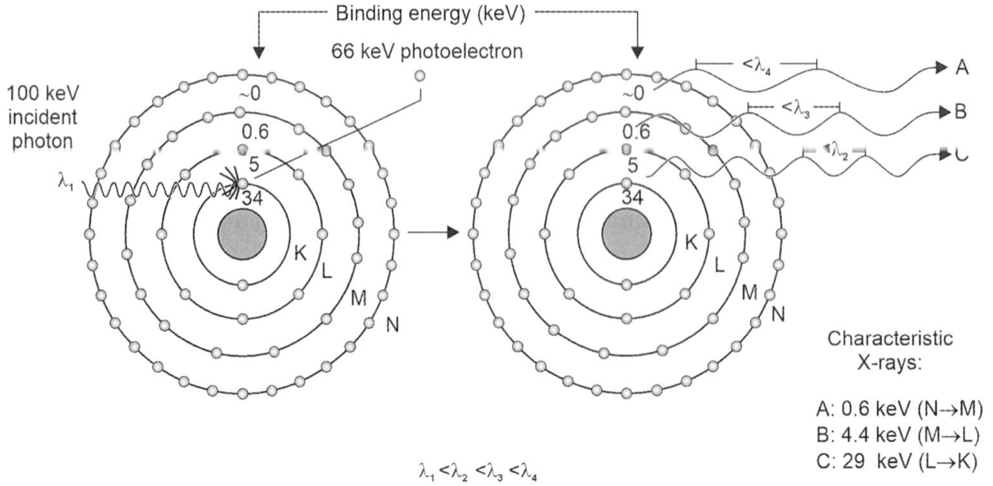

FIG. 22: Photoelectric effect.

K edge: Spike in attenuation due to increased photoelectric absorption that occurs at photon with energy **just greater** than that of k shell binding electron. values vary for each element and increase as the atomic number increases

Role of Photoelectric Effect in X-ray Filters

- Filter out low energy photons from the polyenergetic spectrum, which only contribute to dose.
- Material used is aluminum(Z = 13), as photoelectric effect is directly proportional to atomic number it will attenuate the lower energy photons.
- Atomic number of filter material should be high enough to make PE dominate, not too high else it will absorb useful X-rays.

Ultrasound Imaging

1. What is sonoelastography? Describe the role of sonoelastography in breast and liver diseases. [2+4+4] [MD (WBUHS) 24, MD (WBUHS) 20]

Elastography is also known as virtual palpation, it is a novel imaging technique of measuring stiffness of tissue or lesion. It is measured by movement or deformation (strain) of tissue in response to small applied pressure/stress.

- Stress-force per unit area
- Strain-deformation in response to stress
- Elastography was first described by Krouskop.
- Elastography can be done by MRI or USG, elastography by USG is known as sonoelastography.

It is of mainly two types **(Flowchart 4)**

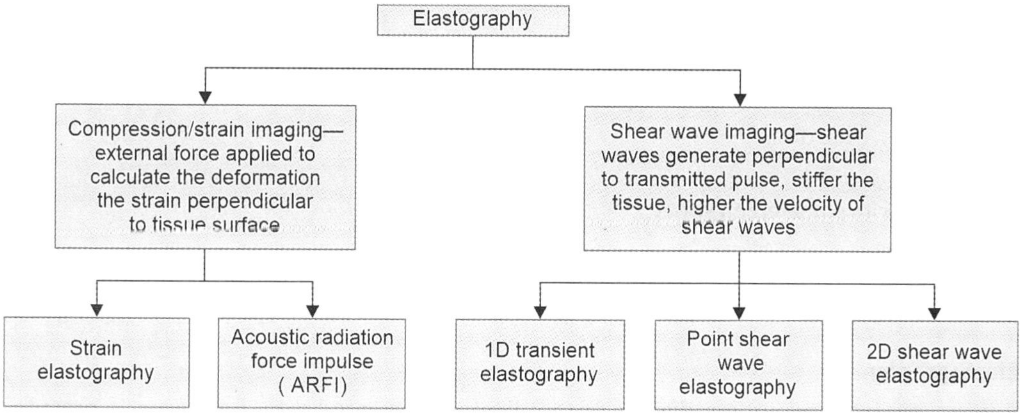

FLOWCHART 4: Types of elastography.

Role in Breast Lesions

- Role of elastography in characterizing breast lesions is now well-established.
- Main concept was to differentiate between benign and malignant lesion which is stiffer and harder.

Additional Role

- Characterization of complex lesion
- May detect more than one lesion when grey scale shows one lesion
- Detection of fat globules
- Help in decision making of biopsy of lesion (adjunct feature in 5th edition of BIRADS US lexicon)
- Recent use in assessment of neoadjuvant chemotherapy. Hard lesion on strain elastography show better response than softer malignancy.
- Both strain and shear elastography can be performed **(Fig. 23)**.

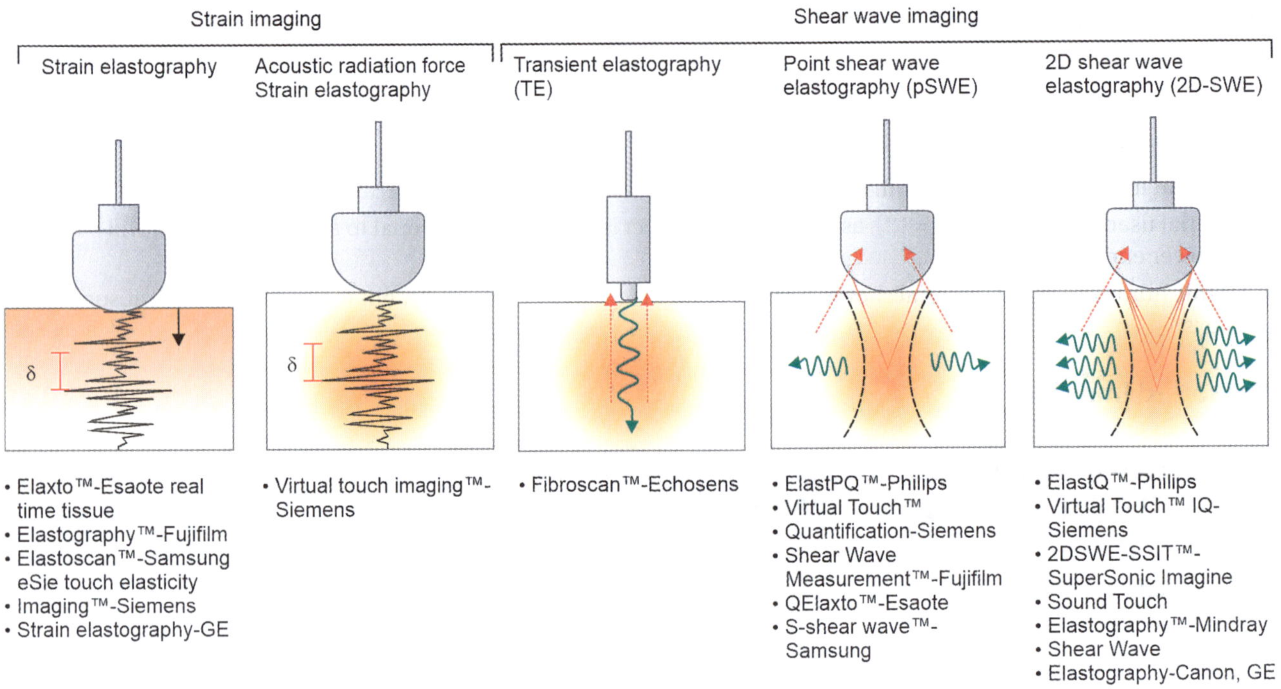

FIG. 23: Strain versus shear wave imaging.

Strain elastography: It is most widely used, different parameters used to differentiate benign vs malignant lesion, most commonly used score is elasticity score.

Color coded maps (TSUKUBA SCORE) display the stiffness of the lesion:

- Score 1-chromatic tristratification (red/blue/green)
- Score 2-green with few blue dots
- Score 3-mainly green
- Score 4-almost blue with some green spots
- Score 5-complete blue

But this method is not quantitative, so semi-quantitative technique **distance ratio** introduced, which measures measurement of lesion in elasto by lesion size in gray scale: more than 1 is cut off for chances of being malignant.

Shear Wave Elastography

Focused USG beam produces acoustic radiation force—displacement produces shear waves—provides information about viscoelastic property.

Measurement in kPA

It allows differentiation of adipose tissue (<3 kPa), dense parenchyma (~45 kPa), benign lesions (<80 kPa), malignant lesion (>100 kPa).

Limitations

1. Benign masses like hyalinized fibroadenoma, and fat necrosis appear hard
2. Medullary, mucinous, papillary carcinomas appear soft.

Nonviscous fluids are incompressible—therefore simple cysts do not display any signal.

Role of Elastography in Liver Lesions

Elastography is novel, easy, reliable technique for the evaluation of diffuse liver disease as well as characterization of focal liver lesions **(Table 6)**.

TABLE 6: Role of elastography in liver lesions.

Diffuse liver disease: Fibrosis, cirrhosis, acute hepatitis, non-alcoholic fatty liver disease	Chronic liver disease changes the stiffness of liver by fibrosis **Metavir Score** • Stage 0-normal • Stage 1-portal fibrosis • Stage 2-septal fibrosis • Stage 3-septal fibrosis with occasional nodules • Stage 4-cirrhosis Acute insult to liver parenchyma or congestive cardiac failure can cause cell edema, swelling with increased stiffness **Techniques** a. Transient elastography/FibroScan-wide range values 2.5-75 kpa, normal ~5.5 kpa, not good in obesity or ascites b. Point shear wave elastography/ARFI-limited range (0.5-4.4 m/s) c. Real time elastography – Useful for grading/staging of fibrosis guiding therapy – Post-treatment assessment—significant drop in stiffness after treatment with antiviral like ribavirin in case of acute viral hepatitis – Portal hypertensions-splenic elasticity shows correlation with hepatic venous pressure gradient (HVPG-invasive)—predictor of variceal bleed – Assessment of transjugular intrahepatic portosystemic stent shunt (TIPSS)-splenic stiffness decreases with Rx – Liver transplant—HCV infected patients show rapid stiffness within 1 year of post treatment – NASH—degree of steatosis can be done
Characterization of focal liver lesions	• Malignant lesions are more stiff than benign • Strain index is higher in malignant lesions than benign lesions. Although hemangiomas can show variable response depending the amount of fibrotic septae • **Cholangiocarcinomas are the stiffest** among all malignant hepatic lesion • Shear wave can differentiate between FNH, adenoma – FNH—radial pattern – Adenoma—homogeneous • Benign lesions appearing stiff are healed abscess, scars of radiofrequency ablation

Limitations

- Ascites, excessive obesity
- False positive—BMI >30, metabolic syndrome, acute hepatitis

2. Write short note on tissue harmonic imaging. [5] [MD (WBUHS) 21, MD (WBUHS) 20, DNB Dec 20]

Nonlinear propagation of ultrasound waves in tissue produces harmonics, which are integer multiples of transmitted frequency. This is the basis of THI.

In conventional grey-scale imaging, image is produced by transmitted frequency, however in THI image is produced by higher frequency waves. **It is the second harmonic used for imaging (Fig. 24)**

- Insonation of tissue with ultrasound waves of a specific transmitted frequency

⇓

- The fundamental wave (*f*) is generated at the transducer surface and attenuates linearly as it is transmitted through the body

⇓

- The harmonic wave (*2f*) is generated as the fundamental wave travels through the body
- The harmonic wave increases exponentially in intensity before attenuating within the deeper tissues.

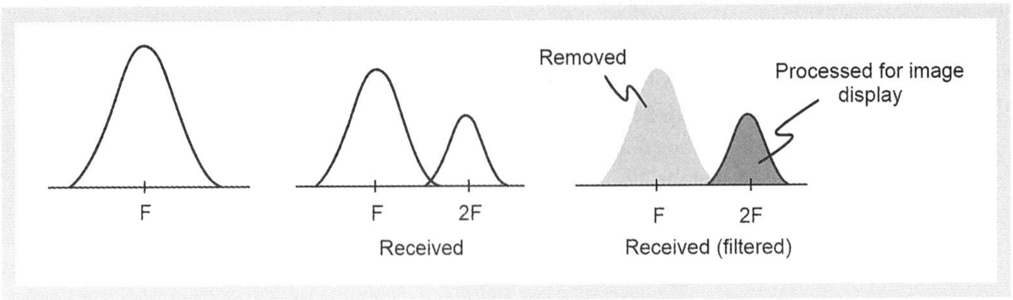

FIG. 24: Tissue harmonic imaging.

Frequency Spectrum of the Transmitted and Received Waves

Harmonic imaging uses only the harmonic frequency in the echo signal received by filtering out the transmitted frequency spectrum in the signal.

Advantages of Harmonic Imaging

- Improved axial resolution due to shorter wavelength.
- Better lateral resolution due to improved focusing with higher frequencies
- THI is specifically useful in obese patients as highest nonlinear coefficient are generated where amount of fat is high, so in obese patient lesion visibility is better with THI.
- Less artifacts than with conventional US—Artifacts are eliminated using harmonic imaging because the artifact—producing signals do not consist of sufficient energy to generate harmonic frequencies and are, therefore, filtered out during image formation.
- Better lesion detection and characterization
- Accentuates subtle shadowing
- Posterior acoustic enhancement-detection and characterization of cystic lesions
- Comet tail artifacts

Clinical uses of THI

- **Liver**: Increased detection of small focal lesions in patients with cirrhosis.
- **GB**: Comet tail artifacts indicative of cholesterol crystals and adenomyomatosis.
- **Kidney**: Differentiation of simple from complex cysts.
- **Uterus**: Improves contrast b/w fibroid and normal uterus.

3. Define Doppler principle. How Doppler principle application is utilized in medical imaging, [10] [MD (WBUHS) 20]

- The Doppler principle is named after the mathematician and physicist named *Christian Johann Doppler* who first described this effect in 1842 by studying light from stars.
- The same doppler effect is applied in ultrasound to detect blood flow by analyzing the relative frequency shifts of received echoes brought about by the movement of red blood cells.

Doppler Shift (Fig. 25)

- It is the difference between the transmitted and received frequencies.
- Transmitted and received frequencies are in the MHZ range.
- Doppler shift frequencies often in audible range.
- **Blood velocity**: As velocity increases, so does the Doppler frequency.

Doppler equation

- Relationship between Doppler shift (or just Doppler) frequency, F_0, and reflector velocity, v:

$$F_D = \frac{2f_0 v \cos\theta}{c}$$

- f_0 is the ultrasound frequency, or the transmitted beam frequency.
- v is the reflector velocity (m/s; cm/s)
- q is the Doppler angle
- c is the speed of sound

FIG. 25: Doppler equation.

- **Ultrasound frequency**: Higher ultrasound frequencies give increased Doppler frequency.
- Angle of insonation **(Fig. 26)**

Continuous Wave (CW) Doppler

- Use two crystals, one to send and one to receive.
- Uses continuous transmission and reception of ultrasound.
- Doppler signals are obtained from all vessels in the path of the ultrasound beam (until the ultrasound beam becomes sufficiently attenuated due to depth).
- Continuous wave Doppler ultrasound is unable to determine the specific location of velocities within the beam and cannot be used to produce color flow images.
- Used in adult cardiac scanners to investigate the high velocities in the aorta.

$$F_D = \frac{2f_0\, v \cos\theta}{c}$$

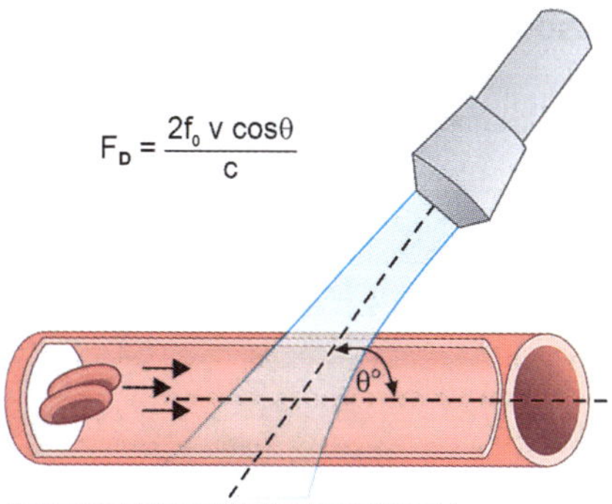

Angle	Cos theta
0	1
45	0.7
60	0.5
90	0

$$V = \frac{F_D \times C}{2f_0 \times \cos\theta}$$

Optimal angle → 30°–60°

FIG. 26: Calculation of angle of insonation.

Pulse Wave Doppler

- Uses brief pulses of ultrasound energy using only one crystal.
- The echo delay time can be converted into distance and the depth of echo source can be determined.
- The sensitive volume from which flow data are sampled can be controlled in terms of shape, depth and position.
    - Pulse repetition frequency (PRF): No. of pulses transmitted per second
    - With increasing scanning depth, PRF must be at least twice the frequency of the Doppler signal to construct the signal successfully.
    - This sets upper limit to the flow velocities to be accurately recorded.
    - Use higher PRF for high flow velocities, low PRF for slow venous flow.

Power Doppler

- New technology of Doppler signal processing, in which its energy instead of its amplitude is recorded
- The energy is related to the square of the amplitude of the signal
- Using this technology, even weak signals (corresponding to low flow rates) can be recorded
- Sensitive to low flows
- No directional information
- Very poor temporal resolution
- Susceptible to noise

Duplex Ultrasound Scanning

These are real time B-mode scanners with built in Doppler capabilities.

- B-mode (for outline anatomic structures)
- Pulsed Doppler (for flow and movement patterns)

4. Write short note on ultrasound contrast agent. [5] [DNB Dec 21]

Ultrasound Contrast Agent

Ultrasound contrast agent is a new introduction in the field of medical imaging with proved result.

Properties

- Us contrast agents are microbubble gas with a shell made of protein, lipid or albumin, etc.
- They stay within the intravascular compartment, unable to go into the interstitium
- Get exhaled by lung and the coat is metabolized in liver
- Helpful in CKD patient, as there is no renal excretion

Low mechanical index of the machine (0.07-0.2) is required for the imaging.

Classification of Ultrasound Contrast Agents (Table 7)

TABLE 7: Classification of ultrasound contrast agents.

First generation: • Ecovist • Levovist • Albunex • Agitated saline	• They are comprised of soluble gas • Mainly used for right hear imaging, cardiac shunts, etc. • Large size
Second generation: • Sonovue • Luminity • Sonazoid • Optison	• Mostly these are used now a days • Contain insoluble gases like perfluorocarbon or sulfur hexafluoride • With different coating • Sonovue—ideal for vascular phase imaging of different organs • Sonazoid—additional phase—reticuloendothelial

Dosage

- Too much will cause too much scatter
- Too low—sub-diagnostic
- For intravenous use—Sonovue-half vial (2.4 mL) for liver lesion imaging
  - For other lesions—1.2 mL is used.
  - For intracavitary use 0.1–1 mL.

Technique: Intravenous cannulation

- Grey scale evaluation with target lesion in focus
- Freshly prepared sonovue administration followed by saline flush

Clinical Application

- **Liver lesions:** characterization of liver lesions
- Contrast enhanced ultrasound (CEUS) can be used in categorizing LI-RADS category
- Also, in post treatment response assessment
  - HCC—non-rim arterial hyperenhancement with washout of a nodule >10 mm—LI-RADS5
  - Benign—
    - Hemangioma—peripheral nodular enhancement
    - FNH—spoke wheel centrifugal pattern of enhancement
    - Adenoma—hyperenhancing
  - Metastases—peripheral rim enhancement
- Pancreatic lesion—detection of pancreatic necrosis in acute pancreatitis
  - Pancreatic adenocarcinoma-hypoenhancing
- Renal—complex cystic lesion vs malignancy, renal pseudo tumor, renal vascular lesion

Recent Advances

1. Hemodynamically stable abdominal trauma
2. Inflammatory aortoarteritis
3. Inflammatory bowel disease

5. Discuss the role of sonoelastography and MR elastography in evaluation of diffuse liver disease. Discuss the role of sonoelastography in evaluation of breast lesion. [6+4] [MD (WBUHS) 22, MD (WBUHS) 20, MD (WBUHS) 17, AIIMS Dec 23, DNB June 22, DNB June 21]

Elastography is also known as virtual palpation, it is a novel imaging technique of measuring stiffness of tissue or lesion. It is measured by movement or deformation (strain) of tissue in response to small applied pressure/stress.

- Stress—force per unit area
- Strain—deformation in response to stress

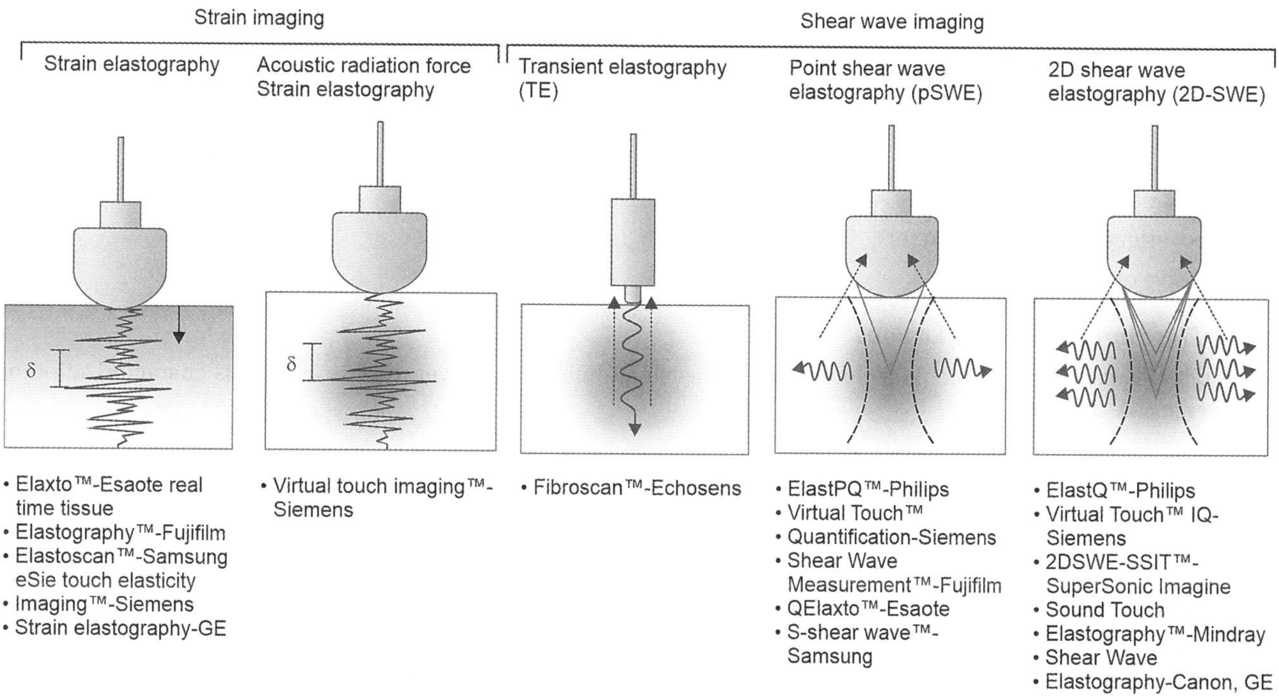

FIG. 27: Strain versus shear wave imaging *(For Color Version Refer Fig. 23).*

- Elastography was first described by Krouskop.
- Elastography can be done by MRI or USG, elastography by USG is known as sonoelastography.

It is of mainly two types **(Fig. 27 and Flowchart 5)**

Mr Elastography

Emerging novel technique to provide information about the stiffness if the tissue or lesion.

Shear waves are transmitted to the tissue or lesion and elasticity of the tissue or lesion are measured using specific motion sensitive MR imaging sequences.

Steps

1. Production of shear waves into the tissue by different types of devices—pneumatic, electromechanical or piezoelectric which are closely placed to body surface. Compression waves RAE produced at skin surface which then generate transverse shear wave at internal tissue.
2. Phase contrast MR sequence to provide phase and magnitude image. Wide variety of sequences—GRE, SE, bSSFP or EPI can be used to obtain image.
3. Elastogram—by inversion algorithm-wave image to map.

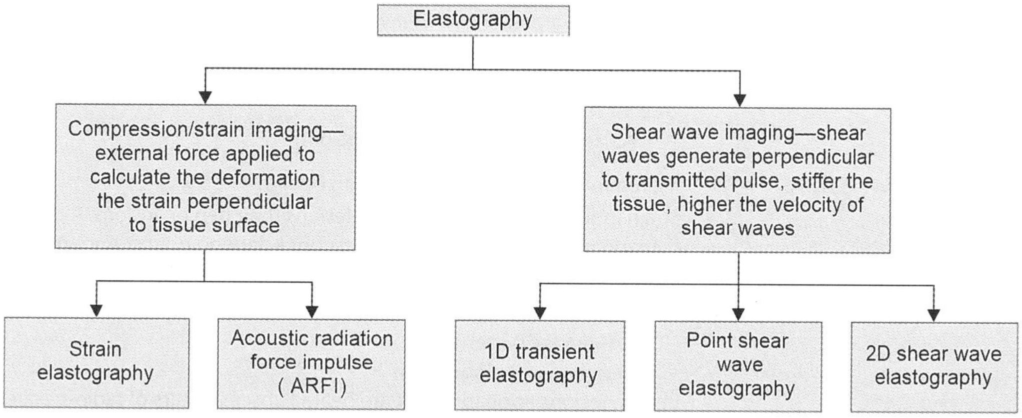

FLOWCHART 5: Types of elastography.

Clinical Applications

- Main role in the evaluation of chronic liver disease to see the degree of fibrosis.
- Alternative to biopsy in areas showing maximum fibrosis
- Differentiating malignant versus benign lesions of liver, kidney, breast, brain, etc.

Limitations

1. Iron overload confounding factor
2. Excessive obesity

Role of Elastography in Liver Lesions

Elastography is novel, easy, reliable technique for the evaluation of diffuse liver disease as well as characterization of focal liver lesions **(Table 8)**.

Limitations

- Ascites, excessive obesity
- False positive—BMI >30, metabolic syndrome, acute hepatitis

Role in Breast Lesions

- Role of elastography in characterizing breast lesions is now well established.
- Main concept was to differentiate between benign and malignant lesion which is stiffer and harder.

TABLE 8: Role of elastography in liver lesions.

Diffuse liver disease: Fibrosis, cirrhosis, acute hepatitis, non-alcoholic fatty liver disease	Chronic liver disease changes the stiffness of liver by fibrosis **Metavir Score** • Stage 0-normal • Stage 1-portal fibrosis • Stage 2-septal fibrosis • Stage 3-septal fibrosis with occasional nodules • Stage 4-cirrhosis Acute insult to liver parenchyma or congestive cardiac failure can cause cell edema, swelling with increased stiffness **Techniques** a. Transient elastography/Fibroscan - wide range values 2.5-75 kpa, normal ~5.5 kpa, not good in obesity or ascites b. Point shear wave elastography/ARFI-limited range (0.5-4.4 m/s) c. Real time elastography – Useful for grading/staging of fibrosis guiding therapy – Post-treatment assessment—significant drop in stiffness after treatment with anti-viral like ribavirin in case of acute viral hepatitis – Portal hypertensions—splenic elasticity shows correlation with hepatic venous pressure gradient (HVPG-invasive)- predictor of variceal bleed – Assessment of TIPSS—splenic stiffness decreases with Rx – Liver transplant—HCV infected patients show rapid stiffness within 1 year of post treatment – NASH-degree of steatosis can be done
Characterization of focal liver lesions	• Malignant lesions are more stiff than benign • Strain index is higher in malignant lesions than benign lesions. Although hemangiomas can show variable response depending the amount of fibrotic septae • **Cholangiocarcinomas are the stiffest** among all malignant hepatic lesion • Shear wave can differentiate between FNH, adenoma – FNH—radial pattern – Adenoma—homogeneous • Benign lesions appearing stiff are healed abscess, scars of radio-frequency ablation

Additional Role

- Characterization of complex lesion
- May detect more than one lesion when grey scale shows one lesion
- Detection of fat globules
- Help in decision making of biopsy of lesion (adjunct feature in 5TH edition of BIRADS US lexicon)
- Recent use in assessment of neo-adjuvant chemotherapy. Hard lesion on strain elastography show better response than softer malignancy.
- Both strain and shear elastography can be performed:

Strain elastography: It is most widely used, different parameters used to differentiate benign vs malignant lesion, most commonly used score is elasticity score.

Color coded maps (TSUKUBA SCORE) display the stiffness of the lesion

- Score 1-chromatic tristratification (red/blue/green)
- Score 2-green with few blue dots
- Score 3-mainly green
- Score 4-almostblue with some green spots
- Score 5-complete blue

But this method is not quantitative, so semi-quantitative technique **distance ratio** introduced, which measures measurement of lesion in elasto by lesion size in grey scale: more than 1 is cut off for chances of being malignant.

Shear Wave Elastography

Focused USG beam produces acoustic radiation force-displacement produces shear waves-provides information about viscoelastic property

Measurement in kPA

It allows differentiation of adipose tissue (<3 kpa), dense parenchyma (~45 kpa), benign lesions (<80 kpa), malignant lesion (>100 kpa).

Limitations

1. Benign masses like hyalinized fibro-adenoma, fat necrosis—appear hard
2. Medullary, mucinous, papillary carcinomas appear soft.

Non-viscous fluids are incompressible—therefore simple cysts do not display any signal

6. Role of sonoelastography in obstetrics and gynecology. [5]

Role of Elastography in Obstetrics and Gynecology (Table 9)

TABLE 9: Role of elastography in obstetrics and gynecology.

Role in Gynecology	
1. Cervical cancer	**TVS elastography** 1. Benign cervical lesions appear less stiff, strain ratio appears less 2. Follow up of cervical cancer 3. Endoluminal growth which may be missed in routine scan can be picked up by elastography **Limitations** • Comparison is done with surrounding myometrium • In case of myometrial invasion result become erroneous • Heterogeneity of cervix
2. Uterine pathology	**Stiffness** • Fibroid > normal myometrium > adenomyoma • Fibrosis with hyaline degeneration appear less stiff
3. Ovarian pathology	Ovaries in PCOS appear stiffer than normal

Continued...

Continued...

Role in Obstetrics	
1. Induction of labor	• Softer internal os is associated with successful induction of labor • Helps in deciding about the requirement of prostaglandins
2. Placenta	Stiffness of placenta can be used as predictor of many maternal and fetal conditions-like pre-eclampsia, IUGR, GDM, etc.

7. Color Doppler artifacts and how to prevent it. [10] [DNB June 22]

Doppler Artifacts and Ways to Reduce them (Table 10)

Although using proper setting, we can reduce artifacts, there are some because of anatomical location. Brief knowledge about these artifacts is very important to avoid misinterpretation. Some of the artifacts also carry diagnostic value.

TABLE 10: Doppler artifacts and ways to reduce them.

Artifact	*Description*	*Way to reduce*
Mirror image artifact	• Similar with grey scale image, interface between high and low acoustic impedance zone produce mirror image. • Example-duplication of subclavian artery or vein by the pleural reflection of apical pleura	Changing the scanning angle
Pseudoflow	• Due to fluid motion rather than movement of blood • Example, ascites, urine, collection of pus	Spectral analysis does not produce any specific pattern
Twinkling artifact	• We get it as alternating red, blue pixels due to turbulent flow seen in urinary calculi, parenchymal calcification, also seen in gallbladder adenomyomatosis	• Spectral analysis—no definite pattern • Increasing the velocity or scale eliminates the flow signal but the twinkling artifact persists
Edge artifact	Smooth reflection along rim of calcified structure-gallbladder stone	Not a true flow as similar flow seen both above and below baseline
Flash artifact	• Random color due to transducer motion or tissue motion • Cyst, fluid collection, left lobe of liver	Specifically seen in power Doppler imaging
Color bruit	• Seen around anastomotic site, area of stenosis, arterio-venous fistula • Seen as color mosaic within the organ adjacent to vessel	Mostly seen in low PRF settings

8. Ultrasound contrast agents. [5] [MD (WBUHS) 19, AIIMS Dec 24]

Ultrasound Contrast Agent

Ultrasound contrast agent is a new introduction in the field of medical imaging with proved result.

Properties

- Ultrasound contrast agents are microbubble gas with a shell made of protein, lipid or albumin, etc.
- They stay within the intra-vascular compartment, unable to go into the interstitium
- Get exhaled by lung and the coat is metabolized in liver
- Helpful in CKD patient, as there is no renal excretion
- Low mechanical index of the machine (0.07-0.2) is required for the imaging

Classification of Ultrasound Contrast Agents (Table 11)

TABLE 11: Classification of ultrasound contrast agents.

First generation: • Ecovist • Levovist • Albunex • Agitated saline	• They are comprised of soluble gas • Mainly used for right hear imaging, cardiac shunts, etc. • Large size
Second generation • Sonovue • Luminity • Sonazoid • Optison	• Mostly these are used now a days • Contain insoluble gases like perfluorocarbon or sulfur hexafluoride • With different coating • Sonovue—ideal for vascular phase imaging of different organs • Sonazoid—additional phase—reticuloendothelial

Dosage

- Too much will cause too much scatter
- Too low—subdiagnostic
- For intravenous use—Sonovue-half vial (2.4 mL) for liver lesion imaging
  - For other lesions-1.2 mL is used.
- For intracavitary use 0.1-1 mL.

Technique: Intravenous cannulation:

- Grey scale evaluation with target lesion in focus
- Freshly prepared sonovue administration followed by saline flush

Clinical Application

- **Liver lesions**: Characterization of liver lesions
- CEUS can be used in categorizing LI-RADS category
- Also, in post treatment response assessment
  - HCC—non-rim arterial hyperenhancement with washout of a nodule >10 mm-LI-RADS5
  - Benign—
    - Hemangioma—peripheral nodular enhancement
    - FNH—spoke wheel centrifugal pattern of enhancement
    - Adenoma—hyperenhancing
  - Metastases—peripheral rim enhancement
- Pancreatic lesion—detection of pancreatic necrosis in acute pancreatitis
  - Pancreatic adenocarcinoma-hypoenhancing
- Renal—complex cystic lesion vs malignancy, renal pseudo tumor, renal vascular lesion

Recent Advances

1. Hemodynamically stable abdominal trauma
2. Inflammatory aortoarteritis
3. Inflammatory bowel disease

9. HIFU—principle and clinical uses. [5] [DNB Dec 21]

High-intensity focused ultrasound is an emerging novel technique with proved therapeutic role.

- It is a non-invasive technique delivering high energy focused ultrasound beam to the target tissue by increasing its temperature or by altering the biological interactions leading to cell death.

- HIFU is usually guided, assessed, and monitored by magnetic resonance imaging (MRI) or ultrasound imaging. Recently, high-intensity focused ultrasound (HIFU) and magnetic resonance-guided focused ultrasound (MRgFUS) have proven clinical implications.

Principle

- HIFU beam pass through skin and tissues without causing harm, and focus on a localized area with a size limit of approximately 3–4 cm in diameter for tumors **(Fig. 28)**.
- US beyond diagnostic range produce various kinds of reactions—thermal, mechanical, acoustic cavitation, shear stress, radiation force, etc.
  - Thermal effect—high-intensity US generally refers to US with an intensity of greater than 5 W/cm^2, which is capable of producing coagulation necrosis of tissue and is most often utilized for HIFU ablation.
  - HIFU thermal effects are secondary to the absorption of US waves. Frictional heat results from vibrations and/or rotations of molecules secondary to the US waves. Protein denaturation and coagulation necrosis typically occur at 56°C with an exposure length of 1 second, whereas a temperature of greater than 43°C for 1 hour may render the tissue more susceptible to chemotherapy and radiation.
  - Shape of thermal lesion resembles a cigar ~1.5 to 2 mm in width and 1.5 to 2 cm in length.

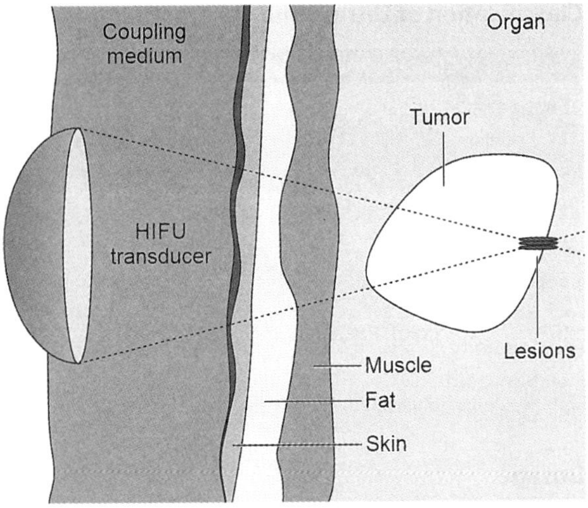

FIG. 28: Principle of HIFU.

Acoustic Cavitation

Defined as formation and activity of a gas or vapor filled cavity in a medium exposed to US field.

Radiation Force

Interface between two medium—acoustic streaming-shear stress

Technique

1. Cheapest—self-focused spherical curved Us source-beam focus fixed
2. Flat US transducer-with interchangeable lens-drawback-sonic attenuation by lens
3. Phased array transducer-beam steering and focusing possible as desired level

Image Guidance

- Both by MR and US, MRI has the advantage of showing the temperature data after seconds of exposure.
- Sonographic technique provides benefit in term of imaging at the same time, lesion which is not well-visualized on USG will not be effective target for HIFU.

Clinical Application

1. Treatment of benign and solid tumors: BCC, HCC, Bladder SOL, pancreatic carcinoma, prostate carcinoma
2. Treatment of primary bone tumor and palliative treatment of pain from bony metastases by denervation of nerves at the periosteum
3. Treatment of uterine myomas
4. MR guided FUS in brain for functional neurosurgery
5. Breast carcinoma
6. Treatment of hypersplenism
7. Ablation of arrhythmic focus
8. Achieve hemostasis in traumatic injury
9. BPH and prostatic carcinomas

10. Drug and gene delivery—cancer drugs, thrombolytics, etc., can be given to target tissue by temperature sensitive liposomes

Limitations

1. As it is ultrasound based, artifacts related to USG will be applicable to this
2. Excessive bowel gas can reflect sound wave causing burns in tissues in between
3. Refraction—deposition of energy adjacent to the target.
4. Dissemination of cancer cells due to shear force generated by the procedure.

10. Principle of color Doppler imaging. [5] [DNB Dec 21]

The Doppler principle is named after the mathematician and physicist named *Christian Johann Doppler* who first described this effect in 1842 by studying light from stars.

The same Doppler effect is applied in ultrasound to detect blood flow by analyzing the relative frequency shifts of received echoes brought about by the movement of red blood cells.

Doppler Shift (Fig. 29)

- It is the difference between the transmitted and received frequencies.
- Transmitted and received frequencies are in the MHZ range.
- Doppler shift frequencies often in audible range.
- **Blood velocity**: as velocity increases, so does the Doppler frequency.
- **Ultrasound frequency**: higher ultrasound frequencies give increased Doppler frequency.
- Angle of insonation **(Fig. 30)**

Doppler equation

- Relationship between Doppler shift (or just Doppler) frequency, F_0, and reflector velocity, v:

$$F_D = \frac{2f_0 v \cos\theta}{c}$$

- f_0 is the ultrasound frequency, or the transmitted beam frequency.
- v is the reflector velocity (m/s; cm/s)
- q is the Doppler angle
- c is the speed of sound

FIG. 29: Doppler equation.

Continuous Wave (CW) Doppler

- Use two crystals, one to send and one to receive.
- Uses continuous transmission and reception of ultrasound.
- Doppler signals are obtained from all vessels in the path of the ultrasound beam (until the ultrasound beam becomes sufficiently attenuated due to depth).
- Continuous wave Doppler ultrasound is unable to determine the specific location of velocities within the beam and cannot be used to produce color flow images.
- Used in adult cardiac scanners to investigate the high velocities in the aorta.

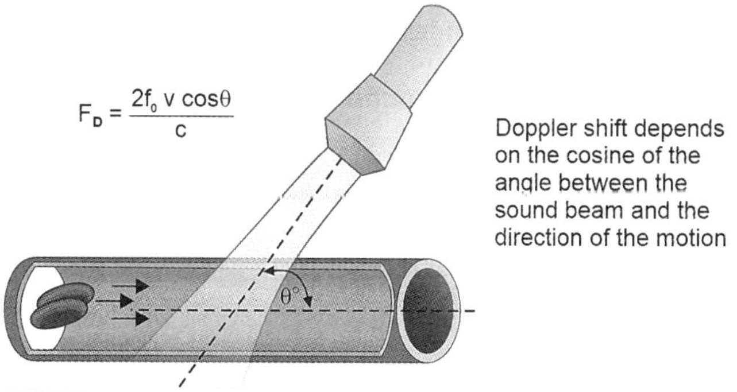

Angle	Cos theta
0	1
45	0.7
60	0.5
90	0

$$V = \frac{F_D \times C}{2f_0 \times \cos\theta}$$

Optimal angle → 30°–60°

FIG. 30: Calculation of angle of insonation *(For Color Version Refer Fig. 26)*.

Pulse Wave Doppler

- Uses brief pulses of ultrasound energy using only one crystal.
- The echo delay time can be converted into distance and the depth of echo source can be determined.
- The sensitive volume from which flow data are sampled can be controlled in terms of shape, depth and position.
  - Pulse repetition frequency (PRF): No. of pulses transmitted per second
  - With increasing scanning depth, PRF must be at least twice the frequency of the Doppler signal to construct the signal successfully.
  - This sets upper limit to the flow velocities to be accurately recorded.
  - Use higher PRF for high flow velocities, low PRF for slow venous flow.

Power Doppler

- New technology of doppler signal processing, in which its energy instead of its amplitude is recorded
- The energy is related to the square of the amplitude of the signal
- Using this technology, even weak signals (corresponding to low flow rates) can be recorded
- Sensitive to low flows
- No directional information
- Very poor temporal resolution
- Susceptible to noise

Duplex Ultrasound Scanning

These are real time B-mode scanners with built in Doppler capabilities.

- B-mode (for outline anatomic structures)
- Pulsed Doppler (for flow and movement patterns)

11. First and second generation of ultrasound contrast agent and its application. [10] [DNB June 21]

Ultrasound Contrast Agent

Ultrasound contrast agent is a new introduction in the field of medical imaging with proved result.

Properties

- Ultrasound contrast agents are microbubble gas with a shell made of protein, lipid or albumin, etc.
- They stay within the intravascular compartment, unable to go into the interstitium
- Get exhaled by lung and the coat is metabolized in liver
- Helpful in CKD patient, as there is no renal excretion
- Low mechanical index of the machine (0.07-0.2) is required for the imaging.

Classification of Ultrasound Contrast Agents (Table 12)

TABLE 12: Classification of ultrasound contrast agents.

First generation • Ecovist • Levovist • Albunex • Agitated saline	• They are comprised of soluble gas • Mainly used for right hear imaging, cardiac shunts, etc. • Large size
Second generation: • Sonovue • Luminity • Sonazoid • Optison	• Mostly these are used now a days • Contain insoluble gases like perfluorocarbon or sulfur hexafluoride • With different coating • Sonovue—ideal for vascular phase imaging of different organs • Sonazoid—additional phase—reticuloendothelial

Dosage

- Too much will cause too much scatter
- Too low—sub-diagnostic
- For intravenous use—Sonovue-half vial (2.4 mL) for liver lesion imaging
  - For other lesions—1.2 mL is used.
  - For intracavitary use 0.1–1 mL.

Technique: Intravenous cannulation

- Grey scale evaluation with target lesion in focus
- Freshly prepared sonovue administration followed by saline flush

Clinical Application

- **Liver lesions**: characterization of liver lesions
- CEUS can be used in categorizing LI-RADS category
- Also, in post treatment response assessment
  - HCC—non-rim arterial hyperenhancement with washout of a nodule >10 mm-LI-RADS5
  - Benign—
    - Hemangioma—peripheral nodular enhancement
    - FNH—spoke wheel centrifugal pattern of enhancement
    - Adenoma—hyperenhancing
  - Metastases—peripheral rim enhancement
- Pancreatic lesion—detection of pancreatic necrosis in acute pancreatitis
  - Pancreatic adenocarcinoma-hypoenhancing
- Renal—complex cystic lesion vs malignancy, renal pseudotumor, renal vascular lesion

Recent Advances

1. Hemodynamically stable abdominal trauma
2. Inflammatory aortoarteritis
3. Inflammatory bowel disease

12. Ultrasound artifacts. [5] [DNB June 20, AIIMS May 23, AIIMS May 24]

- Artifacts is a term used to describe any unwanted information generated in the process of image formation **(Table 13)**.
- The ultrasound equipment relies on physical assumption to assign location and intensity of each received echo.

  The assumptions are:
  - The echo detected arose from within the main US beam.
  - It has returned to the transducer after a single reflection.
  - Sound travels at a constant speed and in a straight line.
  - The acoustic energy in an ultrasound field is uniformly attenuated.
  - While examining patients using ultrasound these assumptions are often not maintained resulting in artifacts.

TABLE 13: Ultrasound artifacts.

Artifacts associated with ultrasound beam characteristics	
1. **Beam width Artifact** 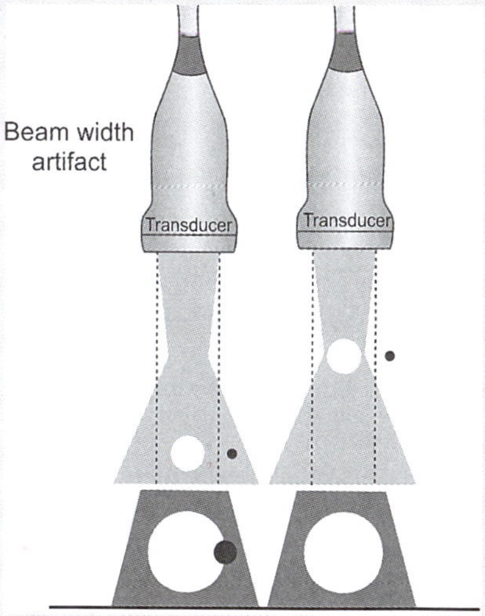	• Ultrasound beam exits the transducer at approximately the same width as the transducer – Narrows as it approaches the focal zone – Widens again distal to focal zone and the distal beam widens beyond the actual width of the transducer. • A highly reflective object located within the widened beam beyond the edges of the transducer may generate detectable echoes. • The system assumes that these echoes arose from within the imaging plane and displays them accordingly.

Continued...

Continued...

Artifacts associated with ultrasound beam characteristics	
2. **Side lobe and grating lobe artifacts** 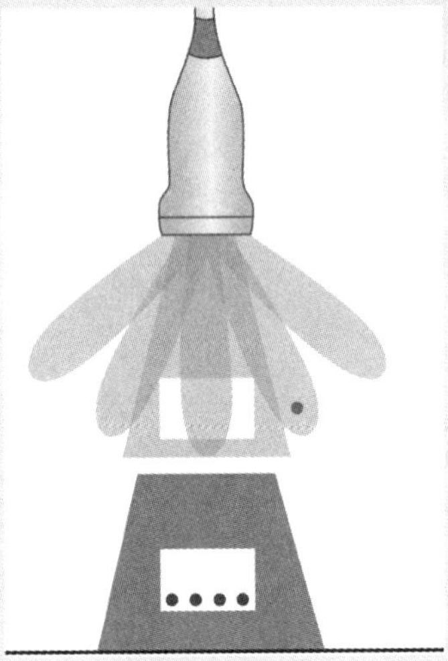	• These are multiple beams of low amplitude ultrasound energy that project radially from the main beam • It is generated from the radial expansion of piezoelectric crystals and is seen primarily in linear array transducers. • Strong reflectors present in the path of these low energy off axis beams may create echoes detectable by the transducer. These echoes will be displayed as having originated from within the main beam in the side beam artifact
Artifacts associated with multiple echoes	
1. **Reverberation artifacts**	• US assumes that an echo returns to the transducer after a single reflection and that the depth of an object is related to the time for this round trip. • However, in the presence of two parallel highly reflective surfaces, the echoes generated from a primary ultrasound beam may be reflected back and forth before returning to the transducer. • The sequential echoes will take longer to return to the transducer and the ultrasound will erroneously place the delayed echoes at an increased distance from the transducer. • Appearance • Series of bright bands • Parallel to sound beam's main axis • Decreasing in intensity • Equidistant from each other
2. **Comet tail**	• It is a form of reverberation artifact • Since the reverberation bands depends on the distance between the reflectors if the reflectors are very closely spaced the sequential echoes may be close that individual bands cannot be seen. • Commonly seen deep to calcifications, surgical clips, IUCD and in adenomyosis of gallbladder. • Surgical clips, staples, sutures and mechanical heart valves
3. **Ringdown (resonance)**	• Another form of reverberation artifact. Occurs due to the resonance (vibration) of the fluid trapped between air bubbles • Displayed as line of series of parallel bands extending posterior gas collection
4. **Mirror image artifact**	• Also called multi-path artifact. • Generated by false assumption that echo return to the transducer after a single reflection. • Commonly seen at the level of the diaphragm with pleural air interface acting as the strong reflector.
5. **Acoustic enhancement**	When ultrasound beam encounters a focal weakly attenuating structure within the imaging field, the amplitude of the beam beyond this structure is greater seen in cystic lesions

Continued...

Continued...

Artifacts associated with multiple echoes	
6. **Artifacts associated with velocity errors** – **Speed-displacement artifact** – **Refraction artifact**	• This artifact is mostly seen when an area of focal fat is encountered. • The returning echoes takes longer to return to the transducer. • The system assumes delay is due to increased distance travelled by the echo. • The echoes are thus displayed deeper on the image than they actually are. • Here non-perpendicular incident ultrasound energy encounters an interface between two materials with different speeds of sound. • When this occurs incident ultrasound beam changes direction. • Usually seen in pelvic imaging occurring deep to the junction of the rectus muscles and midline fat.

13. PC-PNDT Act and its applications. [5] [DNB June 20, AIIMS May 23, AIIMS May 24, MD (WBUHS) 24]

The pre-natal diagnostic technique act came into 20th September, 1994.

This act came after the government realized the rapid decline in the sex ratio predominantly in the northern part of India due to pre-natal termination of female fetus.

- Orthodox mindset of society makes female child unwelcome in many families.
- To combat this, PNDT act came.
- The PNDT law is a prohibitory and regulatory statute in order to check female feticide.
- The Act has undergone 2 amendments—
  1. The pre-natal diagnostic techniques (regulation and prevention of misuse) amendment Act, 2001
  2. The pre-natal diagnostic techniques (regulation and prevention of misuse) amendment Act, 2002

The nomenclature of the Act has been amended and now it stands (wef 14-2-03)-
The pre-conception and pre-natal diagnostic techniques (prohibition of sex selection) Act, 1994

Implications of the 2002 Amendment are:

- Mainly covered bringing the technique of pre-conception sex selection within the ambit of the act
- Bringing ultrasound within its ambit
- Empowering the central supervisory board, constitution of state level supervisory board
- Provision for more stringent punishments
- Empowering appropriate authorities for search, seizure and sealing the machines of the violators
- Regulating the sale of ultrasound machines only to registered bodies.
- **Sex selection includes**:
  - Procedure
  - Technique
  - Test
- Administration/Prescription/Provision of anything for the purpose of ensuring or increasing the probability that an embryo will be of a particular sex

Qualified persons are:

- Radiologist
- Sonologist/imaging specialist
- Gynecologist
- Pediatrician
- Registered medical practitioner having 6 months training or 1 year experience in U/S
- Medical geneticist—degree or diploma in genetic science in the field of sex selection and prenatal diagnostic techniques

Objectives

Prohibition of misuse of PNDT for sex determination

- Prohibition of advertisement
- Permission and regulation of use of PNDT by registered centers under specific circumstances
- Punishment for violation of the provisions of the act

PNDT Act and Rules

Applicable to:

- All Govt./Private hospitals and Nursing homes
- Genetic counselling centers/genetic labs/ USG clinics/Imaging centers
- NGOs
- Vehicles

PNDT Act implementation

Sub-district level

- District level
- State level—State supervisory board
- Central level—Central supervisory board

Appropriate authority (AA) at district is the key person—appointed by central/state governments—advisory committee

Functions of Appropriate Authority

- Grant/suspend/cancel registration
- Enforce the standard prescribed
- To investigate complaints of breach of provision of these Act and Rules
- To seek and consider the advice of Advisory Committee constituted for application or registration and on complaints for suspension or cancellation of registration
- To take appropriate legal action against the use of any sex selection technique
- To create public awareness against the practice of sex selection
- To supervise the implementation of the provisions of the Act

Powers of AA

Summoning of any person who is in possession of any information relating to violations of the provisions of this Act

- Production of any document or material object relating to the above clause
- Issuing search warrant for any place suspected to be indulging in sex determination techniques.

Mandatory Prerequisites for USG Clinic

Registration of the clinic is mandatory.

- Details of all machines and radiologists with copies of their certificates are to be submitted
- In case of portable machines, if USG is to be done in a vehicle, registration of the vehicle is required
- Copy of the registration must be displayed in the machine room and in the waiting room
- Sign board in English and the local language must be displayed, indicating that fetal sex is not disclosed in the clinic

Form F must be filled completely as soon as the USG is done. Signed consent of the patient and radiologist's signature are a must.

- A monthly report should be submitted to the AA regularly by the 5th of every month.
- All records including from F and reference doctor requisition, case record and USG reports must be kept for 2 years. Sonographic plates/films also need to be preserved, if provided to patient.

- In case of any legal dispute till the final disposal of legal proceeding
- PC-PNDT Act book must be available in the department.

Procedure of Registration

What is to be registered—center/USG machine/sonologist/place?

- Submission of form A in duplicate to AA
- **Application fee**:
  - ₹ 25000—Genetic counseling center/clinic/laboratory/ultrasound center/imaging center
  - ₹ 35000—Any combination of above
    - Demand Draft made in favor of AA
    - Affidavit—an undertaking that the center shall not conduct any procedure for sex determination, and that the center shall display a prominent sign board stating the same
- Particulars of the USG machines, qualification/experience certificate of the sonologist are to be attached
- Grant of certificate or rejection within 90 days of submission of the application
- Certificate of registration is nontransferable
- Change of ownership/management—2 copies of registration certificate to be surrendered to the AA.

New owners shall apply afresh

- Validity—5 years from the date of issue

New Registration by AA—Placed before Advisory Committee

- AA—Grants a certificate of registration in duplicate in Form-B within 90 days
- 1 copy displayed in Clinic
- If application rejected—communicate rejection in Form C.
- Form D—Records at genetic counseling centers
- Form E—Records at genetic labs
- Form F—Genetic clinic/ultrasound clinic/imaging center
- Form G—Consent Form
- Form H—Records of AA

Renewal of Registration

Application Form-A in duplicate—30 days before the date of expiry

- 2 copies of earlier certificate to be surrendered
- Fee—half of the new registration fee
- Further renewal for 5 years
- Intimate any change—within 30 days
- Send complete report of all preconception and pregnancy related techniques test by 5th of every month.

Who is Responsible

- Unit owner/manager/individuals/corporate firms/association of people who owns the unit
- Any person doing or seeking sex-selection/determination PNDT Act invites criminal liability

The offences are:

- Cognizable
- Nonbailable
- Noncompoundable

Trial by:

- Metropolitan Magistrate or
- Judicial Magistrate of the 1st Class

Violation Penalty

Minor offences

- Nonavailability of copy of the PNDT Act in the registered center
- Nondisplay of registration certificate
- Nondisplay of Board in the Premises
- Punishment up to 3 months or with fine up to ₹ 1,000 for first offence.
- Additional fine up to ₹ 500 per day for the period of contravention for subsequent offence.
- Or Show cause notice for temporary suspension of registration
- Advertisement relating to preconception and prenatal determination of sex. Imprisonment up to 3 years, fine up to ₹ 10,000.

Any person found guilty of seeking the aid of pre-natal diagnostic techniques for sex selection shall be punishable for a term up to 3 years/fine up to ₹ 50,000 for the first offense and 5 years/1 lakh rupees for subsequent offenses.

Computed Tomography

1. Discuss the principle and utility of dual energy CT. [6+4] [MD (WBUHS) 23, MD (WBUHS) 20, MD (WBUHS) 17, AIIMS Dec 23, DNB Dec 20, DNB June 20]

Principle: Dual energy: 2 X-ray source and 2 detectors

- Simultaneously acquire data sets at two different kVp in single CT acquisition[3]
- Material decomposition possibledue to differential absorption of X-ray at energy depending on its k-edge.
  - Two main interactions of matter with X-ray in clinical imaging: **Photoelectric effect and compton scatter**
  - Photoelectric effect: Incident photon interacts with K-shell electron and generate a photoelectron **(Fig. 31)**
  - Likelihood of photoelectric effect (PE) depends on the atomic number and energy of the beam
  - K-edge: Increase in attenuation of X-ray at incident energy level just greater than K-shell binding energy due to increased PE
  - K-edge value ∝ Atomic number **(Table 14)**

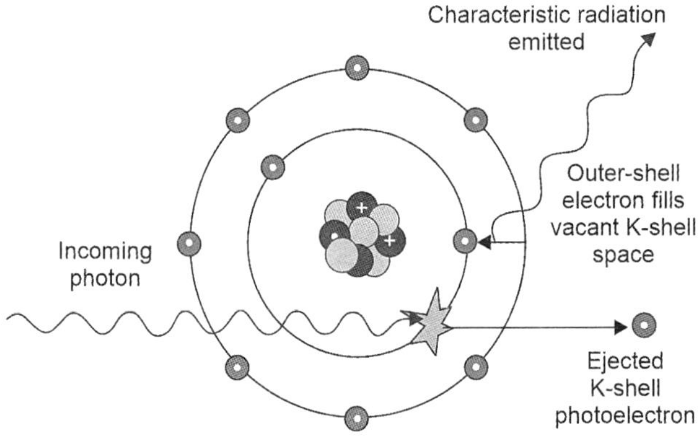

FIG. 31: Photoelectric effect.

TABLE 14: K-edge and atomic number of common substances.

Substance	*K-edge (keV)*	*Atomic Number (Z)*
Hydrogen	0.01	1
Carbon	0.28	6
Nitrogen	0.40	7
Oxygen	0.53	8
Calcium	4.00	20
Iodine	33.20	53
Barium	37.45	56
Gadolinium	50.20	64

In dual energy CT, images are obtained at 80 and 140 kVp.

Detection of enhancing structure or vessels is easily done at 80 kVp image as these structures contain iodine.

On conventional single-energy CT images, two materials can often not be distinguished due to considerable overlap in their CT numbers. On dual-energy CT scans, materials with different elemental compositions can be differentiated and quantified by comparing their CT numbers at two different energy levels **(Fig. 32)**.

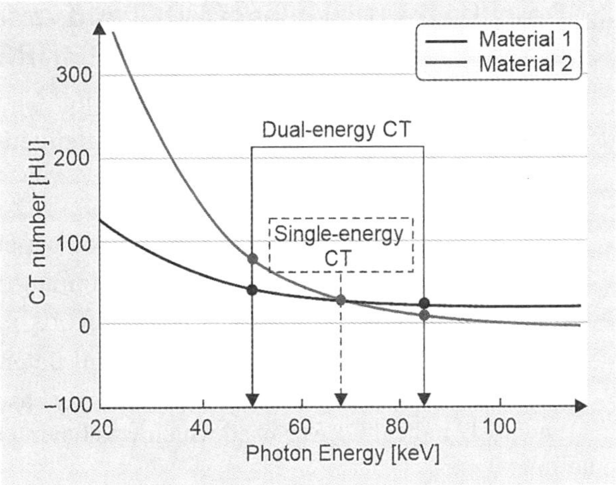

FIG. 32: Principle of dual energy CT.

Applications

Material decomposition, e.g., soft tissue-, fat-, and iodine-is possible with DECT. Another benefit of DECT is virtual unenhanced can be obtained, avoiding the need of taking NCCT.

Applications of dual energy CT **(Table 15)**.

TABLE 15: Applications of dual energy CT.

System	*Description*
Head & neck tumors	1. Differentiate from hyperdense hemorrhage to enhancement in hemorrhagic mass 2. Differentiating mass from other lesions
Brain trauma	Use of virtual NECT—hemorrhage vs contrast extravasation, especially stroke patients
Cardiothoracic imaging	• Thoracic oncology—differentiate benign vs malignant • Ex- thymic cyst vs epithelial tumors • Pulmonary nodules • Cardiac—efficient depiction of myocardial perfusion/infarction • Pulmonary thromboembolism • High iodine density/increased perfusion of the lung parenchyma around the pulmonary opacity in COVID-19
Abdominal imaging	• Hypervascular liver metastasis • Better depiction of pancreatic and renal cell carcinoma • Follow up after hepatic tumor ablation or TACE- caution in case of imaging with lipiodol • Differentiating from fat containing lesion to steatohepatitis in absence of iron deposition • Differentiation between lymphoma vs lymph node metastases • Bowel lesions—mural enhancement-inflammatory bowel lesions-Crohn's disease • Dual-energy CT can detect the presence of transmural necrosis of the appendix /gallbladder- thus helping in planning of surgery • Adrenal adenoma—no need of NCCT for the detection fat within the lesion. • Renal cyst characterization—differentiating simple and complex cyst or solid enhancing lesion or hemorrhagic cyst
Gallstones and renal calculi	1. Identification of composition of gallbladder calculi 2. Dual-energy CT can differentiate non-uric acid calculi from uric acid calculi 3. In DS-DECT, if the dual energy ratio is kept below1.13, uric acid calculi seen to lie below the reference level while non-UA calculi above it.
DECT in vascular imaging	For the evaluation of the carotid and cerebral arteries virtual monoenergetic imaging at 40–60 keV provides excellent result diagnostic accuracy for detection of endoleak is also increased
DECT in musculoskeletal application	• DECT—promising result in the diagnosis of gout. • Non-invasive alternative to synovial fluid aspiration. • Bone marrow edema marker of occult fractures or stress fractures, various studies revealed that DECT virtual non-calcium imaging can detect BME • In patients with trauma, VNC images can be created to differentiate chronic fractures from acute and non-displaced occult fractures.
Metal artifact reduction	Combining metal artifact reduction software with high keV imaging suggested to achieve the greatest artifact reduction in patients

2. Describe the principles of MDCT and various reconstruction methods. What are the techniques of radiation dose reduction? [4+3+3] [RG 18, MD (WBUHS) 22, MD (WBUHS) 21]

Computed tomography is an imaging modality which acquires and reconstructs a cross-sectional image of body depending on precise measurement of X-ray attenuation by computers.

Basic Principle of CT

- Beam of X-ray scans across thin cross section of patient
- On opposite side detectors detect X-ray attenuation
- Multiple scans taken at different orientation of X-ray tube and detectors collection and representation of data.
- Distribution of X-ray attenuation coefficients determined by computer as shades of image
- Followed by image reconstruction and display based on these attenuation coefficient

Previously helical CT was used which was having the limitation of increased scan time and poor coverage of large anatomical area.

There after the concept of MDCT, i.e., multidetector CT was introduced

- These are all third generation rotate—rotate geometry
- Replacing single row of detector by multiple rows along the z-axis **(Fig. 33)**
- **Major advantages**:
    - Reduced time of scan
    - Increased anatomical coverage

Technical Principles

Isotropic data acquisition

- Isotropy—"uniformity in all orientations"
- Each voxel has length, breath, and depth
- In SS-CT, slice thickness cannot be reduced
    - Increase scan time
    - Reduce volume coverage
- Voxel does not have same length in all 3 planes
- With MDCT idea of isotropic data was conceived

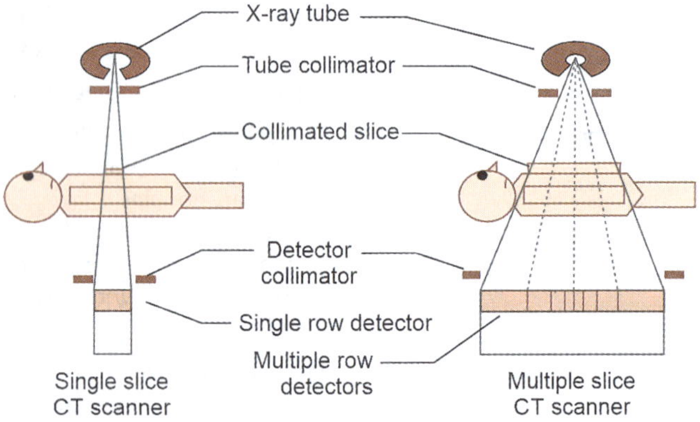

FIG. 33: Basic difference between single and multiple slice CT scanner.

- But with initial MDCT thinnest sections was 1.25 mm (was the smallest length of DE available) so data was still anisotropic
- Higher slice MDCT (16 and higher) used DE with length <1 mm thus reducing slice thickness
- Made isotropic data reconstruction possible
- Now length, breath and width of a voxel became equal in all planes.

Detectors

Detector Row

- **SS-CT**: 1 X-ray tube and 1 row of detectors (contains 500–900 detector elements)
- **MS-CT scanner**: 1 X-ray tube and multiple rows of detectors (each row has multiple detector elements) along z axis of patient
- Each row has multiple detector elements (DE)
- Detector arrays are mounted on electronics module, which includes power supplies for the amplifiers, amplification circuits for the detector module, analog to digital converter systems.

Detector Array Design

Divided into two groups:

1. Detector elements of equal width along the z axis (also called *matrix/mosaic detectors*)
2. Detector elements of unequal width (also called *adaptive/non-uniform array detectors*)

Types of Image Reconstruction

- Image obtained in CT is different from conventional radiography.
- In radiography, X-rays form image directly on image receptor.
- In CT, X-rays form electrical signal which is reconstructed to form image.
- The cross-sectional portion of body which is scanned for the production of CT image has length, breath, and depth.
- So has a volume.

  MATRIX: The cross-section is divided into 3D rectangular blocks (80 × 80 initially now days 512 × 512)

  VOXEL: 3D volume representing each element

  PIXEL: 2D representation of each element (no depth)

Linear Attenuation Coefficient (μ)

"Main objective of CT image reconstruction is to determine the amount of X-ray attenuation in each voxel of reconstruction matrix".

- Is used to quantify the attenuation of X-ray in a voxel.
- For each voxel, attenuation is calculated by—The number of initial photon (Io), transmitted photons (It) and thickness (t).
- The main role of computer is to determine μ of each individual voxel from the total value detected by detectors
- This is done by mathematical computational methods called algorithm
- Most commonly used methods include **(Table 16)**:[4]
  - Filtered back projection
  - Iterative methods

TABLE 16: CT reconstruction algorithms.

Filtered back projection	• Also called summation method • Its principle demonstrates: – When a ray from two projection is superimposed or back projected they produce a reproduction of original object – Most popular reconstruction algorithm used today in CT
Iterative reconstruction	• *Iteration means* act of repeating a process with the aim of approaching a desired goal, target or result • It is a mathematical model based on trial and error • It start with an assumption that all point in matrix have same value • And make correction until values come within acceptable range • Is a newer more robust algorithm-requires lesser amount of data for reconstruction, this helps reduce radiation dose • All X-ray attenuation data must be available before reconstruction can begin

Techniques of Radiation Dose Reduction

Although being an excellent informative modality CT carries the disadvantage of radiation exposure; so we should be highly very cautious in CT imaging to reduce the exposure without losing any diagnostic information.

AERB guideline of safety:

1. Justification
2. Optimization
3. Dose limitation

Strategies to Reduce Exposure in CT (Table 17)

TABLE 17: Techniques of radiation dose reduction.

Before the scan	• Avoid if other imaging modality solves the question • Avoid duplicate imaging • Avoid studies with low yield	
During the scan	Modification of acquisition parameters	• Proper positioning of patient • Reduce Kvp • Reduce mAs • Reduce scan length • Increase pitch • Optimize slice thickness • Taking scan during selected phases • Size dependent protocol • DECT- virtual noncontrast image reconstruction
	• Automated exposure control • Software – Siemens: CARE- target effective mAs – Philips: Reference image concept – GE: Noise index concept	Advanced technology in recent scanner-by which scanner automatically chose the proper kvp and mAs with reference of topogram
After the scan	Iterative reconstruction	Reduce noise and improve image quality

3. Briefly outline the evolution of presentday CT scanners citing the key specific change through different generations. [10] [MD (WBUHS) 24, MD (WBUHS) 19]

First commercial CT scanner introduced in 1971 with a single detector for brain study by Sir Godfrey Hounsfield

Further upgradation was done by modifying the source and detector

Based on

- X-ray beam geometry
- Pencil; fan
- Detector array/shape
- Single; arc; ring
- If X-ray tube-detector complex translates across the cross-section or not

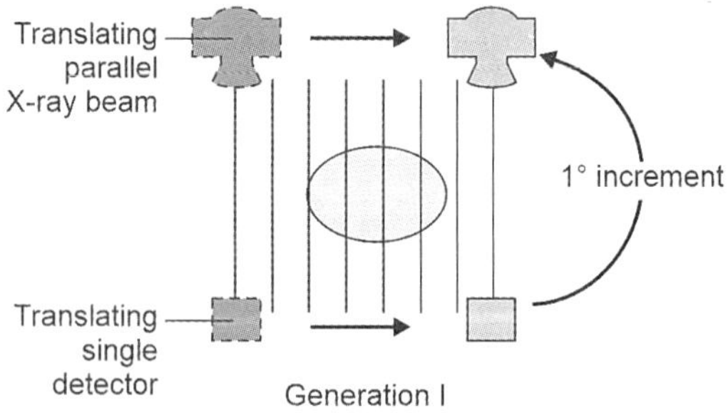

FIG. 34: First generation CT scanner.

First Generation (Fig. 34)

- Pencil—beam
- Single detector
- Translate—rotate configuration
- 4.5 to 5 min scan time per slice (for head scan 25-30 min)

Limitations

- It took longer time
- Only head scan is possible

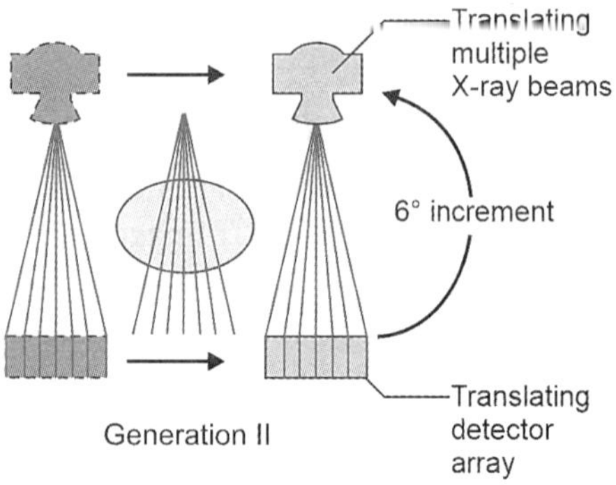

FIG. 35: Second generation CT scanner.

Second Generation (Fig. 35)

- Fan-shaped beam (5°–30°)
- Detector up to 30 in number

- Translate—rotate configuration
- 10–90-second scan time.

Advantage: Reduce scan time-after one translation gantry rotated—5°-30°

Limitations: Increased scattered radiation—fan-shaped beam instead of pencil beam

Third Generation (Fig. 36)

- Fan-shaped beam (5°–30°).
- Detector up to 30 in number
- Translate–rotate configuration
- 10-90-second scan time

Advantage: Reduce scan time—after one translation gantry rotated 5°–30°

Limitations

- Increased scattered radiation—fan-shaped beam instead of pencil beam
- *Designed to overcome ring artifacts*

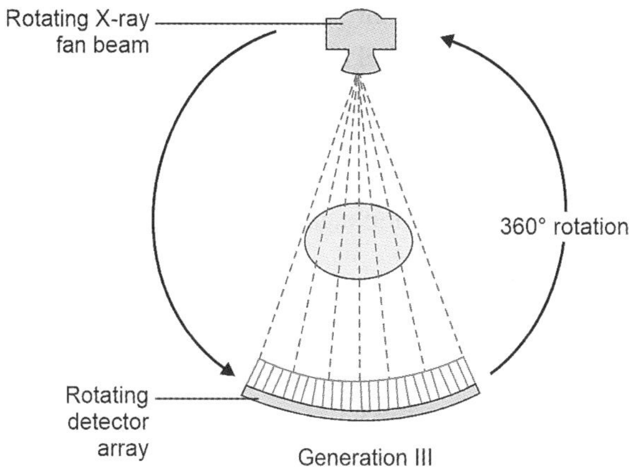

FIG. 36: Third generation CT scanner.

Fourth Generation (Fig. 37)

- Fan-beam.
- Ring of detector array
- Rotate-fixed configuration.
- ≤1-second scan time.

Advantages:
- It eliminated "ring artifacts".
- No fear of cable wear and tear as detector fixed

Disadvantages:
- Costly
- Inefficient use of detectors

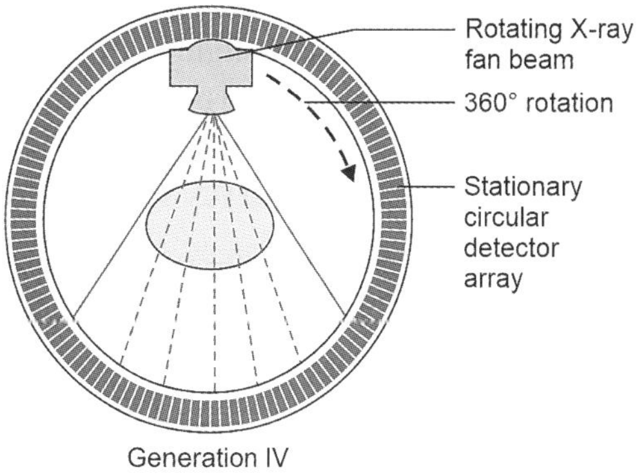

FIG. 37: Fourth-generation CT scanner.

Fifth Generation

- Electron beam CT
- Used for ultra-fast scanning
- Large bell shaped X-ray tube
- Electron beam emitted from cathode is focused into a narrow beam and electronically deflected to fall on a small focal post of anode
- Electron beam is swept along all or part of circumference of the target
- No physical motion of source or detector

Sixth Generation

- Helical or spiral CT
  - Previous to this scanners act in a sequence
  - Tube rotation around patient for 360 degree-then translation of table- then again rotation
- Continuous acquisition of 3D volume of data done by continuous rotation of X-ray tube and detector with simultaneous translation of patient across the gantry with the help of slip ring technology

- Modification of third-generation CT with volumetric data acquisitions.
- Slip-ring technology:
  - Electromechanical Devices
  - Circular contact ring with sliding brushes that allows passage of electric impulses
  - Allows the gantry to rotate continually, untethered by wires.
  - Sets of parallel conducting rings concentric to gantry axis that is connected to tube and detectors by carbon brushes.
- High-power X-ray tubes- high heat capacity with two focal spots
- Interpolation algorithms-produces helical trajectory
- CT reconstruction algorithms assume that the X-ray source has negotiated a circular, and not helical, path around the patient.
- For image reconstruction, helical data sets along z-axis are interpolated into a series of planar image data sets.
- Also allows production of overlapping images with no additional dose to patient (interleaved reconstruction).

Seventh Generation CT

- Multi-row detector CT
- Begins to utilize radiation along z-axis
- All are third-generation rotate—rotate geometry
- Replacing single row of detector by multiple rows along the z-axis
- **Major advantages**:
  - Reduced time of scan
  - Increased anatomical coverage
  - Isotropic data acquisition
  - Pitch does not depend on collimation, depends on detector

4. Mobile CT scan and its applications. [5]

The concept of mobile imaging came in 1980, CT was the first modality to get introduced in Mobile vendor.

- Presence of mobile imaging trailer made these possible
- It is a type of MDCT.

Usage

1. Stroke imaging
2. Imaging of patients whose transportation not possible.
3. Use in covid pneumonia
4. Screening mammography in rural population
5. Screening of tuberculosis
6. Sometimes expansion of hospital not possible, there mobile CT may give a solution.
   - Mobile CT originated in USA but now-a-days has gained popularity all over world
   - Mobile CT is same as fixed CT except it is fixed on a trailer with proper shielding
   - The trailer provides heating and air conditioning, which allows it to operate in many different weather conditions.
   - Mobile units typically withstand in external conditions of -20°F to 110°F, relying on air-conditioning, heating, and humidification units to maintain proper environmental conditions inside the trailer.
   - Maintenance of a mobile CT is a key factor due to the stresses in moving the system in a trailer of torque, vibration, shock, vertical and lateral movement.

Mobile CT Advantages

- Shared costs and services between multiple sites (hospitals/branches)
- Less travel for patients
- Decreased preinstallation costs
- Increased revenue and ability to justify the purchase by receiving revenue from multiple clinics or hospitals
- Ability to alter locations based on patient volume. Flexible fixed schedule and/or on-demand
- Dramatically shorter installation time with fewer logistics issues.
- Lower initial investment

Mobile CT Disadvantages

- More frequent maintenance
- Not advantageous for sites that may need emergency scans because it's possible the unit will be at a different location
- **Transportation costs**: Driver's salary, fuel (including generator fuel), mileage, and insurance, which are not associated with a fixed site
- Increased downtime for site travel and more frequent maintenance and quality assurance checks
- Limited interior space and increased claustrophobia incidents

5. What are the limitations of standard coronary CT scan with a retrospective ECG-gated acquisition? Describe the current and novel imaging strategies to overcome these limitations. [5+5]

MDCT is now widely used for the assessment of coronary artery disease because of its improve spatial and temporal resolution.

- Spatial—currently in range of 0.4 mm in 64-slice scanner.
- Pre-requisite—heart rate control, oral/IV β-blocker, e.g., metoprolol used

Retrospective ECG-gated

- It is one of the two techniques of cardiac CT **(Fig. 38)**
- Here images are acquired throughout the cardiac cycle, making it more informative

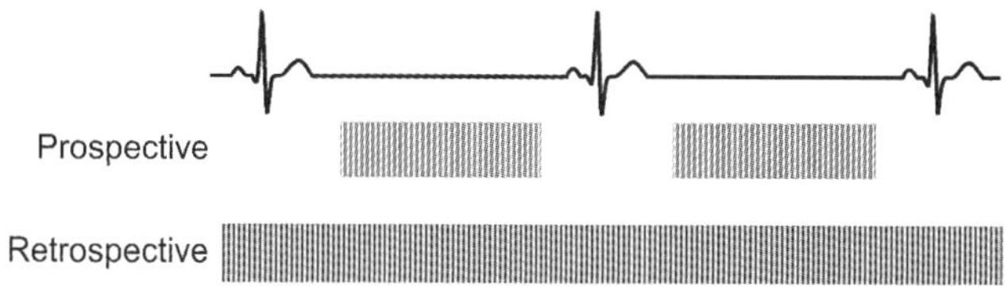

FIG. 38: Prospective and retrospective ECG-gating of cardiac CT.

- Person taking the scan can choose the phase of cardiac cycle for better visualization of coronary arteries and pathology
- It also provides information about ventricular and valvular function

Disadvantages

As the scan is taken for the entire cycle, patient radiation dose is higher

To overcome this,

1. Prospective gating is used—where imaging is done in a specific period of cycle, preferable end diastole
   - Scans are taken after R peak of the ECG/ R-R interval, approximately 75% of RR interval is used for imaging.
   - Prospective CT 3-5 mSV
   - Retrospective CT 12-13 mSV.
2. Electron beam CT—very fast acquisition, not readily available
3. Dual energy CT—radiation less than 1 msv.

6. CT enterography. [5]

CT enterography is an emerging and promising technique for the evaluation of the small bowel pathologies.

Multi-detector CT with thin slice of acquisition and appropriate luminal distension, these are two key components of CT enterography.

Indications

1. Crohn's disease
2. Suspected small bowel pathology
3. Hemodynamically stable case of small bowel bleed
4. Suspected cases of small bowel stricture

Contrast: Neutral oral contrast, preferably mannitol

Procedure

Three percent mannitol solution is used for enterography, about 1500 mL of appropriately dilated solution is given to patient in 4 divided doses in a span of 45–60 mins before study. 200–250 mL of contrast is given just before the scan or on the table for the distension of the stomach.

Acquisition is done 45–60 seconds after the injection of contrast; it can be multiphasic in suspected cased of GI bleed.

Advantages

1. Non-invasive, unlike CT enteroclysis where luminal distension is done by giving contrast via NG tube
2. Well appreciation of strictures, depending on the status of post-contrast enhancement activity of the disease can be commented.

7. CT enteric contrast agents. [5] [DNB Dec 21]

In general, enteric contrast media is used interchangeably with oral contrast media, but rectal contrast also comes under this.

Primarily the use of oral contrast is to distend the bowel loops properly, so that it can be easily differentiated from other abdominal structures.

Mainly oral contrast is of two types:

1. **Neutral oral contrast**: Water, mannitol, polyethylene glycol—low attenuation solution which mimics water, these are very good for depicting the strictures, enteroliths, etc. They are excellent for depicting mural abnormalities.
2. **Positive oral contrast**: Iodinated or barium solution, volumen (0.1% of barium suspension) which are radio-opaque, hence the bowel loops appear distinct from other structure. In case of leaks, these contrasts show better visualization.

For routine abdominal CT 1-1.5 liter of contrast is given to the patient over a period of 45-60 minutes in divided doses with some amount of water on table for the distension of stomach.

- 2-3% of mannitol solution is used for neutral oral contrast.
- In cases of suspected rectal carcinoma, positive oral contrast is given in general.

Disadvantages of Oral Contrast

- Generally, both the contrast is well tolerated
- In suspected cases of perforation barium solutions should not be given due to the chances of peritonitis or mediastinitis.
- In very few cases, mannitol can cause diarrhea as it is osmotically active.

8. Cone beam CT. [5] [DNB June 21]

- X-rays beam is cone shaped not fan shaped
- Volume of images acquired by rotating tube-detector around patient 3D volume acquired, contrary to conventional where both rotation and translation along z-axis is done
- Patient stationary

X-ray tube: Low energy power equipment

Detectors: Recently FPDs–flat panel detector of indirect conversion type based on cesium iodide is used.

Image Reconstruction

- High isotropic spatial resolution
- Volumetric data reconstructed into MPRs and panoramic reconstructions
- Reconstruction algorithm is a modification of filtered back-projection, known as Feldkamp algorithm
- Longer times for acquisition and reconstruction despite acquisition done in single rotation

Advantages

- Reduction of radiation dose relative to MDCT- 0.2 mSv vs 1–2 mSv for CT head.
- Patient upright for scans no need to lie
- Significantly cheaper than MDCT.

Limitations

- Limited anatomic coverage
- Poor contrast resolution—higher scatter
- **CsI FPD limitations**:
  - Greater response time
  - Lower quantum efficiency and dynamic range

Applications

- Maxillofacial imaging includes dental imaging, sinus and temporal bone imaging.
- C-arm based CBCT systems used In Interventional radiology and orthopedic surgeries.
- Surgical planning in head and neck and neurosurgical procedures
- Radiation therapy planning.

Magnetic Resonance Imaging

1. Discuss the principle of MR spectroscopy in brief and its utility in differentiation of brain lesions. [3 + 7] [MD (WBUHS) 23, MD (WBUHS) 19, DNB June 20]

Principle of MR Spectroscopy

Physical and chemical properties of a tissue can be assessed by the spectrum of MR spectroscopy. MR spectroscopy is based on the fact that certain atoms have odd number of protons and neutrons such as H1, P-31, C-3 having a magnetic moment, so they interact with magnetic field.

In case of MRS signal is acquired without a frequency encoding gradient, so the signal obtained differs in frequency corresponding to chemical shift, spatial data is not obtained.[5]

The amplitude of chemical shift depends on the gyromagnetic ration of the atom and also the external magnetic field. In presence of a static magnetic field, every chemically distinct nucleus resonates at a slightly different frequency-giving the spectra.

J coupling or spin coupling is due to interactions with a neighbor atom which provides additional information. It can cause fusion of peaks-lactate at 1.4 ppm.

The water signal needs to be suppressed (either via inversion recovery or chemical shift selective (CHESS) techniques) as its intensity is much higher than the signal intensity of other metabolites due to its high concentration making the other metabolites undetectable on MRS.

- Single voxel spectroscopy—in case of homogeneous pathology
- Pulse sequences used in SVS are—STEAM, PRES ISIS
- Multivoxel spectroscopy—lesion or pathology showing heterogeneity

MRS can detect metabolites or chemicals having concentration more than 0.1 mM.

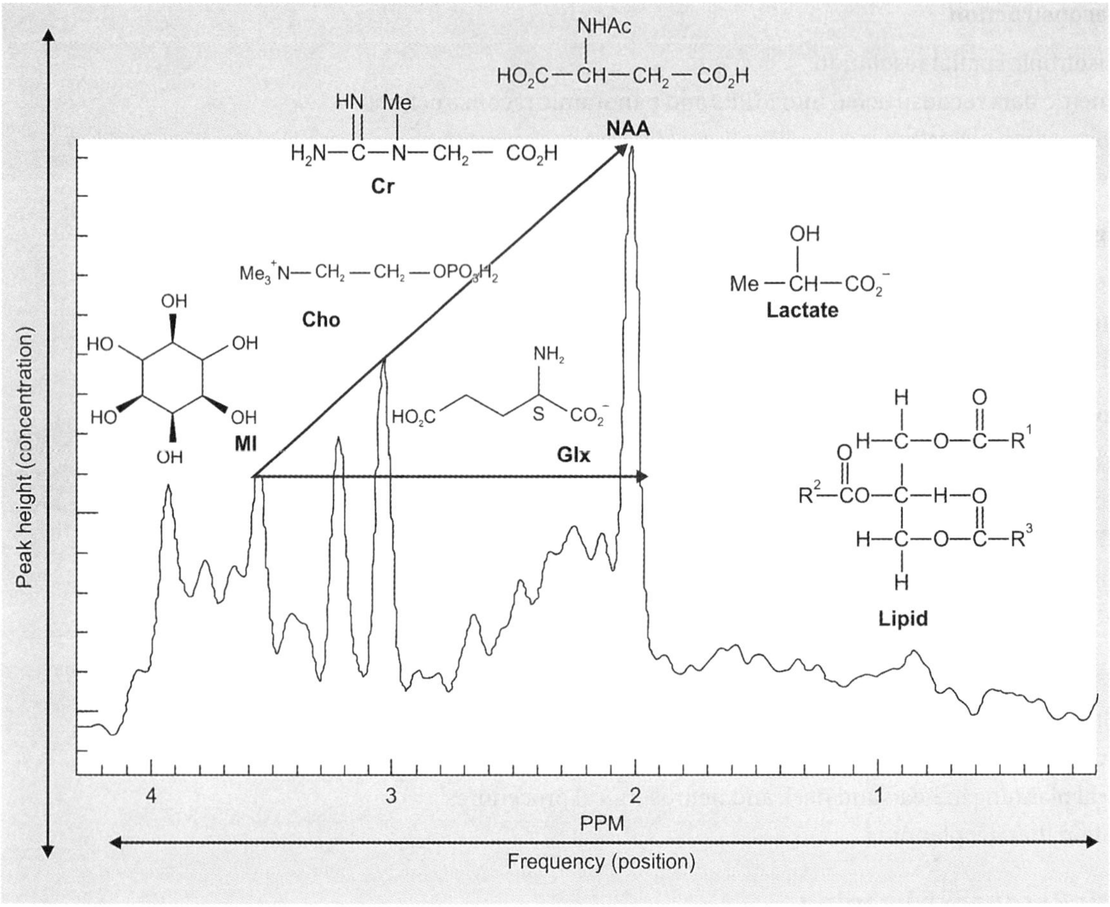

FIG. 39: Hunter's angle.

Hunter's Angle (Fig. 39)

Peaks

Many thousands of metabolite peaks have been described, although most are not identifiable using routing imaging techniques and it is the Time of Echo (TE) that conditions the number of measurable metabolites: long TE (136-272 ms) vs short TE (10-50 ms).

Peaks are plotted from right to left along the x-axis and the y-axis (height) is the degree of chemical shift as expressed in part-per-million (ppm). Normal choline, creatine, and NAA peaks form a straight line that if extended, create an angle of 45 degrees with the x-axis. This is known as Hunter's angle and can be used to determine quickly whether the MRS is most probably normal or not.

- **Lipids**: Resonates at 1.3 ppm
- **Lactate**: Resonates at 1.33 ppm
- **Alanine**: Resonates at 1.48 ppm
- **N-acetylaspartate (NAA)**: Resonates at 2.0 ppm
- **Glutamine/glutamate**: Resonates at 2.2-2.4 ppm
- **GABA**: Resonates at 2.2-2.4 ppm
- **2-hydroxyglutarate**: Resonates at 2.25 ppm
- **Citrate**: Resonates 2.6 ppm
- **Creatine**: Resonates at 3.0 ppm
- **Choline**: Resonates at 3.2 ppm

Application of MRS in Brain Lesion

Brain tumors:

- Noninvasive diagnosis and grading of tumors
- Tumor extent
- Therapeutic planning for gliomas
- Distinction between radiation necrosis and recurrent tumor

Potential uses of magnetic resonance spectroscopy in brain tumor imaging **(Table 18)**

Frequently encountered metabolites and their characteristics and clinical role in evaluating brain tumors **(Table 19)**.[6]

TABLE 18: Potential uses of magnetic resonance spectroscopy in brain tumor imaging.

Clinical applications	*Research applications*
• Differentiating tumor from potential mimics – Metastatic disease – Demyelinating disease – Lymphoma – Infection • Evaluation of treated tumor to differentiate – Recurrent tumor – Pseudoprogression/radiation necrosis	• Three-dimensional evaluation of tumor heterogeneity • Detection of molecular/genetic features – IDH mutation • Treatment planning – Surgical resection/biopsy – Radiation therapy

TABLE 19: Frequently encountered metabolites and their characteristics and clinical role in evaluating brain tumors.

Metabolite	*ppm*	*Elevated in*	*Decreased in*	*Clinical significance in brain tumor imaging*
Choline	3.2 ppm	• Neoplasms • Inflammation • Gliosis	Necrosis	• Grading of gliomas • Distinguishing glioblastomas from metastases • Radiation planning in gliomas • Differentiating tumor progression versus pseudoprogression/radio necrosis
N-acetylaspartate	2.0 ppm		• Gliomas and more so in high grade gliomas • Radiation necrosis • Metastasis • Lymphoma	• Grading of gliomas • Distinguishing gliomas from metastasis
Creatine	3.0 ppm		• High grade gliomas • Necrosis	• Grading of gliomas • Distinguishing metastasis from glioblastoma
Lactate	1.3 ppm	• Glioblastoma • Abscess	Not present in normal spectra	Grading of gliomas
Lipids	1.3 ppm with inversion at intermediate TE	• Glioblastoma • Abscess • Lymphoma • Metastasis		Grading of gliomas
Myo-inositol	3.5 ppm	• Low grade gliomas • Progressive multifocal encephalopathy	High grade gliomas	Grading of gliomas
2-Hydroxyglutarate	2.5 ppm	IDH-1 positive tumors		Detection of IDH-1 positive tumors

- Differentiation of ring enhancing lesion
  - Tubercular granuloma versus NCC-TB—lipid, lactate levels at 1.3 ppm
  - Pyogenic vs tubercular abscess-pyogenic—lactate and amino acid at 0.9 ppm.
  - **Necrotic tumor vs abscess**: pyogenic abscess—lactate, valine, alanine, leucine, necrotic tumor—only lactate
- Prematurity-decreased PCR/Pi ratio
- Metabolic disorder and leukodystrophies—hepatic encephalopathies—elevated glutamine. High NAA in Canavan's disease
- Epilepsy-reduction of NAA/Ch/Cr ratio in temporal lobe epilepsy.
- Neurodegenerative disorder-
  a. Alzheimer's disease-reduced NAA, NAA/Cr in frontoparietal, temporal lobes and in hippocampus.
- Trauma—in case of diffuse axonal injury—reduced NAA, NAA/Cr ration
- Multiple sclerosis—increase in choline creatinine ratio in plaques, decrease NAA/Cr, active plaque shows elevated lipid, lactate, MI
- Stroke—NAA, CR reduced, choline, lactate elevated
- Schizophrenia-reduced NAA in hippocampus
- HIV/AIDS-marked reduction of NAA/Cho and NAA/Cr ratio in HIV encephalopathy, MRS helps to differentiate lymphoma (choline peak, Increase Cho/Cr ratio) from toxoplasma (lipid lactate peak)
- In PML, increased lactate peak.

2. Write short note on DTI. [5] [MD (WBUHS) 24, MD (WBUHS) 20]

Full name: Diffusion tensor imaging

It is an emerging robust technique of imaging of white matter tracts.

Physics: DTI exploits the molecular diffusion of white matters both the magnitude and the direction.

DTI uses the anisotropy property of white matter tracts, i.e., dependency of diffusion along the orientation of tracts due the presence of myelin sheath.

Diffusion Anisotropy

Diffusion of water molecules in white matter is not same all direction

Tensor: Mathematic representation of diffusion (directional vector) in three-dimensional space.

- Anisotropic diffusion can be described in terms of an ellipsoid tensor (D) **(Fig. 40)**
- **Consist of**: Eigen vectors—diffusion direction
  Eigen values—diffusion magnitude
- DWI obtained in 6 directions

The data for tensor must be obtained along six or more directions by gradients.

From this data EIGEN values along the eigen vectors can be calculated.

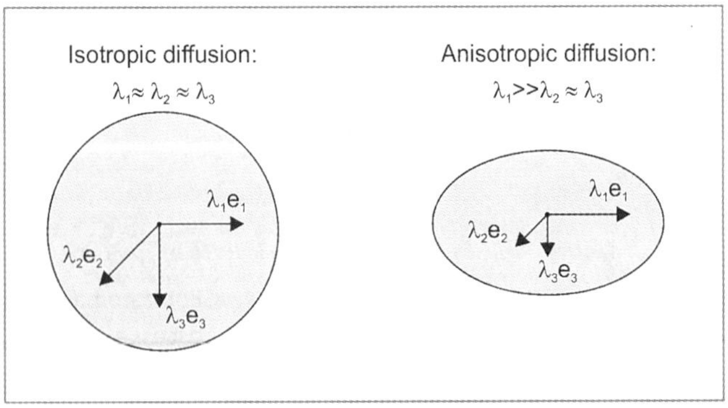

FIG. 40: Isotropic versus anisotropic diffusion.

DTI metrics:

Quantities related to diffusion calculated from the tensor (matrix):

- Fractional anisotropy (FA)—measure of the degree of anisotropy
- Mean diffusivity (MD)—the average diffusivity of water—trace of the diffusion tensor matrix
- Trace—isotropic diffusion
- FA maps with and without color codes
- Tensor image-calculated diffusion data with direction and velocity.

3T MR is preferable for it.

TABLE 20: Different patterns of white matter fiber involvement.

DTI patterns	*FA*	*Location/orientation (FA color-coded maps)*	*Illustration*	*Diagnosis*
Displaced	Normal/slightly decreased	Abnormal (intact tracts)	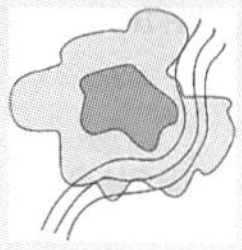	• Low-grade gliomas • Anaplastic astrocytomas • Glioblastoma multiforme • Metastasis
Edematous	Decreased	Normal	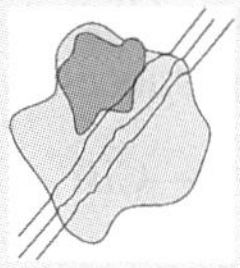	Metastasis
Infiltrated	Decreased	Fiber tracts remain identifiable	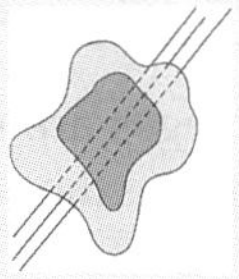	• Anaplastic astrocytomas • Glioblastoma multiforme
Disrupted	Markedly decreased (isotropic or near isotropic diffusion)	Nonidentifiable fiber tracts	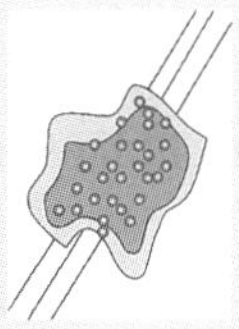	• Anaplastic astrocytomas • Glioblastoma multiforme

Clinical Application

White matter tracts—

a. **Projection fibers**: Cortical to deep gray nuclei color blue
b. **Association fibers**: Connects different white matters in same hemisphere color green
c. **Commissural**: Similar areas in different hemisphere-red.

Patters of fiber involvement **(Table 20)**

- To delineate the anatomy and pathology of white matter tracts
- **Tumors**:
  - Presurgical planning, delineation of tracts around lesion, deviated, infiltrated, edematous, destroyed.
  - Differentiating from benign versus aggressive tumor displaced fibers are more commonly seen in benign tumors
  - Destroyed and infiltrated tracts seen in malignant tumors
  - Edematous pattern of involvement seen in both benign and malignant tumor
  - Pre-operative and intra-operative tracking of white matter tract can be done, prognosis of sensory and motor deficits.
- Trauma—diffuse axonal injury
- Multiple sclerosis—loss of anisotropy in damaged white matter
- Developmental disorders
- Psychiatric disorders like schizophrenia.

3. Write short note on MR perfusion. [5]

Principle: In general perfusion means, volume of blood that flows into the tissue in a specific time period, expressed as mL/100 g/min.

Two main approaches of MR perfusion are **(Flowchart 6)**.

DSC: Most commonly used perfusion technique in day-to-day practice, mostly used for brain, this technique uses the T2 susceptibility effects of gadolinium rather than T1 shortening effect, signal loss in the perfused tissue is assessed to measure the perfusion, it is assumed that contrast remains intravascular with minimal leakage of contrast.

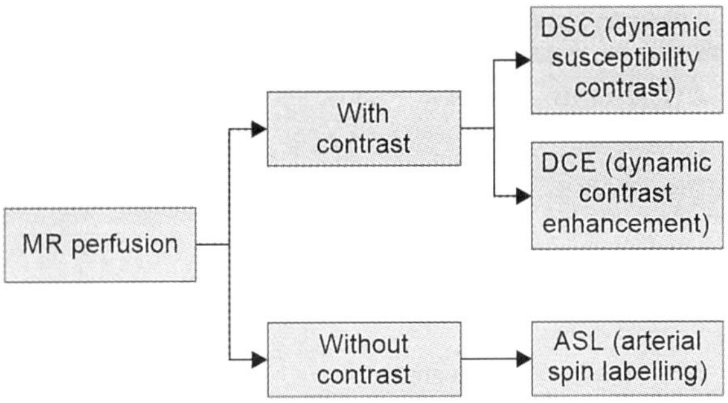

FLOWCHART 6: Approaches of MR perfusion.

Acquisition: Fast imaging technique such as EPI is used to obtain the image.

Standard dose of contrast 0.1 mmol/kg of body weight given, preferably with pressure injector, then successive images obtained.

Data analysis: Parameters measured—CBF, CBV, MTT, and TTP

DCE: T1 shortening effect of gadolinium is used, it is also known as permeability perfusion.

This technique considers two compartmental pharmacokinetics-including the intravascular and interstitial.

Image acquisition: Pre-contrast images are obtained followed by which post contrast images are obtained. Images acquisition is longer than DSC as it allows the contrast to percolate into the interstitium after the equilibrium has reached.

Data analysis

- K^{trans}-transfer constant
- V_{e-} fractional volume of the extracellular space
- V_{p-} fractional volume of plasma
- Most commonly used metric is K trans which denotes the permeability.

ASL: Without use of contrast **(Flowchart 7)**

Principle: Magnetically labeled blood as endogenous contrast agent

Spatially selective excitation pulse or gradient pulse applied to differentiate the static tissue and flowing blood. Time is allowed for the blood to come in tissue, then the signal change in the tissue is measured to calculate the perfusion.

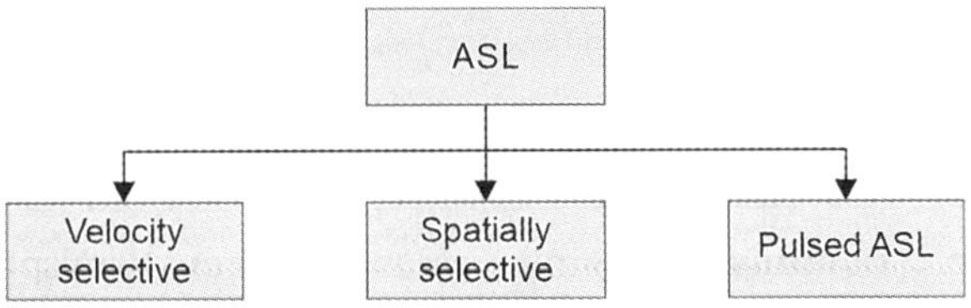

FLOWCHART 7: Types of ASL.

Two sets of images obtained, tag and control

1. **Tag**: LM of arterial blood saturated
2. **Control**: LM of arterial blood relaxed

CBF: magnetization difference between control-tag

4. Discuss the principle of MR perfusion. Elaborate the role of MR perfusion in neuroimaging. [4+6] [MD (WBUHS) 21, MD (WBUHS) 20]

Principle: In general perfusion means, volume of blood that flows into the tissue in a specific time period, expressed as mL/100g/min.

Two main approaches of MR perfusion are there **(Flowchart 8)**.

DSC: Most commonly used perfusion technique in day-to-day practice, mostly used for brain. this technique uses the T2 susceptibility effects of gadolinium rather than T1 shortening effect, signal loss in the perfused tissue is assessed to measure the perfusion, it is assumed that contrast remains intravascular with minimal leakage of contrast.

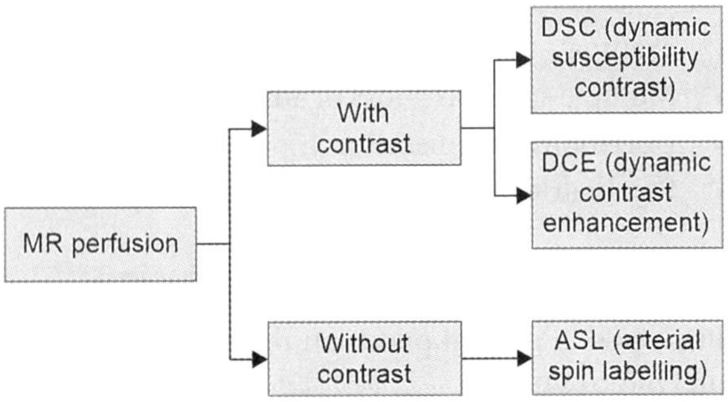

FLOWCHART 8: Approaches of MR perfusion.

Acquisition: Fast imaging technique such as EPI is used to obtain the image.

Standard dose of contrast 0.1 mmol/kg of body weight given, preferably with pressure injector, then successive images obtained.

Data analysis: Parameters measured—CBF, CBV, MTT, TTP

DCE: T1 shortening effect of gadolinium is used, it is also known as permeability perfusion.

This technique considers two compartmental pharmacokinetics-including the intravascular and interstitial.

Image acquisition—pre-contrast images are obtained followed by which post-contrast images are obtained. Images acquisition is longer than DSC as it allows the contrast to percolate into the interstitium after the equilibrium has reached.

Data analysis:

- K^{trans}-transfer constant
- V_{e-}fractional volume of the extracellular space
- V_{p-} fractional volume of plasma
- Most commonly used metric is K trans which denotes the permeability.

ASL: Without use of contrast **(Flowchart 9)**

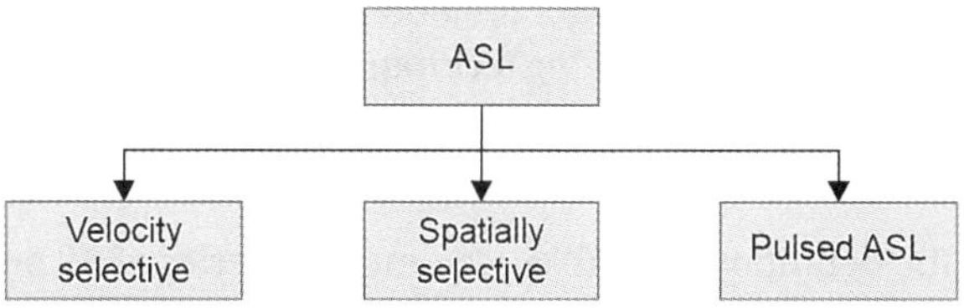

FLOWCHART 9: Types of ASL.

Principle: Magnetically labeled blood as endogenous contrast agent

Spatially selective excitation pulse or gradient pulse applied to differentiate the static tissue and flowing blood. Time is allowed for the blood to come in tissue, then the signal change in the tissue is measured to calculate the perfusion.

Two sets of images obtained, tag and control

- **Tag**: LM of arterial blood saturated
- **Control**: LM of arterial blood relaxed

CBF: Magnetization difference- between control-tag.

Role of MR Perfusion in Neuroimaging

1. **Stroke**: Most popular application of MR perfusion imaging has been in the assessment of cerebral ischemia.

   Perfusion imaging in combination with diffusion imaging can identify surrounding viable ischemic tissue at risk **(the so-called ischemic penumbra**)

   Acute MR Stroke Protocol

   A. Parenchymal imaging:
      - DWI using EPI and parallel imaging
      - FLAIR using EPI and parallel imaging
      - GRE

   B. MR angiography

   C. Perfusion imaging
      - 20 Minutes ⟶ 6 Minutes

        Mismatch between the perfusion and diffusion denotes the salvageable ischemic tissue which respond to thrombolytic and neuroprotective agents.

        In sub-acute infarction, it is possible to identify luxury perfusion, i.e., increased cerebral blood volume, surrounding the infarct core.

2. **Brain tumors**: Cerebral blood volume maps used to assess neovascularity in tumors, believed to be corresponding with tumor grade and malignant histology.

   Cerebral blood volume maps may aid in early evaluation of therapeutic agents, aimed at suppressing growth of tumor blood vessels.

   Noninvasively differentiation of radiation necrosis from recurrent tumor is possible where conventional MR findings are equivocal.

3. **Other disorders**: MR perfusion imaging has been applied to the study of various other neurologic and psychiatric disorders, such as dementia and migraine headaches.

   In the case of migraine headaches, decreases in cerebral blood volume and cerebral blood flow have been seen during the auras compared with the post-aura state

In the case of dementia, decreases in cerebral blood volume in the temporal and parietal lobes of patients with Alzheimer's disease, correlated well with the results of SPECT

4. **Functional brain mapping**: Absolute quantification of cerebral blood flow possible in the area of functional MR brain mapping.

   Cerebral activation is assessed by qualitative assessment of local changes in deoxyhemoglobin concentration.

   Relation between blood neuronal activity to blood oxygenation levels is known as blood oxygenation level dependant (BOLD) effect.

   Quantitative cerebral blood flow changes during motor and working memory tasks have been measured with the arterial spin tagging technique and yield results similar to those obtained with other techniques such as ^{133}Xe SPECT.

5. Write in brief the basic principle and application of various MRI sequence. [10] [MD (WBUHS) 19]

The definition of a pulse sequence is a series of RF pulses, gradient applications and intervening time periods.

The RF pulses are applied for excitation purposes and in the case of spin echo for rephasing purposes. The gradients are applied to spatially encode signal and to rephase and dephase spins depending on the type of pulse sequence and imaging option selected.

The intervening time periods refer to the time intervals between these various functions

Therefore, a pulse sequence is a carefully coordinated and timed sequence of events to generate a particular type of image contrast. It is a time chart of interplay of—

a. Patient's net longitudinal magnetization
b. Transmission of RF pulses (90, 180 degree or any degree)
c. X, Y and Z gradient activation for localization and acquisition of signal
d. K - space filling with acquired signals

Pulse sequences can be broadly divided into two categories:

a. Spin echo sequence
b. Gradient echo sequence

Dephasing caused by inhomogeneities produces a rapid loss of coherent transverse magnetization → signal reaches zero before most tissues attain their T1 or T2 relaxation times

To measure relaxation times and produce an image with good contrast, we need to compensate for T2* dephasing so that T1 and T2 properly measured.

There are two ways of doing this—by using an additional 180-degree RF pulse or by using gradients. Sequences that use a 180-degree pulse to regenerate signal are called spin echo sequences, those that use a gradient are called gradient echo sequences.

Inversion recovery and echo planar imaging (EPI) can be applied theoretically to both spin echo and gradient echo sequences. For practical purposes, four types of sequences can be considered:

a. Spin echo sequence (SE)
b. Gradient echo sequence (GRE)
c. Inversion recovery sequences (IR)
d. Echo planar imaging (EPI)

Spin Echo Sequence (SE) (Fig. 41 and Flowchart 10)

- T2* dephasing occurs almost immediately → signal decays[7]
- FID is weak and insufficient for image formation
- A 180° RF pulse is then used to compensate for this dephasing

In conventional SE sequence:

- Only one 180° pulse is applied after the 90° pulse
- Only one spin echo is formed in one TR **(Fig. 42)**
- Only one line of K-space is filled per TR

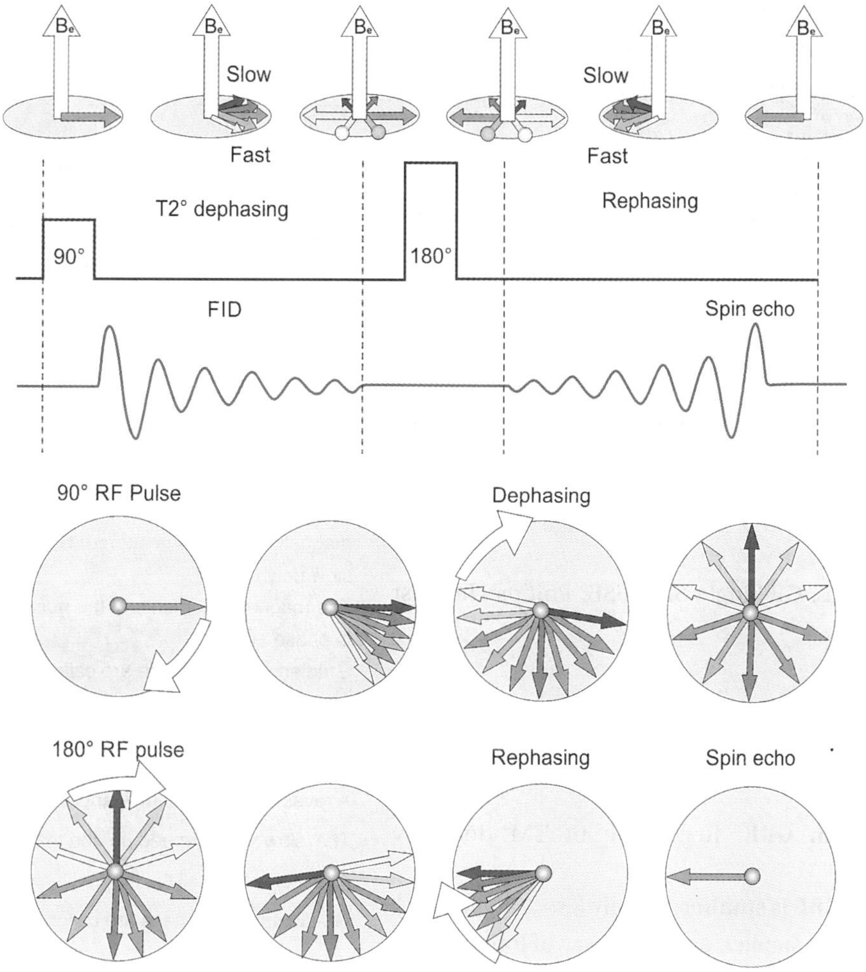

FIG. 41: Signal generation in spin echo sequence.

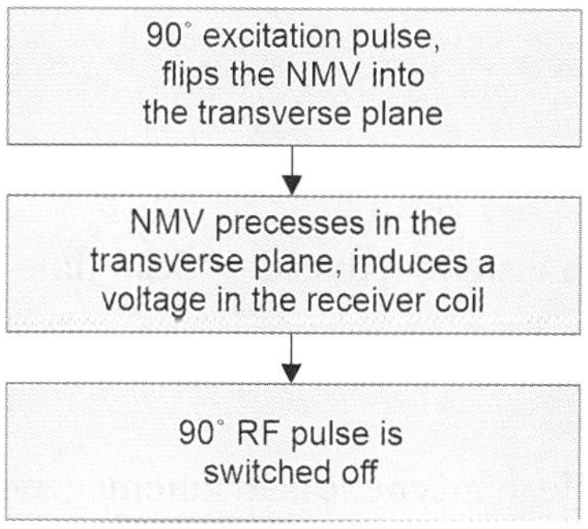

FLOWCHART 10: Spin echo sequence (SE).

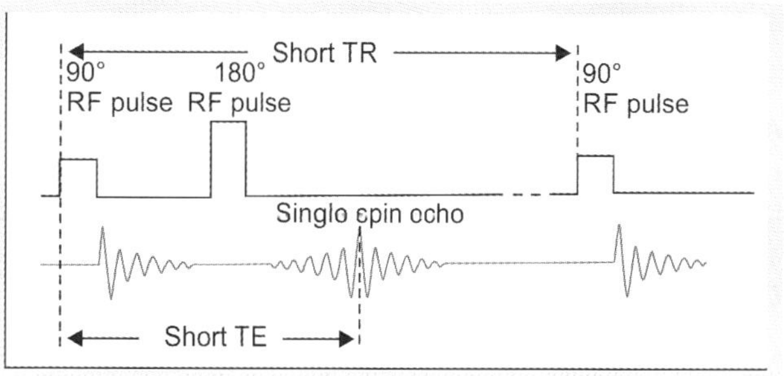

FIG. 42: Standard pulse sequence diagram.

Modifications of SE Sequence

- More than one 180° RF pulse after the excitatory 90° RF pulse
- Each 180° RF pulse obtains one echo

Three routinely used modifications include

- **Dual SE** (two 180° pulses per TR)

  The PD + T2 double echo sequence is a modified SE sequence – widely used in MSK imaging, better detection of bone marrow edema, stress fracture, sub-chondral cyst, cartilage or ligament injury

- **Fast (Turbo) SE** (multiple 180° pulses per TR) - Multiple 180° pulses are sent after each 90° pulse

  K - space is filled much faster with multiple echoes in a single TR

  Scanning speed increases considerably

  Multiple 180° pulses reduce magnetic susceptibility effects, can be used in presence of prosthesis and implants.

Disadvantages

- Fat bright on T2W images
- Image blurring with long echo trains
- **Single-shot fast SE**: Fast SE with only half of the K - space filled, other half of the K - space is mathematically calculated by half-Fourier transformation
  - All the echoes required to form an image are acquired in a single TR
  - Siemens-HASTE, GE-Single Shot FSE, Philips-Ultrafast SE
  - USED in MRCP

Gradient Echo Pulse Sequence

Basic differences between SE and GRE sequences **(Flowchart 11)**

1. **No 180° pulse in GRE**. Rephasing of TM done by gradients
2. The **flip angle in GRE is smaller**, usually less than 90°.
   - Since flip angle is smaller, early recovery of longitudinal magnetization occurs - TR hence the scanning time
   - In GRE sequence, dephasing effects of magnetic field inhomogeneity are not compensated, as there is no 180° pulse
   - T2 relaxation in GRE is actually T2* relaxation.

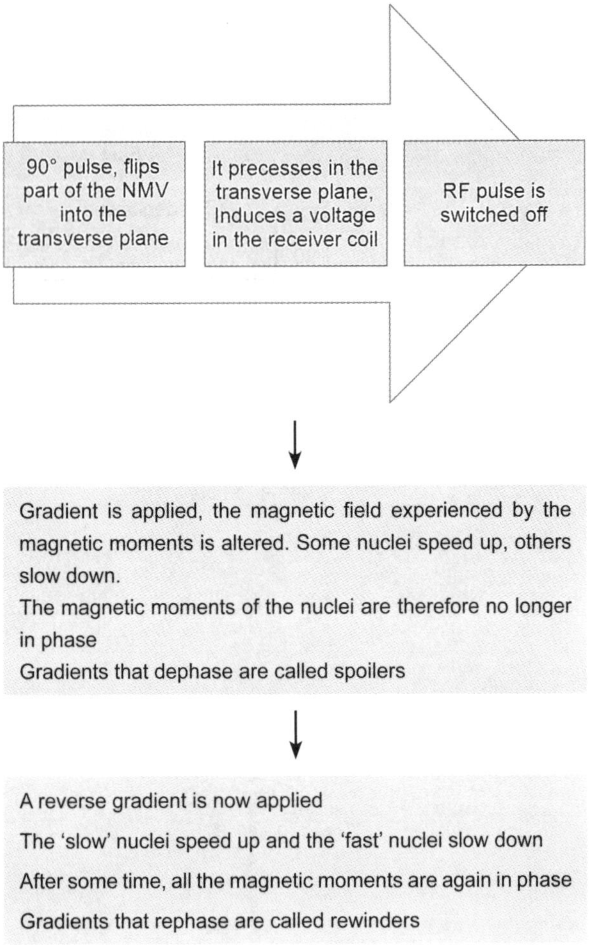

FLOWCHART 11: Signal generation in gradient echo pulse sequence.

Advantages

Gradients rephase much faster than 180° pulses → TE much shorter → TR can also be reduced → Scan time can be reduced

Disadvantages

- No compensation for magnetic field inhomogeneities - hence very susceptible to magnetic field inhomogeneities
- True T2 weighting not seen
- Can be divided into two types depending on what is done with the residual TM after reception of signal.
- **Steady state or coherent GRE sequences**: Residual TM is destroyed by RF pulse or gradient such that it does not interfere with next TR
  1. Pre-excitation—PSIF, SSFP-CSF flow study
  2. Post-excitation—FISP (fast imaging with steady state precession), GRASS (gradient recalled acquisition in the steady state)—orthopedic imaging
  3. Fully refocused steady state sequence-true FISP, FIESTA-cardiac, fetal
  4. CISS—inner ear imaging

- **Spoiled or incoherent GRE sequences**: Residual TM is destroyed by RF pulse or gradient such that it does not interfere with next TR
  1. 2D spoiled-FLASH-MR ANGIO
  2. 3D spoiled-VIBE-body imaging
     - Multiple gradient echo-MERGE, MEDIC-MSK, SPINE
     - 3D ultrafast GRE-MP-RAGE-cerebral imaging, T1W
     - Echo-planner imaging-diffusion, perfusion, functional MRI-T2w
- **Gradient/spin echo hybrid-Turbo GSE**-T2 w imaging of brain and orthopedics

Other Implications

- Abscess
- Highly cellular tumor
- Epidermoid cyst
- Subacute blood
- Acute encephalitis
- Creutzfeldt-Jakob disease

6. Discuss the principle of diffusion weighted imaging and its utility in differentiation of brain lesions. [3+7] [MD (WBUHS) 22, DNB Dec 21, DNB June 21]

Diffusion Weighted Imaging (DWI)

- The concept of DWI was given by Le BIHAN.
- Water molecules in body undergo a random motion, which is called Brownian motion. Mobility of water in different tissues or normal versus pathological tissue depicted by DWI.
- When diffusion is unhindered in all direction, it is called isotropic diffusion, but when it occurs in a preferential direction, it is called anisotropic diffusion, e.g., white matter tract.[8]

Technique—Suggested by Stejskal and Tanner
Two diffusion sensitizing gradients (same magnitude but opposite direction) applied on either side of 180-degree RF pulse

⇓

First one is dephasing and second one is rephrasing gradient

⇓

The 180° RF pulse will eliminate the dephasing due to the inhomogeneity of external magnetic field

Water molecules whose diffusion is unhindered will get dephased by the first dephasing gradient and move into other location having different magnetic field when rephrasing gradient is applied, so no signal is produced.

On the other hand, water molecules having restricted mobility will be subjected to both dephasing and rephasing gradient, neutralizing each other, so their spin will be in phase producing strong signal.

Apparent Diffusion Coefficient (ADC): Magnitude of diffusion is ADC, measured as b factor (mm^2/s). At least two b values needed to calculate ADC, with increase b value SNR is reduced, so for optimal image acquisition there is a balance.

Tissues showing diffusion restriction will be hyperintense on DWI and hypointense on ADC.
DWI sequences: Fast sequences to fill k spaces

1. Echo-planar imaging
2. Turbo spin echo
3. Steady state free precession

Role of DWI in Neuroimaging (Table 21)

TABLE 21: Role of DWI in neuroimaging.

Stroke	• Gold standard for imaging of stroke • Ability to identify infract core prior to any other sequence • Able to detect acute lacunar infarct, other sequence may miss • Hyperintense on both DWI and ADC- gliotic change
Tumor	• Highly cellular tumor show restriction • Lymphoma • Medulloblastoma > Ependymoma • Post-treatment- low cellularity with disrupted cell membrane- no diffusion restriction- marker of response assessment
Epidermoid versus arachnoid cyst	Due to component of epidermoid cysts—g-keratin, cholesterol debris epidermoid cyst shows diffusion restriction
Pyogenic abscess	Due to high cellularity and pus, abscesses show hyperintensity on DWI
Necrotic component of brain tumor	Though it is peripherally enhancing, it does not show diffusion restriction as the cell membrane is leaky and cellularity is less
Herpes encephalitis	Medial temporal lobe-cytotoxic edema—DWI hyperintensity
Creutzfeldt-Jakob disease	DWI hyperintense lesion in cortex and basal ganglia, more sensitive for detection of cortical lesion

7. Briefly describe the techniques of MR neurography and black blood imaging of brain. [5+5]

MR neurography—imaging technique for evaluation of peripheral nerve pathologies

- Nowadays, MRN is possible due to robust improvement in the hardware and also in the imaging technique.
- MRN provides valuable information about the neuropathies which has both diagnostic and therapeutic value.[9]
- Diagnosis is done by direct visualization of pathological nerve, muscle denervated by the nerve, it also provides information about any lesion which can cause neural compression mimicking neuropathy.
- Role in diagnosing hereditary neuropathy.

MRI Protocol

The MRI protocol can vary depending on the indication and body parts to be imaged.

In Majority

- T2W fat-saturated sequence
- T1W with or without contrast
- 3D T2W/STIR SPACE
- 3D DW PSIF
- DWI and DTI
- Use of contrast is done mainly for the assessment of infection or involvement by tumor.
- Dedicated surface coils given better result than surface coils

For Brachial Plexus

- T2 STIR COR
- T2 SAG
- T2 space COR
- T2 axial
- 3D STIR space
- DTI

For Peripheral Nerves

- PDFS axial/COR/SAG
- T2 axial
- T1 COR/axial
- 3D MEDIC
- DWI
- T2 space
- 3D PSIF

Interpretation

- T1W—for anatomy, fascicular pattern
- T2W-abnormal nerve signal or muscle denervation edema
- 3D STIR SPACE—most sensitive sequence

Clinical Application

1. Allowing visualization of fascicles, exact localization of pathology can be done.
2. Differentiation between spinal root compression from pre or post ganglionic nerve discontinuity. As the management of root compression is conservative while others need surgical intervention.
3. Useful in delineating complex pathology
4. Differentiation from mono to polyneuropathy
5. Differentiation of neuropraxia, axonotmesis and neurotmesis **(Table 22)**
6. Post-surgical follow up of nerve repair

Black Blood Imaging of Brain

Vessel wall (VW) MRI is an effective technique to characterize pathologic features involving the VW. The clinical importance lies looking beyond the lumen for low-grade stenosis.

Clinical Application

1. To characterize intracranial vascular disease (e.g., atherosclerotic plaque, vasculitis Moyamoya disease)
2. Detecting angiographically occult atherosclerotic plaques
3. Guiding biopsies of vessels

Technique: This is mainly possible due to optimization of three-dimensional high spatial-resolution VW MRI imaging.

Administration of gadolinium-containing contrast agents has proven to be essential in the detection and characterization of inflammatory vasculopathies on VW MRI scans, but reasons for enhancement on VW MRI scans extend beyond inflammation.

Black blood MRI was established to characterize carotid artery atherosclerotic plaque size and composition.

Challenges

1. 2D—small size and tortuous course of these vessels
2. 3D—long imaging times and suboptimal flow suppression

Technique

Blood flow suppression is achieved by inflow blood saturation, nulling the stationary tissue by an inversion preparation pulse, or dephasing of the moving spins.

DIR—most commonly used for 2D blackblood MRI

- The first 180° pulse is not section selective and inverts all spins within the imaging volume, The second 180° pulse is section selective, thereby effectively cancelling the inversion of spins in that section back to the z direction, mitigating the T1 weighting of the VW and thereby improving its signal-to-noise ratio.

TABLE 22: MR neurography findings of different types of nerve injuries.

	Degree of nerve injury	*Myelin*	*Axon*	*Endoneurium*	*Perineurium*	*Epineurium*	*Tinel sign*	*MRN (signal Intensity)*	*Recovery potential*	*Rate of recovery*	*Surgery*
I	Neurapraxia	±	-	-	-	-	No	Nerve-incr T2 SI, Muscle-Normal	Full	Up to 12 weeks	None
II	Axonotmesis	Yes	Yes	No	No	No	Yes	Nerve-incr T2 SI, and diffusely enlarged	Full	1 mm/day	None
III		Yes	Yes	Yes	No	No	Yes	Fascicles-enlarged or effaced due to edema; Muscles-denervation	Usually slow, incomplete	1 mm/day	None or neurolysis
IV	NIC-neuroma in continuity	Yes	Yes	Yes	Yes	No	Yes but no advancement	Nerve-focally enlarged with heterogeneous SI; Underlying diffuse abnormality ±; Fascicles disrupted with heterogeneous SI-NIC; Muscles-denervation	Poor to none	Poor to none	Nerve repair, graft, or transfer
V	Neurotmesis	Yes	Yes	Yes	Yes	Yes	Yes but no advancement	Complete nerve discontinuity ± hemorrhage and fibrosis in the nerve gap and end-bulb neuroma; Epineurial thickening	None	None	Nerve repair, graft, or transfer
VI	Mixed Injury (I to V)	Variable combination across the cross-section of the nerve					Some fascicles (II, III)	Variable findings along the circumferential segment (I-V) with heterogeneous; SI due to fibrosis; Muscles-denervation	Variable, can be poor to none	Variable, depends on injury (I-V)	Neurolysis, Nerve repair, graft, or transfer

- Mechanism for blood flow suppression on 3D VW MRI scans is intravoxel dephasing of moving protons of blood.
- Protons with laminar flow in the magnetic field cause phase dispersion with signal attenuation. Flow suppression is a function of blood velocity and is more effective when the velocity is more than 5 cm/sec.
- Blood velocity often has a laminar distribution, with the slowest flow adjacent to the VW where inadequate flow suppression may occur when flow is reduced sufficiently.

8. What are the advantages and limitations of 3T over 1.5T MRI? Briefly discuss MRI safety. [6+4] [DNB June 21]

As the name suggests difference between 3T and1.5T is the strength of magnetic field.

Technical Differences (Table 23)

PROS of 3T machine:

A. **Signal to noise ratio**: 3T-associated increase in the signal-to-noise ratio (SNR)
   - Signal is proportional to square of static magnetic field strength (B0) by two mechanisms, firstly the increase in sample magnetization and secondly, the increase in the precessional (Larmor) frequency.
   - In terms of imaging, SNR is proportional to the voxel size and the acquisition time.
   - The main benefit of the increased SNR in 3T system provides improved image quality, including the ability to trade SNR for higher spatial resolution.

B. **Relaxation time**: The longitudinal (T_1) and transverse (T_2) relaxation times of biological tissue depend on the physical and chemical environments of the protons as well as the static magnetic field strength. Whilst there are generally no significant differences between T_2 values at 3T compared to 1.5T, the T_1 values for tissues are generally longer at 3T. At 3T, three-dimensional time-of-flight (3D TOF) MR angiography also benefits from the longer T_1 relaxation times in brain parenchyma resulting in improved saturation of the stationary spins and better vessel-to-background contrast.

- **Higher contrast to noise ratio (CNR)**: The T1 shortening effects of gadolinium chelate based contrast agents are relatively unaffected while longer T1 values at 3T provide better background tissue suppression. As a result, CNR is higher. This leads to more pronounced contrast enhancement effects and increased conspicuity of lesions in solid organs. It may also be used to reduce the dose of gadolinium.
- Greatest technical superiority of 3T over 1.5T by virtue of speed, SNR and resolution gains is in volumetric structural brain imaging, small lesion detection, i.e. multiple sclerosis, evaluation of epilepsy, diffusion tensor imaging, MR angiography, fast spectroscopic imaging and techniques exploiting susceptibility effects, i.e. BOLD and perfusion imaging
- Reduced motion artifacts owing to the shorter TEs possible.

TABLE 23: Comparison between 3T and 1.5T.

Parameter	*1.5T*	*3T*
Larmor frequency	63.9 MHZ	127.8 MHz
Chemical shift	220 Hz	440 Hz
Susceptibility	Less	More
Field Inhomogeneity	Less	Difficult to achieve
T1 relaxation time	Less compared to 3T	Increased by ~25%
T2 relaxation time	More compared to 3T	Decreased by ~10-15%
In and out-of-phase TEs in ms	In-phase: 4.5, 9.5.. Out-phase: 2.3, 6.9..	In-phase: 2.3, 4.5.. Out-phase: 1.1, 3.4..
Specific absorption rate (SAR)	Less	More (fourfold)
Signal-to-noise ratio (SNR)	Less	More (double)
Contrast-to-noise ratio	Less	More

MR Spectroscopy

As the field strength increases the spectral separation of the peaks also increases, so at 3T the shifts would be twice those at 1.5T. The greater the range of frequency shifts the easier it is to identify the multiple peaks in complex molecules.

- Chemical shift increases in proportion to the magnetic field and this is of advantage in MR spectroscopy imaging, fat suppression and opposed phase imaging
- **MRCP**: Improved SNR is very pronounced at T2WI, particularly with single-shot fast spin echo techniques used in MRCP. The long T2 relaxation times of fluid result in increased conspicuity and shorter TEs yield less blurring and motion artifacts.

Susceptibility Effects

The magnetic susceptibility (χ) is a measure of how magnetized a material will become in the presence of an external magnetic field.

The magnetic susceptibility causes a variation in the uniformity of the static magnetic field ($\Delta\beta 0$)

Hence the static field non-uniformity is doubled at 3 T compared to 1.5 T. A greater non-uniformity results in a shortening of the T_2^* relaxation time and a relative decrease in signal in T_2^* -weighted imaging. This is a double-edged sword. Whilst a greater static field non-uniformity is often undesirable in terms of signal loss, there are also applications where magnetic susceptibility is an important contrast mechanism. Example—functional imaging (bold)

- 3T MRI is particularly useful in prostate imaging owing to improved spatial resolution
- MSK imaging—enhanced detection of tears of the articular cartilage of the labrum of the shoulder and hip, triangular fibrocartilage complex tears of wrist, diagnosis and staging of various internal derangements of knee.
- Improved cardiac imaging and breast imaging.

CONS

- Magnetic susceptibility effects double at 3T resulting in more prominent susceptibility artifacts
- Increases in Chemical shift artifacts is a disadvantage for imaging cartilage and bone interfaces
- There is T1 prolongation and T2 shortening on 3T, which reduces grey white matter contrast.
- Increase in SAR leads to increase in tissue heating resulting in safety concerns. Parallel imaging and newer improved coils and magnets can lower the SAR.
- Gradient noise increases with increased magnetic field strength
- More subject to flow artifacts
- Standing wave or Dielectric Shading is more prominent as the RF wavelength approaches the dimensions of the field of view for abdomen and pelvis. There is non-uniform RF distribution to the body and constructive and destructive interference results in large local variation in signal intensity across the image. These effects are more common in pregnant patients (large volume of amniotic fluid) and patients with large volume ascites. This can be reduced by placing dielectric pads, improved shimming, parallel imaging and by using a post-processing normalization filter called Bias Field Correction or BiFiC image filter.
- Cost and design issues

  Rapid gradient switching leads to an increase in the intensity of the acoustic noise, which requires better insulation of both the unit itself and the containing room.
- The main limitations of 3T are the necessity to control the increased RF power deposition, dealing with the RF non-uniformity challenges, particularly in thoracic and abdominal imaging and the appropriate management of patients with implanted devices.

MRI Safety

MR is considered safe as it does not use ionizing radiation, although there are specific and significant risks associated with MR.

All MR scanners are under regulation of FDA which takes care of SAR.

MR Safety Risks

- One should always keep in mind that MR is always on.
- There should be a display portraying this outside the scan room to create awareness.
- Presence of a strong magnetic field can attract any metallic objects producing translational force and torque.
- So, this can dislodge metallic stents or implants.
- Projectile injury can also occur in presence of ferromagnetic object near the bore which can cause human cost and also extensive damage of the machine.

Screening

- Meticulous screening of all individuals and patients by trained personnel and also by metal detector.
- No oxygen tank to enter in MR room.
- Screening of patients by level 2 personnel who cannot give proper history
- Plain film radiography- in suspected cases to detect metallic foreign body

MR Zoning (Fig. 43)

The 5 gauss line: This is the outer limit of pacemaker (including MR conditional) safety, drawn at a distance of 5 gauss from bore magnet. It is seen within the scan room.

Although this does not provide protection against projectile injury.

MR personnel:

- **Level I**: Training about some safety aspects-their own safety, e.g, nurse, technician
- **Level II**: Extensively trained, aware about thermoregulatory and neurostimulatory issue, MR technician, radiologists.

MRI Emergencies

- In case of any emergency patient should be taken out from zone 4 and resuscitation should be done in zone 3.
- Quench occurs when the superconducting coil is heated above the critical temperature with increased resistance.
- In case of a projectile injury, intentional quench is required.

Medical Device Compatibility

FDA has divided medical devices in three categories:

a. MR safe—labeled green
b. MR conditional—safe under specific operational condition labeled yellow
c. MR unsafe, e.g., Cochlear implant-labeled red

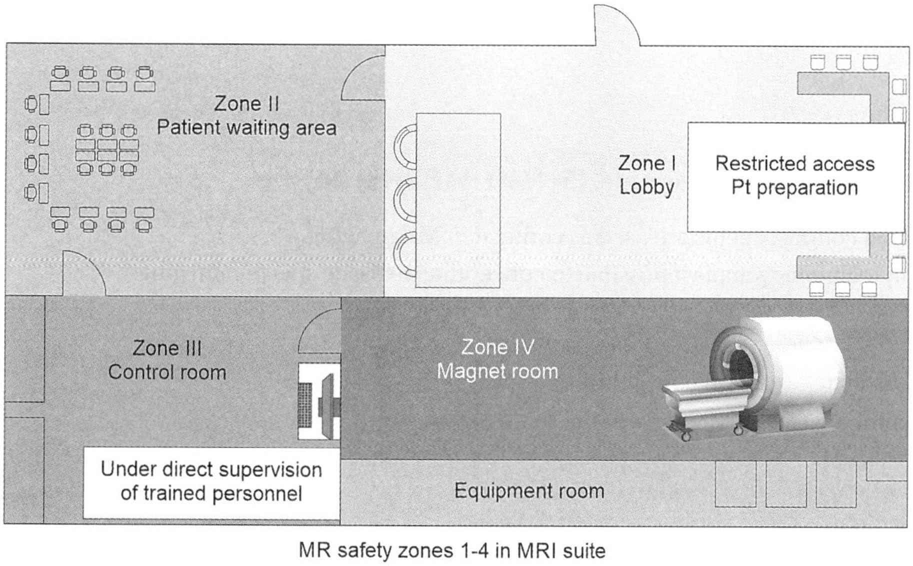

FIG. 43: MR safety zones.

Risks associated with MR gradient and RF coils:

1. Acoustic noise
2. Peripheral nerve stimulation
3. Burns

FDA limit of SAR - 2 to 4 W/kg averaged over 6 minutes.

9. Pulmonary MRI. [5]

Emerging Technique

- Limited use in clinical practice especially compared with CT.
- Can provide structural and quantitative information without ant ionizing radiation making it suitable for pediatric population, pregnant women, patients who require long term follow up.
- Ultrashort echo time, zero echo time has made it possible to obtain images of lung MRI

Indications of pulmonary MRI (Fleischner Society)

1. Current clinical application—
   a. Cystic fibrosis—bronchiectasis, mucus plugging, bronchial wall thickening, MR perfusion defect
   b. Lung cancer staging
   c. Lung nodule characterization—DW MRI most effective
   d. Pulmonary hypertension—DCE similar sensitivity and specificity to SPECT
2. Promising but require validation—
   a. Pulmonary embolism—MR angiography
   b. Pulmonary parenchymal abnormality
   c. Lung nodule detection
3. Investigational
   - COPD
   - Asthma
   - Interstitial lung disease—T1 values of fibrotic lung parenchyma is higher than emphysematous lung

Disadvantages

- Cost ineffective
- Complexity
- Difficulty in reading

10. Hepatobiliary MRI contrast agents. [5] [MD (WBUHS) 24]

- Gadolinium based contrast agents are used as contrast in MR imaging.
- Advancement in technology made it possible to conceptualize tissue specific imaging.

Hepatobiliary Contrast Agents (Table 24)

1. Primovist (Gadoxetate—not available in India)
2. Multihance (gadobenate)

Properties

1. Initial phase of intravascular and interstitial distribution same as other Gd-based contrast
2. Later taken up by functioning hepatocytes and then excreted through bile
3. Some amount of contrast is excreted by kidney.

TABLE 24: Hepatobiliary MRI contrast agents.

	Hepatocyte uptake	Biliary excretion	Renal excretion	Imaging time for liver pathologies
Gd-BOPTA (gadobenate)	2-4%	4-5%	95%	1-2 hours after administration of contrast
Gadoxetate	50%	50%	50%	20-30 minutes

Both are linear GBCAS.

Lesions containing functioning hepatocyte will appear bright while lesions which do not contain functioning hepatocyte will appear dark.

CE: MRCP—better delineation of ductal anatomy.

Clinical Application

1. Focal nodular hyperplasia—contain functioning hepatocytes , so becomes bright after administration of liver specific GBCAS
2. HCC—appear hypointense, ability to detect small lesion

Disadvantage

Expensive

11. What is K-space and various techniques using it? [10] [DNB June 22]

- Imaginary space which represents a raw data matrix
- Represents stage between the reception of signals and image formation **(Fig. 44)**
- After acquisition all signals are stored in the K-space
- This raw data is used reconstruct the image by Fourier transformation

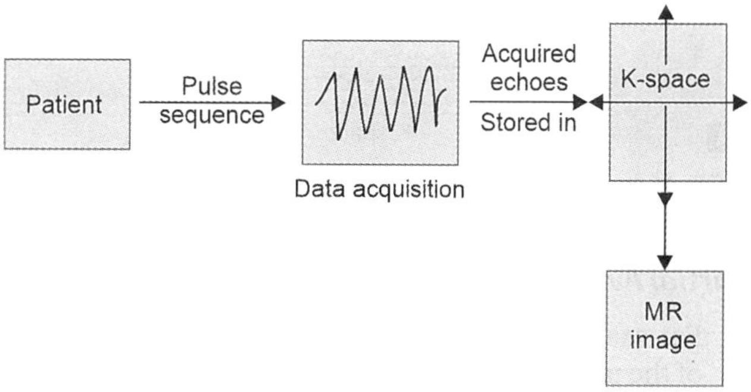

FIG. 44: K-space.

K-space has two axes

- Y axis represents the phase axis
- X axis represents the frequency axis and is perpendicular to the phase axis
- Signals are filled in the K-space as horizontal lines
- In conventional SE imaging one line of K-space is filled every TR **(Fig. 45)**

K-space is not the image

- Data are symmetrical in K-space
- Data acquired in central lines contribute signal and contrast, while data acquired in the outer lines contribute resolution
- The scan time is the time to fill the K-space

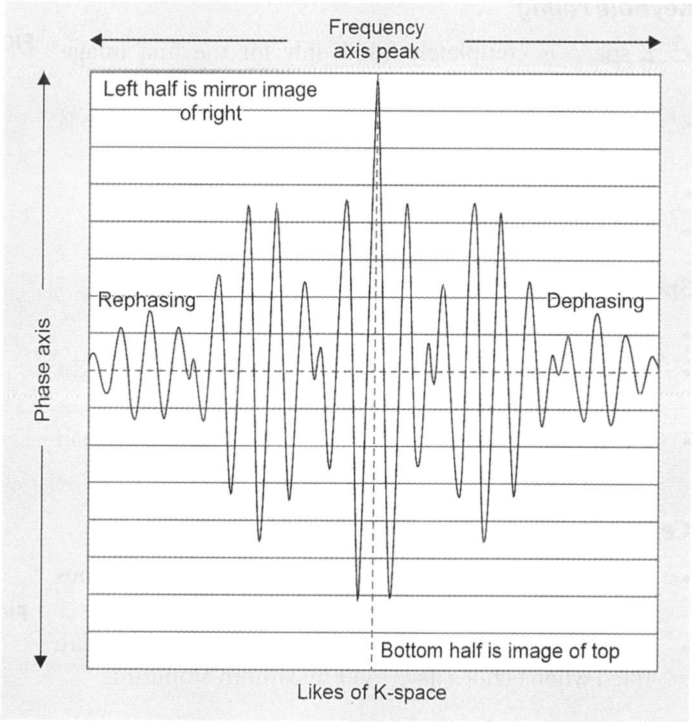

FIG. 45: K-space filling.

Faster Methods of K-space Filling

Partial Echo Imaging (Figs. 46A and B)

- System samples only half the echo
- Only half of the frequency area of k-space is filled
- However, as the remaining is a mirror image, the system can calculate its amplitude accordingly

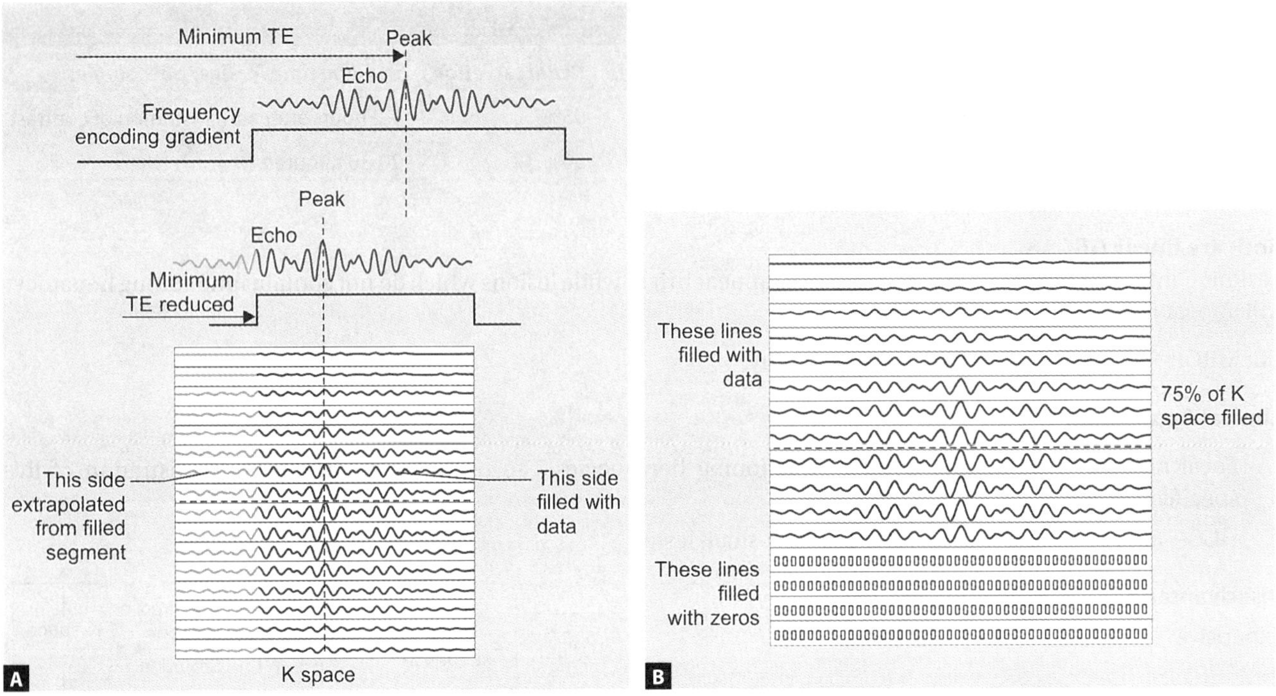

FIGS. 46A and B: Partial echo imaging.

Partial Averaging or Half Fourier

- For example, if only 75% of k-space is filled, only 75% of the phase encoding selected needs to be performed
- Remaining lines are filled with zeroes

Keyhole Filling

- K-space is completely filled only for the first image **(Fig. 47)**
- For subsequent images, only central (~20%) K-space is filled
- Rest 80% is filled from the first image
- Mainly used in CE MR angiography

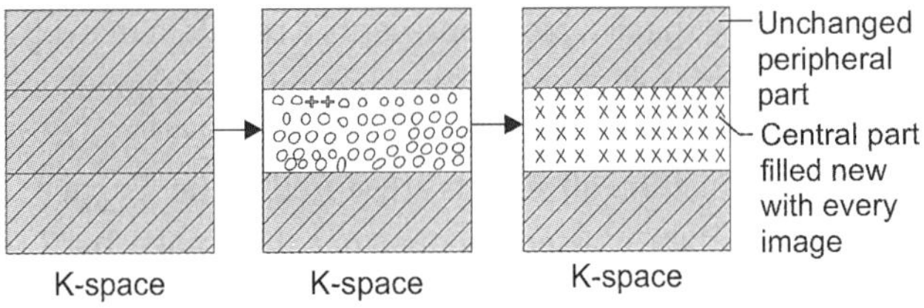

FIG. 47: Keyhole filling.

Spiral K-Space Filling

- K-space filling begins at the center
- Readout gradient oscillates to fill lines from left to right and then right to left
- Phase gradient also oscillates to fill a line in the top half followed by a line in the bottom half

Centric K-space Filling (Fig. 48)

- K-space is filled linearly (line by line) but central lines are filled first
- Signal and contrast are maximized as central lines are filled when echoes have their maximum amplitude

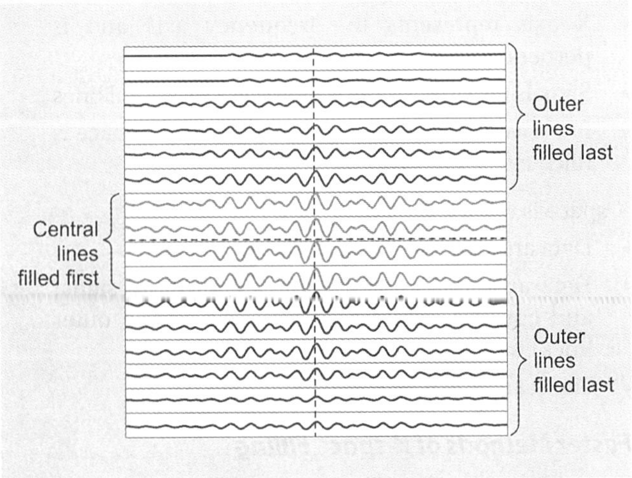

FIG. 48: Centric K-space filling.

12. Chemical shift imaging in MRI—techniques, advantages and disadvantages. [10] [DNB June 22]

Imaging Physics

- Hydrogen protons (H+) precess at a specific frequency when placed in a magnetic field.
- Depending on shielding from electron shell precessional frequency differs for all hydrogen ions **(Fig. 49)**
- Water and fat protons precess at fractionally different frequency
- 1.5 ppm relative to Larmor frequency of water.

Chemical Shift

- Signal intensity difference on MR imaging due to differences in the resonant frequencies of the precessing protons
- It offers the ability to investigate the relative ratio of fat to water content within individual voxels on MR images.
- Chemical shift is directly proportional to the magnetic field strength and is approximately 225 HZ at 1.5 T and 450 HZ at 3T.

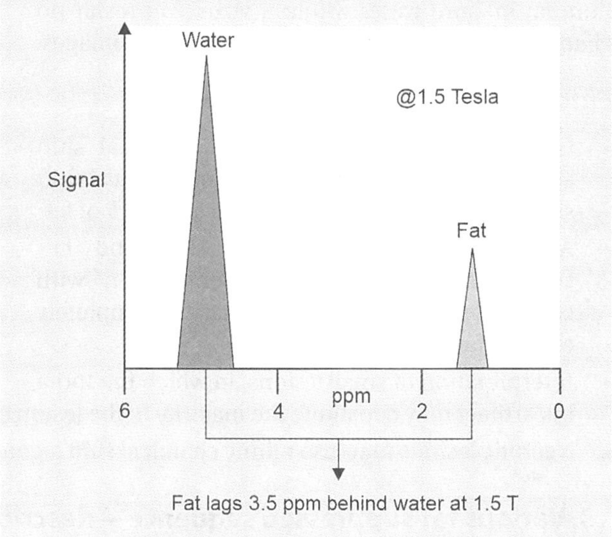

FIG. 49: Chemical shift imaging.

Types of Chemical Shift

Type 1 and Type 2

Type 1 Chemical shift

- Occurs both in spin echo and gradient echo sequences
- Error of spatial localization

Type 2 Chemical shift

- Occurs only with gradient echo imaging
- At 1.5 T , water and fat protons will be in phase at an echo time (TE) of 4.4 ms (1/225 Hz) and will be out of phase 2.2 ms before and after the first in phase TE
- Thus voxels containing both fat and water will have additive signal at the in phase TE and cancellation of signal at the out of phase TE.
- Effect is maximum when the relative ratio of fat and water in a voxel is 1:1
- The in-phase and opposed phase images should be ideally viewed side by side simultaneously **(Fig. 50)**
- Quantitative measurement can be done by carefully selecting region of interest.
- The ROI first should be drawn on the opposed—phase image to avoid measuring a region containing India Ink artifact.
- Then the ROI should be selected on the in-phase image either by using copy and paste function or by carefully drawing it manually.
- The region of interest should encompass the highest signal intensity within a lesion on the in-phase image to minimize selection of necrotic or cystic area.

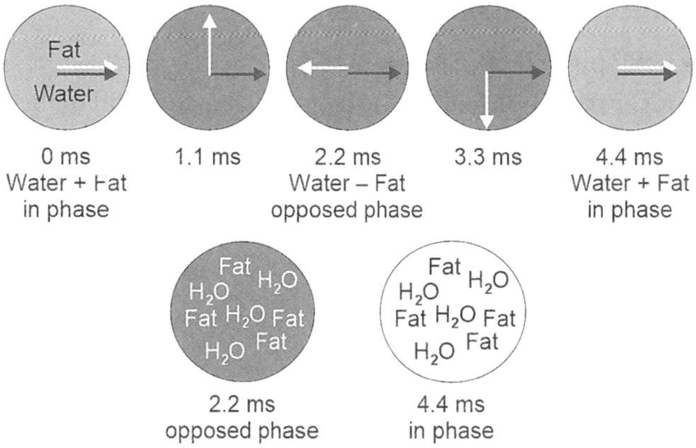

FIG. 50: In-phase and opposed phase images.

Applications of chemical shift signal intensity loss **(Table 25)**

Pure fat or pure water within a voxel will result no change in signal intensity in in and out phase images.

Pitfalls

- Gross fat will not demonstrate chemical shift signal intensity loss, and absence of chemical shift signal intensity loss does not indicate a lack of fat
- Assessment of non-fat suppressed and fat-suppressed MR images, in conjunction with chemical shift imaging, is necessary to completely exclude fat within a lesion.
- Interpretation of small lesions, in which the India ink artifact may constitute the majority of the lesion could lead to an erroneous diagnosis of intravoxel lipid.
- Necrotic lesions may also mimic chemical shift signal intensity loss.

TABLE 25: Applications of chemical shift signal intensity loss.

Benign diagnosis	• Adrenal adenoma • Thymic hyperplasia • Renal AML (fat poor)
Tissue characterization	• Diffuse hepatic steatosis • Infiltrative or mass like hepatic steatosis
Adjunct imaging feature	• Pulmonary hamartoma • Chylothorax • HCC • Xanthogranulomatous cholecystitis • Retroperitoneal lymphangioma • Skeletal metastases

13. Various fat suppressed sequence—describe them. [10] [DNB June 22]

Fat suppression: Nulling the signal from the adipose tissues

- Used to differentiate other short T1 tissues (e.g. enhancing lesion) from fat in any lesion or organ
- The basic techniques of fat suppression are as follows:
  - Frequency selective fat suppression
  - Short tau inversion recovery
  - Out of phase imaging
  - Dixon method

Frequency Selective Fat Suppression (Fig. 51)

- Based on the difference in precessional frequency of protons in water and fat environment
- Frequency selective RF pulse with same resonant frequency as lipids is applied to each slice selection RF pulse
- Followed by homogeneity spoiling gradient pulse to dephase the lipid signal
- The signal received contains no lipid signals
- Sensitive to B_0 inhomogeneities
- Hence, fat suppression is not homogeneous

Short Tau Inversion Recovery

- 90° pulse is applied at short TI
- Corresponds to the time fat takes to recover till halfway stage

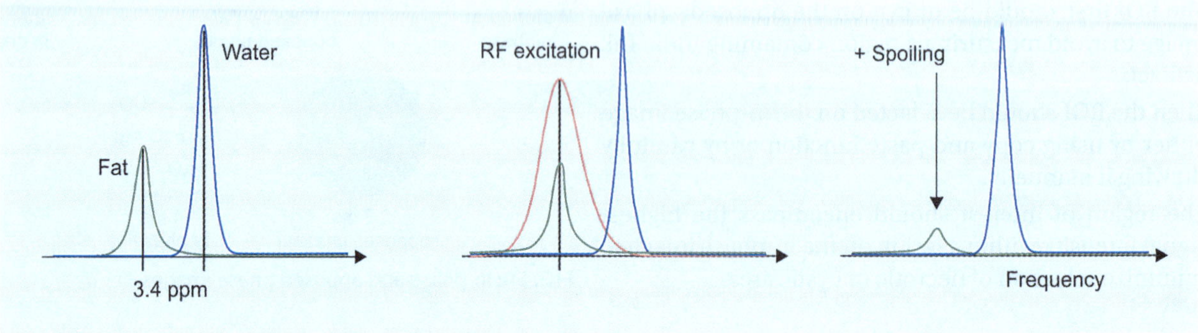

FIG. 51: Frequency selective fat suppression.

- No signal from fat
- Ensures homogeneous suppression of fat
- Also suppresses other tissues with short TI

Out of Phase Imaging

- Difference in precessional frequency of protons in water and fat environment is called chemical shift
- Because of this, they are in-phase at certain echo time (TE) and they are in opposite phase at a certain TE
- At 1.5 Tesla, fat and water protons are in-phase at TE of 4.45 ms, 8.9 ms and so on while they are out of phase at TE of 2.23 ms, 6.69 ms and so on
- Images acquired at in-phase TE have signal from water and fat protons added together
- Images at out-of-phase TE will have signal from water and fat protons subtracted
- On out-of-phase images, fat will appear darker as compared to in-phase images
- Voxels containing only water or only fat will not change in signal
- Hence subcutaneous fat does not become darker on out-of-phase images
- Used for detection of microscopic fat

Dixon Method

- Based on in and out-of-phase imaging
- Two sets of images are acquired, one at in-phase TE and other at out-of-phase TE
- Addition of these two sets gives 'water-only' image
- Subtraction gives 'fat-only' image

14. MR perfusion techniques. [10] [DNB June 22, MD (WBUHS) 24]

MR Perfusion

Principle: In general perfusion means, volume of blood that flows into the tissue in a specific time period, expressed as mL/100g/min.

Tracers

a. Diffusible tracers (H_2O, H_2O^{15} used in PET, xenon used in CT)
b. Intravascular tracers (iodinated contrast in CT and gadolinium and other tracers in MRI)
c. Microsphere type tracers (used in research).

Two main approaches of MR perfusion are there **(Flowchart 12)**.

Contrast-enhanced MR perfusion techniques **(Table 26)**

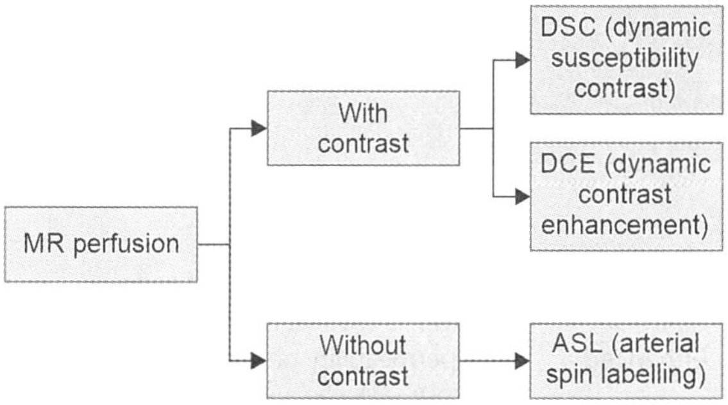

FLOWCHART 12: Approaches of MR perfusion.

TABLE 26: Contrast-enhanced MR perfusion techniques.

Contrast-enhanced MR perfusion techniques	*Principle*	*Parameters measured*
Dynamic Susceptibility Contrast-enhanced MR perfusion (DSCMRP)	• T2* susceptibility effects of gadolinium • The signal loss resulting from passage of the contrast agent bolus on T2* weighted images used to calculate the change in contrast concentration occurring in each pixel.	Time intensity curve • Area under this curve yields relative Cerebral Blood volume (rCBV) • Mean transit time (MTT) • Total blood flow (rCBF) • Time to arrival (TTA) • Time to peak (TPP)

Continued...

Continued...

Contrast-enhanced MR perfusion techniques	***Principle***	***Parameters measured***
	• At least five pre-contrast images • A standard dose of contrast (0.1 mmol/kg) is injected via an 18-20 G cannula at a high rate of 3-7 mL/s, followed by saline flush. Successive images of the region of interest (ROI) are then acquired. • Data analysis: The drop in T2* signal is computed on a voxel-by-voxel basis • Time-versus intensity curve constructed.	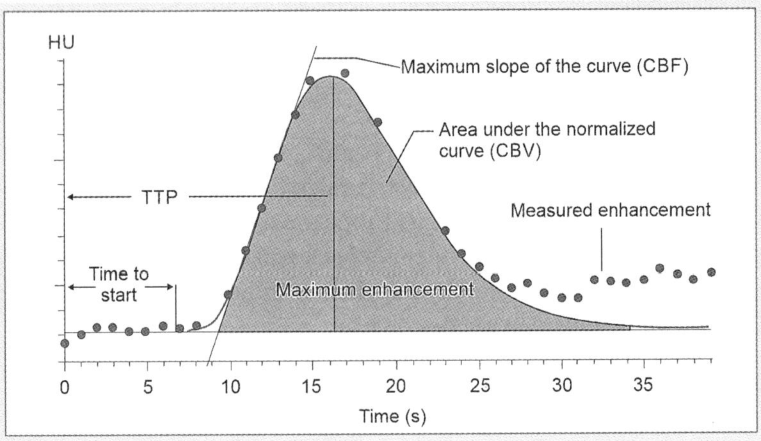 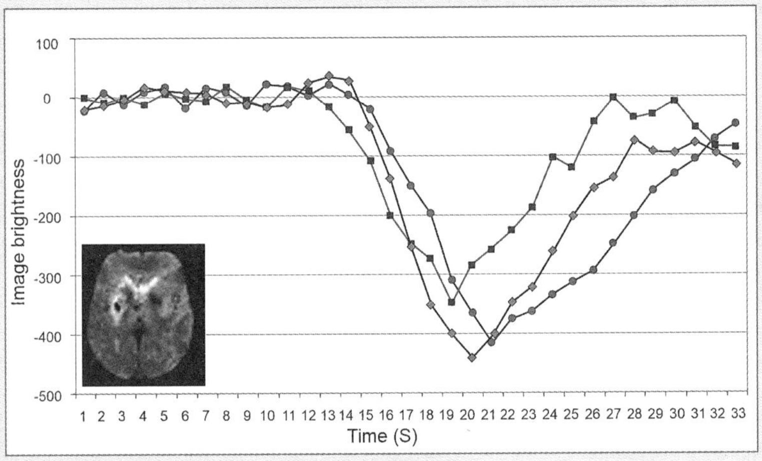
Dynamic contrast enhanced	• T1 shortening effect of gadolinium is used - it is also known as permeability perfusion. • This technique considers two compartmental pharmacokinetics-including the intravascular and interstitial. • Image acquisition- pre-contrast images are obtained followed by which post- contrast images are obtained. Images acquisition is longer than DSC as it allows the contrast to percolate into the interstitium after the equilibrium has reached.	• K^{trans}-transfer constant • V_{e}- fractional volume of the extracellular space • V_{p}- fractional volume of plasma • Most commonly used metric is K^{trans} which denotes the permeability.

15. Parallel imaging and its use. [10] [DNB June 22]

Robust technique for fast acquisition

- Basic principle
- Multiple coil elements

- Information from each coil element combined to produce single image

K-space filling in parallel imaging—the number of phase encoding lines in k-space sampled are reduced.

Reduced Scan Times

- R factor—acceleration factor/pat factor
- The factor by which phase-encoding lines and hence the scan time is reduced.
- Theoretically equal to the number of phased array coil elements. Ex. 2, 3, 4

Parallel Imaging – Simplistic Overview

Coil sensitivity maps + Partial k-space data from 2 coils = Reconstructed image **(Fig. 52)**

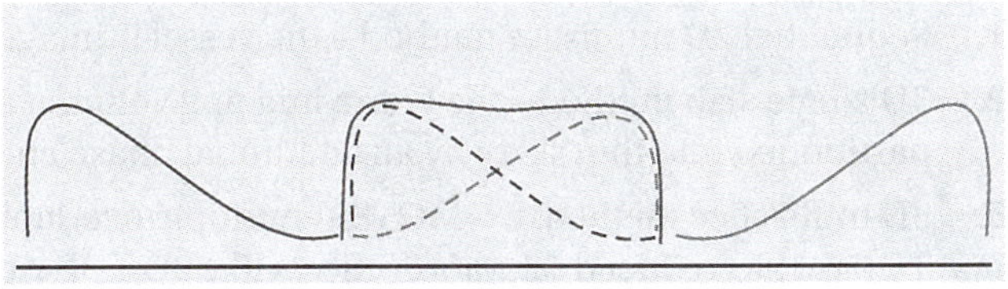

FIG. 52: K-space filling in parallel imaging.

Two image reconstruction techniques

1. SENSE (Sensitivity Encoding)
2. SMASH (SiMultaneous Acquisition of Spatial Harmonics)
   - iPAT (SIEMENS)
   - SENSE (PHILLIPS)
   - ASSET (GE)
   - SENSE- image based
   - Partial images from each coil are reconstructed to produce final image
   - Ex: mSENSE
   - SMASH- k-space based
   - Partial k-spaces (one from each coil) used to reconstruct image
   - Less wrap around artifacts
   - Better suited for single-shot EPI, DWI, perfusion and fMRI
   - Ex: GRAPPA

Applications: Mainly due to increased speed of acquisition and improved spatial resolution

1. Contrast enhanced MRI
2. MR angiography
3. Cardiac imaging
4. Breast imaging
5. CT colonography/enterography

16. Principle and pitfalls of TOF-MRA. [5] [DNB Dec 21]

Time of Flight

It is a type of bright blood imaging

Basic principle: Inflow-related enhancement.

Stationary nuclei receive repeated RF pulses within a short TR period, so they get saturated, having their magnetization in spin down direction. Nuclei flowing perpendicular to the slice have not received these repeated RF pulses and are said to be fresh, as their magnetic moments are mainly oriented in the spin-up direction and give a higher signal.

Fully relaxed blood entering the measured volume behaves as an endogenous contrast agent by producing a bright signal.

To overcome the effects of spin dephasing, flow rephasing techniques (gradient motion rephasing) required.

Advantages of TOF-MRA using GRE sequences:

- Not affected by washout effect
- Permit the use of short TR (<40 ms) needed to saturate stationary tissue
- TE can be kept short (<5 ms) further reducing spin dephasing
- Short acquisition time

TOF-MRA Techniques (Table 27)

TABLE 27: 2D versus 3D TOF-MR angiography.

2D TOF	*3D TOF*
Favored for visualizing slow flow	Good for high flow
Low resolution and SNR	High resolution and SNR
Less susceptible to saturation effect	More susceptible to saturation effect
Better for larger field of views (FOV)	Smaller FOV
Used for cerebral venography, abdominal and peripheral angiography	Cerebral angiography (arteries)

1. Sequential 2D multislice method—the vessel is imaged by sequentially scanning multiple thin slices
2. 3D single slab method—the entire imaging volume, usually 30 to 60 mm thick, is excited simultaneously and then partitioned into thin slices by an additional phase encoding gradient along the slice-selection gradient.
3. 3D multi slice method: Ex- MOTSA (multiple overlapping thin slab acquisition) which retains the advantages of 3D TOF yet has reduced saturation effects like 2D TOF. Adjacent slabs must overlap by 20–30% to compensate for signal attenuations arising at the slab edges.

Optimization

- Orientation of slices or volume is done perpendicular to flow direction
- 2D for slow flow (veins), 3D for fast flow (arteries)
- 3D multislab for larger vessel sections
- Spatial presaturation to isolate arteries and veins
- Use of minimum TE reduces signal loss due to spin dephasing
- TONE pulse reduces saturation effects in 3D TOF
- Magnetization transfer and fat suppression improve vessel contrast

17. (a) What is nephrogenic systemic fibrosis, (b) risk factors for NSF, and (c) method of prevention? [10] [DNB June 21]

Definition: Nephrogenic systemic fibrosis (NSF) is a fibrosing disease, primarily involving the skin and subcutaneous tissues.

Risk Factors (Fig. 53)

- On dialysis (of any form)
- Severe or end-stage CKD (CKD 4 or 5, eGFR <30 mL/min/1.73 m^2) without dialysis

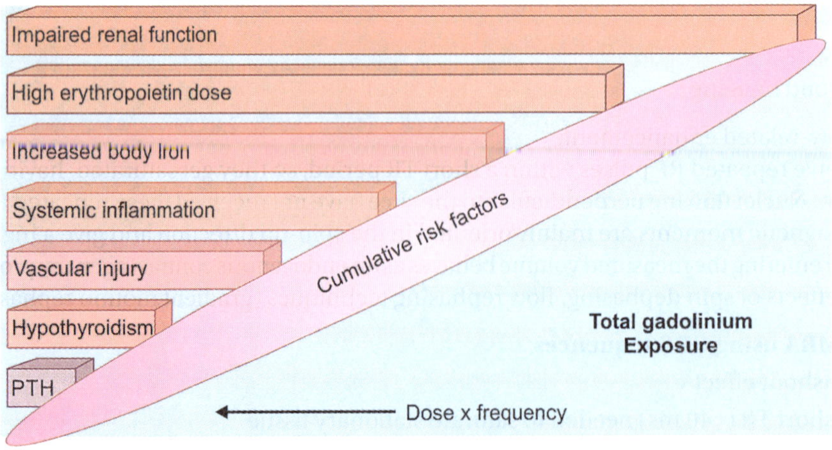

FIG. 53: Risk factors for nephrogenic systemic fibrosis (NSF).

- eGFR 30 to 40 mL/min/1.73m^2 without dialysis
- AKI

Prevalence

- **After single administration**: 3-12% (in pts of impaired renal function) and 36% after two administrations
- 0% in pts with normal renal function.
- Rare in children, no reported cases < 6 years pt

Group I: Agents Associated with the Greatest Number of NSF Cases

- Gadodiamide (Omniscan)
- Gadopentetate dimeglumine (Magnevist)
- Gadoversetamide (OptiMARK)

Group II: Agents Associated with Few, if any, Unconfounded Cases of NSF

- Gadobenate dimeglumine (MultiHance)
- Gadoteridol (ProHance)
- Gadoteric acid (Dotarem)
- Gadobutrol (Gadavist)

Group III: Agents Which have only Recently Appeared on the Market in the US

- Gadofosveset (Ablavar)
- Gadoxetic acid (Eovist)

Signs and Symptoms

- First signs of NSF may be seen within hours of exposure to gadolinium-based contrast agents, but may occur as late as 3 months after exposure
- Begins with subacute swelling of the distal extremities followed in subsequent weeks by severe skin induration
- Constant pain, muscle restlessness, and loss of skin flexibility (contractures)
- Muscle weakness and deep bone pain in the hips and ribs
- Radiography may show soft tissue calcification
- Acute kidney injury

Other systemic effects: Fever, hypotension, acute pancreatitis, vascular thrombosis, sepsis, hepatorenal syndrome

Prevention and T/t:

- Use low dosages of GBCM (preferably macrocyclic agents)
- GBCM is absolutely contraindicated in patients on peritoneal dialysis
- In patients who are on hemodialysis, immediately start dialysis and continue for 3 consecutive days.
- Avoid intravenous iron immediately before or after GBCM exposure

Supportive T/t

Gd and Dialysis: Hemodialysis (at least 3-4 sessions) have a role in preventing NSF. Many studies including ESUR clearly states the definitive role; however, many studies still believe that no definitive role can be established. Peritoneal dialysis has very minimal role, due to slow removal.

18. MR artifacts. [5] [DNB June 21, DNB Dec 20]

- All MRI images contain some degree of artifacts.
- Some artifacts are unavoidable, some can be reduced and some can be completely avoided.
- **MRI artifacts can be dived into three categories**: 1. Related to acquisition technique, 2. Scanner malfunction or interference from outside, and 3. Motion related artifacts.

Motion Related Artifacts

This occurs due to patient movement that can be in form of respiration, swallowing, heartbeat, etc., signal misregistration occurs in the direction of phase encoding gradient.

It occurs in phase encoding direction only because:

- The phase encoding gradient has different amplitude every TR
- As anatomy moves during the scan it is misplaced in phase encoding direction as the phase gradient changes
- There is a time delay between phase encoding and readout

1. **Ghosting or smearing**: Appears as blurring of images

   Ghosting occurs dur to periodic motion (respiration, heartbeat) while smearing is due to aperiodic motion (peristalsis, blood flow).
2. **Pulsatile flow related artifacts**: Periodic motion of any flow perpendicular to the imaging plane produces ghosting of blood vessels, this is frequently seen in abdominal imaging when GRE sequence is used.

Remedy of Motion Artifacts

1. Swapping Phase and Frequency

- As ghosting only occurs along the phase axis
- The direction of phase encoding can be changed
- So that the artifact does not interfere with the area of interest

2. Using presaturation Pulses

- Nulls signal from specified areas
- Placing presaturation volumes over the area producing artifact nullifies signal and reduces the artifact

3. Using Respiratory Compensation Techniques

- Respiratory ordered phase encoding (ROPE)
- Respiratory navigator echoes

4. Cardiac Gating

- Co-ordinates the excitation pulse with the R wave of systole
- Achieved by using an electrical signal generated by the cardiac motion to trigger each excitation pulse

5. Other Motion Reducing Techniques

- Eye movement, can be reduced by asking the patient to focus their eyes
- Bowel motion, is reduced by administering antispasmodic agents
- Voluntary motion can be reduced by making the patient as comfortable as possible
- Immobilizing them with pads and straps
- In extreme cases, sedation of the patient

Artifacts Related to Technique

1. Aliasing or Wrap Around

- Every phase value from 0° to 360° must be mapped into the FOV in the phase encoding direction
- This phase curve is repeated on both sides of the FOV along the phase axis
- As the curve is repeated, signal originating outside the FOV is allocated a phase value that has already been given to signal originating from inside the FOV
- There is, therefore, a duplication of phase values

Remedy:

- increase field of view
- Oversampling
- Swapping the phase and frequency encoding gradient

2. Moiré Artifact

- Especially in the coronal plane
- Large fields of view that are smaller than the object create an interference pattern called the Moiré or Fringe artifact
- Homogeneity of the main field degrades toward the edges of the FOV, causing phase differences between the two edges

Remedy:

- Arms of the patient by side so that they come within FOV
- Spin echo sequence

3. Chemical Shift Artifact

- Due to the differences between resonance frequencies between fat and water
- Difference in precessional frequency is proportional to the strength of magnetic field.
- Occurs in the frequency encode direction
- It produces dark edge at the interface of fat and water.
- At 1.5t , the precessional frequency difference between fat and water is 220 Hz, and fat water protons are mapped few pixels apart, this pixel shift gives rise to chemical shift.

Advantages:

- Basis of MR spectroscopy
- Detection of microscopic fat

Remedy:

- Use the widest receive bandwidth in keeping with good SNR
- Use chemical saturation to saturate out the signal from either fat or water

4. Truncation or Gibbs Artifact

- Banding artifact at the interfaces of high and low signal
- Results from under-sampling of data so that interfaces of high and low signal are incorrectly represented on the image

Remedy: Increase the number of phase encoding steps

5. Magnetic Susceptibility Artifact

- Produces distortion of the image together with large signal voids
- Main causes are metal within the imaging volume, although it can also be seen from naturally occurring iron content of hemorrhage
- More prominent in gradient echo sequences

Remedy: This artifact can, under some circumstances, aid diagnosis. In particular, small hemorrhages are sometimes only seen because they produce a magnetic susceptibility effect.

a. Remove all metal objects
b. Use spin echo sequences instead of gradient echo
c. Decrease the TE: Longer echo times allow for more dephasing between tissues with susceptibility differences, therefore using a short TE reduces this artifact.

Beneficial effects:

a. Used to diagnose hemorrhage, hemosiderin deposition and calcification
b. Forms the basis of post-contrast T2* weighted MR perfusion studies
c. Used to quantify myocardial and liver iron load

Cross-Excitation and Cross-Talk Artifact

- **Appearance**: Adjacent slices in an acquisition have different image contrasts
- **Cause**: An RF excitation pulse is not exactly square. The width of the pulse should be half its amplitude, but this normally varies by up to 10%. As a result, nuclei in slices adjacent to the RF excitation pulse may become excited by it. Adjacent slices receive energy from the RF excitation pulse of their neighbors.

  This energy pushes the NMV of the nuclei towards the transverse plane, so that they may become saturated when they themselves are excited. This effect is called cross-excitation and affects image contrast. The same effect is produced by energy dissipation to adjacent slices, as nuclei within the selected slice relax to B_0. These nuclei lose their energy due to spin lattice relaxation and may dissipate this energy to nuclei in neighboring slices. This is specifically called cross-talk and should not be confused with cross-excitation.

  Remedy:
  - Abnormal loading on Interleaving: Alternate slices are excited and divided into two acquisitions
  - Some systems use software to 'square off' the RF pulses so that the adjacent nuclei are less likely to become excited

Shading Artifact

Appearance: This produces a difference in signal intensity across the imaging volume. More prominent in 3 Tesla MR scanners.

Main cause: Uneven excitation of nuclei.

- Due to RF pulses applied at flip angles other than 90° and 180°
- Abnormal loading on the coil
- Coupling of the coil at one point
- Inhomogeneities in the main magnetic field

External Errors

1. **Artifacts due to magnetic field distortions**
   a. Inhomogeneous magnetic field
   b. Gradient non-linear
   c. RF field inhomogeneity
2. **Spike(Herringbone) artifact**
   - Loose electric connection in Rf coils
   - Leading burst of short duration noise
   - Seen in echo-planar imaging

Zipper artifact: Interference of entromagnetic field from outside sources—mobile, radio, open door, appear as thin line at the center of the image.

19. (a) Describe the principle and technique of phase contrast MR angiography. (b) Discuss its advantages, limitations and clinical applications. [2+2+2+2+2] [DNB June 20]

Phase Contrast Angiography

It is a non-contrast MR angiography technique.

Phase contrast angiography produces information in two ways:

1. For production of angiographic image
2. For quantification of flow

The flow-induced phase shift of the transverse magnetization is employed to image blood vessels.

It is the most sensitive sequence for detection of slow flow and it is the only sequence to provide information about flow, velocity and pressure.

In phase sequence, moving protons experience a changing magnetic field and accumulate a phase which is different from stationary protons, which experience static magnetic field.

Phase shift is proportional to magnitude of gradient, phase shift greater than 180-degree cause aliasing, so adjusting gradient is necessary, which is done in form of velocity encoding (VENC), i.e., velocity encoding.it is define as the highest velocity to get detected before aliasing.

- Bipolar gradients are used to acquire image, two lobes- dephasing and rephrasing lobes are used.
- Stationary protons experience two gradients (same, opposite direction), net phase 0

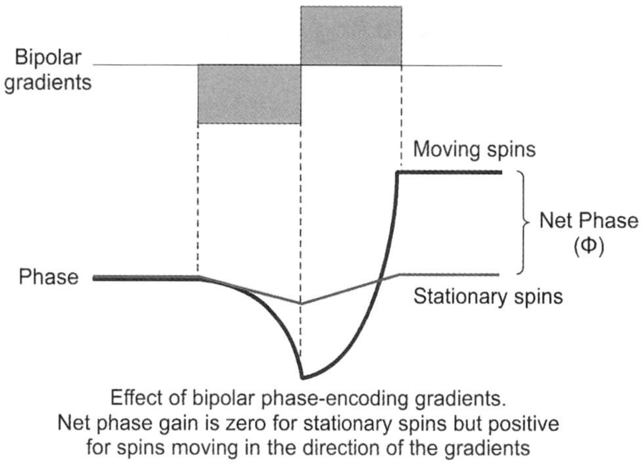

FIG. 54: Principle of phase contrast MR angiography.

- Moving protons accumulate phase as they experience different magnetic field **(Fig. 54)**.
- Time taken is almost double than that of TOF angio as image is obtained after every bipolar gradient.
  A. Complex subtraction yields phase difference and the difference vector.
  B. In phase map images, the phase difference Φ depicts signal intensity and the sign of phase shift encodes flow direction.
  C. Non-moving tissue appear as medium shade of gray while flowing blood is either brighter or darker, according to direction of flow. As the intensity of each pixel is linearly proportional to flow velocity, phase images are suited for flow quantification and identifying flow direction. In magnitude images, the length of the difference vector is used for anatomically image vessels. Velocity encoding (VENC) adapted to different velocity ranges are used for estimating flow velocity and direction.

Clinical Application

1. Cardiovascular study
2. Venography
3. 3D vascular studies
4. CSF flow study.

Advantages

1. Both velocity and flow, cardiac gated through plane images give information throughout the cycle
2. Intraluminal pressure-information about vessel stenosis
3. Good suppression of background

Disadvantages

1. Longer scan time
2. Highly sensitive to motion artifacts
3. Areas showing turbulent flow give signal void
4. Eddy current, gradient non-linearity

Optimization

1. VENC
2. MIP processing
3. ECG gating
4. Arterial and venous separation using different pre-saturation pulse

Digital Subtraction Angiography

1. DSA—basic principles and role in radiological interventions. [5+5] [MD (WBUHS) 23]

Digital Subtraction Angiography (DSA): Basic Principles and Role in Radiological Interventions

Digital Subtraction Angiography (DSA) is an advanced radiological technique primarily used for visualizing blood vessels and detecting vascular abnormalities, such as aneurysms, stenoses, and arteriovenous malformations (AVMs). DSA combines traditional angiographic imaging with digital subtraction to enhance visualization of blood vessels by removing background structures, providing clearer images of the vascular system.

Basic Principles of DSA

1. **Contrast injection**:
   - A contrast medium (usually an iodinated contrast agent) is injected into the bloodstream through a catheter, which is typically placed in an artery (e.g., femoral, radial) or vein (in rare cases) using a technique called catheterization.
   - The contrast agent helps highlight blood vessels on the imaging screen, as it has a high atomic number and absorbs X-rays.
2. **Image acquisition**:
   - The patient is positioned under a fluoroscopy machine, and a series of X-ray images are taken in rapid succession as the contrast flows through the blood vessels.
   - These X-ray images are captured at different time intervals after the injection of contrast to document the dynamic flow of blood through the vascular system.
3. **Subtraction process**:
   - **Digital subtraction**: This is the key feature of DSA. After capturing an initial image (before the contrast injection, known as the "mask" image), additional images are taken during and after contrast injection.
   - The "mask" image (which shows only the bones, tissues, and other structures without the contrast) is digitally subtracted from the subsequent images. This removes the background structures (bones, tissues), leaving only the contrast-filled blood vessels clearly visible.
   - The subtraction process significantly enhances the contrast of blood vessels, making it easier to detect abnormalities and abnormalities that may not be visible on conventional X-ray images.
4. **Real-time imaging**:
   - The process is dynamic, with real-time imaging of blood flow allowing the clinician to assess the vascular structures and abnormalities as the procedure progresses.
   - The technique is particularly useful for evaluating the vascular system in real time and guiding interventions during diagnostic or therapeutic procedures.

Components of a DSA System

- **Fluoroscopy unit**: Provides real-time X-ray imaging and allows the radiologist to guide the catheter into the target area.
- **Contrast injection system**: Delivers the contrast material into the blood vessels at a controlled rate.
- **Digital subtraction software**: Performs the subtraction of the pre-contrast image from the post-contrast images to highlight the vascular structures.
- **Workstation**: Used for viewing, analyzing, and storing the images captured during the procedure.

Role of DSA in Radiological Interventions

DSA has become a cornerstone in the diagnosis and treatment of vascular diseases due to its high resolution, real-time imaging capabilities, and ability to guide minimally invasive interventions. Below are some key roles DSA plays in radiology:

1. Diagnosis of Vascular Conditions

- **Aneurysms**: DSA is highly sensitive in detecting aneurysms, including cerebral, coronary, and peripheral aneurysms. The technique allows for precise visualization of the size, shape, and location of the aneurysm.

- **Stenosis or occlusions**: DSA can identify stenoses (narrowing of blood vessels) or complete occlusions in arteries and veins, such as in cases of coronary artery disease (CAD), peripheral arterial disease (PAD), or carotid artery stenosis.
- **Arteriovenous malformations (AVMs)**: DSA is used to visualize AVMs, where abnormal connections exist between arteries and veins. The imaging helps assess the size, location, and complexity of the AVM.
- **Vascular malformations**: Conditions like hemangiomas or venous malformations are also evaluated using DSA, providing detailed mapping of the abnormal vasculature.

2. Preoperative Planning and Mapping

- **Planning for surgery or interventional procedures**: DSA provides a roadmap of the vascular system, helping to plan surgeries or endovascular procedures (e.g., stent placement, embolization). It helps clinicians assess the anatomy and the location of critical blood vessels, which is crucial for minimizing risks during surgery.
- **Assessment of collateral circulation**: DSA can evaluate the presence and adequacy of collateral blood flow in cases of occlusive disease, such as in the brain (before surgery for brain tumors or carotid artery stenosis) or in the coronary arteries.

3. Guiding Interventional Procedures

DSA is frequently used as a guiding tool for minimally invasive radiological procedures, enabling the interventional radiologist or cardiologist to perform treatments with precision:

- **Angioplasty and stent placement**: In cases of arterial stenosis (e.g., coronary artery disease or peripheral arterial disease), DSA is used to guide catheter-based interventions such as angioplasty (balloon dilation) or stent placement to open up narrowed vessels.
- **Embolization**: DSA is used to guide the delivery of embolic agents (e.g., coils, glue, or particles) to block abnormal blood vessels or stop bleeding (e.g., in trauma, GI bleeding, or to treat uterine fibroids).
- **Thrombolysis**: DSA assists in identifying the location of thrombus (clot) in blood vessels and can be used during catheter-based thrombolysis procedures to deliver clot-busting drugs directly to the affected area.
- **Biopsy guidance**: In some cases, DSA is used to guide a biopsy needle to a specific vascular or organ site when a lesion is located in or near a blood vessel.

4. Endovenous Procedures (for Varicose Veins)

In interventional procedures for treating varicose veins (endovenous laser therapy or sclerotherapy), DSA may be used to visualize the abnormal veins and guide the treatment, ensuring precise localization and treatment of the affected veins.

5. Post-treatment Follow-up

After an interventional procedure (such as stent placement, coil embolization, or angioplasty), DSA is frequently used for post-treatment evaluation to ensure the procedure was successful, confirm proper placement of devices, and check for complications such as restenosis, bleeding, or thrombosis.

Advantages of DSA

- **High sensitivity and specificity**: DSA provides exceptional clarity in visualizing vascular structures, even in complex or difficult-to-assess areas (e.g., brain, coronary arteries).
- **Real-time imaging**: DSA allows for immediate feedback during diagnostic and interventional procedures, helping clinicians make decisions in real time.
- **Minimally invasive**: DSA allows for non-surgical management of many vascular conditions through catheter-based interventions, reducing the need for open surgery.
- **Detailed anatomical information**: Provides accurate information regarding the size, shape, and location of vascular abnormalities, which is essential for planning and guiding treatments.

Limitations of DSA

- **Radiation exposure**: As with all X-ray-based imaging techniques, DSA involves ionizing radiation, so minimizing exposure, particularly for vulnerable patients, is important.

- **Contrast allergies and renal risk**: The use of iodinated contrast agents carries a risk of allergic reactions and potential contrast-induced nephropathy (CIN), particularly in patients with pre-existing kidney disease.
- **Invasiveness**: Although minimally invasive, DSA still involves catheterization, which carries a risk of complications, such as vessel perforation, hematoma, or infection.

Conclusion

Digital Subtraction Angiography (DSA) is a highly effective and versatile tool in both the diagnosis and treatment of a wide range of vascular conditions. Its ability to provide real-time, high-resolution images makes it invaluable in guiding minimally invasive interventions, from angioplasty and stent placement to embolization and biopsy. However, careful consideration of patient-specific factors, such as renal function and contrast sensitivity, is essential to optimize its use in clinical practice.

2. Write short note on Seldinger technique. [5] [MD (WBUHS) 24, MD (WBUHS) 21]

It is a minimally invasive technique to gain access into blood vessels or in a hollow viscus.

History: In 1953, Sven Ivar Seldinger introduced this technique, by this new horizon on interventional radiology has opened up.

This technique allow entry into an area without cut down and minimally damaging the surrounding tissue with a faster recovery.

Equipment

- Seldinger needle
- Guidewire
- Sheath
- Dilatator

Technique (Figs. 55A to F)

- Insert the needle into the vessel forming an acute angle (30-45 degree)
- Stabilize the needle
- Advance guide-wire into the vessel

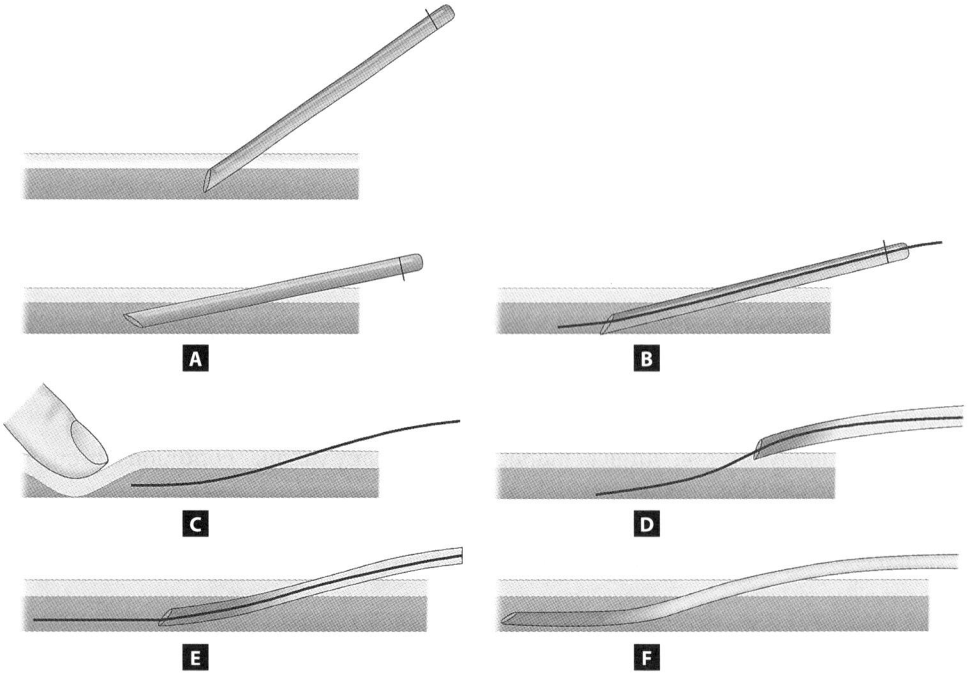

FIGS. 55A to F: Seldinger technique of vascular access.

- Remove needle
- Dilator is advanced over guide wire
- Remove the dilator
- Sheath or catheter is advanced into the vessel
- Removal of guide wire
- Flush and stabilize

The Modified Seldinger Technique (MST) differed from the original concept in that it was used as a tool to insert a tear-away sheath introducer and replace over-the-needle introducers. Interestingly, this technique increased the accuracy of first-time introducer placement to 75% and then, when combined with ultrasound, the accuracy increased to 95–100%.

- Seldinger needle—18-gauge angiographic needle
- Wire—thin, strong, flexible wire made of stainless steel: may be straight or curved-j shaped
- Coating—Teflon, heparin or hydrophilic polymer
- Catheter—thin tubular flexible
- Straight, pigtail, hunter, cobra catheter

Access site:

1. Femoral—most commonly used-large vessel size
   - Lower limb
   - Pelvic area
   - Abdominal aorta and its branches
   - Thoracic aorta and coronary arteries
   - Head, neck angiography
2. Brachial—just above the level of elbow
3. Radial—site of maximum pulsation

Risks/Complications

- Bleeding at puncture site
- Thrombus formation
- Embolus formation—plaque dislodged from vessel wall by catheter
- Dissection of vessel
- Puncture site infection (contaminated sterile field)
- Contrast reaction

3. Write short note on pulse fluoroscopy. [5] [DNB June 22]

In conventional fluoroscopy continuous low energy X-rays are produced (in the range of 4-6 mAs), though the energy is less, continuous X-ray production leads to more radiation dose.

To overcome this problem pulse fluoroscopy was introduced, in which X-rays are produced in pulses either by generator controlled or by grid controlled **(Table 28)**.

TABLE 28: Generator controlled versus grid controlled pulse fluoroscopy.

Generator controlled	• Current is supplied to X-ray tube in short pulses, lasting for 3–10 ms • Due to presence of low resistance cables, low energy X-rays produced initially • Bell-shaped curve if formed, slow rise to fall **Disadvantages**: • Reduced image quality • No significant reduction in radiation dose
Grid controlled	• Negative charge applied between cathode and anode in a pulsatile manner • Without any low energy X-ray

Advantages of Pulse Fluoroscopy

1. Improved temporal resolution
2. Reduction in radiation dose

Disadvantages

1. Noise
2. Speckle
3. Sub-optimal visualization of fine wire, catheters

4. Describe image intensifier with the help of a diagram and briefly discuss its properties and limitations. [5+2+3] [MD (WBUHS) 24, DNB Dec 20]

Image Intensifier: Description, Properties, and Limitations

An **image intensifier** is a device used in fluoroscopic imaging to amplify the brightness of X-ray images in real-time, allowing for clear visualization of structures during diagnostic and interventional procedures. It is commonly used in angiography, fluoroscopy, and other radiological procedures where continuous X-ray imaging is required. The image intensifier enables the radiologist or interventionalist to visualize the internal structures with better contrast and brightness, enhancing clinical decision-making during minimally invasive procedures.

Basic Components of an Image Intensifier

An image intensifier typically consists of the following components:

1. Input phosphor

- The input phosphor is a scintillation screen that absorbs the incoming X-rays and converts them into visible light.
- It is usually made of a phosphor material like **cesium iodide (CsI)** or **gadolinium oxysulfide (Gd_2O_2S)**.
- The input phosphor is circular and is the part of the image intensifier that receives the X-ray photons.

2. Photocathode

- The photocathode is a layer of material (usually made from a compound like **antimony trisulfide** or **cesium-antimony**) that is placed directly on top of the input phosphor.
- It converts the visible light emitted by the phosphor into **electrons**.

3. Electrostatic Lenses

- These are a series of electrodes that focus the electrons emitted from the photocathode toward the output phosphor.
- The electrostatic lenses accelerate and direct the electron flow, increasing the image's resolution and sharpness.

4. Anode

- The anode collects the electrons accelerated by the electrostatic lenses and directs them toward the output phosphor.
- The anode is typically made of a metal such as **aluminum** or **copper**.

5. Output Phosphor

- The output phosphor is a layer of **zinc cadmium sulfide** or similar phosphor material that converts the electrons arriving from the anode back into visible light.
- This visible light is then captured by a camera or viewed directly on a monitor.

6. Video Camera/Monitor

- The light emitted by the output phosphor is used to produce an image on a video screen or monitor, which is viewed by the radiologist or interventionalist.
- The image can also be recorded or processed for further analysis.

Diagram of Image Intensifier (Fig. 56)

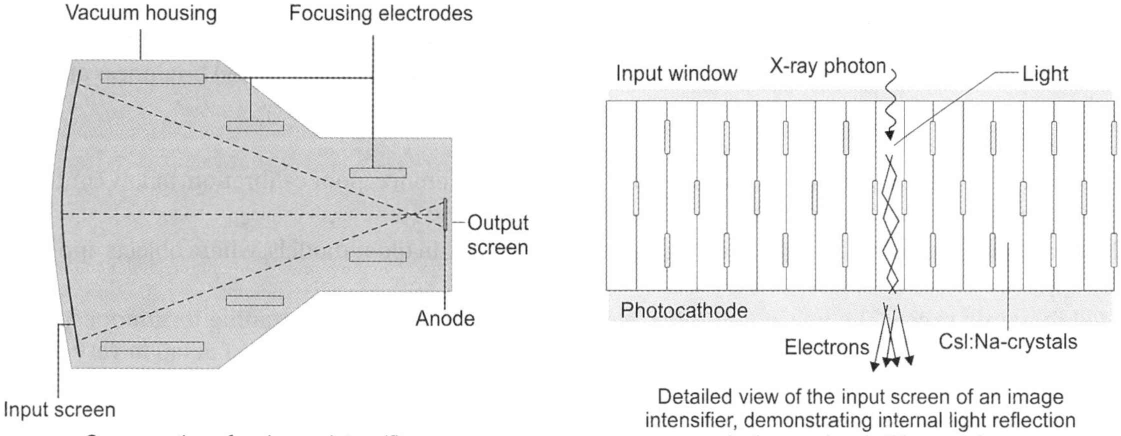

Cross-section of an image intensifier

Detailed view of the input screen of an image intensifier, demonstrating internal light reflection in the caesium iodide crystals

FIG. 56: Image intensifier.

Mechanism of image formation in image intensifier is schematically shown as follows **(Fig. 57)**.

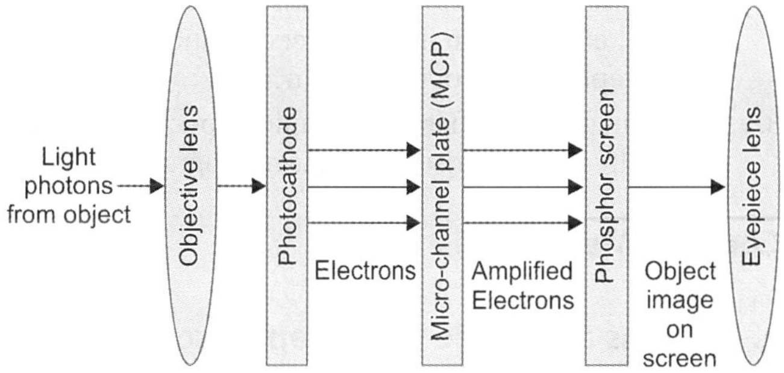

FIG. 57: Mechanism of image formation in image intensifier.

Properties of Image Intensifiers

1. **Image amplification**: The primary function of the image intensifier is to **amplify** the brightness of the X-ray image. The process of converting X-rays into visible light and amplifying the intensity of that light allows for better visualization of internal structures, even in low-light conditions.
2. **Real-time imaging**: Image intensifiers are designed for **real-time** imaging, which is particularly useful in dynamic procedures like fluoroscopy and interventional radiology. This continuous imaging capability allows clinicians to monitor movement or changes during a procedure.
3. **High spatial resolution**: Image intensifiers offer high spatial resolution, meaning they can produce detailed, sharp images. This is crucial when identifying small or complex structures, such as in angiography or catheter guidance.
4. **Improved contrast sensitivity**: The amplification process improves the contrast between structures, allowing for better differentiation of tissues and vessels. This is especially important in low-dose X-ray imaging where conventional radiography might struggle with contrast differences.
5. **Size and portability**: Image intensifiers are relatively compact and can be integrated into mobile fluoroscopic units, making them suitable for a wide range of clinical environments, from operating rooms to emergency departments.
6. **Low radiation dose**: By amplifying the image, the image intensifier allows the use of lower X-ray doses to achieve adequate imaging quality. This is especially important in reducing radiation exposure for both patients and healthcare providers.

Limitations of Image Intensifiers

Despite their usefulness, image intensifiers also have several limitations:

1. **Resolution limitations**:
   - While image intensifiers offer high spatial resolution, the resolution is typically limited by the size of the input and output phosphors. Larger field sizes may reduce image clarity.
   - Over time, the **resolution** may decrease due to aging of the phosphor material, resulting in decreased image quality.
2. **Size and field of view**:
   - The size of the input phosphor determines the field of view (FOV). Larger FOVs result in decreased resolution due to the increased spread of electrons. This is a trade-off when trying to view a larger area.

- Modern systems address this by using **multi-field image intensifiers** that can adjust the FOV for specific procedures, but this still limits the system's flexibility.

3. **Vignetting**: Vignetting is a phenomenon where the image becomes darker toward the edges. This occurs because the electrons are not evenly distributed across the entire field of view, leading to reduced brightness at the periphery of the image.
4. **Noise and distortion**:
   - Noise in the image can occur due to factors like electronic interference, poor calibration, or low contrast imaging, which can make the image less clear.
   - The image may also suffer from geometric distortion, especially in older models, where objects appear stretched or compressed due to imperfections in the focusing system.
5. **Limited dynamic range**: The image intensifier has a limited dynamic range, meaning it cannot capture extreme differences in brightness as well as modern digital detectors. This can result in loss of detail in very bright or dark areas.
6. **Radiation exposure**: Although the image intensifier allows for reduced radiation doses, there is still a significant level of radiation exposure during fluoroscopy and angiography procedures. Prolonged exposure can contribute to radiation-related risks for both patients and healthcare workers.
7. **Aging and degradation**: Over time, components like the input phosphor and photocathode degrade, leading to reduced efficiency in light conversion and amplification. This can result in lower image quality and the need for device replacement or maintenance.
8. **Cost**: Image intensifiers are complex, specialized devices that can be expensive to purchase, maintain, and repair, especially in comparison to digital radiography systems that do not require this amplification technology.

Contrast Media

1. Discuss about the radiographic contrast media. [10] [MD (WBUHS) 22, MD (WBUHS) 21, DNB Dec 18, AIIMS May 24, AIIMS May 23]

Types of Contrast Media

Contrast media (or contrast agents) are substances used in medical imaging to enhance the visibility of internal structures and fluids within the body, helping clinicians identify abnormalities or pathologies. Contrast agents work by altering the way X-rays, ultrasound, MRI, or CT scans interact with tissues, making them appear more distinct on imaging.

The types of contrast media vary depending on the imaging modality (X-ray, CT, MRI, ultrasound), and they are classified based on their **chemical composition**, **mechanism of action**, and **physiological effects**.

Here are the **different types of contrast media** commonly used in diagnostic imaging:

1. X-ray/fluoroscopy Contrast Agents

X-ray and fluoroscopic imaging often rely on **iodinated contrast agents**, which are used to enhance vascular and organ imaging (e.g., angiography, CT scans, and gastrointestinal studies).

a. Iodinated contrast agents

These are the most widely used contrast agents for **X-ray and CT imaging**, and they contain **iodine** (I), which absorbs X-rays and appears white on the X-ray image.

- **High-osmolar contrast media (HOCM)**:
  - *Description:* These are older agents with a higher osmolality (the concentration of particles per unit of solvent). High-osmolar agents can cause more side effects and are less commonly used today.
  - *Example:* **Diatrizoate** (Hypaque), **Iothalamate** (Conray).
- **Properties**:
  - Higher risk of side effects (e.g., nausea, vomiting, allergic reactions).
  - Higher viscosity.
  - Increased risk of contrast-induced nephropathy (CIN).

- **Low-osmolar contrast media (LOCM)**:
  - *Description:* These agents have a lower osmolality than HOCM, making them safer and better tolerated.
  - *Examples:* **Iopamidol** (Isovue), **Iohexol** (Omnipaque), **Iodixanol** (Visipaque).
  - *Properties:*
    - Reduced risk of side effects like allergic reactions.
    - Better for patients with kidney issues.
    - Lower viscosity compared to HOCM.
- **Iso-osmolar contrast media**:
  - *Description:* These agents have an osmolality similar to that of blood, making them the least likely to cause side effects. They are often used in sensitive patients (e.g., those with renal impairment).
  - *Example:* **Iodixanol** (Visipaque).
  - *Properties:*
    - Very low risk of nephrotoxicity.
    - Ideal for patients with poor kidney function.

b. Barium Sulfate ($BaSO_4$)

- **Description**: **Barium sulfate** is used as a contrast agent in **X-ray and fluoroscopic imaging** of the gastrointestinal (GI) tract.
- **Properties**:
  - It is **opaque to X-rays**, meaning it appears white on X-ray images.
  - **Inert** and **non-absorbable**; it stays within the GI tract, making it useful for imaging studies like **barium swallow**, **barium enema**, or **upper GI series**.
  - *Risk:* If the barium sulfate leaks into the peritoneal cavity (e.g., due to a perforation), it can cause serious complications such as peritonitis.

2. Magnetic resonance Imaging (MRI) Contrast Agents

MRI contrast agents usually rely on **gadolinium-based compounds** to enhance tissue differentiation. These agents alter the magnetic properties of certain tissues, improving contrast between healthy and diseased areas.

a. Gadolinium-based contrast agents (GBCA):

- **Description**: These agents contain **gadolinium** (Gd), a rare earth metal that has paramagnetic properties. Gadolinium enhances the magnetic resonance signal, helping to provide detailed images of soft tissues.
- **Examples**:
  - *Gadodiamide* (Omniscan)
  - *Gadopentetate dimeglumine* (Magnevist)
  - *Gadobutrol* (Gadavist)
- **Properties**:
  - **Used for soft tissue imaging**, such as the brain, spine, and blood vessels.
  - Gadolinium agents are typically safe, but patients with **renal impairment** are at higher risk for a rare but serious condition called **nephrogenic systemic fibrosis (NSF)**.
  - Some newer agents (e.g., **Gadobutrol**) have higher relaxivity, which leads to better image quality at lower doses.

b. Superparamagnetic contrast agents:

- **Description**: These agents are based on **iron oxide** particles and are used for specialized MRI techniques like **functional imaging** and **immuno-MRI** (imaging targeting specific biological markers).
- **Example**: **Ferumoxytol**.
- **Properties**: These agents enhance tissue contrast but are less commonly used than gadolinium-based agents.

3. Ultrasound Contrast Agents

Ultrasound contrast agents are primarily used in **contrast-enhanced ultrasound (CEUS)** to enhance the visibility of blood flow, organs, or tumors. These agents usually consist of **microbubbles** or gas-filled spheres that reflect sound waves, enhancing image quality.

Microbubble contrast agents

- **Description**: Microbubbles are tiny gas-filled bubbles that are injected into the bloodstream. They increase the reflection of sound waves and create a strong contrast on ultrasound images.
- **Examples**:
  - **Sulfur hexafluoride microbubbles** (e.g., **Optison**)
  - **Perfluorobutane microbubbles** (e.g., **Sonovue**)
- **Properties**:
  - Primarily used to enhance imaging of **cardiac** and **vascular** studies.
  - Used in **liver imaging** to detect lesions, such as **HCC** (hepatocellular carcinoma).
  - **Minimal risk** of side effects, but precautions are taken in patients with **pulmonary hypertension** or **severe cardiac disease**.

4. Computed Tomography (CT) Contrast Agents

CT contrast agents are similar to **X-ray contrast agents** (usually iodinated), but they are specifically tailored for use in **CT imaging** to provide better tissue differentiation, particularly in high-resolution scans.

Iodinated contrast media for CT

- **Description**: These agents contain iodine, which absorbs X-rays to create images with enhanced contrast.
- **Examples**: The same agents used in **X-ray imaging**, such as **Iohexol** (Omnipaque), **Iopamidol** (Isovue), **Iodixanol** (Visipaque).
- **Properties**:
  - Used to visualize blood vessels, organs, and tissues during CT scans, especially in **angiography**, **CT colonography**, and **abdominal imaging**.
  - **Risk of nephropathy** in patients with pre-existing kidney conditions, especially in high doses.

5. Fluorescence Imaging Contrast Agents

These agents are used in **fluorescence-guided surgery** and **diagnostic imaging**, where the contrast agent fluoresces when exposed to specific light wavelengths.

Fluorescent dyes and agents

- **Description**: These agents emit light in the visible spectrum when excited by a specific wavelength of light.
- **Examples**:
  - **Indocyanine green (ICG)**: Used in **near-infrared fluorescence imaging** for liver, vascular, and cancer surgeries.
  - **5-aminolevulinic acid (5-ALA)**: Used for **fluorescence-guided surgery** in brain tumors.
- **Properties**:
  - Highly sensitive for detecting small tumors, micro-metastasis, or surgical margins.
  - Common in **cancer** and **neurological surgeries**.

6. Other Specialized Contrast Media

There are various other contrast agents designed for niche applications or new imaging techniques.

Oral contrast agents

- **Description**: These are swallowed by the patient before **CT scans** or **X-ray imaging** to help visualize the **gastro-intestinal tract**.
- **Examples**: **Barium sulfate** (for GI series), **Gastrografin** (for water-soluble contrast in bowel imaging).

- **Properties**:
  - **Barium sulfate** is commonly used in **upper GI series**, **barium enema**, and **fluoroscopy** to highlight the stomach and intestines.
  - **Gastrografin** is used in cases where there is a suspicion of bowel perforation, as it is water-soluble and less harmful if leaked.

2. How will you manage a patient with acute radiographic contrast media reaction? [10] [DNB Dec 21, DNB Dec 20, DNB June 20, MD (WBUHS) 19, RG 18, AIIMS Dec 24]

Contrast Reactions: Definition and Types

A **contrast reaction** refers to an adverse or allergic response that occurs after the administration of a contrast agent (also called a contrast medium), which is commonly used in diagnostic imaging procedures such as CT scans, MRIs, angiograms, and fluoroscopy. These reactions can range from mild to severe and can involve a variety of symptoms, depending on the type of reaction and the individual's sensitivity to the contrast material.

Types of Contrast Reactions

1. **Non-allergic (physiologic) reactions**: These are typically mild, self-limiting, and related to the physical properties of the contrast material. They can occur due to the osmolarity, viscosity, or pH of the contrast agent, leading to reactions like:
   - Mild nausea or vomiting
   - Warmth or flushing sensation
   - Metallic taste
   - Mild headache
   - Mild skin reactions (e.g., itching, hives)
2. **Allergic (hypersensitivity) reactions**: These reactions result from an immune-mediated response to the contrast agent, either immediate or delayed. They are less common but can vary in severity:
   - *Immediate (Type I hypersensitivity reactions):* These reactions occur within minutes to hours of contrast administration and may include:
     - Urticaria (hives)
     - Angioedema (swelling of deeper tissues)
     - Anaphylaxis (severe allergic reaction involving airway compromise, hypotension, and potential shock)
   - *Delayed reactions:* These can occur hours to days after administration and are typically less severe. Symptoms may include:
     - Rash
     - Fever
     - Joint pain (arthralgia)
     - Eosinophilia (increased eosinophils in blood)
3. **CIN (contrast-induced nephropathy)**: Contrast-induced nephropathy is a form of kidney injury that can occur after the administration of iodinated contrast agents (commonly used in CT scans and angiography). It presents with an acute increase in serum creatinine levels, typically within 48 to 72 hours after contrast exposure.
4. **Cerebral or cardiovascular effects**:
   - *Contrast-induced cardiotoxicity:* This can lead to arrhythmias or other cardiac symptoms, especially in patients with pre-existing heart conditions.
   - *Seizures:* Rare but serious, often associated with the use of gadolinium-based contrast agents for MRI in patients with a history of epilepsy or seizures.

Management of Contrast Reactions

The management of contrast reactions depends on the severity of the reaction. Here's a breakdown:

1. Mild Reactions (Non-Allergic or Mild Allergic)

- **Management**:
  - *Observation:* Most mild reactions resolve on their own without requiring specific treatment.
  - *Supportive care:* Anti-histamines (e.g., diphenhydramine) or corticosteroids may be used for mild allergic reactions like urticaria or pruritus.
  - *Hydration:* Ensure adequate fluid intake if the patient develops mild nausea or flushing.
- **Follow-up**: Reassure the patient and provide appropriate follow-up care if necessary. These reactions generally do not require discontinuation of further imaging, although a different contrast agent may be considered for future studies.

2. Moderate Reactions (Moderate Allergic Reactions, CIN)

Management:

- **Antihistamines** (e.g., diphenhydramine) and/or **steroids** (e.g., prednisone) for moderate urticaria, rash, or pruritus.
- **Epinephrine** (1:1000) for more severe reactions like moderate angioedema or difficulty breathing. Administer intramuscularly if symptoms progress.
- **Monitoring**: Ensure close monitoring of the patient for up to 30 minutes, especially if respiratory symptoms (e.g., wheezing, shortness of breath) or cardiovascular symptoms (e.g., hypotension) develop.
- **Contrast-induced nephropathy (CIN)**: For patients with impaired renal function, manage CIN by:
  - Ensuring **hydration** before and after contrast administration.
  - Using **N-acetylcysteine (NAC)** or **bicarbonate** infusion to reduce the risk of renal injury.
  - Monitoring **renal function** (e.g., serum creatinine, urine output) for 48-72 hours post-procedure.

3. Severe Reactions (Anaphylaxis, Severe CIN)

Management:

- **Anaphylaxis (Type I Hypersensitivity)**:
  - **Immediate administration of epinephrine** (1:1000) intramuscularly for anaphylaxis.
  - **Oxygen** if needed to maintain adequate oxygen saturation.
  - **IV fluids** to counteract hypotension and shock.
  - **Antihistamines** and **steroids** to treat the inflammation and help with symptoms post-epinephrine administration.
  - **Airway management**: If the patient develops severe respiratory distress, intubation or mechanical ventilation may be necessary.
  - **Severe CIN**:
    - **Dialysis** may be necessary for patients with significant renal impairment or progression to acute renal failure.
    - **Supportive care** (e.g., fluids, monitoring electrolytes, managing hypertension or other complications).

4. Post-reaction Follow-up

- **Documentation**: Document the details of the reaction, including the type of contrast used, the timing, symptoms, and the response to treatment.
- **Reassessment**: A patient with a history of moderate to severe reaction may need premedication (e.g., steroids and antihistamines) if future contrast imaging is necessary.
- **Alternative imaging**: If severe allergic reactions have occurred, non-contrast imaging (e.g., ultrasound, MRI without contrast, or plain X-rays) or alternative contrast agents (e.g., gadolinium for MRIs or different iodinated contrast agents for CT) may be considered.

Prevention of Contrast Reactions

- **History taking**: Identify patients with prior allergic reactions to contrast agents, history of asthma, or renal insufficiency, and tailor the management accordingly.

- **Pre-medication**: For patients with a known history of moderate to severe reactions, pre-medication with steroids (e.g., prednisone 12 hours and 2 hours before the procedure) and antihistamines (e.g., diphenhydramine) is often recommended.
- **Hydration**: Pre-hydrating patients at risk for CIN is a key preventive measure.
- **Use of low-osmolar or iso-osmolar contrast agents**: These are less likely to cause reactions, particularly in patients with kidney disease.

Conclusion

Contrast reactions can vary widely in severity, from mild discomfort to life-threatening anaphylaxis or renal failure. The management of these reactions requires careful assessment of the severity and prompt intervention. Prevention strategies, such as pre-medication and hydration, are key in reducing the risk of contrast-induced adverse events.

Miscellaneous

1. Write short note on PACS. [5] [MD (WBUHS) 20]

Picture archival and communication system is a comprehensive computer system that is responsible for the electronic storage and distribution of medical images.

Aims: To replace conventional analogue film, paper clinical request for and reports with a completely computerized electronic display.

Key components:
- Digital acquisition device
- Network
- Database Server
- Archival Server
- Radiology Information System (RIS)
- Hospital Information System (HIS)
- Softcopy Display Workstation

PACS hardware
- To acquire—Digital DICOM Compatible Acquisition device.
- To display—bright monitor.
- To transport—fast network
- To store—large archive and database.

Components of PACS

Acquisition (CT, MRI, X-ray)

⇓

Storage (DICOM Server) ⇒ Storage and Archive ⇒ Printers

⇓

Display - Diagnostic Workstation/Clinical Workstation

PACS Software Concepts

- **Prefetching and preloading**
  - Retrieval of previous images of a patient from a long-term archive on to short time storage device prior to new imaging examination.
  - Prefetch algorithm—software programs that automatically retrieve historical examination results and reports for correlation with the current study.

- **Worklist and folders**: Subdividing the vast amount of imaging data acquired on to the PACS into clinically relevant subgroups.
- **Default display protocols**: Software for displaying the images of current and related previous examinations in predetermined arrangements on the workstation.
- **Reporting**

  Networking:
  - Computer network is a communication system for a collection of interconnected computer devices.
  - Exchange of information, multiple access of information, resource sharing,

Medium of Transmission

Medium

- Copper—100 m—low cost
- Optical fiber—150 cm—high cost

Bandwidth—maximum rate at which data can pass between 2 points in a network.

- Depends on the medium of transmission
- Number of computers sharing
- Time required for an image to be sent

Database and archive: Store information, identify patient

Redundancy: Medical imaging data are of critical importance. Redundancy refers to storage of multiple copies of data. The RAID is the most frequently used redundancy system.

In RAID, the data are spread over several hard drivers such that if any one drive fails, the data can be reconstructed from these drives.

DICOM

- Digital Image Communication in Medicine
- It is a co-operative standard that allows compatibility between imaging systems
- An international standard for interchange of biomedical image and image related information

Health Level 7 - refers to worldwide standard for data info system such as RIS and HIS

There are at least three information systems in a Radiology Department that requires to handle the data associated with an examination.

These systems include the HIS, RIS and PACS.

HIS: Store demographic data of all patients such as name, date of birth, identification number. Other module of HIS document laboratory data.

RIS: A RIS is a computerized database used by radiology department to store, manipulate and distribute patient radiology data and imaging.

The system generally consists of patient tracking and scheduling, result reporting and image tracking capabilities.

Modern RIS incorporates DICOM such as modality worklist, modality performed, procedure steps, interpretation worklist and structured reporting.

PACS Advantages

- No image can be lost or misplaced.
- Simultaneous multi-location viewing
- Faster image retrieval
- Improved workflow
- Time saving for non-radiology clinicians
- Reduced film storage space

PACS Disadvantages

- Expensive
- Absolute dependency of hospitals
- Requires dedicated maintenance
- Trained hospital staff

2. Write in brief about problem of storage requirements in PACS. Describe its solutions. [5+5] [MD (WBUHS) 22]

Picture Archiving and Communication Systems (PACS) are essential in modern healthcare for storing, managing, and sharing medical images. However, the storage requirements for PACS are a significant challenge due to several factors:

1. **Large volume of data**: Medical images (e.g., X-rays, CT scans, MRIs) are typically large in size. High-resolution images, especially 3D scans and videos, can take up vast amounts of storage.
2. **High frequency of imaging**: Hospitals generate vast quantities of medical imaging daily, leading to continuous growth in storage needs.
3. **Long-term storage**: Medical images are required to be stored for many years, sometimes decades, due to legal, clinical, and regulatory requirements.
4. **Data redundancy**: To ensure data integrity, multiple copies (backup) of images need to be stored, further increasing storage demands.
5. **High availability and reliability**: PACS must ensure immediate access to images, so the system must have high availability and fault tolerance.

Solutions to PACS Storage Requirements

1. **Compression**: Using lossy or lossless compression techniques to reduce the file size of medical images without sacrificing too much quality. This helps lower storage costs and bandwidth usage while maintaining image fidelity.
2. **Tiered storage**: Implementing a multi-tier storage architecture (e.g., using a combination of high-speed SSDs for frequently accessed data and slower, cheaper HDDs or cloud storage for long-term archiving). This allows more efficient use of resources and helps balance cost and performance.
3. **Cloud storage**: Leveraging cloud services for scalable, off-site storage. Cloud solutions provide flexible and virtually unlimited storage capacity, which can be expanded as needed without significant upfront investment in infrastructure.
4. **Data deduplication**: Reducing redundant data storage by identifying and eliminating duplicate copies of the same image across the system. This helps optimize storage utilization and reduces costs.
5. **RAID (redundant array of independent disks)**: Using RAID configurations to protect against data loss and improve performance. RAID can offer both data redundancy (via mirroring) and improved access speed (via striping), ensuring that image data remains safe and accessible.
6. **Archiving solutions**: Implementing specialized archiving solutions for older images that are infrequently accessed. These systems may employ optical media, magnetic tape, or cloud-based archiving to store images more cost-effectively.
7. **AI and image compression algorithms**: Using AI-driven compression and image optimization techniques that reduce storage space while maintaining diagnostic quality, helping to manage the increasing volume of images more efficiently.

By adopting a combination of these solutions, healthcare facilities can effectively address the growing storage requirements of PACS while maintaining fast access, data integrity, and compliance with regulatory standards.

3. Discuss postmortem imaging and its applications. [10] [AIIMS May 24]

Post-Mortem Imaging: Description and Applications

Post-mortem imaging refers to the use of various imaging techniques (such as **X-ray**, **CT**, **MRI**, or **ultrasound**) to examine the body after death. This non-invasive approach can provide valuable insights into the cause of death, the presence of injuries, and other aspects of forensic investigation without the need for a traditional autopsy. Post-mortem imaging has become an increasingly important tool in forensic pathology, offering advantages in terms of speed, repeatability, and the ability to preserve the body for future examination or legal purposes.

Types of Post-Mortem Imaging

1. **Post-mortem X-ray (radiography)**:
   - *Description:* X-ray imaging is used to visualize bones, fractures, foreign objects (such as bullets, knives, or other projectiles), and other abnormalities in the body. It is particularly useful in cases of trauma, blunt force injuries, or firearm-related deaths.
   - *Applications:*
     - Detection of fractures, trauma, and foreign objects (e.g., bullets, sharp objects).
     - Assessing bone fractures in cases of suspected child abuse.
     - Identification of medical devices (e.g., pacemakers, prosthetics).
     - Detection of gas embolism or air in the vascular system.
2. **Post-mortem computed tomography (CT)**:
   - *Description: CT scanning* provides high-resolution, cross-sectional images of the body, allowing for the detailed visualization of both bone and soft tissue structures. It is non-invasive and can be used to create 3D reconstructions of the body.
   - *Applications:*
     - Trauma assessment: CT is widely used in cases of blunt or penetrating trauma to identify fractures, bleeding, and organ damage.
     - Determining the cause of death: CT can identify various pathologies such as myocardial infarction (heart attack), pulmonary embolism, stroke, or aneurysms.
     - Detection of foreign objects: CT scanning can detect foreign objects like bullets, knives, or drugs in the body.
     - Air embolism: CT can show air in the circulatory system, a common sign in drowning or other forms of asphyxiation.
     - Decomposition: CT imaging can sometimes help identify changes in the body due to decomposition, such as gas formation, which might affect organ structure or pose challenges for autopsy.
3. **Post-mortem magnetic resonance imaging (MRI)**:
   - *Description:* **MRI** provides detailed imaging of soft tissues, and it is highly sensitive for detecting brain injuries, soft tissue trauma, and certain pathological changes. It is particularly useful for visualizing the central nervous system, heart, and soft tissues.
   - *Applications:*
     - Neurological conditions: MRI is useful in detecting intracranial hemorrhages, brain injuries, strokes, or tumors.
     - Soft tissue damage: MRI can provide detailed information on damage to organs such as the heart, liver, lungs, and kidneys.
     - Assessment of asphyxiation or drowning: MRI can show changes in the lungs or brain associated with hypoxia, drowning, or suffocation.
     - Post-mortem brain imaging: MRI is increasingly being used to study brain injuries, such as trauma caused by a blow to the head or skull fractures.
4. **Post-mortem ultrasound**:
   - *Description:* **Ultrasound** uses high-frequency sound waves to create images of the body's internal structures. In post-mortem imaging, ultrasound can be used to assess the condition of organs, particularly in cases of suspected trauma or pathology.
   - *Applications:*
     - Abdominal and chest trauma: Ultrasound can detect fluid accumulation, organ injuries, or bleeding in the abdomen or chest, particularly in cases of blunt trauma or stabbing.
     - Fetal death: In cases of maternal death during pregnancy, post-mortem ultrasound can provide information about fetal condition, positioning, and cause of death.

– Assessing organ perfusion: Ultrasound can help determine whether certain organs, such as the heart or kidneys, were properly perfused prior to death.

5. **Dual-energy X-ray absorptiometry (DEXA):**
   - *Description:* **DEXA** scans are primarily used to measure bone mineral density but can also be used in post-mortem imaging to assess bone health and identify skeletal trauma or pathology.
   - *Applications: Bone fragility and fractures:* DEXA can be used to assess bone density in cases of suspected bone-related trauma or pathology, such as osteoporosis or fractures due to blunt force.

Applications of Post-Mortem Imaging in Forensic Medicine

Post-mortem imaging is increasingly integrated into forensic practice, and it has a range of applications in both **forensic investigations** and **legal settings**. Below are some of the key applications:

1. **Cause of death determination**
   - Post-mortem imaging can help establish the cause of death by identifying visible injuries, such as fractures, hemorrhages, or foreign objects.
   - For example, **CT** can detect **myocardial infarction**, **stroke**, **pulmonary embolism**, **trauma**, and **cerebral hemorrhage**.
   - **MRI** can provide more detailed information about soft tissue damage, including brain injuries, internal bleeding, or organ rupture.
   - Imaging can also help identify conditions like **ischemic stroke** or **arterial aneurysms** that might not be apparent during a traditional autopsy.
2. **Non-invasive examination in suspicious deaths**
   - In cases where there are concerns about potential foul play or when an autopsy is not possible due to cultural or religious reasons, post-mortem imaging offers a non-invasive alternative.
   - Imaging can identify **fractures**, **soft tissue injuries**, or **foreign objects**, providing evidence that may suggest **homicide**, **suicide**, or **accidental death**.
   - In some jurisdictions, post-mortem imaging is used in place of traditional autopsy in certain cases, especially when the cause of death is already apparent.
3. **Identification of foreign objects**
   - Post-mortem **X-rays** and **CT scans** are effective for detecting **foreign objects** (e.g., bullets, knives, drugs, or medical devices), which are often crucial for solving cases of **violent death**, **poisoning**, or **accidental injury**.
   - This is particularly important in cases where foreign objects might not be easily detectable in a traditional autopsy due to decomposition or the location of the object.
4. **Trauma assessment**
   - **CT** and **X-ray** imaging are particularly useful in the assessment of **blunt force trauma** (e.g., motor vehicle accidents, falls), **penetrating trauma** (e.g., gunshot wounds, stabbing), and **explosive injuries**.
   - **CT scans** can rapidly identify fractures, internal bleeding, and other trauma-related injuries, which helps guide further investigation into the circumstances surrounding the death.
5. **Assessment of decomposition and post-mortem changes**
   - Post-mortem imaging techniques, particularly **CT** and **MRI**, can be useful in studying the **post-mortem changes** (such as **gas formation** or **decomposition**), which can complicate the autopsy process.
   - For example, **CT scans** can detect **gas embolism** (air bubbles in the vascular system) or **gaseous accumulation** in organs, which can occur in cases of **drowning** or **suffocation**.
6. **Drowning and asphyxiation**
   - **CT** and **MRI** can show changes in the **lungs** and **brain** due to **hypoxia** (lack of oxygen), which can help confirm drowning or asphyxiation as the cause of death.
   - **MRI** can be used to visualize **cerebral edema** (swelling of the brain), which often occurs in cases of drowning or suffocation.

7. **Pediatric forensic imaging**
   - Post-mortem imaging is invaluable in cases of **child abuse** or **suspicious deaths in infants**. For example, **X-rays** and **CT scans** can reveal **multiple fractures** or **skull fractures**, which may be indicative of non-accidental trauma.
   - Imaging techniques can also help identify **shaken baby syndrome** or **internal organ damage** in children, where physical signs may be subtle.
8. **Forensic anthropology**

   Post-mortem imaging is helpful in **forensic anthropology** to assist in the identification of skeletal remains. Imaging techniques such as **CT scans** can help reconstruct bone structures and **identify fractures** or signs of trauma, providing crucial evidence in cases involving **disarticulated bodies** or **skeletons**.

Advantages of Post-Mortem Imaging

- **Non-invasive**: Post-mortem imaging eliminates the need for invasive procedures like traditional autopsies, which is especially important in cases where autopsy is difficult, controversial, or culturally inappropriate.
- **Preservation of evidence**: Imaging can provide permanent, reproducible records that may be needed for legal or investigational purposes.
- **Detailed and precise**: Modern imaging techniques (especially **CT** and **MRI**) offer detailed insights into both soft tissue and bone structures, allowing for more accurate determination of the cause of death.
- **Speed**: Post-mortem imaging can provide rapid results, often more quickly than an autopsy, aiding in the timely investigation

Limitations of Post-Mortem Imaging

- **Limited Soft Tissue Detail (for X-ray and CT)**: While **CT** and **X-ray** are excellent for visualizing bone and fractures, they are less effective in providing detailed information about soft tissue, such as in cases of internal organ damage or brain injuries (where **MRI** is preferred).
- **Cost**: Imaging modalities like **MRI** and **CT** can be expensive, which may limit their availability in certain settings, particularly in resource-limited environments.
- **Decomposition**: Advanced decomposition of the body can affect the accuracy of imaging, particularly with **CT** and **MRI**. However, techniques like **post-mortem CT** have become better at handling such challenges.

4. Technique, indications, contraindications and complications of HSG. [10] [DNB June 21]

Techniques of Hysterosalpingography (HSG)

1. **Preparation**:
   - The patient is usually asked to empty her bladder before the procedure.
   - The procedure is typically scheduled during the **first half of the menstrual cycle** (preferably between days 7 and 10), to avoid the possibility of pregnancy.
   - **Antibiotics** may be prescribed to prevent infection, especially if there is a history of pelvic infections or if the procedure is done after a miscarriage or recent childbirth.
   - **Sterile technique** is used throughout the procedure to minimize the risk of infection.
2. **Procedure**:
   - *Positioning:* The patient is placed in the **lithotomy position** (lying on her back with the legs raised and supported).
   - *Cervical dilatation:* A speculum is inserted into the vagina to visualize the cervix. The cervix is cleaned with an antiseptic solution. In some cases, the cervix may be dilated to facilitate the insertion of the catheter.
   - *Catheter insertion:* A small, flexible catheter is inserted into the cervical canal and positioned within the uterus.
   - *Contrast injection:* A contrast medium (usually an iodine-based solution or oil-based contrast) is injected into the uterine cavity through the catheter. The contrast medium fills the uterus and fallopian tubes, outlining their shape and any abnormalities.

- *X-ray imaging:* X-ray images or fluoroscopy are taken while the contrast medium is injected. The radiologist observes the flow of the contrast through the uterus and fallopian tubes, which can highlight blockages, scarring, or abnormalities.
- *Imaging sequences:* Multiple X-ray images are taken at various angles to ensure adequate visualization of the uterine cavity and fallopian tubes.

3. **Duration**: The entire procedure typically takes about 15 to 30 minutes.
4. **Post-procedure**: After the procedure, the patient may experience some mild cramping or spotting as the contrast medium drains out. Most patients can resume normal activities soon after the procedure.

Indications for Hysterosalpingography (HSG)

HSG is commonly performed to investigate various issues related to **female infertility** and **gynecological abnormalities**. Some of the common indications include:

1. **Infertility evaluation**:
   - *Assessment of fallopian tube patency:* One of the most common reasons for HSG is to determine whether the fallopian tubes are open and functioning. Blocked fallopian tubes can prevent sperm from reaching the egg, leading to infertility.
   - *Tubal pathology:* HSG can reveal **hydrosalpinx** (fluid-filled fallopian tubes) or other tubal abnormalities like **adhesions**, **scarring**, or **tube occlusion.**
2. **Uterine abnormalities**:
   - *Uterine shape abnormalities:* HSG can identify structural abnormalities in the uterus, such as **fibroids**, **polyps**, **septate uterus**, or **adhesions** (Asherman syndrome).
   - *Endometrial cavity:* HSG can provide insights into the shape of the endometrial cavity and assess for abnormalities that could interfere with implantation, such as **polyps** or **fibroids.**
3. **Recurrent miscarriages**: Evaluation of the **uterine cavity** in patients with recurrent pregnancy loss, to check for structural issues that could affect implantation or fetal development.
4. **Post-surgical evaluation**: To assess the uterus and fallopian tubes after surgeries such as **tubal ligation reversal**, **myomectomy**, or **endometrial resection.**
5. **Suspected tubal blockage**: If a woman has been unable to conceive for a prolonged period and no other causes of infertility are found, HSG may be used to evaluate the tubal patency.

Contraindications for Hysterosalpingography (HSG)

While HSG is a relatively safe procedure, there are certain contraindications where it may not be appropriate. These include:

1. **Pregnancy**: HSG should not be performed if the patient is pregnant, as the X-ray radiation could harm the developing fetus. The procedure is typically done after menstruation, when the patient is unlikely to be pregnant.
2. **Active pelvic infections**: Patients with an active pelvic infection (such as **pelvic inflammatory disease** or **vaginitis**) should not undergo HSG, as the procedure can introduce bacteria into the uterus, leading to further infection or complications.
3. **Severe cervical stenosis or vaginal anomalies**: If the cervix is abnormally narrow or there are congenital abnormalities of the cervix or vagina, HSG may not be feasible or may be difficult to perform.
4. **Allergy to iodine contrast media**: HSG involves the injection of iodine-based contrast media. Patients with a known allergy to iodine or contrast agents may experience adverse reactions. In these cases, an alternative contrast agent or imaging modality may be considered.
5. **Active uterine bleeding**: If the patient is experiencing heavy menstrual bleeding or bleeding from other causes, the procedure may be postponed.
6. **Severe uterine or tubal abnormalities**: In certain cases of severe uterine or tubal abnormalities (such as advanced **uterine cancer** or severe **fibroids**), HSG may not be helpful or advisable.

Complications of Hysterosalpingography (HSG)

While HSG is generally considered safe, there are potential complications that should be kept in mind:

1. **Infection**: One of the most common complications is the development of an **infection** following the procedure. The introduction of contrast material and instrumentation into the cervix can potentially introduce bacteria into the uterus, leading to infections such as **pelvic inflammatory disease (PID)**. To reduce this risk, the procedure is done under sterile conditions, and antibiotics may be prescribed.
2. **Contrast reaction**: Although rare, some patients may experience an allergic reaction to the iodine contrast medium. Reactions can range from mild (e.g., rash, nausea) to severe (e.g., anaphylactic shock). Pre-screening for contrast allergies is done to minimize risk.
3. **Uterine perforation**: There is a very small risk of **uterine perforation** during the insertion of the catheter, especially in patients with cervical or uterine abnormalities. If perforation occurs, further intervention may be required.
4. **Tubal spasm**: In some cases, the fallopian tubes may go into **spasm**, which can temporarily obscure the appearance of the tubes on the X-ray images. This can be managed by using medication (such as **antispasmodics**) to relax the tubes.
5. **Pelvic pain or cramping**: Mild **pelvic cramping** or discomfort is common during and after the procedure. This is generally transient and can be managed with over-the-counter pain relievers.
6. **Bleeding**: Some spotting or light bleeding may occur following HSG, especially if the cervix or uterus is irritated during the procedure.
7. **Radiation exposure**: Although the radiation dose during HSG is generally low, there is still a risk of exposure, particularly if the procedure is repeated multiple times. Care is taken to minimize radiation exposure, and the procedure is generally avoided in pregnant women.
8. **Misdiagnosis**: Although HSG is effective in diagnosing many uterine and tubal abnormalities, it may not detect all conditions. For example, some small polyps, submucosal fibroids, or endometrial adhesions might not be visible on HSG. Further imaging or diagnostic methods (such as **laparoscopy** or **sonohysterography**) may be required.

Recent Advances

1. Discuss the principle and clinical application of PET-CT. [3+7] [MD (WBUHS) 23, MD (WBUHS) 21, MD (WBUHS) 20, MD (WBUHS) 18, DNB Dec 18]

Principle of PET-CT

Majority of cancer cells demonstrate high level of glycolysis and hence preferentially use glucose as substrate for their metabolism. Hence, the radiotracer used in PET scan, i.e., ^{18}F-flurodeoxyglucose (FDG) is taken up preferentially by the cancer cells, approximately 4-6 times more than normal cell.

Radiotracer ^{18}F-FDG (fluorodeoxyglucose) injected intravenously

⇓

^{18}F-FDG enters tumor cells in a similar way to glucose using GLUT transporter proteins.
(increased GLUT in membranes of tumor cells)

⇓

FDG is phosphorylated to FDG-6-phosphate

⇓

^{18}F-FDG-6-phosphate cannot be further metabolized and accumulates within the tumor cells

^{18}F-FDG is a positron emitting isotope. It undergoes β^+ decay in the body, with a proton being converted to a neutron, a positron (the antiparticle of the electron, sometimes referred to as a $\beta+$ particle), and a neutrino. The positron travels a short distance and annihilates with an electron. The annihilation reaction results in the formation of two high energy photons which travel in diametrically opposite directions. Each photon has an energy of 511 keV. Two detectors at opposite ends facing each other detect these two photons travelling in opposite directions, and the radioactivity is localized somewhere along a line between the two detectors.

Basic unit of PET scanner is detector scintillation crystal. Three types of crystals are used in PET-CT scanners:

- BGO—Bismuth Germanium Oxide
- GSO—Gadolinium Oxyorthosilicate
- LSO—Lutetium Oxyorthosilicate

The PET scanner detects the pairs of gamma rays and calculates the point of origin of the annihilation event, using the time difference between detection of the photons. This data is then processed to create a 3D image that shows the distribution of the radiotracer within the body. Areas with increased tracer uptake (e.g., tumors or inflamed tissue) appear brighter on the PET scan, indicating higher metabolic activity.

The intensity of FDG uptake is estimated by the Standardized uptake value. It is a semi-quantitative estimate of FDG uptake. It is ratio of activity per unit mass tissue to injected dose per unit body mass.

PET-CT: PET and CT scans are performed sequentially with the patient in the same position to allow co-registration of both sets of images. Images can be displayed side-by-side or fused to overlay the PET data on the CT scan. The integration of PET and CT technologies results in a hybrid imaging system that combines both functional and anatomical data.

Clinical Application of PET-CT

A. **Oncological application**:
   i. Differentiate benign and malignant lesion: SUV value of PET/CT can be used to differentiate between the two.
   ii. Primary staging of malignancy (TNM staging): Local spread, lymph nodes as well as distal metastasis can be reliably detected in one go in PET/CT.
   iii. To guide biopsy
   iv. Treatment planning prior to radiotherapy or surgery: PET/CT helps in planning surgery or radiation therapy by providing precise information about the size, location, and metabolic activity of tumors.
   v. Assessment of disease stability and progression and assessment of treatment response: PET/CT is highly sensitive in detecting changes in metabolic activity, making it valuable for monitoring the response to therapies.
   vi. Detect recurrence: PET/CT is extremely effective in detecting recurrent disease, even when anatomical changes are not apparent on CT alone, due to its ability to detect metabolic activity associated with cancer recurrence.

B. **Cardiology**:
   i. PET imaging is used in myocardial perfusion imaging and the assessment of myocardial viability in patients of myocardial infarction.
   ii. PET permits the measurement of absolute myocardial blood flow and detect areas of ischemia or infarction.
   iii. It can also be used in the evaluation of myocardial inflammation.

C. **Neurology**:
   i. Dementias: In Alzheimer's disease, posterior parietal lobe is hypometabolic. In frontal lobe dementia, frontotemporal lobe is hypometabolic.
   ii. Epilepsy: Helpful in interictal seizure localization of epileptogenic foci.
   iii. Parkinson's disease: PET/CT can evaluate dopaminergic activity in the brain and help diagnose Parkinson's disease

D. **Vasculitis**: In giant cell arteritis: PET-CT uptake is seen in affected arteries, particularly affected large vessels. There may also be concurrent uptake in a pattern consistent with polymyalgia rheumatica, such as within the shoulders and hips.

E. **Infections**:
   i. In paroxysm of unknown origin, to find out the focus of infection. It is useful in diagnosing:
      - Osteomyelitis
      - Endocarditis
      - Soft tissue infections
      - Prosthetic joint infections
   ii. Diagnosis inflammatory disorders like sarcoidosis and inflammatory bowel disease.

2. Write short note on fusion imaging. [5] [MD (WBUHS) 20, AIIMS Dec 24]

Conventional cross-sectional imaging techniques [ultrasound, computed tomography (CT), magnetic resonance (MR), etc.] have important roles in non-invasive diagnosis, and in tumor treatment strategies. The techniques employed have different working principles, consequently complementing each other with respect to the information obtained. The combination (fusion) of two imaging techniques has been developed in recent years, defining the so-called "fusion imaging" or "hybrid techniques".

Fusion imaging involves aligning and overlaying images from two modalities, often in real-time. For example, it can merge the high-resolution anatomical details provided by CT (computed tomography) or MRI (magnetic resonance imaging) with functional or metabolic data from PET (positron emission tomography) or SPECT (single-photon emission computed tomography). The fusion can be achieved through software algorithms or hybrid imaging systems designed to acquire data from multiple modalities simultaneously, such as PET/CT scanners.

Some hybrid imaging modalities are synergistic solely in anatomical details, while others combine structural and molecular imaging.

Existing hybrid imaging modalities include: PET-CT, SPECT-CT, PET-MRI, SPECT-MRI, ultrasound and MRI, ultrasound and CT, MRI and CT and angiography and CT.[10]

One notable anatomical hybrid model is real-time virtual sonography (RVS), a technique that enables the display of an ultrasound B mode image and CT or MR images in real-time. The system includes a magnetic positioning sensor fixed on the convex-shaped probe of the ultrasound scanner, for the creation of images with identical cross-sections in real-time. There are several advantages to this method. Ultrasound exams cannot always identify isoechoic tumors, tumors recurring locally in areas treated with lipiodol following transarterial chemoembolization (TACE), or tumors recurring in areas treated previously by RFA or percutaneous ethanol injection (PEI) procedures. In addition, in ultrasound examinations, there are a few dead angles and it is difficult to examine the whole liver, especially in obese patients. Nodules that are poorly identified on ultrasound are clearly visible on CT/MR. However, interventional treatment is easier to perform under ultrasound-guidance, while the exposure to increased doses of radiation is also avoided. Thus, real-time virtual sonography combines the imaging advantages of both techniques. This is one of many examples.

Other examples are:

- **PET/CT**: In diagnosing and staging disease or monitoring response to therapy, anatomical imaging does not always provide the complete picture. Functional or metabolic changes can and do occur even in the absence of a corresponding anatomical correlate. E.g.: A subcentimetric normal appearing lymph node can be metabolically active requiring biopsy and further management. Isolated CT of post-operative cancer patients may appear normal but reveal precise areas of small recurrence on PET-CT thus allowing early management.
- **MRI/SPECT**: Useful in brain tumor assessment, combining functional imaging from SPECT with the high soft-tissue contrast of MRI for more accurate diagnosis and surgical planning.

In the future, new devices such as whole-body MR/PET and PET/US for breast imaging are highly likely to appear.

3. High-intensity focused ultrasound (HIFU): principle, instrumentation, and its applications. [3+3+4] [MD (WBUHS) 21] [3+3+4] [MD (WBUHS) 21]

High-intensity focused ultrasound (HIFU) is a technique to destroy tissue at depth within the body, selectively and without harming overlying and adjacent structures within the path of the beam because the ultrasonic intensity at the beam focus is much higher than that outside of the focus[11,12]

Principle (Fig. 58)

The intention of a high intensity focused ultrasound (HIFU) treatment is to raise the temperature of a selected, isolated tissue volume above 55°C and to maintain this temperature for 1 s or longer. It is known that 55°C held for this time will lead to coagulative necrosis and immediate cell death. This is possible with a focused ultrasound beam since the short (mm) wavelengths of ultrasound at Megahertz frequencies in soft tissue allows it to be focused into small, clinically relevant, volumes. Ultrasonic energy absorption within the focal volume induces high temperatures locally at the focus, with temperatures outside this region being kept at levels that are not cytotoxic.

Focusing of the ultrasound beam may be achieved in a number of ways.

The simplest method is to use a single element spherical shell of piezo-electric material capable of delivering high power. Whereas quartz was the transducer material of choice in the early days of HIFU, recent developments have seen the use of piezo-ceramics such as PZT (lead zirconate titanate) and piezo-composite materials.

Different focal lengths may be achieved by combining a plane single element transducer with lenses of different specifications. Lenses are usually made from materials having a speed of sound greater than that of water, and thus are of concave shape when a convergent beam is sought.

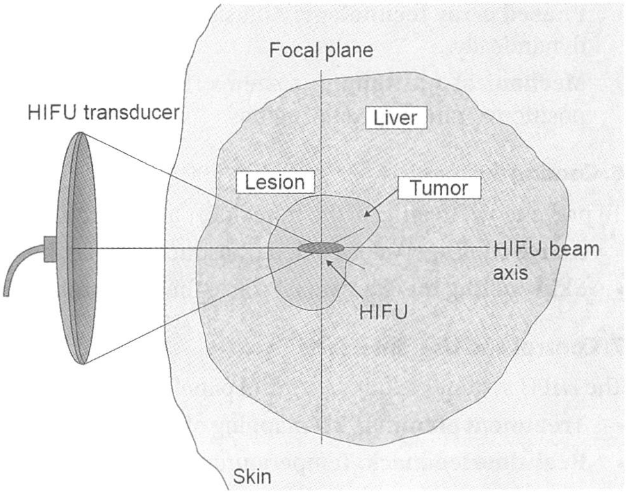

FIG. 58: Basic principle of HIFU.

Instrumentation

Basic parts of a HIFU system are:

1. Ultrasound Transducer

The ultrasound transducer is the central component of a HIFU system, responsible for generating and focusing high-frequency sound waves.

- **Type**: Piezoelectric or capacitive micromachined ultrasonic transducers (CMUTs).
- **Frequency**: Typically operates in the range of 0.5–10 MHz. Lower frequencies penetrate deeper tissues, while higher frequencies target superficial structures.
- **Configuration**:
  - *Focused transducers:* Concave or phased-array designs to focus energy at a specific point.
  - *Single-element or multi-element arrays:* Multi-element arrays provide better control over the focus and beam steering.

Transducers for clinical use fall into three main classes:

1. **Extracorporeal**: Extracorporeal transducers are used for targeting organs that are readily accessible through an acoustic window on the skin.
2. **Transrectal**: Used for the treatment of the prostate.
3. **Endoscopic probes**: Are being developed for the treatment of biliary duct and esophageal tumors.

2. Coupling System

HIFU requires efficient transmission of ultrasound waves from the transducer to the target tissue without significant energy loss.

- **Coupling medium**: Water or gel is used to minimize acoustic impedance mismatches between the transducer and skin.
- **Water baths or balloons**: These systems maintain a stable and thermally regulated coupling environment.

3. Imaging and Monitoring System

Real-time imaging is critical for guiding and monitoring the HIFU procedure.

- **Integrated imaging modalities**:
  - *Ultrasound imaging:* Provides real-time visualization of the target tissue and the focus area.
  - *MRI guidance:* Offers superior soft-tissue contrast and thermal mapping to monitor temperature changes during therapy.
- **Feedback mechanisms**: Imaging systems provide feedback to ensure accurate energy delivery and prevent damage to surrounding tissues.

4. Power Supply and Signal Generator

The power supply drives the ultrasound transducer with the required electrical signals.

5. Beam Steering and Focusing System

Advanced HIFU systems use beam-steering technologies to target multiple areas without moving the transducer mechanically.

- **Phased array technology**: Adjusts the phase and amplitude of individual transducer elements to focus the beam dynamically.
- **Mechanical positioning systems**: For single-element transducers, mechanical systems adjust the transducer position to target specific regions.

6. Cooling System

To prevent overheating of the transducer and surrounding tissues:

- **Active cooling**: Water-cooled transducers and coupling systems maintain stable temperatures during therapy.
- **Skin cooling mechanisms**: Protect the epidermis while focusing energy on deeper tissues.

7. Control and User Interface

The HIFU system includes a control panel or software interface to manage and monitor treatment parameters.

- **Treatment planning**: 3D mapping of the target tissue using imaging data.
- **Real-time feedback**: Temperature monitoring and acoustic intensity adjustments.
- **Safety features**: Automatic shutdown if parameters exceed preset safety thresholds.

During the treatment delivery phase, some indicators of tissue change are looked for. This enables assessment of treatment progress, and may also provide feedback to allow adjustment of exposure parameters in real time. For MR guided HIFU, the temperature rise may be determined using spin-lattice relaxation time (T1), proton resonance frequency (PRF) or proton diffusion (D) related sequences. For US guided treatments, the most commonly used indicator of tissue ablation is the appearance of a hyperechoic region on the image.

Applications

The ability of HIFU to target subcutaneous tissue volumes has made it an attractive potential therapy for deep-seated soft tissue tumors.

1. **Uterine fibroids**: Effectively treats fibroids and maintains fertility.
2. **Adenomyosis**: HIFU has been used as an organ preserving treatment in adenomyosis, with reduction of cyclical pain achieved.
3. **Prostate tumors**: Both benign prostate hyperplasia and prostate cancer.
4. **Ophthalmology**: Treatment of glaucoma, experimental in treatment of intraocular tumors, retinal detachment, vitreous hemorrhage and in sealing of capsular tears. Laser is still the gold standard treatment.
5. **Osteosarcomas with soft tissue components after breaking through bone cortex**: USG HIFU therapeutic ablation of malignant bone tumors is feasible and effective and may eventually become part of a regimen of limb-sparing techniques in patients with malignant bone tumors.
6. **Liver tumors by endoscopic probes**: USG HIFU ablation can be considered as a safe and feasible approach for treating solid liver tumors at difficult locations. HIFU can achieve complete tumor necrosis even when the lesion is located adjacent to the major hepatic blood vessels.
7. Pancreatic cancer.
8. Breast tumors—complete tumor ablation with reduction in blood flow has been achieved.
9. Soft tissue sarcomas
10. Neurology—focused ablation of substantia nigra in Parkinson's disease. Also used in brain tumors.

4. (a) Principle of RFA, (b) application in benign and malignant lesions. [10] [DNB June 21, MD (WBUHS) 18]

Radiofrequency ablation (RFA) is a medical procedure that uses a high-frequency alternating current produced by a radiofrequency generator oscillating in a closed-loop circuit.[13]

Principle

In RFA, the high-frequency alternating current (460-480 kHz) from the electrode generates marked agitation of the ions in the tissue that surrounds the uninsulated tip of the probe. Heat is generated in the tissue surrounding the RFA probe. The frictional heat results in thermal coagulation necrosis of the surrounding tissue.

Roughly the size of ablation correlates with the intensity and duration of energy deposition. The diameter of local coagulation necrosis is a function of the local mean temperature. To achieve an effective heating throughout the tumor 60–100°C have to be achieved and maintained throughout the entire target volume for at least 4–6 min. Due to slow thermal conduction from the electrode surface through the tissue, the duration of application may increase to 10–30 min.

Flow of current and heat absorption depend on tissue characteristics such as electrical and thermal conductivity and tissue perfusion.

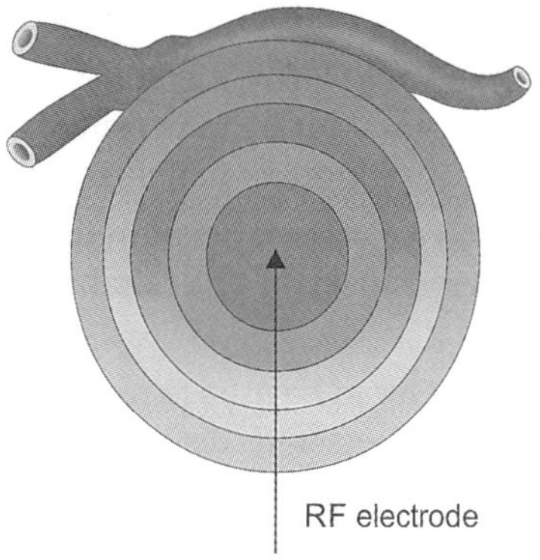

FIG. 59: Heat sink effect.

Oven effect: The size of ablation necrosis is larger in hepatocellular carcinomas (HCCs) than in the surrounding cirrhotic liver tissue because the surrounding fibrous tissue acts as a shell insulating the heat and leading to a temperature increase inside the nodule. However, the oven effect may limit heat diffusion from the tumor into satellite lesions of HCC.

Heat sink effect (Fig. 59): Due to perfusion-mediated tissue cooling (vascular flow) the threshold for coagulation necrosis is 8.5°C higher in living tissue than ex vivo. In addition, the size and shape of coagulation necrosis are smaller and less uniform in vivo compared with ex vivo. This phenomenon is called the 'heat sink effect'. Thus, the coagulation size may be increased by reduction of the hepatic perfusion during RFA by temporary occlusion of the portal vein or the hepatic artery. Portal inflow occlusion (Pringle maneuver) during open or laparoscopic RFA leads to a 10°C increase of temperature around the probe and results in larger diameters of coagulation necrosis. However, it is associated with an increased risk of portal vein thrombosis. For percutaneous RFA the celiac or hepatic artery may be occluded with a balloon catheter, or the feeding arteries may be embolized with gelatine sponge particles.

Applications

Radiofrequency Ablation (RFA) can be used to treat both benign and malignant lesions. It is commonly used for a variety of tumors, including those in the liver, kidney, lung, and thyroid. Below are its applications in benign and malignant lesions:

A. Benign Lesions

RFA is also employed for non-cancerous conditions, offering an alternative to more invasive treatments.

1. **Benign thyroid nodules**: RFA is increasingly used to treat symptomatic benign thyroid nodules that are causing compression symptoms or cosmetic concerns. It is effective in shrinking the nodules and reducing symptoms without requiring surgery.
2. **Fibroids (Uterine leiomyomas)**: RFA can be used to shrink fibroids in the uterus, providing an option for women who want to avoid hysterectomy. It is often used when fibroids cause heavy bleeding or pain.
3. **Breast fibroadenomas**: RFA can be used for the treatment of benign breast lumps (fibroadenomas) that are symptomatic or growing, especially in patients who prefer not to undergo surgical excision.
4. **Prostate hyperplasia (BPH)**: RFA can be used to treat benign prostatic hyperplasia (BPH), where excess tissue in the prostate gland causes urinary symptoms. It can reduce the size of the prostate and alleviate symptoms without surgery.
5. **Osteoid osteoma**: Surgical excision has historically been difficult due to the inability to locate the nidus during surgery. Surgery has largely been replaced by image guided procedures including RFA.
6. Morton neuroma or other nerve plexus ablation neurotomy.
7. **Varicose veins**: Heat causes closure of the effective vein.

B. Malignant Lesions

RFA is particularly beneficial in treating certain types of cancers, especially when surgery is not feasible or in patients who are not surgical candidates.

1. **Liver cancer (hepatocellular carcinoma, HCC)**: RFA is commonly used to treat early-stage liver cancer, especially when the tumor is small (<3-5 cm) or if the patient has liver cirrhosis that precludes surgical resection or liver transplantation. RFA can help shrink tumors and provide symptomatic relief.

2. **Kidney cancer (renal cell carcinoma)**: RFA is used for small, localized kidney tumors, especially in elderly patients or those with multiple comorbidities who are not candidates for traditional surgery. It helps preserve kidney function by targeting the tumor directly.
3. **Lung cancer**: RFA is used for treating primary or metastatic lung cancer, particularly for tumors that are small and peripheral. It's also an option for patients with poor pulmonary function who cannot tolerate surgery.
4. **Thyroid cancer**: RFA has been explored as a treatment for recurrent or small thyroid cancers, especially in cases where surgery is risky or undesirable. It can also be used for benign thyroid nodules to prevent or reduce symptoms.
5. **Bone metastases**: RFA can be used to treat painful bone metastases, providing pain relief and improving the quality of life in patients with metastatic disease.

Benefits of RFA

- **Minimally invasive**: It does not require large incisions or general anesthesia.
- **Quick recovery**: Patients usually experience less pain and a faster recovery compared to traditional surgical approaches.
- **Effective for small to medium-sized lesions**: It is especially useful for lesions that are difficult to access surgically or when the patient's overall health precludes major surgery.

Limitations of RFA

- **Size and location**: RFA is typically most effective for smaller tumors. Tumors larger than 5 cm or those in complex locations may not be amenable to successful treatment.
- **Local recurrence**: There is a risk of recurrence, particularly in malignant tumors, which may require additional treatments.

In conclusion, RFA is a valuable tool in the management of both benign and malignant lesions, offering a less invasive alternative with favorable outcomes in many cases. However, its use depends on tumor size, location, and the overall health of the patient.

5. Recent developments in non-invasive lymphatic imaging techniques for visualizing the central lymphatic anatomy and flow dynamics. [10] [DNB Dec 20]

The thoracic duct in the thorax and the cisterna chyli in the upper abdomen make up the central lymphatic system. The cisterna chyli, which is most commonly found in the retroperitoneum just anterior to the T12-L1 vertebral bodies in a right paramedian location, is where lower extremities and retroperitoneal lymphatics confluence with intra-abdominal lymphatics (hepatic, mesenteric, etc.). The diameter of the cisterna chyli is between 0.5 and 2 cm.

In a left paramedian position just in front of the thoracic vertebral bodies, the thoracic duct runs cephalad along the posterior mediastinum after extending cranially from the cisterna chyli. Numerous lymphatic branches that supply drainage to both lungs are received by the thoracic duct. The cervical segment of the thoracic duct connects to the left central veins after a steady anterior and leftward journey. Most often, the thoracic duct is a single channel with a diameter of 2 to 4 mm.

The anatomy of the central lymphatic system is often varied. Although the cisterna chyli is most frequently seen to the right of the aorta, a median or left paramedian placement may also be a typical variation. About 30% of patients do not have a cisterna chyli.

Lymphangioscintigraphy, CT lymphangiography, and magnetic resonance (MR) lymphangiography are increasingly being used as alternatives to invasive diagnostic lymphangiography

Lymphangioscintigraphy

- Lymphangioscintigraphy demonstrates pathways and patterns of lymphatic drainage.
- It is one of the primary imaging modalities used to diagnose lymphedema and can also be performed to assess the effect of lymphedema treatments.
- More recently, whole body lymphangioscintigraphy without and with SPECT/CT has been used to aid in the diagnosis of lymphatic pathologies that do not cause lymphedema, such as iatrogenic leaks, or those associated with complex congenital heart disease.

Computed Tomography Lymphangiography

CT lymphangiography is performed after injection of ethiodized oil with intranodal lymphangiography or injection of iodized water-soluble contrast material through transperitoneal access to the cisterna chyli.

CT lymphangiography after intranodal lymphangiography can be performed entirely in the CT suite or in a staged fashion.

If performed in a full CT suite, an initial CT scan of the abdomen is performed to identify bilateral inguinal lymph nodes.

Under CT guidance, the target lymph nodes are accessed using a 20-23 gauge needle (depending on the patient size) and a 3 ml syringe connected to a tube. After confirming correct needle placement with CT, approximately 1 mL of water-soluble contrast (300 mg iodine/mL) is injected and the CT is repeated to confirm intranodal contrast injection.

These procedures are then repeated on the contralateral side.

A total of 2 ml of deionized oil is then injected into the inguinal lymph nodes bilaterally. Immediately after injection of the iodized oil, a CT scan is performed to confirm lymph node enhancement.

A CT scan from the mid-neck to the pelvis is performed within 60 minutes.

When the diagnosis is made, intranodal lymphangiography is first performed in the angiography department (as described below in the section "Intranodal Lymphangiography").

The patient is then transferred to the CT department, where a CT scan from the mid-neck to the pelvis is performed within 60 minutes of completing the intranodal lymphangiography. CT lymphangiography after transabdominal access to the cisternal chyle involves accessing the cisternal chyle under CT guidance and injecting a water-soluble contrast agent to opacify the cisternal chyle and thoracic duct.

CT -Lymphangiography is more reliable than the MR -Lymphangiography in patients with metallic implants and a metallic artifact obtained, and also provides a faster acquisition of images for patients who cannot tolerate a complete study of MR images.

In addition, interventions with CT, such as thoracic duct intervention can be carried out immediately after CT lymphangiography.

Magnetic Resonance Lymphangiography

Excellent visualization of the lymphatic system is made possible by magnetic resonance lymphangiography techniques.

Like CT and ultrasonography, MR lymphangiography makes it possible to see the lymph nodes. The thoracic duct, cisterna chyli, and lymphatic vessels can also be seen using MR lymphangiography. Because of this, MR lymphangiography is being utilized more and more as a non-invasive imaging substitute for invasive diagnostic lymphangiography.

Noncontrast-enhanced MR Lymphangiography

Clinical imaging equipment with 1.5-T or 3-T capabilities can be used for non-contrast-enhanced MR lymphangiography. Patients are supine when they are scanned. After cardiac gating with ECG leads on the chest, phased-array coils anterior elements are positioned over the chest, belly, and pelvis. To lessen respiratory motion artifact, respiratory gating monitors are used for every sequence.

After few anatomic images, thoracic duct images are obtained using coronal and sagittal heavy T2 three-dimensional (3D) volume sequence using no angulation.

6. PET-MRI. [5] [DNB June 20, DNB Dec 18]

PET-MRI is a hybrid imaging technique utilizing the functional uptake information of positron emission tomography (PET) with the anatomical and soft tissue detail of magnetic resonance imaging (MRI). Integrated PET-MR scanner was launched in 2010 in Munich, Germany.

It has several advantages over PET-CT:

1. PET-CT is unable to perform simultaneous data acquisition leading to imaging artifacts.
2. Radiation exposure in CT.
3. CT has poor contrast resolution among soft tissues and areas of complex anatomy like head, neck and pelvis.

Certain modification in technology is required to make MRI compatible with PET like:

1. Photomultiplier based PET scanners do not work within the magnetic field of an MR scanner. Avalanche photodiode or silicon PMT based PET detector systems were developed.

2. Metallic surface coils used in MRI interfere with the gamma rays of PET causing unwanted attenuation. Surface coils with lower metallic content are required.

Clinical Applications of PET-MR

A. **Oncology**: The sensitivity and specificity in oncology staging can be significantly improved using PET-MR.
   i. Lesion conspicuity is better on MRI compared to CT in liver lesions due to relatively high physiological FDG activity in liver in PET-CT masking focal liver lesions with only slightly elevated FDG activity.
   ii. PET-MRI is advantageous over PET-CT in assessment of tumor invasion into adjacent structures in rectal, bladder, prostate and gynecological cancers.
   iii. Surrounding soft tissue infiltration is better assessed in head and neck cancers.
   iv. Improved accuracy in the assessment of spread to regional lymph nodes, especially in the pelvis, mediastinum and head-neck region.
   v. Detecting recurrence in areas of poor soft tissue contrast on PET-CT, like brain tumors, metastatic liver disease and head-neck cancer.
   vi. PET-MRI is of particular benefit to pediatric patients with chronic inflammatory conditions or malignancy, where serial follow up examinations following therapy are required.
   vii. For detection and staging of lymphoproliferative disorders.

B. **Neurology**:
   i. Early diagnosis and evaluation of disease progression in Alzheimer's.
   ii. Localization of epileptogenic focus in patients with refractory epilepsy.

C. **Cardiology**: PET-MR may be useful in evaluation of vascular wall and identification of plaques prone to rupture.

REFERENCES

1. Curry TS. Christensen's Physics of Diagnostic Radiology. Philadelphia: Lippincott Williams & Wilkins; 1990.
2. Kuppusamy T. Basic radiological physics. New Delhi: Jaypee Brothers Medical Publishers Pvt Ltd.; 2017.
3. Tatsugami F, Higaki T, Nakamura Y, Honda Y, Awai K. Dual energy CT: minimal essentials for radiologists. Jpn J Radiol. 2022;40:547-59.
4. Allisy-Roberts PJ, Williams J. Farr's physics for medical imaging. Philadelphia: Elsevier Health Sciences; 2007.
5. Chavhan GB. MRI made easy. Jaypee Brothers Medical Publishers Pvt Ltd.; 2013.
6. Weinberg BD, Kuruva M, Shim H, Mullins ME. Clinical applications of magnetic resonance spectroscopy in brain tumors: from diagnosis to treatment. Radiol Clin. 2021;59(3):349-62.
7. Hashemi RH, Bradley WG, Lisanti CJ. MRI: The basics: The Basics. Philadelphia: Lippincott Williams & Wilkins; 2012.
8. Khandelwal N, Gupta AK, Chowdhury V. AIIMS-MAMC-PGI's Comprehensive Textbook of Diagnostic Radiology. Jaypee Brothers Medical Pubishers Pvt Ltd.; 2016.
9. Chhabra A, Ahlawat S, Belzberg A, Andreseik G. Peripheral nerve injury grading simplified on MR neurography: As referenced to Seddon and Sunderland classifications. Indian J Radiol Imaging. 2014;24(03):217-24.
10. Sandulescu DL, Dumitrescu D, Rogoveanu I, Saftoiu A. Hybrid ultrasound imaging techniques (fusion imaging). World J Gastroenterol. 2011;17(1):49.
11. Zhang L, Wang ZB. High-intensity focused ultrasound tumor ablation: review of ten years of clinical experience. Front Med China. 2010;4:294-302.
12. Ter Haar G, Coussios C. High intensity focused ultrasound: physical principles and devices. In J Hyperthermia. 2007;23(2):89-104.
13. Widmann G, Bodner G, Bale R. Tumour ablation: Technical aspects. Cancer Imaging. 2009;9(Special issue A):S63.

CHAPTER

2 Neuroradiology Including Head and Neck Imaging

Soumik Das, Shis Mahammad Pail, Manideepa Maiti, Rohan Dey, Himadri Shee, Saikat Sen, Sayanwita Majumder, Omkar Oraon, Arghya Chattopadhyay, Azhar Molla, Hasibur Rahaman

QUESTIONS

Relevant Anatomy and Imaging Techniques

1. Precath work up and the procedure in DSA intracerebral arteries. Write down the names of intracerebral arteries with a schematic diagram. [5+5] [MD (WBUHS) 21]
2. Briefly discuss the venous circulation of brain with appropriate diagram. [10] [MD (WBUHS) 19]
3. Describe anatomical variations of circle of Willis with the help of a diagram. Enumerate the sites of intracranial aneurysm. [7+3] [MD (WBUHS) 22]

Trauma

1. Radiological anatomy of central skull base and imaging in CSF rhinorrhea. [10] [DNB June 21]
2. A young adult patient has presented with unilateral pulsatile proptosis and chemosis after a road traffic accident. What is the probable etiology and how will you confirm the diagnosis by imaging? Discuss the role of radiologic interventions in managing such a condition. [(1+5)+4] [DNB June 20, MD (WBUHS) 24]

Stroke

1. Mention the stroke protocol. Discuss the role of intervention radiology in management of stroke. [4+6]
2. Role of intervention radiology in subarachnoid hemorrhage. [5]
3. Discuss etiology, radiological imaging features of subarachnoid hemorrhage (SAH) and role of intervention radiology in its management. [2+4+4] [MD (WBUHS) 20, MD (WBUHS) 21]
4. Write a short note on: CT perfusion in acute ischemic stroke. [5] [MD (WBUHS) 19]
5. Discuss the role of imaging and interventional radiology in stroke. [10] [MD (WBUHS) 23, MD (WBUHS) 22, AIIMS May 24]
6. A 30-year-old man is brought to the emergency department with symptoms of acute stroke with onset 1 hour back. Discuss the imaging evaluation in such a case. Describe the role of interventional radiology in acute ischemic stroke. [6+4]
7. Various stages of intracerebral hemorrhage as seen on MRI and the underlying patho-physiological basis for the observed imaging findings. [2+3]
8. Causes of SAH and imaging. [10] [DNB June 22]
9. CT in ischemic stroke. [10] [DNB Dec 21]
10. Discuss in brief, the salient CT and MRI features in an acute ischemic stroke patient arriving to the hospital within 6 hours of onset. Suggest an algorithm-based approach for confirmation of diagnosis and guiding the management of such a patient. [5+5] [DNB Dec 20, DNB June 20, DNB Dec 21]

Infections

1. Discuss CT and MRI features of neurological complications of AIDS. [5+5] [MD (WBUHS) 22]
2. Describe briefly the neuroimaging manifestations of COVID-19. [10]
3. Neuroimaging manifestations of congenital TORCH infections. [5]
4. CNS manifestation in HIV with imaging. [10] [DNB June 22, DNB June 19, AIIMS Dec 24, MD (WBUHS) 17]
5. Manifestations of CNS TB: Clinical findings, pathology, imaging. [10] [DNB Dec 21]

Epilepsy

1. A 37-year-old female presents with history of intractable epilepsy. Discuss the imaging modalities and protocols used in workup of this patient. Describe imaging findings of mesial temporal sclerosis. [(3+3)+4] [MD (WBUHS) 21, AIIMS Dec 23, DNB Dec 20]

Brain Tumors

1. Describe radiological anatomy of sella turcica and imaging features of suprasellar masses. [4+6] [MD (WBUHS) 23, DNB Dec 21]
2. Discuss the MRI findings in common posterior fossa neoplasms in pediatric age. [10] [MD (WBUHS) 23, DNB Dec 20]

Head and Neck Imaging

1. Describe the imaging features of juvenile nasopharyngeal angiofibroma. Discuss the role of radiological intervention in its management. [6+4] [MD (WBUHS) 23, MD (WBUHS) 21]
2. Describe with a neat diagram the anatomy of brachial plexus. [10] [MD (WBUHS) 20]
3. Classify the infrahyoid neck spaces. Mention the imaging findings of carotid body tumor. [4+6] [MD (WBUHS) 24, MD (WBUHS) 20]
4. Imaging modalities in a case of sudden visual loss. [10] [MD (WBUHS) 20]
5. Discuss radiological anatomy of neck spaces and lymph nodes. [6+4] [MD (WBUHS) 21, DNB Dec 19, AIIMS May 23]
6. Discuss the role of ultrasonography in ocular trauma. [10] [MD (WBUHS) 21]
7. Write short notes on: (a) Radiological anatomy of PNS. (b) Retromolar trigone. [5+5] [MD (WBUHS) 21, AIIMS Dec 23]
8. Write a short note on: HRCT of temporal bone in cholesteatoma. [5] [MD (WBUHS) 21]
9. Classify orbital lesions in relation to various orbital spaces. Discuss MR features in orbital pseudo tumors. [4+6] [MD (WBUHS) 24, MD (WBUHS) 21]
10. Discuss the CT anatomy of the temporal bone with a schematic diagram. [10] [MD (WBUHS) 22]
11. Write a short note on: TIRADS. [5] [MD (WBUHS) 24, MD (WBUHS) 22, MD (WBUHS) 19, DNB Dec 20, AIIMS Dec 24]
12. Discuss the cervical lymph node stations and their imaging. [5+5] [MD (WBUHS) 22]
13. Describe in brief the technique and appearances of various anatomical structures on ocular ultrasound. [2+3]
14. Discuss the role of ultrasound in the evaluation of thyroid nodule. [10]
15. Salivary gland tumors and imaging. [10] [DNB June 22, MD (WBUHS) 24]
16. Malignant thyroid lesion and imaging. [10] [DNB June 22]
17. Suprahyoid neck spaces—boundaries and radiological anatomy. Pathologies of masticator space. [10] [DNB June 21, MD (WBUHS) 24]
18. Describe the imaging protocol of paranasal sinuses for functional endoscopic sinus surgery (FESS). What are the important anatomical landmarks and anatomical variants which should be looked for while evaluating for FESS? Discuss the radiological patterns and features of aspergillus infection of paranasal sinuses. [3+3+4] [DNB Dec 20]
19. Discuss the role of HRCT and MRI in the evaluation of congenital sensorineural hearing loss. [5+5] [DNB June 20]

Spine Imaging and Interventions

1. Describe the common CV junction anomalies with their imaging features. [5+5] [MD (WBUHS) 23]
2. Discuss about the radiological anatomy of CV junction. [10] [MD (WBUHS) 21, DNB June 19]
3. Discuss imaging features and various intervention in intracranial and spinal arteriovenous malformation. [4+3+3] [MD (WBUHS) 21]
4. Mention various symptoms out of slipped disc and how the images play the role for assessment. [10] [MD (WBUHS) 19]
5. Describe imaging protocol in traumatic injury of dorsal spine causing paraplegia. [10] [MD (WBUHS) 19]
6. Write a short note on: Diastematomyelia. [5] [MD (WBUHS) 22]
7. Write a short note on: Vertebroplasty. [5] [MD (WBUHS) 22, AIIMS Dec 24]
8. Discuss the various interventional procedures in spinal arteriovenous malformation. [10] [MD (WBUHS) 22, DNB Dec 18]

Congenital and Vascular Diseases

1. Write a short note on imaging features of Sturge Weber Syndrome. [5]
2. What are the imaging modalities and causes of pulsatile tinnitus. [10] [MD (WBUHS) 20]
3. Enumerate causes of unilateral proptosis. Describe briefly imaging findings of optic glioma and caroticocavernous fistula. [4+6] [MD (WBUHS) 20]
4. Write a short notes on: (a) Joubert's syndrome. (b) Tuberous sclerosis. [5+5] [MD (WBUHS) 21]
5. Classify various neural tube closure defects. Briefly describe types of Arnold Chiari malformation and discuss their imaging features. [10] [MD (WBUHS) 18, MD (WBUHS) 21]
6. How DSA of brain performed? Describe role of intervention radiography in the management of intracranial aneurysm and AVM. [10] [MD (WBUHS) 19]
7. Diagnostic criteria of neurofibromatosis type 2 with its imaging findings. [10] [MD (WBUHS) 19, DNB Dec 21]
8. (a) Describe briefly various neurocutaneous syndrome. (b) Describe imaging features of von Hippel Lindau syndrome. [5+5] [DNB June 20]

ANSWERS

Relevant Anatomy and Imaging Techniques

1. Precath work up and the procedure in DSA intracerebral arteries. Write down the names of intracerebral arteries with a schematic diagram. [5+5] [MD (WBUHS) 21]

The advancement of diagnostic imaging is greatly contributed by the recent improvement in X-ray technology. DSA is a radiological angiographic procedure to evaluate blood vessels using fluoroscopic techniques (producing real-time and continuous images).

Principle: Initial images from an angiographic sequence are acquired and stored. Subsequent angiographic images are obtained. Digitally subtract the initial images from subsequent angiographic images.

DSA images = Subsequent angiographic images – initial precontrast images.

DSA technique shows the contrast-filled blood vessels without interference from the background. It helps to visualize the blood vessels in a dense soft tissue environment, as it removes the bones and soft tissues from images.

Indications

A. **Diagnostic Indication**:
- To diagnose the vascular malformations (Arteriovenous malformation).
- Arteriovenous fistula
- To diagnose the vasculitis/occlusive disease.
- Nontraumatic subarachnoid hemorrhage.
- Aneurysm.
- To assess the vascularity of the tumor

B. **Therapeutic Indication**:
- Endovascular management of aneurysm
- Embolization
- Angioplasty
- Thrombolysis/thrombectomy

Contraindication

No absolute contraindication (in absolute indication, the underlying condition should be corrected or preventive measures should be taken).

Relative Contraindication:
- Renal dysfunction
- Abnormal coagulation profile
- Non-co-operative patient
- Congestive heart failure and respiratory failure
- Pregnancy
- History of previous contrast reaction.

Preprocedural Workup

a. **History:** A brief clinical history should be taken before performing DSA.
   - Present complaints
   - Significant past medical or surgical history
   - Current medications.

b. Targeted clinical examination must be performed.

c. Clearly explain the procedure to the patient and informed consent should be taken.
d. **Laboratory report**: PT, INR, platelet count, hemoglobin, and EGFR results should be checked.
e. NPM before procedure (for solid or nonclear fluids—NPM for 6 to 8 hours, for clear fluids—NPM for 2 to 4 hours).
f. Maintained adequate hydration of the patient.
g. Guidelines for specific conditions:
   - Patient on heparin: Heparin infusion should be stopped 2 hours before the procedure. Heparin infusion can be restarted 2 to 4 hours after the manual removal of the catheter sheath. If the patient is on low molecular weight heparin, then hold the dose before the procedure.
   - Patient on warfarin: Discontinuation for 3 to 5 days before the procedure. If INR is persistently elevated, vitamin K (2 to 10 mg) may be administered orally (24–48 hours prepuncture) or intravenously (12–24 hours pre-puncture) for nonurgent cases. For urgent cases, fresh frozen plasma may be administered. The target INR is 1.5 or less.

Procedure

- **Preparation**:
  - Patients must lie in a comfortable position.
  - Antiseptic dressing and draping.
  - The procedure is performed with continuous physiologic monitoring.
  - Local anesthesia should be infiltrated before the puncture.
- **Femoral Artery Puncture**:
  - Localization of the femoral artery puncture site could be performed by palpation, USG, or fluoroscopic guidance.
  - Fluoroscopy guidance localization of puncture site: It prevents high and low arterial entry. The arterial entry site should be over the middle 3rd of the femoral head and the skin entry site should be over the lower 3rd of the femoral head.
  - Puncture the artery by using the Seldinger technique and advancement of the guide wire is performed.
- **Catheterization**:
  - After the advancement of the guide wire into the aorta, serial dilators are introduced over the guide wire. The subsequent exchange of the desired catheter is performed over the wire. Frequent flushing with heparinized saline should be performed to prevent thrombus formation.
  - Confirm the position of the tip of the catheter.
  - Injects the contrast and desired imaging performed.

Intracranial Vasculature: The intracranial arterial system is divided into two parts,

a. **Anterior Circulation**: It consists of internal carotid arteries on both sides and its branches. It has two terminal branches, the anterior cerebral artery and the middle cerebral artery.
b. **Posterior Circulation**: It consists of bilateral vertebral arteries and their branches, basilar artery and its branches, and terminal branches of basilar artery (bilateral posterior cerebral arteries).

   a. **Anterior Circulation**:

   Internal Carotid Artery and its Branches: The internal carotid artery **(Fig. 1)** is a branch of the common carotid artery, originating at the neck. It is divided into seven segments:[1]

   - **Cervical Segment (C1 Segment)**: Extracranial part of the internal cerebral artery. No named branches are present in the cervical segment.
   - **Petrous Segment (C2 Segment)**: Part of the ICA is contained in the carotid canal of the petrous part of temporal bone. Branches are the vidian artery and the caroticotympanic artery.
   - **Lacerum Segment (C3 Segment)**: Lies just above the foramen lacerum. It is a short segment without any branches.
   - **Cavernous Segment (C4 Segment)**: The cavernous segment is traversing through the cavernous sinus. Branches are meningohypophyseal trunk and inferolateral trunk.
   - **Clinoid Segment (C5 Segment)**: The C5 segment has usually no branches.

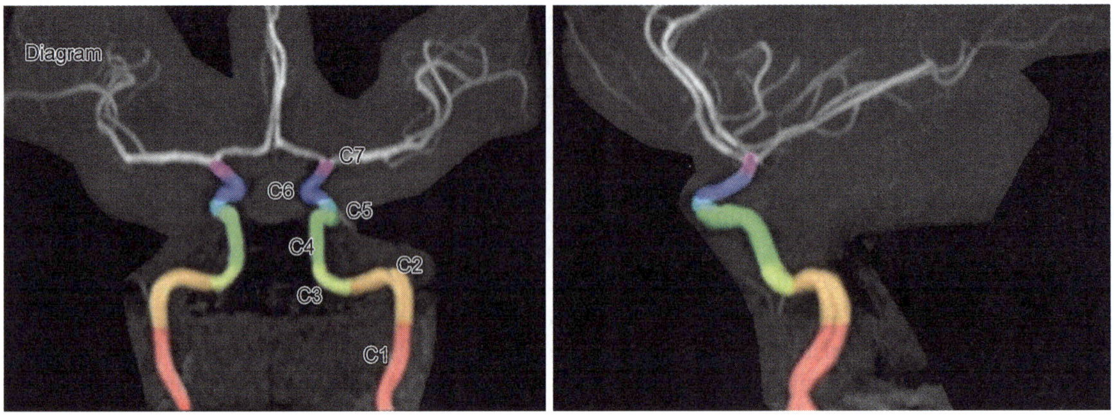

FIG. 1: Colored magnetic resonance angiography (MRA) maximum intensity projection (MIP) images showing the various numbered segments of the internal carotid artery.

- **Ophthalmic Segment (C6 Segment)**: It lies wholly inside the subarachnoid space and extends from the level of the distal dural ring to just proximal to the origin of posterior communicating artery. Branches are ophthalmic artery and superior hypophyseal artery.
- **Communicating Segment (C7 Segment)**: The C7 (communicating) segment represents the terminal segment of the ICA and extends from proximal to the origin of posterior communicating artery to the bifurcation of terminal ICA into the anterior and middle cerebral arteries. Branches are the posterior communicating artery and the anterior choroidal artery.

Anterior Cerebral Artery: Anterior cerebral artery **(Fig. 2)** is one of the terminal branches of the internal carotid artery. It has three segments.

1. **A1 Segment**: Extends from its origin to the anterior communicating (ACoM) artery. It has two groups of branches, the recurrent artery of Heubner and the medial lenticulostriate branches.
2. **A2 Segment**: Extends from the A1-Anterior communicating artery junction to the corpus callosum rostrum. Branches are orbitofrontal and frontopolar arteries.
3. **A3 Segment**: It curves anteriorly along the genu of corpus callosum. The A3 segment is divided into two terminal ACA branches, the callosomarginal and pericallosal arteries.

Middle Cerebral Artery

This is a terminal branch of ICA and has four segments **(Fig. 3)**.

- **Horizontal M1 Segment**: Extends from its origin to bifurcation or trifurcation of MCA. Branches are the anterior temporal artery and the lateral lenticulostriate group of arteries.

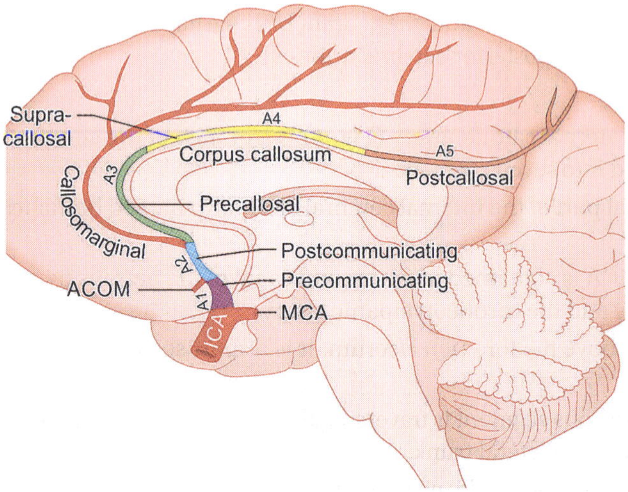

FIG. 2: Segments of anterior cerebral artery.

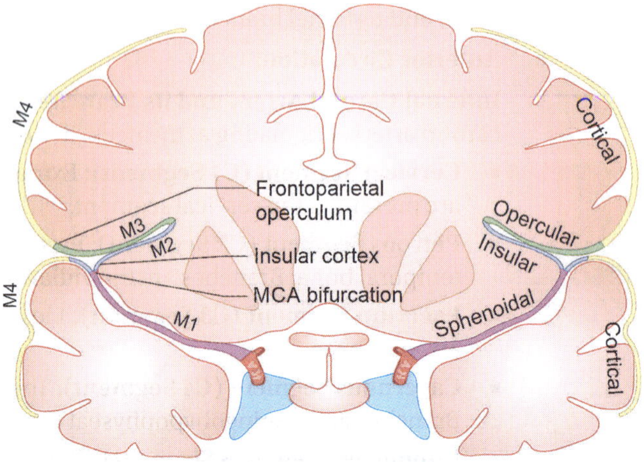

FIG. 3: Segments of middle cerebral artery.

- **Insular M2 Segments**: It is the postbifurcation middle cerebral artery trunks in the Sylvian fissure.
- **Opercular M3 Segments**: Branches at the top of Sylvian fissure and then course laterally along the opercula.
- **Cortical M4 Segments**: It becomes M4 segments as they exit from the Sylvian fissure. M4 segments are ramified over the lateral surface of the cerebral hemisphere.

b. **Posterior Circulation**:

Vertebrobasilar System: It consists of bilateral vertebral arteries that unite with each other to form one basilar artery and its branches **(Fig. 4)**.

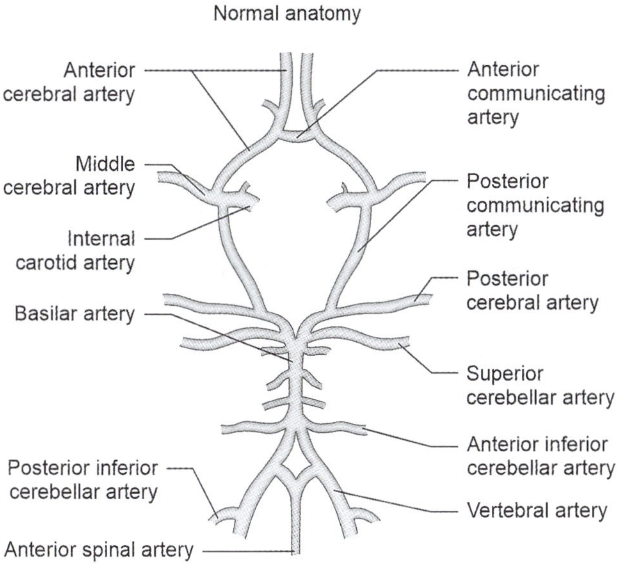

FIG. 4: Normal anatomy of major intracerebral arteries. Posterior cerebral arteries.

Vertebral Arteries

It has four segments.

- **Extraosseous/Preforaminal V1 Segment**: Originates from the ipsilateral subclavian artery and extends up to the transverse foramen of the C6 vertebra.
- **Foraminal V2 Segment**: It courses superiorly from C6 transverse foramina to the C2 transverse foramina.
- **Extradural/extraspinal V3 Segment**: It curves and courses across the top of the C1 vertebra. It extends until enters the skull by piercing the dura.
- **Intracranial/Intradural V4 Segment**: It is the only intracranial segment and extends from the dura (piercing site) to its confluence at the level of the lower border of the pons. Branches are anterior and posterior spinal arteries, medullary perforating branches, and posterior inferior cerebellar artery.

Basilar Artery

The two vertebral arteries unite with each other to form a basilar artery at the level of the pontomedullary junction. It terminates into two posterior cerebral arteries at the interpeduncular fossa. Multiple small perforating branches originate from the entire basilar artery and supply the pons and midbrain. Named branches are, the anterior inferior cerebellar artery (AICA—originates from the proximal BA) and the superior cerebellar artery (SCA—originates from either side of the distal BA).

Posterior Cerebral Arteries

Two posterior cerebral arteries are the terminal branches of basilar artery. Its course can be subdivided into four segments **(Fig. 5)**.

- **Precommunicating/P1 Segment**: It extends from the termination of the basilar artery to the junction with the posterior communicating artery (PCoA).
- **Ambient/P2 Segment**: It extends from the P1-PCoA junction and runs within the ambient cistern around the midbrain. Branches are the anterior and posterior temporal arteries. The medial and lateral choroidal arteries also originate from the P2 segment.
- **Quadrigeminal/P3 Segment**: It extends from behind the midbrain and ends as it enters into calcarine fissure. The P3 segment lies completely within quadrigeminal cistern.
- **Calcarine/P4 Segment**: It lies within the calcarine fissure and divides into medial and lateral terminal trunks. Branches of medial terminal trunks are calcarine artery,

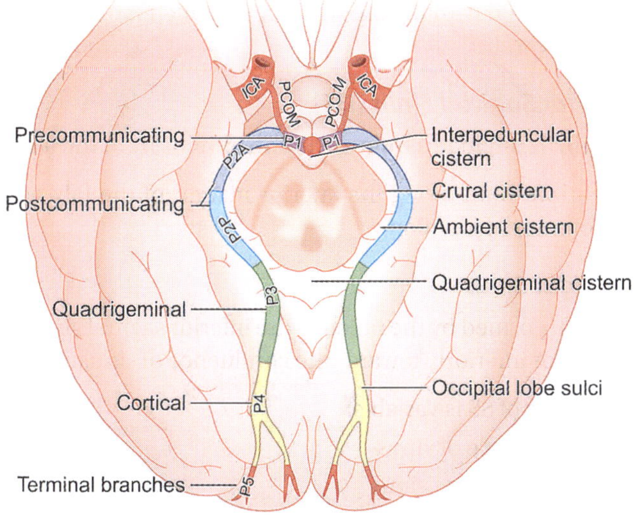

FIG. 5: Segments of posterior cerebral artery.

the medial occipital artery, parieto-occipital artery, and posterior splenial artery. The lateral occipital artery originates from lateral terminal trunk.

2. Briefly discuss the venous circulation of brain with appropriate diagram. [10] [MD (WBUHS) 19]

The intracranial venous system consists of two major components, the cerebral veins and the dural venous sinuses.[2]

Characteristics of Intracranial Venous Srainage

- Does not follow the arteries, so venous territories do not match with arterial territories.
- Cerebral veins have extremely thin walls with no muscular tissue.
- Lack of valves and can have bidirectional flow.
- Runs in subarachnoid space.

Dural Venous Sinuses

Venous plexuses and dural sinuses are thin wall endothelium lined channels, located between the periosteal and meningeal and periosteal layers of the dura matter. Arachnoid granulations are frequently seen projecting into dural venous sinuses. The most common locations of arachnoid granulations are the superior sagittal and transverse sinuses.

It is further subdivided into postero-superior and antero-inferior groups.

The Postero-superior Group: Consists of the inferior sagittal sinus (ISS), superior sagittal sinus (SSS), straight sinus (SS), the sinus confluence (torcular herophili), transverse and sigmoid sinuses, and jugular bulbs.

The Antero-inferior Group: Consists of the cavernous sinus (CS), the superior petrosal sinuses, the inferior petrosal sinuses, clival venous plexus, and the sphenoparietal sinus (SphPS).

Superior Sagittal Sinus (SSS)

It is the largest dural venous sinus.

Origin: Superior sagittal sinus arises anteriorly from the ascending frontal veins.

Course: Courses posteriorly in the midline along the superior aspect of falx cerebri and terminates into sinus of confluence.

The superior sagittal sinus collects many small unnamed superficial cortical venous channels and the relatively larger anastomotic vein of Trolard.

Variant: Hypoplastic/absent anterior (rostral) segment of superior sagittal sinus.

As compared with the SSS, the ISS is a much more inconstant curvilinear channel that lies along the inferior margin of the falx cerebri.

Inferior Sagittal Sinus (ISS)

Origin: It originates from the union of veins from the adjacent part of the falx, corpus callosum, and cingulate gyrus.

Location: Runs along the inferior margin of the falx and joins with the vein of Galen to form a straight sinus at the falcotentorial junction.

Straight Sinus

Origin: Formed by the union of the inferior sagittal sinus (ISS) and vein of Galen (VofG) at the falcotentorial apex. It runs posterior inferiorly towards the confluence of sinus.

Drainage of SS is variable:

- Confluence of sinus
- Left transverse sinus
- Right transverse sinus.

Variant: A persistent falcine sinus is a midline venous structure that connects the inferior sagittal sinus or VofG directly with superior sagittal sinus. It is frequently (approximately two-thirds of patients) associated with absent/rudimentary straight sinus.

Sinus Confluence (Torcular Herophili): Sinus confluence is the junction superior sagittal sinus, straight sinus, transverse sinus, and occipital sinus.

Transverse Sinus: Transverse sinuses (lateral sinuses) are paired structures that originate from the confluence of sinuses. It runs along the lateral border of the tentorium cerebelli and terminates into the sigmoid sinuses.

Variants

- Hypoplastic/absent one transverse sinus.
- Arachnoid granulations/fibrous septa cause filling defects.

Sigmoid Sinuses and the Jugular Bulbs: The sigmoid sinuses are paired structures that run inferiorly in an S-shaped groove behind the petrous temporal bone to the jugular foramen. It is the continuation of the transverse sinus where tentorium cerebelli ends and terminates in the jugular bulb. A common and normal variant is asymmetry of the sigmoid sinuses.

The Jugular Bulbs: It is the focal venous dilatations at the junction of the sigmoid sinuses and IJVs.

Cavernous Sinus: The cavernous sinuses are paired structures located along both sides of the sella turcica. Anteriorly it communicates with the sphenoparietal sinus and ophthalmic vein. Posteriorly it communicates through the superior petrosal sinus with the junction of sigmoid and transverse sinuses and through the inferior petrosal sinus with the sigmoid sinus.

Superior and Inferior Petrosal Sinuses: Both are paired structures. The superior petrosal sinus runs along the superior aspect of petrous temporal bone and connects the sigmoid sinus to the cavernous sinus. The inferior petrosal sinus runs along the inferior border of the petrous temporal bone and connects the CS to the jugular bulb.

Clival Venous Plexus: It is a network of interconnected veins that lies along the clivus.

Sphenoparietal Sinus: It is located around the lesser wing of sphenoid at the rim of middle cranial fossa. Superficial veins from the anterior temporal lobe drain into the sphenoparietal sinus which further drains into the CS.

Cerebral Veins: The cerebral veins are located in the subarachnoid space and drain the brain parenchyma into the dural venous sinus after piercing through the meninges. They are classified into three groups according to their anatomical location:

- Superficial cortical veins
- Deep cerebral veins
- Posterior fossa/brain stem veins

Superficial Cortical Veins

The superficial cortical veins are located on the brain's surface and again subdivided into three groups according to their drainage.

- Superior group.
- Middle group.
- Inferior group.

Superior Cortical Veins/Superior Sagittal Group: Multiple unnamed (Between eight and twelve) superficial cortical veins courses over the superolateral surface of the cerebral hemispheres. They pierce the arachnoid membrane and meningeal layer of dura to drain into SSS.

The vein of Trolard is a dominant anastomotic superior cortical vein that connects the superficial middle cerebral vein with the SSS.

Middle Cortical Veins/Sphenoidal Group: This group drains into the cavernous sinus via the sphenoparietal sinus. In this group, the superficial middle cerebral vein (SMCV) is the dominant vein located in the sylvian fissure. It receives numerous small branches from the superior temporal gyrus, the inferior part of the frontal lobe, and the parietal opercula.

The vein of Labbe is a dominant posterior anastomotic vein that courses over the lateral surface of the temporal lobe to drain into the TS. It receives tributaries from the postero-inferior temporal lobe and adjacent parietal lobes.

Inferior Cortical Veins: The most important vein of this group is the deep middle cerebral vein (DMCV). It collects tributaries from the insula, basal ganglia, parahippocampal gyrus, inferior frontal and temporal lobes. It is located deep to the Sylvian fissure and connects with the basal vein of Rosenthal which is a part of the deep venous system.

The named superficial anastomotic veins are the vein of Labbe, vein of Trolard, and SMCV. They vary in size and maintain a reciprocal relationship with each other.

Deep Cerebral Veins

The deep cerebral veins drain the deep structures of the brain including the gangliothalamic region, corpus callosum, and the posterior part of the limbic system. It consists of three groups:

- Medullary veins,
- Subependymal veins, and
- Deep paramedian veins

Medullary Veins: Numerous small, unnamed medullary veins originate from the subcortical region of both cerebral hemispheres. They course through the white matter toward the ventricles and drain into the ipsilateral subependymal veins.

Subependymal Veins: The subependymal veins are located beneath the ventricular ependyma. It collects the venous drainage from the ipsilateral gangliothalamic region and deep white matter. Two prominent named subependymal veins are the thalamostriate veins and the septal veins.

Septal Vein: It curves around the frontal horn of the ipsilateral lateral ventricle followed by courses posteriorly along the septum pellucidum.

Thalamostriate Vein: It collects tributaries from the ipsilateral caudate nucleus and thalamus, courses medially to join the ipsilateral septal vein near foramen of Monro forming the internal cerebral vein (ICV).

Deep Paramedian Veins: The ICVs are paired paramedian veins, that drain most deep brain structures. It is formed by uniting the ipsilateral septal vein and thalamostriate vein near the foramen of Monro and coursing posteriorly in cavum velum interpositum. The ICVs of both sides and the bilateral basal veins of Rosenthal unite with each other at the rostral quadrigeminal cistern to form the single great vein of Galen.

Basal vein of Rosenthal is a paired deep cerebral vein formed by the union of the anterior cerebral vein, DMCV, and inferior striate veins.

The great vein of Galen courses postero-superiorly under the splenium of corpus callosum in the quadrigeminal cistern. It forms the straight sinus after uniting with the inferior sagittal sinus.

Brainstem/Posterior Fossa Veins

The midbrain and posterior fossa structures drain by these veins. It comprises three groups:

- Superior (galenic) group,
- Anterior (petrosal) group, and
- Posterior group.

The Superior (Galenic) Group: The superior galenic group of veins draining superiorly into VofG. The named veins of this group include the superior vermian vein, precentral cerebellar vein (PCV), and the anterior pontomesencephalic vein (APMV).

Behind the inferior colliculi, the PCV terminates into the VofG. The superior vermian vein courses over the top of the vermis and unites with the PCV draining into the vein of Galen. The APMV is an interconnected venous plexus that covers the anterior surface of the pons and the cerebral peduncles.

The Anterior (Petrosal) Group: The petrosal vein (PV) is the dominant venous trunk in the cerebellopontine angle cistern. It receives numerous tributaries from the pons, cerebellum, and medulla forming a petrosal star (star shaped vascular collection) on CT venography or DSA. The petrosal vein is an important structure for cerebellopontine angle cistern surgeons and forms anastomosis with the lateral mesencephalic vein and sphenoparietal sinus.

The Posterior (Tentorial) Group: The dominant veins in this group include the inferior vermian veins located under the vermis. Inferior vermian veins are paired paramedian structures, that receive tributaries from the inferior surface of the cerebellum and drain into unnamed tentorial sinuses.

Venous Drainage Territories (Fig. 6): Cerebral venous drainage is described in four basic patterns.

Peripheral (Surface) Brain Drainage: Superficial parts of the brain (most of the mid and upper cortex and their subjacent subcortical white matter of the cerebral hemispheres) drain via cortical veins into the superior sagittal sinus.

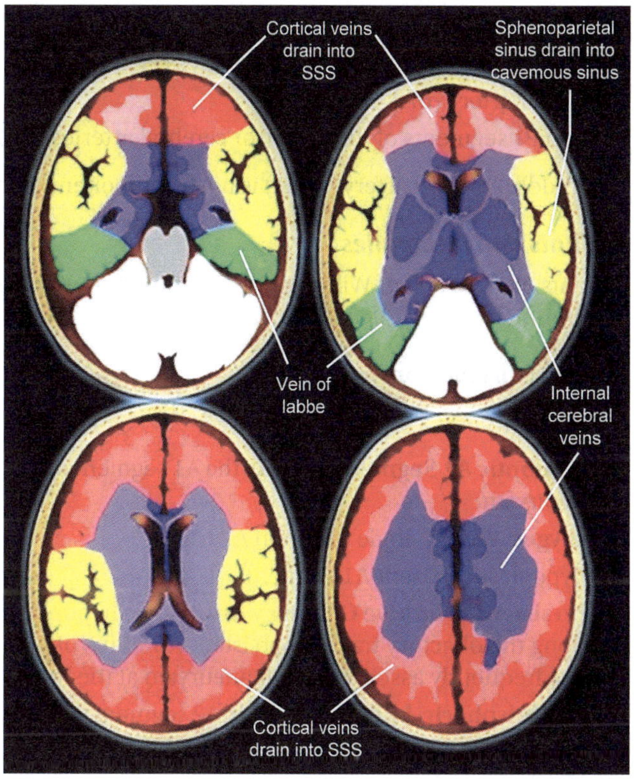

FIG. 6: Venous drainage territories.

Deep (Central) Brain Drainage: The central core of the brain consists of the basal ganglia and thalami, and majority of the white matter is drained into the deep cerebral veins. The anteromedial temporal lobe (uncus and the anteromedial hippocampus) and inferior frontal lobe are drained via the DCMV and BVR into the VofG.

Inferolateral (Perisylvian) Drainage: The perisylvian brain parenchyma comprises the frontal, temporal, and parietal opercula plus the insula are drained via the SMCV into the SphPS and CS.

The Posterolateral (Temporoparietal) Drainage: The posterior temporal and the adjacent infero-lateral parietal lobes are drained via the vein of Labbe into the transverse sinus.

3. Describe anatomical variations of circle of Willis with the help of a diagram. Enumerate the sites of intracranial aneurysm. [7+3] [MD (WBUHS) 22]

Circle of Willis (COW)

The circle of Willis is an arterial anastomotic ring **(Fig. 7)**, connecting the anterior and posterior circulations of the brain. It surrounds the basal brain structures and is the most important potential source of collateral blood flow to the occluded territory.[3]

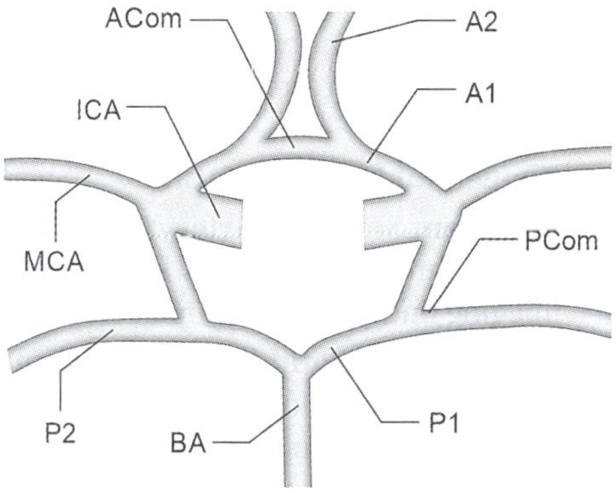

FIG. 7: Components of the circle of Willis.

Components of the Circle of Willis

Anterior Circulation

- Two internal carotid arteries (ICA)
- Two A1 segments of anterior cerebral arteries (ACA)
- Anterior communicating artery (ACOM)

Posterior Circulation

- Two posterior communicating arteries (PCOM)
- Basilar artery (BA)
- Two P1 segments of the posterior cerebral arteries (PCA)

The middle cerebral artery (MCA) is not a component of the circle of Willis.

Variants and Anomalies

Variants of the circle of Willis are very common. In the majority of the cases, one or more components are hypoplastic or absent.

Anterior Circulation Variants

ACA Variants

- **Infraoptic A1 Segment of ACA**: The A1 segment of ACA passes below the optic nerve. It is frequently associated with aneurysm.
- **Azygos ACA**: A single common A2 trunk.
- Hypoplastic/absent A1 segment.
- **Persistent Primitive Olfactory Artery**: It is hypoplastic proximal ACA with a long anterior and inferomedial course along the olfactory tract. A persistent primitive olfactory artery has a hairpin turn and continues as distal ACA. It is also frequently associated with aneurysm at the region of hairpin turn.
- **Bihemispheric ACA**: Hypoplastic A2 segment with contralateral dominant A2 segment. The contralateral dominant A2 segment is supplying the bilateral ACA territories.
- ACA fenestration.
- Duplication of A1 segment.
- ACA trifurcation.

ACOM Variants

- The most common variant is hypoplastic or absent ACOM.
- Duplicated or multichanneled or fenestrated ACOM.

ICA Variants

- **Aberrant ICA**: It is a rare but important vascular anomaly and represents a collateral pathway resulting from agenesis of the first embryonic segment (cervical portion) of ICA. It enters the posterior middle ear cavity and lies just lateral to the cochlear promontory. The rest of the distal ICA has a normal and expected course. Patients are typically presenting with pulsatile tinnitus. It can mimic paraganglioma. It is very important to identify this condition as an inadvertent biopsy may be disastrous. On angiography, the aberrant ICA courses more laterally with a sharp angulation that resembles 7. A stenosis is often present at the reconnection site with the horizontal petrous segment of ICA.
- **Congenital Absence of ICA**
- **Persistent Stapedial Artery**: Persistent stapedial artery originates from the genu of the petrous segment of ICA and passes through the stapes footplate. It is continuing intracranially as the middle meningeal artery. Characteristic imaging findings are, hypoplastic/absent foramen spinosum and an enlarged tympanic segment of facial nerve canal.
- **Embryonic Carotid-basilar Anastomosis**: It is a variant anatomy of arterial communications between anterior and posterior circulations. During embryonic development, there are communications between the primitive carotid artery and two longitudinal neural arteries (future vertebrobasilar artery). These primitive connections exist in the early embryonic period and rapidly involute. Failure to regress these communications leads to the persistence of this carotid-basilar anastomosis.

Types: Four types of embryonic carotid-basilar anastomosis are seen and named according to the cranial nerves with which they run (except for the proatlantal artery).

- **Persistent Trigeminal Artery**: It is the most common embryonic carotid-basilar anastomosis.
  - **Origin**: Proximal cavernous ICA
  - **Types**:
    - **Saltzman Type I**: It supplies the distal basilar artery. Posterior communicating and the proximal basilar arteries are hypoplastic/absent.
    - **Saltzman Type II**: It supplies the superior cerebellar arteries, while the posterior cerebral arteries are supplied by the posterior communicating artery.
    - **Saltzman Type III**: It does not communicate with the basilar artery. Rather, it terminates as superior cerebellar artery (type IIIa), anterior inferior cerebellar artery (type IIIb), and posterior inferior cerebellar artery (type IIIc).
  - **Persistent Otic Artery**: it is the rarest embryonic carotid-basilar anastomosis, as it is the first connection to regress.
    - **Origin**: Petrous ICA.
- **Persistent Hypoglossal Artery**: It is the second most common embryonic carotid-basilar anastomosis.
  - **Origin**: Cervical ICA at C1-C2 level. It passes through the hypoglossal canal and communicates with the basilar artery.
- **Proatlantal (Intersegmental) Artery**: It is the most caudal embryonic carotid-basilar anastomosis.
  - **Types**:
    - Type 1 arises from the cervical ICA, then runs posterosuperiorly, and finally anastomoses with the vertebral artery.
    - Type 2 arises from the external carotid artery, and then follows a similar course.

Posterior Circulation Variants

PCA Variants

- **Fetal Origin of PCA**: It is a common normal variant of the PCA. Proximal PCA originates from ICA. In this condition, the PCOM artery is larger than the P1 segment (hypoplastic/absent) of the PCA.
- **Artery of Percheron**: Artery of percheron is a rare but important variant of posterior circulation characterized by a single dominant arterial trunk that supplies the rostral midbrain and medial thalami bilaterally.

Sites of Intracranial Aneurysm

Aneurysm is an abnormal focal dilatation of blood vessels.

Most intracranial aneurysms occur at the point of maximum hemodynamic stress, especially at the bifurcations of major vessels or branching points. The most common sites are the circle of Willis and MCA bifurcations. It is very uncommon to have aneurysms beyond the circle of Willis.

Anterior Circulation Aneurysms: Most of the aneurysms (approximately 90%) are located in the anterior circulation.

Common sites:

- Anterior communicating artery (30–35%)
- ICA/PCOM junction (30–35%)
- MCA bifurcation (20%).

Posterior Circulation Aneurysms: Approximately 10% of intracranial aneurysms are located in the posterior circulation.

Common Sites: The most common site of posterior circulation aneurysm is the basilar artery bifurcation (approximately 5%). The second most common location is the posterior inferior cerebellar artery.

Other Sites of Aneurysm: Aneurysms are also located in the terminal segment of the ICA, the superior cerebellar artery, the anterior choroidal artery, and the superior hypophyseal artery.

Trauma

1. Radiological anatomy of central skull base and imaging in CSF rhinorrhea. [10] [DNB June 21]

The skull base is a complex anatomical structure forming the floor of the cranial cavity and separates the brain parenchyma with the suprahyoid neck and facial structures. Numerous important structures (especially neurovascular structures) pass through the multiple skull base foramina. The skull base area is inaccessible for direct clinical examination. Without any clear knowledge of anatomy, skull base surgery may lead to devastating complications. Recent advancements in imaging techniques resulted in the improvement of surgical techniques and functional outcomes. CT and MRI can accurately localize the skull base lesion and evaluate the extent and relationship with the adjacent vital structures. CT and MRI complement each other for evaluating skull base lesions.

Anatomy

The skull base is formed by five bones:
- Frontal bone
- Ethmoid bone
- Sphenoid bone
- Occipital bone
- Paired temporal bones.

The endocranial aspect of the skull base is divided into three fossae:
- Anterior cranial fossa
- Middle cranial fossa
- Posterior cranial fossa.

Anterior Skull Base

It separates the anterior cranial fossa structures with orbits and paranasal sinuses.

Boundaries

- **Anteriorly**: Posterior wall of sphenoid sinus
- **Posteriorly**: Lesser wing of the sphenoid bone and anterior clinoid process.
- **Floor**: Roof of the nasal cavity and ethmoid sinuses medially and orbital plates of frontal bones laterally.

Numerous perforations are present in the cribriform plate of ethmoid bone through which olfactory nerves traverse from the olfactory mucosa to the olfactory bulb. Fracture of the cribriform plate (most commonly at lateral lamella where the anterior ethmoidal artery enters into the anterior cranial fossa) is the most common cause of CSF rhinorrhea.

Central Skull Base

The central skull base is the floor of the middle cranial fossa. Few authors denote the central skull base as a poorly defined region centered around the pituitary fossa and surrounding structures.

Boundaries

- **Anteriorly**: Tuberculum sellae, anterior clinoid processes, posterior margin of the lesser wing of the sphenoid bone, and anterior and superior rim of the greater wing of the sphenoid bone.
- **Posteriorly**: Superior border of the petrous temporal bone and dorsum sellae.
- Floor of the central skull base is mostly formed by sphenoid bone.

The central skull base is further subdivided into three compartments by two vertical lines passing medially to the petroclival fissure and just lateral to the foramen ovale.
- **Midline Sagittal Compartment**: Comprises of the body of the sphenoid bone and the portion of the clivus anterior to the spheno-occipital synchondrosis.
- **Off-midline Parasagittal Compartment**: Part of the middle cranial fossa in between the line passing medial to the petroclival suture and the line passing just lateral to the foramen ovale. Comprises of petroclival synchondrosis,

foramen lacerum, and medial aspect of the greater wing of the sphenoid bone. Numerous vital neurovascular structures are seen in this compartment which include cavernous sinus, superior orbital fissure, vidian canal, foramen rotundum, and foramen lacerum.

- **Lateral Compartment**: Part of the middle cranial fossa lateral to the line passing just lateral to the foramen ovale. It comprises of lateral part of the sphenoid bone, the squamous part of the temporal bone, and the temporomandibular joint.

Important Anatomical Landmarks

- Sella turcica
- Cavernous sinus
- **Optic Canal**: It is formed by the lesser sphenoid wing and transmits the optic nerve and the ophthalmic artery.
- **Superior Orbital Fissure**: It lies between the greater and lesser sphenoid wing and transmits cranial nerve III, IV, VI, and ophthalmic divisions of the trigeminal nerve. The superior orbital fissure and the optic canal together form the orbital apex.
- **Foramen Rotundum**: It lies inferior to the superior orbital fissure and transmits the maxillary division of the trigeminal nerve.
- **Foramen Spinosum**: It lies in the greater sphenoid wing posterolateral to the foramen ovale and transmits the middle meningeal artery.
- **Vidian Canal**: The vidian canal lies on the floor of the sphenoid sinus at the junction of the pterygoid process and sphenoid body. It connects the foramen lacerum with the pterygopalatine fossa and transmits the vidian artery (branch of the maxillary artery) and vidian nerve.
- **Pterygopalatine Fossa**:
  - **Boundaries**:
    - Posteriorly: Pterygoid plates
    - Medially: palatine bone
    - Anteriorly: maxillary sinus
    - Laterally: Communicates with infratemporal fossa through the pterygomaxillary fissure.
  - **Contents**:
    - Maxillary nerve
    - Pterygopalatine ganglion
    - Terminal branches of the internal maxillary artery

Posterior Skull Base

Boundaries

- **Anteriorly**: Posterior surface of the clivus
- **Posteriorly**: Squamous occipital bone and mastoid temporal bone.
- **Laterally**: Petrous temporal bone superiorly and condylar part of the occipital bone inferiorly.

Important Landmarks

- Foramen magnum
- Jugular foramen
- Hypoglossal canal
- Internal auditory canal

CSF Rhinorrhea

CSF rhinorrhea is a clinical condition characterized by extracranial leakage of CSF into the adjacent paranasal sinus through an osteodural defect of the skull base. Osteodural defect of the skull base leads to abnormal communication between the subarachnoid space and adjacent paranasal sinus. It increases the risk of the spread of infection from paranasal sinuses leading to meningitis.

Causes

- Traumatic
- Iatrogenic
- Congenital malformations
- Spontaneous leaks.

Relevant Anatomy

Anterior Skull Base

- Anterior skull base separates the anterior cranial fossa structures with orbits and paranasal sinuses.
- **Roof of the Nasal Cavity and the Anterior Ethmoid Sinus**: Medial to laterally formed by cribriform plate, lateral lamella, and fovea ethmoidalis.
- **The Roof of Posterior Ethmoid and Sphenoid Sinus**: Formed by the planum ethmoidale and sphenoidale
- Numerous perforations are present in the cribriform plate of ethmoid bone through which olfactory nerves traverse from olfactory mucosa to the olfactory bulb. Fracture of the cribriform plate (most commonly at lateral lamella where the anterior ethmoidal artery enters into anterior cranial fossa) is the most common cause of CSF rhinorrhea.

Central Skull Base

The central skull base separates the middle cranial fossa from the sphenoid sinus. Hyperpneumatization of sphenoid sinuses is susceptible to bony thinning and vulnerability to iatrogenic injury or erosion leading to spontaneous CSF leaks.

- **Evaluation of Suspected CSF Leak**:
  - Patients are presenting with clear watery nasal discharge.
  - First investigation to be performed: Detection of beta-2-transferrin in the fluid for confirmation of diagnosis. Then imaging studies are performed to localize and characterize the defect.

Imaging

Computed Tomography

HRCT of PNS is the preferred imaging modality in an individual with a CSF leak. It provides excellent delineation of bony anatomy and helps to identify the bony defect.

- **Advantage**: It provides excellent delineation of bony anatomy and helps to identify the bony defect even in patients without active leak
- **Disadvantage**:
  - Not able to detect the concomitant dural defect in a patient with multiple bony defects.
  - Not able to differentiate the mucus secretions from the CSF collection within the paranasal sinuses.

Magnetic Resonance Cisternography

- **Sequence Used**: Heavily T2-weighted sequences with suppression of background signal is used in MR cisternography.
- It is considered as a positive finding when it identifies a CSF track communicating with subarachnoid spaces and extracranial paranasal sinuses with or without herniation of meninges and cerebral parenchyma.
  - **Disadvantage**:
    - Not able to provide clear bony details.
    - Could not able to differentiate the mucus secretions from the CSF collection within the paranasal sinuses.
  - **Advantages**:
    - Excellent soft tissue resolution.
    - Identifies and differentiates a meningocele from an encephalocele with adjacent gliotic brain parenchyma.

CT Cisternography

Procedure: Intrathecal injection of non-ionic iodinated contrast agent (about 8–10 mL).

Keep the patient prone in Trendelenburg position (patient is tilted with foot-end elevation) for about 5 minutes. It leads to cranial migration of contrast and optimal opacification of basal CSF space.

CT of the PNS is performed in a prone position with the head hanging down.

Disadvantage:
- Identifies the site of an active leak only. Could not detect inactive/intermittent leaks.
- Very small leaks can be missed due to non-leakage of high viscosity contrast, adjacent to high-density bone.
- Invasive procedure.
- Increased radiation dose.
- Risks associated with a lumbar puncture and intrathecal administration of iodinated contrast.

Indications:
- Evaluation of CSF leaks in patients with multiple fractures/osseous defects.
- In a patient with suspicious bony defect and clinically confirmed CSF leaks.

Positive Findings: Contrast pooling adjacent to a bony defect on the post-contrast scan.

Contrast-enhanced MRC

Procedure: Intrathecal administration of about 0.5 mL of gadolinium-based contrast agents. Acquisition of two-dimensional (2D)/three-dimensional (3D) thin section T1-weighted images is performed.

Two sets of images are taken:
- About 1–2 hours after contrast administration.
- After 24 hours delay when necessary.

Findings: Hyperintense fistulous track through the osseous defect.

Advantages:
- Identification of meningoceles.
- It has higher sensitivity than CT cisternography for the detection of CSF leak, especially in intermittent leak.
- No difficulty in the detection of leak adjacent to high density bone.

Limitations

Lack of United States Food and Drug Administration approval for the intrathecal instillation of gadolinium-based contrast and recent evidence of gadolinium chelate deposition in the brain following intravenous and intrathecal injection. However, the dose used in MR cisternography is much less than the dose causing adverse effects. So, contrast-enhanced MR cisternography is reserved for problem-solving tools.

Radionuclide Cisternography

Procedure: Intrathecal instillation of the radiotracer agents (usually Technetium—99 or Indium—111) followed by the acquisition of the images.

Findings: Identification of the radiotracer activity in the paranasal sinuses or the nasopharynx. Detection of CSF leak is improved by measuring radiotracer activity in the pledgets placed in the nasal cavity after 24–48 hours. Considered as a positive for CSF leak when pledget-to-serum activity ratio is 1.5–3:1.

Advantages:
- Useful in intermittent CSF leaks.
- It can be performed as an alternative modality especially in cases with intermittent CSF leaks to confirm the presence or absence of a CSF leak.

2. A young adult patient has presented with unilateral pulsatile proptosis and chemosis after a road traffic accident. What is the probable etiology and how will you confirm the diagnosis by imaging? Discuss the role of radiologic interventions in managing such a condition. [(1+5)+4] [DNB June 20, MD (WBUHS) 24]

Causes of Pulsatile Proptosis

- Carotid—cavernous fistula
- Vascular orbital tumors
- Transmitted intracranial pulsations through congenital (NF1 with sphenoid wing dysplasia)/posttraumatic (orbital roof fractures)/postsurgical osseous orbital defects.
- Orbital meningoencephalocele.

For a patient presenting with unilateral pulsatile proptosis after a road traffic accident most probable diagnosis is the carotid-cavernous fistula.

Carotid-cavernous Fistula (CCF)

It is a type of arteriovenous fistula with abnormal communication between the internal carotid artery and/or external carotid artery and the cavernous sinus.

Classification and etiology **(Table 1)**:

TABLE 1: Classification and etiology of carotid-cavernous fistula.

Classification	**Direct**: The cavernous ICA communicates with the cavernous sinus directly It is typically high flow lesion	**Indirect**: Fistulous communication between dural branches of ICA/ECA with the cavernous sinus It is type of slow flow lesion
Etiology	**Trauma**: Most common cause of direct CCF secondary to skull base fractures **Nontraumatic**: Rupture of cavernous ICA aneurysm	Usually, nontraumatic and believe to degenerative in origin

Imaging

General Features: The imaging features of carotid-cavernous fistula reflect the presence of arteriovenous shunting within the CS. Depending on the extent of the shunt, the findings can be variable.

CT Findings

- NECT scans usually demonstrate variable degrees of proptosis, a prominent cavernous sinus with a dilated superior ophthalmic vein (SOV), and prominent extraocular muscles. "Dirty" fat due to venous engorgement and edema may be present.
- CTA shows engorgement of the ophthalmic vein and CS. Dehiscence of the intracavernous ICA is characteristic of direct CCF.

MR Findings: T1 scans may show "bulging" CS and dilated superior ophthalmic vein as well as "dirty" orbital fat. T2W images may show asymmetric signal loss in the affected veins.

Angiography: DSA is the gold standard for diagnosis of CCF. Selective ICA injection with image acquisition at high frame rates is necessary to localize the exact fistula site.

The Barrow classification of carotid-cavernous fistulas is presented in **Table 2** as follows:

TABLE 2: Barrow classification of carotid-cavernous fistulas.

Type A	Direct ICA-CS high-flow shunt
Type B	Dural ICA branches-CS shunt
Type C	Dural ECA-CS shunt
Type D	Both ICA/ECA dural branches shunt to CS

Anatomy: The cavernous sinuses are paired structures located along both sides of the sella turcica and formed by the dural folds.

Extent

- **Anteriorly**: Superior orbital fissure
- **Posteriorly**: Petrous apex
- **Floor and Medial Wall**: Endosteal layer of dura
- **Roof and Lateral Wall**: Meningeal layer of dura

Structural Relations

- **Structures Passing through Cavernous Sinus**:
  - Cavernous segment of internal carotid artery surrounded by venous and sympathetic plexus.
  - Abducens nerve (inferolateral to ICA)
- **Structures at Lateral Wall**: Cranial nerve III, IV, and V1 and V2 divisions of the trigeminal nerve.
- **Tributaries and Communications**:
  - **Anteriorly**:
    - The ophthalmic vein connects with the facial vein
    - Sphenoparietal sinus.
  - **Posteriorly**:
    - The superior petrosal sinus connects with the sigmoid sinus.
    - The inferior petrosal sinus connects with the jugular bulb.
  - **Medially**: Anterior and posterior intercavernous sinuses connect both cavernous sinuses.
  - **Inferiorly**:
    - The emissary vein connects the internal jugular vein through the foramen lacerum.
    - The emissary vein connects the pterygoid venous plexus through the foramen ovale.

Imaging

Detailed clinical history, examination, and imaging can be utilized for diagnosis and as part of preintervention work-up.

CT Findings

NCCT*:*

- May demonstrate mild to marked proptosis.
- Prominent cavernous sinus with an enlarged superior ophthalmic vein.
- Enlarged extraocular muscles with dirty retro-orbital fat due to congestion.
- Evidence of trauma and fractures can be identified.

CECT: Clear demonstration of an enlarged cavernous sinus with an enlarged superior ophthalmic vein.

CTA: Fistulous communication can be identified in most of the cases.

MRI: Due to better soft tissue resolution, the sensitivity of MRI is high. Better visualization of the soft tissue abnormality seen with MRI. Flow voids can be seen within the cavernous sinus and prominent draining veins in high-flow fistulas. MR angiography can detect fistulous communication.

DSA: Digital subtraction angiography is the gold standard for diagnosis of carotico cavernous fistula. With the easy availability of CT angiography, DSA is hardly required as just a diagnostic tool.

Findings: It identifies the fistula with a clear delineation of arterial and venous patterns leading to differentiate between direct and indirect types.

Direct CCFs: Typically demonstrate very rapid flow with very early opacification of the cavernous sinus. Very rapid image acquisition and selective ICA injection are usually necessary to localize the fistula site precisely.

Occasionally, injection into the vertebrobasilar system or in the ICA with manual compression of the ipsilateral common carotid artery is necessary to determine the fistula site. Patterns of venous drainage should be evaluated.

Indirect CCFs: Multiple dural feeders are seen.

Dural Feeder:
- From branches of cavernous ICA (meningohypophyseal and inferolateral trunks).
- Middle meningeal and distal maxillary branches of ECA.

Treatment

Indications of treatment:
- Progressive visual loss
- Uncontrolled glaucoma
- Intolerable headache/bruit/tinnitus
- Enlargement of the fistula
- Epistaxis or signs of cerebral ischemia
- Type A fistulae are high-flow fistulas and almost always require treatment.
- Presence of cortical venous reflux having increased risk of subarachnoid or parenchymal hemorrhage.

The current recommendations for management of indirect CCFs is presented in **Table 3** as follows:

TABLE 3: Current recommendations for indirect CCFs.

Dural CCFs without rapidly progressive visual deterioration, evidence of abnormal cortical venous drainage, hypoxic ocular changes involving the retina and optic nerve or ischemic keratopathy	**Conservative treatment trial**: Trial of manual carotid artery jugular vein compression therapy. (Methods: Manual occlusion of the affected carotid with opposite hand for 10 seconds three times an hour while the patient is awake. The occlusion time is gradually increased. This method induces thrombosis and fistula closure with resolution of symptoms. If patients do not respond to this trial, then embolization therapy is advised

Treatment Methods Depend on the Type of Fistula

- **Conservative Treatment**: Discussed above.
- **Surgical Treatment**: Ligation and proximal embolization have significant risks. Surgical treatment is reserved for patients who do not respond to endovascular treatment.

Endovascular Treatment

Minimally invasive technique with consistently good results. In Traumatic CCFs more life-threating injuries are treated first before the fistula. On every occasion, steroid is administered to reduce the inflammation before the endovascular treatment. Raised intraocular pressure should be treated with medicine.

The Goal of the Treatment: Occlude the fistula without compromising the parent artery.

Angiography is usually the first step of the therapeutic procedure for localization and anatomy of the fistula.

Anesthesia: Try to do the procedure under local anesthesia with mild sedation to allow test occlusion of the ICA. General anesthesia may be necessary in children and uncooperative patients.

Anticoagulation is obtained with a heparin bolus of 3–5,000 units, followed by 1,000 units every hour in an adult.

A. **Transarterial Embolization**:
   - Transarterial placement of detachable balloon/coils through the rent into the cavernous sinus with preservation of ICA flow is performed in most of the direct CCFs.
   - If the rents of the ICA are large or multiple then carotid occlusion is necessary.
   - In children: Difficult to navigate large-size balloons, so coil embolization preferred.

B. **Transvenous Embolization**:
   - The transvenous approach is indicated if the transarterial approach fails because, higher risk of venous rupture and hemorrhage.
   - Increased risk of placing the embolic material away from the fistula site and redirecting flow into cortical veins.

Procedure: The fistula site is accessed through one of its draining veins (which seems to be easiest to catheterize), usually through the IPS or the ophthalmic vein. Advances the microcatheter into the cavernous sinus and towards the fistula. Embolization of the venous drainage of the CS was performed first. The embolic agent of choice for transvenous embolization is Coils.

C. **Parent Artery Reconstruction**: When the artery reconstruction is necessary: Covered stents placement, deployment of flow diverters with coils/in isolation may be performed.

Follow-up

- Residual flow on an angiogram is not an indication of an attempt to achieve a complete angiographic cure.
- The primary goal of the treatment is to alleviate the symptoms.
- Follow-up DSA may be advised after 3–4 months if there is no significant improvement in symptoms.

Stroke

1. Mention the stroke protocol. Discuss the role of intervention radiology in management of stroke. [4+6]

A stroke, also known as a cerebrovascular event (CVA), is characterized by the sudden onset of neurological symptoms due to insufficient blood flow to the brain. Approximately 80% of all strokes are caused by cerebral ischemia or infarction. Due to their speed and availability, nonenhanced computed tomography (NECT) and computed tomography angiography (CTA), with or without CT perfusion, are the most frequently utilized imaging modalities.

Acute stroke protocols depend on factors such as the time elapsed since the onset of symptoms, the availability of urgent imaging with appropriate software reconstructions, preferences of clinicians and radiologists, and access to neurointervention.

The "must know" questions in acute stroke triage that need to be answered are as follows **(Box 1)**.

BOX 1: The "must know" questions in acute stroke triage.

There are four "must know" questions in acute stroke triage that need to be answered rapidly and accurately.

1. Is intracranial hemorrhage or a stroke "mimic" present?
2. Is a large vessel occluded?
3. Is part of the brain irreversibly injured (i.e., is there a core of critically ischemic, irreversibly infarcted tissue)?
4. Is there a clinically relevant "penumbra" of ischemic but potentially salvageable tissue?

Pathophysiology

Brain Ischemia and Stroke Imaging Protocols

Core and Penumbra in Brain Ischemia:

- **Ischemic Core**: The central region of affected brain tissue during a stroke has a cerebral blood flow (CBF) of less than 6–8 cm^3/100 g/min. This area experiences neuronal death and irreversible loss of function.
- **Penumbra**: Surrounding the core, the penumbra is less severely ischemic, with CBF reduced from a normal 60 cm^3/100 g/min to 10–20 cm^3/100 g/min. This tissue is "at risk" but potentially salvageable.

Imaging Goals and Protocols

1. **Primary Objectives**:
   - Differentiate ischemic stroke from intracranial hemorrhage.
   - Select and triage patients for reperfusion therapies.
2. **Imaging Steps**:
   - **NECT**: Emergent nonenhanced CT (NECT) scans determine if intracranial hemorrhage or stroke mimics (e.g., subdural hematoma, neoplasm) are present.
   - **CTA**: CT angiography follows NECT if hemorrhage is excluded, identifying major vessel occlusions and active bleeding (e.g., "spot sign").

- **MRA and DSA**: MR angiography can be affected by motion artifacts, making digital subtraction angiography (DSA) preferable for intra-arterial thrombolysis or mechanical thrombectomy.
- **Perfusion Imaging**: CT or MR perfusion (pCT, pMR) studies assess the extent of irreversible damage and identify salvageable brain tissue (ischemic penumbra).

CT Findings and Protocols

- **Acute Stroke CT Protocol**:
  - Includes NECT, arch-to-vertex CTA, and dynamic first-pass perfusion CT (pCT).
  - Detects hyperattenuating vessels (e.g., "dense MCA" sign) and assesses grey-white matter interfaces.
- **ASPECTS Score**: The Alberta Stroke Program Early CT Score (ASPECTS) evaluates early ischemic changes by subtracting points for affected regions. An ASPECTS score ≤7 indicates increased hemorrhage risk and poor outcomes.
- **CTA and pCT**:
  - **CTA**: Visualizes craniocervical vasculature, localizes thrombus, assesses collateral flow, and characterizes atherosclerosis.
  - **pCT**: Evaluates cerebral blood volume (CBV), cerebral blood flow (CBF), and mean transit time (MTT). The ischemic core shows reduced CBV and CBF, while the penumbra shows mismatched CBV and CBF with prolonged MTT.

Key Imaging Parameters (Table 4)

- **CBV**: Volume of blood in a given brain volume.
- **CBF**: Volume of blood flowing through a brain volume over time.
- **MTT**: Average time for blood to transit through the brain.
- **Color Scales**:
  - **CBV/CBF**: Well-perfused areas appear red/yellow; ischemic areas are blue/purple.
  - **MTT**: Abnormal transit time appears red; normal transit time appears blue.
- **Clinical Implications**: MCA infarct core volume of 70–100 mL predicts poor outcomes. The penumbra, with a mismatch between CBV and CBF, represents potentially salvageable tissue.

TABLE 4: CT perfusion parameters indicating ischemic core and penumbra.

Etiology	*CBF*	*CBV*	*WITT*	*TTP*
Infarct core	↓	↓	≥	↑
Ischemic penumbra	↓	↑	↑	↑

(CBF = cerebral blood flow, CBV = cerebral blood volume, MTT = mean transit time; TTP = time to peak, ↑ indicate increase, ↓ = indicate decrease)

- An important finding in patients having large MCA territorial infarcts is decreased perfusion in the contralateral cerebellar hemisphere with decreased cerebral blood flow, a phenomenon known as crossed cerebellar diaschisis.

MRI Findings in Stroke Preferred Modalities

- **CT/CTA/pCT**: Often chosen due to accessibility and speed. However, rapid stroke protocols using fast FLAIR, T2*, DWI, and pMR are also effective.
- **MRI Advantages**: Superior in detecting small vessel and brainstem ischemia. Useful in identifying the ischemic penumbra when there is a discrepancy between CT/CTA findings and clinical stroke severity.

Specific MRI Techniques and Findings

1. **T2/FLAIR**
   - **Early Detection**: Only 30–50% of acute strokes show cortical swelling and hyperintensity on FLAIR within the first 4 hours. Almost all strokes are FLAIR positive by 7 hours after symptom onset. T2 scans generally become positive within 12–24 hours.
   - **Intraarterial Hyperintensity**: An early stroke sign on FLAIR indicating slow flow, either from delayed antegrade flow or retrograde collateral filling.

- **FLAIR-DWI Mismatch**: When FLAIR is negative, and DWI is positive, it suggests viable ischemic penumbra and eligibility for thrombolysis.

2. ***T2* GRE***
   - **Intraarterial Thrombus Detection**: "Blooming" hypointensity on T2* (GRE, SWI) indicates intraarterial thrombus.
   - **Chronic Hypertension or Amyloid Angiopathy**: "Blooming black dots" in older patients.
   - **Cerebral Microbleeds**: May increase the risk of anticoagulation-related hemorrhage.
3. **DWI and ADC**
   - **Hyperacute Infarcts**: Approximately 95% show diffusion restriction, with hyperintensity on DWI and corresponding hypointensity on ADC.
   - **Sensitivity**: DTI is even more sensitive than DWI, especially for pontine and medullary lesions.
   - **Negative DWI**: Does not rule out stroke, as 2–7% of patients with a final stroke diagnosis are initially DWI negative. Possible reasons include small (lacunar) infarcts, brainstem lesions, clot lysis with recanalization, and moderate or fluctuating hypoperfusion.
4. **pMR**
   - **DWI-PWI Mismatch**: DWI generally reflects the densely ischemic core of the infarct, while pMR shows the surrounding "at-risk" penumbra. A mismatch between DWI and PWI helps determine suitability for intraarterial thrombolysis.

By using these MRI techniques, clinicians can better identify and differentiate between the core and penumbra of an infarct, thereby guiding appropriate treatment decisions.

Stroke Algorithm **(Flowchart 1)**.

Treatment Options

The single most important factor in successful intervention is patient selection, with the two most important considerations being (1) elapsed time from symptom onset and (2) imaging findings on the screening NECT scan.

1. IV thrombolysis is done by recombinant tissue plasminogen activator (rtpa). There are several studies regarding rtpa dose, therapeutic window and effectiveness. The clinically accepted therapeutic window for intravenous recombinant tissue plasminogen activator (rTPA) is less than 3 hours from ictus (the "golden hours"). A dose 0.6 mg/kg is used in Japan and other Asian countries.
2. Intraarterial thrombolysis is typically restricted to less than 6 hours. Exceptions to this general rule include basilar artery thrombosis and patients outside the 6-hour window who have a persistent significant perfusion-diffusion mismatch.
3. Mechanical thrombectomy is suitable in patients beyond the therapeutic window or in whom thrombolytic therapy is contraindicated. However, it is rare that a patient may benefit from thrombectomy if the procedure starts >8 hours after onset in the anterior circulation and >24 hours after onset in the posterior circulation.

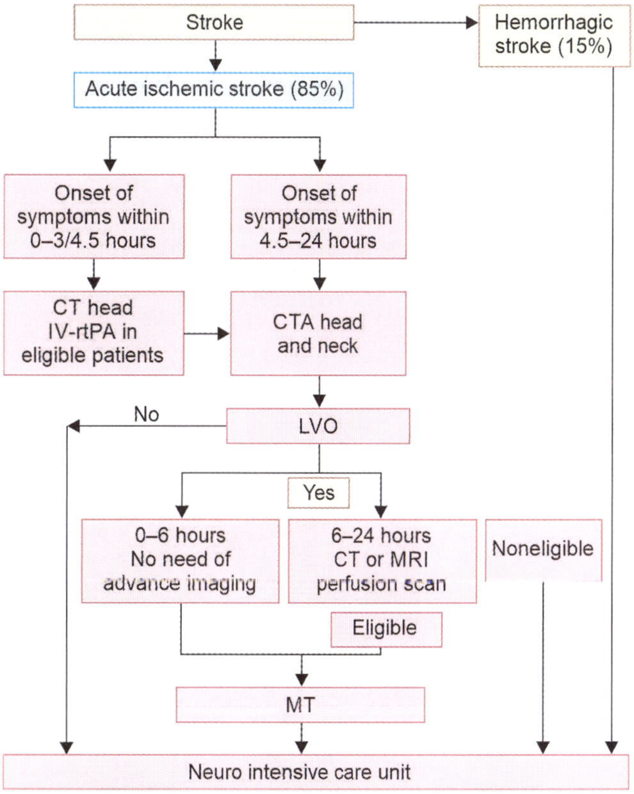

FLOWCHART 1: Stroke algorithm.

Mechanical Thrombectomy Treatment Protocol

Sedation and Anesthesia

- **Conscious Sedation (CS)**: Preferred over general anesthesia (GA) due to faster procedure times and better patient control. CS avoids the hypotension commonly induced by GA, which can be detrimental to acute stroke patients relying on high cerebral perfusion pressure via pial collaterals.

Anticoagulation

Standard Heparin Flushes: No additional anticoagulation or antiaggregation required during thrombectomy, except for standard heparin flushes (e.g., 5 IU/mL). Permanent stenting should be avoided due to the increased risk of reperfusion hematomas or hemorrhagic conversion.

Procedure in Anterior Circulation

- **Stent Retrievers**: Safe to use up to the M2 segments in most patients.
- **Posterior Circulation**: Typically, thrombectomy is not needed beyond the P1 segment.

Procedural Steps (Fig. 8)

1. **Groin Puncture**: Use a long (80 cm) 8 F introducer sheath placed in the common carotid artery (CCA) with a 5 F diagnostic catheter (DC) and a 0.035" (0.89 mm) guidewire (GW).[4]
2. **Balloon Guide Catheter (BGC)**: Position an 8 F BGC in the internal carotid artery. BGC allows for flow reversal, reducing the risk of thrombo-emboli escaping into collateral areas.
3. **Microcatheter Introduction**: After confirming the clot position with contrast injection, introduce a microcatheter with a microguidewire, passing the thrombus if possible while keeping the microguidewire retracted.
4. **Stent Retriever Deployment**: Release the stent retriever centered at the clot, preferably more distal than proximal, covering the proximal clot boundary. Leave it to expand and "incubate" for at least 5 minutes.

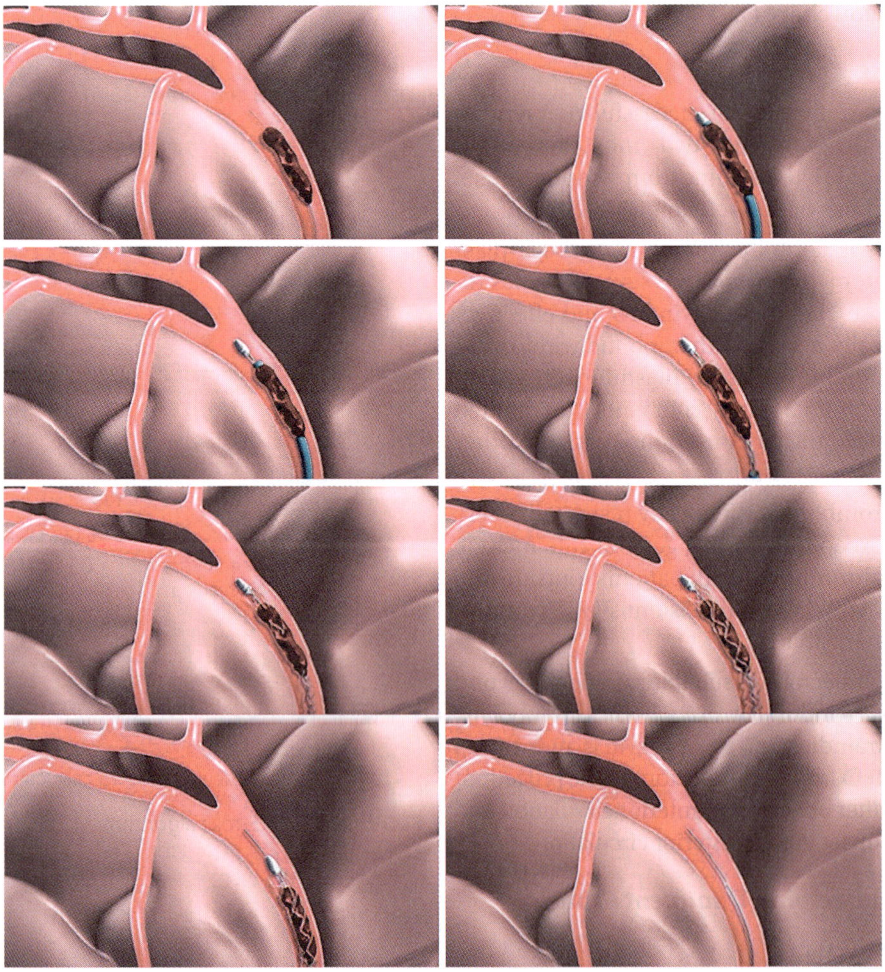

FIG. 8: Schematic diagram representing standard technique of mechanical thrombectomy.

5. **Resheathing and Aspiration**: Readvance the microcatheter, partially resheath the stent retriever to the face of the thrombus, inflate the balloon, and pull back the stent retriever with simultaneous aspiration in the BGC. Gradually escalate and maximize aspiration as the device enters the guide's orifice.
6. **Thrombus Retrieval**: Remove the rotating hemostatic valve (RHV), take out the device to check for thrombus, and apply further aspiration directly to the BGC to clear any remaining small thrombi before deflating the balloon.
7. **Procedure Control**: Verify the procedure's outcome with a contrast injection in the BGC, rinse and clean the device, reconnect the RHV, and repeat the thrombectomy maneuver if necessary. Typically, the same stent retriever can be used up to three times.

Posterior Circulation Adaptations

Guide Catheter: Use a long, soft 6–7 F guide catheter (e.g., Navien, Fargo, Neuron) to advance up to the vertebrobasilar junction, as advancing an 8 F guide catheter into the vertebral arteries can be challenging.

By adhering to this protocol, mechanical thrombectomy can be effectively and safely performed, ensuring optimal outcomes for patients with acute ischemic stroke.

2. Role of intervention radiology in subarachnoid hemorrhage. [5]

Subarachnoid hemorrhage can be classified into traumatic and nontraumatic.

Nontraumatic subarachnoid hemorrhage accounts for approximately 3–5% of all cases of acute stroke. Around 80% of these cases are caused by ruptured intracranial aneurysm.

Imaging in Nontraumatic Subarachnoid Hemorrhage CT Findings:

- **Distribution**: The pattern of subarachnoid hemorrhage depends on the aneurysm location.
  - **Anterior Communicating Artery Aneurysms**: Usually rupture into the anterior interhemispheric fissure.
  - **Middle Cerebral Artery Bifurcation Aneurysms**: Typically rupture into the Sylvian fissure.
  - **Internal Carotid and Posterior Communicating Artery Aneurysms**: Rupture into the suprasellar cistern.
  - **Vertebrobasilar Aneurysms**: Often bleed into the fourth ventricle and prepontine cistern.
- **Intraventricular Hemorrhage**: Present in about 50% of patients with subarachnoid hemorrhage.
- **Focal Parenchymal Hemorrhage**: If present, indicates the rupture site of the aneurysm. Rarely, a focal hematoma within the subarachnoid space is seen as bleeding from the aneurysm.

These imaging findings assist in diagnosing, locating, and managing subarachnoid hemorrhage effectively.

Stepwise increases in modified Fisher grade **(Box 2)** have a moderately linear relationship with the risk of vasospasm, delayed infarction, and poor clinical outcome.

BOX 2: Modified Fisher scale to grade aneurysmal subarachnoid hemorrhage.

A simple scale based on NECT findings, the modified Fisher scale, has been proposed to grade aneurysmal subarachnoid hemorrhage.
Grade 0: No visible SAH or IVH
Grade 1: Focal or diffuse thin (less than 1 mm) layer of subarachnoid blood without IVH
Grade 2: Focal or diffuse thin (less than 1 mm) layer of subarachnoid blood with IVH
Grade 3: Focal or diffuse thick (more than 1 mm) SAH without IVH
Grade 4: Focal or diffuse thick (more than 1 mm) SAH with IVH

MR Findings and Angiography in Subarachnoid Hemorrhage (SAH)

MRI Findings

Acute SAH: Best visualized on FLAIR sequences.

Angiography

- **CT Angiography**: Detects aneurysms 2 mm or larger in 95% of aneurysmal subarachnoid hemorrhage cases.

- **DSA**: Remains the gold standard for identifying and detailing aneurysm angioarchitecture. If initial CT angiography is negative, consider performing DSA. Repeat DSA or CTA is recommended for diffuse-type SAH when initial DSA is negative.

Specific Types of Nonaneurysmal SAH

- **Perimesencephalic SAH (pnSAH)**: Usually found in the interpeduncular, ambient, and prepontine cisterns. Rarely affects the posterior aspect of the suprasellar cistern.
- **Convexal SAH (cSAH)**: Located in superficial cerebral sulci. Possible causes include cortical vein occlusion, vasculitis, amyloid angiopathy, and reversible cerebral vasoconstriction syndrome (RCVS).

Role of Interventional Radiology

Imaging Considerations

- **Aneurysm Details**: Location, size, shape, and neck size.
- **Parent Vessel Anatomy**: Includes the presence or absence of intraluminal thrombus.
- **Access Vessel Anatomy**: Factors such as dominant vs. hypoplastic vertebral artery or ACA, degree of tortuosity, atherosclerosis, or fibromuscular dysplasia.

Procedure Planning

1. **Choice of Access Artery**.
2. **Endovascular Technique**: Options include primary embolization, stent-assisted or balloon-assisted coiling, and flow diversion.
3. **Device Types and Sizes**.

Coiling Technique (Figs. 9A to C)

- **Guide Catheter**: Examples include Neuron™ 0.053 in., Benchmark™ 0.071 in., and Neuron™ MAX 0.088 in. Positioned just below the skull base.[5]
- **Intraprocedure Medication**:
  - **Heparin**: 2,500 IU in the flush bag (500 mL of warmed normal saline).
  - **Systemic Heparin**: 5,000 IU administered during coiling.
  - **Nimodipine**: Administered as a bolus and maintained with an infusion if angiographic vasospasm is detected. Dose: 2 mg per territory, split into 1 mg IA bolus and 1 mg in the flush bag.

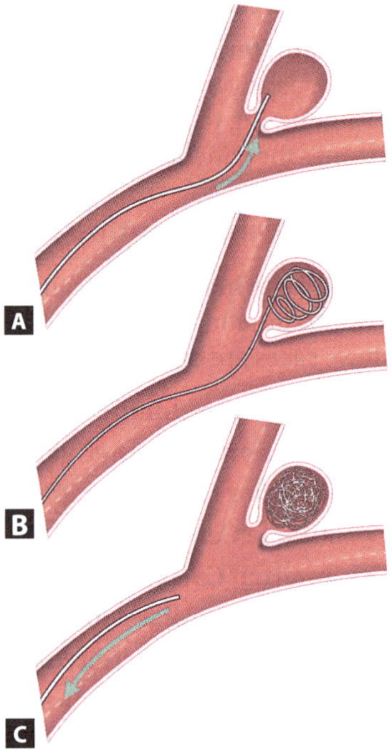

FIGS. 9A TO C: Schematic diagram representing standard technique of aneurysm coiling.

- **Microcatheters**: Options include Excelsior® SL-10, Echelon™ 10, Excelsior® XT-17®, Excelsior® 1018®, and Marksman™.
- **Microwires**: Options include Synchro®-14 0.014 in., Neuroscout®-14 0.014 in., and Transend™ EX 0.014 in. with a floppy tip.

Coil Types

- **Framing Coils**: Diameter should closely match the mean diameter of the aneurysm sac.
- **Filling Coils**.
- **Finishing Coils**.

Catheter Withdrawal: Carefully remove the microcatheter to avoid displacing the deployed coils.

Follow-Up

Conduct follow-up with an MRI (TOF-MRA) or DSA after 6 months.

These detailed imaging findings and procedural steps help ensure accurate diagnosis and effective treatment of subarachnoid hemorrhage.

3. Discuss etiology, radiological imaging features of subarachnoid hemorrhage (SAH) and role of intervention radiology in its management. [2+4+4] [MD (WBUHS) 20, MD (WBUHS) 21]

Subarachnoid Hemorrhage (SAH): Types and Imaging

Types of Subarachnoid Hemorrhage

1. **Traumatic Subarachnoid Hemorrhage**:
   - **Prevalence**: Commonly found in cases of moderate to severe head trauma.
   - **Frequency**: Trauma is the leading cause of subarachnoid hemorrhage.
   - **Associated Condition**: Rarely, intraocular hemorrhage (Terson syndrome) is linked with traumatic subarachnoid hemorrhage.
2. **Nontraumatic Subarachnoid Hemorrhage**:
   - **Prevalence**: Accounts for about 3–5% of all acute stroke cases.
   - **Major Cause**: Approximately 80% are due to ruptured intracranial aneurysms.
   - **Other Causes**: Includes dissections, vasculitis, venous thrombosis, hemorrhage, reversible cerebral vasoconstriction syndrome, and amyloid angiopathy.

Imaging in Traumatic Subarachnoid Hemorrhage

1. **CT Findings**:
   - **Appearance**: Acute traumatic subarachnoid hemorrhage appears as peripheral, linear hyperdensities in the sulci adjacent to cortical contusions or beneath epidural or subdural hematomas.
   - **Rare Presentation**: Isolated traumatic subarachnoid hemorrhage may sometimes be found in the interpeduncular fossa.
2. **MR Findings**:
   - **Acute Stage**: Identifying acute blood on T1-weighted images (T1WI) can be challenging. FLAIR scans reveal hyperintensity in the affected sulci. "Blooming" on T2* scans adjacent to cortical contusions.
   - **Chronic Stage**: Leads to focal superficial siderosis along gyral crests and sulcal spaces.

Differential Diagnosis for Traumatic SAH

1. **Sulcal-Cisternal Hyperintensity**:
   - Can be due to meningitis, artifact (incomplete CSF suppression), neoplasm, contrast leak (e.g., with renal failure), high inspired oxygen during general anesthesia, hyperintense vessels with slow flow (e.g., acute arterial strokes, Sturge-Weber syndrome), pial collaterals post cerebral ischemia-infarction, Moyamoya disease ['Ivy' Sign], and reversible cerebral vasoconstriction syndrome (RCVS).
2. **Pseudosubarachnoid Hemorrhage**: Describes the CT appearance of a brain with severe cerebral edema, where hypodense brain parenchyma makes circulating blood in arteries and veins appear relatively hyperdense.

Imaging in Nontraumatic Subarachnoid Hemorrhage

1. **CT Findings**:
   - **Distribution**: The pattern of subarachnoid hemorrhage depends on the aneurysm location.
     - **Anterior Communicating Artery Aneurysms**: Usually rupture into the anterior interhemispheric fissure.
     - **Middle Cerebral Artery Bifurcation Aneurysms**: Typically rupture into the Sylvian fissure.
     - **Internal Carotid and Posterior Communicating Artery Aneurysms**: Rupture into the suprasellar cistern.
     - **Vertebrobasilar Aneurysms**: Often bleed into the fourth ventricle and prepontine cistern.
   - **Intraventricular Hemorrhage**: Present in about 50% of patients with subarachnoid hemorrhage.
   - **Focal Parenchymal Hemorrhage**: If present, indicates the rupture site of the aneurysm. Rarely, a focal hematoma within the subarachnoid space is seen as bleeding from the aneurysm.

These imaging findings assist in diagnosing, locating, and managing subarachnoid hemorrhage effectively.

Stepwise increases in modified Fisher grade **(Box 3)** have a moderately linear relationship with the risk of vasospasm, delayed infarction, and poor clinical outcome.

BOX 3: Modified Fisher scale to grade aneurysmal subarachnoid hemorrhage.

A simple scale based on NECT findings, the modified Fisher scale, has been proposed to grade aneurysmal subarachnoid hemorrhage

- Grade 0: No visible SAH or IVH
- Grade 1: Focal or diffuse thin (less than 1 mm) layer of subarachnoid blood without IVH Grade 2: Focal or diffuse thin (less than 1 mm) layer of subarachnoid blood with IVH
- Grade 2: Focal or diffuse thin (less than 1 mm) layer of subarachnoid blood with IVH
- Grade 3: Focal or diffuse thick (more than 1 mm) SAH without IVH
- Grade 4: Focal or diffuse thick (more than 1 mm) SAH with IVH

MR Findings and Angiography in Subarachnoid Hemorrhage (SAH)

MRI Findings

Acute SAH: Best visualized on FLAIR sequences.

Angiography

- **CT Angiography**: Detects aneurysms 2 mm or larger in 95% of aneurysmal subarachnoid hemorrhage cases.
- **DSA**: Remains the gold standard for identifying and detailing aneurysm angioarchitecture. If initial CT angiography is negative, consider performing DSA. Repeat DSA or CTA is recommended for diffuse-type SAH when initial DSA is negative.

Specific Types of Nonaneurysmal SAH

- **Perimesencephalic SAH (pnSAH)**: Usually found in the interpeduncular, ambient, and prepontine cisterns. Rarely affects the posterior aspect of the suprasellar cistern.
- **Convexal SAH (cSAH)**: Located in superficial cerebral sulci. Possible causes include cortical vein occlusion, vasculitis, amyloid angiopathy, and reversible cerebral vasoconstriction syndrome (RCVS).

Role of Interventional Radiology

Imaging Considerations

- **Aneurysm Details**: Location, size, shape, and neck size.
- **Parent Vessel Anatomy**: Includes the presence or absence of intraluminal thrombus.
- **Access Vessel Anatomy**: Factors such as dominant vs. hypoplastic vertebral artery or ACA, degree of tortuosity, atherosclerosis, or fibromuscular dysplasia.

Procedure Planning

1. **Choice of Access Artery**.
2. **Endovascular Technique**: Options include primary embolization, stent-assisted or balloon-assisted coiling, and flow diversion.
3. **Device Types and Sizes**.

Coiling Technique (Figs. 10A to C)

- **Guide Catheter**: Examples include Neuron™ 0.053 in., Benchmark™ 0.071 in., and Neuron™ MAX 0.088 in. Positioned just below the skull base.
- **Intraprocedure Medication**:
  - **Heparin**: 2,500 IU in the flush bag (500 mL of warmed normal saline).
  - **Systemic Heparin**: 5,000 IU administered during coiling.

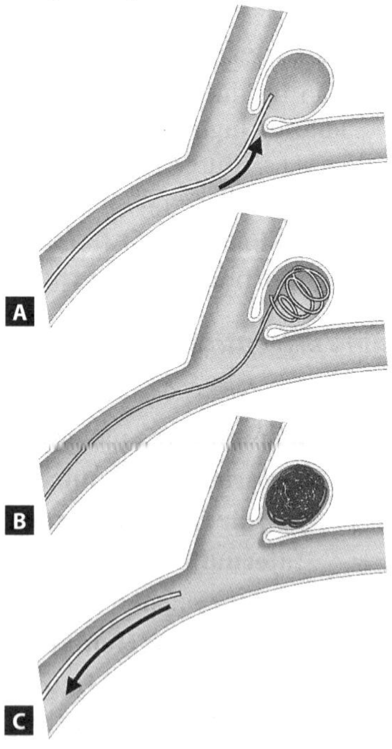

FIGS. 10A TO C: Schematic diagram representing standard technique of aneurysm coiling *(For Color Version Refer Fig. 9).*

- **Nimodipine**: Administered as a bolus and maintained with an infusion if angiographic vasospasm is detected. Dose: 2 mg per territory, split into 1 mg IA bolus and 1 mg in the flush bag.

- **Microcatheters**: Options include Excelsior® SL-10, Echelon™ 10, Excelsior® XT- 17®, Excelsior® 1018®, and Marksman™.
- **Microwires**: Options include Synchro®-14 0.014 in., Neuroscout®-14 0.014 in., and Transend™ EX 0.014 in. with a floppy tip.

Coil Types

- **Framing Coils**: Diameter should closely match the mean diameter of the aneurysm sac.
- **Filling Coils**.
- **Finishing Coils**.

Catheter Withdrawal: Carefully remove the microcatheter to avoid displacing the deployed coils.

Follow-Up: Conduct follow-up with an MRI (TOF-MRA) or DSA after 6 months.

These detailed imaging findings and procedural steps help ensure accurate diagnosis and effective treatment of subarachnoid hemorrhage.

4. Write a short note on: CT perfusion in acute ischemic stroke. [5] [MD (WBUHS) 19]

Brain Ischemia and Stroke Imaging Protocols

Core and Penumbra in Brain Ischemia

- **Ischemic Core**: The central region of affected brain tissue during a stroke has a cerebral blood flow (CBF) of less than 6–8 cm^3/100 g/min. This area experiences neuronal death and irreversible loss of function.
- **Penumbra**: Surrounding the core, the penumbra is less severely ischemic, with CBF reduced from a normal 60 cm^3/100 g/min to 10–20 cm^3/100 g/min. This tissue is "at risk" but potentially salvageable.

Imaging Goals and Protocols

1. **Primary Objectives**:
   - Differentiate ischemic stroke from intracranial hemorrhage.
   - Select and triage patients for reperfusion therapies.
2. **Imaging Steps**:
   - **NECT**: Emergent non-enhanced CT (NECT) scans determine if intracranial hemorrhage or stroke mimics (e.g., subdural hematoma, neoplasm) are present.
   - **CTA**: CT angiography follows NECT if hemorrhage is excluded, identifying major vessel occlusions and active bleeding (e.g., "spot sign").
   - **MRA and DSA**: MR angiography can be affected by motion artifacts, making digital subtraction angiography (DSA) preferable for intra-arterial thrombolysis or mechanical thrombectomy.
   - **Perfusion Imaging**: CT or MR perfusion (pCT, pMR) studies assess the extent of irreversible damage and identify salvageable brain tissue (ischemic penumbra).

CT Findings and Protocols

- **Acute Stroke CT Protocol**:
  - Includes NECT, arch-to-vertex CTA, and dynamic first-pass perfusion CT (pCT).
  - Detects hyperattenuating vessels (e.g., "dense MCA" sign) and assesses grey- white matter interfaces.
- **ASPECTS Score**: The Alberta Stroke Program Early CT Score (ASPECTS) evaluates early ischemic changes by subtracting points for affected regions. An ASPECTS score ≤7 indicates increased hemorrhage risk and poor outcomes.
- **CTA and pCT**:
  - **CTA**: Visualizes craniocervical vasculature, localizes thrombus, assesses collateral flow, and characterizes atherosclerosis.

- **pCT**: Evaluates cerebral blood volume (CBV), cerebral blood flow (CBF), and mean transit time (MTT). The ischemic core shows reduced CBV and CBF, while the penumbra shows mismatched CBV and CBF with prolonged MTT.

Key Imaging Parameters (Table 5)

- **CBV**: Volume of blood in a given brain volume.
- **CBF**: Volume of blood flowing through a brain volume over time.
- **MTT**: Average time for blood to transit through the brain.
- **Color Scales**:
  - **CBV/CBF**: Well-perfused areas appear red/yellow; ischemic areas are blue/purple.
  - **MTT**: Abnormal transit time appears red; normal transit time appears blue.
- **Clinical Implications**: MCA infarct core volume of 70–100 mL predicts poor outcomes. The penumbra, with a mismatch between CBV and CBF, represents potentially salvageable tissue.

TABLE 5: CT perfusion parameters indicating ischemic core and penumbra.

Etiology	*CBF*	*CBV*	*WITT*	*TTP*
Infarct core	↓	↓	≥	↑
Ischemic penumbra	↓	↑	↑	↑

(CBF = cerebral blood flow, CBV = cerebral blood volume, MTT = mean transit time; TTP = time to peak, ↑ indicate increase, ↓ = indicate decrease)

- An important finding in patients having large MCA territorial infarcts is decreased perfusion in the contralateral cerebellar hemisphere with decreased cerebral blood flow, a phenomenon known as crossed cerebellar diaschisis.

5. Discuss the role of imaging and interventional radiology in stroke. [10] [MD (WBUHS) 23, MD (WBUHS) 22, AIIMS May 24]

A stroke, also known as a cerebrovascular event (CVA), is characterized by the sudden onset of neurological symptoms due to insufficient blood flow to the brain. Approximately 80% of all strokes are caused by cerebral ischemia or infarction. Due to their speed and availability, Nonenhanced computed tomography (NECT) and computed tomography angiography (CTA), with or without CT perfusion, are the most frequently utilized imaging modalities.

Acute stroke protocols depend on factors such as the time elapsed since the onset of symptoms, the availability of urgent imaging with appropriate software reconstructions, preferences of clinicians and radiologists, and access to neurointervention.

The "must know" questions in acute stroke triage that need to be answered are as follows **(Box 4)**.

BOX 4: The "must know" questions in acute stroke triage.

There are four "must know" questions in acute stroke triage that need to be answered rapidly and accurately.

1. Is intracranial hemorrhage or a stroke "mimic" present?
2. Is a large vessel occluded?
3. Is part of the brain irreversibly injured (i.e., is there a core of critically ischemic, irreversibly infarcted tissue)?
4. Is there a clinically relevant "penumbra" of ischemic but potentially salvageable tissue?

Pathophysiology

Brain Ischemia and Stroke Imaging Protocols

Core and Penumbra in Brain Ischemia*:*

- **Ischemic Core**: The central region of affected brain tissue during a stroke has a cerebral blood flow (CBF) of less than 6–8 cm^3/100 g/min. This area experiences neuronal death and irreversible loss of function.
- **Penumbra**: Surrounding the core, the penumbra is less severely ischemic, with CBF reduced from a normal 60 cm^3/100 g/min to 10–20 cm^3/100 g/min. This tissue is "at risk" but potentially salvageable.

Imaging Goals and Protocols

1. **Primary Objectives**:
    - Differentiate ischemic stroke from intracranial hemorrhage.
    - Select and triage patients for reperfusion therapies.
2. **Imaging Steps**:
    - **NECT**: Emergent nonenhanced CT (NECT) scans determine if intracranial hemorrhage or stroke mimics (e.g., subdural hematoma, neoplasm) are present.
    - **CTA**: CT angiography follows NECT if hemorrhage is excluded, identifying major vessel occlusions and active bleeding (e.g., "spot sign").
    - **MRA and DSA**: MR angiography can be affected by motion artifacts, making digital subtraction angiography (DSA) preferable for intra-arterial thrombolysis or mechanical thrombectomy.
    - **Perfusion Imaging**: CT or MR perfusion (pCT, pMR) studies assess the extent of irreversible damage and identify salvageable brain tissue (ischemic penumbra).

CT Findings and Protocols

- **Acute Stroke CT Protocol**:
    - Includes NECT, arch-to-vertex CTA, and dynamic first-pass perfusion CT (pCT).
    - Detects hyperattenuating vessels (e.g., "dense MCA" sign) and assesses grey- white matter interfaces.
    - **SPECTS Score**: The Alberta Stroke Program Early CT Score (ASPECTS) evaluates early ischemic changes by subtracting points for affected regions. An ASPECTS score ≤7 indicates increased hemorrhage risk and poor outcomes.
- **CTA and pCT**:
    - **CTA**: Visualizes craniocervical vasculature, localizes thrombus, assesses collateral flow, and characterizes atherosclerosis.
    - **pCT**: Evaluates cerebral blood volume (CBV), cerebral blood flow (CBF), and mean transit time (MTT). The ischemic core shows reduced CBV and CBF, while the penumbra shows mismatched CBV and CBF with prolonged MTT.

Key Imaging Parameters (Table 6)

- **CBV**: Volume of blood in a given brain volume.
- **CBF**: Volume of blood flowing through a brain volume over time.
- **MTT**: Average time for blood to transit through the brain.

TABLE 6: CT perfusion parameters indicating ischemic core and penumbra.

Etiology	*CBF*	*CBV*	*WITT*	*TTP*
Infarct core	↓	↓	≥	↑
Ischemic penumbra	↓	↑	↑	↑

(CBF = cerebral blood flow, CBV = cerebral blood volume, MTT = mean transit time; TTP = time to peak, ↑ indicate increase, ↓ = indicate decrease)

- **Color Scales**:
    - **CBV/CBF**: Well-perfused areas appear red/yellow; ischemic areas are blue/purple.
    - **MTT**: Abnormal transit time appears red; normal transit time appears blue.
- **Clinical Implications**: MCA infarct core volume of 70–100 mL predicts poor outcomes. The penumbra, with a mismatch between CBV and CBF, represents potentially salvageable tissue.
- An important finding in patients having large MCA territorial infarcts is decreased perfusion in the contralateral cerebellar hemisphere with decreased cerebral blood flow, a phenomenon known as crossed cerebellar diaschisis.

MRI Findings in Stroke

Preferred Modalities

- **CT/CTA/pCT**: Often chosen due to accessibility and speed. However, rapid stroke protocols using fast FLAIR, T2*, DWI, and pMR are also effective.
- **MRI Advantages**: Superior in detecting small vessel and brainstem ischemia. Useful in identifying the ischemic penumbra when there is a discrepancy between CT/CTA findings and clinical stroke severity.

Specific MRI Techniques and Findings

1. **T2/FLAIR**
   - **Early Detection**: Only 30–50% of acute strokes show cortical swelling and hyperintensity on FLAIR within the first 4 hours. Almost all strokes are FLAIR positive by 7 hours after symptom onset. T2 scans generally become positive within 12–24 hours.
   - **Intraarterial Hyperintensity**: An early stroke sign on FLAIR indicating slow flow, either from delayed antegrade flow or retrograde collateral filling.
   - **FLAIR-DWI Mismatch**: When FLAIR is negative, and DWI is positive, it suggests viable ischemic penumbra and eligibility for thrombolysis.
2. ***T2* GRE***
   - **Intraarterial Thrombus Detection**: "Blooming" hypointensity on T2* (GRE, SWI) indicates intraarterial thrombus.
   - **Chronic Hypertension or Amyloid Angiopathy**: "Blooming black dots" in older patients.
   - **Cerebral Microbleeds**: May increase the risk of anticoagulation-related hemorrhage.
3. **DWI and ADC**
   - **Hyperacute Infarcts**: Approximately 95% show diffusion restriction, with hyperintensity on DWI and corresponding hypointensity on ADC.
   - **Sensitivity**: DTI is even more sensitive than DWI, especially for pontine and medullary lesions.
   - **Negative DWI**: Does not rule out stroke, as 2–7% of patients with a final stroke diagnosis are initially DWI negative. Possible reasons include small (lacunar) infarcts, brainstem lesions, clot lysis with recanalization, and moderate or fluctuating hypoperfusion.
4. **pMR**
   - **DWI-PWI Mismatch**: DWI generally reflects the densely ischemic core of the infarct, while pMR shows the surrounding "at-risk" penumbra. A mismatch between DWI and PWI helps determine suitability for intraarterial thrombolysis.

By using these MRI techniques, clinicians can better identify and differentiate between the core and penumbra of an infarct, thereby guiding appropriate treatment decisions.

Stroke Algorithm **(Flowchart 2)**.

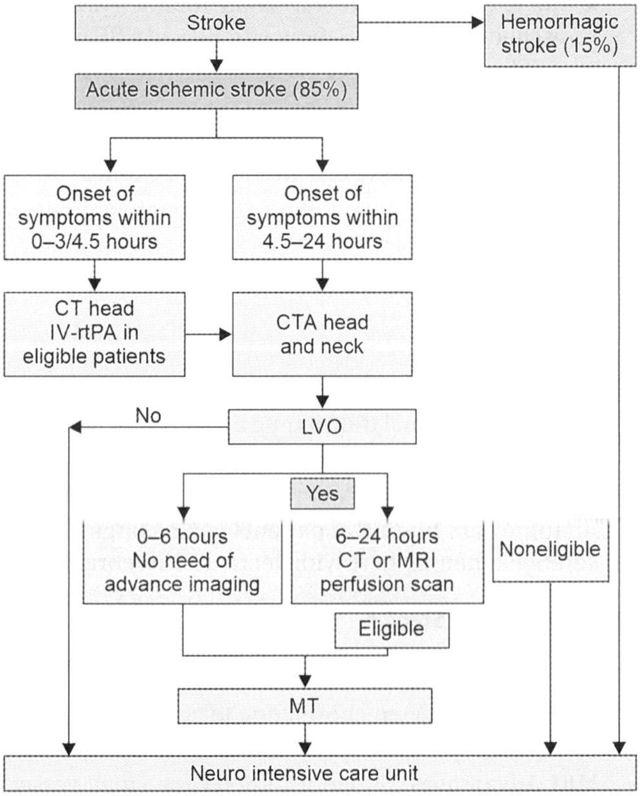

FLOWCHART 2: Stroke algorithm *(For Color Version Refer Flowchart1)*.

Treatment Options

The single most important factor in successful intervention is patient selection, with the two most important considerations being (1) elapsed time from symptom onset and (2) imaging findings on the screening NECT scan.

1. IV thrombolysis is done by recombinant tissue plasminogen activator (rTPA). There are several studies regarding rtpa dose, therapeutic window and effectiveness. The clinically accepted therapeutic window for intravenous recombinant tissue plasminogen activator (rTPA) is less than 3 hours from ictus (the "golden hours"). A dose 0.6 mg/kg is used in Japan and other Asian countries.
2. Intraarterial thrombolysis is typically restricted to less than 6 hours. Exceptions to this general rule include basilar artery thrombosis and patients outside the 6-hour window who have a persistent significant perfusion-diffusion mismatch.

3. Mechanical thrombectomy is suitable in patients beyond the therapeutic window or in whom thrombolytic therapy is contraindicated.[4] However, it is rare that a patient may benefit from thrombectomy if the procedure starts >8 hours after onset in the anterior circulation and >24 hours after onset in the posterior circulation.

Mechanical Thrombectomy Treatment Protocol

Sedation and Anesthesia

Conscious Sedation (CS): Preferred over general anesthesia (GA) due to faster procedure times and better patient control. CS avoids the hypotension commonly induced by GA, which can be detrimental to acute stroke patients relying on high cerebral perfusion pressure via pial collaterals.

Anticoagulation

Standard Heparin Flushes: No additional anticoagulation or antiaggregation required during thrombectomy, except for standard heparin flushes (e.g., 5 IU/mL). Permanent stenting should be avoided due to the increased risk of reperfusion hematomas or hemorrhagic conversion.

Procedure in Anterior Circulation

- **Stent Retrievers**: Safe to use up to the M2 segments in most patients.
- **Posterior Circulation**: Typically, thrombectomy is not needed beyond the P1 segment.

Procedural Steps (Fig. 11)

1. **Groin Puncture**: Use a long (80 cm) 8 F introducer sheath placed in the common carotid artery (CCA) with a 5 F diagnostic catheter (DC) and a 0.035" (0.89 mm) guidewire (GW).
2. **Balloon Guide Catheter (BGC)**: Position an 8 F BGC in the internal carotid artery. BGC allows for flow reversal, reducing the risk of thrombo-emboli escaping into collateral areas.
3. **Microcatheter Introduction**: After confirming the clot position with contrast injection, introduce a microcatheter with a microguidewire, passing the thrombus if possible while keeping the microguidewire retracted.
4. **Stent Retriever Deployment**: Release the stent retriever centered at the clot, preferably more distal than proximal, covering the proximal clot boundary. Leave it to expand and "incubate" for at least 5 minutes.
5. **Resheathing and Aspiration**: Readvance the microcatheter, partially resheath the stent retriever to the face of the thrombus, inflate the balloon, and pull back the stent retriever with simultaneous aspiration in the BGC. Gradually escalate and maximize aspiration as the device enters the guide's orifice.
6. **Thrombus Retrieval**: Remove the rotating hemostatic valve (RHV), take out the device to check for thrombus, and apply further aspiration directly to the BGC to clear any remaining small thrombi before deflating the balloon.
7. **Procedure Control**: Verify the procedure's outcome with a contrast injection in the BGC, rinse and clean the device, reconnect the RHV, and repeat the thrombectomy maneuver if necessary. Typically, the same stent retriever can be used up to three times.

Posterior Circulation Adaptations

Guide Catheter: Use a long, soft 6–7 F guide catheter (e.g., Navien, Fargo, Neuron) to advance up to the vertebrobasilar junction, as advancing an 8 F guide catheter into the vertebral arteries can be challenging.

By adhering to this protocol, mechanical thrombectomy can be effectively and safely performed, ensuring optimal outcomes for patients with acute ischemic stroke.

Among hemorrhagic strokes, interventional radiology plays a vital role in the management of **nontraumatic subarachnoid hemorrhage**.

Imaging in Nontraumatic Subarachnoid Hemorrhage

CT Findings

- **Distribution**: The pattern of subarachnoid hemorrhage depends on the aneurysm location.
  - **Anterior Communicating Artery Aneurysms**: Usually rupture into the anterior interhemispheric fissure.
  - **Middle Cerebral Artery Bifurcation Aneurysms**: Typically rupture into the Sylvian fissure.

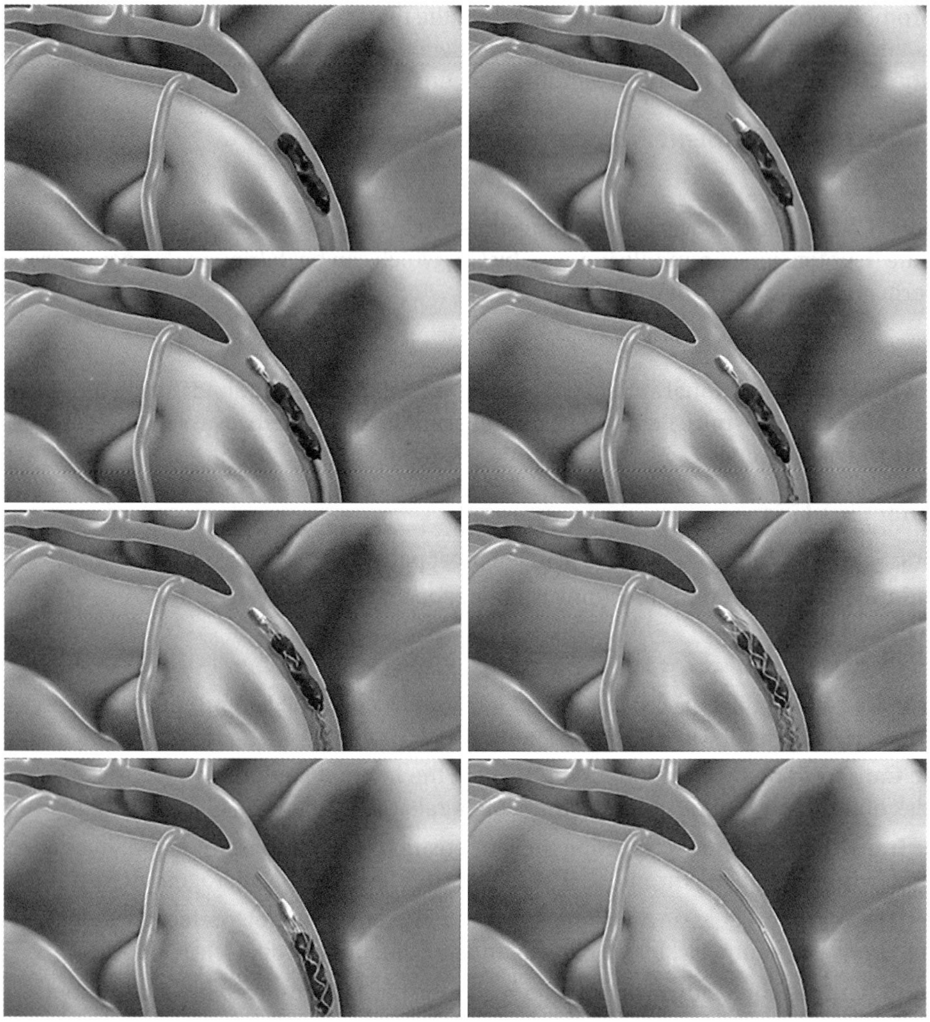

FIG. 11: Schematic diagram representing standard technique of mechanical thrombectomy *(For Color Version Refer Fig. 8)*.

- **Internal Carotid and Posterior Communicating Artery Aneurysms**: Rupture into the suprasellar cistern.
- **Vertebrobasilar Aneurysms**: Often bleed into the fourth ventricle and prepontine cistern.
- **Intraventricular Hemorrhage**: Present in about 50% of patients with subarachnoid hemorrhage.
- **Focal Parenchymal Hemorrhage**: If present, indicates the rupture site of the aneurysm. Rarely, a focal hematoma within the subarachnoid space is seen as bleeding from the aneurysm.

These imaging findings assist in diagnosing, locating, and managing subarachnoid hemorrhage effectively.

Stepwise increases in modified Fisher grade **(Box 5)** have a moderately linear relationship with the risk of vasospasm, delayed infarction, and poor clinical outcome.

BOX 5: Modified Fisher scale to grade aneurysmal subarachnoid hemorrhage.

A simple scale based on NECT findings, the modified Fisher scale, has been proposed to grade aneurysmal subarachnoid hemorrhage.

- Grade 0: No visible SAH or IVH
- Grade 1: Focal or diffuse thin (less than 1 mm) layer of subarachnoid blood without IVH
- Grade 2: Focal or diffuse thin (less than 1 mm) layer of subarachnoid blood with IVH
- Grade 3: Focal or diffuse thick (more than 1 mm) SAH without IVH
- Grade 4: Focal or diffuse thick (more than 1 mm) SAH with IVH

MR Findings and Angiography in Subarachnoid Hemorrhage (SAH)

MRI Findings

Acute SAH: Best visualized on FLAIR sequences.

Angiography

- **CT Angiography**: Detects aneurysms 2 mm or larger in 95% of aneurysmal subarachnoid hemorrhage cases.
- **DSA**: Remains the gold standard for identifying and detailing aneurysm angioarchitecture. If initial CT angiography is negative, consider performing DSA. Repeat DSA or CTA is recommended for diffuse-type SAH when initial DSA is negative.

Specific Types of Non aneurysmal SAH

- **Perimesencephalic SAH (pnSAH)**: Usually found in the interpeduncular, ambient, and prepontine cisterns. Rarely affects the posterior aspect of the suprasellar cistern.
- **Convexal SAH (cSAH)**: Located in superficial cerebral sulci. Possible causes include cortical vein occlusion, vasculitis, amyloid angiopathy, and reversible cerebral vasoconstriction syndrome (RCVS).

Role of Interventional Radiology

Imaging Considerations

- **Aneurysm Details**: Location, size, shape, and neck size.
- **Parent Vessel Anatomy**: Includes the presence or absence of intraluminal thrombus.
- **Access Vessel Anatomy**: Factors such as dominant vs. hypoplastic vertebral artery or ACA, degree of tortuosity, atherosclerosis, or fibromuscular dysplasia.

Procedure Planning

1. **Choice of Access Artery**.
2. **Endovascular Technique**: Options include primary embolization, stent-assisted or balloon-assisted coiling, and flow diversion.[5]
3. **Device Types and Sizes**.

   Coiling Technique (Figs. 12A to C)

   - **Guide Catheter**: Examples include Neuron™ 0.053 in., Benchmark™ 0.071 in., and Neuron™ MAX 0.088 in. Positioned just below the skull base.
   - **Intraprocedure Medication**:
     - **Heparin**: 2,500 IU in the flush bag (500 mL of warmed normal saline).
     - **Systemic Heparin**: 5,000 IU administered during coiling.
     - **Nimodipine**: Administered as a bolus and maintained with an infusion if angiographic vasospasm is detected. Dose: 2 mg per territory, split into 1 mg IA bolus and 1 mg in the flush bag.
   - **Microcatheters**: Options include Excelsior® SL-10, Echelon™ 10, Excelsior® XT-17®, Excelsior® 1018®, and Marksman™.
   - **Microwires**: Options include Synchro®-14 0.014 in., Neuroscout®-14 0.014 in., and Transend™ EX 0.014 in. with a floppy tip.

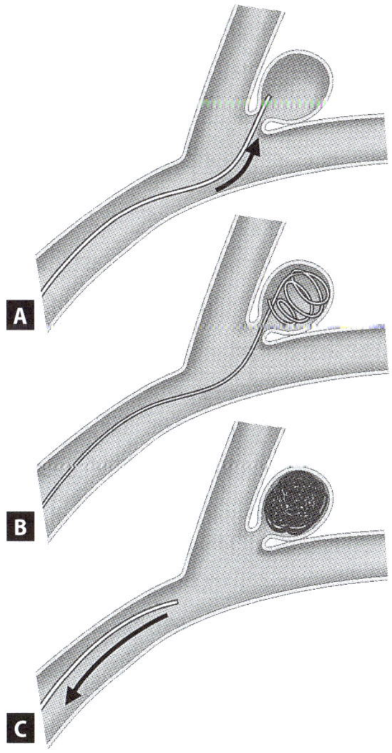

FIGS. 12A TO C: Schematic diagram representing standard technique of aneurysm coiling *(For Color Version Refer Fig. 9)*.

Coil Types

- **Framing Coils**: Diameter should closely match the mean diameter of the aneurysm sac.
- **Filling Coils**.
- **Finishing Coils**.

Catheter Withdrawal: Carefully remove the microcatheter to avoid displacing the deployed coils.

Follow-Up: Conduct follow-up with an MRI (TOF-MRA) or DSA after 6 months.
These detailed imaging findings and procedural steps help ensure accurate diagnosis and effective treatment of subarachnoid hemorrhage.

6. A 30-year-old man is brought to the emergency department with symptoms of acute stroke with onset 1 hour back. Discuss the imaging evaluation in such a case. Describe the role of interventional radiology in acute ischemic stroke. [6+4]

A stroke, also known as a cerebrovascular event (CVA), is characterized by the sudden onset of neurological symptoms due to insufficient blood flow to the brain. Approximately 80% of all strokes are caused by cerebral ischemia or infarction. Due to their speed and availability, nonenhanced computed tomography (NECT) and computed tomography angiography (CTA), with or without CT perfusion, are the most frequently utilized imaging modalities. Acute stroke protocols depend on factors such as the time elapsed since the onset of symptoms, the availability of urgent imaging with appropriate software reconstructions, preferences of clinicians and radiologists, and access to neurointervention.

The "must know" questions in acute stroke triage that need to be answered are as follows **(Box 6)**:

BOX 6: The "must know" questions in acute stroke triage.

There are four "must know" questions in acute stroke triage that need to be answered rapidly and accurately.

- Is intracranial hemorrhage or a stroke "mimic" present?
- Is a large vessel occluded?
- Is part of the brain irreversibly injured (i.e., is there a core of critically ischemic, irreversibly infarcted tissue)?
- Is there a clinically relevant "penumbra" of ischemic but potentially salvageable tissue?

Pathophysiology

Brain Ischemia and Stroke Imaging Protocols

Core and Penumbra in Brain Ischemia

- **Ischemic Core**: The central region of affected brain tissue during a stroke has a cerebral blood flow (CBF) of less than 6–8 cm^3/100 g/min. This area experiences neuronal death and irreversible loss of function.
- **Penumbra**: Surrounding the core, the penumbra is less severely ischemic, with CBF reduced from a normal 60 cm^3/100 g/min to 10–20 cm^3/100 g/min. This tissue is "at risk" but potentially salvageable.

Imaging Goals and Protocols

1. **Primary Objectives**:
   - Differentiate ischemic stroke from intracranial hemorrhage.
   - Select and triage patients for reperfusion therapies.
2. **Imaging Steps**:
   - **NECT**: Emergent nonenhanced CT (NECT) scans determine if intracranial hemorrhage or stroke mimics (e.g., subdural hematoma, neoplasm) are present.
   - **CTA**: CT angiography follows NECT if hemorrhage is excluded, identifying major vessel occlusions and active bleeding (e.g., "spot sign").
   - **MRA and DSA**: MR angiography can be affected by motion artifacts, making digital subtraction angiography (DSA) preferable for intra-arterial thrombolysis or mechanical thrombectomy.
   - **Perfusion Imaging**: CT or MR perfusion (pCT, pMR) studies assess the extent of irreversible damage and identify salvageable brain tissue (ischemic penumbra).

CT Findings and Protocols

- **Acute Stroke CT Protocol**:
  - Includes NECT, arch-to-vertex CTA, and dynamic first-pass perfusion CT (pCT).
  - Detects hyperattenuating vessels (e.g., "dense MCA" sign) and assesses grey- white matter interfaces.

- **ASPECTS Score**: The Alberta Stroke Program Early CT Score (ASPECTS) evaluates early ischemic changes by subtracting points for affected regions. An ASPECTS score ≤7 indicates increased hemorrhage risk and poor outcomes.
- **CTA and pCT**:
  - **CTA**: Visualizes craniocervical vasculature, localizes thrombus, assesses collateral flow, and characterizes atherosclerosis.
  - **pCT**: Evaluates cerebral blood volume (CBV), cerebral blood flow (CBF), and mean transit time (MTT). The ischemic core shows reduced CBV and CBF, while the penumbra shows mismatched CBV and CBF with prolonged MTT.

Key Imaging Parameters (Table 7)

- **CBV**: Volume of blood in a given brain volume.
- **CBF**: Volume of blood flowing through a brain volume over time.
- **MTT**: Average time for blood to transit through the brain.
- **Color Scales**:
  - **CBV/CBF**: Well-perfused areas appear red/yellow; ischemic areas are blue/purple.
  - **MTT**: Abnormal transit time appears red; normal transit time appears blue.

TABLE 7: CT perfusion parameters indicating ischemic core and penumbra.

Etiology	*CBF*	*CBV*	*WITT*	*TTP*
Infarct core	↓	↓	≥	↑
Ischemic penumbra	↓	↑	↑	↑

(CBF = cerebral blood flow, CBV = cerebral blood volume, MTT = mean transit time; TTP = time to peak, ↑ indicate increase, ↓ = indicate decrease)

- **Clinical Implications**: MCA infarct core volume of 70–100 mL predicts poor outcomes. The penumbra, with a mismatch between CBV and CBF, represents potentially salvageable tissue.
  - An important finding in patients having large MCA territorial infarcts is decreased perfusion in the contralateral cerebellar hemisphere with decreased cerebral blood flow, a phenomenon known as crossed cerebellar diaschisis.

MRI Findings in Stroke

Preferred Modalities

- **CT/CTA/pCT**: Often chosen due to accessibility and speed. However, rapid stroke protocols using fast FLAIR, T2*, DWI, and pMR are also effective.
- **MRI Advantages**: Superior in detecting small vessel and brainstem ischemia. Useful in identifying the ischemic penumbra when there is a discrepancy between CT/CTA findings and clinical stroke severity.

Specific MRI Techniques and Findings

1. **T2/FLAIR**
   - **Early Detection**: Only 30–50% of acute strokes show cortical swelling and hyperintensity on FLAIR within the first 4 hours. Almost all strokes are FLAIR positive by 7 hours after symptom onset. T2 scans generally become positive within 12–24 hours.
   - **Intraarterial Hyperintensity**: An early stroke sign on FLAIR indicating slow flow, either from delayed antegrade flow or retrograde collateral filling.
   - **FLAIR-DWI Mismatch**: When FLAIR is negative, and DWI is positive, it suggests viable ischemic penumbra and eligibility for thrombolysis.
2. ***T2* GRE***
   - **Intraarterial Thrombus Detection**: "Blooming" hypointensity on T2* (GRE, SWI) indicates intraarterial thrombus.
   - **Chronic Hypertension or Amyloid Angiopathy**: "Blooming black dots" in older patients.
   - **Cerebral Microbleeds**: May increase the risk of anticoagulation-related hemorrhage.
3. **DWI and ADC**
   - **Hyperacute Infarcts**: Approximately 95% show diffusion restriction, with hyperintensity on DWI and corresponding hypointensity on ADC.
   - **Sensitivity**: DTI is even more sensitive than DWI, especially for pontine and medullary lesions.

- **Negative DWI**: Does not rule out stroke, as 2–7% of patients with a final stroke diagnosis are initially DWI negative. Possible reasons include small (lacunar) infarcts, brainstem lesions, clot lysis with recanalization, and moderate or fluctuating hypoperfusion.

4. **pMR**
   - **DWI-PWI Mismatch**: DWI generally reflects the densely ischemic core of the infarct, while pMR shows the surrounding "at-risk" penumbra. A mismatch between DWI and PWI helps determine suitability for intraarterial thrombolysis.

By using these MRI techniques, clinicians can better identify and differentiate between the core and penumbra of an infarct, thereby guiding appropriate treatment decisions.

Stroke Algorithm **(Flowchart 3)**.

Treatment Options

The single most important factor in successful intervention is patient selection, with the two most important considerations being (1) elapsed time from symptom onset and (2) imaging findings on the screening NECT scan.

1. IV thrombolysis is done by recombinant tissue plasminogen activator (rtpa). There are several studies regarding rtpa dose, therapeutic window and effectiveness. The clinically accepted therapeutic window for intravenous recombinant tissue plasminogen activator (rTPA) is less than 3 hours from ictus (the "golden hours"). A dose 0.6 mg/kg is used in Japan and other Asian countries.
2. Intraarterial thrombolysis is typically restricted to less than 6 hours. Exceptions to this general rule include basilar artery thrombosis and patients outside the 6-hour window who have a persistent significant perfusion-diffusion mismatch.
3. Mechanical thrombectomy is suitable in patients beyond the therapeutic window or in whom thrombolytic therapy is contraindicated. However, it is rare that a patient may benefit from thrombectomy if the procedure starts >8 hours after onset in the anterior circulation and >24 hours after onset in the posterior circulation.

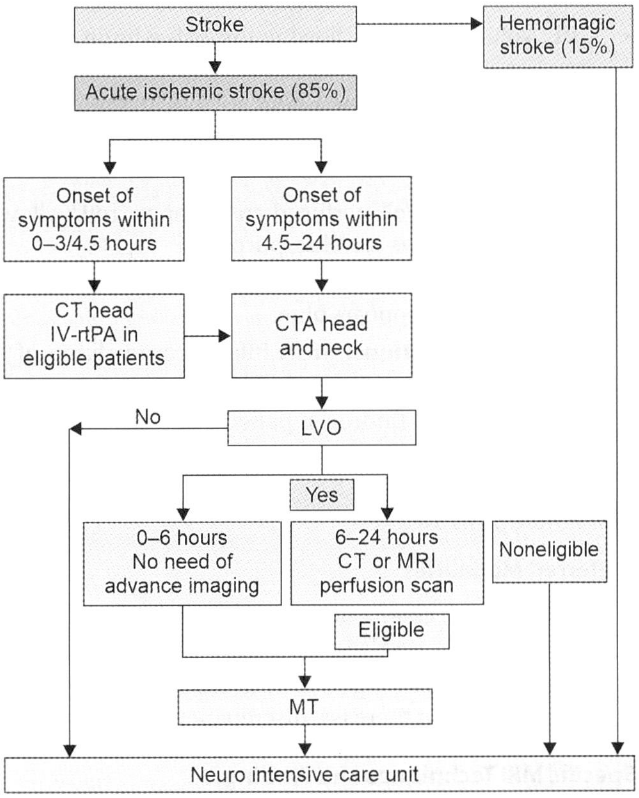

FLOWCHART 3: Stroke algorithm *(For Color Version Refer Flowchart 1)*.

Mechanical Thrombectomy Treatment Protocol

Sedation and Anesthesia

- **Conscious Sedation (CS)**: Preferred over general anesthesia (GA) due to faster procedure times and better patient control. CS avoids the hypotension commonly induced by GA, which can be detrimental to acute stroke patients relying on high cerebral perfusion pressure via pial collaterals.

Anticoagulation

- **Standard Heparin Flushes**: No additional anticoagulation or antiaggregation required during thrombectomy, except for standard heparin flushes (e.g., 5 IU/mL). Permanent stenting should be avoided due to the increased risk of reperfusion hematomas or hemorrhagic conversion.

Procedure in Anterior Circulation

- **Stent Retrievers**: Safe to use up to the M2 segments in most patients.
- **Posterior Circulation**: Typically, thrombectomy is not needed beyond the P1 segment.

Procedural Steps (Fig. 13)

1. **Groin Puncture**: Use a long (80 cm) 8 F introducer sheath placed in the common carotid artery (CCA) with a 5 F diagnostic catheter (DC) and a 0.035" (0.89 mm) guidewire (GW).

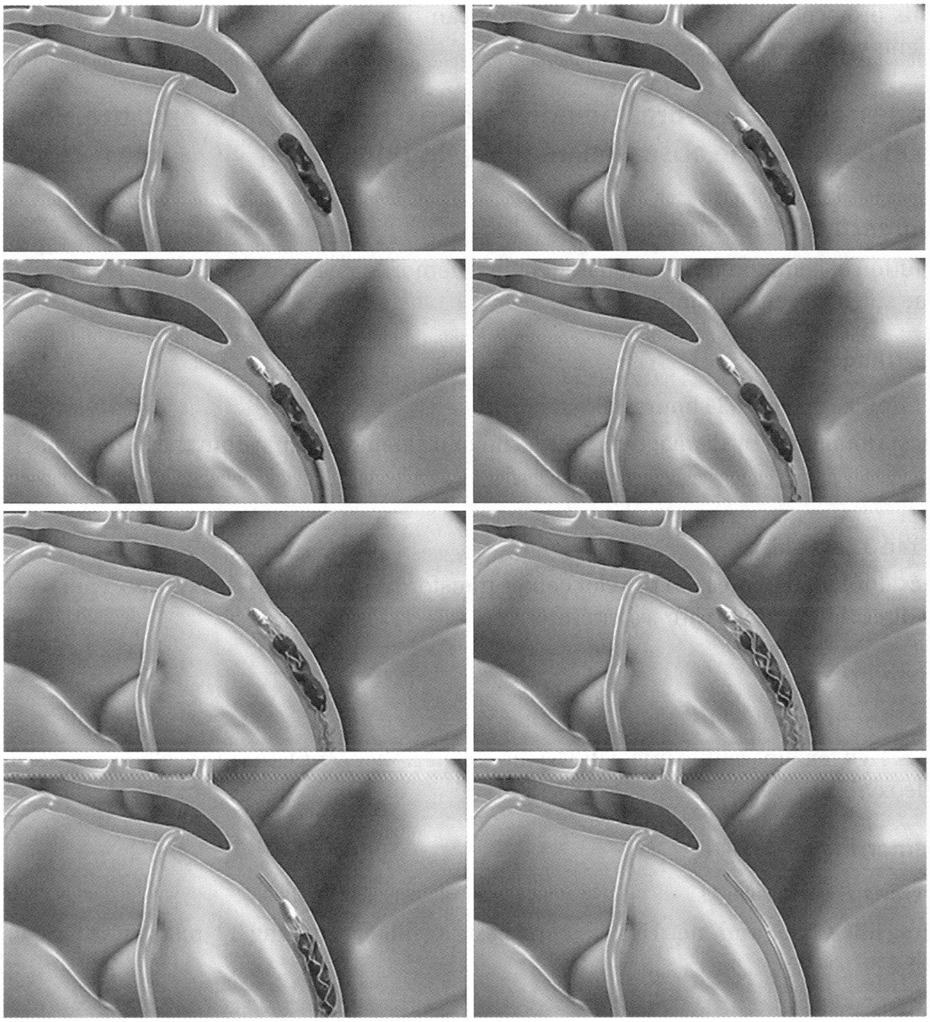

FIG. 13: Schematic diagram representing standard technique of mechanical thrombectomy *(For Color Version Refer Fig. 8).*

2. **Balloon Guide Catheter (BGC)**: Position an 8 F BGC in the internal carotid artery. BGC allows for flow reversal, reducing the risk of thrombo-emboli escaping into collateral areas.
3. **Microcatheter Introduction**: After confirming the clot position with contrast injection, introduce a microcatheter with a microguidewire, passing the thrombus if possible while keeping the microguidewire retracted.
4. **Stent Retriever Deployment**: Release the stent retriever centered at the clot, preferably more distal than proximal, covering the proximal clot boundary. Leave it to expand and "incubate" for at least 5 minutes.
5. **Resheathing and Aspiration**: Readvance the microcatheter, partially resheath the stent retriever to the face of the thrombus, inflate the balloon, and pull back the stent retriever with simultaneous aspiration in the BGC. Gradually escalate and maximize aspiration as the device enters the guide's orifice.
6. **Thrombus Retrieval**: Remove the rotating hemostatic valve (RHV), take out the device to check for thrombus, and apply further aspiration directly to the BGC to clear any remaining small thrombi before deflating the balloon.
7. **Procedure Control**: Verify the procedure's outcome with a contrast injection in the BGC, rinse and clean the device, reconnect the RHV, and repeat the thrombectomy maneuver if necessary. Typically, the same stent retriever can be used up to three times.

Posterior Circulation Adaptations

- **Guide Catheter**: Use a long, soft 6–7 F guide catheter (e.g., Navien, Fargo, Neuron) to advance up to the vertebrobasilar junction, as advancing an 8 F guide catheter into the vertebral arteries can be challenging.

By adhering to this protocol, mechanical thrombectomy can be effectively and safely performed, ensuring optimal outcomes for patients with acute ischemic stroke.

7. Various stages of intracerebral hemorrhage as seen on MRI and the underlying pathophysiological basis for the observed imaging findings. [2+3]

Stages of Intraparenchymal Hemorrhage

The temporal evolution of hematomas in intraparenchymal hemorrhage is classified into five stages: Hyperacute, acute, early subacute, late subacute, and chronic.

Hyperacute Hemorrhage

- **Time Frame**: Minutes to under 24 hours.
- **Characteristics**: Dominated by diamagnetic intracellular oxyhemoglobin within the hematoma.

Acute Hemorrhage

- **Time Frame**: 1 to 3 days old.
- **Characteristics**: Profound hypoxia in the clot center transforms oxy-Hgb to deoxy-Hgb, which is paramagnetic but shielded from direct interactions with water protons.

Early Subacute Hemorrhage

- **Time Frame**: 3 days to 1 week old.
- **Characteristics**: Hgb remains within intact RBCs; the clot periphery contains intracellular met-Hgb, while the center persists with deoxy-Hgb.

Late Subacute Hemorrhage

- **Time Frame**: One to several weeks.
- **Characteristics**: RBCs lyse, and met-Hgb becomes extracellular, reducing T1 relaxation time and prolonging T2 relaxation time.

Chronic Hemorrhage

- **Time Frame**: Months to years.
- **Characteristics**: Heme proteins are stored as ferritin in macrophages or as hemosiderin if storage capacity is exceeded, causing strong magnetic susceptibility.

Imaging of Intracranial Parenchymal Hemorrhage (Table 8)

The imaging appearance of intraparenchymal hemorrhage on MR depends on intrinsic and extrinsic factors:

TABLE 8: Imaging of different stages of intracranial parenchymal hemorrhage.

Imaging the Stages of Intraparenchymal Hemorrhage

Stage	*Time (Range)*	*Blood Products*	*CT*	*T1*	*T2*	*T2**	*DWI*	*ADC*
Hyperacute	<24 hours	Oxy-Hgb	Hyperdense	Isointense	Bright	Rim "blooms"	Bright	Dark
Acute	1–3 days	Deoxy-Hgb	Hyperdense	Isointense	Dark	↑ "blooming"	Dark	Dark
Early subacute	>3 days to 1 week	Intracellular met-Hgb	Isodense	Bright	Dark	Very dark	Dark	Dark
Late subacute	1 week to months	Extracellular met-Hgb	Hypodense	Bright	Bright	Dark rim, variable center	Bright	Dark
Chronic	>14 days (≥months)	Hemosiderin	Hypodense	Dark	Dark	Dark	Dark	Dark

Intrinsic Factors

- **Clot Structure**: Macroscopic structure of the clot.
- **RBC Integrity**: Integrity of red blood cells.
- **Hgb Oxygenation Status**: State of hemoglobin oxygenation.
- **RBC Concentration and Tissue pH**: Influences signal intensity.
- **Bleeding Source**: Arterial or venous origin.
- **Blood-Brain Barrier Integrity**: Affects imaging appearance.

Extrinsic Factors

- **Pulse Sequence and Parameters**: Affects imaging results.
- **Receiver Bandwidth and Magnet Field Strength**: Contributes to image quality.

Specific Imaging Findings

1. **Hyperacute Hemorrhage**:
   - **Oxy-Hgb**: Diamagnetic, dependent on water content.
   - **T1WI**: Isointense to slightly hypointense to gray matter.
   - **T2**: Generally, hyperintense but can be heterogeneous.
2. **Acute Hemorrhage**:
   - **Deoxyhemoglobin**: Paramagnetic with four unpaired electrons.
   - **T2WI**: Hypointense due to deoxyhemoglobin.
   - **T1WI**: Low/intermediate signal intensity.
3. **Early Subacute Hemorrhage**:
   - **Intracellular Methemoglobin**: At the clot periphery.
   - **T1WI**: Hyperintense rim surrounding an isointense to slightly hypointense core.
   - **T2WI**: Hypointense due to paramagnetic methemoglobin.
4. **Late Subacute Hemorrhage**:
   - **Extracellular Methemoglobin**: Determines signal intensity.
   - **T1WI and T2WI**: Clots appear very hyperintense on both sequences.
5. **Chronic Hemorrhage**:
   - **Intracellular Ferritin and Hemosiderin**: Hypointense on T1WI and T2WI.
   - **T2***: Hyperintense cavity with a "blooming" rim may persist.
   - **Residual Scar**: Eventually, a slit-like scar remains.

8. Causes of SAH and imaging. [10] [DNB June 22]

Subarachnoid Hemorrhage (SAH): Types and Imaging

Types of Subarachnoid Hemorrhage

1. **Traumatic Subarachnoid Hemorrhage**:
   - **Prevalence**: Commonly found in cases of moderate to severe head trauma.
   - **Frequency**: Trauma is the leading cause of subarachnoid hemorrhage.
   - **Associated Condition**: Rarely, intraocular hemorrhage (Terson syndrome) is linked with traumatic subarachnoid hemorrhage.
2. **Nontraumatic Subarachnoid Hemorrhage**:
   - **Prevalence**: Accounts for about 3–5% of all acute stroke cases.
   - **Major Cause**: Approximately 80% are due to ruptured intracranial aneurysms.

- **Other Causes**: Includes dissections, vasculitis, venous thrombosis, hemorrhage, reversible cerebral vasoconstriction syndrome, and amyloid angiopathy.

Imaging in Traumatic Subarachnoid Hemorrhage

1. **CT Findings**:
    - **Appearance**: Acute traumatic subarachnoid hemorrhage appears as peripheral, linear hyperdensities in the sulci adjacent to cortical contusions or beneath epidural or subdural hematomas.
    - **Rare Presentation**: Isolated traumatic subarachnoid hemorrhage may sometimes be found in the interpeduncular fossa.
2. **MR Findings**:
    - **Acute Stage**: Identifying acute blood on T1-weighted images (T1WI) can be challenging. FLAIR scans reveal hyperintensity in the affected sulci. "Blooming" on T2* scans adjacent to cortical contusions.
    - **Chronic Stage**: Leads to focal superficial siderosis along gyral crests and sulcal spaces.

Differential Diagnosis for Traumatic SAH

1. **Sulcal-Cisternal Hyperintensity**: Can be due to meningitis, artifact (incomplete CSF suppression), neoplasm, contrast leak (e.g., with renal failure), high inspired oxygen during general anesthesia, hyperintense vessels with slow flow (e.g., acute arterial strokes, Sturge-Weber syndrome), pial collaterals post cerebral ischemia-infarction, Moyamoya disease ['Ivy' Sign], and reversible cerebral vasoconstriction syndrome (RCVS).
2. **Pseudosubarachnoid Hemorrhage**: Describes the CT appearance of a brain with severe cerebral edema, where hypodense brain parenchyma makes circulating blood in arteries and veins appear relatively hyperdense.

Imaging in Nontraumatic Subarachnoid Hemorrhage

CT Findings

- **Distribution**: The pattern of subarachnoid hemorrhage depends on the aneurysm location.
    - **Anterior Communicating Artery Aneurysms**: Usually rupture into the anterior interhemispheric fissure.
    - **Middle Cerebral Artery Bifurcation Aneurysms**: Typically rupture into the Sylvian fissure.
    - **Internal Carotid and Posterior Communicating Artery Aneurysms**: Rupture into the suprasellar cistern.
    - **Vertebrobasilar Aneurysms**: Often bleed into the fourth ventricle and prepontine cistern.
- **Intraventricular Hemorrhage**: Present in about 50% of patients with subarachnoid hemorrhage.
- **Focal Parenchymal Hemorrhage**: If present, indicates the rupture site of the aneurysm. Rarely, a focal hematoma within the subarachnoid space is seen as bleeding from the aneurysm.

These imaging findings assist in diagnosing, locating, and managing subarachnoid hemorrhage effectively.

Stepwise increases in modified Fisher grade **(Box 7)** have a moderately linear relationship with the risk of vasospasm, delayed infarction, and poor clinical outcome.

BOX 7: Modified Fisher scale to grade aneurysmal subarachnoid hemorrhage.

A simple scale based on NECT findings, the modified Fisher scale, has been proposed to grade aneurysmal subarachnoid hemorrhage.

- Grade 0: No visible SAH or IVH
- Grade 1: Focal or diffuse thin (less than 1 mm) layer of subarachnoid blood without IVH
- Grade 2: Focal or diffuse thin (less than 1 mm) layer of subarachnoid blood with IVH
- Grade 3: Focal or diffuse thick (more than 1 mm) SAH without IVH
- Grade 4: Focal or diffuse thick (more than 1 mm) SAH with IVH

MR Findings and Angiography in Subarachnoid Hemorrhage (SAH)

MRI Findings

Acute SAH: Best visualized on FLAIR sequences.

Angiography

- **CT Angiography**: Detects aneurysms 2 mm or larger in 95% of aneurysmal subarachnoid hemorrhage cases.
- **DSA**: Remains the gold standard for identifying and detailing aneurysm angioarchitecture. If initial CT angiography is negative, consider performing DSA. Repeat DSA or CTA is recommended for diffuse-type SAH when initial DSA is negative.

Specific Types of Nonaneurysmal SAH

- **Perimesencephalic SAH (pnSAH)**: Usually found in the interpeduncular, ambient, and prepontine cisterns. Rarely affects the posterior aspect of the suprasellar cistern.
- **Convexal SAH (cSAH)**: Located in superficial cerebral sulci. Possible causes include cortical vein occlusion, vasculitis, amyloid angiopathy, and reversible cerebral vasoconstriction syndrome (RCVS).

9. CT in ischemic stroke. [10] [DNB Dec 21]

Brain Ischemia and Stroke Imaging Protocols

Core and Penumbra in Brain Ischemia

- **Ischemic Core**: The central region of affected brain tissue during a stroke has a cerebral blood flow (CBF) of less than 6–8 $cm^3/100$ g/min. This area experiences neuronal death and irreversible loss of function.
- **Penumbra**: Surrounding the core, the penumbra is less severely ischemic, with CBF reduced from a normal 60 $cm^3/100$ g/min to 10–20 $cm^3/100$ g/min. This tissue is "at risk" but potentially salvageable.

Imaging Goals and Protocols

1. **Primary Objectives**:
   - Differentiate ischemic stroke from intracranial hemorrhage.
   - Select and triage patients for reperfusion therapies.
2. **Imaging Steps**:
   - **NECT**: Emergent nonenhanced CT (NECT) scans determine if intracranial hemorrhage or stroke mimics (e.g., subdural hematoma, neoplasm) are present.
   - **CTA**: CT angiography follows NECT if hemorrhage is excluded, identifying major vessel occlusions and active bleeding (e.g., "spot sign").
   - **MRA and DSA**: MR angiography can be affected by motion artifacts, making digital subtraction angiography (DSA) preferable for intra-arterial thrombolysis or mechanical thrombectomy.
   - **Perfusion Imaging**: CT or MR perfusion (pCT, pMR) studies assess the extent of irreversible damage and identify salvageable brain tissue (ischemic penumbra).

CT Findings and Protocols

- **Acute Stroke CT Protocol**:
  - Includes NECT, arch-to-vertex CTA, and dynamic first-pass perfusion CT (pCT).
  - Detects hyperattenuating vessels (e.g., "dense MCA" sign) and assesses grey- white matter interfaces.
- **ASPECTS Score**: The Alberta Stroke Program Early CT Score (ASPECTS) evaluates early ischemic changes by subtracting points for affected regions. An ASPECTS score ≤ 7 indicates increased hemorrhage risk and poor outcomes.
- **CTA and pCT**:
  - **CTA**: Visualizes craniocervical vasculature, localizes thrombus, assesses collateral flow, and characterizes atherosclerosis.
  - **pCT**: Evaluates cerebral blood volume (CBV), cerebral blood flow (CBF), and mean transit time (MTT). The ischemic core shows reduced CBV and CBF, while the penumbra shows mismatched CBV and CBF with prolonged MTT.

Key Imaging Parameters (Table 9)

- **CBV**: Volume of blood in a given brain volume.
- **CBF**: Volume of blood flowing through a brain volume over time.
- **MTT**: Average time for blood to transit through the brain.
- **Color Scales**:
  - **CBV/CBF**: Well-perfused areas appear red/yellow; ischemic areas are blue/purple.
  - **MTT**: Abnormal transit time appears red; normal transit time appears blue.
- **Clinical Implications**: MCA infarct core volume of 70–100 mL predicts poor outcomes. The penumbra, with a mismatch between CBV and CBF, represents potentially salvageable tissue.

TABLE 9: CT perfusion parameters indicating ischemic core and penumbra.

Etiology	*CBF*	*CBV*	*WITT*	*TTP*
Infarct core	↓	↓	≥	↑
Ischemic penumbra	↓	↑	↑	↑

(CBF = cerebral blood flow, CBV = cerebral blood volume, MTT = mean transit time; TTP = time to peak, ↑ indicate increase, ↓ = indicate decrease)

An important finding in patients having large MCA territorial infarcts is decreased perfusion in the contralateral cerebellar hemisphere with decreased cerebral blood flow, a phenomenon known as crossed cerebellar diaschisis.

10. Discuss in brief, the salient CT and MRI features in an acute ischemic stroke patient arriving to the hospital within 6 hours of onset. Suggest an algorithm-based approach for confirmation of diagnosis and guiding the management of such a patient. [5+5] [DNB Dec 20, DNB June 20, DNB Dec 21]

A stroke, also known as a cerebrovascular event (CVA), is characterized by the sudden onset of neurological symptoms due to insufficient blood flow to the brain. Approximately 80% of all strokes are caused by cerebral ischemia or infarction. Due to their speed and availability, nonenhanced computed tomography (NECT) and computed tomography angiography (CTA), with or without CT perfusion, are the most frequently utilized imaging modalities.

Acute stroke protocols depend on factors such as the time elapsed since the onset of symptoms, the availability of urgent imaging with appropriate software reconstructions, preferences of clinicians and radiologists, and access to neurointervention.

The "must know" questions in acute stroke triage that need to be answered are as follows **(Box 8)**:

BOX 8: The "must know" questions in acute stroke triage.

There are four "must know" questions in acute stroke triage that need to be answered rapidly and accurately.

- Is intracranial hemorrhage or a stroke "mimic" present?
- Is a large vessel occluded?
- Is part of the brain irreversibly injured (i.e., is there a core of critically ischemic, irreversibly infarcted tissue)?
- Is there a clinically relevant "penumbra" of ischemic but potentially salvageable tissue?

Pathophysiology

Brain Ischemia and Stroke Imaging Protocols

Core and Penumbra in Brain Ischemia

- **Ischemic Core**: The central region of affected brain tissue during a stroke has a cerebral blood flow (CBF) of less than 6–8 cm^3/100 g/min. This area experiences neuronal death and irreversible loss of function.
- **Penumbra**: Surrounding the core, the penumbra is less severely ischemic, with CBF reduced from a normal 60 cm^3/100 g/min to 10–20 cm^3/100 g/min. This tissue is "at risk" but potentially salvageable.

Imaging Goals and Protocols

1. **Primary Objectives**:
   - Differentiate ischemic stroke from intracranial hemorrhage.
   - Select and triage patients for reperfusion therapies.

2. **Imaging Steps**:
   - **NECT**: Emergent nonenhanced CT (NECT) scans determine if intracranial hemorrhage or stroke mimics (e.g., subdural hematoma, neoplasm) are present.
   - **CTA**: CT angiography follows NECT if hemorrhage is excluded, identifying major vessel occlusions and active bleeding (e.g., "spot sign").
   - **MRA and DSA**: MR angiography can be affected by motion artifacts, making digital subtraction angiography (DSA) preferable for intra-arterial thrombolysis or mechanical thrombectomy.
   - **Perfusion Imaging**: CT or MR perfusion (pCT, pMR) studies assess the extent of irreversible damage and identify salvageable brain tissue (ischemic penumbra).

CT Findings and Protocols

- **Acute Stroke CT Protocol**:
  - Includes NECT, arch-to-vertex CTA, and dynamic first-pass perfusion CT (pCT).
  - Detects hyperattenuating vessels (e.g., "dense MCA" sign) and assesses grey-white matter interfaces.
- **ASPECTS Score**: The Alberta Stroke Program Early CT Score (ASPECTS) evaluates early ischemic changes by subtracting points for affected regions. An ASPECTS score ≤7 indicates increased hemorrhage risk and poor outcomes.
- **CTA and pCT**:
  - **CTA**: Visualizes craniocervical vasculature, localizes thrombus, assesses collateral flow, and characterizes atherosclerosis.
  - **pCT**: Evaluates cerebral blood volume (CBV), cerebral blood flow (CBF), and mean transit time (MTT). The ischemic core shows reduced CBV and CBF, while the penumbra shows mismatched CBV and CBF with prolonged MTT.

Key Imaging Parameters (Table 10)

- **CBV**: Volume of blood in a given brain volume.
- **CBF**: Volume of blood flowing through a brain volume over time.
- **MTT**: Average time for blood to transit through the brain.
- **Color Scales**:
  - **CBV/CBF**: Well-perfused areas appear red/yellow; ischemic areas are blue/purple.
  - **MTT**: Abnormal transit time appears red; normal transit time appears blue.
- **Clinical Implications**: MCA infarct core volume of 70–100 mL predicts poor outcomes. The penumbra, with a mismatch between CBV and CBF, represents potentially salvageable tissue.
  - An important finding in patients having large MCA territorial infarcts is decreased perfusion in the contralateral cerebellar hemisphere with decreased cerebral blood flow, a phenomenon known as crossed cerebellar diaschisis.

TABLE 10: CT perfusion parameters indicating ischemic core and penumbra.

Etiology	*CBF*	*CBV*	*WITT*	*TTP*
Infarct core	↓	↓	≥	↑
Ischemic penumbra	↓	↑	↑	↑

(CBF = cerebral blood flow, CBV = cerebral blood volume, MTT = mean transit time; TTP = time to peak, ↑ indicate increase, ↓ = indicate decrease)

MRI Findings in Stroke

Preferred Modalities

- **CT/CTA/pCT**: Often chosen due to accessibility and speed. However, rapid stroke protocols using fast FLAIR, T2*, DWI, and pMR are also effective.
- **MRI Advantages**: Superior in detecting small vessel and brainstem ischemia. Useful in identifying the ischemic penumbra when there is a discrepancy between CT/CTA findings and clinical stroke severity.

Specific MRI Techniques and Findings

1. **T2/FLAIR**
   - **Early Detection**: Only 30–50% of acute strokes show cortical swelling and hyperintensity on FLAIR within the first 4 hours. Almost all strokes are FLAIR positive by 7 hours after symptom onset. T2 scans generally become positive within 12–24 hours.

- **Intraarterial Hyperintensity**: An early stroke sign on FLAIR indicating slow flow, either from delayed antegrade flow or retrograde collateral filling.
- **FLAIR-DWI Mismatch**: When FLAIR is negative, and DWI is positive, it suggests viable ischemic penumbra and eligibility for thrombolysis.

2. ***T2* GRE***
   - **Intraarterial Thrombus Detection**: "Blooming" hypointensity on T2* (GRE, SWI) indicates intraarterial thrombus.
   - **Chronic Hypertension or Amyloid Angiopathy**: "Blooming black dots" in older patients.
   - **Cerebral Microbleeds**: May increase the risk of anticoagulation-related hemorrhage.
3. **DWI and ADC**
   - **Hyperacute Infarcts**: Approximately 95% show diffusion restriction, with hyperintensity on DWI and corresponding hypointensity on ADC.
   - **Sensitivity**: DTI is even more sensitive than DWI, especially for pontine and medullary lesions.
   - **Negative DWI**: Does not rule out stroke, as 2–7% of patients with a final stroke diagnosis are initially DWI negative. Possible reasons include small (lacunar) infarcts, brainstem lesions, clot lysis with recanalization, and moderate or fluctuating hypoperfusion.
4. **pMR**
   - **DWI-PWI Mismatch**: DWI generally reflects the densely ischemic core of the infarct, while pMR shows the surrounding "at-risk" penumbra. A mismatch between DWI and PWI helps determine suitability for intraarterial thrombolysis.

By using these MRI techniques, clinicians can better identify and differentiate between the core and penumbra of an infarct, thereby guiding appropriate treatment decisions.

Stroke Algorithm **(Flowchart 4)**.

Treatment Options

The single most important factor in successful intervention is patient selection, with the two most important considerations being (1) elapsed time from symptom onset and (2) imaging findings on the screening NECT scan.

1. IV thrombolysis is done by recombinant tissue plasminogen activator (rTPA). There are several studies regarding rTPA dose, therapeutic window and effectiveness. The clinically accepted therapeutic window for intravenous recombinant tissue plasminogen activator (rTPA) is less than 3 hours from ictus (the "golden hours"). A dose 0.6 mg/kg is used in Japan and other Asian countries.
2. Intraarterial thrombolysis is typically restricted to less than 6 hours. Exceptions to this general rule include basilar artery thrombosis and patients outside the 6-hour window who have a persistent significant perfusion-diffusion mismatch.
3. Mechanical thrombectomy is suitable in patients beyond the therapeutic window or in whom thrombolytic therapy is contraindicated. However, it is rare that a patient may benefit from thrombectomy if the procedure starts >8 hours after onset in the anterior circulation and >24 hours after onset in the posterior circulation.

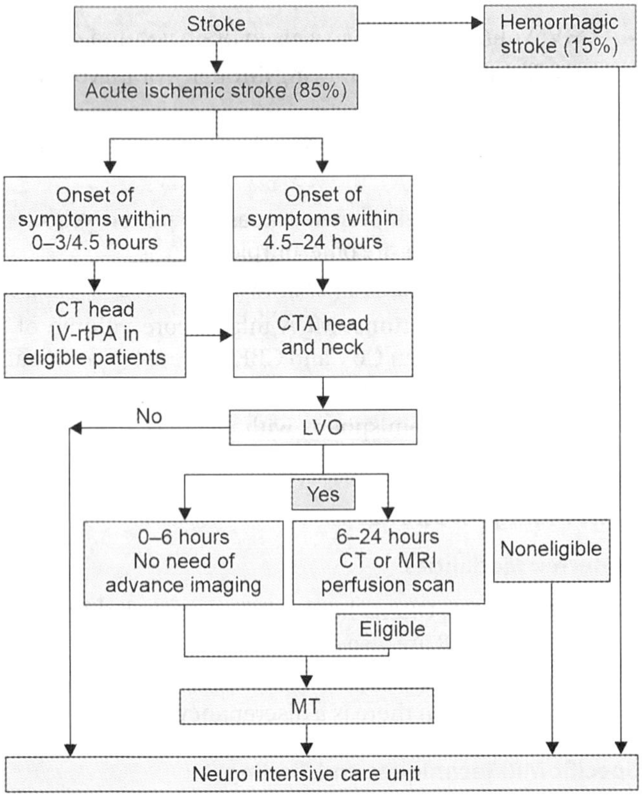

FLOWCHART 4: Stroke algorithm *(For Color Version Refer Flowchart1)*.

Mechanical Thrombectomy Treatment Protocol

Sedation and Anesthesia

Conscious Sedation (CS): Preferred over general anesthesia (GA) due to faster procedure times and better patient control. CS avoids the hypotension commonly induced by GA, which can be detrimental to acute stroke patients relying on high cerebral perfusion pressure via pial collaterals.

Anticoagulation

Standard Heparin Flushes: No additional anticoagulation or antiaggregation required during thrombectomy, except for standard heparin flushes (e.g., 5 IU/mL). Permanent stenting should be avoided due to the increased risk of reperfusion hematomas or hemorrhagic conversion.

Procedure in Anterior Circulation

- **Stent Retrievers**: Safe to use up to the M2 segments in most patients.
- **Posterior Circulation**: Typically, thrombectomy is not needed beyond the P1 segment.

Procedural Steps (Fig. 14)

1. **Groin Puncture**: Use a long (80 cm) 8 F introducer sheath placed in the common carotid artery (CCA) with a 5 F diagnostic catheter (DC) and a 0.035" (0.89 mm) guidewire (GW).
2. **Balloon Guide Catheter (BGC)**: Position an 8 F BGC in the internal carotid artery. BGC allows for flow reversal, reducing the risk of thrombo-emboli escaping into collateral areas.
3. **Microcatheter Introduction**: After confirming the clot position with contrast injection, introduce a microcatheter with a microguidewire, passing the thrombus if possible while keeping the microguidewire retracted.
4. **Stent Retriever Deployment**: Release the stent retriever centered at the clot, preferably more distal than proximal, covering the proximal clot boundary. Leave it to expand and "incubate" for at least 5 minutes.

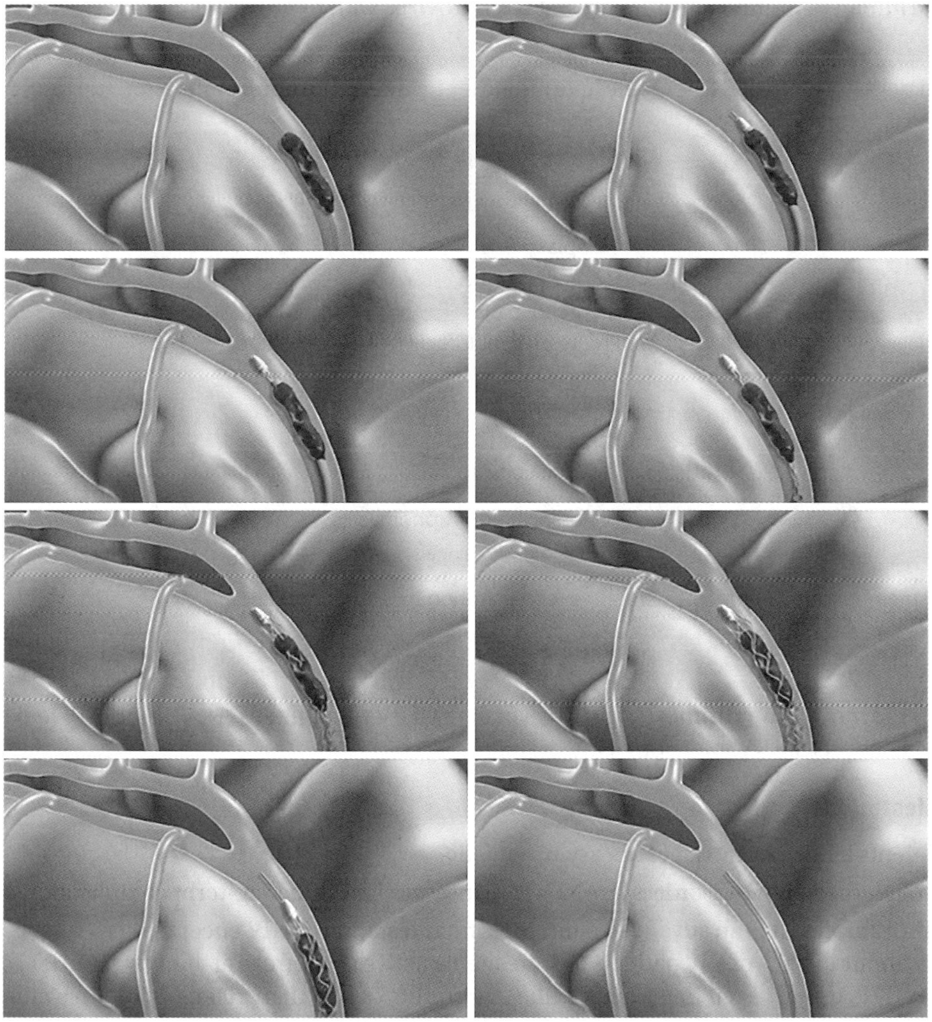

FIG. 14: Schematic diagram representing standard technique of mechanical thrombectomy *(For Color Version Refer Fig. 8)*.

5. **Resheathing and Aspiration**: Readvance the microcatheter, partially resheath the stent retriever to the face of the thrombus, inflate the balloon, and pull back the stent retriever with simultaneous aspiration in the BGC. Gradually escalate and maximize aspiration as the device enters the guide's orifice.
6. **Thrombus Retrieval**: Remove the rotating hemostatic valve (RHV), take out the device to check for thrombus, and apply further aspiration directly to the BGC to clear any remaining small thrombi before deflating the balloon.
7. **Procedure Control**: Verify the procedure's outcome with a contrast injection in the BGC, rinse and clean the device, reconnect the RHV, and repeat the thrombectomy maneuver if necessary. Typically, the same stent retriever can be used up to three times.

Posterior Circulation Adaptations

Guide Catheter: Use a long, soft 6–7 F guide catheter (e.g., Navien, Fargo, Neuron) to advance up to the vertebrobasilar junction, as advancing an 8 F guide catheter into the vertebral arteries can be challenging.

By adhering to this protocol, mechanical thrombectomy can be effectively and safely performed, ensuring optimal outcomes for patients with acute ischemic stroke.

Infections

1. Discuss CT and MRI features of neurological complications of AIDS. [5+5] [MD (WBUHS) 22]

Causative Agent: Human immunodeficiency virus. It is a retrovirus with neurovirulent properties. HIV-1 and HIV-2 are the two subtypes.

AIDS patients can develop neurological manifestations either by direct or indirect effects on the CNS **(Table 11)**.

TABLE 11: Neurological manifestations of AIDS.

HIV infection itself	HIV encephalitis—most common (60%)
Opportunistic infections	• Toxoplasmosis • Cytomegalovirus • Cryptococcosis • Progressive multifocal leukoencephalopathy • Tuberculosis • Neurosyphilis • Varicella zoster • CMV encephalitis
Neoplasms	• HIV-associated lymphomas • Kaposi Sarcoma
Treatment-related metabolic derangements	Immune reconstitution inflammatory syndrome

HIV Encephalitis

HIV encephalitis is the most common infection in AIDS patients. HIV encephalitis (HIVE) and HIV leukoencephalopathy (HIVL) are the direct effects of HIV infection of the brain.

Neurologic Manifestations

- Most of the patients in their early stages are asymptomatic.
- HIV-associated neurocognitive disorders (HANDs) are intermediate and long-term complications.
- **AIDS dementia complex**: It is an advanced neurologic manifestation of HIV encephalitis.

Approximately about 15–20% of HIV patients despite highly active antiretroviral therapy (HAART) can develop AIDS dementia complex. It is usually seen in patients with CD4 counts of less than 200 cells/μL. It is clinically manifested as progressive dementia characterized by cognitive, behavioral, and motor deterioration resulting in death if left untreated.

Imaging

CT Scan: In the early stages, it could be normal. As the disease progresses, mild to moderate brain atrophy with confluency patchy white matter hypodensities is seen. On the postcontrast scan, no enhancement is seen.

MRI: MR is more sensitive than a CT scan. It shows diffuse cerebral atrophy with bilateral patchy relatively symmetric deep and subcortical white matter hyperintensities. With time hyperintensities become confluent and hazy. It reduced medial and superior frontal gyri gray matter volume described as a possible early imaging marker for HIVE. On the postcontrast scan, it does not show any enhancement. Perivenular enhancement may show in fulminant cases and indicate acute demyelination. No diffusion restriction was seen in HIVE.

MR spectroscopy may identify the early metabolic changes before the morphological changes. It shows decreased NAA and elevated choline peak denotes the neuronal loss and presence of gliosis. Increased myoinositol (MI) peak may be seen in the early stage of infection. MRS is also helpful in monitoring the treatment response.

Magnetization transfer ratio and DTI can detect the early changes of HIVE.

Opportunistic Infections: The prevalence of CNS opportunistic infections has decreased after the advent of HAART therapy. However opportunistic infections cause substantial morbidity in a patient of HIV infection.

Toxoplasmosis

- **Causative Agent**: Intracellular parasite *Toxoplasma gondii.*
- **Presentations**: Focal neurologic deficits superimposed on HIVE symptoms. The most common focal deficit is mild hemiparesis.

Imaging

CT Findings: CT shows multiple ill-defined hypodense lesions in the ganglia-thalamic regions with moderate to marked surrounding edema. On a postcontrast scan, it shows rim and punctate enhancement.

MR Findings:

- **T1WI**: Hypointense lesion with occasional demonstration of mild peripheral hyperintensity by coagulative necrosis or hemorrhage.
- **T2WI**: It shows alternating concentric zones of hyper and hypointensity with marked surrounding edema.
- **Central T2 Hyperintensity**: Denotes to a necrotizing abscess.
- As the abscess organizes, T2 intensity decreases and becomes isointense to white matter. Surrounding hyperintensity represents edema.
- **Postcontrast Scan**: The lesions show ring and nodular enhancement. Ring enhancement with an eccentric small nodule represents the eccentric target sign.
- **Disseminated Toxoplasmosis Encephalitis**: Also known as microglial nodule encephalitis. It shows multifocal hyperintensities in the basal ganglia and subcortical white matter on T2-weighted images with absent or minimal enhancement.
- MR spectroscopic findings are nonspecific and often show a lipid-lactate peak.

Cryptococcosis

Causative Agent: Fungus—*Cryptococcus neoformans.* Cryptococcosis usually occurs when CD4 counts drop to below 50–100 cells/μL.

Pathology

- **Three Forms of CNS Cryptococcal Infection**: Meningitis, gelatinous pseudocysts, and focal cryptococcosis.
- **Immunocompetent Patients**: Cryptococcomas and meningitis are the most common forms.
- **Immunocompromised/AIDS Patient**: Meningitis and gelatinous pseudocysts are the most common forms.

Imaging

- **NECT Scan**: Usually shows hypodensity in the basal ganglia. In immunocompromised patients, it usually does not show any enhancement.
- **MRI**: Multiple cryptococcal gelatinous pseudocysts are seen following the CSF signal intensity. Surrounding edema is generally absent. Lack of enhancement on postcontrast scan is typical although mild pial enhancement is occasionally seen.

Progressive Multifocal Leukoencephalopathy

Causative Agent: JC virus (JCV), a member of the Papovaviridae family.

Imaging Findings

- Multifocal white matter lesions, predominantly involve the subcortical white matter.
- Bilateral but asymmetric.
- Involving the subcortical U fibers. Subcortical U fibers are usually spared in HIVE.
- Generally, does not enhance on postcontrast scan. Exception: Hyperacute PML in the setting of IRIS and in MS patients on natalizumab.

Other Opportunistic Infections

Cytomegalovirus

- Acquired CMV infections are commonly manifesting as meningoencephalitis and ventriculitis/epididymitis. Ventricular ependymal enhancement in an immunocompromised patient is highly suggestive of CMV.
- **Extracranial Presentations**: Retinitis and myelitis with radiculitis.

Tuberculosis

- Tuberculosis is one of the most devastating opportunistic infections and the main cause of morbidity and mortality in HIV-infected patients worldwide. Multidrug-resistant and extensively drug-resistant tuberculosis are found almost entirely in patients coinfected with HIV.
- Tubercular co-infection generally exacerbates the severity and accelerates the progression of HIV.
- Tuberculosis should be treated first in HIV-infected patients to increase the effectiveness of HAART and to prevent the development of TB-IRIS.
- **Imaging**: Enhancement of meninges, tuberculomas, and pseudo abscesses are often mild or absent even in the presence of more acid-fast bacilli.

Immune Reconstitution Inflammatory Syndrome

CNS IRIS is a T cell-mediated encephalitis in treated HIV patients or autoimmune disease (multiple sclerosis). It is a dysregulated immune response to infectious or non-infectious antigens.

Underlying Pathogens:

- JC virus (PML-IRIS),
- Tuberculosis (TB-IRIS)
- Fungal infections especially cryptococcus (crypto IRIS).
- Natalizumab associated PML IRIS in patients of multiple sclerosis.

Two forms are recognized:

- **Unmasking IRIS**: When antiretroviral therapy reveals a subclinical, previously unrecognized opportunistic infection.
- **Paradoxical IRIS**: When a patient who has been successfully treated for a recent opportunistic infection deteriorates after initiation of antiretroviral therapy.

The most common presentation of CNS IRIS is clinical deterioration of the patients despite the rising CD4 counts and lower viral loads in a newly treated AIDS patient.

Imaging

- **PML IRIS**: Confluent and linear or "punctate" perivascular hyperintensities on T2/FLAIR images. A punctate pattern of enhancement is typical in the acute stage. Bizarre-looking parenchymal masses and progressively enlarging and enhancing lesions are also common.
- **TB-IRIS**: May develop florid TB pseudo abscesses (TB gone wild) and/or rapidly increasing enhancement in the basilar meninges.

Other Manifestations of HIV/AIDS

- Vasculopathy
- HIV/AIDS-related bone marrow changes
- Benign lymphoepithelial lesions
- Lymphoid hyperplasia.

2. Describe briefly the neuroimaging manifestations of COVID-19. [10]

COVID-19 infection is predominantly respiratory illness. Neurologic involvements in COVID-19 patients are well-recognized. CNS manifestations of COVID-19 infections are also contributed by comorbidities such as hypertension, complications of prolonged illness and hospitalization, and associated supportive treatments.[6]

Long-term neurologic follow-up after recovery from COVID-19 infection may be warranted for emerging evidence of long-term changes in the central nervous system.

Neurological Manifestations

- Acute infarcts with large clot burden and intracranial hemorrhage, including microhemorrhages.
- Leukoencephalopathy
- Global hypoxic injury
- Acute disseminated encephalomyelitis
- Cytotoxic lesions of the corpus callosum
- Olfactory bulb involvement
- Cranial nerve enhancement
- Guillain-Barré syndrome.

Pathogenesis: The above-mentioned CNS manifestations represent the secondary involvement from immune activation that leads to a prothrombotic state and cytokine storm. Evidence for direct neuroinvasion of the virus is very low.

The neurologic manifestations of COVID-19 can be broadly classified into four categories **(Table 12)**:

TABLE 12: Neurologic manifestations of COVID-19 infection.

Category	*Putative pathogenesis*	*Clinical syndromes*
Direct viral effect	Neuroinvasion	Anosmia; possible encephalitis or meningoencephalitis
Direct viral effect	Endotheliopathy	Thromboembolism
Para-infectious	Immune response: Coagulopathy	Thromboembolism; hemorrhage
Para-infectious	Immune response: Cytokine storm	• Acute necrotizing leukoencephalopathy • Encephalitis • Cytotoxic lesions of corpus callosum • Thromboembolism • Hemorrhage
Postinfectious	Delayed immune response	• Guillain-Barré syndrome • Acute demyelinating encephalomyelitis
Complications of prolonged illness or hospitalization	Anticoagulation	Hemorrhage
Complications of prolonged illness or hospitalization	Hypoxic changes	• Diffuse hypoxic damage • Posthypoxic demyelination
Complications of prolonged illness or hospitalization	Drug related	Neurotoxicity
Complications of prolonged illness or hospitalization	Dialysis related	Posterior reversible encephalopathy syndrome

- Direct viral effects
- Para-infectious immune response to the virus
- Postinfectious delayed immune response
- Complications of prolonged illness or hospitalization

Imaging Findings

No specific imaging finding is demonstrated in COVID-19-infected patients.

Thromboembolic Manifestations

It was the most common intracranial manifestation in COVID-19-positive patients during the pandemic. Acute stroke was a poor prognostic indicator. It may be the first presentation of COVID-19 and may associated with increased D-dimer levels and inflammatory markers.

Commonly observed patterns of acute cerebral thromboembolic disease:

- Large vessel occlusion with territorial infarcts
- Branch vessel occlusion
- Small vessel occlusion/small vessel infarcts
- Watershed infarcts
- Extensive bilateral multivessel infarcts.

Patients with COVID-19 infection may show acute thromboembolic manifestations elsewhere in the body, including the carotid artery, vertebral artery, subclavian artery, pulmonary artery, and lower extremity venous system. Limited reports of cerebral venous thrombosis are noted.

Hemorrhages

Intracranial hemorrhage is commonly seen in COVID-19-positive patients.

Patterns of Hemorrhage

- Lobar hemorrhage
- Microhemorrhages
- Subarachnoid hemorrhage
- Subdural hemorrhage
- Hemorrhagic transformation of acute infarcts
- COVID-19 patients may develop disseminated intravascular coagulation leading to intracranial hemorrhage.

Leukoencephalopathy

White matter changes may be observed in COVID-19-positive patients with prolonged ICU stays. This leukoencephalopathy manifested as symmetric confluent white matter T2 hyperintensity and diffusion restriction with relative sparing of juxtacortical and infratentorial white matter. The findings are nonspecific, however, may represent a delayed post-hypoxic status.

Global Hypoxic Injury

Global hypoxic injury can happen in COVID-19-positive patients. Manifests as restricted diffusion of the basal ganglia, thalami, hippocampi, and cortex.

Meningitis/Encephalitis

Meningitis and encephalitis are less common manifestations than thromboembolic events in COVID-19-positive patients.

Presentations:

- **Meningitis**: Leptomeningeal enhancement.
- Brain stem encephalitis.
- Limbic encephalitis

- Acute necrotizing encephalopathy.
- Acute demyelinating encephalomyelitis
- Acute hemorrhagic leukoencephalitis

Reported cases were not confirmed by histopathology. The diagnosis was made on the basis of clinical or radiologic manifestations. Whether these cases represent direct viral invasion or a sequela of cytokine storm is unclear.

Cytotoxic Lesions of the Corpus Callosum

Cytotoxic lesions of the corpus callosum likely represent the inflammatory damage from the cytokine storm. On MRI it shows focal T2/FLAIR hyperintensity with diffusion abnormality at the splenium of the corpus callosum.

Olfactory Bulb Involvement

Anosmia is a clinical marker for COVID-19 infection.

Findings

- T2 hyperintensity and/or enhancement in the olfactory bulbs, tract, and gyrus recti.
- Normal signal intensity and enhancement.
- Olfactory bulb atrophy after COVID-19-induced anosmia was also documented.

Cranial Nerve Enhancement

Apart from olfactory nerve involvement, other cranial neuropathies were also recorded in COVID-19-positive patients.

Cranial Neuropathies

- Optic neuritis
- Oculomotor nerve enhancement
- Miller-Fisher syndrome:
  - **Miller-Fisher Syndrome**: It is an acute peripheral neuropathy that develops after exposure to infectious pathogens.
  - Characterized by a triad of:
    - Ophthalmoplegia
    - Ataxia
    - Areflexia
  - **Findings**: T2 hyperintensity, enlargement, and enhancement of CN III.

Spinal Manifestations

- Guillain Barré syndrome may occur in COVID-19-positive patients.
- **Findings**: T2 hyperintensity in the distal cord and enhancement of the caudal nerve roots.

3. Neuroimaging manifestations of congenital TORCH infections. [5]

Congenital infections of the central nervous system are infections of the developing central nervous system in fetal and neonatal immature immune systems.[7]

Baldwin and Whitley's criteria for congenital infections:

- The onset of symptoms within 48 hours of birth
- Serological confirmation
- The exclusion of other pathologies
- **Infection at early gestational age**:
  - May lead to miscarriage, premature birth, and intrauterine growth restriction (IUGR). May cause microcephaly, parenchymal calcifications, white matter abnormalities, hydrocephalus, and cortical developmental abnormality.

- **Late Infections in the Second and Third Trimesters**: May cause abnormal white matter myelination and usually result in milder outcomes.

TORCH infection: TORCH stands for,

- **T**: *Toxoplasma gondii*
- **O:** Other agents (e.g., Syphilis, Listeria, and parvovirus B19)
- **R**: Rubella,
- **C**: Cytomegalovirus (CMV)
- **H**: Herpes virus

TORCH infections are a group of pathogens transmitted from mother to child through the placenta during the delivery or immediately after the birth.

Toxoplasmosis

Transplacental transmission rate of toxoplasmosis increases with increasing trimester. The transmission rate in the third trimester is higher than in the first trimester.

Triad of congenital toxoplasmosis:

- Hydrocephalus
- Bilateral chorioretinitis
- Intracranial calcifications.

Mortality rates of the congenital toxoplasmosis infection are approximately 1 to 5%. The surviving patient usually has long-term sequelae including developmental delay and seizures.

Imaging Findings

Multifocal calcifications on US, CT, and MR scans are seen involving the periventricular regions, basal ganglia, or cerebral cortex. Hydrocephalus with marked expansion of the atria and occipital horns of the lateral ventricles is frequently seen usually secondary to aqueductal stenosis and associated tissue loss. Toxoplasmosis does not cause migrational anomalies. Nonspecific neuroimaging findings are atrophy, encephalomalacia, hydranencephaly, or microcephaly.

Syphilis

Congenital syphilis can occur regardless of the stage of the maternal infection.

It can cause, spontaneous abortion, stillbirth, nonimmune hydrops, premature delivery, and perinatal death. Approximately 40% of congenital syphilis-infected infants are fatal during the perinatal period. Approximately 33% of congenital syphilis-infected infants presented with disseminated infection at birth.

Clinical signs of disseminated infection:

- Characteristic long bone periostitis
- Hepatosplenomegaly
- Jaundice
- Skin rash
- Persistent rhinitis
- Lymphadenopathy
- Meningitis
- Hydrocephalus
- **Late Manifestations of Congenital Syphilis**: It appears after 2 years of age and consists of:
  - Orodental, facial, and skin deformities
  - Sensorineural hearing loss
  - Hydrocephalus
  - Mental retardation
  - Seizures
  - Hemiplegia

Imaging Findings

Hydrocephalus and leptomeningeal enhancement may be seen. Enhancement may extend in brain parenchyma leading to enhancing parenchymal mass. It may cause arteritis or less commonly phlebitis leads to infarction (most commonly middle cerebral artery territory).

Rubella

The maximum risk of congenital rubella infection is noted during the first trimester of pregnancy.

Characterized by:

- Hepatosplenomegaly
- Congenital heart disease (PDA, pulmonary artery stenosis)
- Growth retardation
- Ocular abnormalities (cataracts, pigmentary retinopathy)
- Jaundice
- Rash
- Sensorineural hearing loss
- Meningoencephalitis
- Microcephaly

Imaging

Ultrasonography: May show nonspecific findings:

- Subependymal cysts in the caudate nucleus and subthalamic region.
- Echogenic foci at basal ganglia suggest mineralizing vasculitis.

CT: May show microcephaly and parenchymal calcifications.

MRI

- Deep and subcortical white matter lesions
- Delayed myelination may be seen
- Cerebellar hypoplasia and neuronal migration abnormalities were also reported.

Cytomegalovirus (CMV)

It is the most common congenital CNS infection. The cytomegalovirus has a predilection for the periventricular subependymal germinal matrix region. Other sites of central nervous system involvement include the cerebral cortex, white matter, brainstem, spinal cord, and cerebellum.

Presentations

- Neuronal migration abnormalities (polymicrogyria, heterotopia)
- Microcephaly
- Hydranencephaly and porencephaly may also be seen
- Long-term sequelae (visual deficits, mental retardation, hearing loss, and seizures may occur)
- Nonhereditary deafness in children

Imaging Findings

Microcephaly with periventricular calcification is the characteristic imaging findings. Intracranial calcification (best seen on CT) is typically located in the periventricular region but basal ganglia, cortical and subcortical calcifications may be noted.

MRI

- Encephalomalacia
- Migrational anomalies (polymicrogyria, lissencephaly, pachygyria, heterotopia)

- Ventricular enlargement
- Delayed myelination
- Subependymal periventricular cysts

The main differences between congenital CMV and toxoplasmosis infection are as follows **(Table 13)**.

TABLE 13: Main differences between congenital CMV and toxoplasmosis infection.

Features	*Congenital CMV*	*Congenital toxoplasmosis*
Calcifications	Periventricular	More peripheral
Head size	Microcephaly	Macrocephaly
Anomalies of cortical development	Common	Rare

Herpes Simplex Virus (HSV)

It is the second most common congenital TORCH infection.

Imaging

CT*:*

- Hypodense lesions at the periventricular white matter.
- Finger-like increased density within the cortical grey matter along with white matter lucency is a characteristic imaging finding in the first 3 weeks after presentation.
- Focal necrosis, cystic encephalomalacia, parenchymal calcification, and diffuse cerebral atrophy may be seen with disease progression.

Emerging Congenital Infections

- Zika Virus
- SARS-CoV-2

The imaging manifestations of important congenital infections are presented in a tabular form as follows **(Table 14)**.

TABLE 14: Imaging manifestations of important congenital infections.

	Calcifications	*Ventricles*	*Cortex*	*White matter*	*Other*
CMV	Periventricular, punctate	Ventriculomegaly	Polymicrogyria, lissencephaly, schizencephaly	• Periventricular delayed myelination • Germinolytic cysts • Temporal cyst	• Hemorrhage (rare) • Cerebellum hypoplasia
Toxoplasmosis	Extensive and most commonly in basal ganglia, thalami, cerebral cortex, and periventricular tissue	• Hydrocephalus • Hydranencephaly (rare)	• Microcephaly • Macrocephaly • Porencephaly	• Microcephaly • Macrocephaly • Porencephaly	Aqueduct occlusion/stenosis secondary to epididymitis
HSV	Less common	Ventriculomegaly, hydranencephaly	• Microcephaly • Porencephaly	• Microcephaly • Porencephaly	Corpus callosum agenesis, microphthalmia, meningeal involvement
Rubella	Basal ganglia and periventricular	Ventriculomegaly	Polymicrogyria	Extensive multifocal white matter hyperintensity, mainly in the frontal lobes	Subependymal cysts, lenticulostriate vasculopathy, myelination delay, cerebellar hypoplasia

Continued...

Continued...

	Calcifications	*Ventricles*	*Cortex*	*White matter*	*Other*
Parvovirus	Less common	Ventricular dilatation	• Ischemic and hemorrhagic strokes • Polymicrogyria (rare) • Heterotopia (rare)	Ischemic and hemorrhagic strokes	Cerebral vasculitis, hydrops
SARS-COVID-19		Intraventricular hemorrhage	Parenchymal hemorrhage, Cerebral ischemia	Periventricular leukomalacia, parenchymal hemorrhage, cerebral ischemia	Cerebral vein thrombosis
Zika virus	Corticomedullary junction in frontal and parietal lobes, less frequently in the thalamus, basal ganglia, cortex, and periventricular regions	Ventriculo megaly	Microcephaly, polymicrogyria, gyral simplification, pachygyria-lissencephaly, opercular dysplasia, heterotopia	Microcephaly, delayed myelination, dysmyelination, hypoplasia of corticospinal tracts	Pseudocysts in the occipital horns, asymmetrical microphthalmia, cataracts, optic nerve atrophy, coloboma, lens defects, herniation of the orbital fat into the cranial vault, thin spinal cord

4. CNS manifestation in HIV with imaging. [10] [DNB June 22, DNB June 19, AIIMS Dec 24, MD (WBUHS) 17]

Causative Agent: Human immunodeficiency virus. It is a retrovirus with neurovirulent properties. HIV-1 and HIV-2 are the two subtypes.

AIDS patients can develop neurological manifestations either by direct or indirect effects on the CNS **(Table 15)**.

Neurologic Manifestations:

HIV Encephalitis

HIV encephalitis is the most common infection in AIDS patients. HIV encephalitis (HIVE) and HIV leukoencephalopathy (HIVL) are the direct effects of HIV infection of the brain.

Neurologic Manifestations

- Most of the patients in their early stages are asymptomatic.
- HIV-associated neurocognitive disorders (HANDs) are intermediate and long-term complications.

AIDS Dementia Complex: It is an advanced neurologic manifestation of HIV encephalitis. Approximately about 15–20% of HIV patients despite highly active antiretroviral therapy (HAART) can develop AIDS dementia complex. It is usually seen in patients with CD4 counts of less than 200 cells/μL. It is clinically manifested as progressive dementia characterized by cognitive, behavioral, and motor deterioration resulting in death if left untreated.

TABLE 15: Neurological manifestations of AIDS.

HIV infection itself	HIV encephalitis—most common (60%)
Opportunistic infections	• Toxoplasmosis • Cytomegalovirus • Cryptococcosis • Progressive multifocal leukoencephalopathy • Tuberculosis • Neurosyphilis • Varicella zoster • CMV encephalitis
Neoplasms	• HIV-associated lymphomas • Kaposi sarcoma
Treatment-related metabolic derangements	Immune reconstitution inflammatory syndrome

Imaging

CT Scan: In the early stages, it could be normal. As the disease progresses, mild to moderate brain atrophy with confluency patchy white matter hypodensities is seen. On the postcontrast scan, no enhancement is seen.

MRI: MR is more sensitive than a CT scan. It shows diffuse cerebral atrophy with bilateral patchy relatively symmetric deep and subcortical white matter hyperintensities. With time hyperintensities become confluent and hazy. It reduced medial and superior frontal gyri gray matter volume described as a possible early imaging marker for HIVE. On the postcontrast scan, it does not show any enhancement. Perivenular enhancement may show in fulminant cases and indicate acute demyelination. No diffusion restriction was seen in HIVE.

MR spectroscopy may identify the early metabolic changes before the morphological changes. It shows decreased NAA and elevated choline peak denotes the neuronal loss and presence of gliosis. Increased myoinositol (MI) peak may be seen in the early stage of infection. MRS is also helpful in monitoring the treatment response.

Magnetization transfer ratio and DTI can detect the early changes of HIVE.

Opportunistic Infections: The prevalence of CNS opportunistic infections has decreased after the advent of HAART therapy. However opportunistic infections cause substantial morbidity in a patient of HIV infection.

Toxoplasmosis

- **Causative Agent**: Intracellular parasite *Toxoplasma gondii.*
- **Presentations**: Focal neurologic deficits superimposed on HIV symptoms. The most common focal deficit is mild hemiparesis.

Imaging

CT Findings: CT shows multiple ill-defined hypodense lesions in the ganglia-thalamic regions with moderate to marked surrounding edema. On a postcontrast scan, it shows rim and punctate enhancement.

MR Findings:

- **T1WI**: Hypointense lesion with occasional demonstration of mild peripheral hyperintensity by coagulative necrosis or hemorrhage.
- **T2WI**: It shows alternating concentric zones of hyper and hypointensity with marked surrounding edema?
- **Central T2 Hyperintensity**: Denotes to a necrotizing abscess.
- As the abscess organizes, T2 intensity decreases and becomes isointense to white matter. Surrounding hyperintensity represents edema.
- **Postcontrast Scan**: The lesions show ring and nodular enhancement. Ring enhancement with an eccentric small nodule represents the eccentric target sign.
- **Disseminated Toxoplasmosis Encephalitis**: Also known as microglial nodule encephalitis. It shows multifocal hyperintensities in the basal ganglia and subcortical white matter on T2-weighted images with absent or minimal enhancement.
- MR spectroscopic findings are nonspecific and often show a lipid-lactate peak.

Cryptococcosis

Causative Agent: Fungus—Cryptococcus neoformans. Cryptococcosis usually occurs when CD4 counts drop to below 50–100 cells/µL.

Pathology

- **Three Forms of CNS Cryptococcal Infection**: Meningitis, gelatinous pseudocysts, and focal cryptococcosis.
- **Immunocompetent Patients**: Cryptococcomas and meningitis are the most common forms.
- **Immunocompromised/AIDS patient**: Meningitis and gelatinous pseudocysts are the most common forms.

Imaging

NECT Scan: Usually shows hypodensity in the basal ganglia. In immunocompromised patients, it usually does not show any enhancement.

MRI: Multiple cryptococcal gelatinous pseudocysts are seen following the CSF signal intensity. Surrounding edema is generally absent. Lack of enhancement on post contrast scan is typical although mild pial enhancement is occasionally seen.

Progressive Multifocal Leukoencephalopathy

Causative Agent: JC virus (JCV), a member of the papovaviridae family.

Imaging Findings

- Multifocal white matter lesions, predominantly involve the subcortical white matter.
- Bilateral but asymmetric.
- Involving the subcortical U fibers. Subcortical U fibers are usually spared in HIVE.
- Generally, does not enhance on postcontrast scan. Exception—hyperacute PML in the setting of IRIS and in MS patients on natalizumab.

Other Opportunistic Infections

Cytomegalovirus

Acquired CMV Infections are commonly manifesting as meningoencephalitis and ventriculitis/epididymitis. Ventricular ependymal enhancement in an immunocompromised patient is highly suggestive of CMV.

Extracranial presentations: Retinitis and myelitis with radiculitis.

Tuberculosis

Tuberculosis is one of the most devastating opportunistic infections and the main cause of morbidity and mortality in HIV-infected patients worldwide. Multidrug-resistant and extensively drug-resistant tuberculosis are found almost entirely in patients coinfected with HIV.

- Tubercular co-infection generally exacerbates the severity and accelerates the progression of HIV.
- Tuberculosis should be treated first in HIV-infected patients to increase the effectiveness of HAART and to prevent the development of TB-IRIS.

Imaging: Enhancement of meninges, tuberculomas, and pseudo abscesses are often mild or absent even in the presence of more acid-fast bacilli.

Immune Reconstitution Inflammatory Syndrome

CNS IRIS is a T cell-mediated encephalitis in treated HIV patients or autoimmune disease (multiple sclerosis). It is a dysregulated immune response to infectious or noninfectious antigens.

Underlying Pathogens

- JC virus (PML-IRIS),
- Tuberculosis (TB-IRIS)
- Fungal infections especially cryptococcus (crypto IRIS).
- Natalizumab associated PML IRIS in patients of multiple sclerosis.

Two forms are recognized:

1. **Unmasking IRIS**: When antiretroviral therapy reveals a subclinical, previously unrecognized opportunistic infection.
2. **Paradoxical IRIS**: When a patient who has been successfully treated for a recent opportunistic infection deteriorates after initiation of antiretroviral therapy.

The most common presentation of CNS IRIS is clinical deterioration of the patients despite the rising CD4 counts and lower viral loads in a newly treated AIDS patient.

Imaging

PML IRIS: Confluent and linear or "punctate" perivascular hyperintensities on T2/FLAIR images. A punctate pattern of enhancement is typical in the acute stage. Bizarre-looking parenchymal masses and progressively enlarging and enhancing lesions are also common.

TB-IRIS: May develop florid TB pseudo abscesses (TB gone wild) and/or rapidly increasing enhancement in the basilar meninges.

Other Manifestations of HIV/AIDS

- Vasculopathy
- HIV/AIDS-related bone marrow changes
- Benign lymphoepithelial lesions
- Lymphoid hyperplasia

5. Manifestations of CNS TB: Clinical findings, pathology, imaging. [10] [DNB Dec 21]

- **Causative Organism**: *Mycobacterium tuberculosis*
- About 5–10% of tuberculosis patients and up to 20% of AIDS-related tuberculosis patients have CNS involvement.

Pathogenesis

A two-step model of CNS TB pathogenesis:

1. Hematogenous spread of bacteria from distant focus (e.g., from lungs to subpial or subependymal region—call called the "Rich" focus).
2. The Rich focus may rupture into the subarachnoid space or into the ventricular system leading to meningitis.

Presentations of CNS Tuberculosis

- **Tubercular Meningitis**: Leptomeningeal and pachymeningeal.
- **Parenchymal Tuberculosis**:
  - Tuberculomas
  - Disseminated tuberculomas (military tuberculosis)
  - Tubercular abscess
  - Tubercular encephalopathy
  - Focal tubercular cerebritis

Tubercular Meningitis (TBM)

The most common presentation of CNS tuberculosis is tubercular meningitis. Children are more frequently affected by tubercular meningitis due to their poor immune response to contain bacteria within the lungs.

Clinical Manifestations

- Insidious onset malaise, low-grade fever, vomiting, intermittent headache, and neck stiffness.
- Cranial nerve palsies (especially third, fourth, and sixth nerves) and seizures are common.
- In severe cases, patients may be presented with confusion, hemiparesis, and coma. The cerebrospinal fluid evaluation shows lymphocytosis, increased protein levels, and decreased glucose levels. Presence of *M. tuberculosis* in cerebrospinal fluid in approximately 90% of cases. Negative finding of bacteria in CSF analysis does not preclude treatment, if there is strong clinical suspicion or radiologic evidence of tuberculous disease.

Imaging

NCCT:

- May show obliteration of the basal cisterns by isoattenuating or hyperattenuating exudates and plaque-like dural thickening.
- May show hydrocephalous.
- May show vasculitic infarct.

CECT

- Basal enhancing exudates and meningeal enhancement. Meningeal enhancement may extend to the convexities and Sylvian fissures.
- If ventricles are involved then postcontrast scan shows ependymal enhancement.

MRI: Better than CT for detection of soft tissue resolution basal exudates, meningeal enhancement, identification of infarct and parenchymal abnormalities.

Magnetization Transfer (MT)

- The quantification of MT ratio (MTR) helps to differentiate tubercular meningitis from other causes. The high lipid content of the tuberculous bacilli accounts for the low MTR in TBM.
- **The MTR of the meninges:** Fungal and pyogenic meningitis > tubercular meningitis > viral meningitis.

Complications of Tubercular Meningitis

- **Hydrocephalus**: Communicating hydrocephalus > noncommunicating hydrocephalus
- **Cranial Neuropathies**
- **Focal Infarction**
- **Focal Atrophy and Syringobulbia**
- **Hydrocephalus**:
  - The basal cisterns and subarachnoid spaces exudates are blocking the CSF circulation and causing hydrocephalus.
  - The mass effect over the aqueduct of Sylvius or over the fourth ventricle from a focal parenchymal lesion may lead to obstructive hydrocephalus.
  - A complex type of hydrocephalus (combination of communicating and noncommunicating hydrocephalus) may be seen due to epididymitis and entrapped ventricles noncommunicating (obstructive) hydrocephalus.
- **Vasculitis**: Intracranial vasculitis may occur due to a direct invasion of the vessel by the pathogenic microorganism or an extension of adjacent arachnoiditis. It is most commonly seen in the basal ganglia, thalamus, and internal capsule due to the involvement of the small perforating branches (the lenticulostriate and thalamo-perforating arteries) supplying these regions.
- **Cranial Neuropathies**:
  - Approximately 17–40% of patients with CNS tuberculosis presented with cranial nerve neuropathies. The most commonly affected cranial nerves are the II, III, IV, VI, and VII nerves
  - Contrast enhancement and thickening may be seen on the contrast scan suggesting the involvement.

Tubercular Pachymeningitis

It is the involvement of pachymeninges by the tuberculous bacilli and can be focal or diffuse. Focal tubercular pachymeningitis: On imaging, it shows focal pachymeningeal thickening and enhancement. Differentials could be meningioma or metastatic deposit.

Parenchymal Tuberculosis

It comprises of:

- Tuberculomas
- Miliary TB
- Abscess
- TB encephalopathy and focal tubercular cerebritis.

Tuberculomas: Tuberculomas are more common in pediatric age group. It may occur anywhere in the brain parenchyma.

CT: It may show isodense to hyperdense solid-enhancing lesions to ring-enhancing lesions with surrounding edema. The target sign (central calcification surrounded by a rim of enhancement) is highly suggestive of tubercular infection.

MR features of tuberculomas vary depending on the nature of the granuloma **(Table 16)**.

TABLE 16: MR features of tuberculomas.

MR sequences	*Noncaseating*	*Caseating with a solid center*	*Caseating with central liquefaction*
T1 and T2 sequences	Hypointense signal on T1 and hyperintense signal on T2-weighted images	Hypointense on T1 and markedly hypointense on T2-weighted images	Peripheral hypointense rim on T2 weighted images
Postcontrast scan	Homogenous enhancement of the lesion	Rim enhancement	Rim enhancement

MT Imaging

Precontrast MT T1-weighted images are better than conventional spin-echo images for the identification of tuberculomas due to their low MT ratio.

MR Spectroscopy

- Show prominent lipid peaks at 0.9 and 1.3 ppm.
- Markedly elevated choline peak is seen in metastasis and glioma which helps to differentiate from tuberculomas.

Disseminated Tuberculomas (Miliary TB)

Multiple small granulomas (<5 mm) scattered throughout the brain parenchyma in disseminated disease. On a postcontrast scan, it shows ring and disc enhancement of the lesions.

Tuberculous Abscess

It is more common in the elderly or immunocompromised patients; however, it is seen in <10% of CUN TB patients. A tuberculous abscess is often indistinguishable from a pyogenic brain abscess or a caseous tuberculoma.

Imaging Features

- Usually solitary lesions and larger (>3 cm).
- Multiloculated with smooth and thin enhancing wall.
- Mass effect with surrounding edema.
- Shows diffusion restriction.
- **Differential diagnosis**: Pyogenic abscess **(Table 17)**.

TABLE 17: Differences between tubercular and pyogenic abscess.

MR sequences	Tuberculous abscess	Pyogenic abscess
MT images	Low MTR	High MTR
MR spectroscopy	Absence of amino acid peak. May show lipid, lactate	Presence of amino acid peak (leucine, isoleucine, valine) at 0.9 ppm

TB Encephalopathy

It usually occurs in infants, preschool and school-age children following pulmonary tuberculosis due to type IV hypersensitivity reaction to the tuberculous antigen. The patients usually succumb to death within 1–2 months of the onset despite antitubercular treatment.

- **Imaging**: Shows a diffuse unilateral/bilateral cerebral edema.
- Death usually occurs within 1–2 months of the onset despite antitubercular treatment.

Focal Tuberculous Cerebritis

It is the focal cerebral involvement by the microorganism. On imaging, it shows a focal gyriform pattern of postcontrast enhancement.

CNS TB and AIDS

Tuberculous infections of CNS show a very rapidly progressive course in HIV-infected patients. Infarction, meningeal enhancement, and parenchymal disease are more common presentations of CNS tuberculosis in HIV-infected patients. However, the differential diagnosis in AIDS patients (opportunistic infections and primary or metastatic CNS lymphoma) must be kept in mind.

Epilepsy

1. A 37-year-old female presents with history of intractable epilepsy. Discuss the imaging modalities and protocols used in workup of this patient. Describe imaging findings of mesial temporal sclerosis. [(3+3)+4] [MD (WBUHS) 21, AIIMS Dec 23, DNB Dec 20]

The causes of intractable epilepsy in this 37-year-old female could be many which are:

1. **Mesial Temporal Sclerosis**
2. **Developmental**: Less likely at this age except focal cortical dysplasia type I
3. **Epileptogenic Tumors**:
   - Ganglioglioma
   - Dysembryoplastic neuroepithelial tumor (DNET)
   - Pleomorphic xanthoastrocytoma
   - Hypothalamic hamartoma
4. **Gliosis due to Scars**
5. **Neurocutaneous Syndromes**:
   - Sturge-Weber
   - Tuberous sclerosis

Imaging modalities that can be used are:

1. **MRI**: MRI is the mainstay imaging modality in case of intractable epilepsy. MRI protocol:
   - Preferably at 3T strength for better image clarity, spatial and contrast resolution.
   - Slice thickness 3 mm, slice spacing 0.5 mm
   - Sequences (epilepsy protocol):
     - Axial T2
     - 3D Axial T1
     - 3D Axial T2 FLAIR
     - Axial DWI
     - Axial GRE/Axial SWI
     - Coronal T2
     - Sagittal T2
     - Coronal Oblique SPGR thin (2 mm) along right and left temporal lobes at right angles to the hippocampus—entire hippocampus must be visualized.
     - Coronal Oblique T2 FLAIR thin (2 mm) along right and left temporal lobes at right angles to the hippocampus
     - 3D double inversion recovery (DIR)
     - Axial T1 pre-and postcontrast if needed in case of tumors.
     - Additional sequences like DTI if needed as in case of tumors
     - Certain sequences have their own benefits:
     - GRE/SWI for hemoglobin breakdown products in posttraumatic changes and cavernomas, or to look for calcifications in tuberous sclerosis, Sturge-Weber, cavernomas and gangliogliomas.
     - SPGR thin along hippocampus to look for mesial temporal sclerosis.
     - 3D Axial T1 for cortical thickness, heterotopias and grey-white interface.
     - 3D Axial T2 FLAIR for cortical and subcortical hyperintensities.
     - 3D DIR are very sensitive for cortical abnormalities.
2. **CT**: It is not the modality of choice but can be used in certain conditions such as in detecting calcifications or hemorrhage.
3. **PET**: Identify epileptogenic foci by identifying areas of hypometabolism and hypermetabolism.

4. **SPECT**: Identify epileptogenic foci by detecting changes in blood flow.
5. EEG with fusion imaging with MRI or functional MRI improves accuracy of localization of seizure focus.

Mesial Temporal Sclerosis (MTS): MTS is the most common association with intractable temporal lobe epilepsy. It is a specific pattern of hippocampal neuronal loss accompanied by gliosis and atrophy.

Its imaging findings on MRI are as follows:
- **Reduced Hippocampal Volume**: Hippocampal atrophy
- **Increased T2 Signal (Represents Gliosis)**
- **Abnormal Morphology**: Loss of internal architecture (interdigitations of hippocampus), stratum radiata, a thin layer of white matter separates the dentate gyrus and Ammon horn.
- Enlargement of the temporal horn of the lateral ventricle—least specific. Comparing one side with the other is the best technique, however care should be taken in case of bilateral pathology when it may be reported as normal.

When severe and long standing, additional associated findings include:
- Atrophy of the ipsilateral fornix and mammillary body
- Increased signal and or atrophy of the anterior thalamic nucleus
- Atrophy of the cingulate gyrus
- Increased signal and/or reduction in the volume of the amygdala
- Reduction in the volume of the subiculum
- Dilatation of temporal horn and temporal lobe atrophy
- Collateral white matter and entorhinal cortex atrophy
- Thalamic and caudate atrophy
- Ipsilateral cerebral atrophy
- Contralateral cerebellar hemiatrophy
- Loss of grey-white matter interface in the anterior temporal lobe
- Reduced white matter volume in the parahippocampal gyrus
- **MR Spectroscopy Findings Typically Represent Neuronal Dysfunction:**
  - Decreased NAA and decreased NAA/Cho and NAA/Cr ratios
  - Decreased MI in ipsilateral temporal lobe
  - Increased lipid and lactate soon after a seizure

Brain Tumors

1. Describe radiological anatomy of sella-turcica and imaging features of suprasellar masses. [4+6] [MD (WBUHS) 23, DNB Dec 21]

The sella-turcica is a spherical depression in the superior surface of the sphenoid bone bounded by the sphenoid sinus antero-inferiorly, the paired cavernous sinuses laterally, the suprasellar cisterns and its contents, diaphragma sellae and hypothalamus superiorly and the dorsum sella and brainstem posteriorly.

The cortical bone of sella varies from few microns to several millimeters in thickness, depending upon the degree of pneumatization of the sphenoid sinus. The carotid artery forms a groove on the posterosuperior wall of the sphenoid sinus. The wall between the artery and the sinus may be very thin, even absent in up to one-third of patients, thus making it vulnerable to injury during transsphenoidal surgery. Localized defects in its bony cortex or asymmetry of the sellar floor are common. The bony sella is invested by a reflection of dura, the outer layer of which lines the floor while the inner layer forms a diaphragm at the roof (diaphragma sellae). A central opening in the diaphragm allows the pituitary infundibulum to pass into the sella. Anteriorly, the sellar floor is continuous with the tuberculum sellae and limbus sphenoidale. The dorsum sella demarcates the posterior sellar border. Cavernous sinuses are two multiseptated, symmetrically paired parasellar venous sinuses with a straight or slightly convex outer wall. The two layers of dura form the roof, outer wall and inner wall of the sinuses. The lateral walls of the cavernous sinuses from superior to inferior contain the cranial nerves III, IV as well as first and second divisions of the Vth nerve (V1 and V2). The VIth nerve passes through the sinus below the internal carotid artery (ICA). The ICA has a variable course within the sinus; however, a more medial location of the artery is a normal variation

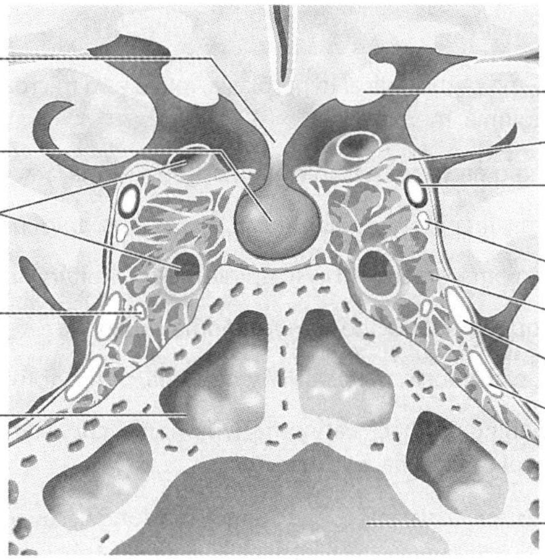

FIG. 15: Schematic diagram showing coronal section of pituitary with adjacent structures.

and is surgically important. The artery may actually indent the gland at times and the distance between the arteries may be as little as 4 mm. The ICA exits the sinus at level of anterior clinoid process to give off its supra cavernous branches. Meckel's cave housing the Gasserian ganglion lies at the posterior part of the cavernous sinus. The third division of Vth nerve (V3) passes inferior from here to foramen ovale. The suprasellar cistern is a six-pointed expansion of the subarachnoid space containing the optic nerves, optic chiasma and the tracts, circle of Willis and the pituitary infundibulum. The optic chiasma lies 4–6 mm posterosuperior to the tuberculum sellae, however, it may be directly above it (prefixed) or lie more posteriorly above the dorsum sella (postfixed). These variations are important for surgeons. The optic and infundibular recesses are downward invaginations of the third ventricle in relation to its floor **(Fig. 15)**.

The hypothalamus is a layer of tissue extending from the anterior commissure to the posterior commissure and forms the floor and the lateral walls of the third ventricle.

The inferior ridge of the tissue from the optic chiasma anteriorly to the paired mammillary bodies posteriorly is called the tuber cinereum. At the lateral margins of the hypothalamus are the optic tracts and the sulci of temporal lobes. The hypothalamus consists of multiple nuclei regulating temperature, water balance, drinking behavior and sexual activity. The hypothalamus and the pituitary gland are functionally and physiologically interlinked contiguous structures and often referred to as the hypothalamic-pituitary-axis (HPA). Release of pituitary hormones is mediated by the hypothalamus. Oxytocin and vasopressin are synthesized in hypothalamus and transported to the posterior pituitary. The pituitary gland is composed of two anatomically and functionally distinct lobes: the anterior lobe (adenohypophysis) and the posterior lobe (neurohypophysis). The anterior lobe comprises 75% of the volume of the gland and consists of pars tuberalis, pars intermedia and pars distalis which develop from Rathke's pouch. Pars intermedia which lies between the adeno and neurohypophysis, is a vestigial structure and common site for developmental cysts. The anterior lobe of pituitary is isointense to brain on both T1 and T2WI. It secretes growth hormone (GH), adrenocorticotropic hormone (ACTH), prolactin (PRL), thyroid stimulating hormone (TSH), luteinizing hormone (LH) and melanocyte-stimulating hormone (MSH). The anterior lobe shares a common blood supply with hypothalamus via the hypophyseal portal system, the pathway by which hypothalamic releasing hormones reach this structure. Alternately the hypophyseal arteries, branches of internal carotid supply the stalk and posterior lobe. The venous drainage is to ipsilateral cavernous sinus predominantly and then to petrosal sinuses. The posterior lobe develops as a downward projection from the neuroectoderm at the base of the brain and along with infundibular stalk, supraoptic and paraventricular hypothalamic nuclei forms the neurohypophysis. Oxytocin and vasopressin synthesized in the hypothalamus are transported to and stored in the posterior pituitary. The posterior lobe appears as a bright spot on T1-weighted images (T1WI) in midline along the dorsum of the sella. The anterior lobe of pituitary gland is larger and rounded and appears hyperintense like posterior lobe in newborns and becomes isointense by 4–6 months of life. The dimensions of pituitary gland are extremely variable, particularly its height. The gland undergoes significant changes in size and shape throughout life and this fact must be kept in mind when assessing it for abnormality. A useful guide to the gland's height in relation to age is the "Elster's rule" of 6, 8, 10, 12. On an average, it is 12 mm in width and 8 mm in anteroposterior diameter. The maximal height is achieved in adolescent girls and during pregnancy. The pituitary stalk tapers inferiorly and has thickness of 2 mm. It should not exceed the width of the basilar artery or a maximum of 4 mm.

TABLE 18: Important sellar and parasellar masses.	
Intrasellar masses	Physiological and pathological hyperplasia, micro and microadenomas, non-neoplastic cyst, craniopharyngioma, meningioma
Suprasellar mass (child)	Craniopharyngioma, hypothalamic glioma, germinoma, arachnoid cyst tuber cinereum hamartoma
Suprasellar mass (adult)	Macroadenoma, meningioma, aneurysm, metastasis, epidermoid/dermoid
Cystic lesions	Craniopharyngioma, arachnoid cyst, epidermoid, pituitary abscess
Infundibular masses (child)	Pituitary hypoplasia, histiocytosis, germinoma, leukemia
Infundibular masses (adult)	Hypophysitis, sarcoidosis, metastasis/lymphoma, pituicytoma
Parasellar lesion (tumors)	Metastasis, meningioma, schwannoma, lymphoma, chordoma, osteocartilaginous tumors, nasopharyngeal carcinoma, plasmacytoma
Parasellar lesions (vascular and inflammatory)	Sarcoidosis, histiocytosis, infections, fungal, nonfungal, cavernous sinus thrombosis, cavernous sinus hemangioma, aneurysm, caroticocavernous fistula, Tolosa-Hunt syndrome

The important sellar and parasellar masses are presented in the following table **(Table 18)**.

Sellar Suprasellar Masses

Pituitary Adenoma

Adenomas arise from the adenohypophysis and are classified by size and hormonal activity; features that determine their clinical presentation. They are the most common tumors of the sellar and parasellar region in adults and constitute 10–15% of all intracranial neoplasms.[8] By definition, adenomas measuring less than 10 mm are called microadenomas while the larger ones are termed macroadenomas. In general, hormonally active lesions are discovered at a smaller size due to endocrinopathy and consequent clinical symptoms. Nonfunctioning adenomas are usually large at the time of diagnosis when they produce symptoms due to mass effect on surrounding structures. Approximately three-fourths of adenomas show signs of hormone excess while the rest are nonfunctioning tumors. Sometimes these nonfunctioning lesions may be discovered incidentally (Incidentalomas). Clinically silent adenomas have been demonstrated in 10% of asymptomatic volunteers. The rest may produce symptoms by compressing adjacent structures, causing various symptoms, i.e., visual field defects (bitemporal hemianopia) due to optic chiasma compression, hypopituitarism due to compression of pituitary gland, cranial nerve deficits due to lateral extension into cavernous sinuses, hydrocephalus/ CSF rhinorrhea due to third ventricular obstruction, or rarely, diabetes insipidus due to mass effect on hypothalamus.

Types of Adenomas

Prolactinomas are the most common functioning adenomas comprising 50% of all adenomas. These tumors clinically present with amenorrhea, galactorrhea and infertility in females and loss of libido and impotence in males. Serum PRL level is usually greater than 100 ng/mL (normal 20 ng/mL). In case serum PRL level is greater than 200 ng/mL, the cause is nearly always a pituitary adenoma.

ACTH secreting adenomas produce early symptoms when they are small, often measuring 1- 2 mm in size and thus are difficult to diagnose. However, an ectopic source of ACTH secretion must also be kept in mind in a patient with hypercortisolism. GH secreting tumors are macroadenomas as they are diagnosed late in the course of disease. They produce acromegaly in adults and gigantism in children. Rarely adenomas arise from the thyrotrophs (TSH secreting) or gonadotrophs (FHS and/or LH secreting). In addition, 10% of secreting adenomas are plurihormonal, the most common combination being the PRL-GH producing adenoma.

Imaging of Adenomas

Imaging is indicated both to confirm the existence of an adenoma and to define its size and location for appropriate surgical or medical therapy. MRI is the preferred modality, though CT is also useful.

Reported sensitivity and specificity of noncontrast MRI and contrast enhanced CT are roughly equal varying from 50% to 90%. However, there is no large blinded prospective study comparing CT and MRI in the same group of patients. Overall, T1WI are more reliable for detection of adenomas. The addition of Gd enhancement increases the detection rate of microadenomas by 10%. Postcontrast dynamic acquisition allows evaluation of temporal changes in signal intensity in intrasellar structures and adds additional 5–20% sensitivity over the nondynamic studies for detection of microadenomas (particularly small ACTH secretors and those which are isointense). Signal intensity increases more rapidly and to a greater degree in normal pituitary gland than in microadenoma, however, 3–5 minutes following the contrast administration the signal of the normal gland and the adenoma may become identical. The maximum contrast difference between the normal gland and the microadenoma occurs at about 30–60 seconds when the distinction between normal pituitary and the adenoma is the best. Microadenomas also demonstrate a slower washout of accumulated contrast that may cause them to appear hyperintense on delayed images (>20 minutes postcontrast). With modern state- of-the art MRI equipment, more than 90% adenomas should be picked up. The prescribed protocol should be high resolution plain scan which if negative should be followed by contrast-enhanced magnetic resonance imaging consisting of both dynamic scanning and regular postcontrast scan. Certain studies have shown that if the conventional and dynamic contrast imaging is combined with an additional 3D volumetric interpolated breath-hold examination, a spoiled-gradient echo 3D T1 sequence (SGE), the accuracy of identifying microadenomas increases significantly. Parasellar extension and invasion of the base of skull are also accurately shown on MRI with dynamic T1 and heavily T2-weighted sequences proving the best. CT scores over MRI in showing subtle cortical involvement, however, this may not be surgically important.

Microadenomas (<10 mm in size) typically appear hypointense compared to the normal adenohypophysis on T1WI (80–90%) and iso to hyperintense on T2WI. The signal intensity of adenomas and normal gland are comparable to the grey and white matter of the temporal lobe respectively on T1WI. They may sometimes appear hyperintense on T1WI. This is attributable to hemorrhage. Occasionally they may be isointense and can only be detected on enhanced scans (particularly dynamic study) where they stand out as hypointense areas within the enhancing gland.

On contrast-enhanced CT (CECT) adenomas are seen as discrete, hypodense regions within the enhancing gland. Imaging has little to offer for differentiating different types of microadenomas, however, the PRL and GH secreting adenomas tend to be located more laterally in the gland and ACTH and gonadotropin secretors tend to be more central. Indirect signs for the presence of adenoma include enlargement of gland and a bulge in the gland outline.

Tilt of the pituitary stalk and asymmetry of the sellar floor though helpful signs may sometimes occur physiologically due to developmental asymmetry of the brain or stalk insertion. Inferior petrosal sinus sampling may be extremely useful for localizing adenoma and distinguishing Cushing's disease from ectopic ACTH secretion and autonomous adrenal disease when imaging fails to show the site of adenoma. Lateralization of the lesion to either half of the pituitary gland is also possible. However, in larger lesions, lateralization may not be accurate due to venous drainage occurring in either direction i.e. both cavernous sinuses.

Macroadenomas (>10 mm), being larger, are easier to diagnose. They usually enlarge the sella, erode the sphenoid sinus, encroach upon the suprasellar cistern and may displace the chiasma. Solid adenomas enhance uniformly, while others may show heterogeneous hypodense areas within it on CECT. Macroadenomas are frequently hyperintense on T2WI. Hyperintense macroadenomas may be soft and necrotic while hypointense lesions may be more fibrous; a finding that may be of help to the surgeon. Apparent diffusion coefficient values on diffusion- weighted imaging may be higher in softer variety. Hemorrhage and necrosis are common particularly following bromocriptine therapy, majority of these being subclinical. In large lesions, residual pituitary tissue may not be visible. Most microadenomas enhance late as compared to the adenohypophysis while macroadenomas enhance early. This reflects the difference in their blood supply. With suprasellar extension, the adenomas acquire a typical "figure-of-eight", appearance. Early cavernous sinus involvement by adenoma is often difficult to diagnose. The most reliable signs of cavernous sinus invasion are encasement of cavernous carotid arteries, presence of tumor lateral to them, delayed enhancing soft tissue in sinus, a lateral bulge of the outer dura and a serum PRL level of 1,000 ng/mL or more (in case of prolactinomas). In one study MDCT was found to better delineate the lateral margin of tumor.

MR has been shown to be useful in precisely demonstrating the cavernous sinus invasion. Many grading schemes have been proposed to prognosticate the effect of cavernous sinus extension on the surgical outcomes of these patients. Knosp grading **(Fig. 16)** has been widely used and has proven to show good correlation with outcomes. The grading is defined by the relation of carotid lines with the

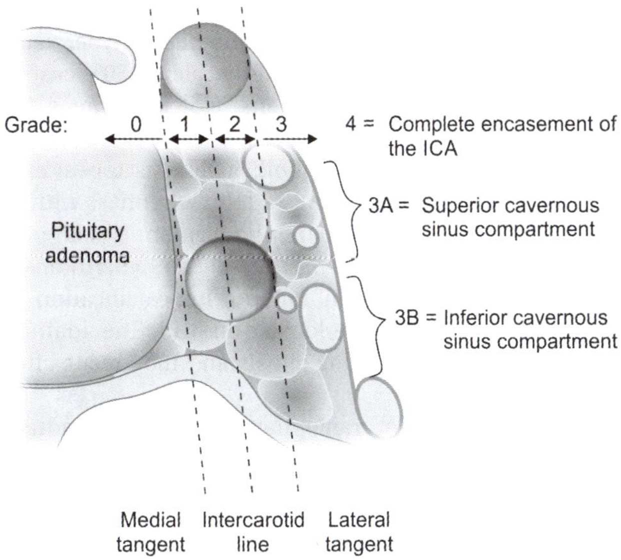

FIG. 16: Knosp grading of pituitary invasion of cavernous sinus.

limits of invasion. These lines pass through supra- and intracavernous parts of ICA in coronal view. There are medial, median and lateral carotid lines.

Atypical Presentations of Adenomas

Their blood supply being marginal, pituitary adenomas may present acutely with infarction and hemorrhage, a condition called pituitary apoplexy. However, these events may be silent and only detected at pathology or imaging. Hemorrhage/infarction may be spontaneous or following bromocriptine therapy (in more than half of the treated patients). The gland may show areas which appear hyperdense on noncontrast CT, dark on T2WI (acute blood) or bright on T1WI (subacute blood). Massive hemorrhage may have subarachnoid/intracerebral extension. Diffusion imaging may show restriction.

Although pituitary adenomas are generally benign slow growing neoplasms, malignant variants exist. These tend to infiltrate dura, bone and surrounding structures. As histology and imaging do not allow distinction between the two, the presence of metastatic disease is the only definite clue to diagnosis.

The term invasive pituitary adenomas represent an intermediate part of the spectrum. These infiltrate surrounding structures but grow slowly and by definition do not cause metastasis.

An aggressive subtype of ACTH producing adenoma is seen in Nelson's syndrome, a condition in which the adenoma enlarges in the absence of regulatory mechanisms after bilateral adrenalectomy.

Ectopic adenomas can arise from infundibulum or in suprasellar cistern from pars tuberalis.

Postoperative Sella

It may be difficult to differentiate residual/recurrent tumor from scarring and a variety of graft materials in the post-operative bed, i.e., fat, gelfoam, muscle, etc. Gadolinium-enhanced scan may be helpful in such cases. It is recommended that postoperative scanning be done 4–6 months after surgery to allow resorption of gelfoam, hemorrhagic material and debris. Comparison with preoperative scans, progressive growth of lesion and correlation with endocrinological markers are important. Development of empty sella, CSF leaks and sinusitis are some of the sequel of surgery.

Positron emission tomography potentially appears useful for assessing tumor response to therapy and for differentiating postsurgical changes from recurrent tumors.

Craniopharyngioma

These are benign, slowly growing, locally invasive, hormonally inactive lesions accounting for 2–4% of all intracranial lesions. They are derived from Rathke's pouch. Twenty percent of craniopharyngiomas may be purely intrasellar, while 80% have their epicenter in the suprasellar cistern. Rarely, they may be intraventricular or infrasellar. There is a bimodal age distribution, majority of lesions presenting in the 5–10 years age group with a second small peak in sixth decade. The children usually have features of raised intracranial pressure while visual disturbances and endocrinopathy are the usual presentation in 70–90% of adults. There are two histological subtypes of the lesions—adamantinomatous and papillary types. They are distinct in terms of clinical presentation, imaging features and treatment outcome. The more common classic form is adamantinomatous type, usually seen in children. They are almost always cystic with small solid components which frequently calcify (80% cases). Characteristically, these tumors appear as a combination of hypodense (cystic) and hyperdense (calcified) areas on CT. The solid portion appears isodense/isointense to brain on CT and MRI. The cyst fluid contains wet keratin, cholesterol crystals, proteinaceous fluids, hemorrhages and necrotic debris and is likened to motor oil. Such cysts appear extremely bright on both T1 and T2-weighted images.

In the suprasellar region is a lobulated mass with cystic signal and high peripheral T1, the latter seen as calcium on the previous CT. Irregular enhancement is seen peripherally. The pituitary is seen separately. The optic chiasm is displaced. The other cysts may be slightly hyperintense to CSF on T1WI, more so, on FLAIR and may show peripheral enhancement. CT is useful for showing calcification, particularly if the tumor is only a small solid calcified nodule, which may be totally overlooked on MRI. The adamantinomatous type is more likely to be locally invasive, encase vessels, cause surrounding gliosis and may recur after surgery. Contrast enhancement of the solid portions of the tumor may be seen.

Papillary variety of craniopharyngioma seen in adults are solid, often located within third ventricle and do not calcify. They are encapsulated and easily removable and hence have a lesser tendency to recur.

Craniopharyngiomas cause fibroinflammatory adhesions with surrounding tissues and tend to recur after surgery.

Pituicytoma

These arise from pituicyte, a glial cell in neurohypophysis and infundibulum and are also called granular cell tumors and myoblastoma. The location is usually posterior intrasellar with suprasellar extension.

Size ranges from 1 mm to 2 mm to 4 cm. On CT a hyperdense sellar/suprasellar mass is seen which enhances homogeneously. On T1WI, the lesion is iso to hypointense with absent bright spot and on T2 it is usually heterogeneous.

Meningioma

Ten percent of meningiomas occur in sellar and parasellar region. The site of origin is commonly tuberculum sella, the other locations being clinoid processes, the dorsum, medial sphenoid wing and cavernous sinuses. Tumors originating from optic sheath, olfactory groove and planum sphenoidale may also extend into supra/parasellar regions. They are slow growing lesions causing mass effect, i.e., visual loss, ophthalmoplegia or proptosis due to venous congestion at the orbital apex.

On MRI, they are usually isointense to grey matter on T1WI. T2WI images show isointensity in 50% and hyperintensity in 30–40%.[10] Meningiomas show bright contrast enhancement on both CT and MRI. It is important to differentiate meningioma from adenoma as the surgical approach varies in the two. MR signal intensity and enhancement pattern do not allow this differentiation. However, morphological features like a broad base with dural tail, hyperostosis rather than erosion, calcification (better shown on CT), a cleft demarcating the lesion from brain and pituitary gland, greater propensity for arterial encasement and normal sized sella favor a diagnosis of meningioma. 31P-spectroscopy may show higher phosphate monoester in meningioma.

Germinoma and Teratoma

Twenty percent of these germ cell tumors may be seen in suprasellar cistern or pituitary fossa in children and young adults. They may arise here or may be metastatic lesions from a pineal tumor. There is no sex predilection unlike pineal tumors, which have a strong male predominance. Patients present with endocrinopathy, visual field defects, hydrocephalus, etc., as is common to all suprasellar neoplasms. However, diabetes insipidus is the earliest symptom due to invasion of hypothalamus.

Germinomas tend to be large noncapsulated solid lesions, centered on or behind stalk that infiltrate into surrounding structures. They are homogenous lesions without cystic components (unlike craniopharyngioma). On CT they are hyperdense like lymphoma. On MRI, they are slightly hypointense on T1 and hyperintense on T2WI. They show strong contrast enhancement on CT/MRI. There is also a high tendency of CSF dissemination. The posterior pituitary bright spot is often absent. Teratomas show evidence of fat or calcification and are more heterogeneous.

Dermoid and Epidermoid Tumors

These are slow growing benign inclusion tumors due to trapping of ectodermal cells during neural tube closure. Epidermoids are five times more common than dermoids and usually are parasellar in location; the second most common site in the head after the CP angles. They are seen in adults of 20–40 years of age. Dermoids are more common in children, tend to occur in the midline and in posterior fossa but may occur in the suprasellar cistern. Epidermoid cysts are composed of desquamated keratin while the dermoids contain dermal appendages. Both show slow growth, tend to insinuate in the available space and produce symptoms by compression of the adjacent structures. Rarely, chemical meningitis may occur due to rupture. Epidermoids appear heterogeneous and slightly hyperdense to CSF on CT and usually slightly hyperintense to CSF on T1WI. They rarely enhance but occasionally calcify peripherally.

FLAIR and diffusion images are extremely useful in showing these lesions as is CT cisternography. Dermoids are more heterogeneous and often show fat density (fat fluid levels sometimes) or calcification. Fat droplets may be visualized in the subarachnoid space in ruptured dermoids. However, epidermoids, dermoids and other purely cystic lesions may be indistinguishable on imaging.

Chiasmatic/Hypothalamic Glioma

Seventy five percent of these tumors occur in first decade of life. This diverse group of neoplasms often present with different behavior and response to therapy and are referred to together as chiasmatic hypothalamic gliomas. The site of origin is often difficult to decide, as the lesions are usually large when detected and are infiltrative in nature. Neurofibromatosis 1 (NF-1) is present in 20–50% patients with optic chiasmatic lesions. The chiasmatic lesions tend to infiltrate the hypothalamus leading to hypothalamic dysfunction and hydrocephalus. They also tend to infiltrate along the optic tracts, hence the importance of imaging the entire brain. The tumors confined to the chiasma can be differentiated from optic neuritis by clinical presentation or resolution of neuritis on steroids.

The lesions appear isointense to brain on T1WI and hyperintense on T2WI. Calcification and hemorrhages are not seen but cystic component can occur. Contrast enhancement is seen in 50% lesions. Lack of serial growth and enhancement differentiate benign hamartomatous NF lesions from glioma.

Hypothalamic gliomas are aggressive and present with hypothalamic dysfunction. Diencephalic syndrome almost always indicates this diagnosis and refers to a clinical state of cachexia in an alert/euphoric child who often has a good appetite.

In general, chiasma/hypothalamic lesions are more aggressive compared to the optic nerve lesions. Lesions arising above 20 years and below 5 years of age also show a more aggressive behavior compared to those arising between 5 years and 20 years. Similarly sporadic lesions also are more aggressive.

Schwannoma

Parasellar schwannomas most commonly arise from branches of Vth nerve. The lesions present with sensory deficit, problems of mastication, facial pain or diplopia. Imaging shows asymmetry and expansion of cavernous sinus. They are encapsulated lesions isointense to brain on T1WI and bright on T2WI. They are isodense on CT and enhance strongly. Larger tumors may be heterogeneous with a tigroid appearance. The 3rd to 6th nerve schwannomas follow the course of respective nerves but are rare lesions.

The dumb-bell configuration of Vth nerve schwannoma straddling the petrous apex is characteristic but less common than a Meckel's cave or posterior fossa mass.

Skull base Lesions

Primary, secondary and metastatic tumors of the skull base can involve the parasellar area. The primary lesions include chondroma, chondrosarcoma, and plasmacytoma. Secondary tumors are often from nasopharynx and paranasal sinuses. Common metastasis comes from lung, breast and prostate primaries. These are difficult to differentiate from chordoma.

Chordoma

They are locally malignant tumors derived from notochordal remnants; 35% of them arise in the clivus (spheno-occipital synchondrosis) though occasionally they may present in Meckel's cave and petrous bone. Mean age of presentation is 20–40 years though no age is exempt. Imaging shows lobular lesions iso to hypointense on T1WI and heterogeneous on T2WI replacing the clival marrow. They appear hyperintense on postcontrast studies with septations of fibrous connective tissue. CT shows a destructive mass with fragments of bone and calcification. Localization of the epicenter of the lesion within the clivus and identification of normal or displaced pituitary gland differentiates chordomas from invasive adenomas.

Metastasis

Anterior lobe dysfunction or diabetes insipidus in a patient with known malignancy (carcinomas of lung, GI tract, breast, leukemia/lymphoma and skull base tumors) may indicate pituitary metastasis. However, most of these lesions are detected on autopsy. Presumably, most patients succumb to advanced disseminated malignancy before these lesions produce symptoms. The routes of spread may be hematogenous, by CSF seeding or by direct extension. Imaging may show an enhancing intrasellar, suprasellar or combined lesion. Although difficult to differentiate from adenoma by imaging, endocrinopathy in a patient with known malignancy, rapid growth/disproportionate invasion and destruction of surrounding structures by a small-sized lesion, a dumbbell shape with constriction at diaphragm in a normal sized sella, associated brain edema and enhancement and thickening of infundibulum suggest the diagnosis of metastasis.

2. Discuss the MRI findings in common posterior fossa neoplasms in pediatric age. [10] [MD (WBUHS) 23, DNB Dec 20]

The infratentorial tumors are classified based on topography and age as follows **(Table 19)**.

Medulloblastoma

Medulloblastoma (MB) is a malignant primitive ectodermal tumor and is the most common infratentorial tumor in children, accounting for one-third of childhood pediatric tumors. About three-quarters of MBs occur in children 5–15 years old. In adults, though much less common, MBs usually occur in the third and fourth decades of life. MBs are typically midline infratentorial tumors and the most common location is in the region of the vermis and the inferior medullary velum. Cerebellar hemispheric MBs are less frequent and occur primarily in adults. Approximately 80% of patients with MB present with features of raised intracranial pressure. CSF seeding occurs in 10–30% of patients with MB.

Pathology

Histologically MBs are classified as classic; nodular or desmoplastic; MB with extensive nodularity; or as anaplastic/large cell variants. Over the past 5 years, considerable advances have been made in understanding MB biology and the 2016 WHO update has incorporated histological and molecular schemes into the classification of MBs. Based on

TABLE 19: Classification of infratentorial tumors based on topography and age.

Location	*Age-group*	*Tumor*
Cerebellar hemisphere and vermis	Pediatric	Medulloblastoma, ependymoma, astrocytoma, atypical teratoid/rhabdoid tumor
	Adult	Metastasis, hemangioblastoma, dysplastic cerebellar gangliocytoma, medulloblastoma
Brainstem	Pediatric	Diffuse midline glioma
	Adult	Diffuse midline glioma, GBM
Cerebellopontine angle	Pediatric	Atypical teratoid/rhabdoid tumor, medulloblastoma, ependymoma
	Adult	Vestibular schwannoma, meningiomas, epidermoid, arachnoid cyst, endolymphatic sac tumor
Fourth ventricle	Pediatric	Medulloblastoma, ependymoma
	Adult	Choroid plexus papilloma, epidermoid, subependymoma

genomic characterization, MBs can be subdivided into 4 distinct molecular subgroups: Wingless (WNT), sonic hedgehog (SHH), group 3, and group 4. These molecular subgroups are more predictive of clinical behavior and outcome than the tumor histology (classic or "variants") or the clinical staging system. Distribution of the different molecular subtypes between adult MB (50–60% SHH subgroup, 20–30% group 4 and 10–15% WNT) and pediatric MB (50–60% group 3 tumors, 10–30% group 4 tumors, 10–15% WNT and 10–15% SHH) are significantly different.

Imaging

Most pediatric MBs arise in the cerebellar vermis and often extend into the roof of the fourth ventricle and the brain stem. On imaging, MB appears as a well-circumscribed fourth ventricular mass. On CT scan, MBs are isodense to hyperdense due to their high cellularity and show variable enhancement after contrast administration. Approximately 20% of MBs have intratumoral calcification. Cystic and necrotic degeneration are most commonly found in adult MBs.

On MRI, typically they are hypointense to isointense on T1- and T2-WI; and show avid contrast enhancement **(Figs. 2A to F)**. The tumors are mostly homogeneous, although some display T2 heterogeneous signal due to the presence of intratumoral cysts, hemorrhage, calcification and necrotic foci. MBs show evidence of restricted diffusion (bright on DWI and dark on ADC maps) in their solid components presumably due to their high cellularity and high nucleus-to-cytoplasm ratio.

Postgadolinium brain and the spine MR imaging may show evidence of leptomeningeal metastatic spread in 33% of cases at the time of diagnosis or during the course of the disease.

At MR spectroscopy, MBs characteristically show taurine, detectable at short TE, and a high choline peak.

Compared to pediatric MBs, adult MBs are more likely to be located in cerebellar hemispheres and have an atypical presentation with more hyperintense signal on T1-WI, more hypointense signal on T2-WI and inhomogeneous contrast enhancement.

Recently, there have been attempts to predict the molecular subtype of MBs based on imaging phenotype; a new emerging field of imaging known as radiogenomics. This is quite helpful when advanced molecular subtyping is not available. Wingless-type–subgroup MBs are likely to be off midline tumors arising from the dorsal brainstem and cerebellum around the foramen of Luschka.

This subtype of MBs may present as an isolated CP angle mass, a mass in region of foramen of Luschka or as a midline fourth ventricle mass. These tumors are likely to contact the dorsal brainstem. SHH subgroups of MBs typically occurs in adults and appear as off-midline intracerebellar tumors without any contact with the brainstem. Group 3 MBs are likely to present as midline intraventricular tumors especially in children with small tumor size and prominent enhancement. In addition, diffuse leptomeningeal spread at the time of first presentation is also more likely to occur in Gp 3 MBs. Group 4 MBs are likely to present as midline intraventricular tumors which show no or minimal enhancement.

Ependymoma

Ependymomas are an infrequent group of glial tumors that typically arise from ependymal cells in supratentorial, infratentorial and spinal cord regions. Ependymomas are common tumors in children, comprising 10% of pediatric

CNS neoplasms and 15% of infratentorial tumors. The peak age at presentation is 1–5 years, with a smaller peak in adults in their fourth decade. Nearly two-thirds of intracranial ependymomas are present in the infratentorial compartment, arising from the ependymal lining of the fourth ventricle and the foramina of Luschka. Supratentorial lesions can be either intraventricular, typically in the lateral ventricles; or parenchymal. Approximately 60% of these tumors develop infratentorial, 30% supratentorially and 10% in the spinal cord. Infratentorial ependymomas usually present with symptoms of raised intracranial pressure. Cranial nerve palsies are also common, especially involving cranial nerves VI to X.

Pathology

Ependymomas are glial tumors arising from the ependymal lining of the ventricles and the central canal. The WHO classifies ependymal tumors into four types: (1) ependymoma (grade II), which include variants such as cellular, papillary, epithelial, clear-cell and mixed; (2) anaplastic ependymoma (grade III), (3) subependymoma (grade I), and (4) myxopapillary ependymoma (grade I). Anaplastic ependymomas have a greater incidence of leptomeningeal spread at the time of diagnosis and have poorer prognosis. Typical gross pathology shows a well-defined lobulated mass with areas of calcification, hemorrhage, and cysts. The tumor cells usually form ependymal rosettes, which are diagnostic but not always present.

Comprehensive genomic studies have divided infratentorial ependymomas into 2 prognostically different subgroups, PF-A and PFB.[14] The poor prognostic subgroup (group A), found predominantly in infants, exhibited a CpG island methylator phenotype and transcriptional silencing of the polycomb repressive complex 2, leading to repressed expression of differentiation genes.

Imaging

At CT, ependymomas appear as irregular and lobulated heterogeneous midline intraventricular masses with calcification (up to 45%). At MRI, they appear heterogeneous with T1 hypointensity, T2 iso/hyperintensity and iso-to-hyper FLAIR signal intensity due to presence of calcification, hemorrhage and cystic changes within the tumor. Following contrast administration, they usually show intense mixed heterogeneous enhancement; however, rarely, ependymomas do not enhance. The presence of calcifications within a lobulated heterogeneous fourth ventricular mass is highly suggestive but not diagnostic of ependymoma. Diffuse leptomeningeal spread is seen in less than 10% of patients at diagnosis when ependymoblastoma (ETANTR) are excluded.

On DWI, ADC of ependymomas is generally intermediate between that of pilocytic astrocytomas and MBs, however, ADC values are not completely reliable in differentiation between various infratentorial parenchymal masses. On Dynamic Susceptibility Contrast (DSC) perfusion MRI, ependymomas typically have markedly elevated perfusion (rCBV) and marked leakiness of contrast with poor return to baseline presumably due to presence of fenestrated blood vessels and an insufficient blood–brain barrier.

This behavior, although very characteristic of ependymomas, is not entirely pathognomonic and also may be demonstrated in other tumors, such as embryonal tumors. Typically, ependymomas show tumor extension through the fourth ventricular outflow foramina; however, this feature is not entirely pathognomonic, as some MBs may also extend through the fourth ventricular exit foramina. The extensions through the foramina in MBs is more bulbous and have more restricted diffusion compared to the thin tongues of tissue and intermediate diffusion in ependymomas. Rarely, ependymoma can present as an isolated mass within the cerebellopontine angle, presumably arising from the rests of ependymal cells. Proton MR spectroscopy typically demonstrates elevated high myoinositol (MI) levels in classic grade II ependymomas.

Treatment for EPN to this date remains maximal-safe surgical resection followed by adjuvant radiotherapy in order to reduce the likelihood of recurrence in the tumor bed. The survival rates have seen limited improvement (~80%) in the last decade, with survivors suffering from the debilitating side effects of radiation induced severe neurocognitive impairment and other radiation-induced complications.

Cerebellar Pilocytic Astrocytoma

Pilocytic astrocytomas (PA) are well-defined, slow growing, WHO Grade I tumors of CNS arising from astrocyte precursor cells. They typically present between 5 and 15 years of age. They generally arise from the cerebellum (60%), hypothalamus-optic chiasm region, brainstem and less commonly from cerebral hemispheres. Classically, cerebellar astrocytoma manifests with waxing and waning headache, truncal ataxia, dysdiadochokinesia are other cerebellar signs. They have an excellent prognosis with 90% of patients having a 10-year survival after total resection.

Pathology

PAs may be vermian or hemispheric in origin. Grossly, the cerebellar PA is usually sharply circumscribed, with a very narrow zone of microscopic infiltration. Approximately 50% of tumors are cystic with an enhancing mural nodule. Enhancement of the cyst wall is possible, but is not pathognomonic.[25] Nearly 40% of tumors are mixed solid with cystic or necrotic components and the rest are purely solid mass lesions. The tumor is supplied by capillaries that lack a complete blood-brain barrier (BBB). It has open tight junction in the endothelial cells with fenestration and therefore differs from low grade astrocytoma. This fact and the lack of BBB is the cause of both intense enhancement, as well as the source of production of the proteinaceous fluid that accumulates in the "cyst" of the tumor.

Imaging

Classically, cerebellar PA appears as a cystic mass with an enhancing mural nodule or a mixed solid-cystic mass. Solid portion is hypointense on T1WI (higher than CSF intensity) and hyperintense on T2W1 and show variable enhancement. Typically, diffusion is facilitated in the solid enhancing portion of the tumor in comparison to MB and AT-RT.

Peritumoral edema and intratumoral calcifications are usually absent. Hemorrhage can be present but rare. MR spectroscopy is quite tricky. Choline is typically very high in pilocytic tumors, despite the benign clinical course for tumors of this type. In addition, lipids and lactate are also usually demonstrated in the spectra of PAs. Despite being low grade (grade I tumors), PAs may present with high blood volumes on MR perfusion studies. This finding is not related to aggressiveness in these lesions.

Atypical Teratoid/Rhabdoid Tumor

CNS AT/RTs are highly malignant neoplasms which account for 1–3% of all primary CNS tumors in the pediatric population and 6.7% of all primary CNS tumors in children <3 years of age.

Although by definition they contain rhabdoid cells, ATRTs have widely divergent cell populations, including mesenchymal, epithelial, glial, and neuronal cell lines accounting for the "teratoid" descriptor.

About two-thirds of ATRTs occur in the cerebellum, typically in the cerebellopontine angle, with invasion of the surrounding structures. About one-fourth are supratentorial and 8% are multifocal. The primary AT-RT of the brain can present between 1 month to 12 years of age (average age 24.5 months), and have with a male predominance (M:F, 3:1).

Pathology

Histologically, ATRTs are characterized by rhabdoid cells and are similar to that of other small round blue cell tumors; up to 70% also contain cell fields typical of a primitive neuroectodermal tumor.

Necrosis and a high MIB-index are common.

Nearly all ATRTs demonstrate bi-allelic inactivation of SMARCB1 (or INI1) on chromosom,[22]. whereas a very small percentage show inactivation of SMARCA4 (or BRG1).[30] Having one of these genetic alterations is now formally required for diagnosis.

Imaging

On imaging, lesions are usually large at presentation, with moderate-to-marked surrounding edema.

On CT, these tumors are hyperdense or mixed density lesions attributed to the presence of areas of necrosis, cyst formation, hemorrhage and calcification and show varying pattern of enhancement following contrast administration. On MR, they are T1-hypointense, T2-iso to hypointense with restricted diffusion and inhomogeneous enhancement. These imaging findings overlap with those described for MBs and are likely secondary to high cell density and high nucleus-to-cytoplasm ratio. Diffuse leptomeningeal dissemination is common, hence the spine should also be imaged. MRS shows elevated Cho, reduced NAA and a prominent lipid peak.

The main differential diagnosis for posterior fossa ATRT is MB and both show restricted diffusion. If a posterior fossa tumor occurs in a child less than 3 years of age, located off-midline, has intratumoral blood products and extends to the CPA, it is more likely to be an AT-RT than a MB. Very young children presenting with cranial nerve deficits and masses involving the CPA with restricted diffusion are more likely to have an ATRT.

Hemangioblastoma

Hemangioblastomas are uncommon, slow-growing tumors of CNS (WHO grade 1) that occur in the cerebellum (83–86%), brainstem (2–5%), spinal cord (3–13%) and cerebrum (1.5%).[35] They may occur either sporadically (75%) or as a manifestation of von Hippel-Lindau (VHL) disease in 25% along with retinal angioma, renal cell carcinoma, adrenal pheochromocytoma, as well as benign cysts in the lungs, liver, kidneys, and pancreas. The hemangioblastomas in VHL disease develop at an earlier age and are often multifocal in 20%.

Pathology

Hemangioblastomas typically appear as well-demarcated masses with smooth margins. The tumor can be either entirely solid (40%) or cystic with a hypervascular enhancing mural nodule with prominent blood vessels (60%). VHL-associated and some sporadic hemangioblastomas are caused by inactivation of the VHL tumor suppressor gene, located on chromosome 3p.

Imaging

On NCCT, hemangioblastoma typically appears as a well-defined, either entirely solid or hypodense cystic lesion with an iso-hyperdense mural nodule. Solid hemangioblastomas appear hyperdense on NCCT and show strong homogeneous enhancement. The iso-hyperdense mural nodule abuts the pial surface and shows strong homogeneous contrast enhancement.

On MRI the cystic component of hemangioblastoma is either iso- or slightly hyperintense relative to CSF on T1WI and hyperintense on T2WI.[35] The nodule is T1 hypointense, T2 hyperintense and enhances avidly following gadolinium administration.

Vascular flow-voids may be present within and at the periphery of the tumor. The peritumoral edema is usually minimal or absent. Perfusion MR imaging reveals high rCBV ratios in these lesions (around 11), values significantly higher than those of metastases (around 5) and pilocytic astrocytomas. Cerebral angiography is reserved for preoperative tumor embolization and shows dilated feeding arteries and a prolonged tumoral blush corresponding to the solid portion. The other differential diagnosis of a cyst with enhancing mural nodule in the infratentorial compartment is pilocytic astrocytoma which generally occurs at a younger age, is not associated with intratumoral flow-voids and show less increase in rCBV and permeability.

Metastases

Metastases are the most common infratentorial intra-axial neoplasms in the adult population. They are usually well-defined round masses, often with nodular or ring enhancement (due to central necrosis).

Multiple masses are usually seen and help to confirm the diagnosis. However, even if solitary, the lesion is still more commonly metastasis than a primary intracranial neoplasm. In adults, lung and breast carcinoma account for the majority of metastatic disease, followed by melanoma, renal cell carcinoma, thyroid carcinoma, and gastrointestinal malignancies.

Unknown primaries account for 10–15% of patients with brain metastases.

Imaging

Metastases are typically hypodense on CT; they are hypointense on T1WI and hyperintense on T2WI; and show varying pattern of enhancement. Most metastases have considerable surrounding edema. Metastases with increased T1 signal intensity before contrast administration include melanoma, renal cell carcinoma, lung carcinoma, choriocarcinoma, and gastrointestinal adenocarcinoma (because of the presence of mucin). Metastases with areas of hemorrhage and calcification have variable signal on T2WI. MR spectroscopy shows significantly elevated choline and very low NAA (the presence of NAA in many metastases represents contamination from adjacent tissues due to partial averaging). Lactate and lipids are usually high. The tissues surrounding the enhancing mass usually are normal by spectroscopy (unlike high grade gliomas).

Embryonal Tumor with Multilayered Rosettes C19MC-altered

A new entity, embryonal tumor with multilayered rosettes (ETMR) C19MC-altered, was recently described in children younger than 4 years.[4] The term, primitive neuroectodermal tumor (PNET), has been removed and they are classified according to the presence of amplification of the C19MC region on chromosome 19 (19q 13.42). The presence of C19 MC amplification results in a diagnosis of ETMRs (ETMR-C19MC-altered). In its absence, the tumor is called ETMR-NOS.

These are usually large masses, more than 5 cm in size at the time of presentation in the supratentorial compartment, but may also be found in the infratentorial compartment. They are well delineated masses with absent or minimal peritumoral edema despite their large size. Typically, they are heterogeneous isodense to hyperdense masses on CT.

Calcifications are seen in 70% of cases. On MRI, the signal on T1/T2 is variable due to the presence of blood products, calcifications, and cystic changes. FLAIR shows areas of necrosis (hyperintense) and cystic components (hypointense). On diffusion-weighted imaging, the tumor shows restricted diffusion presumably due to its high cellularity and nucleus-to-cytoplasm ratio. The solid components demonstrate avid heterogeneous contrast enhancement. Perfusion MRI shows increased relative cerebral blood volume. ETMRs develop subarachnoid dissemination in 40% of cases; thus, the entire neuroaxis should be imaged. The presence of metastases changes management, requiring chemotherapy and increased radiation dose. Prognosis is dismal despite radiation therapy.

Brainstem and Cervicomedullary Junction

Brainstem Gliomas

Brainstem gliomas are a heterogeneous group of tumors that differ significantly in their growth characteristics, histology, and response to therapy. They represent 10–20% of pediatric CNS tumors and three-fourths of these occur before 20 years of age. In adults, they represent less than 2% of brain tumors and usually occur in younger adults and tend to be of low grade (WHO I or II).

The majority (85%) are composed of high-grade fibrillary gliomas, which arise predominantly in the pons and less frequently in the medulla. There is no sex predilection, and children between 7 and 10 years of age are commonly affected. Multiple cranial nerve palsies, pyramidal tract signs, ataxia and nystagmus are the usual presentation. Except in tectal gliomas, hydrocephalus is uncommon in brain stem gliomas. Diffuse pontine gliomas have the worst prognosis.

Pathology

Brainstem gliomas can be divided into the diffuse brainstem glioma and focal glioma (including dorsal exophytic, tectal, and cervicomedullary).

Recent molecular studies have revealed that diffuse brainstem gliomas in children most likely harbor a highly specific point mutation, K27M, in histone 3.3, 3.2, or 3.1.3–7. In the revised 2016 update of the WHO brain tumor classification, these neoplasms constitute a new entity termed as diffuse midline glioma, H3 K27M-mutant characterized by a diffuse growth pattern, and a midline location (e.g., thalami, brainstem, spinal cord, and other midline structures, including the third ventricle, hypothalamus, and pineal region). The majority of histone H3 K27M-mutant tumors are high-grade astrocytomas with high proliferative potential, often with contiguous extension of tumor from the brainstem into the thalami and upper cervical spinal cord. Most of these tumors have poor prognosis but exceptions have been reported.

Imaging

MR imaging is useful for diagnosis and localization of the tumor. Diffuse brainstem glioma appears as poorly defined T1 hypointense and T2 hyperintense regions.

Intratumoral heterogeneity is occasionally present, but cysts are not common. The signal changes may extend into the cerebellum and/or the adjacent brainstem. There is often exophytic spread laterally and ventrally with basilar artery encasement. An undulating ventral border of the brainstem on sagittal image may be an indirect clue to the presence of the mass lesion. Contrast enhancement has been reported in approximately one half of the cases and is often focal and nodular **(Fig. 14C)**. Areas of restricted diffusion may be present, indicating higher cell density and providing targets for biopsy. No significant differences are seen in the characteristics of enhancement, infiltration, or peritumoral edema in patients with diffuse pontine glioma with or without the histone H3 K27M mutation.

Focal brainstem gliomas are often well circumscribed and sometimes markedly exophytic. Exophytic component is readily identified on MR, due to its multiplanar imaging capability. The dorsally exophytic lesions are grossly multicystic and often enhance intensely. The presence of enhancement has not been correlated reliably with type or grade of malignancy. The other subtypes of focal gliomas are tectal plate glioma and cervicomedullary glioma.

Ganglioglioma

Ganglioglioma (GG) is another diagnostic consideration for tumors located in the brainstem and upper cervical cord. Infratentorial GGs are less common than supratentorial GGs.[57] On imaging, infratentorial GGs are typically infiltrative and expansile solid masses with dorsal predominant "paintbrush" enhancement.

Infratentorial GGs are difficult to resect completely and have poor progression-free survival and high mortality, in comparison to supratentorial GGs.

Rosette-forming Glioneuronal Tumor (RGNT)

RGNT of the fourth ventricle is a rare, benign, mixed neuronal-glial primary brain tumor primarily affecting young adults.[80] It is recognized as a distinct entity since the 2007 WHO Classification of Tumors of the Central Nervous System.[81] RGNT often occupies the fourth ventricle but occasionally it shows cerebellar (vermian) invasion or may involve the aqueduct. Rare extraventricular locations have been reported, including the cerebellar hemispheres, cerebellopontine angles, pineal gland, tectum, thalami, third ventricle, optic chiasm, spinal cord, and a recent case in the septum pellucidum. Symptoms are nonspecific and include headache, gait disturbances, vertigo, and visual disturbances, which develop over months to years. The tumor may be incidentally discovered.

Head and Neck Imaging

1. Describe the imaging features of juvenile nasopharyngeal angiofibroma. Discuss the role of radiological intervention in its management. [6+4] [MD (WBUHS) 23, MD (WBUHS) 21]

Juvenile nasopharyngeal angiofibroma is a rare, benign but locally aggressive vascular tumor that primarily affects adolescent males.

Computed Tomography (CT)

1. **Location and Extent**: JNA typically originates in the sphenopalatine foramen extending into the nasopharynx, nasal cavity and possibly into the pterygopalatine fossa, infratemporal fossa and orbit.
2. **Bone Involvement**: Bone remodeling and erosions are common, particularly of the posterior wall of maxillary sinus, pterygoid plate and base of the skull.

   Expansile growth with smooth margin and the presence of bone destruction is often noted.
3. **Density**: The mass usually appears iso to hyperdense compared to the surrounding muscles on noncontrast CT due to high vascularity and fibrous content. There might be calcifications within the tumor in some cases.
4. **Contrast Enhancement**: Intense enhancement is observed postcontrast administration, indicating vascular nature of the tumor.
5. **Holman Miller Sign (Antral Sign)**: Seen on lateral skull radiographs or CT, indicating anterior bowing of the posterior wall of the maxillary sinus due to the mass effect of the tumor.

MRI

1. **T1 Weighted Imaging**: Isointense or slightly hypointense compared to muscles.
2. **T2 Weighted Imaging**: Heterogeneous high signal intensity due to presence of multiple vascular channels and stroma.
3. **Contrast Enhancement (Gadolinium Enhanced T1 Weighted Imaging)**: Strong and homogeneous enhancement is characteristic, reflecting tumors high vascularity.
4. **Specific Signs**: Salt and pepper appearance due to presence of small serpentine flow voids against a hyperintense background on T2 weighted imaging.

Cerebriform Pattern: Sometimes observed on enhanced T1 weighted images, showing a convoluted brain like appearance due to enhancing vascular channels.

Angiography

1. **Vascular Supply**: JNA is highly vascular and angiography typically demonstrates it's extensive blood supply, primarily from the external carotid branches, specially internal maxillary artery. Feeder arteries: External carotid artery:
   a. Internal maxillary artery
   b. Ascending pharyngeal artery
   c. Palatine arteries internal carotid artery: Less common, usually in larger tumors
   d. Sphenoidal branches
   e. Ophthalmic artery

   Of note, enlargement of feeding vessels is not a common finding.

2. **Tumor Blush**: A dense persistent tumor blush is seen during the arterial phase, indicating the high vascular nature of the tumor.
3. **Feeder Vessels**: Detailed delineation of the feeding vessels and their contribution, crucial for preoperative embolization planning, which is often performed to reduce intraoperative bleeding.

Radiographic Features

Plain Radiography

- Plain X-rays are generally not very useful but might show a soft tissue mass in the nasopharyngeal region.
- Signs of bone remodeling or erosion can sometimes be seen, but CT or MRI provide far superior details.

Management

- Interventional radiology plays a critical role in the management of JNA (particularly in the preoperative setting).
- The primary intervention is preoperative embolization which significantly aids in reducing intraoperative blood loss and improving surgical outcomes.

Preoperative Embolization

Purpose and Benefits

1. Reducing blood loss
2. Improvement of surgical field
3. Reducing tumor size

Procedure

1. Vascular mapping to identify tumors blood supply.
2. **Catheterization:** Super selective catheterization of feeding arteries using microcatheters.
3. **Embolic Agents:** Poly vinyl alcohol particles, coils and liquid embolic agents (N butyl cyanoacrylate). The choice depends on the vessel size, flow characteristics and need for permanent or temporary occlusion.
4. **Postoperative Angiography:** To confirm the successful reduction or cessation of blood flow to the tumor.
5. **Timing:** 24–48 hours before surgery.
6. **Role in Nonsurgical Candidates:** In cases where surgery is not feasible or the patient is a poor surgical candidate, embolization may be used as a stand-alone palliative treatment to control symptoms and reduce tumor growth.

2. Describe with a neat diagram the anatomy of brachial plexus. [10] [MD (WBUHS) 20]

The brachial plexus **(Fig. 17)** is a complex network of nerves that originates from the spinal cord and provides motor and sensory innervation to the upper limb. Here's a detailed overview of its anatomy:

Roots

The brachial plexus begins with the anterior rami of the spinal nerves C5, C6, C7, C8, and T1. These roots emerge from the spinal cord and travel through the intervertebral foramina.[2]

Trunks

The roots converge to form three trunks:

- **Superior Trunk**: Formed by the union of C5 and C6 roots.
- **Middle Trunk**: Continuation of C7.
- **Inferior Trunk**: Formed by the union of C8 and T1 roots.

Divisions

Each trunk splits into an anterior and a posterior division:

- **Anterior Divisions**: These move towards the front of the body.
- **Posterior Divisions**: These move towards the back of the body.

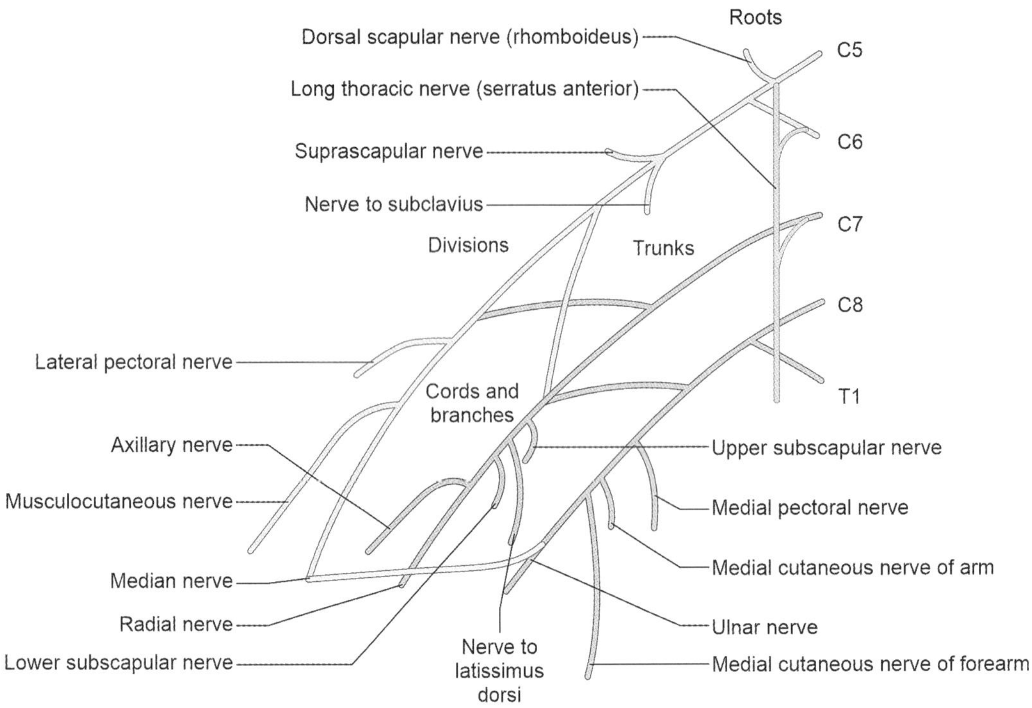

FIG. 17: Schematic diagram of anatomy of brachial plexus.

Cords

The divisions then regroup to form three cords, named according to their position relative to the axillary artery:

- **Lateral Cord**: Formed by the anterior divisions of the superior and middle trunks (C5-C7).
- **Posterior Cord**: Formed by the posterior divisions of all three trunks (C5-C8, T1).
- **Medial Cord**: Formed by the anterior division of the inferior trunk (C8-T1).

Terminal Branches

The cords give rise to five main terminal branches, which provide motor and sensory innervation to the upper limb:

- **Musculocutaneous Nerve**: Arises from the lateral cord and innervates the muscles of the anterior arm.
- **Axillary Nerve**: Arises from the posterior cord and innervates the deltoid and teres minor muscles.
- **Radial Nerve**: Arises from the posterior cord and innervates the posterior arm and forearm.
- **Median Nerve**: Formed by the union of the lateral and medial cords, it innervates most of the flexor muscles in the forearm and some muscles of the hand.
- **Ulnar Nerve**: Arises from the medial cord and innervates the intrinsic muscles of the hand and some forearm muscles.

Supraclavicular Branches

In addition to the terminal branches, the brachial plexus gives rise to several preterminal branches, including:

- **Dorsal Scapular Nerve**: Innervates the rhomboid muscles.
- **Long Thoracic Nerve**: Innervates the serratus anterior muscle.
- **Suprascapular Nerve**: Innervates the supraspinatus and infraspinatus muscles.

Clinical Relevance

Understanding the anatomy of the brachial plexus is crucial for diagnosing and managing nerve injuries and conditions affecting the upper limb. Damage to any part of the plexus can result in motor and sensory deficits, impacting the function of the arm and hand.

3. Classify the infrahyoid neck spaces. Mention the imaging findings of carotid body tumor. [4+6] [MD (WBUHS) 24, MD (WBUHS) 20]

The infrahyoid neck spaces **(Fig. 18)** are anatomical compartments within the neck, delineated by the deep cervical fascia. These spaces are crucial for understanding the spread of infections, tumors, and other pathologies1. Here's a detailed classification of the infrahyoid neck spaces:

1. **Visceral Space**
   - **Location**: Central compartment containing several viscera.
   - **Contents**: Larynx, thyroid gland, hypopharynx, and cervical esophagus.
   - **Boundaries**: Enclosed by the visceral layer of the deep cervical fascia.
2. **Carotid Space**
   - **Location**: Paired space just lateral to the visceral compartment.
   - **Contents**: Internal carotid artery, internal jugular vein, and several neural structures.
   - **Boundaries**: Defined by the carotid sheath, which is a part of the deep cervical fascia.
3. **Retropharyngeal Space**
   - **Location**: Midline space behind the pharynx.
   - **Contents**: Lymph nodes, fat, and connective tissue.
   - **Boundaries**: Anteriorly by the pharynx, posteriorly by the prevertebral fascia.

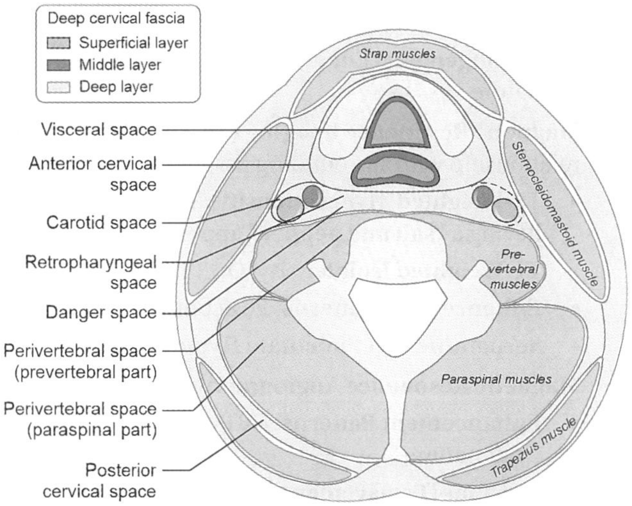

FIG. 18: Schematic diagram of infrahyoid neck spaces.

4. **Posterior Cervical Space**
   - **Location**: Lateral to the retropharyngeal space.
   - **Contents**: Lymph nodes, fat, and connective tissue.
   - **Boundaries**: Anteriorly by the prevertebral fascia, posteriorly by the vertebral column.
5. **Perivertebral Space**
   - **Location**: Surrounds the vertebral column.
   - **Contents**: Prevertebral muscles, vertebral column, and associated structures.
   - **Boundaries**: Enclosed by the prevertebral fascia.
6. **Anterior Cervical Space**
   - **Location**: Lateral to the visceral space.
   - **Contents**: Lymph nodes, fat, and connective tissue.
   - **Boundaries**: Anteriorly by the investing layer of the deep cervical fascia, posteriorly by the visceral fascia.
7. **Danger Space**
   - **Location**: Extends from the skull base to the diaphragm.
   - **Contents**: Lymph nodes, fat, and connective tissue.
   - **Boundaries**: Anteriorly by the alar fascia, posteriorly by the prevertebral fascia.

These spaces are essential for understanding the spread of infections and tumors in the neck, as well as for planning surgical interventions.

Imaging Findings of Carotid Body Tumor

Carotid body tumors (CBTs), also known as carotid body paragangliomas, are typically diagnosed and evaluated using various imaging modalities. Here are the key imaging findings:

1. **Ultrasound (US)**:
   - **Initial Screening**: Doppler ultrasound is often the first imaging modality used to detect a carotid body tumor.
   - **Findings**: It can show a well-defined, hypoechoic mass at the carotid bifurcation, often with increased vascularity on color Doppler imaging.

2. **Computed Tomography (CT) Scan**: **CT** scans are valuable for evaluating the anatomical details and extent of carotid body tumors (CBTs). Here are the key findings:
   - **Hypervascular Mass**: The tumor typically appears as a well-defined, enhancing mass at the level of the carotid bifurcation.
   - **Splaying of Carotid Arteries**: The tumor often causes splaying of the internal and external carotid arteries, a characteristic known as the **"Lyre Sign"**.
   - **Displacement of Adjacent Structures**: The mass may displace the internal jugular vein and other nearby structures.
   - **Homogeneous Enhancement**: The tumor shows avid enhancement with contrast, indicating its hypervascular nature
3. **Magnetic Resonance Imaging (MRI)**: **MRI** provides detailed information about the tumor's characteristics and its relationship with surrounding tissues. Key findings include:
   - **T2-Weighted Hyperintensity**: The tumor appears hyperintense on T2-weighted images, often described as having a **"salt and pepper" appearance** due to the presence of flow voids from intratumoral vessels.
   - **T1-Weighted Isointensity**: On T1-weighted images, the tumor is usually isointense to muscles.
   - **Enhancement Patterns**: Postcontrast T1-weighted images show intense enhancement of the tumor.
   - **Serpentine and Punctuate Hypointense Foci**: These are related to the signal voids from intratumoral vessels
4. **Magnetic Resonance Angiography (MRA)**:
   - **Enhancement Patterns**: CBTs show intense enhancement on arterial phase images, indicating their hypervascular nature.
   - **Vascular Displacement**: The tumor typically displaces the internal and external carotid arteries, often described as the **"Lyre Sign"**.
   - **Flow-Related Enhancement**: MRA helps in visualizing the flow-related enhancement of feeding vessels and the tumor's relationship with the carotid bifurcation.
   - **Intratumoral Vessels**: The presence of serpentine and punctuate hypointense foci on T2-weighted images, related to signal voids from intratumoral vessels.
   - **Early Enhancement**: The tumor shows early enhancement on arterial phase images, which helps in distinguishing it from other neck masses.
5. **3D Reconstruction**:
   - **Advanced Visualization**: 3D reconstruction techniques can provide a detailed visualization of the tumor and its anatomical context.
   - **Findings**: It helps in understanding the extent of the tumor and planning surgical interventions.

These imaging modalities are crucial for diagnosing carotid body tumors, assessing their extent, and planning appropriate treatment strategies.

4. Imaging modalities in a case of sudden visual loss. [10] [MD (WBUHS) 20]

Sudden visual loss can result from various causes, including vascular, retinal, inflammatory, traumatic, infectious, neurological, and other factors:

1. **Vascular Causes**:
   - **Retinal Artery Occlusion**: Blockage of the central retinal artery.
   - **Retinal Vein Occlusion**: Blockage of the central retinal vein.
   - **Ischemic Optic Neuropathy**: Reduced blood flow to the optic nerve, often related to giant cell arteritis.
2. **Retinal Causes**:
   - **Retinal Detachment**: The retina pulls away from its normal position.
   - **Vitreous Hemorrhage**: Bleeding into the vitreous humor.
   - **Macular Hole**: A break in the macula.
3. **Inflammatory Causes**:
   - **Optic Neuritis**: Inflammation of the optic nerve, often associated with multiple sclerosis.
   - **Uveitis**: Inflammation of the middle layer of the eye.

4. **Traumatic Causes**:
   - **Eye Injury**: Direct trauma to the eye.
   - **Blunt Force Trauma**: Impact to the head or eye affecting visual pathways.
5. **Infectious Causes**:
   - **Endophthalmitis**: Infection inside the eye.
   - **Keratitis**: Infection of the cornea.
6. **Neurological Causes**:
   - **Stroke**: Interruption of blood flow to the brain.
   - **Transient Ischemic Attack (TIA)**: Temporary blockage of blood flow to the brain.
7. **Other Causes**:
   - **Ocular Migraine**: Temporary visual disturbances associated with migraines.
   - **Giant Cell Arteritis**: Inflammation of the arteries.

When evaluating sudden visual loss, several imaging modalities are used to identify the underlying cause. Here are the key imaging techniques and their findings:

Computed Tomography (CT) Scan

Role

- **Rapid Evaluation**: CT scans are often the first-line imaging modality in the acute setting due to their availability and rapid image acquisition.
- **Detection of Hemorrhage**: CT is highly sensitive for detecting acute hemorrhages, which can cause sudden visual loss.
- **Assessment of Structural Abnormalities**: It can detect fractures, foreign bodies, and other structural anomalies that might affect vision.

Indications

- Suspected intracranial hemorrhage or trauma.
- Evaluation of bony structures in the orbit.
- Initial assessment in emergency settings.

Advantages

- Quick and widely available.
- Excellent for detecting acute hemorrhage and bone abnormalities.

Computed Tomography Angiography (CTA)

Role

- **Vascular Assessment**: CTA provides detailed images of blood vessels, crucial for evaluating vascular causes of sudden visual loss.
- **Detection of Occlusions**: It can identify occlusions, aneurysms, dissections, and other vascular abnormalities.

Indications

- Suspected vascular occlusion or aneurysm.
- Evaluation of carotid and cerebral arteries.

Advantages

- Noninvasive and quick.
- Provides detailed images of blood vessels.

Magnetic Resonance Imaging (MRI)

Role

- **Detailed Soft Tissue Evaluation**: MRI provides high-resolution images of the brain, orbits, and optic nerves.
- **Detection of Ischemic Strokes**: It is sensitive for detecting ischemic changes that might lead to sudden visual loss.
- **Assessment of Demyelinating Diseases**: MRI can detect conditions like multiple sclerosis that affect the optic nerves.

Indications

- Suspected optic neuritis, ischemic stroke, or demyelinating disease.
- Detailed assessment of the brain and optic pathways.

Advantages

- Superior soft tissue contrast.
- No radiation exposure.
- Excellent for detailed evaluation of brain and optic nerve pathology.

Ultrasound

Role

- **Orbital Evaluation**: Ultrasound is used to assess the eye and orbit, especially useful in the emergency setting.
- **Detection of Masses**: It can identify orbital masses, retinal detachments, and other abnormalities affecting vision.

Indications

- Assessment of orbital masses, retinal detachment, and vitreous hemorrhage.
- Useful in patients who cannot undergo CT or MRI.

Advantages

- Noninvasive and quick.
- Provides real-time images.
- No radiation exposure.

Summary

- **CT Scan**: Best for initial evaluation, detecting hemorrhages and bony abnormalities.
- **CTA**: Ideal for vascular assessment, detecting occlusions and aneurysms.
- **MRI**: Best for detailed soft tissue evaluation, detecting ischemic strokes, and demyelinating diseases.
- **Ultrasound**: Useful for orbital evaluation and detecting retinal detachments and masses.

Other modalities are:

Fluorescein Angiography (FA)

- **Retinal Evaluation**: FA is used to assess the retinal circulation.
- **Findings**: It can detect retinal vascular occlusions, diabetic retinopathy, and other retinal pathologies.

Optical Coherence Tomography (OCT)

- **Retinal Imaging**: OCT provides high-resolution images of the retina.
- **Findings**: It can detect macular edema, retinal thinning, and other retinal abnormalities.

5. Discuss radiological anatomy of neck spaces and lymph nodes. [6+4] [MD (WBUHS) 21, DNB Dec 19, AIIMS May 23]

Detailed Radiological Anatomy of Neck Spaces

Understanding the neck spaces **(Fig. 19)** is crucial for diagnosing and treating various pathologies, including infections and tumors. These spaces are delineated by the deep cervical fascia and are divided into suprahyoid (above the hyoid bone) and infrahyoid (below the hyoid bone) regions. Here's a detailed breakdown:

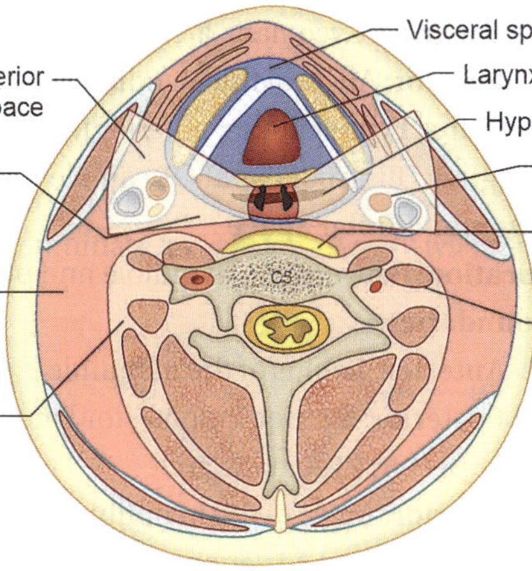

FIG. 19: Schematic diagram of neck spaces.

Suprahyoid Neck Spaces

These spaces are located above the hyoid bone:

1. **Parotid Space**
   - **Location**: Contains the parotid gland, bounded by the superficial layer of the deep cervical fascia.
   - **Boundaries**:
     - **Anterior**: Ramus of the mandible
     - **Posterior**: Sternocleidomastoid muscle
     - **Superior**: Zygomatic arch
     - **Inferior**: Angle of the mandible
   - **Contents**: Parotid gland, external carotid artery, retromandibular vein, and facial nerve.
   - **Imaging**: CT and MRI can show parotid gland masses, abscesses, and tumors.
2. **Masticator Space**
   - **Location**: Encompasses the muscles of mastication.
   - **Boundaries**:
     - **Anterior**: Ramus of the mandible
     - **Posterior**: Sternocleidomastoid muscle
     - **Superior**: Zygomatic arch
     - **Inferior**: Angle of the mandible
   - **Contents**: Masseter, temporalis, medial and lateral pterygoids, mandibular ramus, and mandibular nerve.
   - **Imaging**: MRI and CT reveal masses, infections, and neoplasms affecting these muscles.
3. **Submandibular Space**
   - **Location**: Beneath the mandible, bounded by the superficial and middle layers of the deep cervical fascia.
   - **Boundaries**:
     - **Anterior**: Ramus of the mandible
     - **Posterior**: Sternocleidomastoid muscle
     - **Superior**: Zygomatic arch
     - **Inferior**: Angle of the mandible
   - **Contents**: Submandibular gland, facial artery and vein, lymph nodes.
   - **Imaging**: Ultrasound, CT, and MRI detect submandibular gland stones, infections, and tumors.
4. **Submental Space**
   - **Location**: Below the chin, bounded by the anterior belly of the digastric muscles.

- **Boundaries**:
  - **Anterior**: Ramus of the mandible
  - **Posterior**: Sternocleidomastoid muscle
  - **Superior**: Zygomatic arch
  - **Inferior**: Angle of the mandible
- **Contents**: Lymph nodes, anterior jugular vein, and fat.
- **Imaging**: Ultrasound and CT can identify lymphadenopathy, abscesses, and cysts.

5. **Pterygomandibular Space**
   - **Location**: Between the mandible and pterygoid muscles.
   - **Boundaries**:
     - **Anterior**: Ramus of the mandible
     - **Posterior**: Sternocleidomastoid muscle
     - **Superior**: Zygomatic arch
     - **Inferior**: Angle of the mandible
   - **Contents**: Pterygoid venous plexus and mandibular nerve branches.
   - **Imaging**: CT and MRI are used to detect infections and hematomas.
6. **Infrazygomatic Space**
   - **Location**: Above the zygomatic arch.
   - **Boundaries**:
     - **Superior**: Zygomatic arch
     - **Inferior**: Maxilla
     - **Anterior**: Buccal space
     - **Posterior**: Parotid space
   - **Contents**: Fat, minor salivary glands, and lymph nodes.
   - **Imaging**: MRI and CT can show tumors and inflammatory conditions.
7. **Suprahyoid Pharyngeal Space**
   - **Location**: Central compartment above the hyoid bone.
   - **Boundaries**:
     - **Superior**: Zygomatic arch
     - **Inferior**: Maxilla
     - **Anterior**: Buccal space
     - **Posterior**: Parotid space
   - **Contents**: Pharyngeal mucosal space.
   - **Imaging**: MRI and CT to visualize masses and inflammatory conditions.

Infrahyoid Neck Spaces

These spaces are located below the hyoid bone:

1. **Carotid Space**
   - **Location**: Paired space lateral to the visceral compartment.
   - **Boundaries**:
     - **Anterior**: Visceral space
     - **Posterior**: Prevertebral space
     - **Medial**: Retropharyngeal space
     - **Lateral**: Sternocleidomastoid muscle
   - **Contents**: Carotid artery, internal jugular vein, vagus nerve, and lymph nodes.
   - **Imaging**: CTA and MRI/MRA assess vascular abnormalities, such as carotid artery dissection, aneurysms, and tumors.

2. **Visceral Space**
    - **Location**: Central compartment.
    - **Boundaries**:
        - **Anterior**: Visceral space
        - **Posterior**: Prevertebral space
        - **Medial**: Retropharyngeal space
        - **Lateral**: Sternocleidomastoid muscle
    - **Contents**: Thyroid gland, trachea, esophagus, parathyroid glands, and larynx.
    - **Imaging**: Ultrasound, CT, and MRI reveal thyroid nodules, tracheal stenosis, and esophageal lesions.
3. **Retropharyngeal Space**
    - **Location**: Midline space behind the pharynx.
    - **Boundaries**:
        - **Anterior**: Buccopharyngeal fascia
        - **Posterior**: Alar fascia
        - **Lateral**: Carotid sheath
    - **Contents**: Lymph nodes, fat, and connective tissue.
    - **Imaging**: CT and MRI can identify abscesses, lymphadenopathy, and tumors.
4. **Perivertebral Space**
    - **Location**: Surrounding the vertebral column.
    - **Boundaries**:
        - **Anterior**: Buccopharyngeal fascia
        - **Posterior**: Alar fascia
        - **Lateral**: Carotid sheath
    - **Contents**: Prevertebral muscles, vertebrae, spinal cord.
    - **Imaging**: MRI is ideal for detecting spinal infections, fractures, and tumors.
5. **Posterior Cervical Space**
    - **Location**: Lateral and posterior to the carotid space.
    - **Boundaries**:
        - **Anterior**: Buccopharyngeal fascia
        - **Posterior**: Alar fascia
        - **Lateral**: Carotid sheath
    - **Contents**: Fat, lymph nodes, and the accessory nerve.
    - **Imaging**: Ultrasound, CT, and MRI reveal lymphadenopathy and soft tissue tumors.
6. **Anterior Cervical Space**
    - **Location**: Anterior to the visceral space.
    - **Boundaries**:
        - **Anterior**: Buccopharyngeal fascia
        - **Posterior**: Alar fascia
        - **Lateral**: Carotid sheath
    - **Contents**: Lymph nodes, fat, and connective tissue.
    - **Imaging**: Ultrasound and CT assess lymphadenopathy and inflammatory conditions.
7. **Danger Space**
    - **Location**: Extends from the skull base to the diaphragm.
    - **Boundaries**:
        - **Anterior**: Buccopharyngeal fascia
        - **Posterior**: Alar fascia
        - **Lateral**: Carotid sheath
    - **Contents**: Fat, connective tissue, and lymph nodes.
    - **Imaging**: CT and MRI detect deep neck infections and abscesses.

The cervical lymph nodes are divided into several anatomical stations **(Fig. 20)**, each with specific boundaries and functions. These stations are crucial for diagnosing and treating head and neck cancers, infections, and other conditions. Here's a detailed overview:

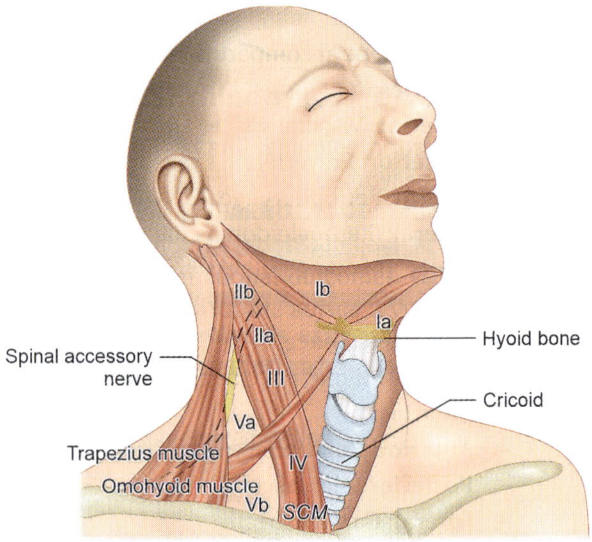

FIG. 20: Cervical lymph node stations.
(SCM: sternocleidomastoid muscle)

Cervical Lymph Node Stations

1. **Level I: Submental and Submandibular**
   - **Location**: Below the chin and jawline.
   - **Boundaries**:
     - **Superior**: Mylohyoid muscle and mandible.
     - **Inferior**: Inferior border of the hyoid bone.
     - **Anterior**: Platysma muscle.
     - **Posterior**: Posterior border of the submandibular gland.
   - **Sublevels**:
     - **Level Ia**: Submental nodes, located between the anterior bellies of both digastric muscles.
     - **Level Ib**: Submandibular nodes, located between the inner side of the mandible and the digastric muscle.
2. **Level II: Upper Internal Jugular (Deep Cervical) Chain**
   - **Location**: Along the upper part of the internal jugular vein.
   - **Boundaries**:
     - **Superior**: Base of the skull at the jugular foramen.
     - **Inferior**: Inferior border of the hyoid bone.
     - **Anterior**: Posterior border of the submandibular gland.
     - **Posterolateral**: Posterior border of the sternocleidomastoid muscle.
     - **Medial**: Medial border of the internal carotid artery.
   - **Sublevels**:
     - **Level IIa**: Inseparable from or anterior to the posterior edge of the internal jugular vein (includes jugulodigastric nodes).
     - **Level IIb**: Posterior to and separable by a fat plane from the internal jugular vein.
3. **Level III: Middle Internal Jugular (Deep Cervical) Chain**
   - **Location**: Along the middle part of the internal jugular vein.
   - **Boundaries**:
     - **Superior**: Inferior border of the hyoid bone.
     - **Inferior**: Inferior border of the cricoid cartilage.
     - **Anterior**: Anterior border of the sternocleidomastoid muscle.
     - **Posterolateral**: Posterior border of the sternocleidomastoid muscle.
     - **Medial**: Medial border of the common carotid artery.
4. **Level IV: Lower Internal Jugular (Deep Cervical) Chain**
   - **Location**: Along the lower part of the internal jugular vein.
   - **Boundaries**:
     - **Superior**: Inferior border of the cricoid cartilage.
     - **Inferior**: Level of the clavicle.
     - **Anterior**: Anterior border of the sternocleidomastoid muscle.
     - **Posterolateral:** Oblique line drawn through the posterolateral edge of the sternocleidomastoid muscle and the lateral edge of the anterior scalene muscle.
     - **Medial**: Medial border of the common carotid artery.
   - **Includes**: Medial supraclavicular nodes (Virchow's node).

5. **Level V: Posterior Triangle**
   - **Location**: Posterior triangle of the neck.
   - **Boundaries**:
     - **Superior**: Skull base at the apex of the convergence of sternocleidomastoid and trapezius muscles.
     - **Inferior**: Level of the clavicle.
     - **Anteromedial**: Posterior border of the sternocleidomastoid muscle.
     - **Posterolateral**: Anterior border of the trapezius muscle.
   - **Sublevels**:
     - **Level Va**: Superior half, superior to the inferior border of the cricoid cartilage (posterior to levels II and III).
     - **Level Vb**: Inferior half, inferior to the inferior border of the cricoid cartilage.
6. **Level VI: Anterior Cervical**
   - **Location**: Anterior to the trachea and esophagus.
   - **Boundaries**:
     - **Anterior**: Investing layer of deep cervical fascia.
     - **Posterior**: Pretracheal fascia.
     - **Lateral**: Carotid sheath.
     - **Inferior**: Clavicle.
7. **Level VII: Retropharyngeal and Retrostyloid**
   - **Location**: Posterior to the pharynx.
   - **Boundaries**:
     - **Anterior**: Buccopharyngeal fascia.
     - **Posterior**: Alar fascia.
     - **Lateral**: Carotid sheath.
     - **Inferior**: Extends down to the superior mediastinum.
8. **Level VIII: Parotid**
   - **Location**: Around the parotid gland.
   - **Boundaries**:
     - **Anterior**: Facial nerve.
     - **Posterior**: Sternocleidomastoid muscle.
     - **Superior**: Zygomatic arch.
     - **Inferior**: Mandible.
9. **Level IX: Buccofacial**
   - **Location**: Around the buccal region.
   - **Boundaries**:
     - **Anterior**: Buccal mucosa.
     - **Posterior**: Masseter muscle.
     - **Superior**: Zygomatic arch.
     - **Inferior**: Mandible.
10. **Level X: Retroauricular and Occipital**
    - **Location**: Around the ear and occipital region.
    - **Boundaries**:
      - **Anterior**: Auricle.
      - **Posterior**: Mastoid process.
      - **Superior**: Zygomatic arch.
      - **Inferior**: Mandible.

6. Discuss the role of ultrasonography in ocular trauma. [10] [MD (WBUHS) 21]

Ultrasonography plays a crucial role in the evaluation and management of ocular trauma. Here's a detailed look at its applications:

Role of Ultrasonography in Ocular Trauma

1. **Detection of Posterior Segment Pathologies**:
   - **Retinal Detachment**: Ultrasonography helps in identifying retinal detachments, which are common in ocular trauma.
   - **Vitreous Hemorrhage**: It can detect vitreous hemorrhages, which may obscure the view of the retina.
   - **Foreign Bodies**: Ultrasonography can locate intraocular foreign bodies that might not be visible through hazy media.
2. **Assessment of Anterior Segment**:
   - **Lens Dislocation**: It helps in identifying lens dislocations or subluxations.
   - **Corneal Abrasions**: Ultrasonography can assess the extent of corneal injuries.
   - **Anterior Chamber Depth**: It measures the depth of the anterior chamber, which is important in cases of trauma.
3. **Evaluation of Optic Nerve**:
   - **Optic Nerve Avulsion**: Ultrasonography can detect avulsions of the optic nerve, which are rare but serious injuries.
   - **Optic Nerve Sheath Diameter**: It can measure the optic nerve sheath diameter to assess for increased intracranial pressure, which may accompany head trauma.
4. **Guidance for Surgical Intervention**:
   - **Preoperative Planning**: It aids in planning surgical interventions by providing detailed images of the ocular structures.
   - **Intraoperative Use**: Surgeons can use real-time ultrasonography to guide their procedures.
5. **Noninvasive and Safe**:
   - **No Radiation**: Unlike CT scans, ultrasonography does not involve radiation, making it safer for repeated use.
   - **Quick and Accessible**: It provides quick results and can be performed at the bedside, which is crucial in emergency situations.

USG Findings in Ocular Trauma

1. **Globe Rupture**:
   - **Findings**: Decrease in size of the globe, anterior chamber collapse, vitreous hemorrhage, disruption of normal globe architecture.
   - **Presentation**: Painful vision loss after high-impact blunt or penetrating trauma.
2. **Retrobulbar Hematoma**:
   - **Findings**: Hypoechoic fluid collection posterior to the globe.
   - **Presentation**: Proptosis (bulging eye), elevated intraocular pressure, decreased visual acuity after trauma.
3. **Foreign Body**:
   - **Findings**: Hyperechoic object, possibly producing a shadow or comet tail artifact.
   - **Presentation**: May present with or without pain and vision loss.
4. **Lens Dislocation**:
   - **Findings**: Abnormal lens positions, which may be associated with trauma.
   - **Presentation**: Decreased vision with a normal pupillary response and without signs of open globe injury.
5. **Vitreous Hemorrhage**:
   - **Findings**: Echogenic (bright) areas within the vitreous body.
   - **Presentation**: Vision loss, eye pain, or floaters.
6. **Retinal Detachment**:
   - **Findings**: Hypoechoic (dark) area floating within the vitreous cavity.
   - **Presentation**: Sudden onset of floaters, flashes of light, or a shadow in the visual field

Types of Ultrasonography Used in Ocular Trauma

1. **B-Scan Ultrasonography**:
   - **Cross-Sectional Imaging**: Provides a cross-sectional view of the eye, useful for detecting posterior segment pathologies.
   - **Nonoptical Method**: Useful when the optical media are opaque due to hemorrhage or other opacities.
2. **A-Scan Ultrasonography**:
   - **Distance Measurement**: Measures the distance between structures within the eye, useful for lens thickness and axial length measurements.
3. **Ultrasound Biomicroscopy (UBM)**:
   - **High-Resolution Imaging**: Provides high-resolution images of the anterior segment, useful for detecting anterior segment injuries.

Clinical Relevance

Ultrasonography is invaluable in the management of ocular trauma as it allows for the early detection of hidden pathologies, guides treatment decisions, and improves patient outcomes. It is a versatile, noninvasive tool that complements other imaging modalities like CT and MRI.

7. Write a short notes on: (a) Radiological anatomy of PNS (b) Retromolar trigone. [5+5] [MD (WBUHS) 21, AIIMS Dec 23]

(a) Radiological Anatomy of PNS

The paranasal sinuses (PNS) are a group of air-filled spaces located within the bones of the skull and face. They are named for their proximity to the nasal cavity and include the maxillary, frontal, ethmoid, and sphenoid sinuses. Here's a detailed overview of their radiological anatomy:

1. **Maxillary Sinuses**:
   - **Location**: Within the maxillary bones, below the orbits.
   - **Radiological Features**: Appears as a large, radiolucent (dark) area on X-rays and CT scans. The floor is the floor of the nasal cavity, and the roof is the orbital floor.
2. **Frontal Sinuses**:
   - **Location**: Within the frontal bone, above the orbits.
   - **Radiological Features**: Appears as a pair of radiolucent areas above the orbits. The frontal sinuses are variable in size and shape.
3. **Ethmoid Sinuses**:
   - **Location**: Between the eyes, within the ethmoid bone.
   - **Radiological Features**: Appears as multiple small air cells, which can be seen in the coronal plane on CT scans. The ethmoid sinuses are divided into anterior, middle, and posterior groups.
4. **Sphenoid Sinuses**:
   - **Location**: Within the sphenoid bone, behind the ethmoid sinuses.
   - **Radiological Features**: Appears as a radiolucent area in the center of the skull base on CT scans. The sphenoid sinuses are close to important structures like the optic nerve and internal carotid artery.

Imaging Techniques for Paranasal Sinuses

1. **Computed Tomography (CT)**:
   - **Preferred Modality**: CT scans are the primary imaging modality for evaluating the paranasal sinuses.
   - **Techniques**: Axial, coronal, and sagittal planes are used to provide detailed images of the bony anatomy and any pathological changes.
   - **Findings**: CT scans can detect sinusitis, polyps, tumors, fractures, and anatomic variants.
2. **Magnetic Resonance Imaging (MRI)**:
   - **Preferred Modality**: MRI is used for soft tissue evaluation within the sinuses.
   - **Techniques**: T1- and T2-weighted images, diffusion-weighted imaging (DWI), and contrast-enhanced T1-weighted images with fat suppression.

   - **Findings**: MRI can detect soft tissue masses, inflammatory changes, and complications like intracranial or orbital involvement.
3. **Plain Radiographs**:
   - **Limited Use**: Plain radiographs are less commonly used due to their limited ability to delineate complex bony anatomy.
   - **Techniques**: Waters' view, Caldwell's view, and submentovertex view are common projections used to visualize the sinuses.

(b) Retromolar Trigone

The retromolar trigone is a significant anatomical area in the oral cavity, particularly relevant in dental and maxillofacial practices. Understanding its radiological anatomy is crucial for various diagnostic and therapeutic procedures. Here is a detailed overview:

Anatomical Location

The retromolar trigone is a small triangular area located posterior to the last molar in the mandible. It lies in the region where the mandible's body transitions into the ramus.

Boundaries

- **Anterior Boundary**: The distal aspect of the third molar (wisdom tooth).
- **Posterior Boundary**: The anterior border of the ascending ramus of the mandible.
- **Medial Boundary**: The medial pterygoid muscle and soft tissues of the oral cavity.
- **Lateral Boundary**: The buccal mucosa and the buccinator muscle.

Contents and Structures

- **Retromolar Foramen**: An occasional anatomical variation that may contain branches of the inferior alveolar nerve and blood vessels. It is important to identify this foramen to avoid complications during dental extractions and implant placements.
- **Buccal Nerve**: This nerve passes through the retromolar trigone, providing sensory innervation to the cheek and mucosa.
- **Fibrous Tissue and Fat**: The retromolar trigone is composed of fibrous tissue interspersed with fat, contributing to its radiolucent appearance on radiographs.

Radiological Imaging

- **Panoramic Radiographs**: Commonly used in dental practice to provide a comprehensive view of the jaw. The retromolar trigone appears as a radiolucent area posterior to the third molar.
- **Cone-beam Computed Tomography (CBCT)**: Provides detailed 3D images of the retromolar trigone, allowing for precise assessment of bone structures and the identification of the retromolar foramen.
- **CT Scans**: Conventional CT scans offer high-resolution images and are used to evaluate the extent of pathology involving the retromolar trigone.
- **MRI**: Although less commonly used for evaluating the retromolar trigone, MRI can provide detailed images of soft tissue structures, which may be useful in assessing soft tissue tumors or infections.

Clinical Relevance

1. **Dental Extractions**: The retromolar trigone's anatomy is essential during the extraction of third molars to avoid damaging the buccal nerve or encountering the retromolar foramen.
2. **Implant Placement**: Knowledge of the retromolar trigone's anatomy ensures safe implant placement, avoiding injury to nerves and blood vessels.
3. **Pathology**: The area can be involved in various pathologies, including benign and malignant tumors, cysts, and infections. Radiological imaging helps in the early detection and management of these conditions.

Radiological Findings

- **Radiolucency**: Due to the presence of soft tissues and fat, the retromolar trigone typically appears radiolucent (dark) on radiographs.
- **Bone Structure**: CBCT and CT scans provide detailed visualization of the bone structure, helping in the identification of any bony abnormalities or lesions.

- **Soft Tissue Evaluation**: MRI can assess soft tissue structures, identifying any masses or inflammatory changes.

Summary

The retromolar trigone is a critical area in the oral cavity with significant clinical implications in dental and maxillofacial procedures. Understanding its radiological anatomy through various imaging modalities helps in the accurate diagnosis and management of pathologies, ensuring safe and effective treatment outcomes.

8. Write a short note on: HRCT of temporal bone in cholesteatoma. [5] [MD (WBUHS) 21]

High-resolution Computed Tomography (HRCT) of the temporal bone is a crucial imaging modality for evaluating cholesteatoma. Here's a detailed look at its role and findings:

Role of HRCT in Cholesteatoma

1. **Preoperative Assessment**:
   - **Location and Extent**: HRCT provides detailed images of the temporal bone, helping to determine the exact location and extent of the cholesteatoma.
   - **Bony Changes**: It identifies bony erosions, dehiscences, and the status of ossicles (malleus, incus, stapes).
   - **Hidden Areas**: Detects cholesteatoma in areas not easily visible during clinical examination, such as the sinus tympani and facial recess.
2. **Intraoperative Guidance**:
   - **Surgical Planning**: Helps surgeons plan the procedure by providing a clear map of the disease extent and bony anatomy.
   - **Avoiding Complications**: Identifies critical structures like the facial nerve, lateral semicircular canal, and internal carotid artery to avoid intraoperative complications.
3. **Postoperative Evaluation**:
   - **Recurrence Detection**: Assesses for residual or recurrent cholesteatoma after surgery.
   - **Complications**: Monitors for complications, such as intracranial or extracranial spread.

HRCT Findings in Cholesteatoma

1. **Cholesteatoma Characteristics**:
   - **Hypoechoic Mass**: Appears as a soft tissue mass with low attenuation on HRCT.
   - **Keratin Debris**: Contains keratin debris, which may appear as calcified areas within the mass.
2. **Bony Erosions**:
   - **Tegmen Tympani**: Erosion of the tegmen tympani, which is the thin bone separating the middle ear from the brain.
   - **Ossicles**: Erosion of ossicles, particularly the long process of the incus and the stapes superstructure.
   - **Labyrinthine Dehiscence**: Dehiscence of the bony labyrinth, which can lead to inner ear complications.
3. **Complications**:
   - **Intracranial Spread**: Extension of cholesteatoma into the intracranial cavity, which can be life-threatening.
   - **Facial Nerve Involvement**: Erosion or dehiscence of the facial canal, which can lead to facial nerve palsy.
   - **Lateral Semicircular Canal**: Erosion of the lateral semicircular canal, which can cause vertigo and balance issues.

Clinical Relevance

HRCT is invaluable in the management of cholesteatoma due to its high sensitivity and specificity in detecting the extent of the disease and associated complications. It aids in accurate preoperative planning, intraoperative guidance, and postoperative monitoring, ensuring better patient outcomes.

9. Classify orbital lesions in relation to various orbital spaces. Discuss MR features in orbital pseudo tumors. [4+6] [MD (WBUHS) 24, MD (WBUHS) 21]

Lesions of the orbit can be broadly subdivided into two groups: Ocular (limited to the globe) and orbital (rest of the orbit excluding globe). The orbital lesions can be further subdivided according to their predominant location in respective spaces.

Orbital Lesions

These can be discussed under the following broad categories: tumors, developmental cysts, inflammatory lesions, endocrine exophthalmos, parasitic infestations, vascular lesions and trauma.

Radiological Features by Lesion Type

1. **Congenital Lesions**
   - **Dermoid/Epidermoid Cyst**:
     - **CT**: Well-defined, low-density lesion; may show calcifications.
     - **MRI**: Hyperintense on T2, may show fat suppression.
   - **Encephalocele**:
     - **CT**: Bony defect with herniation of brain tissue.
     - **MRI**: Soft tissue isointense to the brain with CSF signal.
2. **Inflammatory Lesions**
   - **Orbital Cellulitis**:
     - **CT**: Diffuse soft-tissue swelling, possibly extending from the sinuses.
     - **MRI**: Enhancement of inflamed tissues; abscesses may appear as rim-enhancing collections.
   - **Thyroid Eye Disease**:
     - **CT/MRI**: Enlargement of extraocular muscles (spares tendons), commonly inferior rectus and superior rectus.
3. **Vascular Lesions**:
   - Hemangioma: It could be either capillary or cavernous in type. Both are different lesions differing in clinical presentation, location and age of presentation.

Capillary Hemangioma

- Most common intraorbital tumors of childhood.
- Usually extraconal, situated in the superomedial quadrant with associated cutaneous malformation over the face.
- Present at birth, grow rapidly in the first year of life and usually regress by 7–10 years of age.
- Most commonly arise anteriorly, are unencapsulated and less well-defined than the cavernous forms.
  - **CT**: Well-circumscribed, enhancing lesion in children.
  - **MRI**:
    - **T1**: Iso- to hyper intense.
    - **T2**: Moderately hyperintense with avid postcontrast enhancement.
      - Signal intensity is determined by the amount of fibrosis, calcification and hemosiderin deposition after hemorrhage.
      - Flow voids may be identified within and on the surface on T2W images, which is a helpful distinguishing feature from lymphangioma.

Cavernous Hemangioma

- Most common intraorbital tumors in adults.
- Usually occur as isolated intraconal masses.
- Well encapsulated tumors and tend to be round to oval in shape.
- 4th and 5th decade of life.
- Usually spare the orbital apex.
  - **USG**: Hyperechoic or mixed hypo- and hyperechoic appearance.
  - **CT**: Well demarcated, smoothly marginated, homogeneous, rounded, ovoid or lobulated soft tissue masses of increased density with a variable degree of contrast enhancement owing to slow intratumoral circulation.
  - Uncommonly phleboliths may be seen.

- **MRI**:
  - **T1**: Iso- to hypointense
  - **T2**: Homogeneously hyperintense on T2W image, showing marked enhancement that becomes homogeneous in delayed phase.

Lymphangioma

- Unencapsulated and represent hamartomas. Large majority of these lesions are extraconal in location.
- **CT and MRI**: On CT and MRI, lymphangiomas appear as irregularly marginated, multilobulated, poorly defined lesions that may be heterogenous and enhance partially.
- Ultrasound is useful to evaluate the internal architecture of lymphangioma, especially as intralesional sclerotherapy of its macrocystic variants is now becoming an increasingly popular and effective treatment.

Lacrimal Gland Tumors

- Pleomorphic adenoma (benign mixed tumor) is the most common benign epithelial tumor of the lacrimal gland.
- Involve the orbital part of the gland and are seen as well-defined masses with rounded configuration, displacing and deforming the globe.
  - **CT**: Smooth outline, round to oval.
  - **MRI**:
    - **T1**: Low signal intensity.
    - **T2**: Heterogeneous, high signal intensity. Contrast enhancement is moderate to intense.

4. **Neoplastic Lesions**
   - **Optic Nerve Glioma**:
     - **CT**: Fusiform enlargement of the optic nerve.
     - **MRI**: T2 hyperintensity, may extend intracranially.
   - **Optic Nerve Meningioma**:
     - **CT**: Calcifications with optic nerve sheath thickening ("tram-track" sign).
     - **MRI**: Intense contrast enhancement.

Rhabdomyosarcoma

- The usual clinical presentation is the rapidly progressive painless proptosis and displacement of the globe or motility disturbance.
- The tumor arises in the orbit from extraocular muscles and generally occupies both intra- and extraconal compartments.
- These are aggressive bone destroying and bone pushing lesions.
- The most common site of rhabdomyosarcoma (RMS) is considered to be superonasal quadrant of the orbit.
  - **CT**: Ill-defined, enhancing soft-tissue mass, often causing bone destruction.
  - **MRI**: Isointense on T1, hyperintense on T2 with marked enhancement.
  - **Lymphoma**:
    - **CT**: Homogeneous soft-tissue mass; moulds around structures.
    - **MRI**: T1 isointense, T2 slightly hyperintense, homogeneous enhancement.

5. **Infectious Lesions**
   - **Fungal Infections (e.g., Mucormycosis)**:
     - **CT**: Bony erosion with sinus involvement.
     - **MRI**: Non-enhancing, necrotic tissue with surrounding inflammatory enhancement.
6. **Cystic Lesions**
   - **Mucocele**:
     - **CT**: Expansile, well-defined lesion with remodeling of adjacent bone.
     - **MRI**: T1 variable, T2 hyperintense, enhances if infected.

Imaging-based Differential Diagnosis

Radiological patterns are critical for narrowing down the diagnosis:

- **Well-circumscribed, enhancing lesions**: Cavernous hemangioma, schwannoma.
- **Diffuse orbital involvement**: Thyroid eye disease, lymphoma.
- **Bone erosion/destruction**: Rhabdomyosarcoma, fungal infections.
- **Cystic lesions with fluid-fluid levels**: Lymphangioma.

Idiopathic orbital inflammation, also known as **orbital pseudotumor**, or **idiopathic orbital inflammatory syndrome** and **nonspecific orbital inflammation**, is an idiopathic inflammatory condition that most commonly involves the extraocular muscles. Less commonly there is inflammatory change involving the uvea, sclera, lacrimal gland, and retrobulbar soft tissue.

Associations

The condition has been associated with other inflammatory and autoimmune conditions:

- IgG4-related disease, now recognized as a separate entity: IgG4-related orbital disease
- Sarcoidosis
- Granulomatosis with polyangiitis
- Systemic lupus erythematosus (SLE)
- Polyarteritis nodosa (PAN)
- Dermatomyositis
- Rheumatoid arthritis (RA)
- Sclerosing cholangitis
- Riedel thyroiditis
- Mediastinal fibrosis

Presentation

Patients typically present with rapid-onset, usually unilateral, painful proptosis and diplopia. In a minority of cases (8–20%) bilateral involvement may occur either simultaneously or metachronously. Idiopathic orbital inflammation is a diagnosis of exclusion; atypical presentation, poor response to treatment with corticosteroid and recurrence should prompt biopsy to exclude other diseases.

Pathology

Histologically acute lesions demonstrate lymphocytes (which can be mistaken for orbital lymphoma), plasma cells, and giant cell infiltration.

Classification

Division into a number of subgroups according to location has been proposed:

- Lacrimal pseudotumor (dacryoadenitis)
- **Anterior Pseudotumor**: In the immediate retrobulbar fat
- **Posterior Pseudotumor**: In the fat at the orbital apex; distinguished from Tolosa- Hunt syndrome in that the cavernous sinus is spared.
- **Myositic Pseudotumor (myositis)**: Predominantly involves the extraocular muscles and therefore mimic thyroid-associated orbitopathy (TAO) but unlike TAO it also involves the tendons.
- **Optic Perineuritis**: Involvement of the optic nerve sheath
- **Diffuse Pseudotumor**: Affecting multiple compartments

Radiographic Features

Imaging demonstrates enlargement of the muscle belly of one (or more) extraocular muscles typically with the involvement of tendinous insertions. Involvement of the tendinous insertion distinguishes the idiopathic orbital inflammation from thyroid-associated orbitopathy in which the insertion point is spared. However, sparing of the anterior tendon does not exclude the diagnosis of idiopathic orbital myositis.

Additional inflammation can be seen in surrounding tissues, including the orbital fat, lacrimal gland, and optic nerve sheath.

It can appear as an infiltrative mass and extends outside of the orbit via superior or inferior orbital fissures. Extension into the cavernous sinus, meninges, and dura can occur. It is most commonly unilateral but can be bilateral (either at the same time or sequentially) in 8–20% of cases.

MRI

Reported signal characteristics include:

- **T1**: Affected region typically isointense (to extraocular muscles) but can also be hypointense
- **T2**: Affected region typically hypointense due to fibrosis and with more progression of fibrosis it becomes more hypointense, but the signal can also be iso- to hyperintense to extraocular muscles
- **T1 C+ (Gd)**: Moderate to a marked diffuse enhancement

Differential Diagnosis

One of the main differential diagnoses of idiopathic orbital inflammation is orbital lymphoma. There is considerable overlap between these entities both clinically and radiologically. However, orbital lymphoma usually presents as a progressive orbitopathy rather than acutely, is more often bilateral, shows lower values on ADC, and does not respond to corticosteroid.

10. Discuss the CT anatomy of the temporal bone with a schematic diagram. [10] [MD (WBUHS) 22]

CT anatomy of the temporal bone is best visualized using high-resolution computed tomography (HRCT), which provides detailed imaging of the complex bony structures. Below is an overview of the important structures and their appearance on a CT scan:

1. **CT Planes for Temporal Bone Imaging**

   Temporal bone CT is typically acquired in thin slices (0.5–1 mm) and reformatted into multiple planes:

   - Axial plane: Best for evaluating the inner ear, ossicles, mastoid air cells, and external auditory canal.
   - Coronal plane: Useful for assessing the middle ear, eustachian tube, and mastoid process.
   - Oblique plane: May be used for specific structures like the cochlea or semicircular canals.

2. **Key Anatomical Structures on CT**

   - External Ear
     - External acoustic meatus (EAM):
       - Bony canal extending from the outer ear to the tympanic membrane.
       - Seen as a round or oval canal lateral to the middle ear.
   - Middle Ear
     - Tympanic Cavity:
       - Air-filled space containing ossicles.
       - Anteriorly connected to the eustachian tube.
   - Ossicles:
     - Malleus: Head articulates with the incus; handle attaches to the tympanic membrane.
     - Incus: Connects the malleus to the stapes.
     - Stapes: Its footplate sits in the oval window, transmitting vibrations to the cochlea.
   - Tegmen Tympani: Thin bony roof separating the middle ear from the middle cranial fossa.
   - Inner Ear
     - Cochlea:
       - Spiral-shaped bony structure.
       - Visible as a small rounded structure medial to the middle ear.
   - Vestibule:
     - Central part of the bony labyrinth, between the cochlea and semicircular canals.
     - Oval window is visible connecting to the stapes.

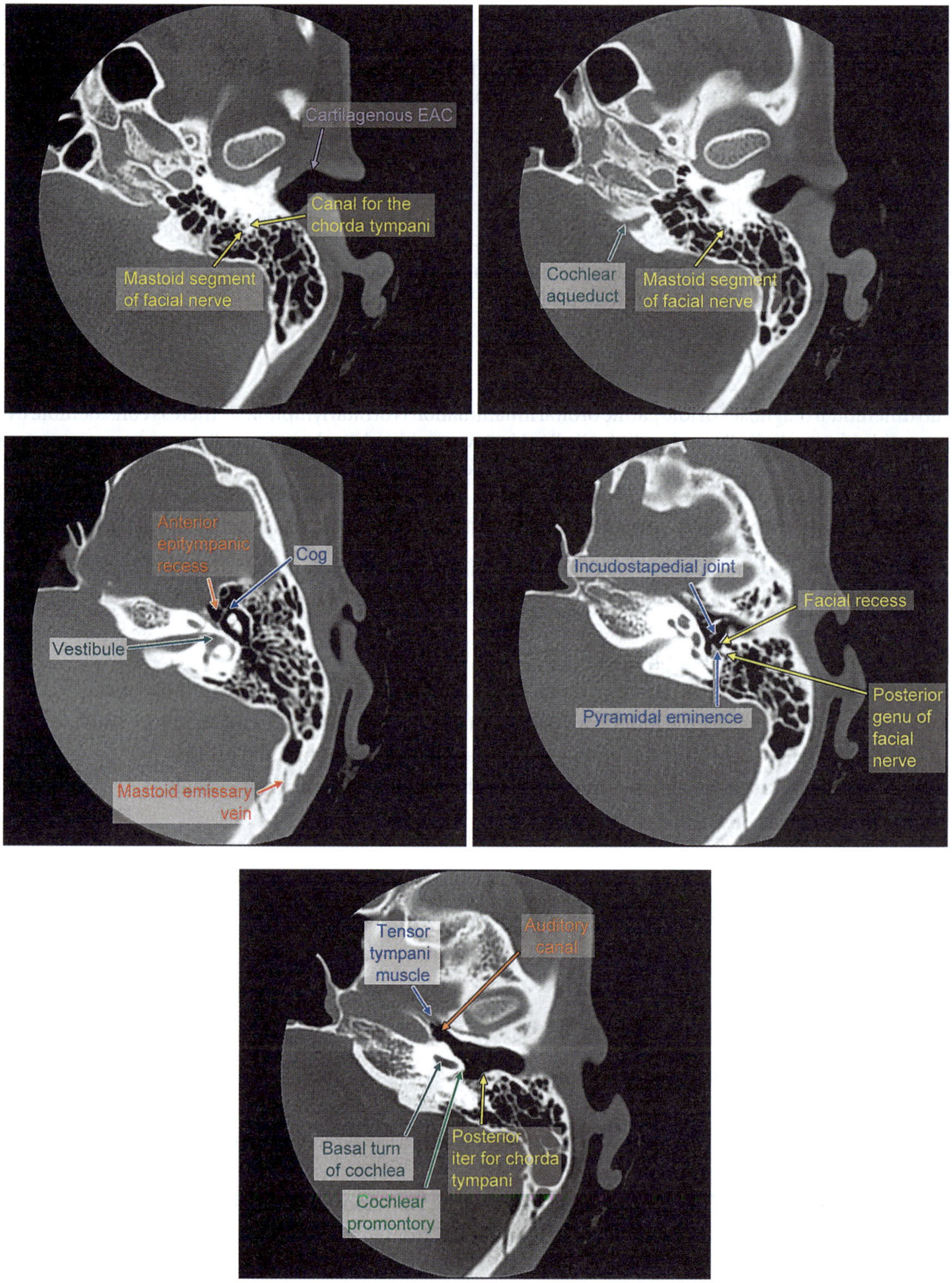

FIG. 21: HRCT anatomy of temporal bone.

- Semicircular canals: Three bony loops oriented in different planes (anterior, posterior, lateral).
    - Internal acoustic meatus (IAM): Contains cranial nerves VII (facial) and VIII (vestibulocochlear) along with the labyrinthine artery.

- Facial Nerve Canal
  - Labyrinthine Segment: From the IAM to the geniculate ganglion.
  - Tympanic Segment: Runs horizontally across the middle ear.
  - Mastoid Segment: Runs vertically to exit through the stylomastoid foramen.
- Mastoid Region
  - Mastoid Air Cells:
    - Honeycomb-like appearance posterior to the middle ear.
    - Communicates with the middle ear via the aditus ad antrum.
- Mastoid Process:
  - Inferior part of the mastoid region, providing muscle attachment.
  - Vascular Structures
- Jugular Foramen: Posterior to the carotid canal; transmits the internal jugular vein and cranial nerves IX, X, and XI.
- Carotid Canal: Anterior and medial to the jugular foramen, containing the internal carotid artery.
- Sigmoid Sinus Groove: Curved groove seen posterior to the mastoid air cells.
- Other Landmarks
  - Stylomastoid Foramen: Exit point for the facial nerve.
  - Eustachian Tube: Bony and cartilaginous structure connecting the middle ear to the nasopharynx.

3. **CT Findings in Common Pathologies**
   - Temporal Bone Fractures:
     - Longitudinal fractures: Parallel to the long axis of the petrous bone; involves the EAM and middle ear.
     - Transverse fractures: Perpendicular to the petrous bone; involves the cochlea, vestibule, or facial nerve canal.
   - Otitis Media and Mastoiditis: Fluid or opacification in the middle ear and mastoid air cells.
   - Cholesteatoma: Non-enhancing, soft-tissue mass in the middle ear with bony erosion.
   - Otosclerosis: Dense or lucent areas around the oval window (fenestral) or the cochlear promontory (retrofenestral).

Advantages of CT in Temporal Bone Imaging

- High-resolution imaging for fine bony details.
- Evaluation of fractures, ossicular chain integrity, mastoid air cells, and otosclerosis.
- Complementary to MRI, which better visualizes soft tissue structures like nerves and inner ear fluid pathways.

Accurate knowledge of the CT anatomy of the temporal bone **(Fig. 21)** ensures effective evaluation of otologic and neurotologic conditions.

11. Write a short note on: TIRADS. [5] [MD (WBUHS) 24, MD (WBUHS) 22, MD (WBUHS) 19, DNB Dec 20, AIIMS Dec 24]

ACR TI-RADS is a reporting system for thyroid nodules on ultrasound proposed by the American College of Radiology (ACR).

This uses a standardized scoring system for reports providing users with recommendations for when to use fine needle aspiration (FNA) or ultrasound follow-up of suspicious nodules, and when to safely leave alone nodules that are benign/not suspicious.

Radiographic Features

Ultrasound

Scoring is determined from five categories of ultrasound findings. The higher the cumulative score, the higher the TR (TI-RADS) level and the likelihood of malignancy.

One score is assigned from each of the following categories:

- **Composition**: (choose one)
  - Cystic or completely cystic: 0 point
  - Spongiform: 0 point
  - Mixed cystic and solid: 1 point
  - Solid or almost completely solid: 2 points
- **Echogenicity**: (choose one)
  - Anechoic: 0 point
  - Hyper- or isoechoic: 1 point
  - Hypoechoic: 2 points
  - Very hypoechoic: 3 points
- **Shape**: (choose one) (assessed on the transverse plane)
  - Wider than tall: 0 point
  - Taller than wide: 3 points
- **Margin**: (choose one)
  - Smooth: 0 point
  - Ill-defined: 0 point
  - Lobulated/irregular: 2 points
  - Extrathyroidal extension: 3 points

Any and all findings in the final category are also added to the other four scores.

- **Echogenic Foci**: (choose one or more)
  - None: 0 point
  - Large comet-tail artifact: 0 points
  - Macrocalcifications: 1 point
  - Peripheral/rim calcifications: 2 points
  - Punctate echogenic foci: 3 points

The findings in each category were detailed in the ACR committee's 2015 publication on a reporting lexicon. If multiple nodules are present only the four highest-scoring nodules (not necessarily the largest) should be scored, reported, and followed up.

Scoring and Classification

- **TR1**: 0 points
  - Benign
- **TR2**: 2 points
  - Not suspicious
- **TR3**: 3 points
  - Mildly suspicious
- **TR4**: 4-6 points
  - Moderately suspicious
- **TR5**: ≥7 points
  - Highly suspicious

Recommendations

- **TR1**: No FNA required
- **TR2**: No FNA required
- **TR3**: ≥1.5 cm follow up, ≥2.5 cm FNA
  - Follow up: 1, 3 and 5 years

- **TR4**: ≥1.0 cm follow up, ≥1.5 cm FNA
  - Follow up: 1, 2, 3 and 5 years
- **TR5**: ≥0.5 cm follow up, ≥1.0 cm FNA
  - Annual follow up for up to 5 years

FNA biopsy is recommended for suspicious lesions (TR3-TR5) with the above size criteria. If there are multiple nodules, the two with the highest ACR TI-RADS scores should be sampled (rather than the two largest), with largest size being used a tie-breaker if there are multiple nodules of the same classification.

Interval enlargement on follow-up is significant if there is an increase of >20% and >2 mm in two dimensions or a >50% increase in volume. If the ACR TI-RADS level increases between scans, an interval scan the following year is again recommended.

Risk of Malignancy

The projected risk of malignancy in the original 2017 paper was based on partial analysis of 3,433 nodules with cytological results. Partial analysis at the time of publication showed rates of <2% for TR1/TR2, 5% for TR3, 5–20% for TR4 and >20% for TR5 nodules. The final analysis demonstrated a stepwise increase for each point awarded by ACR TI-RADS, with each category validated. The published malignancy rates are:

- **TR1**: 0.3%
- **TR2**: 1.5%
- **TR3**: 4.8%
- **TR4**: 9.1%
- **TR5**: 35%

12. Discuss the cervical lymph node stations and their imaging. [5+5] [MD (WBUHS) 22]

The cervical lymph nodes are divided into several anatomical stations (**Fig. 22**), each with specific boundaries and functions. These stations are crucial for diagnosing and treating head and neck cancers, infections, and other conditions. Here's a detailed overview:

Cervical Lymph Node Stations

1. **Level I: Submental and Submandibular**
   - **Location**: Below the chin and jawline.
   - **Boundaries**:
     - **Superior**: Mylohyoid muscle and mandible.
     - **Inferior**: Inferior border of the hyoid bone.
     - **Anterior**: Platysma muscle.
     - **Posterior**: Posterior border of the submandibular gland.
   - **Sublevels**:
     - **Level Ia**: Submental nodes, located between the anterior bellies of both digastric muscles.
     - **Level Ib**: Submandibular nodcs, locatcd be tween the inner side of the mandible and the digastric muscle.

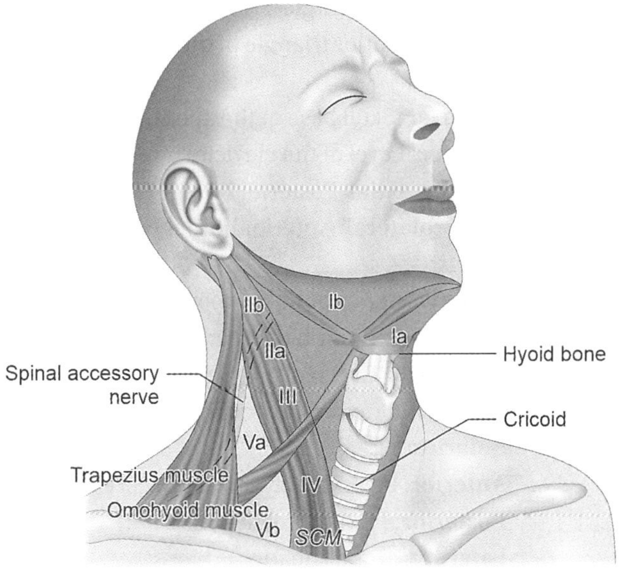

FIG. 22: Cervical lymph node stations *(For Color Version Refer Fig. 20).* (SCM: sternocleidomastoid muscle)

2. **Level II: Upper Internal Jugular (Deep Cervical) Chain**
   - **Location**: Along the upper part of the internal jugular vein.
   - **Boundaries**:
     - **Superior**: Base of the skull at the jugular foramen.
     - **Inferior**: Inferior border of the hyoid bone.
     - **Anterior**: Posterior border of the submandibular gland.

    - **Posterolateral**: Posterior border of the sternocleidomastoid muscle.
    - **Medial**: Medial border of the internal carotid artery.
  - **Sublevels**:
    - **Level IIa**: Inseparable from or anterior to the posterior edge of the internal jugular vein (includes jugulodigastric nodes).
    - **Level IIb**: Posterior to and separable by a fat plane from the internal jugular vein.
3. **Level III**: **Middle Internal Jugular (Deep Cervical) Chain**
  - **Location**: Along the middle part of the internal jugular vein.
  - **Boundaries**:
    - **Superior**: Inferior border of the hyoid bone.
    - **Inferior**: Inferior border of the cricoid cartilage.
    - **Anterior**: Anterior border of the sternocleidomastoid muscle.
    - **Posterolateral**: Posterior border of the sternocleidomastoid muscle.
    - **Medial**: Medial border of the common carotid artery.
4. **Level IV**: **Lower Internal Jugular (Deep Cervical) Chain**
  - **Location**: Along the lower part of the internal jugular vein.
  - **Boundaries**:
    - **Superior**: Inferior border of the cricoid cartilage.
    - **Inferior**: Level of the clavicle.
    - **Anterior**: Anterior border of the sternocleidomastoid muscle.
    - **Posterolateral**: Oblique line drawn through the posterolateral edge of the sternocleidomastoid muscle and the lateral edge of the anterior scalene muscle.
    - **Medial**: Medial border of the common carotid artery.
  - **Includes**: Medial supraclavicular nodes (Virchow's node).
5. **Level V**: **Posterior Triangle**
  - **Location**: Posterior triangle of the neck.
  - **Boundaries**:
    - **Superior**: Skull base at the apex of the convergence of sternocleidomastoid and trapezius muscles.
    - **Inferior**: Level of the clavicle.
    - **Anteromedial**: Posterior border of the sternocleidomastoid muscle.
    - **Posterolateral**: Anterior border of the trapezius muscle.
  - **Sublevels**:
    - **Level Va**: Superior half, superior to the inferior border of the cricoid cartilage (posterior to levels II and III).
    - **Level Vb**: Inferior half, inferior to the inferior border of the cricoid cartilage.
6. **Level VI**: **Anterior Cervical**
  - **Location**: Anterior to the trachea and esophagus.
  - **Boundaries**:
    - **Anterior**: Investing layer of deep cervical fascia.
    - **Posterior**: Pretracheal fascia.
    - **Lateral**: Carotid sheath.
    - **Inferior**: Clavicle.
7. **Level VII**: **Retropharyngeal and Retrostyloid**
  - **Location**: Posterior to the pharynx.
  - **Boundaries**:
    - **Anterior**: Buccopharyngeal fascia.
    - **Posterior**: Alar fascia.

  - **Lateral**: Carotid sheath.
  - **Inferior**: Extends down to the superior mediastinum.

8. **Level VIII: Parotid**
   - **Location**: Around the parotid gland.
   - **Boundaries**:
     - **Anterior**: Facial nerve.
     - **Posterior**: Sternocleidomastoid muscle.
     - **Superior**: Zygomatic arch.
     - **Inferior**: Mandible.
9. **Level IX: Buccofacial**
   - **Location**: Around the buccal region.
   - **Boundaries**:
     - **Anterior**: Buccal mucosa.
     - **Posterior**: Masseter muscle.
     - **Superior**: Zygomatic arch.
     - **Inferior**: Mandible.
10. **Level X: Retroauricular and Occipital**
    - **Location**: Around the ear and occipital region.
    - **Boundaries**:
      - **Anterior**: Auricle.
      - **Posterior**: Mastoid process.
      - **Superior**: Zygomatic arch.
      - **Inferior**: Mandible.

13. Describe in brief the technique and appearances of various anatomical structures on ocular ultrasound. [2+3]

The superficial location of the eye, its cystic composition, and the advent of high-frequency ultrasound make sonography ideal for imaging the eye. MRI is favored by radiologists, so there are few reports on ocular sonography in the radiology literature. Sonography is used more commonly by ophthalmologists to evaluate the eye, particularly when direct examination by slit-lamp and funduscopy is not sufficient. Detailed cross-sectional anatomy of the entire globe is possible with conventional sonographic equipment anterior chamber visualization requires a dedicated sonographic biomicroscope. Color Doppler and A-mode sonography are reported to be useful in characterizing masses. The sonography examination is rapid and cost-efficient, without the contraindications, such as pacemakers, that MRI has. Sonography avoids the irradiation associated with CT and the need for sedation in children. Therefore, it can be used repeatedly during treatment of tumors to assess response to therapy.

Technique

Conventional gray-scale sonographic equipment (Elegra, Siemens Medical Solutions; ATL, Philips Medical Systems) and 7.5–15-MHz transducers were used by the radiology department, scanning through the closed eyelid. The ophthalmology department used a 10-MHz B-mode probe and an 8–10-MHz A-mode probe (Innovative Imaging Systems), scanning through the open eye after paralyzing the blink reflex. A dedicated ocular sonographic biomicroscope, using frequencies up to 50 MHz, was available for a limited time.

The radiology transducers were linear and the images are axial in a traditional anterior-to-posterior orientation. Ophthalmology used sector transducers, and their images are also axial but rotated in a left-to-right orientation to show the A-mode echo patterns. The term "reflectivity" is used in some figure legends to describe A-mode echo patterns and is similar to the term "echogenicity," but in addition describes amplitude of tissue interface reflection.

Normal Anatomy (Fig. 23)

The cornea, conjunctiva, anterior chamber, posterior chamber and iris rarely require sonography and are not well visualized with conventional sonography, but they are excellently detailed with newer sonographic biomicroscopes. The lens is best inspected directly, with no need for sonography. A mature cataract of the lens may obscure the retina on fundoscopy, necessitating sonography. The vitreous body is gelatinous and anechoic, with loose attachments to the retina, and it stabilizes the eyeball. The choroid is part of the uveal tract, which also includes the ciliary body and iris, and is the site of many intraocular tumors. The choroid has a rich vascular supply from the long and short posterior ciliary arteries. Because the retina is pigmented, direct inspection of the choroid by fundoscopy is limited, and sonography plays an important role in diagnosing choroidal melanoma and metastatic tumors. The retina and choroid are sonographically perceived as one layer in the normal eye; the sclera is a highly reflective outer layer.

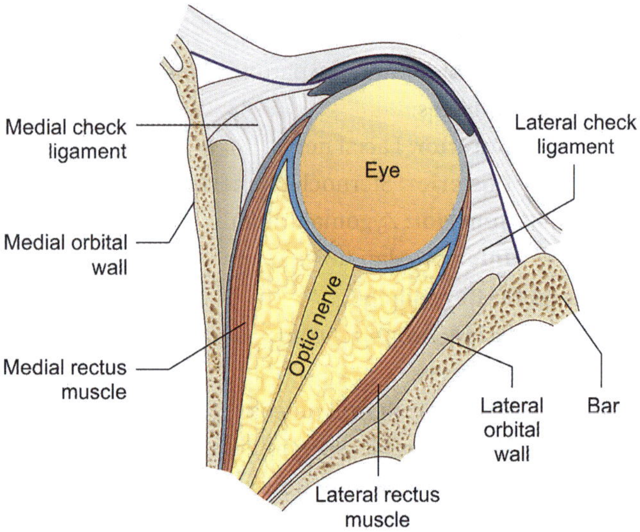

FIG. 23: Schematic diagram showing normal orbital anatomy.

14. Discuss the role of ultrasound in the evaluation of thyroid nodule. [10]

Introduction

Thyroid nodules are any discrete lesion that can be delineated on imaging studies from the adjacent thyroid parenchyma. They can represent a range of benign or malignant conditions.

Up to 67% of the population evaluated with US will have an incidental thyroid nodule.

Epidemiology

More common in females (4:1 F:M)

Etiology

There are many causes of thyroid nodules, some of the more common causes are as follows:

- **Benign nodules**
  - Follicular adenoma
    - Colloid nodule
  - Hurthle cell adenoma
  - Thyroid cyst: Simple, hemorrhagic
  - Focal/asymmetrical thyroiditis
    - Lymphocytic (Hashimoto) thyroiditis
    - Granulomatous (de Quervain) thyroiditis
- **Malignant nodules**
  - Primary thyroid cancer
    - Papillary thyroid carcinoma
    - Follicular thyroid carcinoma
    - Hurthle cell carcinoma
    - Poorly differentiated thyroid carcinoma
    - Medullary thyroid carcinoma
    - Anaplastic thyroid carcinoma

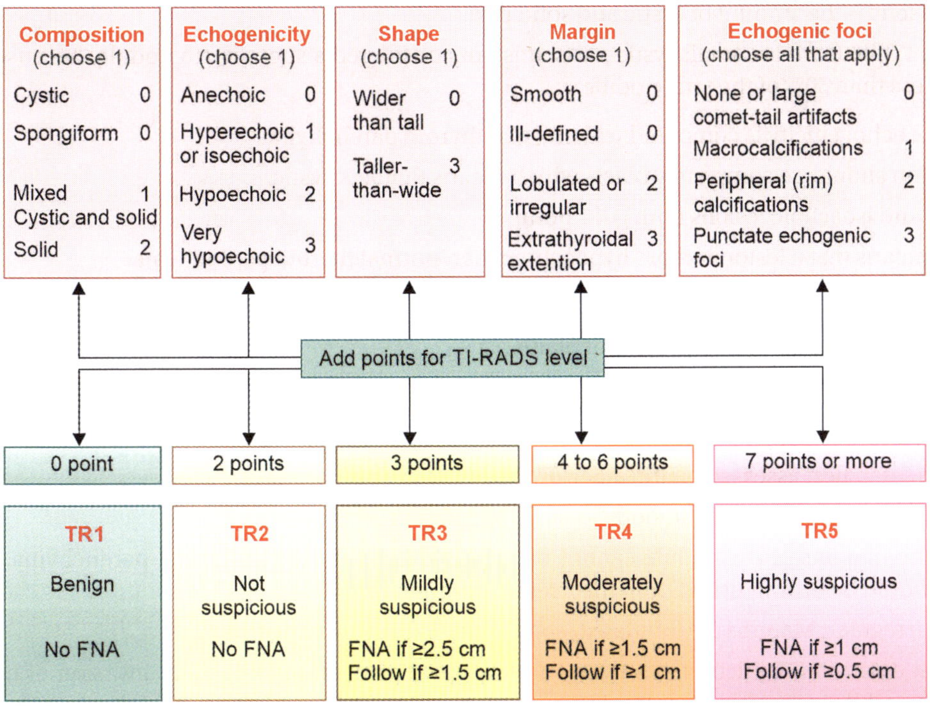

FIG. 24: Ultrasound features of thyroid nodules used in TI-RADS.

- Thyroid lymphoma: Primary or secondary
- Metastases to the thyroid

Role of US in Evaluation of Thyroid Nodule

The Thyroid Imaging Reporting and Data System (TI-RADS) of the American College of Radiology (ACR) was designed in 2017 with the intent to decrease biopsies of benign nodules and improve overall diagnostic accuracy.

The five ultrasound features **(Fig. 24)** of thyroid nodules used in TI-RADS are: Composition, echogenicity, shape, margin and punctate echogenic foci. Each item is given points.

The points are added from all categories to determine the TI-RADS level, each with a recommendation.

There are several exceptions for TI-RADS, where this system cannot be used for. Each of these exceptions have a greater risk of thyroid cancer than the otherwise normal adult population:

- Children
- FDG-PET avid thyroid nodules
- Lymphadenopathy
- Known risk factors for thyroid malignancy, like MEN type 2

Follow-up

Nodules smaller than 5 mm do not need any follow-up, even if they are TI-RADS 5. This is because it is very unlikely that nodules smaller than 5 mm will become a clinically significant malignancy.

The cutoff point of 2.5 cm for fine needle aspiration (FNA) in mildly suspicious TR3 lesions is based on studies showing that thyroid carcinomas don't have a decreased survival until they reach this threshold value.

The ACR-TIRADS category has been shown to have good correlation with the malignancy risk in large studies.

The risk of malignancy is:

TR1: 0.3%, TR2: 1.5%, TR3: 4.8%, TR4: 9.1%, TR5: 35%

Composition

i. Cystic-lesions that are almost completely cystic are benign (TI-RADS 1).
ii. Spongiform: Spongiform nodules have a sponge-like appearance, with at least 50% cystic composition of tiny cystic parts.

iii. Mixed cystic/solid—the amount of cystic and solid part.
iv. Solid lesions: While there are small cystic parts, it is not considered a spongiform nodule, because the small cystic parts are far less than 50% of the total nodule.

Echogenicity: The echogenicity is compared with normal thyroid parenchyma.

i. Anechoic lesion should be completely black, which means that it is cystic.
ii. Hyperechoic and isoechoic lesions both get 1 point.
iii. Hypoechoic means that a lesion is more hypoechoic than normal thyroid parenchyma.
iv. Very hypoechoic—lesion is more hypoechoic than normal muscle.

Shape: The shape should be assessed in the axial plane.

i. Wider-than tall
ii. Taller-than wider: A taller-than-wide shape is a strong predictor of malignancy, and therefore gets 3 points

Margin: Margin is often best assessed on the anterior side.

i. Smooth: The margin is completely smooth
ii. Ill-defined: The margins of the nodule cannot be clearly defined from the thyroid parenchyma. This is a benign feature and should be distinguished from the irregular margin.
iii. Lobulated or irregular: Margins are lobulated, spiculated, irregular or angulated.
iv. Extrathyroidal extension: Difficult to analyze on ultrasound, there should be clear invasion of nearby structures. Bulging of the nodule in nearby structures is not enough.

Echogenic foci: Echogenic foci is the only category where multiple options are possible.

i. None or large comet tail artifacts.
ii. Macrocalcifications: Nodule has large macrocalcifications with acoustic shadowing.
iii. Rim calcification: Peripheral rim calcifications can be complete or incomplete.
iv. Microcalcifications: Punctate echogenic foci are also knows as microcalcifications. They are a strong predictor of malignancy and therefore get 3 points.

Growth: Growth of a nodule according to TI-RADS is also defined, and is in accordance with the ATA guidelines. There should be either:

- ≥20% increase in at least two nodule dimensions, with a minimal increase of 2 mm or
- ≥50% or greater increase in volume

If there is no change in size for 5 years, the nodule can be considered as having a benign behavior, and further follow up is not needed. Comparison should be made with the oldest study available, and not (only) the last one.

Multiple nodules:

- When there are multiple nodules, there should be no more than 4 nodules classified. FNA is not recommended of more than 2 nodules.
- In the case of multiple nodules, the nodule fulfilling the TI-RADS FNA criteria should be sampled, which is not necessarily the dominant or largest nodule.

15. Salivary gland tumors and imaging. [10] [DNB June 22, MD (WBUHS) 24]

Introduction: The ratio of benign to malignant tumors is proportional to the gland size, i.e., the parotid gland tends to have benign neoplasms, the submandibular gland 50:50, and the sublingual glands and accessory glands are mostly malignant.

Location

- **Parotid gland**: 70%
- **Minor salivary glands (including sublingual)**: 22% with the palate being most frequent
- **Submandibular gland**: 8%

Overall ~80% of all parotid masses are benign and the majority of these are pleomorphic adenomas.

Subtypes

Benign

- Epithelial
  - Pleomorphic adenoma: This is the most common (≈50%) tumor of the parotid
  - Warthin tumor: Essentially only found in the parotid, in older, usually male patients; it is bilateral in 10–15%
  - Intraductal papilloma of salivary glands
  - Oncocytoma of salivary glands
  - Myoepithelioma: Considered a subtype of pleomorphic adenoma; they can also originate in breast and bronchus
- Nonepithelial
  - Hemangioma
  - Lymphangioma
  - Lipoma

Malignant

- **Mucoepidermoid carcinoma**: Most of the malignant lesions
- **Adenoid cystic carcinoma**
  - Myoepithelioma
  - Adenocarcinoma (not otherwise specified)
  - Acinic cell carcinoma of salivary glands
  - Squamous cell carcinoma of salivary glands
  - Lymphoepithelial carcinoma
  - Malignant mixed tumors of the salivary glands
    - Carcinoma ex pleomorphic adenoma
    - Carcinosarcoma (true mixed tumor of the salivary glands)
    - Metastasizing pleomorphic adenoma
  - Salivary duct carcinoma
  - Metastases (mostly to intraparotid lymph nodes)
    - Cutaneous squamous cell carcinoma
    - Malignant melanoma
    - Testicular seminoma (rare)
  - Lymphoma (rare)
    - Primary: Arising from the parotid gland as a MALToma
    - Secondary: Involving the intraparotid lymph nodes

Imaging

1. **Pleomorphic Salivary Adenoma of Salivary Glands**

   Well-defined, "bosselated" or "polylobulated" borders (many small undulations, not truly lobulated). They are most commonly located within the parotid gland, particularly the superficial lobe.

   - USG: Typically hypoechoic and may show posterior acoustic enhancement
   - CT: Homogeneous attenuation and prominent enhancement. They can be heterogeneous with less prominent enhancement, foci of necrosis, and possible delayed enhancement. Small regions of calcification are common.
   - MRI:
     - T1: usually of low intensity
     - T2:
       - Characteristically of very high intensity (especially myxoid type)
       - Often have a rim of decreased signal intensity on T2-weighted images representing the surrounding fibrous capsule
       - T1 C+ (Gd): Usually demonstrates homogeneous enhancement

2. **Warthin Tumor** essentially only found in the parotid, in older, usually male patients; it is bilateral in 10–15%.

   The tendency to undergo cystic change is greater than any other salivary gland tumor.

   - USG: Well-defined margins and multiple irregulars, small, sponge-like anechoic areas. They tend to have a higher proportion of cystic content.
   - CT:
     - Well defined, cystic changes appear as intralesional lower attenuation
     - Moderate enhancement, no calcification
     - Presence of a mural nodule is strongly suggestive of Warthin tumor
   - MRI:
     - T1: Low to intermediate signal with cyst containing cholesterol components containing focal high signal
     - T2: Heterogeneous and variable signal intensity
     - T1 C+ (Gd): Cystic components do not take up contrast while solid parts usually enhance
3. **Mucoepidermoid Carcinoma** most common malignant primary parotid gland tumor. Most frequently arise in the parotid gland followed by the hard palate, and present as a painless swelling.
   - USG: A well-circumscribed hypoechoic lesion, with a partial or completely cystic appearance.
   - MRI: Low-grade tumors have similar appearances to pleomorphic adenomas:
     - T1: Low to intermediate signal; low signal cystic spaces
     - T2: Intermediate to high signal; cystic areas will be high signal
     - T1 C+ (Gd): Heterogeneous enhancement of solid components

   High-grade tumors, on the other hand, have lower signal on T2 and poorly defined margins, and infrequent cystic areas:

   - T1: Low to an intermediate signal
   - T2: Intermediate to low signal
   - It is essential to image the cranial nerves with fat-saturated post-contrast T1 sequences to assess for perineural spread, and as such the base of the skull should be imaged up to and including the cavernous sinus and inner ear.
4. **Adenoid Cystic Carcinoma** arise more commonly in the minor salivary glands (~55%) than in the major salivary glands. They are the most common sinonasal tumors of salivary origin. They are locally aggressive with a propensity for perineural spread.

   MRI:

   - T1: Hypo- to isointense
   - T2: Slightly hyperintense, with higher grades being markedly hypointense
   - T1 C+ (Gd): Homogeneous enhancement

16. Malignant thyroid lesion and imaging. [10] [DNB June 22]

- **Introduction**: Thyroid nodules are commonly found during neck ultrasound examinations. Most of these nodules are benign, which leads to a significant number of biopsies being performed to identify the few that are malignant or require surgical intervention for a definitive diagnosis.
- **Risk factors for malignant lesions**
  - Head and neck irradiation
  - Family history of thyroid cancer
  - Age <30 or >60 years
  - Male >2 cm
- **Pathological classification**:
  1. Primary thyroid cancers
     - Papillary thyroid carcinoma: 60–80% of carcinomas
     - Follicular thyroid carcinoma: 10–20%
     - Medullary thyroid carcinoma: 5%

- Hurthle cell thyroid carcinoma: 5%
- Anaplastic thyroid carcinoma : 1–2%
- Poorly differentiated carcinoma: 5%

2. Thyroid lymphoma: ~2.5%
   - Primary thyroid lymphoma
   - Secondary thyroid involvement with lymphoma
3. Metastases to the thyroid: 1% squamous cell carcinoma (rare)
   - Primary
   - Secondary
     - Direct invasion from head and neck squamous cell carcinoma
     - Metastatic disease
4. Carcinoma showing thymus-like elements (CASTLE) (rare)

Imaging Features

a. **Papillary Thyroid Cancer**
   - USG: Papillary carcinoma within the thyroid usually appears as a solitary mass usually with an irregular outline, located in the subcapsular region and demonstrating vascularity. Small punctate regions of echogenicity representing microcalcifications (psammoma bodies) may be present.
   - CT: CT is best at staging lymph node involvement (see thyroid cancer staging). Involved lymph nodes tend to have:
     - Cystic components: ~35%
     - Thick nodular walls: ~40%
     - Septa: ~60%
     - Purely cystic nodes are uncommon and more frequent in young patients
     - Calcification may be seen occasionally
     - The so-called lateral aberrant thyroid is actually a lymph node metastasis from papillary thyroid carcinoma
     - Follicular thyroid cancer
   - USG: Lesions are typically hypoechoic and usually lacks cystic change

b. **Medullary Thyroid Carcinoma**
   - USG: Punctate high echogenic foci resembling calcification may be seen both within the primary thyroid lesion as well as metastatic regional lymph nodes and distant metastatic sites. Involved lymph nodes typically calcify.
   - CT: Both primary and metastatic lesions usually have irregular dense calcific foci within.
   - In the chest, bullae formation and pulmonary fibrosis may develop as a result of a desmoplastic reaction.

c. **Hurthle Cell Carcinoma**
   - USG: Lesions are typically hypoechoic solid (rather than cystic)
   - One study reported that TI-RADS was unreliable in predicting malignancy in Hurthle cell neoplasms.

d. **Anaplastic Thyroid Carcinoma**
   - USG: May show microcalcification. Usually seen as an infiltrative lesion.

17. Suprahyoid neck spaces—boundaries and radiological anatomy. Pathologies of masticator space. [10] [DNB June 21, MD (WBUHS) 24]

Suprahyoid Neck Spaces—Boundaries

The suprahyoid neck space includes several distinct anatomical spaces, each with specific radiological boundaries defined by fascial planes and adjacent structures. Here's a detailed overview of the radiological boundaries:

1. **Pharyngeal Mucosal Space (PMS)**
   - Superior boundary: Skull base.
   - Inferior boundary: Hyoid bone.

- Anterior boundary: Oral cavity and oropharynx mucosa.
- Posterior boundary: Retropharyngeal space.
- Lateral boundary: Parapharyngeal space.

2. **Parapharyngeal Space (PPS)**
   - Superior boundary: Skull base.
   - Inferior boundary: Hyoid bone.
   - Medial boundary: Pharyngeal mucosal space.
   - Lateral boundary: Masticator space and parotid space.
   - Anterior boundary: Pterygoid muscles.
   - Posterior boundary: Carotid space.
3. **Masticator Space (MS)**
   - Superior boundary: Skull base.
   - Inferior boundary: Inferior border of the mandible.
   - Medial boundary: Parapharyngeal space.
   - Lateral boundary: Buccal space.
   - Anterior boundary: Buccal fat pad.
   - Posterior boundary: Parotid space.
4. **Parotid Space (PS)**
   - Superior boundary: Zygomatic arch.
   - Inferior boundary: Mandibular angle.
   - Medial boundary: Parapharyngeal space.
   - Lateral boundary: Skin and subcutaneous tissues.
5. **Carotid Space (CS)**
   - Superior boundary: Jugular foramen at skull base.
   - Inferior boundary: Thoracic inlet (extends below hyoid bone).
   - Medial boundary: Retropharyngeal space.
   - Lateral boundary: Sternocleidomastoid muscle.
6. **Retropharyngeal Space (RPS)**
   - Superior boundary: Skull base.
   - Inferior boundary: Upper mediastinum (T4 vertebral level).
   - Anterior boundary: Pharyngeal mucosal space.
   - Posterior boundary: Prevertebral space.
   - Lateral boundary: Carotid space.
7. **Submandibular Space (SMS)**
   - Superior boundary: Mandibular body.
   - Inferior boundary: Hyoid bone.
   - Medial boundary: Mylohyoid muscle (separates from the sublingual space).
   - Lateral boundary: Inferior mandible and skin.
8. **Sublingual Space (SLS)**
   - Superior boundary: Floor of the mouth.
   - Inferior boundary: Mylohyoid muscle (separates from submandibular space).
   - Medial boundary: Lingual mucosa.
   - Lateral boundary: Mandibular body.

These boundaries provide a framework for localizing and identifying pathologies in the suprahyoid neck spaces based on their radiological appearance and spatial involvement.

Suprahyoid Neck Spaces—Radiological Anatomy

The suprahyoid neck space refers to the region above the hyoid bone in the neck and contains several anatomically distinct spaces important in radiology. Each space is defined by specific fascial layers and contains critical anatomical structures. Here is an overview of its radiological anatomy:

1. **Spaces in the Suprahyoid Neck**

   The suprahyoid neck can be divided into several spaces, each identifiable on imaging:

   a. Parapharyngeal Space (PPS)
      - Location: Between the pharyngeal mucosal space and the carotid space.
      - Contents:
        - Fat (key distinguishing feature)
        - Ascending pharyngeal artery
        - Venous plexus
      - Imaging Features:
        - Appears as a fat-filled space on CT and MRI.
        - Displacement of this space is a crucial clue to identifying the origin of surrounding pathology.

   b. Pharyngeal Mucosal Space (PMS)
      - Location: Surrounds the oropharynx, nasopharynx, and hypopharynx.
      - Contents:
        - Pharyngeal muscles
        - Palatine tonsils
        - Mucosa
        - Minor salivary glands
      - Imaging features: Enhances strongly on contrast CT/MRI due to vascular mucosa.

   c. Parotid Space (PS)
      - Location: Lateral to the mandible.
      - Contents:
        - Parotid gland
        - Facial nerve
        - External carotid artery
        - Retromandibular vein
      - Imaging features: Homogeneous parotid gland signal on MRI; tumors (e.g., pleomorphic adenoma) often alter this pattern.

   d. Masticator Space (MS)
      - Location: Around the ramus of the mandible.
      - Contents:
        - Muscles of mastication (masseter, temporalis, pterygoids)
        - Mandibular division of the trigeminal nerve
      - Imaging features: Symmetry of muscles; abnormal masses or infections cause asymmetry.

   e. Carotid Space (CS)
      - Location: Extends from the base of the skull to the aortic arch.
      - Contents:
      - Internal carotid artery
      - Internal jugular vein
      - Cranial nerves IX–XII
      - Lymph nodes
      - Imaging Features:
        - Appears as a vertical column on axial imaging.
        - Enlarged nodes or vascular abnormalities (e.g., carotid dissection) are detectable.

f. Retropharyngeal Space (RPS)
   - Location: Posterior to the pharyngeal mucosal space, anterior to the prevertebral space.
   - Contents:
     - Fat
     - Lymph nodes
   - Imaging features:
     - Seen as a fat-filled space on imaging.
     - Infections (e.g., abscess) and lymphadenopathy are common pathologies.

g. Submandibular Space (SMS)
   - Location: Below the mandible, extending to the floor of the mouth.
   - Contents:
     - Submandibular glands
     - Facial artery and vein
     - Lymph nodes
     - Imaging features: Submandibular gland shows uniform enhancement; stones or sialadenitis may alter the pattern.

2. **Imaging Modalities**
   - CT (Computed Tomography):
     - Excellent for bone structures, detecting calcifications, and acute infections.
     - Contrast-enhanced CT delineates vascular structures and soft tissue spaces.
   - MRI (Magnetic Resonance Imaging):
     - Superior for soft tissue contrast.
     - Identifies fat, lymph nodes, and tumors in detail.
     - Useful sequences include T1-weighted (for anatomy) and T2-weighted (for edema/infection).
3. **Pathologies**
   - Neoplasms:
     - Benign (e.g., pleomorphic adenoma in parotid space).
     - Malignant (e.g., squamous cell carcinoma in pharyngeal mucosal space).
   - Infections:
     - Ludwig's angina (submandibular space).
     - Retropharyngeal abscess (retropharyngeal space).
   - Vascular Issues: Carotid dissection or aneurysm (carotid space).
   - Lymphadenopathy: Metastatic nodes often involve retropharyngeal and carotid spaces.

Understanding the radiological anatomy of the suprahyoid neck is critical for accurately diagnosing pathologies based on their spatial involvement and imaging features.

Pathologies of Masticator Space

The masticator space is a fascial compartment in the suprahyoid neck that contains the muscles of mastication (masseter, temporalis, medial, and lateral pterygoids), portions of the mandible, and associated structures like the mandibular division of the trigeminal nerve (V3). It can be involved in a variety of pathologies, often identified through radiological imaging (CT or MRI).

1. **Infectious and Inflammatory Conditions**
   - Odontogenic Infections:
     - Cause: Spread from infected teeth or dental procedures.
     - Imaging: Soft tissue swelling, fluid collections, and abscess formation around the mandible or in the muscles of mastication.
   - Ludwig's Angina:
     - Can spread to the masticator space from the submandibular space.
     - Imaging: Diffuse enhancement, edema, or abscess formation.

- Myositis:
  - Inflammatory involvement of the masticatory muscles, sometimes post-infectious.
  - Imaging: Muscle swelling with T2 hyperintensity on MRI.

2. **Neoplastic Conditions**
   - Benign Tumors:
     - Hemangiomas:
       - Vascular tumors involving muscles of mastication.
       - Imaging: Hyperintense on T2, enhance with contrast on MRI.
     - Lipomas:
       - Arising from fat in the space.
       - Imaging: Fat-density lesion on CT; bright on T1-weighted MRI.
     - Malignant Tumors:
     - Sarcomas (e.g., rhabdomyosarcoma):
       - Can arise in the muscles.
       - Imaging: Heterogeneous soft tissue masses, often enhancing with contrast.
       - Squamous Cell Carcinoma:
         - » Can invade the masticator space from nearby structures like the oropharynx.
         - » Imaging: Enhancing mass with possible bony invasion.
3. **Mandibular Pathologies**
   - Mandibular Tumors: Osteosarcoma, chondrosarcoma, or ameloblastoma can expand into the masticator space. Imaging: Bone destruction, periosteal reaction, and soft tissue involvement.
   - Fractures:
     - Can disrupt the masticator space due to trauma.
     - Imaging: Discontinuity of the mandible, associated hematoma.
4. **Perineural Spread**

   Tumors such as adenoid cystic carcinoma or squamous cell carcinoma can invade cranial nerves, including the mandibular nerve (V3), causing perineural spread.

   Imaging:
   - Thickened, enhancing nerves.
   - Tumor tracking along neural pathways on MRI.
5. **Vascular Lesions**
   - Arteriovenous malformations (AVMs):
   - Vascular anomalies involving the mandibular or masticator region.
   - Imaging: Flow voids on MRI, enhancement on CT angiography.
6. **Trauma**
   - Hematoma:
     - Due to blunt or penetrating trauma to the jaw or face.
     - Imaging: Non-enhancing fluid collections on CT or T2 hyperintensity on MRI.
7. **Fibrous Dysplasia**
   - Benign bony overgrowth involving the mandible or maxilla, potentially encroaching on the masticator space.
   - Imaging: Ground-glass appearance of bone on CT.
8. **Neurological Conditions**
   - Trigeminal Neuralgia:
     - May involve the mandibular division of the trigeminal nerve (V3) within the masticator space.
     - Imaging: Often normal but can show nerve compression (e.g., by vascular loops).

9. **Metastatic Disease**
   - Secondary tumors from primary sites (e.g., lung, breast) may involve the masticator space lymphatics or muscles.
   - Imaging: Enhancing soft tissue lesions with potential adjacent bone involvement.

Key Imaging Features

CT

- Excellent for bony lesions and calcifications.
- Contrast enhances abscesses, tumors, and vascular anomalies.

MRI

- Superior for soft tissue and muscle involvement.
- T1: Anatomical detail; T2: Edema and fluid collections.
- Contrast-enhanced MRI for tumor characterization.

Understanding the underlying pathology and utilizing imaging findings in the context of clinical presentation are crucial for accurate diagnosis and management of masticator space conditions.

18. Describe the imaging protocol of paranasal sinuses for functional endoscopic sinus surgery (FESS). What are the important anatomical landmarks and anatomical variants which should be looked for while evaluating for FESS? Discuss the radiological patterns and features of Aspergillus infection of paranasal sinuses. [3+3+4] [DNB Dec 20]

The imaging protocol for paranasal sinuses in preparation for functional endoscopic sinus surgery (FESS) is typically focused on high-resolution CT scanning. This imaging is crucial for surgical planning, as it provides detailed information about sinus anatomy, variants, and disease extent. Here is a detailed description of the protocol:

CT Protocol for Paranasal Sinuses (FESS Planning)

1. **Patient Preparation**:
   - No fasting or contrast is usually required.
   - Remove all metal objects (e.g., glasses, jewelry) to avoid artifacts.
   - Ensure patient cooperation to minimize motion artifacts.
2. **Patient Positioning**:
   - The patient is placed supine on the CT scanner table.
   - The head is positioned to align the scanning plane parallel to the hard palate (occlusal plane).
   - Immobilization devices may be used to ensure stability during the scan.
3. **Imaging Parameters**:
   - Modality: Non-contrast high-resolution CT (HRCT).
   - Scan Coverage: Include the frontal, ethmoid, sphenoid, and maxillary sinuses, extending from the roof of the frontal sinus to the hard palate and posteriorly to the sphenoid sinus.
   - Slice Thickness: Thin slices (typically 0.5–1 mm) for optimal resolution.
   - Field of View (FOV): Narrow, focused on the paranasal sinuses to avoid unnecessary exposure.
   - Plane of Acquisition:
     - Axial Plane: Initial images acquired parallel to the hard palate.
     - Multiplanar Reconstructions (MPR): Coronal and sagittal reconstructions from the axial dataset are essential for evaluating sinonasal anatomy and surgical landmarks.
4. **Technical Parameters**:
   - Bone Window Settings:
     - Window Width: 2000–2500 HU.
     - Window Level: 200–500 HU.

Soft Tissue Window Settings: Adjusted as needed to evaluate mucosal thickening, polyps, or other soft tissue abnormalities.

Radiation dose: Utilize low-dose protocols (e.g., iterative reconstruction techniques) to minimize exposure without compromising image quality.

When evaluating for FESS using imaging (typically high-resolution CT), it is crucial to carefully examine anatomical landmarks and variants to guide safe and effective surgery. These structures help avoid complications and ensure optimal outcomes. Below is a comprehensive list:

Key Anatomical Landmarks

1. **Ostiomeatal Complex (OMC)**: The central drainage pathway for the maxillary, anterior ethmoid, and frontal sinuses. Evaluate for obstruction, polyps, or mucosal thickening.
2. **Uncinate Process**:
   - A thin bony structure critical for the drainage of the maxillary sinus.
   - Assess its attachment site (medial wall of orbit, skull base, or middle turbinate).
3. **Ethmoid Sinuses**: Anterior and posterior ethmoid air cells are key areas for dissection. Evaluate for pneumatization and disease extent.
4. **Frontal Recess**:
   - The drainage pathway of the frontal sinus.
   - Look for anatomical obstructions like agger nasi cells or variations in frontal cells.
5. **Middle Turbinate**:
   - Important for orientation during surgery.
   - Assess for concha bullosa (pneumatization) or paradoxical curvature.
6. **Sphenoid Sinus and its Surroundings**:
   - Located near vital structures such as the internal carotid artery, optic nerve, and pituitary gland.
   - Look for sphenoid sinus pneumatization and septations.
7. **Lamina Papyracea**: The thin bony wall separating the ethmoid sinus from the orbit. Evaluate for dehiscence or erosion to avoid orbital injury.
8. **Cribriform Plate**:
   - Part of the skull base, separating the ethmoid sinus from the anterior cranial fossa. Assess for Keros classification (depth of the olfactory fossa):
   - Type I: 1–3 mm (shallow, safer).
   - Type II: 4–7 mm (moderate risk).
   - Type III: 8–16 mm [deep, high risk of cerebrospinal fluid (CSF) leak].
9. **Maxillary Sinus Ostium**: Identify the natural ostium to avoid creating a false passage during surgery.
10. **Posterior Ethmoid Sinus**: Evaluate for its proximity to the sphenoid sinus and optic nerve.

Important Anatomical Variants

1. **Concha Bullosa**:
   - Pneumatization of the middle turbinate.
   - Can contribute to narrowing of the nasal airway or obstructing the OMC.
2. **Agger Nasi Cells**:
   - The most anterior ethmoid air cell, often near the frontal recess.
   - Can block frontal sinus drainage.
3. **Haller Cells**:
   - Infraorbital ethmoid air cells located along the floor of the orbit.
   - Can narrow the maxillary sinus ostium or encroach on the orbit.

4. **Onodi Cells**:
   - Posterior ethmoid cells that are in close proximity to the optic nerve and sphenoid sinus.
   - Important to identify to avoid optic nerve damage.
5. **Paradoxical Middle Turbinate**: A turbinate that curves laterally rather than medially, potentially narrowing the OMC.
6. **Septal Deviation**: Can contribute to asymmetrical sinus ventilation and drainage.
7. **Accessory Maxillary Ostium**: An additional opening in the maxillary sinus wall that may affect sinus ventilation.
8. **Sphenoid Sinus Septations**:
   - Septations within the sphenoid sinus often attach to critical structures such as the internal carotid artery or optic nerve.
   - Important to map to avoid complications.
9. **Pneumatization of Unusual Areas**: Excessive pneumatization of the frontal sinus, ethmoid sinuses, or sphenoid sinus, increasing surgical complexity.
10. **Dehiscent Lamina Papyracea or Skull Base**: Look for thinning or absence of bony structures, increasing the risk of orbital or cranial complications.

Key Pathological Features to Assess

- Mucosal thickening, polyps, or masses.
- Complete or partial sinus opacification.
- Bony erosion, indicative of invasive disease.
- Fluid levels suggesting acute infection.

By systematically evaluating these anatomical landmarks and variants, surgeons can anticipate challenges and mitigate risks such as orbital injury, optic nerve damage, CSF leak, or vascular complications.

Aspergillus infection of the paranasal sinuses, also known as aspergillosis of the paranasal sinuses, presents in several forms, each with distinct radiological patterns. These forms include non-invasive aspergillosis (e.g., fungal ball or mycetoma), allergic fungal rhinosinusitis (AFRS), and invasive aspergillosis (acute or chronic). Below is a detailed discussion of their radiological features:

1. **Noninvasive Aspergillosis (Fungal Ball or Mycetoma)**
   - **Radiological Pattern:**
     - Modality: High-Resolution CT is the primary modality, with MRI used for soft tissue characterization.
     - Features:
       - Unilateral sinus involvement, typically the maxillary sinus.
       - Dense, heterogenous, and irregularly shaped hyperattenuating lesion (high density due to calcium, fungal hyphae, or metal deposition).
       - No bone erosion but may cause remodeling due to chronic pressure.
       - Adjacent mucosal thickening or fluid levels due to secondary inflammation.
     - Differentiating Feature: Hyperattenuation on CT without contrast enhancement is a hallmark.
2. **Allergic Fungal Rhinosinusitis (AFRS)**
   - **Radiological Pattern:** Seen in patients with chronic allergic sinusitis.
     - Modality: CT for bony and sinus involvement, MRI for soft tissue and fungal elements.
     - CT Findings:
       - Hyperdense areas within sinuses:
         - » Representing allergic mucin with fungal debris.
         - » Mixed density with low-density mucin and high-density inspissated secretions.
       - Sinus expansion:
         - » Causing thinning and remodeling of bony walls (but typically no erosion).
         - » Polypoid mucosal thickening or complete opacification of affected sinuses.
         - » Multisinus involvement, often bilateral.

- **MRI Findings:**
  - T1-weighted images: Hypo- to isointense signal for fungal debris or mucin.
  - T2-weighted images: Signal voids within hyperintense mucin due to paramagnetic fungal elements.
  - Postcontrast T1: No enhancement of the fungal debris; adjacent mucosa may enhance due to inflammation.

3. **Invasive Aspergillosis**
   - **Types:** Acute Invasive Aspergillosis: Seen in immunocompromised individuals (e.g., post-transplant or cancer patients).
   - **Radiological Pattern:**
     - CT Findings:
       - Diffuse sinus opacification, often bilateral.
       - Bone destruction: Aggressive erosion of sinus walls and adjacent structures (orbit or skull base).
       - Possible orbital invasion or intracranial extension.
   - **MRI Findings:** Hypointense fungal debris on T1- and T2-weighted images.
     - Contrast Enhancement:
       - Thickened mucosa with enhancement.
       - Lack of enhancement in necrotic areas (indicating tissue infarction).
       - Involvement of orbital fat, muscles, or intracranial structures.
   - **Chronic Invasive Aspergillosis**: Occurs in immunocompetent individuals but with chronic sinus disease.
     - **Radiological Pattern**:
     - **CT Findings**:
       - Chronic sinus opacification with progressive bone erosion or thinning.
       - Mixed density within sinuses due to chronic fungal debris.
   - **MRI Findings**:
     - Signal voids on T2 due to fungal debris.
     - Contrast enhancement in adjacent inflamed tissues, indicating chronic inflammation.

Differential Diagnosis

When evaluating aspergillosis, consider the following:

1. Chronic bacterial sinusitis: Less likely to show hyperdense fungal debris or extensive bone erosion.
2. Mucoceles: Uniformly hypointense on CT with no fungal components.
3. Neoplastic lesions (e.g., squamous cell carcinoma): Often show more aggressive bone destruction and soft tissue mass with enhancement.

19. Discuss the role of HRCT and MRI in the evaluation of congenital sensorineural hearing loss. [5+5] [DNB June 20]

The evaluation of congenital sensorineural hearing loss (SNHL) often involves imaging to identify structural abnormalities of the inner ear and associated neural pathways. Both high-resolution computed tomography (HRCT) and magnetic resonance imaging (MRI) play complementary roles in the diagnostic workup, helping to determine etiology, plan for interventions (e.g., cochlear implantation), and predict prognosis. Here's a detailed discussion:

- **Gross anatomy**: The temporal bone is situated on the sides and the base of the cranium and lateral to the temporal lobe of the cerebrum. The temporal bone is one of the most important calvarial and skull base bones. The temporal bone is divided into several main parts/portions 1-3: squamous part (temporal squama) petrous part (petrous pyramid) tympanic part mastoid part (usually considered a separate part but it is formed by both the squamous and petrous parts) mandibular fossa (formed anteriorly by the squamous part and posteriorly by the tympanic part of temporal bone).

- In addition, there are several bony projections: styloid process (considered a separate part or a component of the petrous part) zygomatic process (a component of the squamous part) mastoid process (considered a component of the mastoid part or synonymous with it).
- **The temporal bone can also be divided into otologic zones**: the medial third of the external auditory canal (part of the external ear) middle ear (tympanic cavity) inner ear internal auditory canal.
- **Articulations**: There are four intrinsic fissures between the divisions of the temporal bone—petrosquamous fissure, petrotympanic (Glaserian) fissure, tympanosquamous fissure and tympanomastoid fissure.

Role of HRCT in Congenital SNHL

HRCT protocol: The HRCT temporal bone protocol is designed to provide high-resolution imaging of the intricate bony structures of the temporal bone. It is optimized to identify congenital anomalies, trauma, infections, or preoperative evaluation for procedures like cochlear implantation.

Scanning Parameters

1. **Patient Positioning**:
   - Supine position with the head immobilized.
   - The gantry should be aligned parallel to the orbitomeatal line to minimize radiation exposure to the eyes.
2. **Equipment and Technique**:
   - Multidetector CT scanner (64-slice or higher recommended).
   - Thin collimation for high-resolution imaging.
3. **Key Parameters**:
   - Slice Thickness: 0.5–1 mm (thin slices are crucial for fine details).
   - Reconstruction Interval: 0.1–0.5 mm.
   - Field of View (FOV): Small FOV to focus on the temporal bone.
   - Matrix Size: 512 × 512 for high spatial resolution.
   - Algorithm: Bone algorithm for optimal visualization of osseous structures.
   - Tube Voltage (kVp): 120 kVp.
   - Tube Current (mAs): Adjusted per patient size, typically 150–200 mAs.
   - Rotation Time: ~1 second.
   - Pitch: Close to 1 for isotropic resolution.
4. **Plane of Acquisition**:
   - Axial Plane: Primary acquisition parallel to the hard palate.
   - Coronal Plane: Reconstructed perpendicular to the axial plane.
   - Oblique Planes: Additional reconstructions along specific axes for structures like the semicircular canals.

Reconstruction Techniques

- **Multiplanar Reconstruction (MPR)**: Generates axial, coronal, and sagittal images.
- **3D Volume Rendering**: Useful for preoperative planning or for a detailed view of complex anatomy.
- **High-resolution Focus**: Enhance visualization of cochlea, ossicles, facial nerve canal, vestibular aqueduct, and semicircular canals.
- HRCT is valuable for assessing the bony anatomy of the temporal bone and inner ear structures.

Advantages of HRCT

- High-resolution images of bone structures.
- Superior for identifying ossification, cochlear anomalies, and temporal bone fractures.
- Shorter scan time and widely available.

Key Findings on HRCT

1. **Inner Ear Malformations**:
   - Cochlear Dysplasia (based on the Mondini classification):
     - Mondini Malformation: Incomplete partitioning with fewer than 2.5 cochlear turns.
     - Common Cavity: A single cavity representing the cochlea and vestibule.
     - Cochlear Hypoplasia: Small cochlea with reduced turns.
     - Vestibular Abnormalities:
       - Enlarged vestibule or absence of semicircular canals.
         - Enlarged Vestibular Aqueduct (EVA):
       - Defined as >1.5 mm at the midpoint.
       - Commonly associated with Pendred syndrome.
2. **Bony Abnormalities**:
   - Narrow or aplastic internal auditory canal (IAC), indicating hypoplasia of the cochlear nerve.
   - Otosclerosis or other ossification disorders.
3. **Middle and External Ear**: Assess for any coexisting conductive hearing loss due to middle ear abnormalities.
4. **Cochlear Implant Planning**:
   - Evaluate the patency of the cochlear lumen.
   - Identify aberrant facial nerve courses or other anomalies affecting implantation.

Role of MRI in Congenital SNHL

MRI Temporal Bone Protocol

Patient Preparation

1. **Positioning**:
   - Supine position with the head in a neutral position.
   - Secure the head to minimize motion artifacts.
2. **Patient Instructions**:
   - Inform the patient to remain still during the scan.
   - Earplugs or headphones to minimize discomfort from noise

Imaging Parameters

1. **Equipment**:
   - High-field MRI scanner (1.5T or 3T for better resolution).
   - Dedicated head or surface coil for high signal-to-noise ratio.
2. **Sequence Selection**: The protocol includes both basic sequences for general evaluation and specialized sequences for fine detail.

Key Parameters

1. **Slice Thickness**:
   - 3D Sequences: 0.5–1 mm (isotropic for reconstruction).
   - 2D Sequences: 3–5 mm.
2. **Field of View (FOV)**: Focused on the temporal bone (~18–20 cm).
3. **Matrix Size**: High-resolution (e.g., 256 × 256 or 512 × 512).
4. **Echo Time (TE)**: Short for T1W; long for T2W sequences.
5. **Repetition Time (TR)**: Short for T1W; longer for T2W.
6. **Fat Saturation**: Applied to post-contrast T1W images to highlight lesions.

Planes of Imaging

1. **Axial Plane**: Primary imaging for bilateral temporal bone and brainstem structures.
2. **Coronal Plane**: Evaluate the vertical extent of lesions and their relationship to surrounding structures.
3. **Oblique Plane**: Custom planes aligned to specific structures (e.g., internal auditory canal, semicircular canals).

MRI is essential for visualizing soft tissue structures, particularly the neural pathways and membranous inner ear components.

Advantages of MRI

- Excellent soft tissue contrast.
- Preferred for assessing the cochlear nerve and brainstem auditory pathways.
- No ionizing radiation, safer for children.

Key Findings on MRI

1. **Cochlear Nerve Evaluation**:
    - Use thin-slice T2-weighted sequences in the internal auditory canal (IAC).
    - Evaluate the presence, size, and signal of the cochlear nerve in the IAC.
    - Cochlear Nerve Aplasia or Hypoplasia: A small or absent cochlear nerve is a contraindication for cochlear implants.
2. **Inner Ear Structures**:
    - Confirm abnormalities seen on HRCT, such as: Mondini malformation, common cavity, or cochlear hypoplasia.
    - Membranous labyrinth abnormalities like signal changes in the endolymph or perilymph.
    - Assess for inflammation or fibrosis in the inner ear in cases of post-infectious congenital SNHL.
3. **Enlarged Vestibular Aqueduct (EVA)**:
    - MRI can assess the associated endolymphatic sac and duct enlargement.
    - Helps in distinguishing EVA from other conditions.
4. **Central Nervous System (CNS) Abnormalities**:
    - Brain anomalies associated with syndromic SNHL (e.g., Chiari malformations, hypoplasia of the brainstem or cerebellum).
    - White matter changes in conditions like congenital CMV infection.
    - Detects lesions or atrophy of the auditory brainstem or cortex.

Common Syndromic Associations Identified on Imaging

- **Pendred Syndrome**: EVA with inner ear malformations.
- **Waardenburg Syndrome**: May show hypoplastic cochlea or vestibule.
- **CHARGE Syndrome**: Hypoplasia of semicircular canals and cochlear anomalies.
- **Congenital CMV Infection**:
    - Periventricular calcifications on CT.
    - White matter hyperintensities and cochlear damage on MRI.

Clinical Applications

- **Initial Diagnosis**: HRCT to evaluate bony anatomy and MRI to assess the cochlear nerve.
- **Cochlear Implant Planning**:
    - HRCT for electrode insertion feasibility.
    - MRI for cochlear nerve presence and CNS evaluation.

Prognosis

Presence of cochlear nerve on MRI predicts the success of cochlear implantation.

Summary

- HRCT and MRI are complementary tools.
- HRCT is ideal for detailed evaluation of the bony structures of the temporal bone and middle ear.
- MRI provides superior imaging of soft tissues, neural structures, and the brain.

Their combined use ensures a comprehensive understanding of congenital SNHL, enabling accurate diagnosis, intervention planning, and prognosis estimation.

Spine Imaging and Interventions

1. Describe the common CV junction anomalies with their imaging features. [5+5] [MD (WBUHS) 23]

The craniovertebral junction (CVJ) refers to the area where the skull (cranium) meets the cervical spine, specifically between the occipital bone and the first cervical vertebra (atlas), and between the atlas and the second cervical vertebra (axis). Anomalies at this junction can lead to significant neurological and mechanical problems. Imaging is crucial for diagnosing and understanding these conditions. Common CVJ anomalies and their imaging features include:

1. **Atlantoaxial Dislocation**
   - Description: This occurs when there is abnormal displacement between the atlas (C1) and the axis (C2). It may be due to congenital conditions, trauma, or inflammatory diseases.
   - Imaging Features:
     - X-ray: Lateral and open-mouth odontoid views can show displacement of the odontoid process (dens) relative to the atlas.
     - CT: High-resolution CT can show the degree of dislocation or subluxation between C1 and C2, with detailed bony involvement.
     - MRI: MRI is used to assess the impact on the spinal cord, soft tissue, and ligaments (e.g., atlantoaxial ligament disruption).
2. **Chiari Malformation (Type I)**
   - Description: A condition where the cerebellar tonsils herniate downward through the foramen magnum into the cervical canal, often associated with syringomyelia (fluid-filled cysts in the spinal cord).
   - Imaging Features:
     - MRI: The hallmark feature is cerebellar tonsillar herniation below the foramen magnum (more than 5 mm below the foramen magnum). MRI is also used to identify associated syringomyelia.
     - CT: CT is not as sensitive for detecting the herniation but can be useful in assessing bony abnormalities like platybasia (flattening of the skull base).
3. **Platybasia**
   - Description: Flattening of the skull base, which can alter the normal angle between the clivus and the cervical spine. It is often associated with Chiari malformation or other CVJ abnormalities.
   - Imaging Features:
     - X-ray: The McGregor's line (line from the hard palate to the occipital bone) and the Basion-Atlantic Line can be used to assess for abnormal skull base angulation. A platybasia is typically indicated by a flattening of the normal curve of the skull base.
     - MRI/CT: MRI and CT can show a flattened clivus and may help assess associated anomalies like Chiari malformation.
4. **Occipitocervical Fusion (Cranial-Cervical Junction Fusion)**
   - Description: A congenital or acquired fusion of the occipital bone to the cervical spine, often seen in conditions like Klippel-Feil syndrome or following trauma or surgery.
   - Imaging Features:
     - X-ray/CT: CT is the best imaging modality to identify the bony fusion between the occiput and cervical spine. X-ray can show limited movement at the junction.

  - MRI: MRI is useful in evaluating the neurological structures in these cases, particularly to detect compression of the spinal cord or brainstem.

5. **Basilar Invagination**
   - Description: The upward displacement of the odontoid process (dens) into the skull base, often associated with conditions like rheumatoid arthritis, achondroplasia, or congenital anomalies.
   - Imaging Features:
     - X-ray/CT: The odontoid process may be seen invading the foramen magnum on lateral X- rays or CT scans. The Chamberlain's line (a line drawn from the posterior edge of the hard palate to the opisthion) helps in assessing the degree of invagination.
     - MRI: MRI is essential for evaluating the brainstem and spinal cord for any compression or syringomyelia.
6. **Klippel-Feil Syndrome**
   - Description: A congenital condition characterized by the fusion of cervical vertebrae, which can affect the CVJ and lead to neurological issues.
   - Imaging Features:
     - X-ray: X-ray shows cervical vertebral fusion, most often between C2 and C3, though multiple levels can be involved.
     - CT: High-resolution CT can demonstrate the degree of bony fusion and the associated structural anomalies.
     - MRI: MRI is used to assess any associated spinal cord abnormalities or syringomyelia.
7. **Torticollis (Congenital and Acquired)**
   - Description: Abnormal head tilt due to muscular or neurological causes that affect the CVJ, often leading to secondary cranial deformities.
   - Imaging Features:
     - X-ray: Lateral views can show abnormal positioning of the cervical spine, particularly in congenital forms.
     - MRI: MRI is helpful in identifying the cause, such as basilar invagination, atlantoaxial instability, or spinal cord compression.
8. **Atlanto Occipital Fusion**
   - Description: A congenital or acquired fusion of the atlas (C1) to the occiput, leading to restricted motion at the craniovertebral junction.
   - Imaging Features:
     - X-ray: X-ray can show the fusion, often seen as a bony bridge between the occipital bone and C1.
     - CT/MRI: These modalities are more effective in assessing the degree of fusion and identifying any associated neurological involvement.
9. **Spinal Cord Compression (Due to CVJ Anomalies)**
   - Description: Anomalies like basilar invagination, Chiari malformation, and atlantoaxial dislocation can lead to compression of the brainstem or spinal cord, causing neurological symptoms.
   - Imaging Features: MRI is the gold standard for detecting spinal cord compression at the CVJ and assessing the extent of compression on neural structures.
10. **Syringomyelia**
    - Description: A cyst or cavity within the spinal cord, commonly associated with Chiari malformation and craniovertebral junction anomalies.
    - Imaging Features: MRI is the modality of choice for diagnosing syringomyelia. It will show a fluid-filled cavity in the spinal cord, often associated with Chiari malformation.

Imaging Modalities in CVJ Anomalies

- **X-ray**: Often used to assess bony abnormalities, alignment, and joint spaces. It provides initial assessment and can help identify gross anomalies.
- **CT Scan**: Offers excellent bone detail and is often the modality of choice for evaluating bony structures and alignment at the CVJ.

- **MRI**: Provides detailed soft tissue contrast, making it ideal for assessing the spinal cord, brainstem, and any compression or herniation in the craniovertebral junction.

Conclusion

The craniovertebral junction is a complex and critical area of the body, and abnormalities at this junction can lead to serious neurological and structural problems. Imaging, especially MRI and CT, is key to diagnosing these anomalies, assessing their impact on the central nervous system, and planning appropriate management strategies.

2. Discuss about the radiological anatomy of CV junction. [10] [MD (WBUHS) 21, DNB June 19]

The craniovertebral junction (CVJ) encompasses the anatomical region where the skull base articulates with the upper cervical spine, specifically involving the occiput, atlas (C1), and axis (C2). This region is highly specialized to provide a balance of stability and mobility, while also protecting critical neural and vascular structures. Radiological imaging plays a pivotal role in understanding and evaluating the CVJ.

Key Components and Their Radiological Features

1. **Occiput**
   - Bony Structures:
     - Clivus: Sloping bone extending from the dorsum sellae to the foramen magnum.
     - Foramen Magnum: Large opening at the skull base through which the medulla and spinal cord pass.
     - Occipital Condyles: Paired structures articulating with the atlas (C1) to form the atlanto-occipital joint.
   - Imaging:
     - CT: Sharp details of the clivus, occipital condyles, and margins of the foramen magnum.
     - MRI: Evaluation of the soft tissues passing through the foramen magnum (e.g., brainstem, spinal cord, and vertebral arteries).
2. **Atlas (C1)**
   - Bony Features:
     - Anterior and Posterior Arches: Connect at lateral masses.
     - Lateral Masses: Articulate with the occipital condyles superiorly and the axis inferiorly.
     - No Vertebral Body or Spinous Process: Unique among cervical vertebrae.
   - Imaging:
     - CT: Clear visualization of the ring-like structure and articulation with adjacent bones.
     - MRI: Assessment of surrounding ligaments and neural structures, including the spinal cord.
3. **Axis (C2)**
   - Bony Features:
     - Odontoid Process (Dens): Projects upward to articulate with the anterior arch of the atlas.
     - Body and Spinous Process: More robust compared to C1.
   - Superior Articular Facets: Articulate with the lateral masses of C1.
     - Imaging:
       - CT: Essential for evaluating the dens and its articulation.
       - MRI: Useful for ligamentous and neural evaluations.
4. **Ligaments**

   Key Ligaments and Their Radiological Importance:
   - Transverse Ligament: Encircles the dens and stabilizes the atlantoaxial joint. Best evaluated with MRI.
   - Alar Ligaments: Extend from the dens to the occipital condyles, limiting rotation. Visualized on MRI.
   - Tectorial Membrane: Continuation of the posterior longitudinal ligament, covering the dens. Best seen on MRI.
   - Apical Ligament: Extends from the dens tip to the foramen magnum. Visualized on MRI.

5. **Neural Structures**
   - Components:
     - Medulla Oblongata: Exits the foramen magnum and transitions into the spinal cord.
     - Spinal Cord: Encased within the cervical vertebral canal.
     - Cranial Nerve Roots: Lower cranial nerves exit through foramina near the CVJ.
   - Imaging:
     - MRI: Crucial for assessing compression or abnormalities involving the brainstem, spinal cord, or nerve roots.
6. **Vascular Structures**
   - Components:
     - Vertebral Arteries: Pass through the transverse foramina of C1–C6 and enter the foramen magnum.
     - Venous Plexuses: Surround the vertebral arteries.
   - Imaging:
     - CT Angiography (CTA): Detailed evaluation of the vertebral arteries.
     - MR Angiography (MRA): Assessment of vascular flow and anomalies.
7. **Atlanto-occipital and Atlantoaxial Joints**
   - Atlanto-occipital Joint: Between occipital condyles and atlas.
   - Primary motion: Flexion-extension ("yes" motion).
   - Atlantoaxial Joint: Between atlas and axis.
     - Primary Motion: Rotation ("no" motion).
   - Imaging:
     - Dynamic X-rays: Useful for assessing instability.
     - CT and MRI: Evaluate joint alignment, ligament integrity, and associated soft tissues.

Key Imaging Modalities

1. **X-ray**:
   - Useful for initial evaluation of alignment and basic anatomical relationships.
   - Dynamic views can assess instability.
2. **CT**:
   - Best for osseous anatomy, fractures, and congenital anomalies.
   - Provides high-resolution images of the occiput, atlas, and axis.
3. **MRI**:
   - Gold standard for soft tissue, neural structures, and ligaments.
   - Detects spinal cord compression, syringomyelia, and vascular anomalies.
4. **CT Angiography (CTA)/MR Angiography (MRA)**: Evaluate vertebral artery integrity and anomalies.

Normal Measurements

- **Chamberlain's Line**: Tip of the dens should not project more than 3 mm above this line.
- **McRae's Line**: Dens should not extend above this line at the foramen magnum.
- **Atlanto-Dens Interval (ADI)**:
  - Normal: ≤3 mm in adults, ≤5 mm in children.
  - Increased ADI indicates instability.

Conclusion

The radiological anatomy of the CVJ includes complex interactions between osseous, ligamentous, neural, and vascular structures. Accurate imaging and understanding of this region are critical for diagnosing congenital and acquired anomalies, trauma, and degenerative conditions affecting the CVJ.

3. Discuss imaging features and various intervention in intracranial and spinal arteriovenous malformation. [4+3+3] [MD (WBUHS) 21]

Arteriovenous malformations (AVMs) are abnormal connections between arteries and veins without an intervening capillary bed, and they can occur both intracranially (within the brain) and in the spinal cord. These lesions can lead to significant clinical problems such as hemorrhage, neurological deficits, and increased pressure in surrounding tissues. The imaging features of these malformations are crucial for diagnosis, and interventions can vary depending on the location, size, and symptoms caused by the AVM.

Intracranial Arteriovenous Malformations (AVMs)

Imaging Features of Intracranial AVMs

1. **Computed Tomography (CT) Scan**:
   - Acute Hemorrhage: A CT scan can quickly identify acute intracerebral hemorrhage, which is a common presentation of AVMs.
   - Chronic Hemorrhage or Calcification: Over time, AVMs can show areas of calcification or hemosiderin deposits on CT.
   - AVM Nidus: It may not always be visible on CT, but a CT angiogram (CTA) can help highlight the abnormal blood vessels.
2. **Magnetic Resonance Imaging (MRI)**:
   - AVM Nidus: MRI is more sensitive than CT for detecting the nidus (the central area of the AVM where the abnormal blood vessels are concentrated).
   - Flow Voids: On MRI, areas of abnormal flow in arteries and veins may appear as flow voids (areas with low signal) within the AVM.
   - Hemosiderin Deposits: MRI can identify chronic hemorrhage or hemosiderin (iron deposits) around the AVM, which are markers of previous bleeding.
   - T2-weighted Imaging: Shows the abnormal vascular network and surrounding tissue changes.
3. **Angiography [Digital Subtraction Angiography— (DSA)]**:
   - Gold Standard for Diagnosis: DSA provides the most detailed visualization of intracranial AVMs, including the feeding arteries, nidus, and draining veins.
   - Arterial Phase: During the arterial phase of angiography, early filling of the abnormal vascular network (nidus) is seen.
   - Venous Phase: In the venous phase, draining veins can be identified, which may show early venous congestion or venous ectasia (dilated veins).
   - Spetzler-Martin Grading: DSA is used to classify AVMs according to their size, location, and venous drainage, which helps determine treatment options.

Interventions for Intracranial AVMs

1. **Surgical Resection**:
   - If the AVM is accessible and in a non-eloquent area of the brain, surgical excision can be considered. This is often the treatment of choice for smaller AVMs.
   - The goal is to completely remove the AVM, but the surgery can be risky due to the potential for significant hemorrhage.
2. **Endovascular Embolization**:
   - A minimally invasive procedure where a catheter is inserted through the arteries to deliver embolic agents (e.g., coils, liquid embolic agents like Onyx) into the AVM's feeding arteries to block blood flow and reduce the size of the lesion.
   - Endovascular embolization is often used as a preoperative adjunct or for inoperable AVMs to reduce the risk of bleeding.

3. **Stereotactic Radiosurgery (SRS)**:
   - SRS (e.g., using a Gamma Knife or CyberKnife) uses focused radiation to destroy the AVM. It is ideal for small, deep, or surgically inaccessible AVMs.
   - This is often a long-term solution, as the AVM gradually shrinks over months to years, and the risk of bleeding decreases.
4. **Conservative Management**: Some AVMs, especially if asymptomatic or if located in a very high-risk area (e.g., near critical brain structures), may be managed conservatively with regular monitoring through imaging to assess any changes in the AVM's size or behavior.

Spinal Arteriovenous Malformations (Spinal AVMs)

Imaging Features of Spinal AVMs

1. **Magnetic Resonance Imaging (MRI)**:
   - Spinal Cord Involvement: MRI is the most sensitive imaging modality for detecting spinal AVMs. It can identify the abnormal vascular network within or adjacent to the spinal cord.
   - Flow Voids: As in intracranial AVMs, flow voids are visible in the arterial and venous structures of the AVM.
   - Intramedullary signal changes: The spinal cord may show T2 hyperintensities, which can be due to edema or ischemia from abnormal blood flow.
   - Dilated Veins: MRI can show dilated, tortuous veins that are typical of spinal AVMs, often near the dorsal aspect of the spinal cord.
2. **CT Angiography (CTA)**: CTA can provide a detailed image of the feeding arteries and draining veins of the spinal AVM. It is especially helpful for detecting perimedullary veins or arterial feeders that might not be visible on MRI alone.
3. **Digital Subtraction Angiography (DSA)**:
   - Gold Standard for Spinal AVMs: DSA is crucial for evaluating the exact nidus, feeding arteries, and draining veins of spinal AVMs.
   - Arterial Phase: DSA highlights early enhancement of the abnormal vessels and the nidus.
   - Venous Phase: Spinal AVMs often show early venous drainage, leading to venous congestion or dilated perimedullary veins.

Interventions for Spinal AVMs

1. **Endovascular Embolization**:
   - First-line Treatment: Endovascular embolization is often the preferred treatment for spinal AVMs, particularly when the lesion is located in the thoracic or lumbar spine.
   - Embolization agents like Onyx or coils are delivered through a catheter to block the feeding arteries and reduce the size of the AVM. This helps control bleeding risks and may alleviate neurological symptoms.
2. **Surgical Resection**:
   - In cases where the AVM is surgically accessible, complete resection of the nidus may be attempted. However, this is technically challenging due to the proximity of the spinal cord and associated vascular structures.
   - Surgery is more commonly considered when endovascular techniques are not successful or when there are complications like significant hemorrhage.
3. **Radiosurgery**: Stereotactic radiosurgery can be used in rare cases where the spinal AVM is inaccessible via surgery or embolization. It involves delivering targeted radiation to the AVM to reduce its size over time.
4. **Conservative Management**: If the spinal AVM is asymptomatic or presents with mild symptoms, conservative management with periodic imaging follow-up may be considered. The goal is to monitor for any progression or new symptoms.

Summary of Imaging Modalities

- MRI is the primary imaging modality for both intracranial and spinal AVMs, providing detailed visualization of the abnormal vasculature and associated effects on the surrounding tissue (e.g., spinal cord or brain).

- CT and CTA are helpful in assessing the bony structures and identifying feeding vessels, especially in cases where the AVM is not fully visualized on MRI.
- Digital Subtraction Angiography (DSA) remains the gold standard for detailed mapping of the vascular anatomy of AVMs, essential for pre-intervention planning.

Conclusion

- Intracranial and spinal AVMs present significant challenges due to their abnormal blood flow patterns and potential for serious complications like hemorrhage or neurological deficits.
- Imaging techniques, especially MRI and DSA, are essential in diagnosis and guiding treatment strategies. Interventions such as endovascular embolization, surgical resection, and radiosurgery are tailored based on the AVM's location, size, and associated risks.
- Conservative management may be considered for asymptomatic lesions, but regular follow-up imaging is crucial to detect any progression.

4. Mention various symptoms out of slipped disc and how the images play the role for assessment. [10] [MD (WBUHS) 19]

A slipped disc, also known as a herniated disc or disc prolapse, occurs when the gel-like center (nucleus pulposus) of an intervertebral disc bulge or leaks out through a tear or weakness in the outer ring (annulus fibrosus) of the disc. This condition can press on nearby nerves, causing a variety of symptoms, depending on the location of the herniation.

Symptoms of a Slipped Disc

1. **Back Pain**:
   - Location: Pain is often felt in the lower back or neck (depending on the region of the herniated disc).
   - Characteristics: The pain can range from mild to severe and may be aggravated by certain movements like bending, twisting, or lifting.
2. **Sciatica**:
   - Description: Pain that radiates from the lower back down through the buttocks and legs, usually on one side of the body.
   - Cause: This occurs when the herniated disc compresses the sciatic nerve.
3. **Numbness and Tingling**:
   - Location: This can occur in the area of the body affected by nerve compression. For example, a slipped disc in the lower back can cause numbness or tingling in the legs, feet, or toes, while one in the neck can affect the arms or hands.
   - Characteristics: Often described as a "pins-and-needles" sensation.
4. **Weakness in Muscles**:
   - Location: Weakness may develop in the muscles controlled by the compressed nerve, such as the legs or arms.
   - Effect: This can lead to difficulty walking, standing, or performing certain activities (e.g., lifting objects).
5. **Loss of Reflexes**:
   - Cause: Compression of nerve roots can lead to diminished or absent reflexes, particularly in the knees or ankles.
6. **Pain that Worsens with Certain Activities**:
   - Examples: Sitting, coughing, sneezing, or bending forward may worsen the pain, depending on the location of the herniated disc.
7. **Bladder or Bowel Problems**:
   - Serious Complication: In rare cases, a herniated disc can cause cauda equina syndrome, which is a medical emergency that can lead to loss of bowel or bladder control, as well as sexual dysfunction.

Role of Imaging in the Assessment of a Slipped Disc

Imaging plays a critical role in diagnosing a slipped disc, assessing its severity, and guiding treatment decisions. The following imaging modalities are commonly used:

1. **X-rays**:
   - Role: X-rays are useful for assessing the overall alignment of the spine, identifying issues like spinal degeneration, fractures, or misalignment. However, X-rays cannot directly visualize the soft tissues, such as the intervertebral discs or nerves.
   - Limitations: While X-rays can rule out other causes of back pain (e.g., fractures, tumors, infections), they are not helpful in directly diagnosing a slipped disc.
2. **Magnetic Resonance Imaging (MRI)**:
   - Gold Standard: MRI is the most effective imaging modality for diagnosing a slipped disc because it provides detailed images of the soft tissues, including the discs, nerves, and spinal cord.
   - How It Helps:
     - MRI can clearly show a herniated disc and its exact location (e.g., whether the disc is bulging posteriorly, laterally, or medially).
     - It can also reveal nerve compression, swelling around the nerve roots, and other associated soft tissue changes.
     - MRI helps assess the severity of the herniation, whether there is nerve root impingement, and if there are any associated conditions like degenerative disc disease.
     - T2-weighted MRI images are typically used to visualize the disc herniation because they show the disc's water content and any compression on the nerves.
3. **Computed Tomography(CT) Scan**:
   - Role: CT scans provide detailed cross-sectional images of the spine and can be helpful in identifying herniated discs when MRI is not available or not suitable for the patient (e.g., in the case of pacemakers or other contraindications for MRI).
   - How It Helps: A CT myelogram, where contrast dye is injected into the spinal canal, can enhance visualization of nerve roots and disc herniations.
   - Limitations: CT scans are less effective than MRI for evaluating soft tissues like discs and nerves, but they are useful for assessing the bony structures of the spine.
4. **Discography**:
   - Role: Discography involves injecting contrast dye into the disc space to assess pain sources in the spine.
   - How It Helps: It is mainly used when the diagnosis is unclear and helps confirm whether a specific disc is the cause of pain.
   - Limitations: Discography is invasive and is typically used in complex cases where non- invasive imaging has not provided a clear diagnosis.
5. **Myelography**:
   - Role: Myelography involves injecting contrast dye into the spinal fluid and taking X-rays or CT scans to visualize the spinal cord and nerve roots.
   - How It Helps: This method can show compression of the spinal cord and nerve roots caused by a herniated disc.
   - Limitations: This technique has largely been replaced by MRI, but it can still be useful in specific situations.

Summary of Imaging Roles

- **X-rays**: Useful for detecting bony abnormalities or fractures, but not for visualizing herniated discs directly.
- **MRI**: Gold standard for identifying herniated discs and nerve root compression, offering detailed soft tissue imaging.
- **CT Scan**: Alternative when MRI is not available; useful for assessing bony structures and performing myelography for better nerve visualization.
- **Discography**: Used to confirm the specific disc causing pain when other imaging studies are inconclusive.
- **Myelography**: Can provide additional information on nerve root and spinal cord compression, but has been largely replaced by MRI.

Conclusion

A slipped disc can present with a variety of symptoms, ranging from localized back pain to severe neurological deficits like sciatica or muscle weakness. Imaging plays a crucial role in diagnosing the condition, understanding the extent of the herniation, and guiding treatment. MRI is the most effective tool for visualizing the soft tissue and nerve involvement, whereas X-rays, CT scans, and other diagnostic tests provide supportive information. Early diagnosis and appropriate intervention, based on imaging findings, are key to managing the symptoms and preventing further complications.

5. Describe imaging protocol in traumatic injury of dorsal spine causing paraplegia. [10] [MD (WBUHS) 19]

In the context of traumatic injury to the dorsal spine resulting in paraplegia, an imaging protocol typically involves a combination of modalities to assess the extent of the injury, spinal cord involvement, and possible associated fractures or deformities. The protocol can be broken down into several stages, depending on the clinical presentation and the urgency of the situation.

Initial Assessment (Emergency Setting). When paraplegia is suspected, the primary goal is to quickly assess the spinal injury and rule out life-threatening conditions.

This can include:

1. **X-ray (Radiographs)**
   - Purpose: To quickly identify gross skeletal injuries, such as fractures or dislocations, and provide an initial assessment of spinal alignment.
   - Standard views: Anteroposterior (AP) and lateral views of the spine (thoracic and lumbar if relevant).
   - Limitations: While X-rays are fast and widely available, they are not sensitive enough to detect soft tissue injury or subtle fractures (e.g., ligamentous injury, compression fractures).
2. **Computed Tomography (CT)**
   - Purpose: Provides detailed evaluation of bony structures and is more sensitive than X-rays for identifying fractures, dislocations, and other osseous abnormalities.
   - Protocol:
     - Thin slice CT of the entire thoracic and lumbar spine.
     - 3D reconstructions are helpful for assessing fracture patterns, dislocations, and spinal canal compromise.
     - Indication for CT: If X-rays are inconclusive or if there is suspicion of significant bony injury, CT is used as the next step to clarify the fracture type and severity.
3. **Magnetic Resonance Imaging (MRI)**
   - MRI is the gold standard for evaluating soft tissue injuries in the spinal cord, ligaments, intervertebral discs, and surrounding structures.
     - Protocol: Sagittal and Axial T2-weighted images for detailed assessment of the spinal cord, nerve roots, and soft tissues.
   - T1-weighted images for better evaluation of anatomical structures.
   - Fat-saturated sequences to evaluate for edema or hemorrhage in the spinal cord and surrounding tissues.
   - Contrast-enhanced imaging may be used if there is concern for acute cord injury, post-traumatic hemorrhage, or infection (e.g., abscess, epidural hematoma).
   - Findings:
     - Spinal Cord Injury: Contusions, edema, hemorrhage, or transection can be visualized, indicating the degree of injury.
     - Fractures or Dislocations: Vertebral fractures and alignment abnormalities, as well as the degree of spinal canal compromise, are evaluated.
     - Ligamentous injury: MRI can detect rupture of ligaments (e.g., anterior or posterior longitudinal ligament), which may be subtle on CT.
     - Herniated discs or fracture fragments compressing the spinal cord or nerve roots.
   - Timing of MRI: MRI should ideally be performed within the first 48 hours of injury if the patient is stable. Delayed imaging may still provide valuable information on long-term prognosis and surgical planning.
4. **Functional Imaging** (if indicated) In some cases, additional imaging may be required to assess the degree of functional injury to the spinal cord.

5. **Spinal Angiography**
   - Purpose: If there is concern for vascular compromise (e.g., spinal cord ischemia), angiography can assess blood supply to the spinal cord, particularly in cases of severe traumatic injury.

CT or MRI Myelography: If there is suspected cerebrospinal fluid (CSF) leak or complex spinal cord injury, myelographic imaging may be performed.

Post-traumatic Monitoring (Follow-up Imaging)

- **Purpose**: To monitor progression or resolution of spinal cord edema, hemorrhage, and recovery, as well as to evaluate for secondary complications such as syringomyelia (fluid- filled cavities within the spinal cord) or post-traumatic cysts.
- MRI is typically used for follow-up imaging at regular intervals (e.g., 1-3 months post-injury) to track changes in the spinal cord and vertebral structures.

6. Write a short note on: Diastematomyelia. [5] [MD (WBUHS) 22]

Diastematomyelia, also called **split cord malformation**, is a type of spinal dysraphism showing a longitudinal split in spinal cord.

Pathology

Genesis of this condition is thought to occur during the stage of gastrulation due to abnormal movement and separation of precursor cells. It has been postulated that an abnormal adhesion in between the endoderm and ectoderm creates an additional neuroenteric canal which leads to the eventual development of notochord into two hemicords.

Classification

- **Type I**: dural sac duplicated, with rigid cartilaginous or osseous spur in the midline
- **Type II**: dural sac single, with non-rigid fibrovascular or fibrous septum in the midline

Radiographic Features

Split cord malformation is common in the lower spinal cord but can also occur at other levels.

- 50% occur in between L1 and L3 levels
- 25% occur in between T7 and T12 levels

Associated cartilaginous or bony spur projecting forwards from the vertebral arch through the dura mater is seen in 33% of cases.

Vertebral segmentation anomalies (spina bifida, hemivertebrae, or butterfly vertebra) may also be seen.

Ultrasound

Antenatal ultrasound reveals the presence of an extra echogenic focus in the midline in between the fetal spinal posterior elements.

Plain Radiograph

- Associated scoliosis
- Multilevel spina bifida
- Increased interpedicular distance
- Anteroposterior narrowing of vertebral body

Computed Tomography (CT)

CT can show the bony septum better.

Magnetic Resonance Imaging (MRI)

MRI is the best imaging modality for assessing diastematomyelia.

7. Write a short note on: Vertebroplasty. [5] [MD (WBUHS) 22, AIIMS Dec 24]

Vertebroplasty is imaging-guided procedures that involve percutaneous injection of surgical polymethylmethacrylate (PMMA) cement into a diseased vertebral body. Vertebroplasty provides pain relief and strengthens the bone of vertebrae weakened by disease

Indications

It can be used as a treatment or as a palliative measure for:

- Insufficiency fracture
- Aggressive hemangioma
- Vertebral multiple myeloma
- Vertebral metastases

Contraindications

Absolute Contraindications

- Septicemia
- Active infection (osteomyelitis, discitis, cellulitis, etc.) of the vertebra or paravertebral tissues
- Uncorrectable coagulopathy
- Allergy to bone cement or opacifying agent

Relative Contraindications

- Chronic fractures (variable relief and therefore not often covered by insurance payers in the US.)
- Radiculopathy beyond local vertebral pain, caused by a compressive syndrome unrelated to vertebral collapse
- Occasionally, preoperative vertebroplasty can be performed before a spinal decompressive procedure.
- Retropulsion of a fracture fragment or epidural tumor extension causing signs and symptoms of neurological compromise.
- Current systemic infection
- Patient improving on medical therapy
- Prophylaxis in osteoporotic patients
- Myelopathy or cauda equina syndrome originating at the fracture level.

Complications

- **Leakage of Vertebroplasty**:
  - Compression of adjacent structures
  - Inferior vena cava syndrome
  - Note that kyphoplasty has shown lower rates of cement leakage
- **Cement Intravasation**: Cement pulmonary embolism: Via intravasation into paravertebral veins or IVC
- **Neurologic Injury**:
  - Nerve root traversal
  - Spinal cord injury (unlikely in lumbar levels)
- **Fracture**:
  - Iatrogenic
  - Higher rates of adjacent level fracture postprocedure
- **Bleeding**:
  - IVC or aorta injury if anterior vertebral cortex is traversed
  - Epidural hematoma
  - Paravertebral
  - Intercostal
- Pneumothorax

8. Discuss the various interventional procedures in spinal arteriovenous malformation. [10] [MD (WBUHS) 22, DNB Dec 18]

Endovascular Treatment of Spinal AVMs Extradural AVFs

Extradural AVFs may be treated endovascularly, usually through a transarterial approach. Occasionally a transvenous approach may provide improved access to the fistula.

Intradural Dorsal AVFs

Intradural dorsal AVFs may be treated by embolization, surgery or both. Prior to embolization, microcatheter injections are used to verify the absence of normal spinal cord supply. If a spinal artery is visualized, surgical treatment is recommended.

The goal of embolization is obliteration of the fistulous site as well as the proximal portion of the intradural arterialized draining vein. n-Butyl cyanoacrylate (nBCA) was historically preferred as it provides a more permanent occlusion than particles. Several recent reports have described ethylene-vinyl alcohol copolymer embolization for sDAVF.

Following fistula embolization, collateral supply must be ruled out by microcatheter injections at the same level on the contralateral side, as well as two levels above and below the fistula.

Intradural Ventral AVFs

Treatment of intradural ventral AVFs differs depending on the lesion subtype. In type A fistulas, the ASA is minimally dilated and arteriovenous transit is slow. Effective embolizate penetration is limited by the small caliber of the ASA, and surgical treatment is generally favored. In type B fistulas, supraselective catheterization of feeding vessels near the fistulous point is often possible, and embolization is feasible. In type C lesions the fistulous pouch may be accessed either transarterially or transvenously. Fistula occlusion is then performed using liquid embolics with or without coil embolization.

Extradural-intradural ACMs

Extradural-intradural AVMs typically exhibit multiple high-flow feeders and encompass both intramedullary and extramedullary components. Complete obliteration of these lesions is associated with a significant risk of neurological morbidity, and treatment goals thus generally include reducing the malformation size to minimize mass effect and ameliorate symptoms of ischemic steal. Staged embolization using coils, particles or liquid embolic agents is often followed by surgical resection.

Intramedullary AVMs

Intramedullary AVMs are treated by a combination of embolization and surgery. Almost all of these lesions exhibit a main feeder from the ASA; however, the posterior spinal artery also contributes supply in many cases. Many authors believe, as with brain AVMs, that surgical resection is the mainstay of treatment for these lesions. However, many centers advocate presurgical embolization and embolization may represent definitive treatment in select cases. Endovascular cure requires catheterization close to the nidus, with significant intranidal embolizate penetration.

Conus Medullaris AVMs

Optimal treatment of conus medullaris AVMs involves aggressive embolization followed by microsurgical resection.

Intradural Dorsal AVFs

Early series used polyvinyl alcohol (PVA) but, in general, patients treated in this manner demonstrated a high rate of recanalization. Given these high recurrence rates, most authors currently favor liquid embolics. Although most modern series have reported acrylic embolization, Onyx embolization is currently emerging as an effective treatment option for DAVFs.

Intradural Ventral AVFs

- Type A and B fistulas have traditionally been treated by microsurgery and endovascular reports are limited.
- Type C lesions pose a particular treatment challenge. Surgical treatment is high-risk given the risk of intraoperative hemorrhage, and endovascular treatment is generally favored. Both transarterial and transvenous treatment routes as well as direct venous puncture have been described.

Extradural-intradural AVMs

The endovascular treatment of extradural-intradural AVMs is limited to single case reports. Although these lesions have historically been considered incurable, in select cases preoperative embolization followed by microsurgical resection can result in acceptable outcomes.

Congenital and Vascular Diseases

1. Write a short note on imaging features of Sturge Weber Syndrome. [5]

Sturge-Weber syndrome, also known as **encephalotrigeminal angiomatosis** or **encephalofacial angiomatosis**, is a phakomatosis characterized by facial port-wine nevus (capillary malformation) and pial angiomas. It is part of a wide spectrum of possible cerebrofacial arteriovenous metameric syndrome (CAMS) phenotypes.

Epidemiology

Sturge-Weber syndrome is rare, with an incidence estimated at 1 in 20,000–50,000.

Associations

- Coarctation of aorta
- Paragangliomas

Pathology

The leptomeningeal angiomatosis results in a vascular steal affecting the subjacent cortex and white matter producing localized ischemia. In about 80% of the cases, there is unihemispheric involvement.

Classification

According to Roach et al., Sturge-Weber syndrome can be classified according to the presence/absence of facial and leptomeningeal angiomas:

- **Type I**: Represents the classic syndrome, with both facial and leptomeningeal angiomas; may have glaucoma.
- **Type II**: Facial angioma without evidence of intracranial disease; may have glaucoma.
- **Type III**: Isolated leptomeningeal angioma; usually no glaucoma.

However, this classification system has been criticized as it suggests that all patients with facial capillary malformations have Sturge-Weber syndrome, even in the absence of brain or eye involvement (type II), which does not appear to be the case.

Radiographic Features

Plain Radiograph

Skull radiographs were historically useful and capable of identifying the gyriform calcification of the subcortical white matter although they no longer play a significant role in the diagnosis or management of this condition. The finding usually becomes evident between 2–7 years of age.

CT

- Subcortical calcification (seen at an earlier age than plain film) and associated parenchymal volume loss
- Tram-track sign of cortical and subcortical calcification
- Calvarial and regional sinus enlargement may be evident
- Ipsilateral choroid plexus may be enlarged
- In severe cases, a Dyke-Davidoff-Masson appearance may be seen
- Orbital choroidal hemangiomas may be present
- Asymmetric cavernous sinus enlargement

MRI

- **T1**: Signal of the affected region is largely normal, with anatomic volume loss evident at an older age

- **T1 C+ (Gd)**
  - Prominent leptomeningeal enhancement in the affected area (due to congested internal cerebral veins, a manifestation of the so-called "pial angiomatosis", resulting in venous congestive ischemia with infarction and obliteration of cerebral parenchyma)
  - Much later in life, the angioma may "burn out", losing enhancement
  - Enlarged ipsilateral choroid plexus
  - Dilatation of transparenchymal veins that communicates between the superficial and deep venous systems
- **T2**
  - Low signal in white matter subjacent to angioma representing
    - Postulated accelerated myelination in neonate
    - Calcification later in life
    - Abnormal deep venous drainage seen as flow voids
- **GE/SWI/EPI**: Sensitive to calcification, seen as regions of signal dropout
- **MR spectroscopy**: Decreased NAA.

Angiography (DSA)

In most cases (82%), angiography is abnormal and demonstrates absent superficial cortical veins with abnormal and enlarged deep venous drainage.

Treatment and Prognosis

Treatment revolves primarily around seizure control, with surgical resection only indicated rarely in refractory cases. An ophthalmological examination is also essential to identify and treat ocular involvement.

2. What are the imaging modalities and causes of pulsatile tinnitus. [10] [MD (WBUHS) 20]

Causes of Pulsatile Tinnitus

- **Normal Vascular Variants**:
  - **Arterial Variants**: Aberrant/laterally displaced carotid artery, persistent stapedial artery, persistent trigeminal artery, anomalous artery in the stria vascularis of the cochlea.
  - **Venous Variants**: Large jugular bulb, large emissary veins, idiopathic venous tinnitus, jugular bulb diverticulum.
- **Pathological Vascular Causes**:
  - **Arterial Causes**: Carotid artery dissection, aneurysms of the petrous carotid/anterior communicating artery aneurysms, atherosclerosis, fibromuscular dysplasia, arteritis.
  - **Arteriovenous Vascular Causes**: Glomus tympanicum/glomus jugulare AVMs intracranial arteriovenous malformation, e.g., cerebral AVMs, dural AV fistulas and direct AV fistulas, otosclerosis, Paget's disease of bone, miscellaneous vascular tumors, such as hemangiomas, jugular meningiomas histiocytosis and cholesterol granulomas.
  - **Venous Causes**: Pregnancy, anemia, thyrotoxicosis, hypertension, transverse sinus stenosis.

Normal Vascular Variants

Aberrant position of the internal carotid artery is thought to be due to abnormal regression of the cervical ICA during embryogenesis resulting in opening of and enlargement of collateral arteries, such as the anastomosis between the carotid tympanic artery anastomosis between the caroticotympanic artery and the inferior tympanic artery. The aberrant artery, therefore, courses through the middle ear over the cochlear promontory to join the horizontal carotid canal via a dehiscence in the carotid plate. The findings on HRCT are characteristic in that the posterior carotid plate is absent and that the horizontal part of the carotid canal appears to merge with the lateral cochlear promontory. Variations of the jugular bulb include a very high riding jugular bulb. This normal variant is associated with well-defined bony margins of the jugular foramen. When the caroticojugular plate is deficient, the condition is termed as dehiscent jugular bulb.

Jugular bulb diverticulum is a finger like extension of the jugular bulb in the cephalad direction. Ecstatic loops of AICA/PICA or tortuous course of vertebral artery going into the internal auditory meatus may cause tinnitus due to compression on the VIII nerve complex.

Pathological Vascular Causes

Arterial Causes

Dissection of the internal carotid artery can be spontaneous or traumatic. Angiographic appearances include intimal flaps, with or without occlusion. MRI will show loss of flow void which suggest occlusion of the artery. If there is intraluminal hemorrhage, a hyperintense signal will be observed in the affected artery. Petrous carotid aneurysms and AVMs can be detected on digital subtraction angiography (DSA). Atherosclerosis of the carotid artery at times produces pulsatile tinnitus. Atherosclerotic plaques may produce turbulence of carotid flow which manifests as pulsatile tinnitus. Fibromuscular dysplasia (FMD) is a segmental noninflammatory, nonatheromatous vasculopathy. It is seen in 0.5–0.6% of carotid angiograms and autopsies. It is a disease which affects medium-size muscular arteries. Vertebral and renal arteries can also be affected apart from the extracranial arteries. It is associated with intracranial berry aneurysms. Middle-aged females are most commonly affected. Unlike atherosclerotic plaques fibromuscular dysplasia affects the cervical internal carotid arteries at the level of the first two cervical vertebrae. Hence, these patients generally present with symptoms of vascular tinnitus more frequently unlike those with atherosclerosis. The classical angiographic appearance of FMD is the string of beads appearance which is seen in 85% of patients. Successful treatment of FMD by transluminal angioplasty has been reported.

Arteriovenous Causes

The diagnosis of cerebral AVMs and dural AV fistulas and direct AV fistulas depends upon the clinical presentation apart from that of pulsatile tinnitus. Angiography is the gold standard in demonstration of the vascular lesions which may be partly delineated on CT scans and MRI. Paget's disease and otosclerosis are representative bony pathologies associated with neovascularization and AV shunting, resulting in pulsatile tinnitus.

Amongst the group of arteriovenous causes, paraganglionomas or glomus tumors are the typical lesions which require radiographic evaluation.[32] Glomus tumors of the temporal bone are the most common neoplastic cause of pulsatile tinnitus and vascular tympanic membrane. Tumors commonly involve the jugular bulb and/or the tympanic cavity. CT scan will help to delineate whether the lesion is confined within the tympanic cavity or involves the jugular bulb. If the lesion is confined within the tympanic cavity, no further investigation is required. If the lesion is seen to extend to involve the jugular foramen and beyond, CT examination is continued up to the carotid bifurcation to see the complete extent of the lesion and to rule out multicentricity. An MR examination will help in assessing the involvement of internal jugular vein. On MR high resolution T1WI, a flow void pattern can be appreciated. On postcontrast T1WI, intense enhancement is seen. Postcontrast MR angiography shows relatively low signal of the tumor with high signal intensity spots inside due to high flow in feeding vessels.

Venous Tinnitus

Venous tinnitus unlike arterial tinnitus is heard as a continuous murmur accentuated during systole. It is caused by turbulent flow in the venous structures around the ear. It is usually heard on the side of the dominant jugular vein which is usually on the right side. A venous hum is physiological and can be elicited in an 80% of pregnant women and in the lower jugular vein in 50% of normal individuals. Venous tinnitus is also observed in patients of thyrotoxicosis, anemia and hypertension.

Venous tinnitus may be the presenting symptom of intracranial hypertension. It is believed that tinnitus in conditions of raised intracranial tension is related to CSF pressures and compression of dural sinuses by transmitted intracranial arterial pulsations. Raised intracranial hypertension can manifest as pulsatile tinnitus as well. Conditions, such as aqueduct stenosis, Chiari I malformation, pneumocephalus and idiopathic intracranial hypertension can present with tinnitus which can be the role symptoms of the underlying pathology.

3. Enumerate causes of unilateral proptosis. Describe briefly imaging findings of optic glioma and caroticocavernous fistula. [4+6] [MD (WBUHS) 20]

Differential diagnosis of proptosis by laterality and age.

Differential Diagnosis by Laterality

Unilateral Proptosis

- Orbital cellulitis
- Developmental anomalies
- Inflammatory conditions

- Vascular anomalies
- Neoplasms
- Metabolic disease

The differential diagnoses of causes of unilateral proptosis based on age are presented in the following table **(Table 20)**.

TABLE 20: Differential diagnosis of causes of unilateral proptosis based on age.

Differential diagnosis by age			
1–5 years of age	***5–10 years of age***	***10–30 years of age***	***30–50 years of age***
• Dermoid • Metastatic neuroblastoma • Rhabdomyosarcoma • Epithelial cyst • Glioma of the optic nerve • Sphenoid wing meningioma • Hemangioma	Pseudotumor, orbital extension of retinoblastoma, malignant lymphoma and leukemias, dermoid, hemangioma	Pseudotumor, mucocele, meningioma, TED, lacrimal gland tumor, malignant lymphoma/leukemia, dermoid, hemangioma	Pseudotumor, mucocele, malignant lymphoma/leukemia, hemangioma, TED, lacrimal gland tumors

Imaging Findings of Optic Nerve Glioma

Classification

The most widely accepted classification of optic pathway gliomas is the Dodge classification that was first proposed by Dodge et al., in 1958. The Dodge classification divides these tumors into just three groups based on anatomical localization:

- **Stage 1**: Optic nerves only
- **Stage 2**: Chiasm involved (with or without optic nerve involvement)
- **Stage 3**: Hypothalamic involvement and/or other adjacent structures

A modification of the Dodge classification has been proposed which further subdivides each stage.

Radiographic Features

Plain Radiograph

Radiographs no longer have any real role to play in the diagnosis of orbital masses, however, if performed enlargement of the optic canal may be demonstrated if a tumor is not confined to the orbit. Additional findings of neurofibromatosis type 1 may also be visible.

CT

CT is often the first investigation performed and although not as sensitive as MRI, the diagnosis can often be made, especially if thin slice imaging through the orbits is performed, or coronal and sagittal reconstructions obtained from volumetric data.

- Enlargement of the optic nerve and the mass may either be fusiform or exophytic in appearance.
- Enlargement of the optic canal
- The optic nerve may be elongated with kinking or buckling

MRI

MR imaging is optimal for showing the relationship of the mass to the hypothalamus, optic chiasm, and infundibulum as well as the intraorbital and intercanalicular components of the mass. Large tumors are typically heterogeneous with cystic and solid components.

- **T1**: Enlargement, often iso to hypointense compared to the contralateral side
- **T2**:
  - Hyperintense centrally
  - Thin low-signal at the periphery representing the dura.
  - **T1 C+ (Gd)**: Enhancement is variable.

Imaging Findings in Carotidocavernous Fistula

Radiographic Features

CT: CT angiography is the noninvasive imaging modality of choice for evaluation of suspected caroticocavernous fistula. Features include:

- **Orbital congestion**:
  - Proptosis/exophthalmos
  - Retrobulbar fat stranding/edema
  - Enlargement of extraocular muscles
- **Venous engorgement and enhancement**:
  - Enlarged superior ophthalmic vein
  - Bulging cavernous sinus
  - Asymmetric enhancement of cavernous sinus with attenuation similar to that of internal carotid artery and higher than that of transverse sinus
- **Dehiscent internal carotid artery (for direct type fistulas)**: Snowman appearance of fistula tract involving the feeding carotid artery and draining venous pouch.
- Intracranial hemorrhage from a ruptured cortical vein

Angiography (DSA)

Catheter-based digital subtraction angiography is the gold standard imaging technique due to its superior spatial and temporal resolution.

- Rapid shunting from internal carotid artery to cavernous sinus
- Enlarged draining veins
- Retrograde flow from cavernous sinus, most commonly into the ophthalmic veins

Ultrasound

Doppler assessment may show arterialized enlarged ophthalmic veins.

4. Write a short notes on: (a) Joubert's syndrome. (b) Tuberous sclerosis. [5+5] [MD (WBUHS) 21]

(a) Joubert anomaly, also known as **vermian aplasia or molar tooth midbrain-hindbrain malformation**, is an autosomal recessive disorder where there is a variable degree of cerebellar vermal agenesis.

Epidemiology

The prevalence of Joubert syndrome is approximately 1 in 100,000. There are numerous associations which are variably present:

- **Ocular abnormalities**
  - Coloboma
  - Retinal dysplasia: 50% (some authors advocate dividing Joubert syndrome patients into two groups according to the presence or absence of retinal dysplasia)
- Nephronophthisis
- Multicystic dysplastic kidneys (MCDK): 30%
- **Hepatic fibrosis**: Usually as part of COACH syndrome
- **Polydactyly**: 15%
- Occipital (meningo) encephalocele

Pathology

Joubert syndrome patients are a genetically heterogeneous population with some having a mutation of chromosome 9q34.3 however many do not. At least 10 genes relating to subcellular organelles (including the primary cilium and basal body) have been implicated; as such Joubert syndrome is one of a number of related disorders known as ciliopathies.

Radiographic Features

Cross-sectional axial imaging demonstrates isolated abnormality of the cerebellum consisting of:

- Small dysplastic or aplastic cerebellar vermis (with characteristic median cleft)
- Absence of fiber decussation in the superior cerebellar peduncles and pyramidal tracts, which can be assessed by diffusion tensor imaging
- Abnormal inferior olivary nucleus
- Dysplasia and heterotopia of cerebellar nuclei

The posterior fossa typically shows a bat wing 4th ventricle and prominent thickened elongated superior cerebellar peduncles giving a characteristic molar tooth sign appearance.

In a minority of cases minor lateral ventriculomegaly (6–20% of cases) and corpus callosal dysgenesis (6–10% of cases) is also present.

(b) Tuberous sclerosis (TS), also called as **tuberous sclerosis complex (TSC)** or **Bourneville disease,** is a neurocutaneous disorder (phakomatosis) characterized by development of benign tumors in organs derived from embryonic ectoderm (e.g., eyes, skin, and the central nervous system).

Pathology

- **TSC1 Gene**: Encoding hamartin, located on chromosome 9q32–34
- **TSC2 Gene**: Encoding tuberin, located on chromosome 16p13.3 (this gene accounts for most of the cases).

Radiographic Features

The commonest radiographic manifestations are:

- Cortical tubers, subependymal tubers and also white matter abnormalities
- Cardiac rhabdomyomas
- Renal angiomyolipomas

Neurological

- **Cortical/Subcortical Tubers**: Low T1 and high T2 and with few tubers showing postcontrast enhancement; most calcify after 2 years.
- **Subependymal Hamartomas**:
  - Most are associated with calcification, although calcification is usually absent in early childhood
  - Enhancement is variable, so it is not a useful feature to distinguish them from subependymal giant cell astrocytomas; only growth on serial imaging is reliable.
- **Subependymal Giant Cell Astrocytomas (SGCA)**:
  - Usually large in size and demonstrate serial growth
  - Show intense postcontrast enhancement
- **White Matter Abnormalities**:
  - Rradial bands—specific for tuberous sclerosis
- Retinal phakomas
- **Rarer Findings**:
  - Infarcts
  - Cerebellar atrophy
  - Cerebral aneurysms
  - Chiari malformations

    - Corpus callosum dysgenesis
    - Microcephaly
    - Chordoma
    - Arachnoid cysts

Abdominal

- **Renal Angiomyolipoma (AML)**:
    - Tuberous sclerosis accounts for approximately 20% of all AMLs
    - Tend to be multiple and bilateral
    - May be associated with aneurysms
- **Renal Cysts**:
    - Seen in 18–53% of patients with TS
- **Renal Cell Carcinoma and Oncocytomas**.
    - Renal cell carcinoma occurs at a younger age
- Gastrointestinal polyps
- **Retroperitoneal Lymphangiomyomatosis (LAM)**:
    - Cystic lesions in the retroperitoneum
    - Chylous ascites, thoracic duct dilatation
- Pancreatic neuroendocrine tumors
- Hepatic angiomyolipoma(s)

Thoracic

- **Lymphangioleiomyomatosis (LAM)**:
    - Identical to sporadic LAM
    - Chylous pleural effusions and pneumothorax common
- **Cardiac Rhabdomyomas**:
    - Benign striated muscle tumor characterized by the presence of spider cells
    - Multiple or single
    - Usually involve the interventricular septum
    - 75% cases occur prior to 1 year of age
- Aortic/pulmonary artery aneurysm

Musculoskeletal

- Periosteal new bone
- **Sclerotic Bone Lesions**: ~55% (range 40–66%)
- Calvarial hyperostosis involving the inner table
- Bone cysts
- Scoliosis

Skin

- **Hypopigmented Macules (Ash Leaf Spots)**: Found in 90% of patients
- **Facial Angiofibromas (Adenoma Sebaceum)**: Found in 75% of patients
- **Periungual Angiofibroma or Koenen Tumors**: Seen in 20% of patients.
- **Shagreen Patches**: Found in 20–30% of patients.

5. Classify various neural tube closure defects. Briefly describe types of Arnold Chiari malformation and discuss their imaging features. [10] [MD (WBUHS) 18, MD (WBUHS) 21]

The classification of spinal dysraphism is presented in **Flowchart 5** as follows:

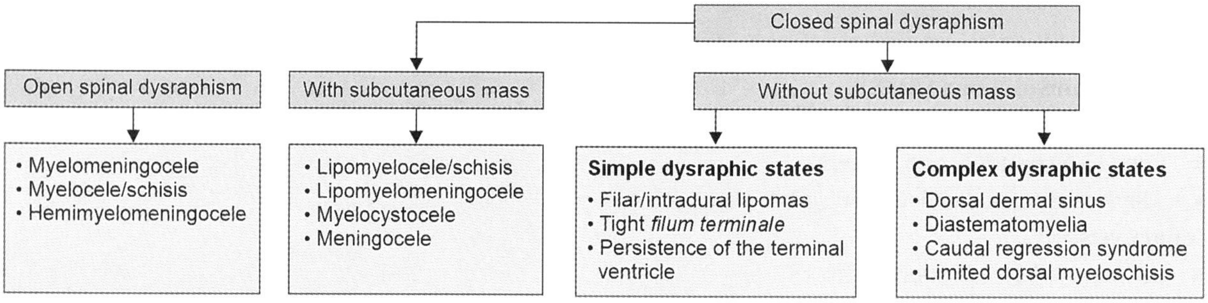

FLOWCHART 5: Classification of spinal dysraphism.

Types of Arnold Chiari Malformation with Imaging Findings

Initial descriptions were based on autopsy observations. Three types were described, with others added later. Chiari 2 (Chiari II) and 3 (Chiari III) are thought to be related to each other while Chiari 1 (Chiari I) represents a distinct entity.

- **Chiari 0**
  - No cerebellar tonsillar descent (<5 mm caudal descent in relation to the foramen magnum) but presence of a syrinx and presence of typical Chiari symptoms
  - Infrequently used and confusing term to be avoided, based on reports of syrinx improvement after posterior fossa decompression
- **Chiari 0.5**
  - No cerebellar tonsillar descent (<5 mm caudal descent in relation to the foramen magnum) but the tonsillar position is ventral to a line bisecting the medulla
- **Chiari 1 (Chiari I)**
  - Most common
  - Cerebellar tonsillar herniation (>5 mm caudal herniation in relation to the foramen magnum) alone
  - There may or may not be an associated syrinx
- **Chiari 1.5**
  - Cerebellar tonsillar herniation (>5 mm caudal herniation in relation to the foramen magnum) with herniation of the obex inferior to the foramen magnum
  - Described in the literature as both a condition in its own right as well as a variant of Chiari I malformation
- **Chiari 2 (Chiari II)**
  - Cerebellar tonsillar (>5 mm caudal herniation), brainstem, and fourth ventricle herniation in relation to the foramen magnum, with an associated lumbosacral myelomeningocele
- **Chiari 3 (Chiari III)**
  - Similar features to Chiari II, but with an occipital and/or high cervical encephalocele instead of a lumbosacral myelomeningocele
- **Chiari 3.5**
  - Similar features to Chiari III, but with an occipitocervical myeloencephalocele and foregut communication
- **Chiari 4 (Chiari IV)**
  - Severe cerebellar hypoplasia without displacement of the cerebellum through the foramen magnum, associated with an occipital encephalocele probably a variation of cerebellar hypoplasia
- **Chiari 5 (Chiari V)**
  - Absent cerebellum with myelomeningocele and herniation of the occipital lobe through the foramen magnum.

6. How DSA of brain performed? Describe role of intervention radiography in the management of intracranial aneurysm and AVM. [10] [MD (WBUHS) 19]

Digital Subtraction Angiography (DSA) is a fluoroscopic technique used extensively in interventional radiology for visualization of blood vessels.

Procedure

Preprocedural evaluation:

- The patient is informed about the procedure and any necessary preprocedural assessments are performed (e.g., blood tests, renal function tests, etc.).
- The patient is usually asked to fast for several hours before the procedure.

Positioning/Room Set Up

- The angiography suite must be equipped with a crash cart and monitoring equipment all procedures should be performed under strict aseptic conditions.
- Depending on the procedure and the patient's condition, an anesthesiologist may be required to administer conscious sedation or even general anesthesia.
- The patient can be positioned with their head on either end of the bed to facilitate convenience of vascular access and maneuvering for the interventional radiologist.

Equipment

The fluoroscopy unit consists of a C-arm unit that can be rotated axially and sagittally around the floating-top table. The distance between the X-ray tube and the image intensifier can be adjusted, as can collimation and several other parameters.

The image is at least a 1024 × 1024-pixel matrix. Most modern medical displays are flat screens; some of the detectors are flat panel.

DSA Technique

- The noncontrast or mask image of the region of interest is taken prior to injection of the contrast material and therefore shows only the anatomy and any radiopaque foreign bodies (such as stents, surgical clips, etc.).
- Contrast opacified images are acquired in succession as the contrast material is injected. These images show the contrast opacified vessels superimposed on anatomy and are saved in the computer.
- Then the mask image is subtracted, pixel by pixel from the contrast images. The resulting subtracted images show only the contrast-opacified vessels.
- The subtraction images can be viewed in real-time. Even if the patient lies still, there is bound to be some degree of misregistration of images due to movement between the acquisition of the mask image and the subsequent contrast images. Pixel shifting (either manual or automatic), i.e., moving the mask retrospectively, can minimize misregistration, but focal movement such as bowel peristalsis, will not be corrected.

Procedural Technique

- The patient lies on the angiography table.
- Local anesthesia is administered at the intended puncture site (usually lidocaine hydrochloride 1% or 2% w/v). In certain procedures (e.g., a child undergoing cerebral angiography), general anesthesia is performed.
- The Seldinger technique is used to gain access to a blood vessel.
- A standard diagnostic DSA kit consists of an 18-gauge puncture needle and .035″ guidewires, over which the diagnostic catheters are threaded.
- On completion of procedure, hemostasis at the puncture site is ensured.

Postprocedural Care

- This depends whether the procedure was performed on an outpatient or inpatient basis.
- Patient should remain immobilized for around 4–6 hours and lie on supine position. Close observation is mandated to look out for development of puncture site hematomas.

Role of Intervention Radiography in the Management of Intracranial Aneurysm and AVM

Interventional radiology plays a critical role in the management of intracranial aneurysms and AVMs through minimally invasive techniques that can reduce morbidity and mortality associated with these conditions:

1. **Management of Intracranial Aneurysms**
   i. **Endovascular Coiling**:
      - **Procedure**: A microcatheter is navigated to the aneurysm through a blood vessel. Detachable coils made of soft metal are then deployed into the aneurysm sac, promoting clotting and reducing blood flow into the aneurysm.
      - **Benefits**: This method is less invasive than traditional surgical clipping and can be performed under local anesthesia. It has a shorter recovery time and lower complication rates.

   ii. **Flow Diversion**:
      - **Procedure**: A flow-diverting stent is placed across the neck of the aneurysm, redirecting blood flow away from it while allowing normal flow through the parent artery.
      - **Benefits**: This technique can be particularly useful for large or complex aneurysms that may not be amenable to coiling.
2. **Management of Arteriovenous Malformations (AVMs)**
   i. **Embolization**:
      - **Procedure**: Similar to aneurysm treatment, a catheter is used to deliver embolic agents (such as glue or particles) directly into the feeding arteries of the AVM. This reduces blood flow to the malformation, potentially decreasing its size and associated risks.
      - **Benefits**: Embolization can be used as a standalone treatment or as a preoperative measure to reduce intraoperative bleeding during surgical resection of the AVM.

   ii. **Stereotactic Radiosurgery**:
      - **Procedure**: High-dose radiation is precisely targeted at the AVM over a period of time, causing endothelial damage and eventual closure of the abnormal vessels.
      - **Benefits**: This noninvasive method can be effective for AVMs that are difficult to access surgically or are located in eloquent brain regions.

Conclusion

Interventional radiography has revolutionized the management of intracranial vascular conditions such as aneurysms and AVMs. By utilizing minimally invasive techniques, it provides effective treatment options that minimize risks and improve patient outcomes.

7. Diagnostic criteria of neurofibromatosis type 2 with its imaging findings. [10] [MD (WBUHS) 19, DNB Dec 21]

Diagnostic Criteria of Neurofibromatosis Type 2

Definite NF2

- Bilateral vestibular schwannomas (VSs)
- First-degree relative with NF2 and unilateral VS diagnosed before 30 years of age
- Or first degree relative with NF2 and any 2 of the following:
  - Meningioma
  - Glioma
  - Schwannoma
  - Juvenile posterior subcapsular lenticular opacities or cataracts

Probable NF2

- **Unilateral VS diagnosed <30 years of age and 1 of the following**:
  - Meningioma
  - Glioma

  - Schwannoma
  - Juvenile posterior subcapsular lenticular opacities or cataracts
- **≥2 Meningiomas and 1 of the Following**:
  - 1 VS diagnosed <30 years of age
  - 1 meningioma, glioma, schwannoma, or lens opacity

Imaging Findings

Neurofibromatosis type 2 (NF2) is a rare autosomal dominant neurocutaneous disorder (phakomatosis) manifesting as a development of multiple CNS tumors.

The *NF2* gene is located on the long arm of chromosome 22 (22q12) and encodes the merlin protein (also known as "schwannomin"). It plays a role in contact inhibition of growth and has tumor suppressor function at least in part according to this mechanism. Mutations in *NF2* cause loss of protein function, resulting in a predisposition to tumor formation throughout the nervous system.

Imaging Features

- The cardinal imaging feature of NF2 is bilateral vestibular schwannomas.
- **CT Findings**: NECT scans typically demonstrate a mass in one or both cerebellopontine angle (CPA) cisterns. Both schwannomas and meningiomas are typically iso- to slightly hyperdense on NECT and exhibit strong enhancement following contrast administration.
- Nonneoplastic choroid plexus calcifications in atypical locations (e.g., temporal horn) are a rare manifestation of NF2 but can be striking. Bone CT typically shows that one or both internal auditory canals are widened, whereas schwannomas of other cranial nerves may demonstrate enlargement and remodeling of their exit foramina.
- **MR Findings**: MR findings of NF2-related schwannomas and meningiomas are similar to those of their sporadic counterparts.
- **Schwannomas have Fairly Predictable Signal Characteristics on MRI**:
  - **T1**: Isointense or hypointense
  - **T1 C+ (Gd)**: Intense enhancement
  - **T2**: Heterogeneously hyperintense cystic degenerative areas may be present, especially in larger tumors
  - **T2***: Larger tumors often have areas of hemosiderin

  Signal Characteristics of Typical Meningiomas Include:
  - **T1**
    - Usually isointense to grey matter
    - Hypointense to grey matter: Particularly in fibrous, psammomatous variants
  - **T1 C+ (Gd)**: Usually intense and homogeneous enhancement
  - **T2**
  - Usually isointense to grey matter (~50%)
  - Hyperintense to grey matter (35–40%)
    - Usually correlates with a soft texture and hypervascular tumors
    - Seen in microcystic, secretory, cartilaginous (metaplastic), chordoid and Angiomatous variants
  - **Hypointense to Grey Matter (10–15%)**: Compared to grey matter and usually correlates with harder texture and more fibrous and calcified contents
  - **DWI/ADC**: Grade 2 and 3 tumors may show greater than expected restricted diffusion although this is not universally useful in prospectively predicting histological grade
  - A number of imaging signs that have been described to be very helpful in diagnosing a meningioma includes:
    i. CSF cleft sign, which is not specific for meningioma, but helps establish the mass to be extra-axial; loss of this can be seen in grade II and grade III which may suggest brain parenchyma invasion
    ii. Dural tail is seen in 60–72% (note that a dural tail is also seen in other processes)
    iii. Sunburst or spoke-wheel appearance of the vessels

iv. White matter buckling sign

v. Arterial narrowing:

a. Typically seen in meningiomas which encase arteries

b. Useful sign in parasellar tumors, in distinguishing a meningioma from a pituitary macroadenoma; the latter typically does not narrow vessels

vi. Peripheral rim of enhancement between meningioma and brain parenchyma in postcontrast 3D-FLAIR can help in distinguishing meningioma from other dural based tumor.

If NF2 is suspected on the basis of brain imaging, the entire spine and spinal cord should be screened. High-resolution T2WI and contrast-enhanced sequences disclose asymptomatic tiny schwannomas and intramedullary ependymomas (39-25) in at least half of all individuals with NF2.

Dural enhancement at the porus acusticus is present in approximately 10% of extracanalicular VSs. Although it may represent dural reaction, hypervascularity, or neoplastic infiltration, it portends increased tumor adherence and greater likelihood of subtotal resection and should be considered in surgical planning.

8. (a) Describe briefly various neurocutaneous syndrome. (b) Describe imaging features of von Hippel Lindau syndrome. [5+5] [DNB June 20]

Neurocutaneous Syndromes

Neurocutaneous syndromes, a/k/a phakomatoses, are a group of disorders characterized by the association of neurological symptoms with skin lesions. They are a heterogeneous group of disorders most characterized by the involvement of structures that arise from the embryonic ectoderm (thus central nervous system, skin, and eyes are predominantly involved), although other systems may also be involved.

The concept of the phakomatoses was originated by Dutch ophthalmologist Jan van der Hoeve in 1921, who originally used the term 'phakoma' (from Greek 'lentil') to describe similar retinal lesions seen in von Recklinghausen disease (then an umbrella term for both NF1 and NF2) and tuberous sclerosis, later expanding the grouping to include Sturge-Weber and von Hippel-Lindau (VHL).

Separately, in 1931 the term 'neurocutaneous syndromes' was proposed by American neurologist Paul Yakovlev and psychiatrist Riley Guthrie, to describe the same conditions.

Here are some of the most common types:

1. **Neurofibromatosis Type 1 (NF1)**:
   - Characterized by café-au-lait spots, neurofibromas, and Lisch nodules (iris hamartomas).
   - Patients may have learning disabilities and an increased risk of certain tumors like neurofibromas, optic nerve gliomas, etc.
2. **Neurofibromatosis Type 2 (NF2)**:
   - Characterized by bilateral vestibular schwannomas (acoustic neuromas) and other central nervous system tumors.
   - Skin manifestations include meningiomas and schwannomas.
3. **Tuberous Sclerosis Complex (TSC)**:
   - Features include facial angiofibromas, ash leaf spots, and shagreen patches.
   - Neurological manifestations can include seizures, intellectual disability, and tumors in the brain (hamartomas).
4. **Sturge-Weber Syndrome**:
   - Characterized by a facial capillary malformation (port-wine stain) and leptomeningeal angiomas.
   - Associated with neurological deficits, seizures, and developmental delays.
5. **Ataxia-Telangiectasia**:
   - Features include ataxia, immunodeficiency, and telangiectasias (small dilated blood vessels).
   - Increased risk of lymphoid malignancies.

6. **VHL**: Less common ones include:
   i. Incontinentia pigmenti (Bloch-Sulzberger syndrome)
   ii. Basal cell nevus syndrome (Gorlin-Goltz syndrome)
   iii. Wyburn-Mason syndrome (Bonnet-Dechaume-Blanc syndrome)
   iv. Encephalocraniocutaneous lipomatosis
   v. Hypomelanosis of Ito
   vi. Nijmegen breakage syndrome
   vii. Neurocutaneous melanosis
   viii. CHILD (congenital hemidysplasia with ichthyosiform erythroderma and limb defects) syndrome.

Imaging Features of von Hippel-Lindau Syndrome

VHL is an autosomal dominant familial tumor syndrome with marked phenotypic variability and age dependent penetrance. VHL syndrome predisposes individuals to various tumors and cysts.

VHL can be classified according to clinical phenotypes, and the classification correlates with particular genotypes:

- **Type 1**: Low-risk for pheochromocytoma but higher-risk for CNS hemangioblastoma, renal cell carcinoma, pancreatic cyst, and pancreatic neuroendocrine tumor
- **Type 2A**: High-risk for pheochromocytoma; low-risk for renal cell carcinoma
- **Type 2B**: High-risk for pheochromocytoma and renal cell carcinoma
- **Type 2C**: High-risk for pheochromocytoma only

Imaging modalities used to evaluate VHL syndrome include: MRI (for brain, spine, abdomen, etc.), CT (for brain, abdomen, pelvis, etc.), ultrasound (for abdomen, pelvis, etc.), PET-CT (for detecting metastatic disease)

The imaging features typically observed in VHL include:

1. **CNS Hemangioblastomas**:
   - These are often found in the cerebellum and can appear as well-defined, vascular lesions on MRI with characteristic "cystic" appearances due to associated cysts. NCCT typically demonstrates isodense cysts with isodense mural nodule that abuts the pial surface of the cerebellum. The tumor nodule enhances intensely on CECT. They appear hyperintense to CSF on T1WI and Hyperintense on T2/FLAIR. Hemorrhage is common and peritumoral edema varies.
   - Nearly half of all VHL associated HBs occur in spinal cord. Intraspinal HBs are often multiple and are frequently associated with a syrinx.
2. **Retinal Hemangioblastomas**:
   - Most common presenting feature
   - Detected via fundoscopic examination; these appear as yellowish-white lesions on the retina, often with associated exudates.
   - On NCCT, posterior globe appears hyperdense compared to normal vitreous. Tiny enhancing nodules may be seen on T1 CEMRI. They may lead to hemorrhagic retinal detachments.
3. **Renal Cell Carcinoma**:
   - MRI or CT may reveal renal masses, which can be solid or cystic, often with calcifications or hemorrhage.
   - Usually of the clear cell type and frequently bilateral
   - Renal cell carcinomas present at an earlier age
4. **Pancreatic Cysts and Tumors**: Imaging may show multiple pancreatic cysts or solid tumors, which may be benign or malignant.
5. **Pheochromocytomas**:
   - These adrenal tumors can be visualized on CT or MRI as hypervascular masses, often with associated calcifications.
   - They are considered as hallmark of Type 2 VHL.

6. **Endolymphatic Sac Tumors**: Imaging hallmark of ELST is that of a retrolabyrynthine mass associated with osseus erosion. Bone CT shows an infiltrative, poorly circumscribed lytic lesion with central intramural bony spicules. On MRI, hyperintense foci are seen on T1WI, Hypo-hyperintense mixed signal intensity are seen on T2WI. Heterogenous enhancement is seen on CEMRI with prolonged tumor blush on DSA.
7. **Epididymal cystadenomas**
8. **Broad ligament cystadenomas**

   VHL diagnostic criteria:

   a. No family history:
      i. >/= 2 CNS hemangioblastomas or
      ii. 1 CNS hemangioblastoma + Visceral tumor
   b. Positive family history for VHL:
      i. 1 CNS hemangioblastoma or
      ii. Pheochromocytoma or
      iii. Clear cell RCC

Overall, imaging plays a crucial role in the diagnosis and management of VHL syndrome, allowing for early detection of associated tumors and cysts.

REFERENCES

1. Osborn AG, Hedlund GL, Salzman KL. In: Price EB, Moss HE (Eds). Osborn's Brain: Imaging, Pathology, and Anatomy. Philadelphia: Elsevier; 2017.
2. Egemen E, Solaroglu I. Anatomy of cerebral veins and dural sinuses. In: Egemen E, Solaroglu I. Primer on cerebrovascular diseases, 2nd edition. Philadelphia: Academic Press; 2017. pp. 32-36.
3. Khandelwal N, Gupta AK, Chowdhury V. In: Khandelwal N, Gupta AK, Chowdhury V (Eds). AIIMS-MAMC-PGI's Comprehensive Textbook of Diagnostic Radiology. New Delhi: Jaypee, The Health Sciences Publisher; 2016.
4. Murphy K, Robertson F (Eds). Interventional neuroradiology. Springer Science & Business Media; 2013.
5. Harrigan MR, Deveikis JP. Handbook of cerebrovascular disease and neurointerventional technique. Luxembourg: Springer Science & Business Media; 2012.
6. Moonis G, Filippi CG, Kirsch CF, Mohan S, Stein EG, Hirsch JA, et al. The spectrum of neuroimaging findings on CT and MRI in adults with COVID-19. Am J Roentgenol. 2021;217(4):959-74.
7. Lucignani G, Guarnera A, Rossi-Espagnet MC, Moltoni G, Antonelli A, Figà Talamanca L, et al. From fetal to neonatal neuroimaging in TORCH infections: a pictorial review. Children. 2022;9(8):1210.

CHAPTER 3

Chest and Cardiovascular Imaging

Lipika Afroz, Mehtaab Alam

QUESTIONS

CHEST IMAGING

Techniques, Normal Anatomy, and Basic Patterns in Chest Diseases

1. Write a short note on radiographic differences between PA and AP view of chest radiograph. [5] [MD (WBUHS) 22]
2. CT and radiographic anatomy of bronchopulmonary segments. Hilum overlay sign and hilum convergence sign. [10] [DNB June 21]
3. MDCT reconstruction methods in airway. Imaging in intraluminal lesions of tracheobronchial tree. [10] [DNB June 21]
4. (a) Hilum overlay sign and its significance on diagnostic radiology. (b) Cervicothoracic sign and its significance on diagnostic radiology. [5+5] [DNB June 20]
5. Describe various types of lung collapse. Discuss radiologic features of collapse in general and the specific imaging features which help in localization of collapse. [4+6] [DNB June 20]
6. Discuss the imaging evaluation of various catheters, tubes and lines seen on a chest radiograph in an ICU setting. [10] [DNB June 20, MD (WBUHS) 24]

Pulmonary Infections and Pulmonary Interstitium

1. Write short note on pulmonary aspergilloma. [5] [MD (WBUHS) 23, AIIMS May 24]
2. Describe HRCT findings of pulmonary involvement in different stages of COVID-19 infection and CT severity index of COVID-19 infection. [10] [MD (WBUHS) 21]
3. Classify different types of Emphysema. Discuss the role of HRCT in evaluation of types of emphysema. [10] [MD (WBUHS) 19]
4. Classify the diffuse lung diseases. Discuss in brief the salient imaging findings of diffuse cystic lung diseases. [5+5] [MD (WBUHS) 22]
5. Discuss the role of radiography in COVID-19 patients. [10] [MD (WBUHS) 22]
6. Describe anatomy of secondary pulmonary lobule on HRCT. Describe role of HRCT in the diagnosis of interstitial lung disease. [3+7] [DNB Dec 19, AIIMS Dec 23]
7. Discuss the thoracic imaging manifestations in Collagen vascular diseases. [10]
8. Pathophysiology of covid pulmonary infection. Chest CT protocol. Chest CT findings. [10] [DNB Dec 21]
9. Lifecycle of *Echinococcus granulosus*. Pulmonary findings in hydatid cyst. [10] [DNB Dec 21]

10. Discuss the indications of imaging in a suspected COVID-19 patient. Describe imaging features and pattern of involvement of respiratory system in COVID-19. [4+6] [DNB June 20]
11. (a) Radiological patterns of pneumonias on chest computed tomography in immunocompromised patients. (b) Imaging features of fungal infections. [5+5] [DNB Dec 20]

Mediastinum, Lung Nodules, and Masses

1. Discuss the imaging features of the common anterior mediastinal lesions. [10] [MD (WBUHS) 23]
2. Define solitary pulmonary nodule (SPN). Enumerate its causes. Discuss the radiological work up of a solitary nodule highlighting the features which enable to differentiate between benign and malignant nodules. [1+2+7] [MD (WBUHS) 23, DNB June 21]
3. Briefly discuss the radiological divisions of Mediastinum with their contents. [10] [MD (WBUHS) 19]
4. Write short note on Pancoast Tumor. [5] [MD (WBUHS) 19]
5. Describe imaging features and differential diagnosis of Silicosis. [10] [MD (WBUHS) 19]
6. Multinodular pulmonary lesions and its imaging. [10] [DNB June 22]
7. Cystic lesions of lung and imaging. [10] [DNB June 22]
8. Radiographic compartments of mediastinum. Pediatric mediastinal masses. Posterior mediastinal masses in 1-year-old [10] [DNB Dec 21]
9. Causes of hilar node enlargement. How to differentiate causes on imaging? [10] [DNB Dec 21]
10. Pathologies of lung carcinoma. TNM staging in lung carcinoma. FDG PET role in lung carcinoma. [10] [DNB June 21, RG 18, AIIMS May 24]
11. ITMIG classification of mediastinum. Thymoma-imaging features and approach. Imaging features thymoma vs hyperplasia. [10] [DNB June 21]
12. Solitary pulmonary nodule definition. Discuss the etiologies/differential diagnosis. Benign vs malignant SPN. [10]
13. Describe anatomy of mediastinum with the help of diagram. Discuss imaging features of anterior mediastinum masses. [5+5] [DNB Dec 20, AIIMS May 23, AIIMS Dec 24]

Emergency Chest

1. Describe bolus tracking technique used during MDCT pulmonary angiography. Discuss the MDCT findings in a case of acute pulmonary thromboembolism. [5+5] [AIIMS Dec 23]
2. Lung ultrasound in emergency department. [5] [AIIMS Dec 23]
3. Describe in brief, protocol for CT pulmonary angiography for a suspected case of pulmonary thromboembolism. Describe plain radiographic and CT features of pulmonary thromboembolism. [4+3+3] [AIIMS Dec 23, DNB June 20]

Pediatric Chest

1. Discuss in brief the causes and radiographic features of respiratory distress in newborn. [5+5] [MD (WBUHS) 23]
2. Enumerate causes of neonatal respiratory distress. Describe in detail pathophysiology and imaging findings in hyaline membrane disease. [2+(2+6)] [DNB Dec 20, AIIMS May 24]
3. The role of imaging in a newborn with respiratory distress. [10] [MD (WBUHS) 19]
4. Describe the congenital anomalies of the lung. [10] [MD (WBUHS) 20]
5. Describe the classification of developmental lung anomalies. Discuss CT findings in any three common developmental lung anomalies. [4+6]
6. Write short note on pulmonary sequestration. [5] [MD (WBUHS) 20]
7. Write short note on Scimitar syndrome. [5] [MD (WBUHS) 20, MD (WBUHS) 19]

Pleura and Diaphragm

1. Classify pleural tumors. Briefly discuss chest radiographic and CT findings of malignant mesothelioma. [3+3+4] [MD (WBUHS) 23]
2. Discuss various imaging signs of diaphragmatic injury. Describe the differences between blunt and penetrating diaphragmatic injury. Discuss signs to differentiate diaphragmatic hernia from eventration and paralysis. [5+2+3] [DNB June 20]
3. Draw a schematic diagram describing anatomy of diaphragm and imaging features of diaphragmatic injury on chest X-ray, ultrasound, CT and MRI. [2+2+2+2+2] [DNB Dec 20]
4. What role radiologist plays in the diagnosis of patient who has pleural effusion. [10] [MD (WBUHS) 19]

Miscellaneous

1. Enumerate causes of unilateral opaque hemithorax. Describe the role of imaging in the evaluation of unilateral opaque hemithorax in an adult. [3+7]
2. Describe the chest radiographic findings in rheumatic heart disease. [5]
3. USG in pleural and parenchymal pathology. [10] [DNB June 22]
4. Differentials of calcifications on chest X-ray. [5] [DNB Dec 21]
5. Differentials of cavitary pulmonary lesions. [5] [DNB Dec 21]

Interventions in Chest

1. Role of intervention radiology in massive hemoptysis. [5] [MD (WBUHS) 20]
2. What are the causes of massive hemoptysis? Describe the process of Bronchial artery embolization in case of intractable hemoptysis. [10] [MD (WBUHS) 24, MD (WBUHS) 19, AIIMS May 23]
3. Enumerate the causes of hemoptysis in adult patient. Briefly discuss indications, techniques and complications of radiological interventions in them. [2+2+4+2] [DNB Dec 20]
4. (a) Anatomy of bronchial artery. (b) Indications, technique and complications of bronchial artery embolization. [4+(2+2+2)] [DNB Dec 20]
5. Enumerate causes of massive hemoptysis? Role if intervention radiology in management of hemoptysis. [2+8] [MD (WBUHS) 22]
6. Hemoptysis—role of radiology and intervention [10] [DNB June 22]

CARDIOVASCULAR IMAGING

Cardiac Imaging

1. Discuss the radiological anatomy of coronary arteries. Describe the technique of CT coronary angiography. Discuss the recent advances in assessment of coronary artery stenosis by CT angiography. [3+3+4] [MD (WBUHS) 23, [MD (WBUHS) 18, DNB June 20]
2. Write short note on Ebstein anomaly. [5] [MD (WBUHS) 23]
3. Classify congenital heart disease. Discuss PDA. [10] [MD (WBUHS) 20]
4. Describe advantages and pitfalls of cardiac MRI. [10] [MD (WBUHS) 19, AIIMS Dec 23]
5. Mitral stenosis, etiology, and radiographic findings. [10] [MD (WBUHS) 19]
6. Discuss the plain radiographic findings in congenital heart diseases. [10]
7. Triple rule out CT coronary angiography—technique, its principle and protocol. [10] [DNB June 22]
8. Cardiac tumors and imaging. [10] [DNB June 22, RG 18]

9. Imaging protocol in 50-year-old with acute chest pain. Likely causes and Imaging findings. [10] [DNB Dec 21]
10. MR in ischemic heart disease. [5]
11. Radiographic findings in congenital cyanotic heart disease. [5] [DNB Dec 21]
12. Imaging findings mitral stenosis. [5] [DNB Dec 21]
13. Dark and white blood cardiac MRI. Viability scans in IHD. [10] [DNB June 21]
14. Constrictive pericarditis—CT imaging. Radiographic Imaging of mitral valve diseases. [10] [DNB June 21]
15. Describe the imaging protocol and role of MRI in evaluation of ischemic heart disease. [5+5] [DNB June 20, DNB June 18]
16. Role of nuclear imaging, cardiac MRI and MDCT in evaluation of ischemic heart disease patient. [2+4+4] [MD (WBUHS) 17, DNB Dec 20]
17. Define pulmonary edema and describe its pathophysiology. Enumerate causes and imaging features in pulmonary edema. [2+2+(2+4)] [DNB Dec 20, RG 18]

Nuclear Medicine

1. Scintigraphy in cardiac imaging. [5] [DNB Dec 21]

Vascular Imaging

1. Discuss various types of aortic aneurysms and their radiological evaluation. [10] [MD (WBUHS) 20]
2. Describe briefly the imaging of aortic aneurysm, rupture and dissection. [10] [MD (WBUHS) 19, MD (WBUHS) 17]
3. Imaging in patent ductus arteriosus. [10] [MD (WBUHS) 19]
4. Enumerate the causes of superior vena cava obstruction with their imaging features. [10] [MD (WBUHS) 19]
5. Classify aortic dissection. Enumerate the salient radiological findings to differentiate true lumen and false lumen. [4+6] [MD (WBUHS) 22]
6. Imaging in varicose veins. [5] [DNB Dec 21]
7. Imaging in chronic PTE. [5] [DNB Dec 21]
8. Peripheral arterial disease—imaging with advantages and disadvantages. [10] [DNB June 21]
9. Describe various types of aortic dissection. Discuss the role of imaging in evaluation of aortic dissection. [5+5] [DNB June 20, MD (WBUHS) 24]
10. Discuss the imaging approach to acute limb ischemia. Discuss the interventional radiological treatment options for it. [5+5] [DNB June 20]
11. (a) Enumerate causes of inferior rib notching. (b) Describe X-ray, CT, and MRI findings in Coarctation of aorta. (c) Briefly discuss role of interventional radiology in its management. [2+(2+2+2)+2] [DNB Dec 20, MD (WBUHS) 17, AIIMS Dec 23]
12. (a) Arterial and venous anatomy of lower limb with help of diagram. (b) Imaging features of deep venous thrombosis. [5+5] [DNB Dec 20]
13. Define acute aortic syndrome. Classify aortic dissection. Describe its imaging features on CT angiography and its management. [1+2+(4+3)] [DNB Dec 20, MD (WBUHS) 24]

ANSWERS

CHEST IMAGING

Techniques, Normal Anatomy, and Basic Patterns in Chest Diseases

1. Write a short note on radiographic differences between PA and AP view of chest radiograph. [5] [MD (WBUHS) 22]

The main radiographic differences between PA and AP view of chest radiograph are as follows **(Table 1)**:[1]

TABLE 1: Radiographic differences between PA and AP view of chest radiograph.[1]

	PA view	*AP view*
FFD/FRD	180 cm	120 cm
Type of radiography	DDR, CR	Mainly DDR
Position of patient	Mostly erect	Mostly supine, portable and used mainly in ICU settings
Scapulae	Outside the lung fields	Overlapping lung fields
Clavicles	Overlying lung apices	Projected cranially, lie above the apices
Heart size	No magnification	Apparent cardiomegaly due to magnification
Ribs	More oblique	More horizontal
Diaphragms	Near the level of 9th posterior rib or 5–6th anterior rib	Higher in position
Fundal air fluid level	Seen	Not seen
Spine	Spinous process better seen	Vertebrae and disc spaces better seen

2. CT and radiographic anatomy of bronchopulmonary segments. Hilum overlay sign and hilum convergence sign. [10] [DNB June 21]

Bronchopulmonary segments: Each segmental bronchus passes to a structurally and functionally independent unit of lung lobe called bronchopulmonary segments.2 These are functional, anatomical and surgical units of lung.

Illustrated image **(Figs. 1 and 2)** of bronchopulmonary segments:

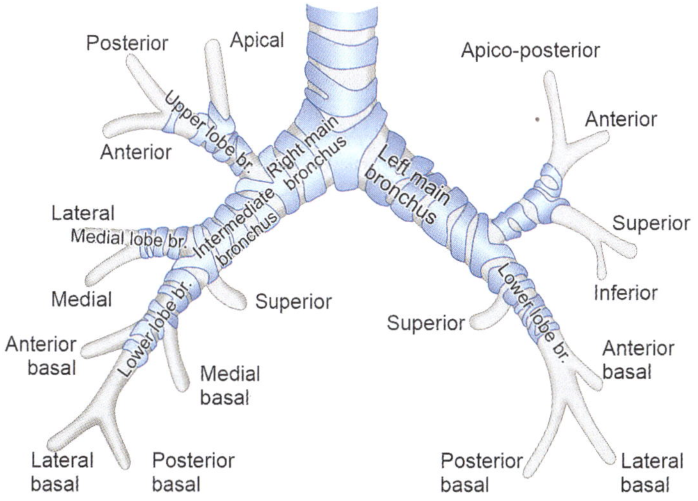

FIG. 1: Normal anatomy of tracheobronchial tree.

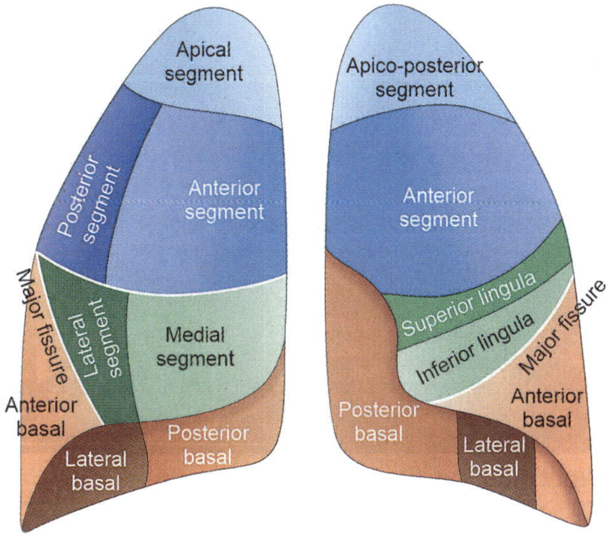

FIG. 2: Normal anatomy of bronchopulmonary segments.

Hilum Overlay Sign

Introduction

Visualization of the hilar vessels through a mediastinal mass—means that mass does not arise from the hilum.

This sign differentiates whether an opacity on a frontal chest radiograph in the region of the lung hilum is located within the hilum versus anterior or posterior to it. The sign refers to preserved visualization of the hilar vessels—mass arising from anterior or posterior mediastinum.
An opacity—from hilum, silhouette normal pulmonary vessels.

Causes of hilar opacity are:

1. Middle mediastinal tumors
2. Hilar adenopathy
3. Pericardial effusion
4. Vascular and cardiac enlargement

If the edges of the vessels are seen through the opacity and not in contact with the hilum that means the opacity is either anterior or posterior mediastinum. Most of these opacities are masses in the anterior mediastinum.

Causes of anterior mediastinal masses are:

1. Thymic lesion
2. Thyroid and parathyroid lesion
3. Germ cell tumor
4. Vascular lesion (lymphangioma, hemangioma)

Hilum Convergence Sign

Introduction

Distinguish a bulky hilum due to pulmonary artery dilatation from a juxtahilar mass/nodal enlargement.

If pulmonary artery branches are visible through the opacity and converge towards the waist of the heart (positive hilum convergence sign), then the opacity is due to a juxtahilar mediastinal mass.

If pulmonary vessels appear to converge centrally towards the lateral margin of the abnormal "bump", then the hilar opacity is an enlarged pulmonary artery **(Figs. 3 and 4)**.

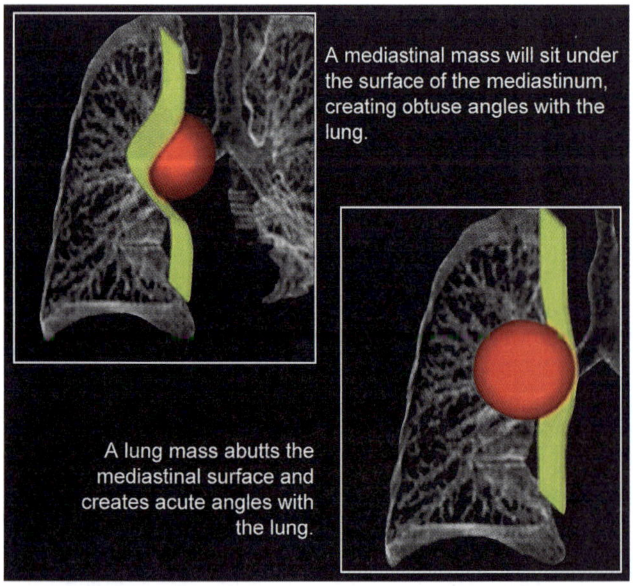

FIG. 3: Hilum convergence and hilum overlay sign.

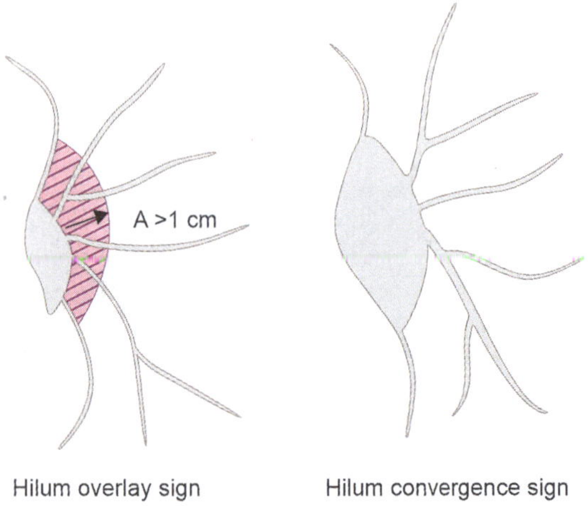

FIG. 4: Schematic representation of hilum convergence and hilum overlay sign.

3. MDCT reconstruction methods in airway. Imaging in intraluminal lesions of tracheobronchial tree. [10] [DNB June 21]

The multidetector computed tomography (MDCT) reconstruction is an imaging technique used for detailed evaluation of the anatomy and pathology of the airways, including the trachea, bronchi, and smaller airway.[3]

Parameters for Multidetector CT (Table 2)

TABLE 2: Acquisition parameters for multidetector CT.

kVp, mAs	110–140, 50–80
Pitch	≥1
Field of view	Lung apices to bases or to the first or second branching of the main bronchi
Acquisition	End-inspiration; end-expiration with lower kV and mA settings; forced expiration with lower kV and mA settings'

Postprocessing Reconstruction (Table 3)

TABLE 3: Postprocessing reconstruction algorithm for multidetector CT.

2D reconstructions	1 mm thickness—axial, coronal, and sagittal
2D thick MPRs	1–10 mm thickness, coronal, ± MinIP algorithm
3D surface rendering	Surface rendering of trachea and main bronchi
3D virtual bronchoscopy	Internal surface rendering of the trachea and main bronchi

Steps of MDCT reconstruction methods are:
Data acquisition: *MDCT scanning*: uses multiple rows of detectors to acquire high-resolution, volumetric images of the respiratory airways in thin slices. Modern MDCT scanners can obtain submillimeter slices.

Helical scanning: Used to minimizing respiratory motion artifacts.

- **Image reconstruction algorithms**: Methods are:
  - *Filtered back projection (FBP)*: Reconstructing CT images by converting raw data from multiple projections into a 2D or 3D image.
  - *Iterative reconstruction (IR)*: Enhance image quality by reducing noise and improving resolution.
  - *Model-based iterative reconstruction (MBIR)*: Improves the signal-to-noise ratio and spatial resolution while reducing radiation dose.
- **Multiplanar reconstruction (MPR)**: After the acquisition of axial images then data is reconstructed into sagittal, coronal, and oblique views. This multiplanar reconstruction helps assess the airways in multiple dimensions, improving the detection of airway narrowing, obstruction, or malformations.
- **3D Reconstruction and visualization**:
  - *Volume rendering*: A 3D image of the airways can be reconstructed and provides detailed view of the bronchial tree.
  - *Virtual bronchoscopy*: Endoscopic view of the airways, allowing for noninvasive visualization of the internal airway lumen.
- **Quantitative airway analysis**: Quantitative analysis of the airways like airway wall thickness, lumen diameter, and cross-sectional area.
- **Respiratory motion and gating**: Used to reduce motion artifacts caused by breathing.

Application of MDCT

- **Obstructive Airway Diseases**: COPD, asthma, bronchiectasis, and bronchial stenosis.
- Evaluation of airway tumor, involvement, and plan interventions.

- **Congenital Anomalies**: Tracheomalacia or bronchomalacia, where airways collapse or narrow, can be visualized with MDCT, aiding in diagnosis and treatment planning.

Advantages of MDCT in airways:

- High resolution which helps to detailed evaluation of both central and peripheral airways.
- MDCT is fast, minimizing the impact of respiratory motion.
- Virtual bronchoscopy provides a noninvasive which better visualize the airway.

Imaging in intraluminal lesions of tracheobronchial tree:

- **Chest X-ray**: Initial imaging that can reveal large lesions or airway obstruction.
- **CT Scan**: HRCT is the gold standard for evaluating intraluminal lesions. It provides detailed images of the airway structure, lesion's size, location, and relationship to surrounding structure.
- **Bronchoscopy**: Direct visualization of the tracheobronchial tree and used for biopsy, brushing, or lavage of the lesion for histopathological examination.
- **MRI**: Assessing adjacent structures, soft tissue but is less common for airway lesions.
- **PET Scan**: Used for metabolic activity of the lesion.

4. (a) Hilum overlay sign and its significance on diagnostic radiology. (b) Cervicothoracic sign and its significance on diagnostic radiology. [5+5] [DNB June 20]

a. Hilum Overlay Sign

Introduction

Visualization of the hilar vessels through a mediastinal mass—means that mass does not arise from the hilum.[4]

This sign differentiates whether an opacity on a frontal chest radiograph in the region of the lung hilum is located within the hilum versus anterior or posterior to it. The sign refers to preserved visualization of the hilar vessels—mass arising from anterior or posterior mediastinum.

An opacity—from hilum, silhouette normal pulmonary vessels.
Causes of hilar opacity are:

- Middle mediastinal tumors
- Hilar adenopathy
- Pericardial effusion
- Vascular and cardiac enlargement

If the edges of the vessels are seen through the opacity and not in contact with the hilum that means the opacity is either anterior or posterior mediastinum. Most of these opacities are masses in the anterior mediastinum.

Causes of anterior mediastinal masses are:

- Thymic lesion
- Thyroid and parathyroid lesion
- Germ cell tumor
- Vascular lesion (lymphangioma, hemangioma).

b. Cervicothoracic Sign

- By Felson—"If a thoracic lesion is in anatomical contact with the soft tissues of the neck—its contiguous border is lost".
- Used to determine whether a lesion is in posterior/middle mediastinum or anterior mediastinum.
- The anatomic basis for the sign is the obliquity of the thoracic inlet. The thoracic inlet is bounded by T1 vertebral body posteriorly, the first ribs on both sides, and the superior border of the manubrium anteriorly.
- In the posterior aspect, the thoracic inlet is higher up, and the lungs thus are present superior to the level of the clavicle. So, any posterior mediastinal mass will be surrounded by lung tissue laterally and superiorly. So, any soft

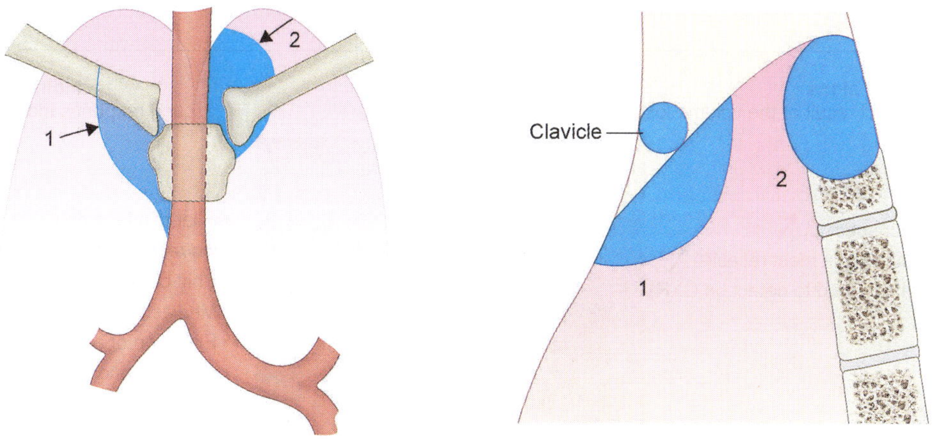

FIG. 5: Cervicothoracic sign.

tissue density mass, seen a sharp demarcation between the mass and the air-density lungs, and superior border of the mass will be appreciated above the clavicle **(Fig. 5)**.

- Examples include posterior mediastinal masses like neurofibroma.
- On the other hand, at the anterior aspect, a soft tissue density mass in the mediastinum merge with the soft tissue density of the neck anteriorly as there is no inferior air-density lung parenchyma to provide a silhouette. Thus, the superior border of the mass will not be appreciable above the clavicle in an anterior mediastinal mass.
- Examples of anterior mediastinal masse are—cystic hygroma, left superior vena cava, right aortic arch, and thymic cyst.
  - *Anterior mediastinum*: Ends at the level of clavicle
  - *Middle and posterior mediastinum*: Projects above the clavicle

5. Describe various types of lung collapse. Discuss radiologic features of collapse in general and the specific imaging features which help in localization of collapse. [4+6] [DNB June 20]

Introduction

Collapse indicates loss of lung volume, associated with a decrease in the amount of air within alveoli.[5]

Types of collapse:

- **Obstructive**: Due to blockage of airways. Causes are:
  - Foreign body obstruction
  - Bronchogenic carcinoma
  - Bronchial carcinoid
  - Lymphoma
  - Tuberculosis
  - Left atrial enlargement from mitral stenosis
  - Main stem bronchus dilatation
- **Nonobstructive**: This includes
  - *Passive atelectasis*: Parenchymal compression due to pleural effusion/pneumothorax/mass.
  - *Adhesive atelectasis*: Due to loss of surfactant. Causes are
    - Respiratory distress syndrome of newborn
    - Adult respiratory distress syndrome
    - Radiation pneumonitis

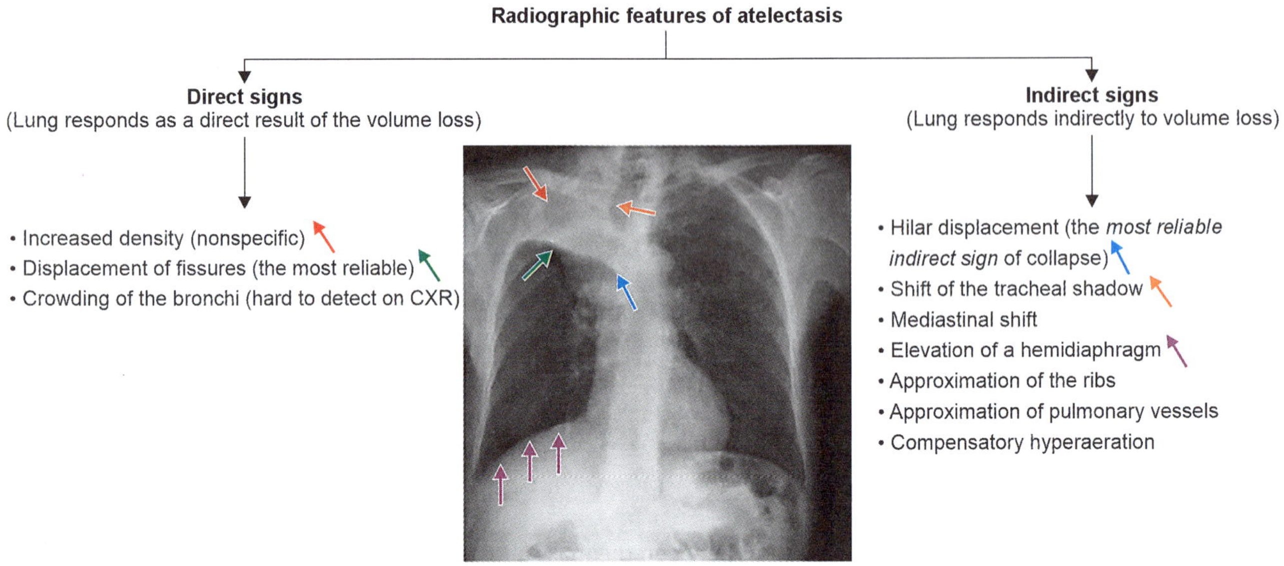

FIG. 6: Signs of direct and indirect signs of atelectasis.

- *Cicatricial atelectasis*: Replacement of lung tissue by scarring or infiltrative diseases. Causes are:
  - Granulomatous disease
  - Late sequelae of tuberculosis
  - Necrotizing pneumonia
  - Radiation
  - Collagen vascular disease
  - Pneumoconiosis
- *Compression atelectasis*: Caused by any space occupying lesions.

Radiographic Signs of Collapse (Fig. 6)

Direct Signs

- Displacement of fissures
- Crowding of vessels

Indirect Signs

- Diaphragmatic elevation
- Mediastinal shift
- Compensatory overinflation of normal lung
- Hilar displacement
- Reorientation of the hilum
- Approximation of ribs
- Increased lung opacity
- Shifting granuloma sign
- Absence of air bronchogram

Right upper lobe collapse frontal radiograph (Fig. 7A):

- Ill-defined increased opacity in the upper thorax
- Apparent right mediastinal widening
- Silhouetting of right upper mediastinum
- Tracheal shift to right

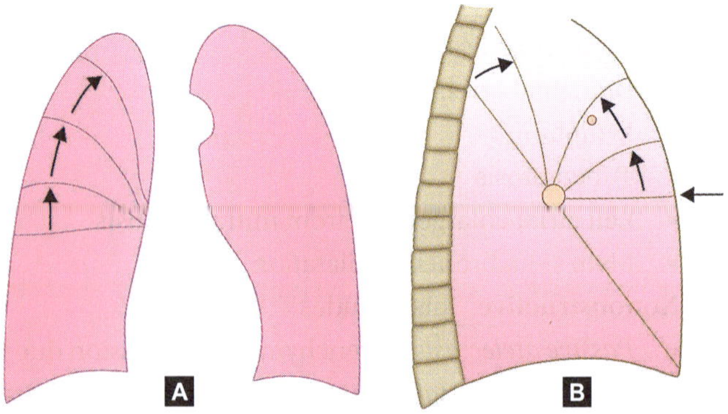

FIGS. 7A and B: Right upper lobe collapse (A) PA and (B) lateral views: Horizontal fissure is drawn upward and curves towards the apex and mediastinum on PA view. On the lateral view there is upward displacement of the horizontal fissure with forward displacement of the oblique fissure above the hilum.

- Upward bowing of minor fissure
- Golden S sign

Right upper lobe collapse lateral radiograph (Fig. 7B):

- Upward displacement and bowing of minor fissure
- Anterior displacement and bowing of the upper major fissure

Right upper lobe collapse CT scan (Fig. 8)

- Minor fissure rotates anteriorly and medially.
- The major fissure outlines the posterior margin of the collapsed lobe and may bowed anteriorly.
- In presence of hilar mass the appearance will be similar to Golden S sign.

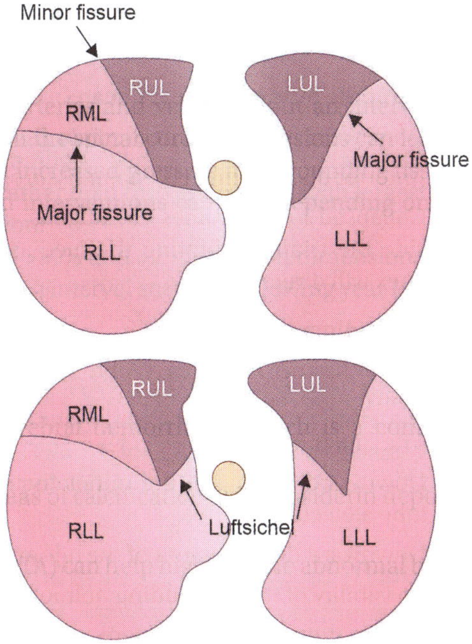

FIG. 8: Right upper lobe collapse.

Left upper lobe collapse frontal radiograph (Fig. 9A):

- Ill-defined increase in opacity in upper thorax
- Silhouetting of the left upper mediastinum
- Tracheal shift to the left
- LUFTSICHEL sign
- Apical gap
- Outward rotation of the bronchus
- Elevation of hilum
- Juxtaphrenic peak

Left upper lobe collapse lateral radiograph **(Fig. 9B)**:
Anterior bowing and displacement of the major fissure

Left upper lobe collapse CT scan:

- The major fissure rotates anteromedially with upper lobe collapse.
- The luftsichel sign is associated with a V shaped appearance at the posterior margin of the collapsed lobe as the superior segment of the lower lobe extending medial to the collapsed lobe.

Right middle lobe collapse (Figs. 10A and B): Frontal radiograph

- Minor fissure is invisible Increase lung opacity
- Silhouetting of the right heart border

Lateral radiograph

- Downward bowing and displacement of the minor fissure
- Anterior bowing and displacement of the major fissure

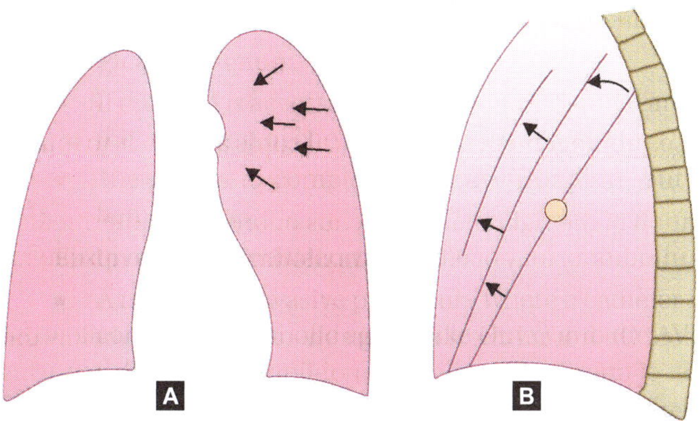

FIGS. 9A and B: Left upper lobe collapse on (A) PA and (B) lateral views: Increased density is seen with increasing severity of collapse on PA view. The fissure moves forward on lateral view.

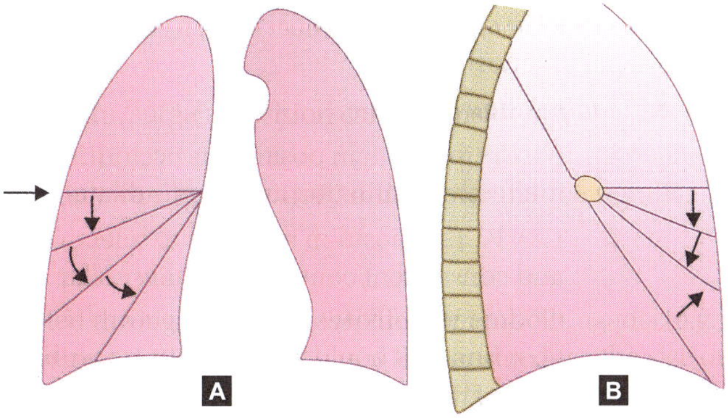

FIGS. 10A and B: Right middle lobe collapse (A) PA and (B) lateral views: The horizontal fissure is displaced downwards on both views, on the lateral view there is forward displacement of the lower part of the oblique fissure.

- Wedge shaped consolidated lung anchored at the hilum

Right middle lobe collapse CT scan:

1. Downward displacement of minor fissure.
2. Anterior displacement of major fissure.
3. Collapsed lobe assumes a triangular shape with one side the triangle abutting the mediastinum and the apex will direct laterally.

Frontal radiograph

1. Major fissure becomes visible (upper portion best seen)
2. Triangular opacity
3. Downward bowing of the minor fissure (right lower lobe atelectasis)
4. Downward displacement of the hilum
5. Invisibility of the descending pulmonary artery
6. Obscuration of the diaphragm
7. Shift of the heart
8. "Flat-waist sign"

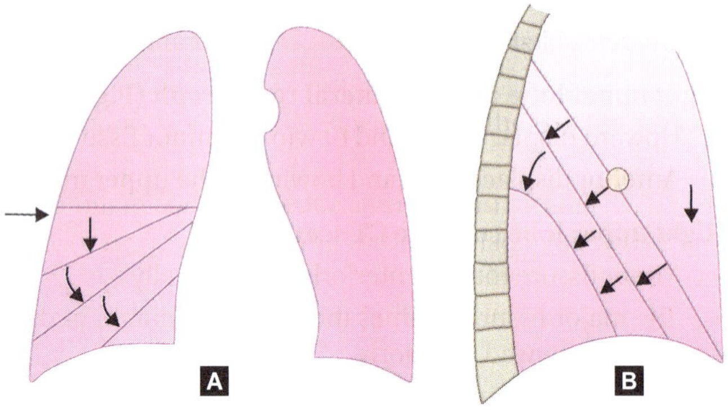

FIGS. 11A and B: Right lower lobe collapse on (A) PA and (B) lateral views: Downward displacement of horizontal fissure is noted on PA view. The oblique fissure is displaced backwards on lateral view.

Lower lobe atelectasis (both lung) (Figs. 11 and 12): Lateral radiograph

- Obscuration of the posterior diaphragm.
- Posterior bowing of the major fissure.

Lower lobe atelectasis (both lung) CT scan

- Major fissure rotates posteromedially from the hilum with collapse.
- This displacement will be more with increased atelectasis.

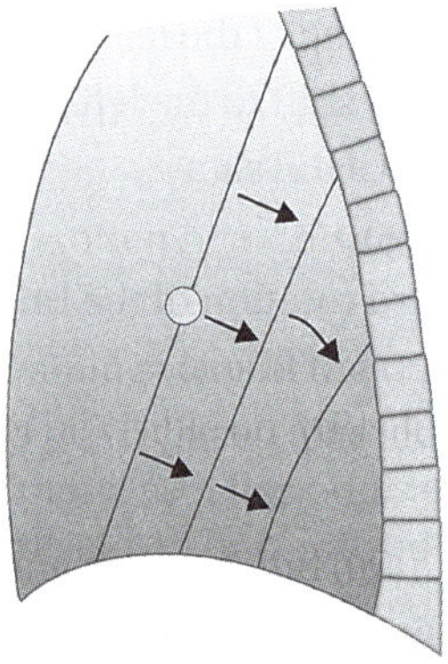

FIG. 12: Left lower lobe collapse on lateral view—No fissure is seen on the PA projection. Lateral view shows the oblique fissure to be displaced posteriorly.

6. Discuss the imaging evaluation of various catheters, tubes and lines seen on a chest radiograph in an ICU setting. [10] [DNB June 20, MD (WBUHS) 24]

Imaging evaluation of catheters, tubes, and lines on chest radiographs in an ICU setting is crucial for assessing placement, complications, and ongoing management.[6,7] The commonly used tubes, lines are:

1. **Endotracheal tube (ETT):**
   a. *Aim*: To maintain airway patency and facilitate ventilation.
   b. *Location of tip*: mid tracheal level, 5 cm above the carina and at least 3 cm distal to the vocal cords, with head in neutral position.
   c. *Malposition of the tip*:
      i. If ETT tip is high in position its occluding cuff causes impingement over the vocal cords and leads to injury, ineffective ventilation and gastric dilatation.
      ii. Low ETT tip position may lead to selective ventilation of the right main bronchus or bronchus intermedius and consequent contralateral lung collapse. Pneumothorax may occur in low positioning due to ipsilateral lung/lobar hyperinflation.
      iii. Esophageal placement of the ETT is potentially fatal. On frontal chest radiograph - the tip will be below the level of the carina and the air column lateral to that of trachea. Right posterior oblique radiograph confirms the position of ETT outside the tracheal walls and along the esophageal wall.
      iv. Over inflation of the ETT cuff beyond 1.5 times the diameter of trachea predisposes to tracheal injury in the form of rupture in acute setting, which occurs within 7 cm of carina and usually involves the posterior membranous wall.

d. *Complications*:
   i. In cases of high airway rupture at the level of hypopharynx, cervical subcutaneous emphysema is seen.
   ii. Nontraumatic complications of ETT include aspiration pneumonitis, airway obstruction due to mucus plugs or clots and consequent lobar or segmental lung collapse.
   iii. Air leak: Air leak due to barotrauma is a known complication of positive pressure ventilation. The radiographic features include emphysema, pneumothorax and pneumomediastinum.
   iv. Chronic injury may cause tracheomalacia or stenosis.

2. **Tracheostomy tube (TT)**:
   a. *Aim*: To provide airway and remove secretions from lungs.
   b. *The ideal location*: Is such that the tip is located 1/2 of the distance from the stoma to carina, and its position is unaffected by neck flexion or extension.
   c. *Complications*:
      i. Small subcutaneous emphysema or pneumomediastinum may be recognized on radiographs after placement of TT.
      ii. Tracheal stenosis at the stoma site may occur due to fibrosis.

3. **Intercostal drainage tube (ICT/ICD)**:
   a. *Aim*: Drainage of pleural effusions or pneumothorax or hemothorax.
   b. *Position of the ICT tip*: Should be in the apical or basal region depending on the drainage of air or fluid respectively from the pleural cavity.
      i. Presence of a radiopaque stripe along the length and tip of the tube allows the position of tip and side holes to be recognized on radiographs.
      ii. The tube should be positioned such that side holes should be medial to the inner margins of ribs.
      iii. As air/fluid outlines both sides of an appropriately positioned tube, an obscured outline of the tube suggests subcutaneous placement.
   c. *Malposition*: Leads to incomplete drainage or accumulation of the air or fluid along the chest wall.
      i. A horizontally or obliquely oriented tube in frontal chest radiograph suggests tube placement in the fissure. The same can be confirmed on a lateral radiograph of the chest.
      ii. Malposition of the ICT in the pulmonary parenchyma may cause lung laceration, hematoma or a bronchopleural fistula. It is usually better visualized on a CT.
      iii. Other rare misplacement of the ICT includes mediastinal placement with injury to the mediastinal structures and transdiaphragmatic course of the tube to cause injury to the infra- diaphragmatic structures. These are also better evaluated on cross sectional imaging like CT.
   d. *Complications*:
      i. Extra pleural hematoma due to intercostal vessel injury.
      ii. Pulmonary oedema due to rapid drainage of the pleural contents.
      iii. Residual thickening of the pleura may be seen along the tube tract after its removal.

4. **Nasogastric nasoenteric tube**:
   a. *Aim*: Nutritional support and gastric decompression.
   b. *Position of tube*: The tip of the nasogastric tube is ideally positioned beyond the cardia so that the side port is located distal to the gastroesophageal junction.

      If a small-bore NE tube is used, its tip should be located in the second part of duodenum, so as to reduce the risk of aspiration.
   c. *Malposition*: The tube lies coiled within the hypopharynx or esophagus, trachea or the bronchial tree, with resultant pleural, pulmonary parenchymal or diaphragmatic injury.
   d. *Complications*: Pneumothorax, hydropneumothorax, pulmonary parenchymal opacities due to malposition of the tube.

Perforation of viscuslike esophagus and stomach may present on radiograph with mediastinal abnormalities like widening, pneumomediastinum, air fluid levels and pneumoperitoneum.

5. **Central venous catheters**
   a. *Aim*: For medication administration, fluid management, and monitoring.
   b. *Position of catheter*: The tip of a central venous catheter should be positioned in the superior vena cava just superior to the right atrium.
   c. *Malposition*: Malposition of the catheter may occur in as high as 40% cases, and the tip may lie in the right atrium, azygos vein or the internal jugular vein.
   d. *Complications*:
      i. Right atrial placement of the tip of the catheter-arrhythmia, myocardial rupture and cardiac tamponade.
      ii. Pneumothorax is the next most common complication
      iii. Inadvertent vascular perforation—Extra pleural hematoma, hemothorax and mediastinal hematoma
      iv. Vascular perforation—identified by injecting contrast medium through the catheter
      v. Twisted/kinked catheter forming a loop
      vi. Rarely, it may fragment due to compression of the catheter between the clavicle and the first rib, called "pinch-off syndrome"
6. **Other devices**:
   a. *Dialysis catheters*: Check for proper positioning within the SVC or right atrium and assess for signs of thrombosis.
   b. *Pulmonary artery catheters (Swan-Ganz)*: Ensure the catheter tip is within the pulmonary artery and not in a bronchus or pulmonary vein.
   c. *Pacemakers*: Temporary pacing in ICU setting—best achieved by transvenous pacing, via either internal jugular or subclavian veins.

Pulmonary Infections and Pulmonary Interstitium

1. Write short note on pulmonary aspergilloma. [5] [MD (WBUHS) 23, AIIMS May 24]

Pulmonary Aspergilloma

- Aspergillomas (mycetomas) are mass-like fungus balls (mycetomas)—typically saprophytic infection that are composed of *Aspergillus fumigatus*.
- Noninvasive form of pulmonary aspergillosis.
- Pathologically, aspergilloma consists of a combination of fungal hyphae, cellular debris, and mucus within a cavity.
- Aspergillomas occur in patients with normal immune status but structurally abnormal lungs, with pre-existing cavitation like-
  - Pulmonary tuberculosis (most common)
  - Pulmonary sarcoidosis
  - Bronchiectasis from any cause
  - Other pulmonary cavities
    - Bronchogenic cyst
    - Pulmonary sequestration
    - Pneumocystis pneumonia associated pneumatoceles.

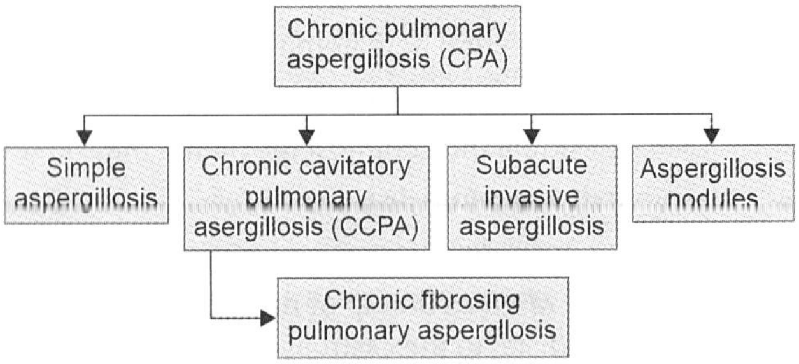

FLOWCHART 1: Classification of chronic aspergillosis.

Classification of chronic aspergillosis is given in **Flowchart 1**:

Clinical Presentations Include

Generally asymptomatic. When symptoms are present, cough, weight loss, and hemoptysis are common.

Imaging findings:

- **Chest X-ray**: Aspergilloma usually appears as a round or oval mass (the "fungus ball") partially filling a cavity and creating the characteristic finding of the air-crescent sign, commonly in the upper lobes. If the fungus ball completely fills the pulmonary cavity, the air-crescent sign may not be discernible.[8] Aspergillomas often show mobility with decubitus imaging.
- **CT scan**: Provides more details, findings are
  - A dense, homogeneous opacity.
  - A surrounding air crescent sign (air surrounding the mass).
  - Possible associated bronchial obstruction or consolidation can be evaluated.

2. Describe HRCT findings of pulmonary involvement in different stages of COVID-19 infection and CT severity index of COVID-19 infection. [10] [MD (WBUHS) 21]

The HRCT findings of pulmonary involvement in different stages of COVID- 19 infections are:[9]

1. **Early Stage (0-4 Days)**:
   a. Ground-glass Opacities (GGO): The most common finding in the early phase, often peripheral and subpleural in distribution.
   b. Unilateral or Bilateral Involvement: Lesions may initially be unilateral but can become bilateral.
   c. No or Minimal Crazy-paving Pattern: The crazy-paving pattern (thickened interlobular septa within areas of GGO) is not typically seen.
2. **Progressive Stage (5-8 Days)**:
   a. Increasing Ground-glass Opacities: The areas of GGO tend to increase in size and number.
   b. Consolidation: Areas of consolidation may begin to appear in combination with GGO.
   c. Crazy-paving Pattern: This becomes more evident, with thickened interlobular and intralobular septa superimposed on GGO.
3. **Peak Stage (9–13 Days)**:
   a. Diffuse Ground-Glass Opacities: GGOs are typically diffuse and bilateral, involving multiple lobes.
   b. Consolidation: Consolidation becomes more prominent and widespread.
   c. Crazy-Paving Pattern: prominent.
   d. Pleural Effusion: Can be seen in severe cases.
4. **Absorption or Late Stage (≥14 Days)**:
   a. Gradual Decrease in Ground-Glass Opacities and Consolidation: As the infection resolves, the GGOs and areas of consolidation begin to decrease.
   b. Fibrotic Changes: Reticulation and subpleural fibrotic bands may develop, leading to potential long-term pulmonary fibrosis in severe cases.
   c. Residual Lesions: Some patients may have long-lasting GGO or fibrotic streaks.

The typical features on CT imaging of COVID-19 **(Table 4)**:

TABLE 4: Typical findings of COVID-19 on CT.

Parameter	*Characteristic manifestations on CT imaging*
Density	Ground glass opacity and consolidation, possible interlobular septal thickening
Shape	Patchy, sub-segmental, or segmental
Distribution	Mid and lower lungs along the bronchovascular bundles with bilateral involvement
Location	Peripheral and subpleural areas of the lung parenchyma
Concomitant signs (variable)	Air bronchogram, a small amount of pleural effusion, no obvious lymphadenopathy

CT involvement Score

The severity of the lung involvement on the CT correlates with the severity of the disease.

Visual Assessment

- The severity on CT can be estimated by visual assessment. This is the easiest way to score the severity.
- The CT images show a 25% involvement by visual assessment.

Severity Score

Another method is by scoring the percentages of each of the five lobes that is involved:
- <5% involvement
- 5–25% involvement
- 26–49% involvement
- 50–75% involvement
- >75% involvement.

The total CT score is the sum of the individual lobar scores and can range from 0 (no involvement) to 25 (maximum involvement), when all the five lobes show more than 75% involvement.

Some say that the percentage of lung involvement can be calculated by multiplying the total score times 4.

This, however, is not true. Suppose that all lobes have a 10% involvement, then this would lead to an overall score of 10, which could lead to the impression that 40% of the lungs are involved.

CT Severity Grading

Score	*CT severity*
<8	Mild
9–15	Moderate
>15	Severe

3. Classify different types of Emphysema. Discuss the role of HRCT in evaluation of types of emphysema. [10] [MD (WBUHS) 19]

Introduction: Emphysema is defined as a condition characterized by permanent abnormal enlargement of airspaces with destruction of walls, distal to terminal bronchioles, without associated fibrosis.[10]

Types of emphysema:
- Centrilobular emphysema
- Paraseptal emphysema
- Panlobular emphysema
- Bullous emphysema
- Paracicatricial emphysema

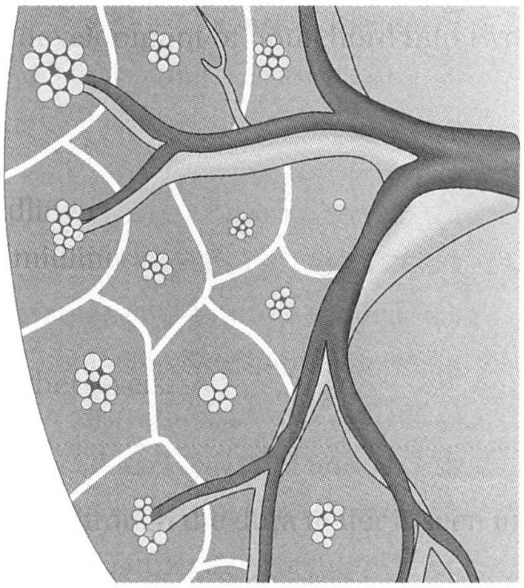
FIG. 13: Centrilobular emphysema.

The HRCT findings of various types of emphysema:
- **Centrilobular emphysema (Fig. 13)**:
    - Well defined round centrilobular lucencies, mainly in upper lobe
    - Well-defined margin differentiating emphysematous lung from normal lung giving heterogenous appearance
    - Margin of secondary pulmonary lobule is preserved.
    - *Features of pulmonary arterial hypertension*: Enlargement of central pulmonary arteries with peripheral pruning
- **Panlobular emphysema (Fig. 14)**.
    - Affects whole secondary pulmonary lobule uniformly
    - Ill-defined areas of decreased CT attenuation
    - Paucity of vessels
    - Vascular distortion
    - Homogenously distributed
    - Mainly in lower lobe
    - Features of hyperinflation
    - Bronchiectasis ±

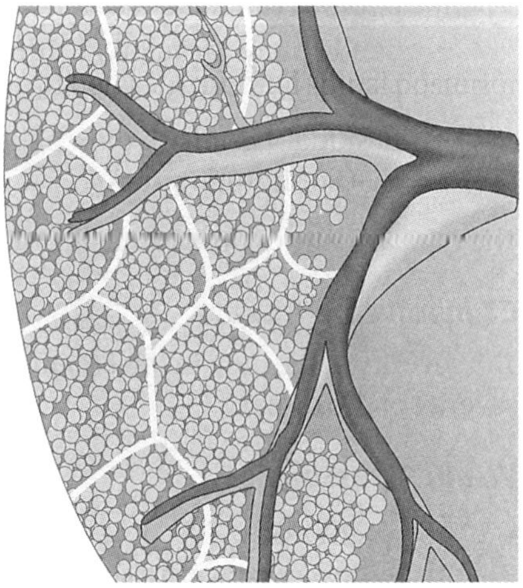
FIG. 14: Panlobular emphysema.

- Associated with alpha 1 antitrypsin deficiency and smokers in advanced stage
- **Paraseptal emphysema (Fig. 15)**:
  - Small subpleural and peribronchovascular cystic spaces arranged in a linear fashion, separated by interlobular septa
  - Large bulla which may rupture to cause pneumothorax
  - Mainly in upper lobe

MinIP images—better detection of emphysema

CT Densitometry: For quantification of emphysema

- *Paracicatricial or irregular emphysema*:
  - Secondary to pulmonary fibrosis, focal and diffuse
  - Secondarily in pneumoconiosis.

The different types of emphysema and their imaging features and clinical history are presented in a tabular form **(Table 5)**.

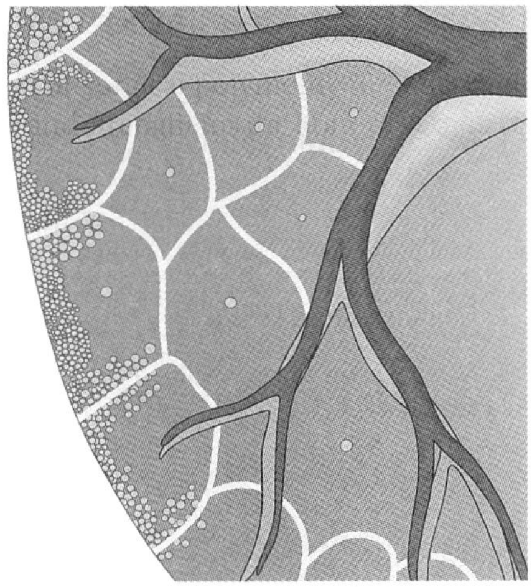

FIG 15: Paraseptal emphysema.

TABLE 5: Types of emphysema and their imaging features and clinical history.

Emphysema			
Mild centrilobular emphysema	Multiple small lucencies without a wall	Upper lobe predominance: uneven distribution. Centrilobular; centrilobular arteriole may be visible	Smoking history
Advanced, confluent centrilobular emphysema	Irregular, confluent lucencies; walls can often be recognized	Upper lobe predominance: uneven distribution	Smoking history. Lung destruction is evident
Mild panlobular emphysema	Overall decrease in king attenuation and size reduction of vessels	Generalized or lower lobe predominance	May be associated with alpha-1-antitrypsin deficiency. Sometimes difficult to differentiate from decreased perfusion
Advanced panlobular emphysema	Overall decrease in lung attenuation and size reduction of vessels with areas of evident lung destruction	Generalized or lower lobe predominance	May be associated with alpha-l-antitrypsin deficiency. Sometimes difficult to differentiate from advanced confluent emphysema
Paraseptal emphysema	Single layer of subplural lucencies often with visible thin wall	Upper lobe predominance: subpleural location. Thin walls corresponding with interlobular septa	
Bullous emphysema	Large air-containing areas (1 cm to several centimeters) Thin wall	Predominantly subpleural upper lobes, Often asymmetric	Bullae may increase progressively. Smokers and nonsmokers. Often associated with centrilobular and paraseptal emphysema

4. Classify the diffuse lung diseases. Discuss in brief the salient imaging findings of diffuse cystic lung diseases. [5+5] [MD (WBUHS) 22]

Diffuse lung diseases: Also known as interstitial lung diseases are group of lung diseases that are characterized by inflammation, fibrosis and scarring affecting the interstitium and surrounding alveoli.[11,12]

Classification of diffuse parenchymal lung diseases (DPLDs):

Category	*Examples*
1. DPLD of known cause or association	Drug toxicity Associated connective tissue disease (CTD) Hypersensitivity pneumonitis Pneumoconiosis
2. Granulomatous DPLD	Sarcoidosis
3. Rare DPLD with well-defined features	Lymphangioleiomyomatosis (LAM) Langerhans' cell histiocytosis (LCH) Respiratory bronchiolitis interstitial lung disease Cryptogenic organizing pneumonia (COP)
4. Idiopathic interstitial pneumonia (IIP)	Idiopathic pulmonary fibrosis (IPF) Nonspecific interstitial pneumonia (NSIP) Acute interstitial pneumonia (AIP) Desquamative interstitial pneumonia (DIP)

Imaging Findings in Diffuse Cystic Lung Diseases

Introduction: Cysts are well defined parenchymal spaces containing air and surrounded by thin wall (thickness <3 mm).

The diagnostic algorithm for evaluating cystic lung diseases is presented in **Flowchart 2** as follows:

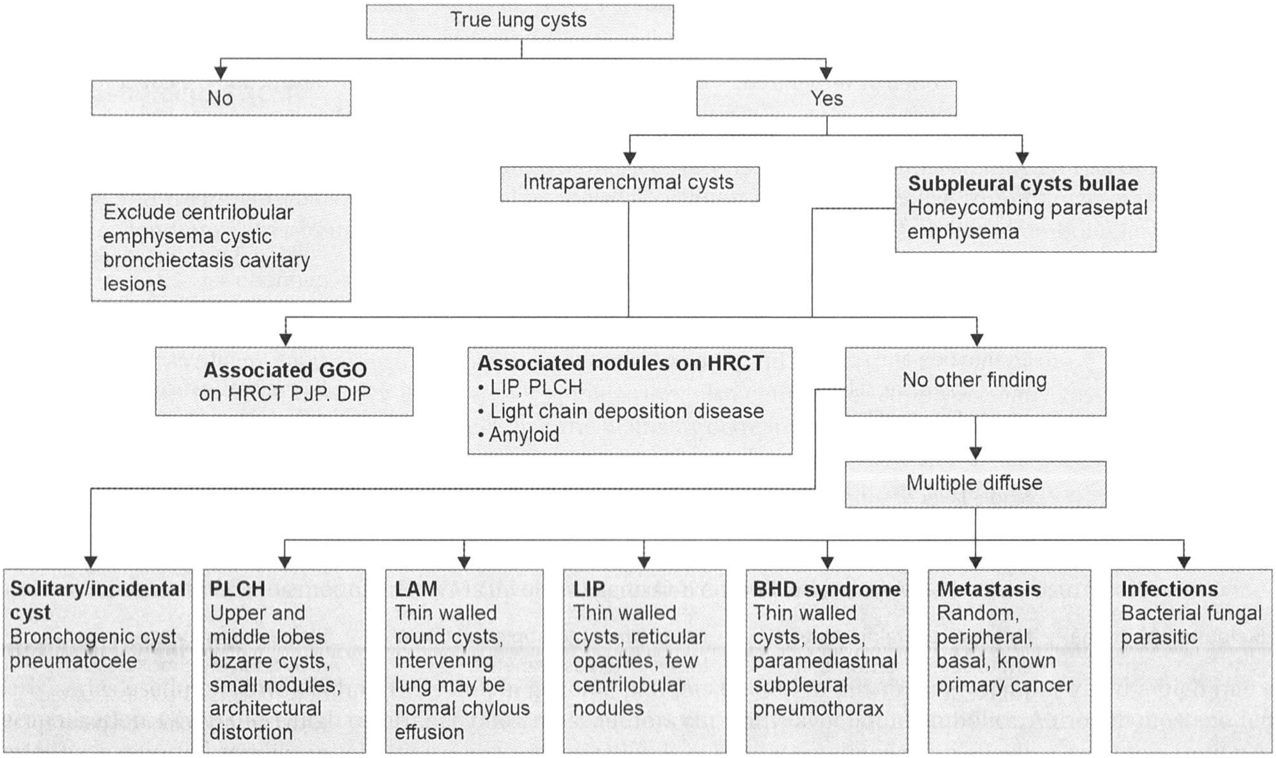

FLOWCHART 2: Diagnostic algorithm for evaluating cystic lung diseases.
(GGO: ground-glass opacity; LCH: Langerhans cell histiocytosis; LAM: lymphangioleiomyomatosis; LIP: lymphoid interstitial pneumonia)

The differentiating features of important cystic lung diseases are presented in **Tables 6 and 7**, and **Figure 16**. Mimickers of cystic lung diseases are shown in **Table 8**.

TABLE 6: Differentiating features of important cystic lung diseases.

Disease	*Imaging*	*Distribution*	*Additional findings*
PLCH	Nodules with cysts (Irregular bizarre-shaped cysts)	Predominantly upper zones, spares basal zones	Lung volume normal or hyperinflated
LAM	Thin-walled cysts (uniform round cyst)	Random, diffuse	Chylous effusion
Tuberous sclerosis	Thin-walled cysts	Randomly distributed	Angiomyolipomas of kidneys and liver; other features of TS
LIP	Well-defined cysts	Predominantly in basal zones	Ground glass haze

TABLE 7: Difference between PLCH and LAM.

	PLCH	*LAM*
Age	20–40 years M=F	30–35 years Female
Cysts	Cysts are irregular and are of varying shapes such as bilobed, cloverleaf shaped or bizarre shaped. Nodules may be seen in the intervening lung parenchyma between the cysts	Cysts are round and uniform May show features similar to tuberous sclerosis
Location	Upper and mid zones, relatively sparing lower zones and CP angles	No zonal predominance Uniformly distributed
Lung volume	Preserved	Preserved
Intervening lungs	Nodular with mild architectural distortion	Usually normal
Other findings	Pneumothorax	Chylous effusion Pneumothorax

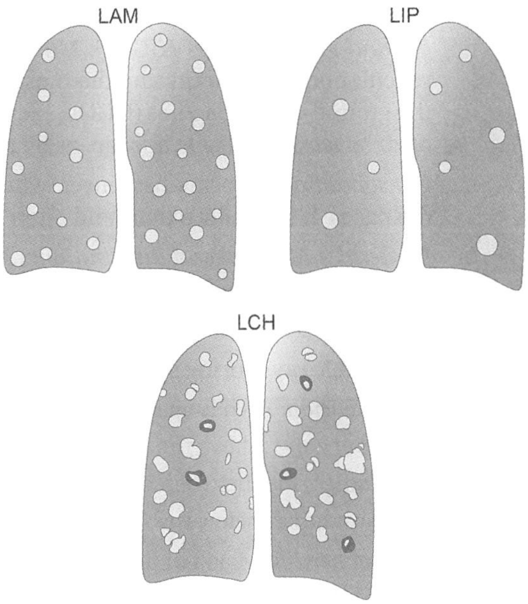

FIG. 16: Different characteristics of cysts in LCH, LAM and LIP.

TABLE 8: Few conditions mimicking of cystic lung diseases.

Conditions	*Imaging*	*Distribution*	*Additional findings*
Honeycombing	Multilayered honeycomb cysts	Subpleural, peripheral, basal zones	Intra-and interlobular interstitial thickening, ground glass haze
Cystic bronchiectasis	Cysts continuous with bronchial structures	Focal or diffuse, depending on etiology	Signet ring sign
Centri lobular emphysema	Cystic airspaces without wall	Upper lobe predominance	Vessels coursing through the cyst
Paraseptal emphysema	Cystic air spaces without wall	Subpleural, more in upper lobes	Cysts adjacent to pleural surface
Bullae	Round focal lucency or decreased attenuation >1 cm in size	Focal or diffuse	Adjacent lungs show emphysematous changes
Cavity	Often thick walled (>4 mm), irregular shaped gas-filled space/lucency within pulmonary consolidation or mass, or nodule	Distribution depending on the etiology	Consolidation or mass seen

5. Discuss the role of radiography in COVID-19 patients. [10] [MD (WBUHS) 22]

Role of Radiography in COVID-19 Patients

Radiography helps in diagnosing, assessing, and managing COVID-19 patients, especially during the early stages of the disease. The imaging modalities used are chest X-rays (CXR) and computed tomography (CT) scans, both of which help in assessing the extent of lung involvement in COVID-19 and monitoring disease progression.[13,14]

1. Diagnosis by Imaging and Assessment

a. **Chest X-rays (CXR) findings**: Although chest radiograph is not routinely used in clinical settings because they are insensitive to detect COVID-19 in the early stage, however chest radiography is typically the first-line imaging modality used for patients with suspected COVID-19 patients. In cases where the patient's physical condition does not allow for transport to the radiology department for CT scan of thorax, in such cases chest X-ray is used. Findings are:

   i. *Ground-glass opacities (GGOs)*: Most common findings reported are interstitial abnormalities, reticular and reticulonodular patterns and the most common alveolar findings include hazy pulmonary opacities similar to the ground-glass opacities (GGOs) identified on CT. Hazy areas of opacities on the lungs indicate partial filling of air spaces. It typically appears as bilateral, posterior and peripheral locations.

   ii. *Consolidation*: Appears as denser, white areas on the CXR and represents fluid or solid material filling the airspaces. It is usually patchy and often bilateral.

   iii. *Bilateral and peripheral distribution*: CXR findings are typically bilateral and are more frequently observed in the lower lung zones and peripheral locations.

   iv. Even pleural fluid (in a severe case) has been found on the chest radiographs.

   Brixia Chest X-ray scoring system for COVID-19:

   1. *Lung division*: Each lung is divided into three zones:
      - Upper zone (above the carina)
      - Middle zone (between carina and inferior pulmonary vein)
      - Lower zone (below the inferior pulmonary vein)
   2. *Scoring per zone*: Each of the six lung zones is scored based on the extent and nature of the lung abnormalities:
      - 0: No lung abnormalities.
      - 1: Interstitial infiltrates.
      - 2: Interstitial and alveolar infiltrates (mixed pattern).
      - 3: Predominantly alveolar infiltrates.
   3. *Total score*: Scores from all six zones are summed to give a total score, ranging from 0–18. Higher scores indicate more severe lung involvement.
      - *Mild (Score 0–6)*: Typically associated with mild symptoms or asymptomatic cases.
      - *Moderate (Score 7–12)*: Indicates moderate lung involvement, often requiring close monitoring and possibly supplemental oxygen.
      - *Severe (Score 13–18)*: Severe lung involvement, often correlating with hypoxia and potential need for intensive care.

b. **HRCT findings**: HRCT have a sensitivity and detects early lung involvement in COVID-19 patients. Findings are:

   - *Ground-glass opacities (GGOs)*: GGOs are seen as areas of increased opacity, described as hazy, which partially obscure the lung's normal structure. They are usually multifocal, bilateral and peripheral, but in the early phase it may present as a unifocal lesion, most commonly located in the inferior lobe of the right lung.
   - *Crazy-paving pattern*: GGOs with interlobular septal thickening, resembling paving stones. It indicates disease progression.
   - Air space consolidation
   - Bronchovascular thickening
   - Traction bronchiectasis
   - *Air bronchograms*: Air-filled bronchi within areas of lung consolidation or GGOs.
   - *Vascular enlargement*: Associated with increased vessel caliber in areas of GGOs.

- *Subpleural and peripheral locations*: Predominantly subpleural and peripheral, often affecting multiple lobes and both lungs.
- *Fibrotic changes*: In more advanced or severe cases, patients may show fibrotic bands or reticulations, which can indicate the formation of scar tissue.

CT Manifestations of Different Stages of COVID-19 (Table 9)

TABLE 9: Stagewise lung involvement in COVID-19.

Early stage	*Advanced stage*	*Severe stage*	*Dissipation stage*
Single or multiple scattered patchy ground-glass opacities, predominately distributed in the peripheral and subpleural area of the lung. A crazy-paving pattern, secondary to intralobular and interlobular septal thickening can be seen in this stage.	Increased extent and density of bilateral lung parenchymal opacities. In this image, there are both areas of ground glass opacification and areas of consolidation in both lungs, which coexist and have varying sizes and presence of air bronchogram.	Diffuse consolidation of the lung parenchyma with uneven density, air bronchi and bronchial dilation, which maybe present as "whited out lung" on a corresponding chest radiograph.	Areas of ground glass opacity and consolidation have nearly completely resolved, leaving some residual curvilinear areas of density.

The HRCT findings of pulmonary involvement in different stages of COVID-19 infections **(Table 9)** are:

- **Early Stage (0–4 Days)**:
  - *Ground-glass opacities (GGO)*: The most common finding in the early phase, often peripheral and subpleural in distribution.
  - *Unilateral or bilateral involvement*: Lesions may initially be unilateral but can become bilateral.
  - *No or minimal crazy-paving pattern*: The crazy-paving pattern (thickened interlobular septa within areas of GGO) is not typically seen.
- **Progressive Stage (5–8 Days)**:
  - *Increasing ground-glass opacities*: The areas of GGO tend to increase in size and number.
  - *Consolidation*: Areas of consolidation may begin to appear in combination with GGO.
  - *Crazy-paving pattern*: This becomes more evident, with thickened interlobular and intralobular septa superimposed on GGO.
- **Peak Stage (9–13 Days)**:
  - *Diffuse Ground-glass Opacities*: GGOs are typically diffuse and bilateral, involving multiple lobes.
  - *Consolidation*: Consolidation becomes more prominent and widespread.
  - *Crazy-paving Pattern*: Prominent
  - *Pleural effusion*: Can be seen in severe cases
- **Absorption or Late Stage (≥14 Days)**:
  - *Gradual decrease in ground-glass opacities and consolidation*: As the infection resolves, the GGOs and areas of consolidation begin to decrease.
  - *Fibrotic changes*: Reticulation and subpleural fibrotic bands may develop, leading to potential long-term pulmonary fibrosis in severe cases.
  - *Residual LESIONS*: Some patients may have long-lasting GGO or fibrotic streaks.

The Typical Features on CT Imaging of COVID-19 (Table 10)

TABLE 10: Typical findings of COVID-19 on CT.

Parameter	*Characteristic manifestations on CT imaging*
Density	Ground glass opacity and consolidation, possible interlobular septal thickening
Shape	Patchy, sub-segmental, or segmental
Distribution	Mid and lower lungs along the bronchovasular bundles with bilateral involvement
Location	Peripheral and subpleural areas of the lung parenchyma
Concomitant signs (variable)	Air bronchogram, a small amount of pleural effusion, no obvious lymphadenopathy

CT involvement score: The severity of the lung involvement on the CT correlates with the severity of the disease.

Visual Assessment

The severity on CT can be estimated by visual assessment. This is the easiest way to score the severity.

The CT images show a 25% involvement by visual assessment.

Severity Score

Another method is by scoring the percentages of each of the five lobes that is involved:

1. <5% involvement
2. 5–25% involvement
3. 26–49% involvement
4. 50–75% involvement
5. >75% involvement.

The total CT score is the sum of the individual lobar scores and can range from 0 (no involvement) to 25 (maximum involvement), when all the five lobes show more than 75% involvement.

Some say that the percentage of lung involvement can be calculated by multiplying the total score times 4.

This however is not true. Suppose that all lobes have a 10% involvement, then this would lead to an overall score of 10, which could lead to the impression that 40% of the lungs are involved.

CT Severity Grading

Score	*CT severity*
<8	Mild
9–15	Moderate
>15	Severe

c. **USG findings**: Ultrasound have advantages that it does not expose patients to ionizing radiation and is easily accessible in terms of its portability and the ability to perform bedside examinations. Findings are:
   a. Multiple B-lines: vertically oriented hyperechoic artifacts that originate from the pleura or from areas of consolidation. These lines indicate accumulation of fluid in the pulmonary interstitial space or alveoli.
   b. A-lines can then be seen in the recovery phase of the disease.
   c. Irregular, thickened pleural line with scattered discontinuities.
   d. Subpleural and alveolar consolidations
   d. Other imaging modalities like MRI and nuclear medicine rarely used.

Monitoring Disease Progression

- Follow-up imaging: Radiography used to monitor the progression of COVID-19 pneumonia in hospitalized patients, especially in intensive care and planned treatment according to imaging changes.
- Severity scoring: Both X-rays and CT scans were used to quantify the extent of lung involvement by grading severity scores.

Complication Detection

Identifies COVID-19-related complications such as acute respiratory distress syndrome (ARDS), pulmonary embolism, and secondary infections. CT accurately diagnosed thrombotic events, which is a known as a significant complication in COVID-19 patients and required immediate intervention.

Guiding Treatment Decisions

Help in treatment decisions like whether antiviral therapies, corticosteroids, or respiratory support (such as ventilators) were needed.

6. Describe anatomy of secondary pulmonary lobule on HRCT. Describe role of HRCT in the diagnosis of interstitial lung disease. [3+7] [DNB Dec 19, AIIMS Dec 23]

Secondary Pulmonary Lobule (Fig. 17)

1. Smallest unit of lung.
2. Polyhedron in shape.
3. Bonded by connective tissue.
4. Incorporating 3–24 acini.
5. 5–30 mm in diameter.
6. Terminal bronchiole and pulmonary artery in the center and pulmonary vein and lymphatics in the periphery.
7. When there is thickening of the septa then only it is visible.

Role of HRCT in the Diagnosis of Interstitial Lung Disease

Introduction: Interstitial lung diseases (ILDs) are defined as a group of diffuse lung parenchymal disorder that affects the interstitium, and space around the alveoli from varying degrees of inflammation and fibrosis.

Modality of Choice for Diagnosis: HRCT Thorax

- Radiological features and differential diagnosis of the idiopathic interstitial pneumonias **(Table 11)**:
- The HRCT chest findings associated with specific clinical diseases **(Table 12)**:
- Difference between UIP pattern and idiopathic NSIP is given in **Table 13.**
- Different types of UIP pattern and their diagnostic criteria according to Fleischner society **(Table 14)**:

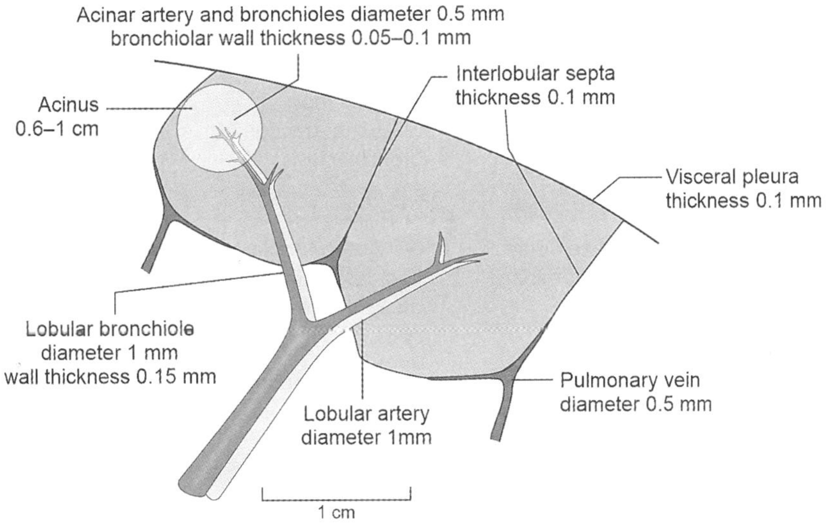

FIG. 17: Normal anatomy of pulmonary lobule.

TABLE 11: Radiological features and differential diagnosis of interstitial pneumonias.

IIP Group and clinical radiologic pathologic diagnosis	*HRCT patterns*	*Typical HRCT distribution*	*Typical HRCT findings*	*HRCT differential diagnosis*
Chronic fibrosing IIPs				
Idiopathic pulmonary fibrosis	Usual Interstitial pneumonia	Peripheral, subpleural, basal	Reticular opacities, honeycombing, traction bronchiectasis, architectural distortion	Collagen vascular disease, hypersensitivity pneumonitis, asbestosis, sarcoidosis

Continued...

Continued...

IIP Group and clinical radiologic pathologic diagnosis	*HRCT patterns*	*Typical HRCT distribution*	*Typical HRCT findings*	*HRCT differential diagnosis*
Idiopathic nonspecific interstitial pneumonia	Nonspecific interstitial pneumonia	Peripheral, basal, symmetric	GGO, Irregular lines, traction bronchiectasis, consolidation	Usual interstitial pneumonia, cryptogenic organizing pneumonia, desquamative interstitial pneumonia, hypersensitivity pneumonitis
Smoking IIPs				
Desquamative interstitial pneumonia	Desquamative interstitial pneumonia	Lower zone, peripheral predominance in most cases	GGO, reticular lines, cysts	Respiratory bronchiolitis—interstitial lung disease, nonspecific interstitial pneumonia, hypersensitivity pneumonitis
Respiratory bronchiolitis-associated interstitial lung disease	Respiratory bronchiolitis	Upper lung predominant	Centrilobular nodules, bronchial wall thickening, patchy GGO	Nonspecific interstitial pneumonia, desquamative interstitial pneumonia, hypersensitivity pneumonitis
Acute or Subacute IIPs				
Cryptogenic organizing pneumonia	Organizing pneumonia	Subpleural or peribronchial	Patchy consolidation or nodules, perilobular pattern, reverse halo sign	Infection, aspiration pneumonia, eosinophilic pneumonia, nonspecific interstitial pneumonia, vasculitis, sarcoidosis, neoplasms, lymphoma
Acute interstitial pneumonia	Diffuse alveolar damage	Bilateral or patchy	Consolidation, GGO, later traction bronchiectasis	Hydrostatic edema, pulmonary hemorrhage, acute eosinophilic pneumonia
Rare IIPs				
Lymphoid interstitial pneumonia	Lymphoid interstitial pneumonia	Lower lung predominant	GGO, centrilobular nodules, peribronchial thickening, thin-walled cysts	Nonspecific interstitial pneumonia, sarcoidosis, Langerhans cell histiocytosis, lymphangioleiomyomatosis
Idiopathic pleuroparenchymal fibro-elastosis	Idiopathic pleuroparenchymal fibroelastosis	Peripheral, upper lung predominant	Pleural thickening, subpleural fibrotic changes or consolidation	Sarcoidosis, pneumoconiosis, postinfective pulmonary fibrosis, connective tissue disease, hypersensitivity pneumonitis

TABLE 12: HRCT chest findings associated with specific clinical diseases.

Thin-section CT finding	*Common clinical disease*
Reticular opacities	• Idiopathic pulmonary fibrosis • Nonspecific interstitial pneumonia • Asbestosis drug-related fibrosis • Fibrotic hypersensitivity pneumonitis • Connective tissue disease, interstitial lung disease
Honeycombing	• Idiopathic pulmonary fibrosis • Fibrotic nonspecific interstitial pneumonia • Fibrotic hypersensitivity pneumonitis • Sarcoidosis (rare)

Continued...

Continued...

Thin-section CT finding	***Common clinical disease***
Ground-glass opacities	• Nonspecific interstitial pneumonia • Acute interstitial pneumonia • Respiratory bronchiolitis, interstitial lung disease • Desquamative interstitial pneumonia • Lymphoid interstitial pneumonia • Organizing pneumonia • Hypersensitivity pneumonitis
Consolidation	• Organizing pneumonia • Acute interstitial pneumonia • Drug toxicity polymyositis • Dermatomyositis • Antisynthetase • Sarcoidosis (rare)
Cysts (nonhoneycomb)	• Pulmonary langerhans cell histiocytosis • Lymphangioleiomyomatosis • Lymphoid interstitial pneumonia • Desquamative interstitial pneumonia • Birt-Hogg-Dubé • Light-chain deposition disease *Pneumocystis jirovecii pneumonia*

TABLE 13: Differentiating features of UIP pattern and idiopathic NSIP.

UIP	***NSIP***
Older age of presentation (>50 years)	40–50 years
Honeycombing is diagnostic	Honeycombing absent
GGO less common and less extensive than reticular abnormalities	GGO predominance favors NSIP
Peripheral distribution	Peribronchovascular/peripheral distribution
Subpleural areas involved	Immediate subpleural sparing in cases of peripheral distribution
Can progressively involve upper lobes	Lower lobe predominance is almost always there
Patchy heterogeneous involvement	Homogeneous involvement

TABLE 14: Different type of UIP pattern and their diagnostic features.

Diagnostic category		***Fleischner society statement***
	Distribution	***Features***
Typical UIP	Subpleural and basal-predominant abnormality Often heterogeneous, can be diffuse	Honeycomb cyst formation Reticulation with traction bronchiectasis or bronchiolectasis Absence of features to suggest an alternative diagnosis
Probable UIP	Subpleural and basal predominant Often heterogeneous	Reticulation with traction bronchiectasis or bronchiolectasis Absence of honeycombing Absence of features to suggest an alternative diagnosis
Indeterminate for UIP	Variable or diffuse; not predominantly sub-pleural or basal	Reticulation with some inconspicuous or minor findings chat suggest an alternative, non-IPF diagnosis
CT features most consistent with a non-IPF diagnosis or alternative diagnosis	Upper or mid lung predominant Areas of subpleural sparing with peribronchovascular predominance	Predominant consolidation Widespread pure GGO (without acute exacerbation) Widespread mosaic attenuation with substantially sharply defined lobular expiratory air trapping Diffuse nodules or cysts

7. Discuss the thoracic imaging manifestations in Collagen vascular diseases. [10]

Introduction: Connective tissue disorders also called collagen vascular disease are autoimmune disorders involving multiple systems. Pulmonary manifestations can happen due to the disease per se or due to the medical therapy.

Diseases included are:

- Rheumatoid arthritis
- Progressive systemic sclerosis
- Systemic lupus erythematosus
- Polymyositis, dermatomyositis
- Sjogren syndrome
- Mixed connective tissue disease

Thoracic manifestations of the diseases on HRCT are as follows:

1. **Rheumatoid Arthritis**
   a. *Interstitial pneumonia and fibrosis*:
      i. Most common pulmonary manifestation. Histologically, it may represent UIP, NIP, OP, or LIP.
      ii. Findings are
      iii. Ground-glass opacity, fine reticulation or coarse reticulation or irregular reticulation, honeycombing.
      iv. Basal and peripheral predominance.
      v. Immediate and subpleural sparing may be present in NSIP pattern.
      vi. OP–. patchy consolidation, nodules, or the "reversed halo or atoll sign"
      vii. Cystic lucencies in LIP may mimic honeycombing.
      viii. Predominance in the posterior and subpleural lung and at the lung bases is typical of reticular opacities and ground-glass opacity in patients with RA.
      ix. Sometimes present with overlap of various interstitial pneumonia patterns, with features of NSIP, OP, and LIP superimposed.

   b. *Pleura*:
      i. Aseptic pleural effusion having cholesterol crystals, unilateral>bilateral
      ii. Coexistent with rheumatoid nodules
      iii. Pneumothorax and bronchopleural fistula

   c. **Airways Large airway**
      i. Cricoarytenoid arthritis due to cricoarytenoid joint involvement
      ii. Compromised upper airway
      iii. Bronchiectasis

   d. *Small airway*: Follicular and constrictive bronchiolitis due to the disease or recurrent infections

   e. *Rheumatoid nodules*:
      i. Size few millimeters to 5 cm or more.
      ii. May be solitary or multiple and numerous.
      iii. Predominate in the lung periphery and are typically well defined.
      iv. They may cavitate, having thick walls that become thin with healing.

   e. *Caplan's syndrome*:
      i. Rare presentation of RA.
      ii. Occur in coal miners or patients with occupational exposures to silicates.
      iii. Caplan's syndrome is characterized by single or multiple lung nodules ranging from a few millimeters to 5 cm in diameter, similar to rheumatoid nodules. The nodules may cavitate. An upper lobe predominance may be seen, resembling silicosis or coal worker's pneumoconiosis.

   f. *Pulmonary hypertension*: Pulmonary hypertension usually occurs secondary to pulmonary fibrosis.

2. **Systemic Sclerosis**

   Lung:
   - Most common pattern—NSIP
     - *Early phase*: Ground glass opacities
     - *Later phase*: Intra and interlobular septal thickening
     - Traction bronchiectasis
     - Bronchiolectasis
     - Honeycombing
     - Microcysts
   - Second most common pattern—UIP
     - Honeycombing seen
     - Worse prognosis
     - Overlap of NSIP and UIP patterns may be seen

   Other findings:
   - Dilated esophagus
       - Aspiration pneumonitis
       - Features of pulmonary hypertension
       - Right ventricular strain
       - Superior surface of ribs eroded
       - Pneumothorax
3. **Systemic Lupus Erythematosus**
   - *Pulmonary hemorrhage*: Bilateral; ground glass opacities and consolidation
   - *Infections*: Community acquired or atypical pneumonia, TB
   - *Pulmonary edema*: Due to renal disease
   - *Pulmonary embolism*: Due to hypercoagulable state
   - *Lupus pneumonitis*: Multifocal consolidation with basal predominance
   - Pleural effusion, thickening, fibrosis
   - Interstitial lung disease—UIP/NSIP
   - Lung fibrosis

   Shrinking Lung Syndrome
   - Dysfunction of respiratory muscle
   - Progressive volume loss
   - Basal atelectasis
   - Ill-defined opacities in juxta diaphragmatic locations
4. **Sjögren syndrome**
   - *Lungs*:
     - NSIP more common
     - LIP more specific
     - UIP, COP, amyloidosis
   - *Airways*:
     - Bronchiectasis with wall thickening
     - Follicular and constrictive bronchiolitis
     - Air trapping
   - ***Pleura***: Pleural effusion and thickening

The following signs suggest the diagnosis of CTD related ILD:

- *Straight-edge sign*: It is seen in usual interstitial pneumonia, signifies the distinct boundary between fibrotic areas inferiorly and relatively unaffected lung parenchyma superiorly.

- *Four-corner sign*: It is axial CT feature seen in systemic sclerosis , where affected regions disproportionately involve the bilateral anterolateral upper lobes and posterosuperior lower lobes. Reticular opacities, ground-glass attenuation and/or honeycombing appear distributed in all four corners of the thorax on the same image.
- *Exuberant honeycombing*: It is an HRCT finding typically observed in usual interstitial pneumonia. This sign is characterized by the presence of extensive honeycomb- like cyst formation within the lungs, comprising more than 70% of the fibrotic portions of the lungs.

Summary of HRCT findings of various conditions of connective tissue diseases is given in **Table 15.**

TABLE 15: HRCT pattern of connective tissue disorder.

Type of GD	*Most common HRCT pattern*	*Less common HRCT patterns*
Systemic sclerosis	NSIP	UIP, OP
MCTD	NSIP	UIP, OP
RA	UIP	SAD, NSIP, LIP, OP
PM-DM	NSIP/OP	DAD
SLE	Diffuse alveolar hemorrhage, serositis, infections	NSIP, DAD
Sjögren syndrome	NSIP, LIP, SAD	UIP, DAD

(DAD, diffuse alveolar damage; LIP lymphocytic interstitial pneumonia; NSIP, nonspecific interstitial pneumonia; OP: organizing pneumonia; SAD: small airway disease; UIP: usual interstitial pneumonia)

8. Pathophysiology of covid pulmonary infection. Chest CT protocol. Chest CT findings. [10] [DNB Dec 21]

Pathophysiology of COVID Pulmonary Infection

Pathophysiology of COVID-19 pulmonary infection **(Flowchart 3)** is complex, it involves direct viral damage to lung tissues, an exaggerated immune response, and alterations in blood vessels.[13,14] Mechanisms are:

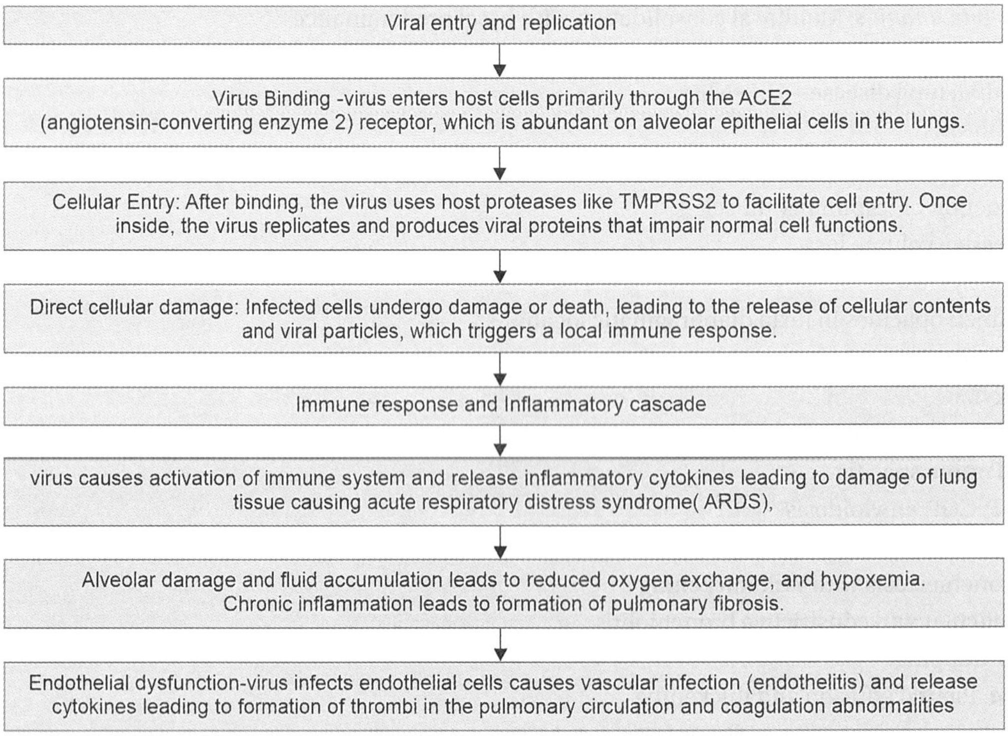

FLOWCHART 3: Pathophysiology of COVID-19 pulmonary infection.

Mechanism of SARS-CoV-2 Invasion into Host Cells

The life cycle of the virus within the host consists of the following five steps:

- Attachment
- Penetration (viral entry to the cell)
- Biosynthesis (viral replication)
- Maturation (assembly and accumulation)
- Release (through cell destruction)

The ACE2 has been identified as a functional receptor for SARS-COV-2. In the human body. ACE2 expression is high in the lung (expressed on lung epithelial cells), heart, gastrointestinal system, kidney, pancreas, spleen, bladder, cornea, and blood vessels. SARS- COV-2 enters a human cell by binding its spike or S protein to the ACE2 receptor of the host, with subsequent fusion of the viral and cell membranes (endocytosis), resulting in viral cell entry and depletion of ACE2 receptors on the cell surface. Once within a cell, the virus activates the intracellular immune system, which causes immune and nonimmune cells to release large amounts of proinflammatory cytokines that activate a cytokine storm and result in damage to the host **(Fig. 18)**.

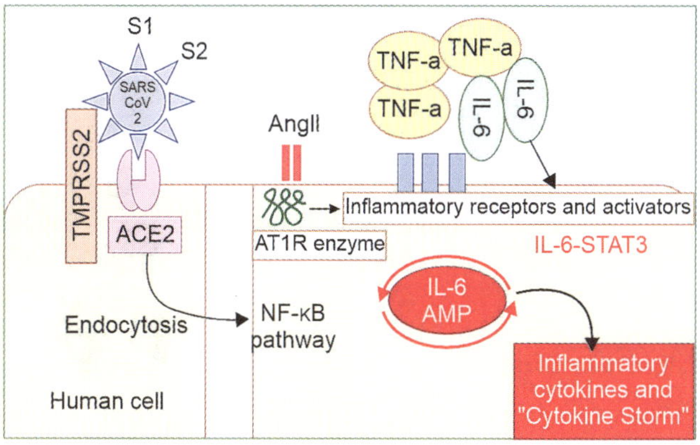

FIG. 18: Illustration shows the proposed mechanism of SARS-CoV-2 cell entry and activation of the immune system. SARS-CoV-2 enters human cells by attaching to a cell surface receptor (ACE) and by utilizing a human enzyme called transmembrane serine protease 2 (TMPRSS2). Once bound to the receptor, SARS-COV-2 undergoes endocytosis and enters into the cell, along with the ACE2 receptor. This process reduces the number of ACE2 receptors on cells, leading to an increase of angiotensin II (Angi) levels in the blood. Angiotensin II triggers an inflammatory pathway involving NF-kB and interleukin 6-signal transducer and activator of transcription 3 protein (IL- 6-STAT3), particularly in nonimmune cells including endothelial and epithelial cells. This pathway forms a positive feedback cycle, named IL-6 amplifier (IL-6 AMP), resulting in its excessive activation and therefore the cytokine storm and ARDS. Part of this pathway involving NF-kB. IL-6-STAT3, or both is enhanced with age, which could be the reason why older patients are more at risk for death following COVID-19 diagnosis compared with other age groups. 51 viral spike protein subunit 1.52 = viral spike protein subunit 2, TNF-a tumor necrosis factor-a.

Chest CT Protocol

The main scanning parameters are given in **Table 16**:

TABLE 16: Chest CT protocol.

Tube voltage	120 kvp
Automatic tube current modulation (tube current)	140–200 mAs
Pitch	0.99–1.22 mm
matrix	512–512
Slice thickness	5 mm
Field of view	350 x 350 mm

HRCT findings: HRCT have a sensitivity and detects early lung involvement in COVID-19 patients **(Fig. 19)**. Findings are:

- **Ground-glass opacities (GGOs)**: GGOs are seen as areas of increased opacity, described as hazy, which partially obscure the lung's normal structure. They are usually multifocal, bilateral and peripheral, but in the early phase it may present as a unifocal lesion, most commonly located in the inferior lobe of the right lung.
- **Crazy-paving Pattern**: GGOs with interlobular septal thickening, resembling paving stones. It indicates disease progression.
- Air space consolidation
- Bronchovascular thickening
- Traction bronchiectasis
- **Air bronchograms**: Air-filled bronchi within areas of lung consolidation or GGOs.
- **Vascular enlargement**: Associated with increased vessel caliber in areas of GGOs.
- **Subpleural and peripheral locations**: Predominantly subpleural and peripheral, often affecting multiple lobes and both lungs.
- **Fibrotic changes**: In more advanced or severe cases, patients may show fibrotic bands or reticulations, which can indicate the formation of scar tissue.

Imaging classification and CT features of COVID 19 pneumonia are given in **Table 17**.

Summary of COVID-RADS **is given in Box 1**:

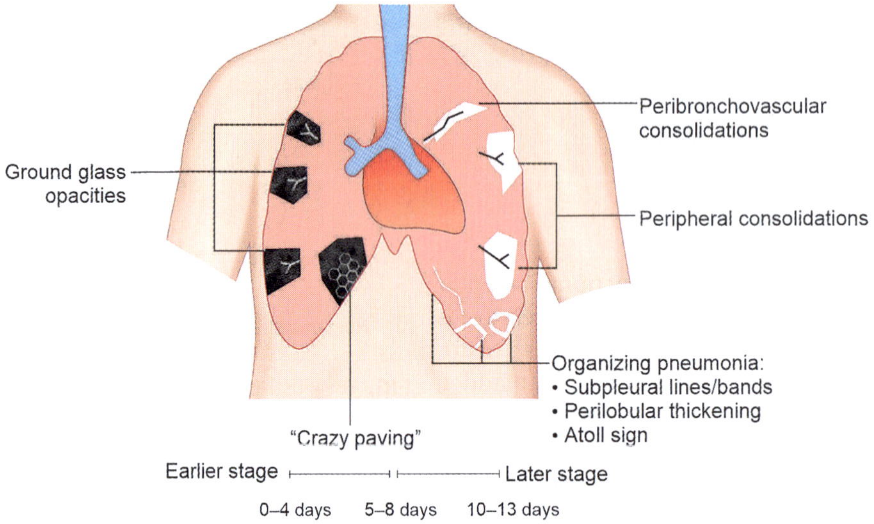

FIG. 19: Chest CT findings in COVID-19.

TABLE 17: Types of COVID 19 pneumonia according to CT imaging features.

Imaging		
Classification	***Rationale***	***CT Features***
Typical appearance	Commonly reported imaging features of greater specificity for COVID-19 pneumonia	Peripheral bilateral GGOs with or without consolidation or visible interlobular lines ("crazy-paving" pattern) Multifocal GGOs or rounded morphology with or without consolidation or visible interlobular lines (crazy-paving pattern) Reverse halo sign or other findings or organizing pneumonia (seen later in the disease)
Indeterminate appearance	Nonspecific imaging features of COVID-19 pneumonia	Absence of typical features AND the presence of the following features: multifocal, diffuse, perihilar, or unilateral GGO with or without consolidation lacking a specific distribution and that are nonrounded or nonperipheral Few small GGOs, with a nonrounded and nonperipheral distribution
Atypical appearance	Uncommonly or not reported features of COVID-19 pneumonia	Absence of typical or indeterminate features AND the presence of the following features: isolated lobar or segmental consolidation without GGOs; discrete small nodules (centrilobular; "tree-in-bud" appearance); lung cavitation; smooth interlobular septal thickening with pleural effusion

BOX 1: COVID-RADS.

Category and description

3: High suspicion
- Typical findings
- Multifocal GGO
- GGO with superimposed consolidation

Continued...

Continued...

Consolidation predominant pattern (late or complicated)
Linear opacities (late or complicated)
Crazy-paving pattern (late or complicated)
Melted sugar sign (late or remission)

2A: Moderate suspicion
Fairly typical findings
Single GGO (early)
Consolidation without GGO (late or complicated)
Focal pleural thickening associated with GGO or consolidation
Vascular dilation or mural thickening
Air bronchogram
Bronchial wall thickening
White long stage (late or complicated)
Parenchymal fibrotic bands (late or remission)

2B: Moderate suspicion
Combination of atypical findings with typical or fairly typical findings

1: Low suspicion
Atypical findings:
Pleural effusion
Cavity
Pulmonary nodule(s)
Nodular pattern
Lymphadenopathy
Peribronchovascular distribution
Halo sign
Tree-in-bud sign
Bronchiectasis
Airway secretions
Pulmonary emphysema
Pulmonary fibrosis
Isolated pleural thickening
Pneumothorax
Pericardial effusion

0: Low suspicion
Normal

(COVID RADS: COVID-19 Imaging Reporting and Data System; GGO: ground-glass opacity)

9. Lifecycle of *Echinococcus granulosus*. Pulmonary findings in hydatid cyst. [10] [DNB Dec 21]

Life Cycle of Echinococcus Granulosus (Fig. 20)

Pulmonary Findings in Hydatid Cyst

Common imaging techniques used are chest X-rays and computed tomography (CT) scans.15 CT is superior to the Chest X-ray.

Radiographic and CT features may differ in complicated and uncomplicated cysts.

Chest X-ray Findings

- **Uncomplicated cyst**:
  - Round, well-defined, homogeneous mass, typically in the lower lobes of the lung and peripheral location.
  - Variable in size, often ranging from a few centimeters to larger masses.

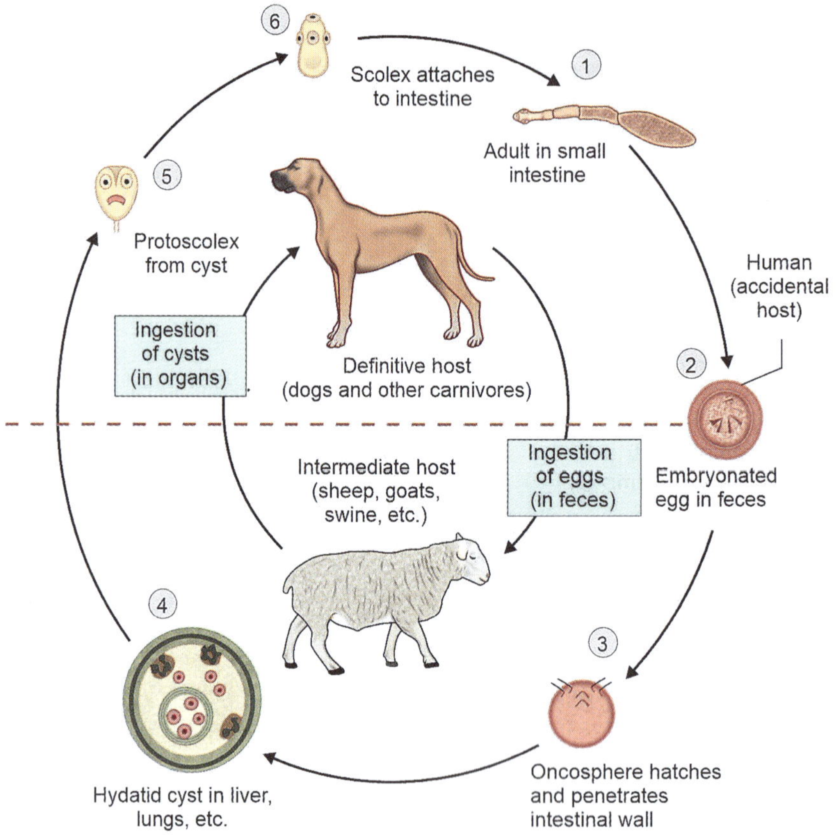

FIG. 20: Life cycle of *Echinococcus granulosus.*

- **Complicated (Ruptured cyst)**:
  - An air-fluid level may be seen inside the cyst, referred to as the "water-lily sign" or "camalote sign".
  - Multiple small cysts may appear within a larger one (daughter cysts).
  - Collapse or consolidation of lung tissue surrounding the cyst may occur'

CT Findings

- Multiple or solitary cystic lesion (most common)
- Diameter of 1–20 cm
- Unilateral or bilateral
- Predominantly found in the lower lobes

Uncomplicated Cysts

- Round or oval masses with well-defined borders
- Enhancement after contrast injection
- Hypodense content relative to the capsule complicated cysts may show:
- Meniscus sign or air crescent sign
- Cumbo sign or onion-peel sign
- Water-lily sign
- Consolidation adjacent to the cyst (ruptured cyst)
  The radiological findings of pulmonary hydatid cyst are presented in **Flowchart 4.**

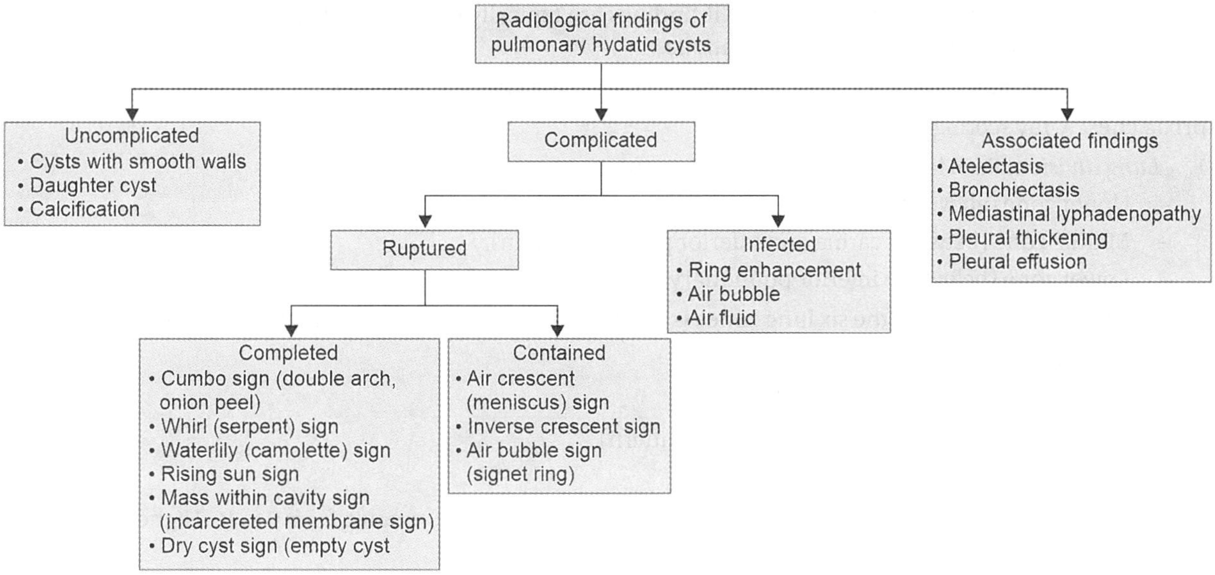

FLOWCHART 4: Radiological findings of hydatid cyst.

10. Discuss the indications of imaging in a suspected COVID-19 patient. Describe imaging features and pattern of involvement of respiratory system in COVID-19. [4+6] [DNB June 20]

According to a Fleischner Society consensus statement published on 7 April 2020:

- Imaging is not indicated in patients with suspected COVID-19 and mild clinical features unless they are at risk for disease progression.
- Imaging is indicated in a patient with COVID-19 and worsening respiratory status.
- In a resource-constrained environment, imaging is indicated for medical triage of patients with suspected COVID-19 who present with moderate-severe clinical features and a high pretest probability of disease.

In suspected cases of COVID-19 imaging studies can be used to assess the severity of lung involvement when symptoms worsen or clinical deterioration occur. Indications are:

- Initial evaluation for moderate to severe disease
- Clinical deterioration in case of increased oxygen requirements, mechanical ventilation or unexplained/sudden worsening of symptoms.
- Monitoring disease progression
- Ruling out complications like pulmonary embolism, secondary bacterial pneumonia, or pneumothorax, evaluation of extrapulmonary complications (e.g., cardiac involvement or thromboembolism).
- Preexisting lung conditions like COPD, asthma.
- Uncertainty in diagnosis like atypical presentations, or when PCR testing results are delayed, imaging may help identify COVID-19-related pneumonia or rule out alternative diagnoses.

Imaging features and pattern of involvement of respiratory system in COVID-19:

a. **Chest X-rays (CXR) findings**: Although chest radiograph is not routinely used in clinical settings because they are insensitive to detect COVID-19 in the early stage, however chest radiography is typically the first-line imaging modality used for patients with suspected COVID-19 patients. In cases where the patient's physical condition does not allow for transport to the radiology department for CT scan of thorax, in such cases chest X-ray is used. Findings are:
   i. *Ground-glass opacities (GGOs)*: Most common findings reported are interstitial abnormalities, reticular and reticulonodular patterns and the most common alveolar findings include hazy pulmonary opacities similar to the ground-glass opacities (GGOs) identified on CT. Hazy areas of opacities on the lungs indicate partial filling of air spaces. It typically appears as bilateral, posterior and peripheral locations.
   ii. *Consolidation*: Appears as denser, white areas on the CXR and represents fluid or solid material filling the airspaces. It is usually patchy and often bilateral.

iii. *Bilateral and peripheral distribution*: CXR findings are typically bilateral and are more frequently observed in the lower lung zones and peripheral locations.

iv. Even pleural fluid (in a severe case) has been found on the chest radiographs.

Brixia chest X-ray scoring system for COVID-19

1. *Lung division*: Each lung is divided into three zones:
   - Upper zone (above the carina),
   - Middle zone (between carina and inferior pulmonary vein),
   - Lower zone (below the inferior pulmonary vein).
2. *Scoring per zone*: Each of the six lung zones is scored based on the extent and nature of the lung abnormalities:

   0: No lung abnormalities.

   1: Interstitial infiltrates.

   2: Interstitial and alveolar infiltrates (mixed pattern).

   3: Predominantly alveolar infiltrates.
3. *Total score*: Scores from all six zones are summed to give a total score, ranging from 0 to 18. Higher scores indicate more severe lung involvement.
   - *Mild (score 0–6)*: Typically associated with mild symptoms or asymptomatic cases.
   - *Moderate (score 7–12)*: Indicates moderate lung involvement, often requiring close monitoring and possibly supplemental oxygen.
   - *Severe (score 13–18)*: Severe lung involvement, often correlating with hypoxia and potential need for intensive care.

b. **HRCT findings**: HRCT have a sensitivity and detects early lung involvement in COVID-19 patients. Findings are:

i. *Ground-glass opacities (GGOs)*: GGOs are seen as areas of increased opacity, described as hazy, which partially obscure the lung's normal structure. They are usually multifocal, bilateral and peripheral, but in the early phase it may present as a unifocal lesion, most commonly located in the inferior lobe of the right lung.

ii. *Crazy-paving pattern*: GGOs with interlobular septal thickening, resembling paving stones. It indicates disease progression.

iii. Air space consolidation

iv. Bronchovascular thickening

v. Traction bronchiectasis

vi. *Air bronchograms*: Air-filled bronchi within areas of lung consolidation or GGOs.

vii. *Vascular enlargement*: Associated with increased vessel caliber in areas of GGOs.

viii. *Subpleural and peripheral locations*: Predominantly subpleural and peripheral, often affecting multiple lobes and both lungs.

ix. *Fibrotic changes*: In more advanced or severe cases, patients may show fibrotic bands or reticulations, which can indicate the formation of scar tissue.

CT manifestations of different stages of COVID-19 are given in **Table 18**:

TABLE 18: CT manifestations of different stages of COVID-19.

Early stage	*Advanced stage*	*Severe stage*	*Dissipation stage*
Single or multiple scattered patchy ground-glass opacities, predominately distributed in the peripheral and subpleural area of the lung. A crazy-paving pattern, secondary to intralobular and interlobular septal thickening can be seen in this stage.	Increased extent and density of bilateral lung parenchymal opacities. In this image, there are both areas of ground glass opacification and areas of consolidation In both lungs, which coexist and have varying sizes and presence of airbronchogram.	Diffuse consolidation of the lung parenchyma with uneven density, air bronchi and bronchial dilation, which may be present as "whited out lung on a corresponding chest radiograph."	Areas of ground glass opacity and consolidation have nearly completely resolved, leaving some residual curvilinear areas of density.

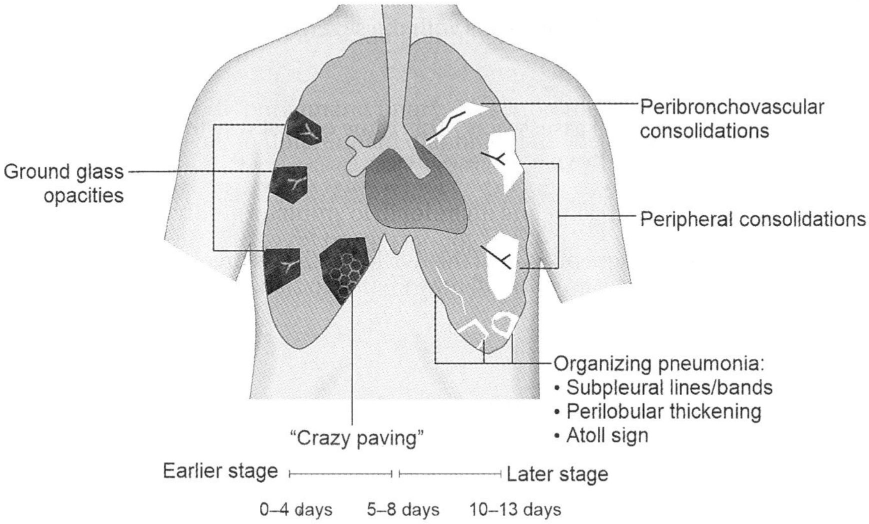

FIG. 21: Chest CT findings in COVID-19 *(For Color Version Refer Fig. 19).*

The HRCT findings of pulmonary involvement in different stages of COVID-19 infections **(Fig. 21)** are:

1. **Early Stage (0–4 Days)**:
   - *Ground-glass opacities (GGO)*: The most common finding in the early phase, often peripheral and subpleural in distribution.
   - *Unilateral or bilateral involvement*: Lesions may initially be unilateral but can become bilateral.
   - *No or minimal crazy-paving pattern*: The crazy-paving pattern (thickened interlobular septa within areas of GGO) is not typically seen.
2. **Progressive Stage (5–8 Days)**:
   - *Increasing ground-glass opacities*: The areas of GGO tend to increase in size and number.
   - *Consolidation*: Areas of consolidation may begin to appear in combination with GGO.
   - *Crazy-paving pattern*: This becomes more evident, with thickened interlobular and intralobular septa superimposed on GGO.
3. **Peak Stage (9–13 Days)**:
   - *Diffuse ground-glass opacities*: GGOs are typically diffuse and bilateral, involving multiple lobes.
   - *Consolidation*: Consolidation becomes more prominent and widespread.
   - *Crazy-paving pattern*: Prominent
   - *Pleural effusion*: Can be seen in severe cases.
4. **Absorption or Late Stage (≥14 Days)**:
   - *Gradual decrease in ground-glass opacities and consolidation*: As the infection resolves, the GGOs and areas of consolidation begin to decrease.
   - *Fibrotic changes*: Reticulation and subpleural fibrotic bands may develop, leading to potential long-term pulmonary fibrosis in severe cases.
   - *Residual lesions*: Some patients may have long-lasting GGO or fibrotic streaks.

The typical features on CT imaging of COVID-19 are given in **Table 19**.

TABLE 19: Typical features on CT imaging of COVID-19.

Parameter	*Characteristic manifestations on CT imaging*
Density	Ground glass opacity and consolidation, possible interlobular septal thickening
Shape	Patchy, sub-segmental, or segmental
Distribution	Mid and lower lungs a long the bronchovascular bundles with bilateral involvement
Location	Peripheral and subpleural areas of the lung parenchyma
Concomitant signs (variable)	Air bronchogram, a small amount of pleural effusion, no obvious lymphadenopathy

CT involvement Score

The severity of the lung involvement on the CT correlates with the severity of the disease.

Visual Assessment

The severity on CT can be estimated by visual assessment. This is the easiest way to score the severity.

The CT images show a 25% involvement by visual assessment.

Severity Score

Another method is by scoring the percentages of each of the five lobes that is involved:

1. <5% involvement
2. 5–25% involvement
3. 26–49% involvement
4. 50–75% involvement
5. >75% involvement.

The total CT score is the sum of the individual lobar scores and can range from 0 (no involvement) to 25 (maximum involvement), when all the five lobes show more than 75% involvement.

Some say that the percentage of lung involvement can be calculated by multiplying the total score times 4.

This however is not true. Suppose that all lobes have a 10% involvement, then this would lead to an overall score of 10, which could lead to the impression that 40% of the lungs are involved.

CT Severity Grading

Score	*CT severity*
<8	Mild
9–15	Moderate
>15	Severe

a. **USG findings**: Ultrasound have advantages that it does not expose patients to ionizing radiation and is easily accessible in terms of its portability and the ability to perform bedside examinations. Findings are:
   - Multiple B-lines: Vertically oriented hyperechoic artifacts that originate from the pleura or from areas of consolidation. These lines indicate accumulation of fluid in the pulmonary interstitial space or alveoli.
   - A-lines can then be seen in the recovery phase of the disease.
   - Irregular, thickened pleural line with scattered discontinuities.
   - Subpleural and alveolar consolidations

b. Other imaging modalities like MRI and nuclear medicine rarely used.

Monitoring Disease Progression

- **Follow-up imaging**: Radiography used to monitor the progression of COVID-19 pneumonia in hospitalized patients, especially in intensive care and planned treatment according to imaging changes.
- **Severity scoring**: Both X-rays and CT scans were used to quantify the extent of lung involvement by grading severity scores.

Complication Detection

Identifies COVID-19-related complications such as acute respiratory distress syndrome (ARDS), pulmonary embolism, and secondary infections. CT accurately diagnosed thrombotic events, which is a known as a significant complication in COVID-19 patients and required immediate intervention.

Guiding Treatment Decisions

Help in treatment decisions like whether antiviral therapies, corticosteroids, or respiratory support (such as ventilators) were needed.

11. (a) Radiological patterns of pneumonias on chest computed tomography in immunocompromised patients. (b) Imaging features of fungal infections. [5+5] [DNB Dec 20]

Introduction

In immunocompromised patients, pneumonias can present with a wide range of imaging features on chest CT, according to causative agents and the underlying immune suppression (e.g., chemotherapy, HIV/AIDS, post-transplant, etc.).16 Different types of pneumonias are:

Viral Pneumonia

Causative organisms: Cytomegalovirus (CMV), herpes group virus, respiratory syncytial virus (RSV), influenza, and COVID-19.

CT Findings

- Diffuse ground-glass or patchy opacities (GGO), particularly bilateral, often in parahilar or subpleural locations and a few nodules with halo are seen, which may later coalesce to form subsegmental or lobar consolidation.
- Peribronchial and septal thickening with superimposed ground-glass opacification is characteristic and is known as "crazy paving" appearance.
- Pulmonary nodules and airway disease like bronchiectasis, bronchial wall thickening may be seen one third cases.

Bacterial Pneumonia

Causative organisms: *Streptococcus pneumoniae, Staphylococcus aureus* (including MRSA), *Klebsiella pneumoniae, and Pseudomonas spp.*

CT findings:

- **Lobar consolidation**: May involve one or more segments. Involvement of multiple adjoining segments can lead to "round pneumonia."
- Staphylococcal and Klebsiella infection typically cause consolidation accompanied by bulging of fissures.
- Staphylococcal consolidation is usually accompanied by cavitation, bilateral pleural effusions, empyema, pneumatoceles and pyopneumothorax.
- **Pseudomonas infection**: Shows lower lobe involvement with mixed features of multilobar consolidation, air bronchogram, and multiple areas of ground glass opacities (GGO).
- *H influenzae* infection manifests as a subsegmental or segmental consolidation with peripherally located GGOs, centrilobular nodules, and bronchial wall thickening.
- Mycoplasma presents with patchy nonsegmental consolidation, ground glass opacities (GGOs), bronchial wall thickening, and centrilobular nodules.
- **Abscess formation**: Seen in necrotizing pneumonia, especially with *Staphylococcus aureus* or *Klebsiella pneumonia*.

Fungal Pneumonia

Causative organisms: Aspergillosis, cryptococcosis, candidiasis, histoplasmosis, *Pneumocystis jirovecii* pneumonia (PJP).

Invasive Aspergillosis

CT findings:

- **Halo sign**: A nodule surrounded by ground-glass opacity, indicating hemorrhage around the fungal infection.
- Nodular or wedge-shaped opacities frequently abutting the pleural surface, often cavitate reflecting the angioinvasive nature of fungus and may show central low density areas or the air crescent sign.
- **Cavitation**: Nodule may cavitate, forming a central cavity with thick or thin walls.
- **Nodules**: Multiple, often scattered pulmonary nodules.

Cryptococcosis

CT findings:

- The lung CT pattern shows various types of peripherally located lesions: either only nodular masses or only pneumonic infiltrates, or GGOs or a mixed one.
- Consolidation: Patchy or lobar consolidation may occur.
- Pleural effusion may be seen.

Pneumocystis Jirovecii pneumonia (PJP)

Seen in: HIV/AIDS, patients on chronic immunosuppressants (e.g., steroids), or transplant recipients.
CT findings:

- **Ground-glass opacities (GGO)**: Bilateral, perihilar or diffuse, symmetrical, affecting the central or perihilar lung regions. The GGO attenuation shows a patchy or geographical distribution with sparing of subpleural region.
- There is a stark contrast between the partially opacified lung and the air-filled bronchus, which is seen as a "dark bronchus" sign.
- **Crazy-paving pattern**: Ground-glass opacities with superimposed interlobular septal thickening.
- **Cysts or pneumatoceles**: Seen in some cases, particularly in recurrent or treated PJP. Rupture of cysts is likely, and manifests as pneumothorax and/or pneumomediastinum.

Nocardiosis

CT Findings:

- **Nodules and masses**: These can be solitary or multiple and may cavitate.
- **Consolidation**: Often lobar or multifocal.
- **Pleural involvement**: Pleural effusion or empyema can be present.
- **Abscess formation**: Nocardiosis can cause necrotizing infection, leading to abscess formation.

Tuberculosis (TB) and Atypical Mycobacterial Infections

Causative organisms: Mycobacterium tuberculosis, Mycobacterium avium complex (MAC). *CT findings*:

- **Cavitary lesions**: Seen in postprimary/reactivation tuberculosis, thick-walled cavitary lesions in the upper lobes.
- **Tree-in-bud pattern**: Seen in endobronchial TB, characterized by small centrilobular nodules with a branching appearance.
- Appearances are of nonlocalized, cavitating consolidation of lower lobes, often surrounded by centrilobular "tree-in-bud" nodules.
- **Nodules**: Small nodules or calcified granulomas may be seen, especially in healed or dormant TB.
- Mediastinal lymphadenopathy is often associated with faint peripheral or rim enhancement and central nonenhancing necrotic areas.

Parasitic Pneumonia

Causative organisms: Strongyloidiasis, Toxoplasmosis.
CT Findings:

- Lower lobe predominant bilateral peripheral GGOs with atelectasis are usually present (Toxoplasmosis).
- Parahilar or diffuse GGOs with interlobular septal thickening, resulting in a "crazy-paving" appearance. Less commonly micronodules/military opacities may be seen. Bilateral pleural effusion is common (Strongyloidiasis).

Imaging Features of Pulmonary Manifestation of Fungal Infections

Causative organisms are involving lungs are Aspergillus, Blastomycosis, Cryptococcus, Histoplasma, Coccidioidomycosis, *Pneumocystis jirovecii,* and Candida

Radiographic imaging modalities used for diagnosis are CT and X-ray.

Aspergillosis

Invasive aspergillosis (usually seen in immunocompromised patients):

CT findings:

- Nodules, often surrounded by a "halo sign" (ground-glass opacity surrounding a nodule).
- Progression to cavitation with an "air crescent sign" during recovery.
- Consolidations or dense segmental opacities.

Aspergilloma (fungus ball in a preexisting lung cavity):

CT/X-ray findings:
A mobile, round mass within a cavity, often with a crescent of air surrounding it.

Pneumocystis Jirovecii Pneumonia (PJP)

Seen in: HIV/AIDS, patients on chronic immunosuppressants (e.g., steroids), or transplant recipients.

X-ray findings: Diffuse, bilateral, symmetrical, interstitial infiltrates.

CT findings:

- **Ground-glass opacities (GGO)**: Bilateral, perihilar or diffuse, symmetrical, affecting the central or perihilar lung regions. The GGO attenuation shows a patchy or geographical distribution with sparing subpleural region.
- There is a stark contrast between the partially opacified lung and the air-filled bronchus, which is seen as a "dark bronchus" sign.
- **Crazy-paving pattern**: Ground-glass opacities with superimposed interlobular septal thickening.
- **Cysts or pneumatoceles**: Seen in some cases, particularly in recurrent or treated PJP. Rupture of cysts is likely, and manifests as pneumothorax and/or pneumomediastinum.

Cryptococcosis

CT findings:

- Single or multiple peripheral, circumscribed nodules, usually without cavitation (in healthy individual).
- Bilateral linear and ground-glass opacity with a miliary pattern may occur as may single or multiple nodules occasionally with cavitation. (HIV pt)
- **Consolidation**: Patchy or lobar consolidation may occur.
- Pleural effusion may be seen.

Histoplasmosis

X-ray/CT findings:

- Nonspecific multifocal areas of consolidation.
- Diffusely distributed, variably sized but usually small (occasionally small enough to resemble a miliary pattern) nodules may be seen. These nodules may undergo calcification when healing occurs.
- Solitary pulmonary nodule contain central "bull's-eye" or "target" calcification with adjacent satellite nodules may be present.
- Lymphadenopathy is common, but pleural effusions are not.
- Granulomatous or fibrosing mediastinitis.

Coccidioidomycosis

X-ray/CT findings:

- Air-space consolidation or GGO, often in the lower lobe.
- Single or multiple pulmonary nodules, either of which may cavitate. Occasionally, such nodule undergoes progressive cavitation into a thin-walled (grape-skin) cyst.

Blastomycosis

Imaging findings

- Focal, multifocal, or diffuse areas of consolidation and ground-glass opacity with variably sized nodules seen.
- Areas of low attenuation and interlobular septal thickening also seen. In few patients, a "reversed halo" sign (the "atoll"sign) may be seen.

Candidiasis

Imaging findings:

- Focal or multilobar consolidation.
- A miliary pattern may occur. Multiple nodules with areas of ground-glass opacity and consolidation; the nodules may be poorly defined or circumscribed.

Mediastinum, Lung Nodules, and Masses

1. Discuss the imaging features of the common anterior mediastinal lesions. [10] [MD (WBUHS) 23]

Imaging features of anterior mediastinal lesions: Anterior mediastinum:

Extent: Posterior to the sternum and anterior to a line drawn along the anterior tracheal wall in the upper mediastinum and the posterior border of the heart in the lower mediastinum.

Contents: Thymus, heart, ascending aorta and great vessels, anterior portion of the main pulmonary artery, pericardium, fat, lymph vessels, and nodes.

Thymus

- Thymic Hyperplasia
- Thymic cysts
- Thymolipoma
- **Thymic Epithelial neoplasm**:
  - Thymoma
  - Thymic carcinoma
- **Neuroendocrine tumors of thymus**
  - Thymic carcinoid
  - Small cell Ca of thymus

Thyroid: Retrosternal thyroid *Parathyroid*: Ectopic parathyroid. *Germ cell tumor*

- Teratoma
  - Dermoid cyst (mature teratoma)
  - Immature teratoma
- Seminoma
- Nonseminomatous germ cell tumors

Vascular lesion:

- Lymphangioma
- Hemangioma

Common anterior mediastinal masses include thymomas, teratomas, thyroid masses, and lymphomas, often summarized by the mnemonic "4 T's" (thymoma, teratoma, thyroid, and terrible lymphoma).

Thymoma

Most common primary tumor of anterior mediastinum.

CT findings:

- Thymomas are well-marginated, smooth or lobulated, encapsulated, unilateral mediastinal masses.
- Show homogenous attenuation and enhancement.
- Soft tissue density mass with possible areas of calcification.
- Invasive thymomas may demonstrate infiltration into adjacent structures.

MRI findings:
- **T1**: Isointense to slightly hyperintense signal compared to muscle
- **T2**
  - Heterogeneous signal, slightly higher than muscle.
  - Cystic areas may be seen, especially in larger tumors.
  - Fibrous septa crossing the mass are of low signal intensity.
- **In/out phase imaging**: Typically, no signal drop out, i.e., no chemical shift.
- **T1 C + (Gd)**: Linear regions of enhancement may be seen coursing through the mass, thought to represent fibrous septa.

Teratoma

- Mature teratomas or dermoid cysts
- Immature or malignant teratomas

The combination of fluid, soft tissue, calcium, and fat is diagnostic of teratoma. The finding of a fat-fluid level within a mass on CT is also diagnostic of teratoma.

CT Findings

- Mature teratomas manifest on CT as smooth or lobulated mediastinal masses with heterogeneous components, including fat, soft tissue, fluid, and calcifications, that typically have cystic and solid components; in contrast, malignant teratomas are usually poorly marginated masses containing areas of necrosis.
- Normal serum levels of β-human chorionic gonadotropin hormone (β-hCG) and α-fetoprotein (AFP).

MRI

- Fat components are hyperintense on T1-weighted images, and cystic areas show high signal intensity on T2-weighted images.
- **Complications**: Can rupture into adjacent structures like the pleura or pericardium, causing inflammation or infection.

Seminoma

Occurs almost entirely in men, with a mean age at presentation of 29 years. Most common malignant mediastinal germ-cell tumor.

CT findings.
- Seminomas present as large, smoother lobulated, homogeneous soft tissue attenuation masses, although small areas of low attenuation can be seen. Obliteration of fat planes is common.
- Pleural or pericardial effusion may be present.

Nonseminomatous Germ Cell Tumors

This are embryonal carcinoma, endodermal sinus (yolk sac) tumor, choriocarcinoma, and mixed types.
- **CT findings**:
  - Large poorly marginated masses often show heterogeneous opacity, including ill- defined areas of low attenuation secondary to necrosis and hemorrhage or cystic areas.
  - May be infiltrative, with obliteration of fat planes, and may be spiculated. Calcification may be seen.
- **MR findings**: Also reflect the inhomogeneous nature of these lesions.

Thyroid Mass (Ectopic or Substernal Goiter)

- **CT findings**: A substernal goiter is typically contiguous with the thyroid gland, extending into the mediastinum. It may have areas of calcification and appear heterogeneous due to varying degrees of iodine content or cystic changes.
- **MRI findings**: Shows a low to intermediate signal on T1 and T2-weighted images, with avid enhancement post-contrast.
- **Nuclear Medicine**: Iodine uptake studies or technetium scans can help confirm thyroid tissue origin.

Thymic Cyst

- Uncommon.
- CT can suggest the diagnosis of thymic cyst if the lesion (a) appears *thin walled,* (b) is unassociated with a mass lesion, (c) contains fluid with a density close to that of water, and (d) remains *unopacified following contrast infusion.*

Lymphoma

- **CT findings**: Mediastinal lymphomas typically present as large, homogeneous, soft tissue masses with lobulated borders. Unlike thymomas, lymphomas rarely contain calcifications or fat. These masses can encase adjacent structures like the great vessels but usually without causing vascular obstruction.
- **MRI findings**: Appears hypointense on T1-weighted images and hyperintense on T2-weighted images, with variable contrast enhancement.
- **PET-CT**: FDG avidity is usually high in lymphomas, making PET-CT a useful tool for staging and monitoring response to treatment.

Vascular Lesion

Lymphangioma

- Rare benign congenital lesions. In <2-year-old child.
- On CT these lesions manifest as lobular multicystic tumors that surround and infiltrate adjacent mediastinal structures.

Hemangioma

- Large interconnecting vascular spaces with varying amounts of interposed stromal elements such as fat and fibrous tissue.
- Focal areas of organized thrombus can calcify as phleboliths.
- CECT and T1 CE MRI: multiple tortuous serpentine enhancing structures may be present.

2. Define solitary pulmonary nodule (SPN). Enumerate its causes. Discuss the radiological work up of a solitary nodule highlighting the features which enable to differentiate between benign and malignant nodules. [1+2+7] [MD (WBUHS) 23, DNB June 21]

Solitary Pulmonary Nodule (SPN)

Definition: A solitary pulmonary nodule (SPN) usually is defined as a focal opacity,17 visible on chest radiographs or computed tomography (CT), which fits the following criteria:

1. Well-defined round or oval lesion
2. <3 cm (>3 cm = mass)
3. Surrounded at least partially by the lung parenchyma
4. With no associated lymphadenopathy, collapse or consolidation.

Causes of solitary pulmonary nodules:

1. **Granulomatous**
   - Tuberculoma
   - Histoplasmoma
   - Others
2. **Malignant tumors**
   - Lung cancer
   - Solitary metastasis
   - Rare malignant lung tumors
3. **Benign tumors**
   - Carcinoid tumor
   - Hamartoma

4. **Infectious/inflammatory**
   - Pneumonia
   - Rounded atelectasis
   - Hydatid
   - Wegener's granulomatosis
   - Sarcoidosis
   - Organizing pneumonia
5. **Congenital**
   - Intrapulmonary lymph node
   - Sequestration
   - Bronchogenic cyst 6.Vascular
   - Hematoma
   - Arteriovenous malformation

Radiological workup of a solitary nodule highlighting the features which enable to differentiate between benign and malignant nodules are given in **Flowchart 5**.

Benign and malignant radiological features of pulmonary nodules are given in **Table 20**.

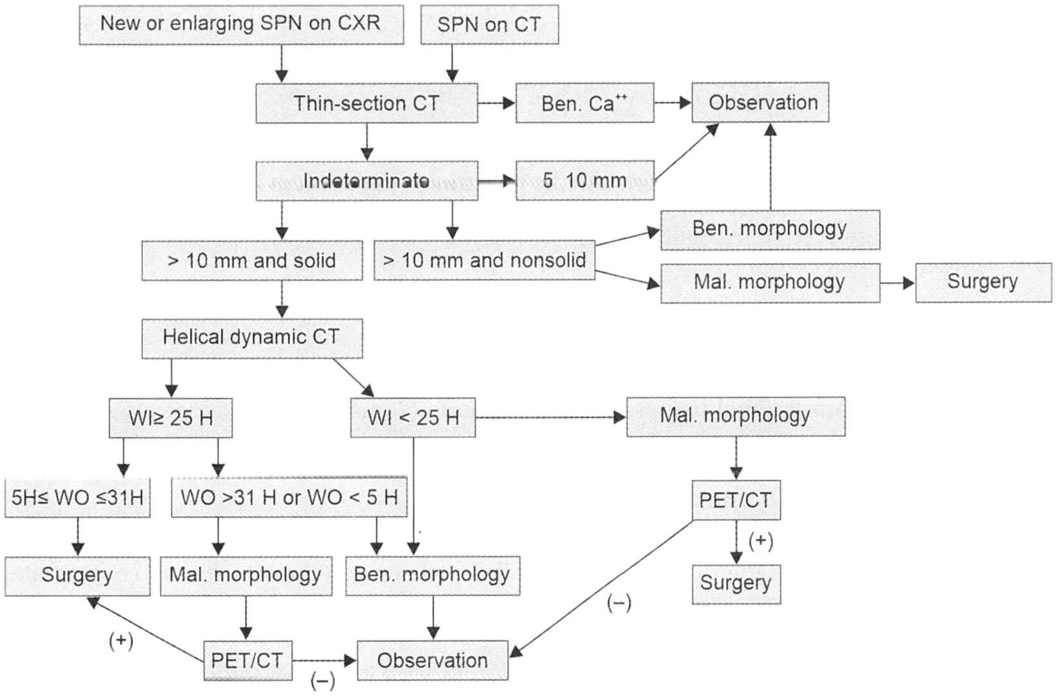

FLOWCHART 5: Algorithm for differentiating features between benign and malignant nodules.

TABLE 20: Benign and malignant radiological features of pulmonary nodules.

Radiological feature	***Benign***	***Malignant***
Size	≤3	>3
Growth rate	Stable over 2 years	Doubling time of 1–18 months
Margins	Well-defined, smooth	Ill-defined, spiculated, undulated
Calcification within nodule	Dense, solid, laminated, popcorn	Fine, dendriform, punctate
Fat within nodule	Yes	No
Cavitation within nodule	Less likely. If so thin walled and round	Increases risk; thick walled and irregular
Enhancement	<15 HU	Average of 40 HU

Perifissural Nodules (Fig. 22) are Mostly Benign

Additional Features of Malignant Nodules

- Upper lobe predominance.
- Pleural retraction.
- Part solid part ground glass nodule.
- Cavitation with a thick wall (>15 mm) and a nodular wall.
- Containing air bronchogram or bubble-like lucency.

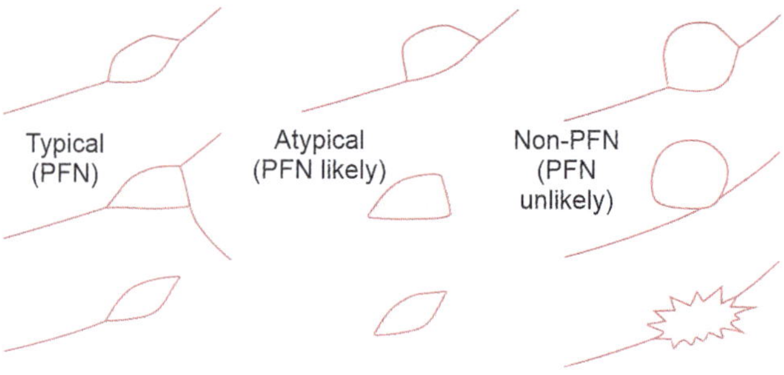

FIG. 22: Types of pulmonary nodules.

3. Briefly discuss the radiological divisions of mediastinum with their contents. [10] [MD (WBUHS) 19]

Plain radiographic divisions (Felson's mediastinal division): On plain radiographs, the divisions of mediastinum are anterior, middle, and posterior mediastinal compartments which were redefined by Felson.

Anterior Compartment

Extent: Posterior to the sternum and anterior to a line drawn along the anterior tracheal wall in the upper mediastinum and the posterior border of the heart in the lower mediastinum.

Contents: Thymus, heart, ascending aorta and great vessels, anterior portion of the main pulmonary artery, pericardium, fat, lymph vessels, nodes.

Middle Compartment

Extent: Between the anterior compartment in front and the posterior compartment behind.

Contents: The trachea and main bronchi, superior vena cava, midportion of the aortic arch, azygos arch, lymph nodes, esophagus, descending aorta (sometimes).

Posterior Compartment

Extent: Posterior to a line 1 cm behind the anterior margin of the vertebral column and anterior to the chest wall.

Contents: Vertebral bodies, paravertebral tissues, descending aorta (sometimes), posterior azygos vein, hemiazygos vein, and lymph nodes.

ITMIG Definition of Mediastinal Compartments

The three-compartment cross-sectional imaging model of the mediastinal compartments developed by ITMIG **(Table 21 and Fig. 23)** includes prevascular (anterior), visceral (middle), and paravertebral (posterior) compartments. Specific compartment boundaries and the anatomic structures they contain can be readily identified at multidetector CT.[18]

TABLE 21: CT based radiological division of mediastinum. ITMIG multidetector CT-based classification of mediastinal compartments.

Compartment	*Boundaries*	*Major contents*
Prevascular	Superior thoracic inlet Inferior: diaphragm Anterior: sternum Lateral: parietal mediastinal pleura Posterior: anterior aspect of the pericardium as it wraps around the heart in a curvilinear fashion	Thymus Fat Lymph nodes Left brachiocephalic vein
Visceral	Superior: thoracic inlet Inferior: diaphragm Anterior: posterior boundaries of the prevascular compartment	Nonvascular: trachea, carina, esophagus. lymph nodes

Continued...

Continued...

Compartment	Boundaries	Major contents
	Posterior: vertical line connecting a point on each thoracic vertebral body 1 cm posterior to its anterior margin	Vascular: heart, ascending thoracic aorta, aortic arch, descending thoracic aorta, superior vena cava, intra pericardial pulmonary arteries, thoracic duct
Paravertebral	Superior: thoracic inlet Inferior; diaphragm Anterior: posterior boundaries of the visceral compartment Posterolateral: vertical line against the posterior margin of the chest wall at the lateral margin of the transverse process of the thoracic spine	Thoracic spine Paravertebral soft tissues

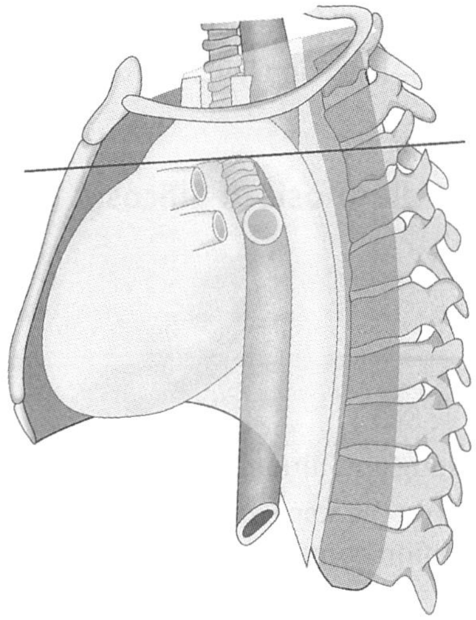

FIG. 23: Illustrated image of mediastinum division.

4. Write short note on Pancoast Tumor. [5] [MD (WBUHS) 19]

Introduction: Also called superior sulcus tumor or lung apex tumor or thoracic inlet carcinoma. Location: superior sulcus at the lung apex

Clinical features: Pain, paresthesia of the ipsilateral upper limb

Pancoast syndrome: Brachial plexus and sympathetic ganglia involvement

- Shoulder pain
- Radicular pain due to plexopathy and consequent wasting of muscles of upper limb
- **Horner's syndrome**: Miosis, ptosis, and anhidrosis
- **Histological type**: Mostly adenocarcinoma

Modality of choice: CECT thorax
An MRI is done to look for involvement of nerve roots and mediastinal extension to great vessels.

Imaging Features

Chest radiograph: Asymmetrical pleural thickening at lung apex >5mm, suggestive of Pancoast tumor.

CECT:

- Soft tissue density mass at lung apex with unilateral or asymmetrical pleural thickening and involving the adjacent structures.

- **Chest wall invasion**: CT is good at showing the extent of invasion into the chest wall, including ribs, vertebrae, and muscles.
- **Bone involvement**: Osteolysis or destruction of the first rib or nearby thoracic vertebrae can be seen.

MRI

- **Soft-tissue extension**: MRI is superior for evaluating soft tissue involvement, especially into the brachial plexus and subclavian vessels.
- **Neurovascular invasion**: MRI is helpful for assessing tumor invasion into the brachial plexus, subclavian artery, and other critical neurovascular structures.
- **Chest wall and spinal involvement**: MRI can better delineate the extent of chest wall invasion and detect early spinal cord compression.

Management

- **Involvement of T1 and T2**: Resectable
- **Involvement of C8 or higher nerve roots**: Unresectable
- **For resectable tumor**: Neoadjuvant chemotherapy followed by resection
- **For unresectable tumor**: Neoadjuvant chemotherapy—resection if it becomes resectable. If it is still unresectable—chemoradiotherapy.

5. Describe imaging features and differential diagnosis of Silicosis. [10] [MD (WBUHS) 19]

Silicosis

- Most common occupational lung disease
- Fibrotic pneumoconiosis.
- Inhalation of dust containing silica (silicon dioxide or SiO_2)
  - Heavy metal mining, quarrying, denim sandblasting and tunnelling are associated with silicosis.
- The radiographic imaging findings of silicosis depend on the stage of the disease and the duration of exposure to silica dust. Imaging modality—chest X-ray and high-resolution computed tomography (HRCT) are used for diagnosis.
  - Two clinical forms of silicosis:
    - *Acute silicosis* or alveolar silicoproteinosis.
    - *Classic silicosis or* chronic interstitial reticulonodular disease - Most common form.
  - According to the radiographic findings, silicosis is divided into:
    - *Simple or uncomplicated silicosis*: small and round or irregular opacities.
    - *Complicated silicosis*: large conglomerate opacities leading to progressive massive fibrosis.

Simple or Uncomplicated Silicosis

Chest X-ray

1. **Multiple nodular opacities which are**:
   - Well-defined and uniform in shape and attenuation
   - 1–10 mm in diameter
   - Involving predominantly the upper lobe and posterior portion of the lung but can be present throughout both lungs.
   - Calcification may be seen.
2. Eggshell calcification of the lymph nodes (thin, peripheral calcification) is a characteristic finding but occurs in about 5–20% of cases.

HRCT Findings

- Multiple small pulmonary nodules
- Ranging from (1–5 mm)

- Usually well-defined
- Often associated with calcifications
- Predominantly located in the upper lung zones with perilymphatic distribution, subpleural nodules that coalesce, termed "candle wax" lesions or pseudoplaques.
- Eggshell calcification of lymph nodes seen, typically occurring at the periphery of the node.

Complicated Silicosis [Progressive Massive Fibrosis (PMF)] Chest X-ray

- Coalescence of the small nodules into large opacities, which are greater than 1 cm in diameter and with an irregular margin.
- Commonly seen in the midportion or periphery of the upper lung zones.
- Progressively migrate toward the hila with time, leaving emphysematous lung tissue between fibrous tissue and the pleural surface.
- On the lateral radiograph, these masses may appear lenticular in shape, often oriented posteriorly, paralleling the major fissure.
- The large masses or opacities can cause distortion of lung architecture.
- Cavitation within the large opacities may occur with superimposed tuberculosis.

HRCT

- Focal soft-tissue conglomerate masses.
- Usually oval and often with irregular or ill-defined margins and calcifications.
- Areas of necrosis, visible as low attenuation, with or without cavitation may be present.
- Eggshell calcification of the hilar or mediastinal lymph nodes are seen.
- Paraseptal emphysema seen due to adjacent parenchymal fibrosis particularly in the upper lobes.
- Areas of mosaic attenuation seen due to air trapping secondary to small airway involvement.
- Traction bronchiectasis seen as fibrosis progresses.

Differential Diagnosis of Silicosis

1. **Coal Worker's pneumoconiosis (CWP)**:
   - Similar nodular pattern in as silicosis predominantly upper lobes.
   - Can differentiate between them with the help of occupational history (coal dust exposure).
   - Massive fibrosis is more central and less likely to have eggshell calcification of lymph nodes.
2. **Talcosis**
   - Type of lung disease related to talc, inhalation or intravenous injection.
   - Multiple numerous discrete nodules 1 mm or less in diameter.
   - Ground-glass opacities may be seen.
   - Later shows gradual coalescence of the nodules toward the parahilar regions of the upper lobes leads to formation of conglomerate masses, similar to progressive massive fibrosis of silicosis.
3. **Sarcoidosis**
   - Bilateral hilar lymphadenopathy (common in sarcoidosis but rare in silicosis).
   - Nodules are more commonly along bronchovascular bundles and subpleural regions rather than upper lobe predominance.
   - Eggshell calcification can occur but is less common compared to silicosis.
4. **Tuberculosis (TB)**:
   - Nodular opacities in the upper lobes, often with cavitation.
   - From clinical history of active TB or positive TB test help to differentiate.
   - Silicosis can predispose to TB, and the two can coexist.

5. **Langerhans Cell Histiocytosis (LCH)**:
   - Associated with smoking.
   - Multiple pulmonary nodules and cysts predominantly involving the upper lobe.
   - LCH often shows bizarre-shaped cysts.
6. **Idiopathic Pulmonary Fibrosis (IPF)**:
   - Diffuse reticular opacities and honeycombing, involving the lower lobes, whereas silicosis is upper lobe-predominant.
   - Does not have nodular opacities.
7. **Asbestosis**:
   - Predominantly involving lower lobe disease with pleural plaques or thickening.
8. **Chronic Beryllium Disease**:
   - Upper lobe fibrosis and nodules may resemble silicosis, but occupational history and beryllium sensitization test help in diagnosis.
9. **Hypersensitivity Pneumonitis**:
   - Diffuse, multiple, small nodules, more in centrilobular locations.
   - Involves the middle and lower lung zones and is associated with exposure to organic dust.

6. Multinodular pulmonary lesions and its imaging. [10] [DNB June 22]

Introduction

Multinodular pulmonary lesions are the presence of multiple nodules within the lung parenchyma.19,20

The occurrence clinical symptoms, occupational history, number of nodules, and their particular imaging characteristics (location, shape, presence and type of calcifications, and presence of spiculation or cavitation) narrow the differential diagnosis **(Flowchart 6)**.

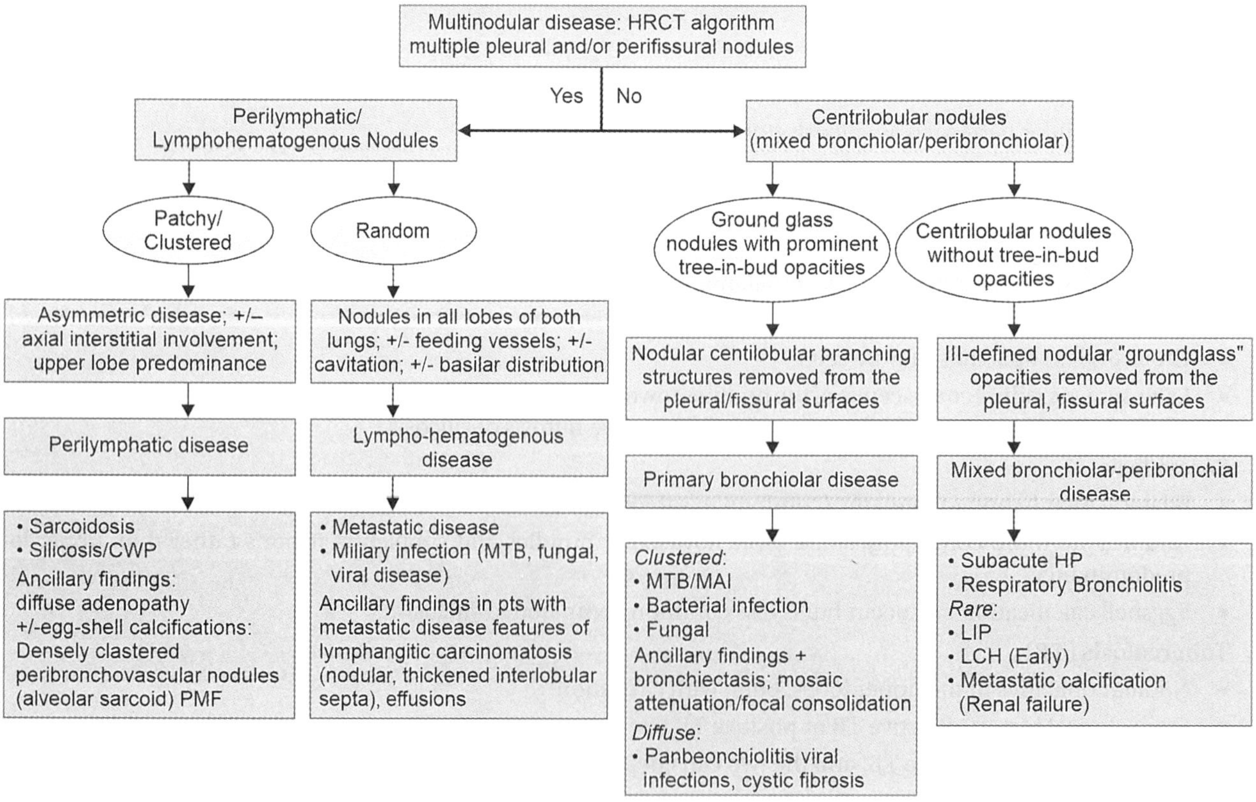

FLOWCHART 6: Algorithm of multinodular diseases.

The differential diagnosis of multiple pulmonary nodules is broad, but includes:

- Sarcoidosis
- Silicosis
- Respiratory bronchiolitis (infective or non-infective)
- Infections
  - Tuberculosis: bronchogenic disseminated tuberculosis
  - Nontuberculous mycobacterial infection
  - Other infective bronchiolitis
    - Pulmonary *Hemophilus influenzae* infection
    - Pulmonary *Mycoplasma pneumoniae* infection
  - Fungal infections such as forms of aspergillus infection
  - Septic emboli from infective endocarditis or infected tube
- Small airway disease
- Hypersensitivity pneumonitis
- Malignant entities
  - Nodular metastases
  - Adenocarcinoma
  - Forms of pulmonary lymphoma
  - Kaposi sarcoma
- Miscellaneous conditions
  - Granulomatosis with polyangiitis
  - *Alveolar microlithiasis*: Very dense
  - Diffuse panbronchiolitis
  - Diffuse idiopathic pulmonary neuroendocrine cell hyperplasia (DIPNECH)
  - Pulmonary amyloidosis: nodular forms

Imaging Findings

1. **Metastatic disease (malignant)**:
   - Multiple nodules of variable size noted throughout lungs parenchyma. These may be well-defined, round, and vary in number and distribution. Depending on their growth, they can vary from diffuse micronodular shadows resembling military disease to multiple large, well-defined "cannonballs". Cavitation may be seen in about 4% of metastases.
   - Example: Breast, colon, renal cell carcinoma, and melanoma.
2. **Pulmonary hamartomas**:
   - Benign, well-defined nodules that may contain fat or calcifications, often described as "popcorn-like".
3. **Granulomatous diseases (e.g., tuberculosis, sarcoidosis)**:
   - Small, well-defined nodules, which can be calcified, especially in healed tuberculosis.
   - Nodules may cluster and often have a perilymphatic distribution in sarcoidosis, particularly along the bronchovascular bundles, septa, and pleura.
4. **Infections (e.g., fungal infections like histoplasmosis or septic emboli)**:
   - Nodules can be random in distribution, often cavitate, and are associated with other signs of infection (e.g., consolidation, pleural effusions).
   - Cavitation is more common with fungal infections or septic emboli.
   - Cavitary lesions: Seen in postprimary/reactivation tuberculosis, thick-walled cavitary lesions in the upper lobes.
   - Tree-in-bud pattern: Seen in endobronchial TB, characterized by small centrilobular nodules with a branching appearance.

5. **Pneumoconiosis (e.g., silicosis, coal worker's pneumoconiosis)**:
   - Upper-lobe predominant nodules.
   - Associated with progressive massive fibrosis in advanced stages.
   - Nodules may be calcified in chronic cases.
6. **Respiratory bronchiolitis**:
   - Faint micronodular nodules (3–5 mm) and patchy ground-glass opacities
   - Predominantly tend to involve the upper lobes.
7. **Vasculitis (e.g., granulomatosis with polyangiitis)**:
   - Multiple nodules, which may cavitate, usually in a random distribution.
   - Cavitation is common in Wegener's granulomatosis.

7. Cystic lesions of lung and imaging. [10] [DNB June 22]

Introduction

Cysts are round parenchymal lucency or low attenuating area with a well-defined interface with normal lung parenchyma, having variable wall thickness but are usually thin-walled (<2 mm) and occur without associated pulmonary emphysema.[21]

Differentials of cystic lesions of lung include:

1. **Postinfective**
   - Bacterial pneumonia
   - *Pneumocystis jirovecii* pneumonia
   - Hydatid cyst
2. **Posttraumatic lung laceration**
3. **Congenital**
   - CPAM
   - Bronchogenic cyst
4. **Neoplastic**
   - Cystic lung metastasis—colonic adenocarcinoma, endometrial stromal sarcoma, epithelioid sarcoma
   - Lung metastasis after treatment
5. **Diffuse lung disease**
   - Tuberous sclerosis
   - Neurofibromatosis
   - Lymphangioleiomyomatosis
   - Langerhans cell histiocytosis
   - Birt-Hogg-dubé syndrome
   - Desquamative interstitial pneumonia
   - Hypersensitivity pneumonitis
   - End stage of fibrotic interstitial lung disease
     - Gold standard for evaluating cystic lung diseases: HRCT **(Flowchart 7)**
     - Provides detailed images of the cysts' size, number, and distribution.

Imaging Findings of Various Cystic Lung Diseases

Imaging Findings in Diffuse Cystic Lung Diseases

Introduction: Cysts are well defined parenchymal spaces containing air and surrounded by thin wall (thickness <3 mm) **(Flowchart 8)**.

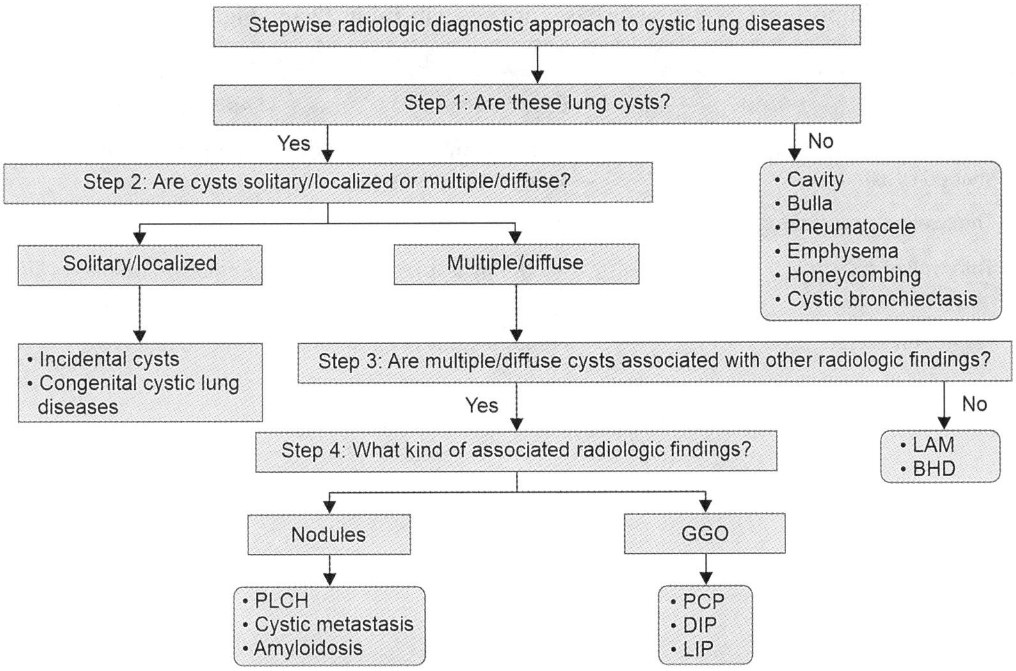

FLOWCHART 7: Algorithm for diagnostic approach of cystic lung diseases.

(BHD: Birt–Hogg–Dubé syndrome; DIP: desquamative interstitial pneumonia; GGO: ground-glass opacity; LAM: lymphangioleiomyomatosis; LIP: lymphoid interstitial pneumonia; PCP: *pneumocystis jirovecii* pneumonia; PLCH: pulmonary Langerhans cell histiocytosis)

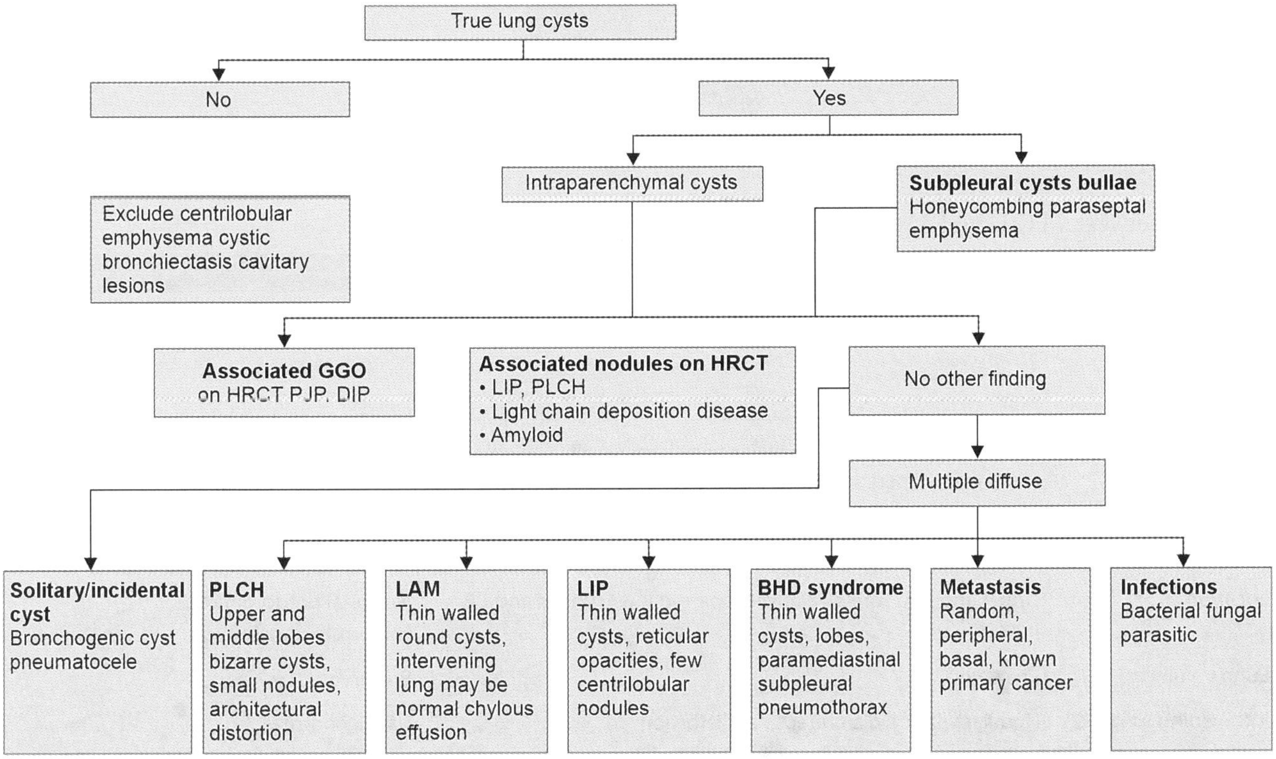

FLOWCHART 8: Diagnostic algorithm for evaluating cystic lung diseases.

(GGO: ground-glass opacity; LAM: lymphangioleiomyomatosis; LCH: Langerhans cell histiocytosis; LIP: lymphoid interstitial pneumonia)

Differentiating features of important cystic lung diseases are given in **Table 22** and **Fig. 24**).

TABLE 22: Differentiating features of important cystic lung diseases.

Disease	*Imaging*	*Distribution*	*Additional findings*
PLCH	Nodules with cysts (Irregular bizarre shaped cysts)	Predominantly upper zones, spares basal zones	Lung volume normal or hyperinflated
LAM	Thin walled cysts (uniform round cyst)	Random, diffuse	Chylous effusion
Tuberous sclerosis	Thin walled cysts	Randomly distributed	Angiomyolipomas of kidneys and liver; other features of TS
LIP	Well-defined cysts	Predominantly in basal zones	Ground glass haze

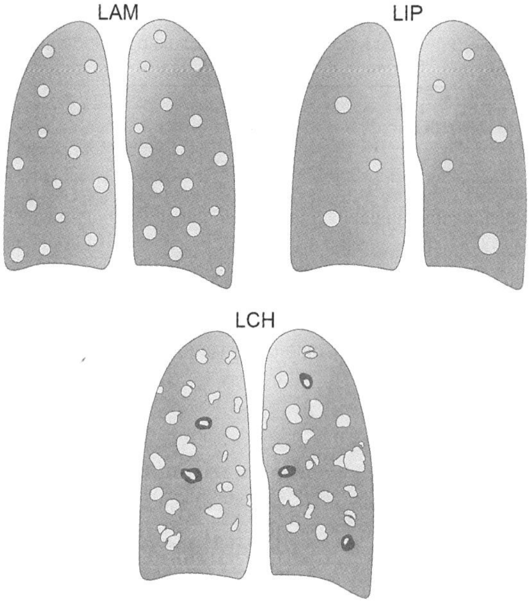

FIG. 24: Different characteristics of cysts in LCH, LAM and LIP.

Difference between PLCH and LAM is given in **Table 23.**

TABLE 23: Difference between PLCH and LAM.

	PLCH	*LAM*
Age	20–40 years	30–35 years
	M=F	Female
Cysts	Cysts are irregular and are of varying shapes such as bilobed, cloverleaf shaped or bizarre shaped.	Cysts are round and uniform
	Nodules may be seen in the intervening lung parenchyma between the cysts	May show features similar to tuberous sclerosis
Location	Upper and mid zones, relatively sparing lower zones and CP angles	No zonal predominance Uniformly distributed
Lung volume	Preserved	Preserved
Intervening lungs	Nodular with mild architectural distortion	Usually normal
Other findings	Pneumothorax	Chylous effusion
		Pneumothorax

Few conditions mimicking cystic lung diseases are given in **Table 24.**

TABLE 24: Mimicker of cystic lung diseases.

Conditions	*Imaging*	*Distribution*	*Additional findings*
Honeycombing	Multilayered honeycomb cysts	Subpleural, peripheral, basal zones	Intra-and interlobular interstitial thickening, ground glass haze
Cystic bronchiectasis	Cysts continuous with bronchial structures	Focal or diffuse, depending on etiology	Signet ring sign
Centrilobular emphysema	Cystic air spaces without wall	Upper lobe predominance	Vessels coursing through the cyst
Paraseptal emphysema	Cystic air spaces without wall	Subpleural, more in upper lobes	Cysts adjacent to pleural surface
Bullae	Round focal lucency or decreased attenuation >1 cm in size	Focal or diffuse	Adjacent lungs show emphysematous changes
Cavity	Often thick walled (>4 mm), irregular shaped gas-filled space/lucency within pulmonary consolidation or mass, or nodule	Distribution depending on the etiology	Consolidation or mass seen

8. Radiographic compartments of mediastinum. Pediatric mediastinal masses. Posterior mediastinal masses in 1-year-old child. [10] [DNB Dec 21]

1. Plain Radiographic Divisions (Felson's Mediastinal Division)

On plain radiographs, the divisions of mediastinum are anterior, middle, and posterior mediastinal compartments which were redefined by Felson.

Anterior Compartment

Extent: Posterior to the sternum and anterior to a line drawn along the anterior tracheal wall in the upper mediastinum and the posterior border of the heart in the lower mediastinum.

Contents: Thymus, heart, ascending aorta and great vessels, anterior portion of the main pulmonary artery, pericardium, fat, lymph vessels, nodes.

Middle Compartment

Extent: Between the anterior compartment in front and the posterior compartment behind.

Contents: The trachea and main bronchi, superior vena cava, midportion of the aortic arch, azygos arch, lymph nodes, esophagus, descending aorta (sometimes).

Posterior Compartment

Extent: Posterior to a line 1 cm behind the anterior margin of the vertebral column and anterior to the chest wall.

Contents: Vertebral bodies, paravertebral tissues, descending aorta (sometimes), posterior azygos vein, hemiazygos vein, and lymph nodes.

2. ITMIG Definition of Mediastinal Compartments

The three-compartment cross-sectional imaging model of the mediastinal compartments developed by ITMIG includes prevascular (anterior), visceral (middle), and paravertebral (posterior) compartments. Specific compartment boundaries and the anatomic structures they contain can be readily identified at multidetector CT (**Table 25** and **Fig. 25**).

TABLE 25: CT-based radiological division of mediastinum.

ITMIG multidetector CT-based classification of mediastinal compartments		
Compartment	***Boundaries***	***Major Contents***
Prevascular	• Superior: Thoracic inlet • Inferior: Diaphragm • Anterior: Sternum • Lateral: Parietal mediastinal pleura • Posterior: Anterior aspect of the pericardium as it wraps around the heart in a curvilinear fashion	• Thymus • Fat • Lymph nodes • Left brachiocephalic vein
Visceral	• Superior: Thoracic inlet • Inferior: Diaphragm • Anterior: Posterior boundaries of the prevascular compartment • Posterior: Vertical line connecting a point on each thoracic vertebral body 1 cm posterior to its anterior margin	• Nonvascular; trachea, carina, esophagus. • Lymph nodes • Vascular: Heart, ascending thoracic aorta, aortic arch, descending thoracic aorta, superior • Vena cava, intrapericardial pulmonary arteries, thoracic duct
Paravertebral	• Superior: Thoracic inlet • Inferior: Diaphragm • Anterior: Posterior boundaries of the visceral compartment • Posterolateral: Vertical line against the posterior margin of the chest wall at the lateral margin of the transverse process of the thoracic spine	• Thoracic spine • Paravertebral soft tissues

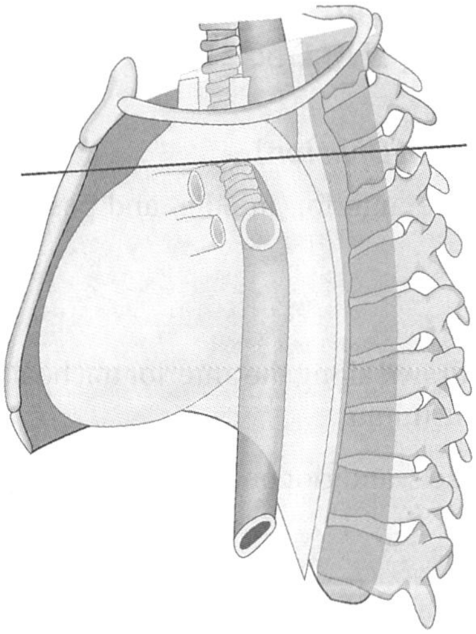

FIG. 25: Illustrated image of mediastinum division.

Pediatric Mediastinal Masses

Pediatric mediastinal masses are the most common chest masses in children **(Table 26** and **Fig. 26)**.[22,23]

Anterior mediastinum (45%) is the most common location.

TABLE 26: Pediatric mediastinal masses.

Mediastinal masses in children		
Mass type	***Lesion(s)***	***Pertinent finding(s)***
Prevascular compartment		
Thymic	Thymic cyst	Cyst, no internal vascularity
	Thymic hyperplasia	Microscopic fat
	Thymolipoma	Macroscopic fat, nodular appearance

Continued...

Continued...

Mediastinal masses in children		
Mass type	***Lesion(s)***	***Pertinent finding(s)***
Prevascular compartment		
Vascular	Lymphatic malformation	Multiseptated cyst, no internal vascularity
	Venous malformation	Slowly enhancing vascular channels communicating with venous system
	Infantile hemangioma	Briskly and intensely enhancing with large feeding arteries and draining veins, homogeneous enhancement, sharply demarcated borders
	KHE	Briskly and intensely enhancing with large feeding arteries and draining veins, heterogeneous enhancement, ill-defined borders
OCT	Teratomas	Imaging findings of fat, fluid, and calcification
	Seminomas, NSGCT	Poorly defined margins with local invasion, often metastatic at manifestation
Lymphoma	HL	Lobulated mass
	NHL	Nodular thymic enlargement, no macroscopic fat
Visceral compartment		
FDC	-	Cyst, no internal vascularity, may be indistinguishable from pericardial cyst
Lymphadenopathy	TB	Lymphadenopathy with lung consolidation, calcification
	Castleman disease	High-attenuation nodes at noncontrast CT
	Sarcoid	Rare in children; a diagnosis of exclusion
Paravertebral compartment		
Neurogenic tumor	NB	Aggressive, displacing other structures, more likely to have calcification
	GNB, GN	Benign features, more likely to have calcification
Nerve sheath tumor	Neurofibroma, schwannoina	History of neurofibromatosis, target sign, spi it-fat sign

(FDC: foregut duplication cyst; GCT: germ cell tumor; GN: ganglioneuroma; GNB: ganglioneuroblastoma; HL: Hodgkin lymphoma; KHE: kaposiform hemangioendothelioma; NB: neuroblastoma; NHL: non-Hodgkin lymphoma; NSGCT: nonseminomatous GCT; TB = tuberculosis)

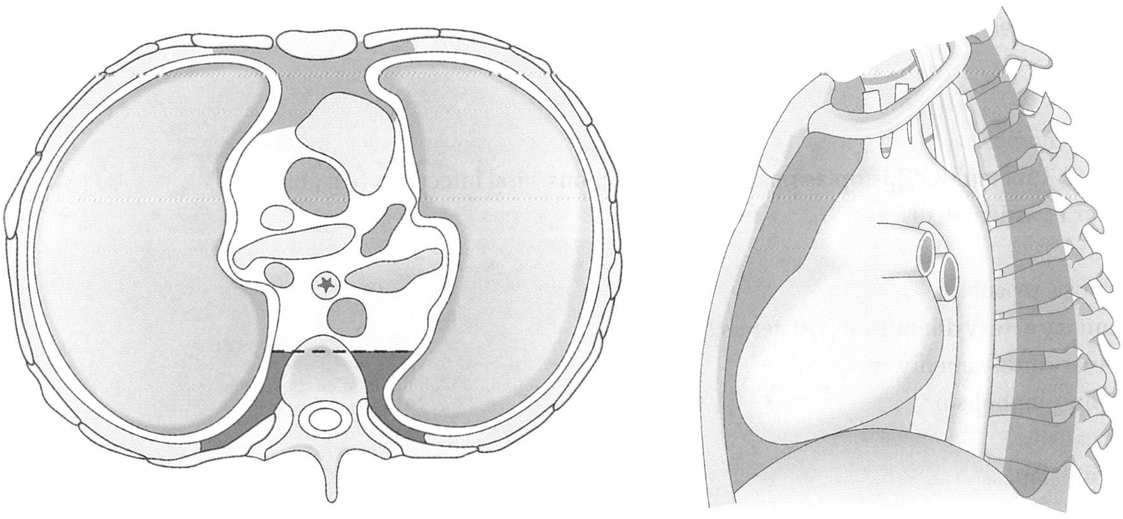

FIG. 26: Diagram illustrates ITMIG based depiction of prevascular (blue), visceral (yellow), and paravertebral (green) compartments.

Posterior Mediastinal Masses in 1-year-old

30% to 405 of pediatric masses are in the posterior compartment and 955 of this are neurogenic origin. Masses are categorized into:

1. **Neoplastic**
   a. Ganglion cell tumors
      i. Neuroblastoma:
         - Malignant tumor arising from the primitive neural crest.
         - Most common pediatric extracranial solid tumor.
         - Chest radiographs show soft-tissue opacity in the paravertebral region associated with rib or vertebral erosion or destruction or widening of intercostal spaces.
         - Calcification is common.
         - CT demonstrate margins of the tumor and internal calcification as well as local extension and distant metastases.
         - On MRI, T2WI—high signal, T1WI— low signal, Postcontrast-enhance early, reflecting the high vascularity of the tumor
      ii. Ganglioneuroblastoma and ganglioneuroma:
         - Less aggressive tumors than neuroblastomas.
         - Ganglioneuroma is a benign, whereas ganglioneuroblastoma considered malignant.
         - Radiologically, they are difficult to differentiate from neuroblastomas because of similar imaging characteristics.
         - Ganglioneuroblastoma and ganglioneuroma may have a more fusiform configuration than neuroblastoma.
         - Ganglioneuroblastomas and ganglioneuromas occur in older children.
   b. Nerve sheath tumor:
      – Benign-schwannoma, neurofibroma
      – Malignant-peripheral nerve sheath tumor (MPNST).
      – Round or oblong posterior mediastinal mass with dumbbell-shaped extension into the spinal canal seen on CT or MRI.
      – On CT, these show decreased attenuation because of their lipid contents or cystic degeneration and have variable enhancement.
2. **Others**: Bochdalek hernia and extramedullary hematopoiesis may be seen posterior mediastinum.

9. Causes of hilar node enlargement. How to differentiate causes on imaging. [10] [DNB Dec 21]

Causes of Unilateral Hilar Enlargement[24]

Lymph Nodes

- Lung carcinoma
- **Infection**: Tuberculosis, histoplasmosis, fungal infections, viral infections (e.g., EBV, CMV).
- Unicentric castleman disease
- Lymphoma
- Sarcoidosis vascular
- **Pulmonary artery dilatation**: Poststenosis
- Pulmonary artery aneurysm
- Pulmonary embolism
- **Other causes**:
- Mediastinal mass

- Carcinoid tumor
- Perihilar pneumonia

Causes of Bilateral Hilar Enlargement

Lymph Nodes

- Sarcoidosis
- Lymphoma
- Lymph node metastasis
- Multicentric Castleman disease
- **Infective**: Virus, histoplasmosis, coccidioidomycosis
- Silicosis Vascular
- Pulmonary artery hypertension

How to Differentiate Causes of Hilar Enlargement on Imaging?

1. **Unilateral versus bilateral**
   - Unilateral hilar node enlargement generally seen in localized diseases like- lung cancer or infection (e.g., tuberculosis).
   - Bilateral hilar lymphadenopathy is seen in systemic conditions like sarcoidosis or lymphoma.
   - Hodgkin's lymphoma, is often associated with mediastinal or supraclavicular lymph node enlargement.
2. **Symmetrical versus asymmetrical**:
   - *Symmetrical enlargement*: sarcoidosis.
   - *Asymmetrical*: Malignancy or infection.
3. **Size and shape**:
   - Larger, bulky nodes with irregular or lobulated margins seen in lymphoma or metastatic disease.
   - Smaller nodes with smoother borders—benign or reactive.
4. **Associated lung parenchymal changes**:
   - *Pulmonary mass or nodules*: Primary lung cancer or metastatic disease. Cavitating lesions: Tuberculosis or fungal infections.
   - *Ground-glass opacities or interstitial changes*: Sarcoidosis, infections, or pneumoconioses. Pneumoconioses (silicosis or berylliosis) present with lung nodules or fibrosis.
5. **Calcifications**:
   - *Eggshell calcification*: Silicosis or coal worker's pneumoconiosis.
   - *Punctate or coarse calcification*: Postinfectious (e.g., tuberculosis or histoplasmosis) or treated lymphoma.
   - *No calcification*: Malignancy or an active inflammatory process (sarcoidosis, lymphoma).
6. **Enhancement on CT/MRI**:
   - *Homogeneous enhancement*: Lymphomas or benign inflammatory causes.
   - *Heterogeneous enhancement*: May indicate necrotic or metastatic lymph nodes.
   - CT angiography identifies hilar enlargement due to vascular causes like pulmonary artery enlargement.
7. **Associated findings**:
   - *Mediastinal lymphadenopathy*: Systemic diseases like lymphoma or sarcoidosis.
   - *Pleural effusion*: Malignancy (lung cancer or lymphoma) or infection (tuberculosis).

10. Pathologies of lung carcinoma. TNM staging in lung carcinoma. FDG PET role in lung carcinoma. [10] [DNB June 21, RG 18, AIIMS May 24]

Pathologies of lung carcinoma are given in **Flowchart 9.**

TNM staging of lung carcinoma is given in **Table 27.**

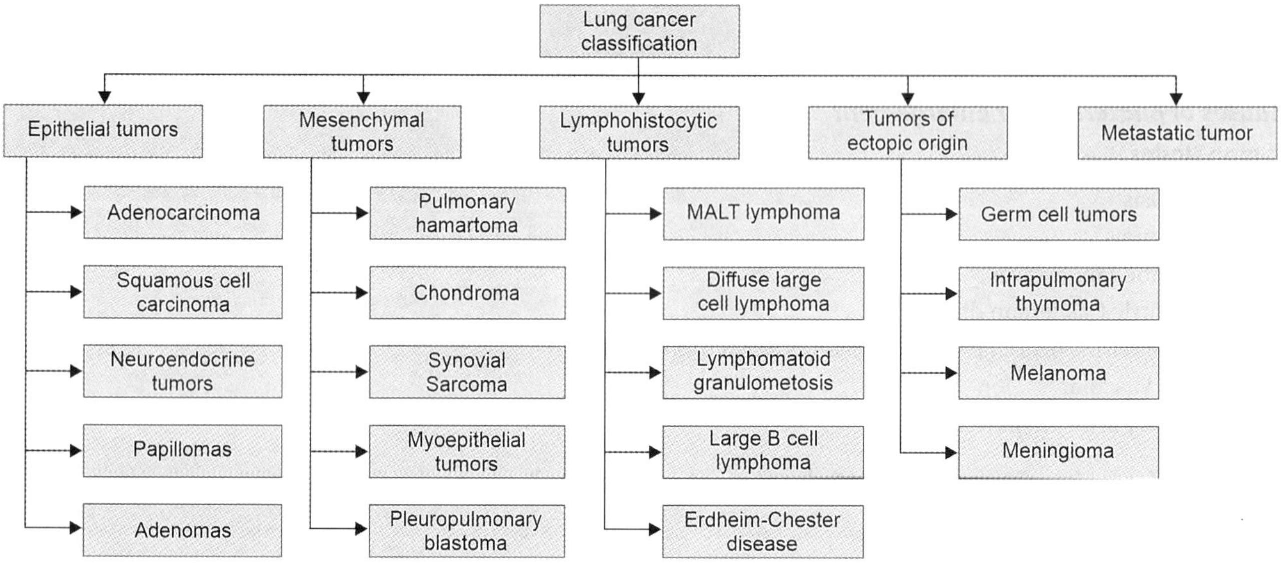

FLOWCHART 9: Classification of lung cancer.

TABLE 27: TNM staging of lung CA.

T_x	Tumor in sputum/bronchial washings but not be assessed in imaging or bronchoscopy
T_0	No evidence of tumor
T_{is}	Carcinoma in situ
T_1	≤3 cm surrounded by lung/visceral pleura, not involving main bronchus
$T_{1a(mi)}$	Minimally invasive carcinoma
T_{1a}	≤1 cm
T_{1b}	>1 to ≤2 cm
T_{1c}	>2 to ≤3 cm
T_2	>3 to ≤5 cm or involvement of main bronchus without carina, regardless of distance from carina or invasion visceral pleural or atelectasis or post obstructive pneumonitis extending to hilum
T_{2a}	>3 to ≤4 cm
T_{2b}	>4 to <5 cm
T_3	>5 to ≤7 cm in greatest dimension or tumor of any size that involves chest wall, pericardium, phrenic nerve or satellite nodules in the same lobe
T_4	>7 cm in greatest dimension or any tumor with invasion of mediastinum, diaphragm, heart, great vessels, recurrent laryngeal nerve, carina, trachea, esophagus, spine or separate tumor in different lobe of ipsilateral lung
N_1	Ipsilateral peribronchial and/or hilar nodes and intrapulmonary nodes
2	Ipsilateral mediastinal and/or subcarinal nodes
3	Contralateral mediastinal or hilar; ipsilateral/contralateral scalene/supraclavicular
M1	Distant metastasis
M1a	Tumor in contralateral lung or pleural/pericardial nodule/malignant effusion
M_{1b}	Single extrathoracic metastasis, including single non-regional lymphnode
M_{1c}	Multiple extrathoracic metastases in one or more organs

Role of PET CT in Lung Carcinoma is given in Tables 28 and 29

- Metabolic status of the mass and lymph nodes.
  - Measured in standardized uptake value (SUV)
  - >2.5: Indicates malignancy.
- For accurate size measurement if atelectasis is also present

TABLE 28: Criteria for using PET CT in nonsmall cell lung CA.			
Lung Cancer	***Initial Workup***	***Restaging/Response/Recurrence***	***Surveillance***
Nonsmall cell lung Cancer	Indicated for inittal staging in all cases	To exclude disease progression or interval development of metastatic disease after induction therapy	Not recommend ed routinely Recommended for RT planning

TABLE 29: Criteria for using PET CT in small cell lung CA.			
Lung cancer	***Initial workup***	***Restaging/response/recurrence***	***Surveillance***
Small cell lung cancer	If limited stage expected Optional tor low or intermediate NET PET/CT has replaced bone scan in NCCN guidelines Recommended for RT planning	Not recommended for routine follow up	Not recommended routinely

- For lesion characterization
  - Differentiation of scar from tumor or atelectasis
  - Differentiation of satellite nodules from post obstructive changes
- For detection of pleural invasion and malignant pleural effusion
- For detecting synchronous tumors or other malignancies
- For staging
  - TNM staging
  - Treatment-response evaluation
  - Restaging
  - Determining the prognosis of lung cancer
- Planning of radiotherapy
  Accuracy of combined PET: CT is significantly higher than PET or CT alone.

Limitations of PET CT

Infections may show avidity (false-positive result)

- TB
- Histoplasmosis
- Aspergillosis
- Cryptococcosis;
- Postsurgical changes
- Postradiotherapy changes
- Flare phenomenon

Low-grade malignancies may not show avidity (false-negative result)

- Bronchoalveolar carcinoma
- Carcinoid tumor

11. ITMIG classification of mediastinum. Thymoma-imaging features and approach. Imaging features thymoma vs hyperplasia. [10] [DNB June 21]

ITMIG Definition of Mediastinal Compartments

The three-compartment cross-sectional imaging model of the mediastinal compartments developed by ITMIG includes prevascular (anterior), visceral (middle), and paravertebral (posterior) compartments. Specific compartment boundaries and the anatomic structures they contain can be readily identified at multidetector CT **(Table 30 and Fig. 27)**.

TABLE 30: Criteria for using PET CT in small cell lung CA.

ITMIG Multidetector CT-based classification of mediastinal compartments		
Compartment	***Boundaries***	***Major contents***
Prevascular	Superior: Thoracic inlet Inferior: Diaphragm Anterior: Sternum Lateral: Parietal mediastinal pleura Posterior: Anterior aspect of the pericardium as it wraps around the heart in a curvilinear fashion	Thymus Fat Lymph nodes Left brachiocephalic vein
Visceral	Superior: Thoracic inlet Inferior: Diaphragm Anterior: Posterior boundaries of the prevascular compartment Posterior: Vertical line connecting a point on each thoracic vertebral body 1 cm posterior to its anterior margin	Nonvascular: Trachea, carina, esophagus, lymph nodes Vascular: Heart, ascending thoracic aorta, aortic arch, descending thoracic aorta, superior vena cava, intrapericardial pulmonary arteries, thoracic duct
Paravertebral	Superior: Thoracic inlet Inferior: Diaphragm Anterior: Posterior boundaries of the visceral compartment Posterolateral: Vertical line against the posterior margin of the chest wall at the lateral margin of the transverse process of the thoracic spine	Thoracic spine Paravertebral soft tissues

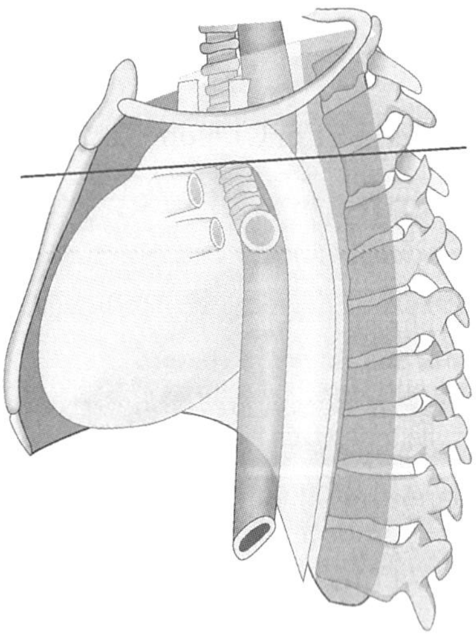

FIG. 27: Illustrated image of mediastinum division.

Approach to a Case of Thymoma

Includes step-by-step use of multiple imaging modalities, starting with the most basic chest X-ray to CT, MRI, and biopsy.

1. **Initial chest x-ray**: Quick and noninvasive but may miss small lesions or poorly defined masses.
2. **CT scan (gold standard)**: Evaluate mass characterization, enhancement pattern, invasion, calcifications and staging.
3. **MRI**: Used when there's suspicion of invasion or vascular involvement not fully confirmed by CT.
4. **PET/CT**: For suspected metastasis or aggressive thymoma variants.
5. **Biopsy**: If imaging features are ambiguous, biopsy under CT/USG guidance may be considered.

Thymoma-imaging Features

Thymoma is the most common tumors of the anterior mediastinum.

1. **Chest X-ray**:
   - Well-defined, sharply marginated and smooth or lobulated mass usually project to one side of the mediastinum and adjacent to the heart or large vessels but may be missed in early stages or small tumors.
   - Dense calcification may be seen throughout the mass or in its periphery.
   - On lateral radiographs, thymoma appear as a lucent triangular opacity in the inferior aspect of the retrosternal clear space.
2. **CT Scan**:
   - Gold standard investigation.
   - Well-circumscribed, smooth or lobular mass involving one lobe of the thymus and do not conform to the normal shape of the thymus.
   - Thymoma shows homogeneous contrast enhancement, however one third cases show heterogeneous enhancement due to areas of hemorrhage, necrosis, or cystic change with punctate, linear capsular, or coarse intratumoral calcifications.
   - In cases of invasive thymoma, local invasion into adjacent structures such as the pericardium, pleura, or large vessels noted.
   - Noninvasive thymoma: Confined to the thymus with a well-defined capsule.
   - Invasive thymoma: Breaks the capsule and invades nearby tissues, requiring careful assessment of adjacent structures.
   - Staging with CT: Masaoka-Koga Staging: Evaluates tumor extent:

     Stage I: Encapsulated tumor.

     Stage II: Tumor invades surrounding fat or pleura.

     Stage III: Tumor invades neighboring structures like the pericardium or great vessels.

     Stage IV: Metastatic spread (pleural, pericardial, or distant metastases).
3. **MRI findings**:
   - *T1*: Isointense to slightly hyperintense signal compared to muscle
   - T2
     - Heterogeneous signal, slightly higher than muscle.
     - Cystic areas may be seen, especially in larger tumors.
     - Fibrous septa crossing the mass are of low signal intensity.
   - *In/out phase imaging*: Typically, no signal drop out, i.e., no chemical shift.
   - *T1 C+ (Gd)*: Linear regions of enhancement may be seen coursing through the mass, thought to represent fibrous septa.
   - MRI is particularly useful for distinguishing between thymoma and other masses like cysts or lipomas.
4. **Positron emission tomography (PET) CT**
   - Low-to-moderate FDG uptake in most thymomas.
   - Higher FDG uptake suggest a more aggressive tumor like thymic carcinoma or recurrent disease.

Imaging Features of Thymic Hyperplasia

Thymic hyperplasia: Thymic hyperplasia is an enlargement of the thymus without true neoplasm formation and is commonly seen in younger patients.

Imaging features:

- Enlargement of the thymus but with preservation of the normal shape
- Often bilateral and symmetric
- Homogeneous, typically without any necrosis or calcifications

- Sometimes, the thymus shows fat-containing tissue
- Mild enhancement with intravenous contrast but not as marked as thymomas
- **On MRI T1WI**: Similar to muscle with fat signals
- **T2WI**: Hyperintense compared to normal thymus

Distinguishing features between thymoma and thymic hyperplasia:
Thymoma usually presents as a well-circumscribed mass, with calcifications or invasion of adjacent structures.

Thymic hyperplasia tends to show a more uniform and symmetric enlargement of the thymus without invasion or calcification.

12. Solitary pulmonary nodule definition. Discuss the etiologies/differential diagnosis. Benign vs. malignant SPN. [10]

Solitary Pulmonary Nodule (SPN)

Definition

A SPN usually is defined as a focal opacity, visible on chest radiographs or CT, which fits the following criteria:

1. Well-defined round or oval lesion
2. <3 cm (>3 cm = mass)
3. Surrounded at least partially by the lung parenchyma
4. With no associated lymphadenopathy, collapse or consolidation.

Causes of solitary pulmonary nodules:

1. **Granulomatous**
   - Tuberculoma
   - Histoplasmoma
   - Others
2. **Malignant tumors**
   - Lung cancer
   - Solitary metastasis
   - Rare malignant lung tumors
3. **Benign tumors**
   - Carcinoid tumor
   - Hamartoma
4. **Infectious/inflammatory**
   - Pneumonia
   - Rounded atelectasis
   - Hydatid
   - Wegener's granulomatosis
   - Sarcoidosis
   - Organizing pneumonia
5. **Congenital**
   - Intrapulmonary lymph node
   - Sequestration
   - Bronchogenic cyst
6. **Vascular**
   - Hematoma
   - Arteriovenous malformation

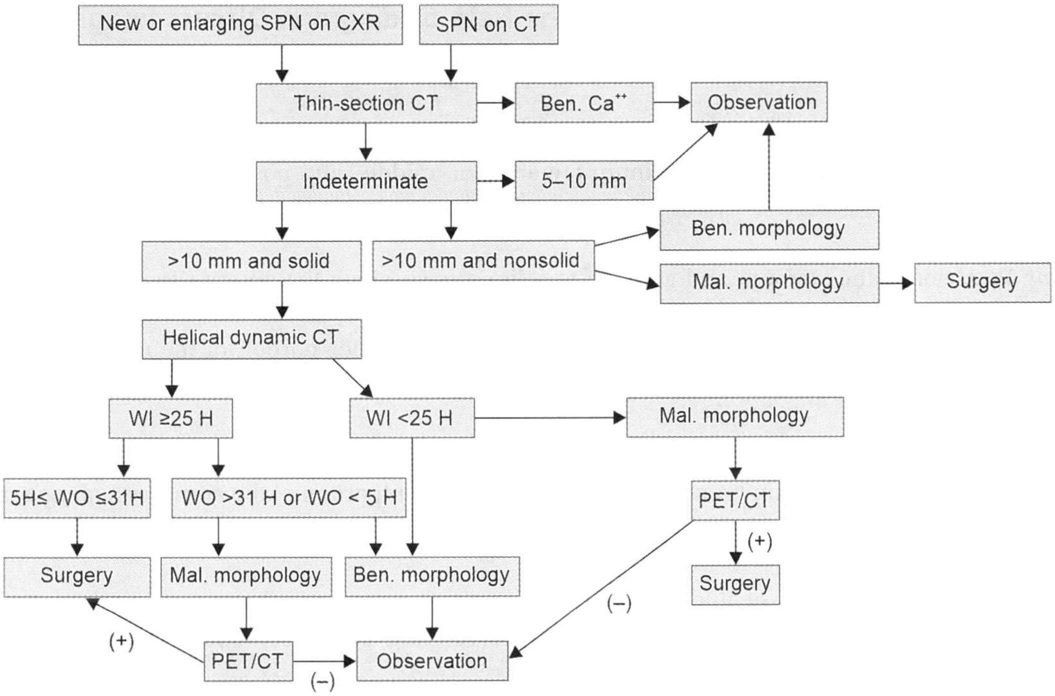

FLOWCHART 10: Algorithm for differentiating features between benign and malignant nodules.

TABLE 31: Benign and malignant radiological features of pulmonary nodules.

Radiological feature	***Benign***	***Malignant***
Size	≤3	>3
Growth rate	Stable over 2 years	Doubling time of 1–18 months
Margins	Well-defined, smooth	Ill-defined, spiculated, undulated
Calcification within nodule	Dense, solid, laminated, popcorn	Fine, dendriform, punctate
Fat within nodule	Yes	No
Cavitation within nodule	Less likely. If so thin walled and round	Increases risk; thick walled and irregular
Enhancement	<15 HU	Average of 40 HU

Radiological workup of a solitary nodule highlighting the features which enable to differentiate between benign and malignant nodules are given in **Flowchart 10**:

Benign and malignant radiological features of pulmonary nodules are given in **Table 31.**

Perifissural Nodules (Fig. 28) are Mostly Benign

Additional features of malignant nodules:

- Upper lobe predominance
- Pleural retraction
- Part solid part ground glass nodule
- Cavitation with a thick wall (>15 mm) and a nodular wall
- Containing air bronchogram or bubble-like lucency

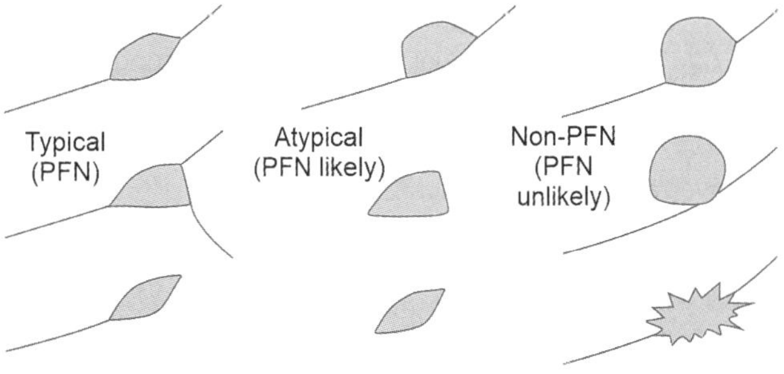

FIG. 28: Types of pulmonary nodules *(For Color Version Refer Fig. 22).*

13. Describe anatomy of mediastinum with the help of diagram. Discuss imaging features of anterior mediastinum masses. [5+5] [DNB Dec 20, AIIMS May 23, AIIMS Dec 24]

1. Plain Radiographic Divisions (Felson's mediastinal division)

On plain radiographs, the divisions of mediastinum are anterior, middle, and posterior mediastinal compartments which were redefined by Felson.

- **Anterior compartment**:
  - *Extent*: Posterior to the sternum and anterior to a line drawn along the anterior tracheal wall in the upper mediastinum and the posterior border of the heart in the lower mediastinum.
  - *Contents*: Thymus, heart, ascending aorta and great vessels, anterior portion of the main pulmonary artery, pericardium, fat, lymph vessels, nodes.
- **Middle compartment**:
  - *Extent*: Between the anterior compartment in front and the posterior compartment behind.
  - *Contents*: The trachea and main bronchi, superior vena cava, midportion of the aortic arch, azygos arch, lymph nodes, esophagus, descending aorta (sometimes).
- **Posterior compartment**:
  - *Extent*: Posterior to a line 1 cm behind the anterior margin of the vertebral column and anterior to the chest wall.
  - *Contents*: Vertebral bodies, paravertebral tissues, descending aorta (sometimes), posterior azygos vein, hemiazygos vein, and lymph nodes.

2. ITMIG Definition of Mediastinal Compartments

The three-compartment cross-sectional imaging model of the mediastinal compartments developed by ITMIG includes prevascular (anterior), visceral (middle), and paravertebral (posterior) compartments. Specific compartment boundaries and the anatomic structures they contain can be readily identified at multidetector CT **(Table 32 and Fig. 29)**.

TABLE 32: CT-based radiological division of mediastinum.

ITMIG multidetector CT-based classification of mediastinal compartments		
Compartment	***Boundaries***	***Major contents***
Prevascular	Superior: Thoracic inlet Inferior: Diaphragm Anterior: Sternum Lateral: Parietal mediastinal pleura Posterior: Anterior aspect of the pericardium as it wraps around the heart in a curvilinear fashion	Thymus Fat Lymph nodes Left brachiocephalic vein
Visceral	Superior: Thoracic inlet Inferior: Diaphragm Anterior: Posterior boundaries of the prevascular compartment Posterior: Vertical line connecting a point on each thoracic vertebral body 1 cm posterior to its anterior margin	Nonvascular: Trachea, carina, esophagus, lymph nodes Vascular: Heart, ascending thoracic aorta, aortic arch, descending thoracic aorta, superior vena cava, intrapericardial pulmonary arteries, thoracic duct
Paravertebral	Superior: Thoracic inlet Inferior: Diaphragm Anterior: Posterior boundaries of the visceral compartment Posterolateral: Vertical line against the posterior margin of the chest wall at the lateral margin of the transverse process of the thoracic spine	Thoracic spine Paravertebral soft tissues

Imaging Features of Anterior Mediastinal Lesions

Anterior mediastinum:

- **Extent**: Posterior to the sternum and anterior to a line drawn along the anterior tracheal wall in the upper mediastinum and the posterior border of the heart in the lower mediastinum.
- **Contents**: Thymus, heart, ascending aorta and great vessels, anterior portion of the main pulmonary artery, pericardium, fat, lymph vessels, nodes.

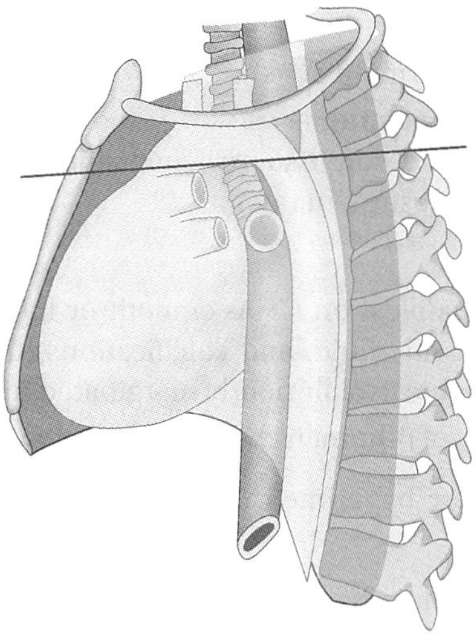

FIG. 29: Illustrated image of mediastinum division.

Thymus:

- Thymic hyperplasia
- Thymic cysts
- Thymolipoma
- Thymic epithelial neoplasm:
  - Thymoma
  - Thymic carcinoma
- Neuroendocrine tumors of thymus
  - Thymic carcinoid
  - Small cell Ca of thymus

Thyroid: *Retrosternal thyroid*

Parathyroid: *Ectopic parathyroid.*

Germ cell tumor

- Teratoma
  - Dermoid cyst (mature teratoma)
  - Immature teratoma
- Seminoma
- Nonseminomatous germ cell tumors

Vascular lesion:

1. Lymphangioma
2. Hemangioma

Common anterior mediastinal masses include thymomas, teratomas, thyroid masses, and lymphomas, often summarized by the mnemonic "4 T's" (thymoma, teratoma, thyroid, terrible lymphoma).

1. Thymoma

Most common primary tumor of anterior mediastinum. CT findings:

- Thymomas are well-marginated, smooth or lobulated, encapsulated, unilateral mediastinal masses.
- Show homogenous attenuation and enhancement.
- Soft-tissue density mass with possible areas of calcification.
- Invasive thymomas may demonstrate infiltration into adjacent structures. MRI findings:
- **T1**: Isointense to slightly hyperintense signal compared to muscle
- **T2**
  - Heterogeneous signal, slightly higher than muscle.
  - Cystic areas may be seen, especially in larger tumors.
  - Fibrous septa crossing the mass are of low signal intensity.
- **In/out phase imaging**: Typically, no signal drop out, i.e., no chemical shift.
- **T1 C+ (Gd)**: Linear regions of enhancement may be seen coursing through the mass, thought to represent fibrous septa.

2. *Teratoma*

- Mature teratomas or dermoid cysts
- Immature or malignant teratomas

The combination of fluid, soft tissue, calcium, and fat is diagnostic of teratoma. The finding of a fat-fluid level within a mass on CT is also diagnostic of teratoma.

CT findings:

- Mature teratomas manifest on CT as smooth or lobulated mediastinal masses with heterogeneous components, including fat, soft tissue, fluid, and calcifications, that typically have cystic and solid components; in contrast, malignant teratomas are usually poorly marginated masses containing areas of necrosis.
- Normal serum levels of β-human chorionic gonadotropin hormone (β-hCG) and α-fetoprotein (AFP).

MRI: Fat components are hyperintense on T1-weighted images, and cystic areas show high signal intensity on T2-weighted images.

Complications: Can rupture into adjacent structures like the pleura or pericardium, causing inflammation or infection.

3. *Seminoma*

Occurs almost entirely in men, with a mean age at presentation of 29 years. Most common malignant mediastinal germ-cell tumor.

CT findings:

- Seminomas present as large, smoother lobulated, homogeneous soft tissue attenuation masses, although small areas of low attenuation can be seen. Obliteration of fat planes is common.
- Pleural or pericardial effusion may be present.

4. *Nonseminomatous Germ Cell Tumors*

This are embryonal carcinoma, endodermal sinus (yolk sac) tumor, choriocarcinoma, and mixed types.

CT findings:

- Large poorly marginated masses often show heterogeneous opacity, including ill-defined areas of low attenuation secondary to necrosis and hemorrhage or cystic areas.
- May be infiltrative, with obliteration of fat planes, and may be spiculated. Calcification may be seen.

MR findings: *Also reflect the inhomogeneous nature of these lesions.*

5. *Thyroid Mass (Ectopic or Substernal Goiter)*

- **CT findings**: A substernal goiter is typically contiguous with the thyroid gland, extending into the mediastinum. It may have areas of calcification and appear heterogeneous due to varying degrees of iodine content or cystic changes.
- **MRI findings**: Shows a low to intermediate signal on T1 and T2-weighted images, with avid enhancement post-contrast.
- **Nuclear medicine**: Iodine uptake studies or technetium scans can help confirm thyroid tissue origin.

6. *Thymic Cyst*

- Uncommon.
- CT can suggest the diagnosis of thymic cyst if the lesion (a) appears *thin walled*, (b) is unassociated with a mass lesion, (c) contains fluid with a density close to that of water, and (d) remains *unopacified following contrast infusion.*

7. *Lymphoma*

CT findings:

Mediastinal lymphomas typically present as large, homogeneous, soft tissue masses with lobulated borders. Unlike thymomas, lymphomas rarely contain calcifications or fat. These masses can encase adjacent structures like the great vessels but usually without causing vascular obstruction.

MRI findings:
Appears hypointense on T1-weighted images and hyperintense on T2-weighted images, with variable contrast enhancement.

PET-CT: FDG avidity is usually high in lymphomas, making PET-CT a useful tool for staging and monitoring response to treatment.

8. Vascular Lesion

a. **Lymphangioma**
- Rare benign congenital lesions. In <2-year-old child.
- On CT these lesions manifest as lobular multicystic tumors that surround and infiltrate adjacent mediastinal structures.

b. **Hemangioma**
- Large interconnecting vascular spaces with varying amounts of interposed stromal elements such as fat and fibrous tissue.
- Focal areas of organized thrombus can calcify as phleboliths.
- *CECT and T1 CE MRI*: Multiple tortuous serpentine enhancing structures may be present.

Emergency Chest

1. Describe bolus tracking technique used during MDCT pulmonary angiography. Discuss the MDCT findings in a case of acute pulmonary thromboembolism. [5+5] [AIIMS Dec 23]

Bolus Tracking Technique

- It is used in multidetector computed tomography pulmonary angiography for detecting pulmonary embolism.
- It is sequential axial slices at a set region of interest conducted during real time monitoring of contrast arrival, peak enhancement in the target vessel and helps in starting the scan with an appropriate predecided time delay.
- The contrast density in bolus tracking in target vessel may not always be linear, variation in contrast arrival time and time to reach the trigger value because of individual cardiac and hemodynamic variations **(Fig. 30)**.

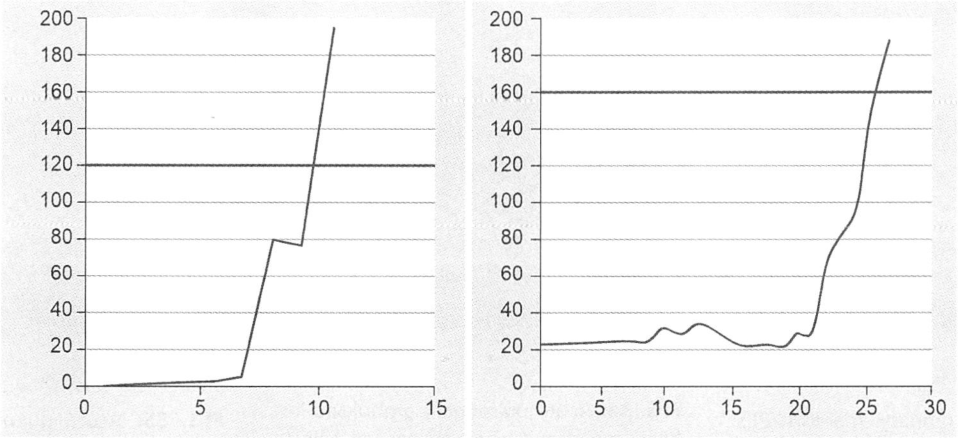

FIG. 30: Contrast arrival time and time to peak vary from patient to patient (illustrated in two different cases) highlighting the importance of the bolus tracking method.

Technique

- Patient position
  - Supine with their arms above their head
- Scout
  - Apices to diaphragm
- Scan extent
  - Apices to diaphragm
- Scan direction
  - Caudocranial
- Contrast injection considerations
  - Monitoring slice (region of interest)
    - Below the carina at the level of the pulmonary trunk with an ROI on the pulmonary artery
  - Threshold: 100 HU
  - Volume: 60 mL of non-ionic contrast with a 100 mL saline chaser at 4.5/5 mL/s
- Scan delay
  - Minimal scan delay
- Respiration phase
  - Inspiration

MDCT findings in a case of acute pulmonary thromboembolism **(Figs. 31 to 35)**.

Findings are acute embolus appears as a hypodense (low attenuation) area within the contrast-filled pulmonary arteries.[25,26]

1. Filling Defects in Pulmonary Arteries

- Central filling defect within a vessel surrounded by contrast material produce "polo-mint" sign.
- Linear intraluminal filling defect within the vessels surrounded by contrast material called "railroad-track" sign.
- Saddle Embolus: An embolus straddling the bifurcation of the main pulmonary artery, often involving both sides.

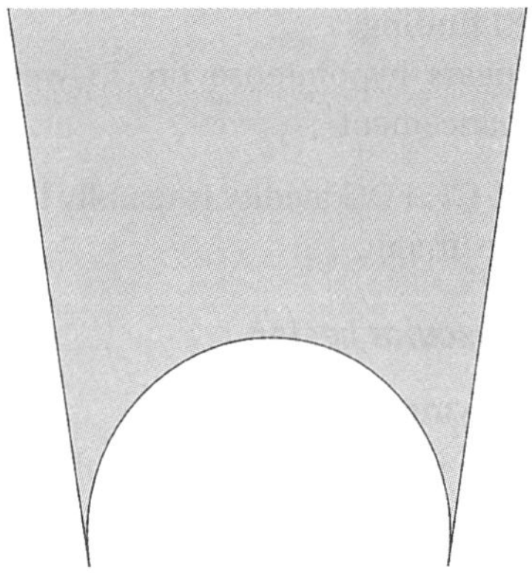

FIG. 31: Acute pulmonary embolism (PE). Illustration of complete obstruction due to acute PE as seen on angiography. Trailing edge of thrombus forms concave filling defect within column of contrast material at level of obstruction.

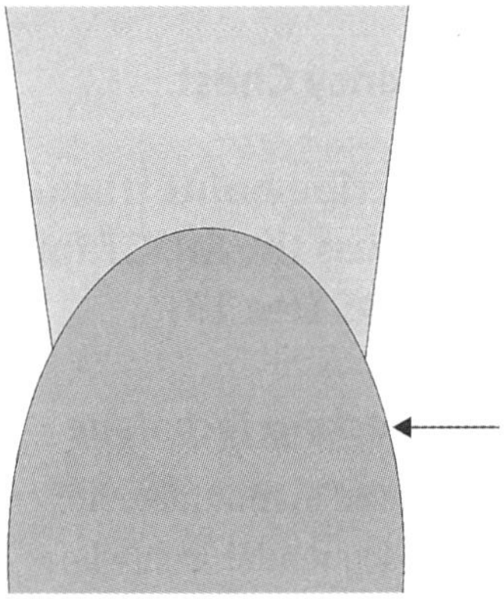

FIG. 32: Acute pulmonary embolism (PE). Illustration of coronal reformatted CT image of acute PE shows expansion of diameter of involved vessel distal to point of obstruction (*arrow*).

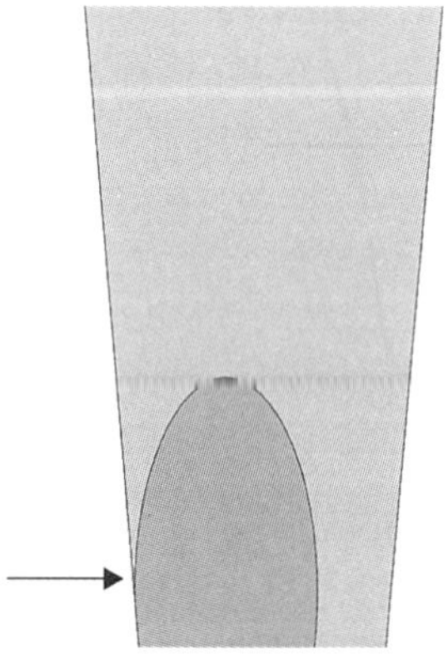

FIG. 33: Acute pulmonary embolism (PE). Illustration shows that eccentric acute thrombus (*arrow*) makes acute angles with vessel wall.

FIG. 34: Acute pulmonary embolism. Illustration shows acute PE central filling defect on CT image viewed perpendicular to plane of thrombus; well-defined central thrombus is completely surrounded by contrast material.

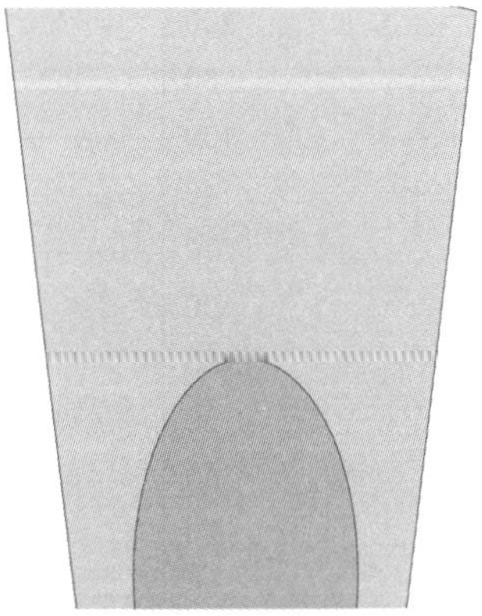

FIG. 35: Acute pulmonary embolism. Illustration shows acute PE central filling defect on CT image viewed in long axis of thrombus. Contrast material can be seen on either side of well- defined thrombus forming the "railroad-track sign."

2. Other Findings

- A wedge-shaped, peripheral opacity representing pulmonary infarcts.
- **Enlarged pulmonary arteries**: Reflects increased pressure within the pulmonary circulation.
- **Right ventricular strain**: Signs of right ventricular enlargement or flattening of the interventricular septum.
- Ground-glass opacities due to hemorrhage.
- Small pleural effusions may be present, often unilateral and on the side of the infarct.

2. Lung ultrasound in emergency department. [5] [AIIMS Dec 23]

Lung ultrasound in the emergency department is used for rapid diagnosis and management of acute respiratory conditions **(Flowchart 11)**.

Uses of lung ultrasound in the emergency department are:

1. Pleural Effusion

- Anechoic space above the diaphragm or adjacent to the lungs
- Detect minimal and mild pleural effusions
- To differentiate between mild effusion and thickening
- To quantify effusions, characterize effusion
- Guided drainage
- Detect nodules/mass

2. Pneumothorax

- Absence of lung sliding, "lung point" (the point where normal lung sliding and pneumothorax alternate), and absence of B-lines.
- Bilateral A-lines
- Used in trauma patients or those on mechanical ventilation

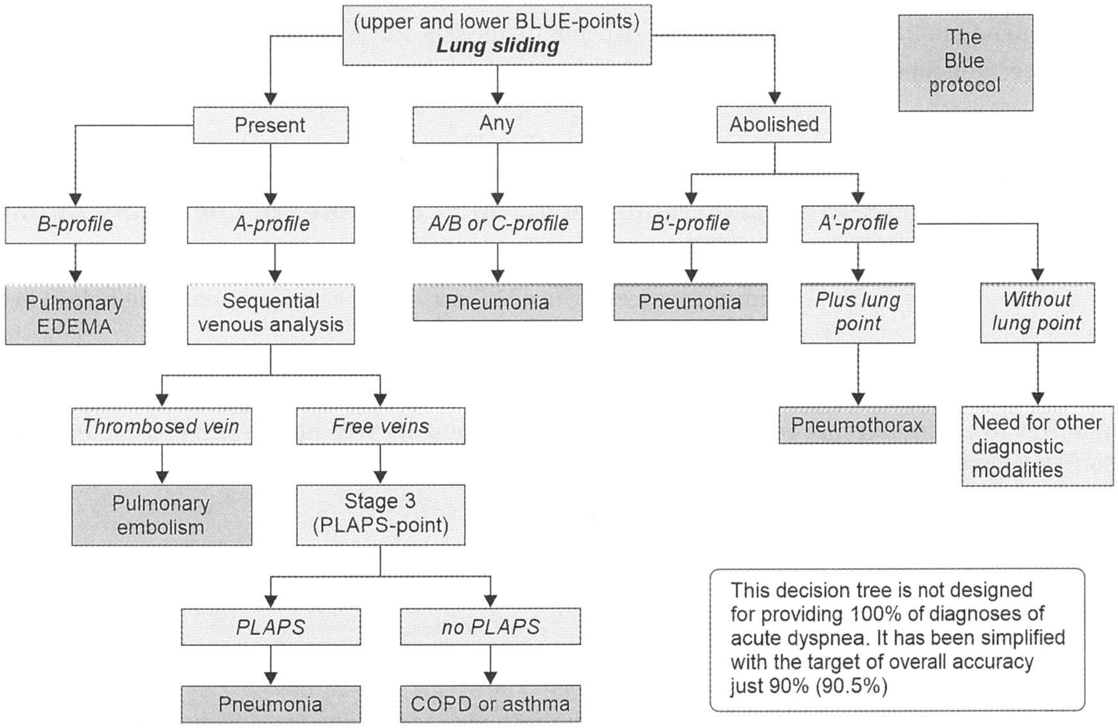

FLOWCHART 11: The blue protocol of USG in lung emergency.

3. Pulmonary Edema

Presence of multiple B-lines (which are vertical, hyperechoic lines, comet-tail artifacts that arise from the pleural line and extend downwards and move with respiration).

4. Pneumonia and Consolidation

- **Consolidation or hepatization of the lung**: Hypoechoic regions of lung with a tissue-like echotexture, often compared to the liver (hepatization of the lung). Subpleural consolidations
- **Shred sign**: Consolidated lung tissue appears as a subpleural hypoechoic region that has an irregular deep border which abuts normally aerated lung, which has echogenic artifacts.
- Unilateral B-lines or bilateral B-lines
- Possible small pleural effusion
- Reduced lung sliding due to thickened pleura in severe cases - Dynamic air bronchograms (atelectasis has static bronchograms)

5. Acute respiratory distress syndrome (ARDS)

- Normal lung sliding.
- Bilateral B-lines, consolidations, pleural thickening, and small subpleural consolidations.

6. COVID-19 Pneumonia

Diffuse B-lines, thickened pleural lines, subpleural consolidations, and irregular pleura.

Advantages:

- Rapid diagnosis
- **Portable and repeatable**: Ideal for critically ill patients in ICU settings
- No radiation exposure
- **Guides procedures**: Useful for guiding thoracentesis or chest tube placement in cases of pleural effusion or pneumothorax

Limitations:

- **Operator dependent**: The accuracy of diagnosis depends on the skill and experience of the operator.
- **Limited in certain conditions**: Air in the lungs (as seen in emphysema) can limit the visualization of deeper structures.

3. Describe in brief, protocol for CT pulmonary angiography for a suspected case of pulmonary thromboembolism. Describe plain radiographic and CT features of pulmonary thromboembolism. [4+3+3] [AIIMS Dec 23, DNB June 20]

CT Pulmonary Angiography (CTPA) is a imaging procedure used in case of suspected pulmonary embolism to visualize the pulmonary arteries.

1. Patient Preparation

History of allergy to contrast agents, needs 4–6 hours fasting before scan to minimize risk of aspirations, ensure IV cannulation, explanation of the procedure.

2. Scan Parameters

- **Patient position**: Supine, arms raised above the head
- **Scout**: Apices to diaphragm
- **Scan extent**: Apices to just below the diaphragm to ensure complete coverage of pulmonary arteries
- **Scan direction**: Caudocranial
- **Breath-hold**: Instruct the patient to hold their breath during image acquisition to avoid motion artifacts

3. Contrast Injection

- Nonionic iodinated contrast
- 80–120 mL of contrast depending on the patient's weight
- **Rate**: 4–5 mL/sec.

4. Bolus Tracking/Timing

- Bolus tracking with trigger at 120 (100) HU in MPA.
- Empirical delay 12–15 sec/15–18 sec

5. Scan Acquisition

- 100–120 kVp used.
- 200–300 mAs tube current used.
- **Reconstruction slice thickness**: Thin slices (1–2 mm) are typically used for optimal spatial resolution.

6. Postprocessing

- Multiplanar Reconstructions (MPR) used for detailed evaluation.
- Maximum Intensity Projections (MIP) used for better visualization of vessels.
- 3D Rendering (optional) often used.

Radiographic features of pulmonary thromboembolism **(Figs. 36 and 37)**

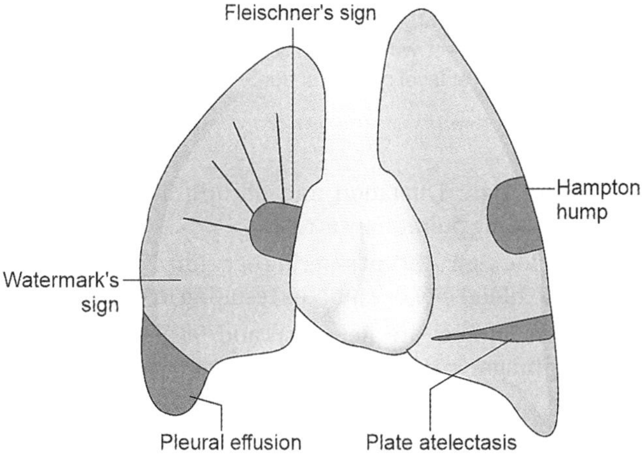

FIG. 36: Signs of pulmonary thromboembolism.

1. Plain Radiographic Features

Chest radiography is neither sensitive nor specific for a pulmonary embolism, however the findings are:

- **Westermark sign**: It is a focal area of oligemia distal to a large vessel that is occluded by thrombus.
- **Hampton's hump**: A well-defined wedge-shaped pleural-based area of increased opacity with a convex medial border—infarction.
- **Fleischner sign**: It is a enlarged pulmonary artery that can be caused either by pulmonary hypertension.
- **Palla's sign**: Enlarged right descending pulmonary artery on the chest radiograph.

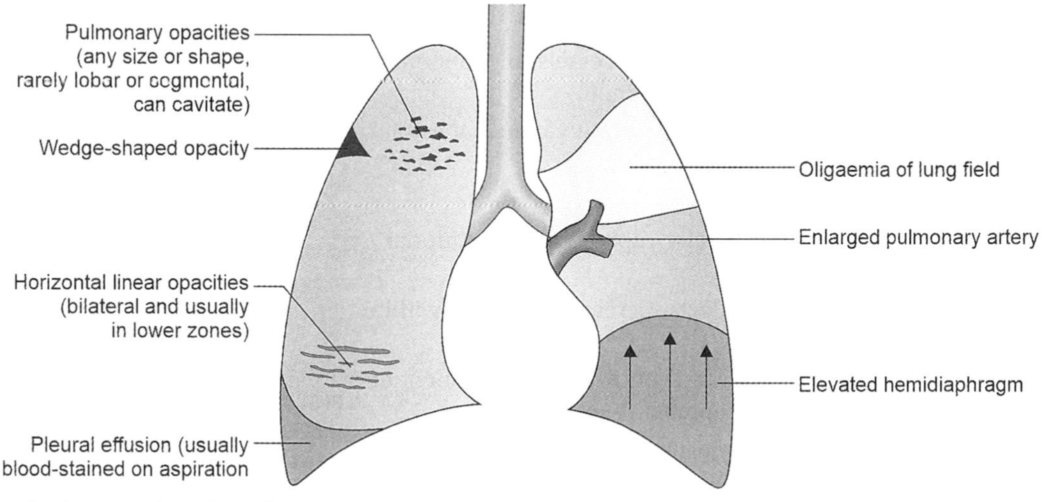

FIG. 37: Signs of pulmonary thromboembolism.

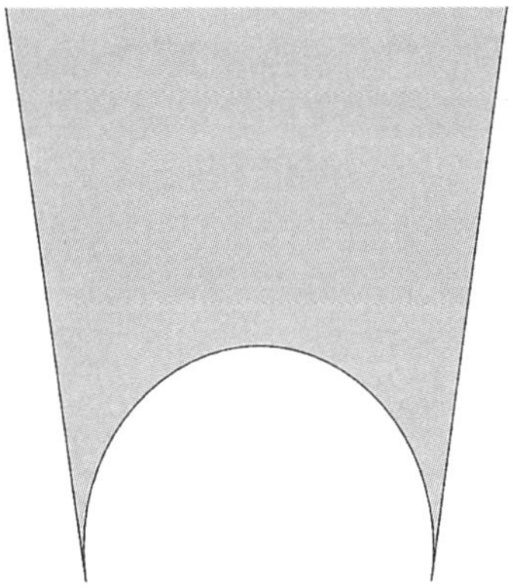

FIG. 38: Acute pulmonary embolism (PE). Illustration of complete obstruction due to acute PE as seen on angiography. Trailing edge of thrombus forms concave filling defect within column of contrast material at level of obstruction.

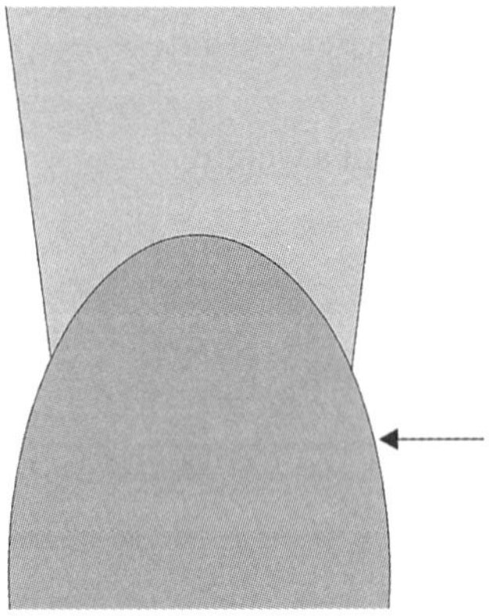

FIG. 39: Acute pulmonary embolism (PE). Illustration of coronal reformatted CT image of acute PE shows expansion of diameter of involved vessel distal to point of obstruction (arrow).

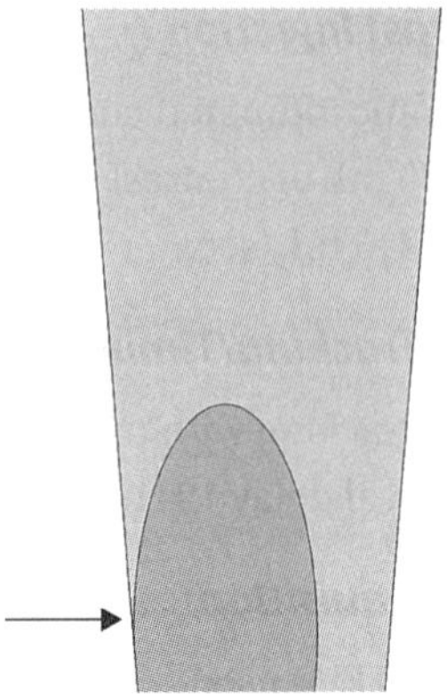

FIG. 40: Acute pulmonary embolism (PE). Illustration shows that eccentric acute thrombus (*arrow*) makes acute angles with vessel wall.

- **Chang sign**: Dilatation and abrupt change in caliber of the right descending pulmonary artery.
- **Knuckle sign**: Abrupt tapering or cutoff of a pulmonary artery segment due to blood clot or embolus resulting in a "knuckle" appearance.
- Others findings are atelectasis and/or pleural effusion, elevated hemidiaphragm, cardiomegaly.

FIG. 41: Acute pulmonary embolism. Illustration shows acute PE central filling defect on CT image viewed perpendicular to plane of thrombus; well-defined central thrombus is completely surrounded by contrast material.

2. CTPA Findings

Acute pulmonary thromboembolism:

MDCT findings in a case of acute pulmonary thromboembolism **(Figs. 38 to 42)**:

Findings are acute embolus appears as a hypodense (low attenuation) area within the contrast-filled pulmonary arteries.

1. **Filling defects in pulmonary arteries**:
   - Central filling defect within a vessel surrounded by contrast material produce "polo-mint" sign .
   - Linear intraluminal filling defect within the vessels surrounded by contrast material called **"**railroad track" sign.
   - *Saddle embolus*: An embolus straddling the bifurcation of the main pulmonary artery, often involving both sides.
2. **Other findings**:
   - A wedge-shaped, peripheral opacity representing pulmonary infarcts.
   - Enlarged pulmonary arteries: Reflects increased pressure within the pulmonary circulation.
   - Right ventricular strain: Signs of right ventricular enlargement or flattening of the interventricular septum.
   - Ground-glass opacities due to hemorrhage.
   - Small pleural effusions may be present, often unilateral and on the side of the infarct.

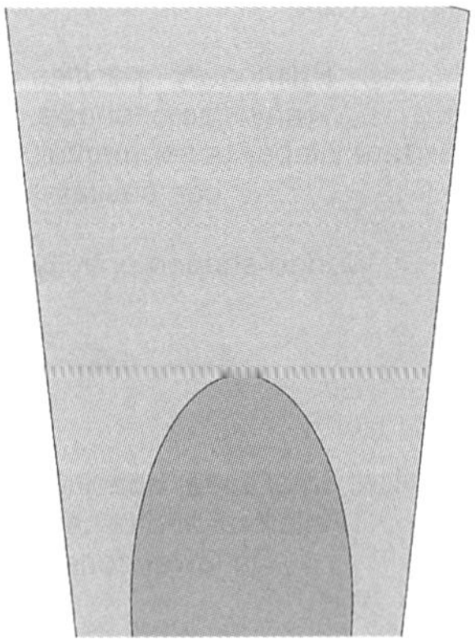

FIG. 42: Acute pulmonary embolism. Illustration shows acute PE central filling defect on CT image viewed in long axis of thrombus. Contrast material can be seen on either side of well- defined thrombus forming the "railroad-track sign."

Chronic pulmonary thromboembolism **(Table 33 and Figs. 43 to 46)**:

TABLE 33: Signs of chronic pulmonary thromboembolism.

1. Vascular signs	• Complete occlusion—vessel cutoff.
	• Partial occlusion—webs, bands, focal stenotic vessel segment and areas of post-stenotic dilatation, irregular thickening of the vessel wall and reduced caliber, calcified residual thrombus, peripheral crescent-shaped defect.
2. Collateral vessels	• Bronchial artery dilation (>2 mm) and tortuosity.
	• Nonbronchial arteries: pleural, intercostal, phrenic, internal mammary.
3. Pulmonary hypertension signs	• Main pulmonary artery dilation (>33 mm).
	• Ratio main pulmonary artery diameter to ascending aorta diameter >1.1:1.
	• Right ventricle enlargement and hypertrophy.
	• Ratio right ventricle diameter to left ventricle diameter >1:1.
	• Bowing of the interventricular septum toward the left ventricle.
	• Right ventricular hyper trabeculation/hypertrophy.
4. Lung parenchymal signs	• Scars from prior pulmonary infarctions: bands, irregular peripheral linear opacities, wedge-shaped opacities with pleural thickening.
	• Mosaic lung attenuation.

FIG. 43: Chronic pulmonary embolism. Line drawing shows complete obstruction of vessel with convex margin with respect to contrast material. This is the "pouch" defect of chronic PE seen on angiography.

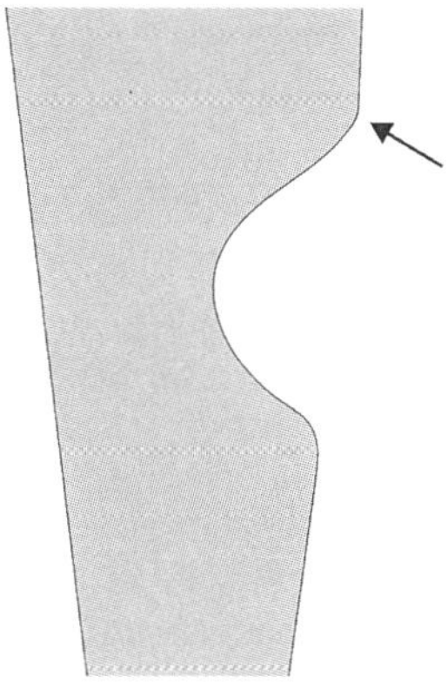

FIG. 44: Chronic pulmonary embolism. Illustration of intimal irregularity of chronic PE as seen on angiography. This broad-based, smooth, margined abnormality can affect one or both sides of vessel; it forms obtuse angles with vessel wall (*arrow*).

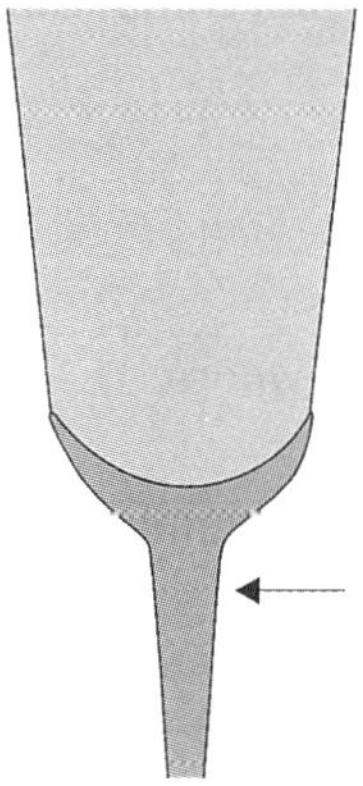

FIG. 45: Chronic pulmonary embolism illustration of reformatted CT image of complete obstruction in chronic PE shows contracted thrombus (*arrow*) distal to pouch defect.

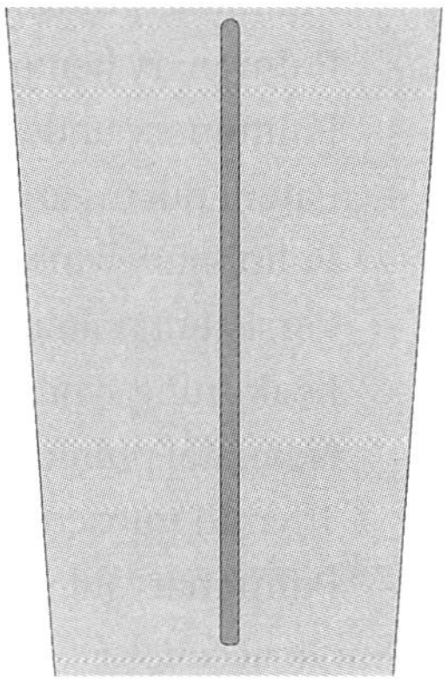

FIG. 46: Chronic pulmonary embolism. Illustration of nonobstructive filling defect of chronic PE. Band or web can be identified as thin dark line surrounded by contrast material, often orientated in direction of blood flow.

The main differences between acute and chronic pulmonary thromboembolism are as follows **(Table 34)**:

TABLE 34: Differences between acute and chronic pulmonary thromboembolism.

Differentiation of acute and chronic pulmonary thromboembolism—CT pulmonary angiography findings		
CTPA findings	***Acute***	***Chronic***
Vascular signs	Central or eccentric filling defect: acute angle with vessel wall: preserved caliber of the artery or expanded secondary to pulsatile flow	Peripheral, crescent-shaped filling defect: obtuse angle with vessel wail; webs, bands, calcified thrombus: vessel narrowing or amputation, intimal irregularities
Collateral vessels	Absent	Bronchial and nonbronchial systemic arteries dilatation
Pulmonary hypertension signs	May be present: however, without right ventricle hypertrophy	Commonly present
Parenchymal signs	Pulmonary infarction ("reversed halo sign")	Pulmonary scars from prior infarction: mosaic lung attenuation

Pediatric Chest

1. Discuss in brief the causes and radiographic features of respiratory distress in newborn. [5+5] [MD (WBUHS) 23]

Causes of Respiratory Distress in Newborn

1. **Intrathoracic**:
   a. Medical causes:
      - Respiratory distress syndrome (RDS)
      - Transient tachypnoea of the Newborn (TTN)
      - Meconium aspiration syndrome
      - Bronchopulmonary dysplasia (BPD)
      - Pulmonary interstitial emphysema (PIE) and complications.
      - Pulmonary hemorrhage
      - Pulmonary underdevelopment
      - Patent ductus arteriosus (PDA)
      - Pulmonary lymphangiectasia
      - Persistent pulmonary hypoplasia of the newborn
      - Leaky lung syndrome
      - Neonatal pulmonary infection/neonatal pneumonia
      - Thyroid transcription factor-1 deficiency
      - Pulmonary interstitial glycogenosis

   b. Surgical causes:
      - Esophageal atresia and tracheoesophageal fistula
      - Congenital diaphragmatic hernia (CDH)
      - Diaphragmatic eventration
      - Congenital pulmonary airway malformation (CPAM)
      - Pulmonary sequestration
      - Congenital Lobar Overinflation (CLO)
      - Enteric duplication cyst
      - Bronchogenic cyst

2. **Extra thoracic**:
   a. Central nervous system
      - Hemorrhage
      - Vein of Galen malformation
      - Increased pressure including hydrocephalus
   b. Neuromuscular and MSK
      - Werdnig-hoffman disease
      - Skeletal abnormality
        - Osteogenesis imperfecta
        - Thanatophoric dwarfism
        - Asphyxiating thoracic dystrophy of Jeune.
   c. Tumor
   d. Trauma
   e. Extrathoracic airway obstruction
   f. Abdominal:
      - Perforation
      - Necrotizing enterocolitis
      - Obstruction
      - Mass/Visceromegaly
      - Ascites.
3. **Systemic causes**:
   a. Sepsis
   b. Profound anemia
   c. Hypothermia
   d. Hypovolemic shock
   e. Electrolyte imbalance
   f. Adrenal insufficiency
   g. Severe acidosis

Radiographic features of Respiratory distress in newborn:

1. **Respiratory Distress Syndrome (RDS) (Fig. 47)**: Insufficient production of surfactant (type 2) in preterm. Also called hyaline membrane disease/lungs of prematurity.

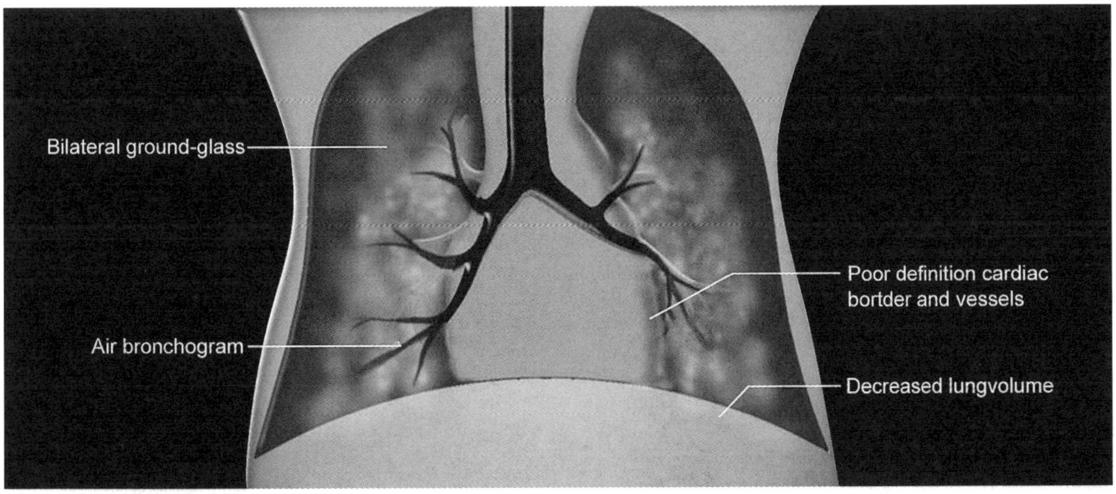

FIG. 47: Illustrated imaging features of RDS.

Chest X-ray:
- Low-lung volumes.
- Diffuse, bilateral, and symmetrical granular opacities in early stages.
- Air bronchograms may be seen.
- Consolidation/alveolar opacity-silhouetting cardiomediastinal and diaphragmatic contours (advanced stages).
- Complete white out lungs due to extensive consolidations.
- Bell-shaped thorax.

USG findings:
- "Solid capping" lung due to coalescent of B-lines.
- Retrodiaphragmatic hyperechogenicity seen.

2. **Transient Tachypnoea of the Newborn (TTN) (Fig. 48)**: Retained fetal fluid or delayed clearance of fetal lung fluids. Also called wet lung diseases.

   Full term neonates by caesarean section/precipitous labor.

   Chest X-ray findings:
   - Diffuse interstitial edema predominantly perihilar seen as perihilar streakiness
   - Small pleural effusions—fluid in fissures.
   - Lung volume may be normal or increased.
   - Perihilar alveolar opacities in severe cases.
   - Normal chest radiograph by 48–72 hours postpartum.

   USG findings: "Double lung point sign"—a sharp boundary between aerated superior lung fields and coalescent "B-lines" (representing interstitial edema) in the basal lung fields.

3. **Meconium Aspiration Syndrome (MAS) (Fig. 49)**:

   Occurs in full term/post-term neonates.

   Due to inhalation of meconium-stained amniotic fluid. *Chest X-ray findings*:
   - Increased lung volumes due to hyperinflated lungs with flattened hemidiaphragms.
   - Asymmetric patchy pulmonary opacities.
   - Areas of air trapping (due to small airway obstruction).
   - Pleural effusions can be seen.
   - Pneumothorax or pneumomediastinum seen in 20–40% of cases.
   - Multifocal consolidation due to chemical pneumonitis.
   - Pulmonary interstitial emphysema.

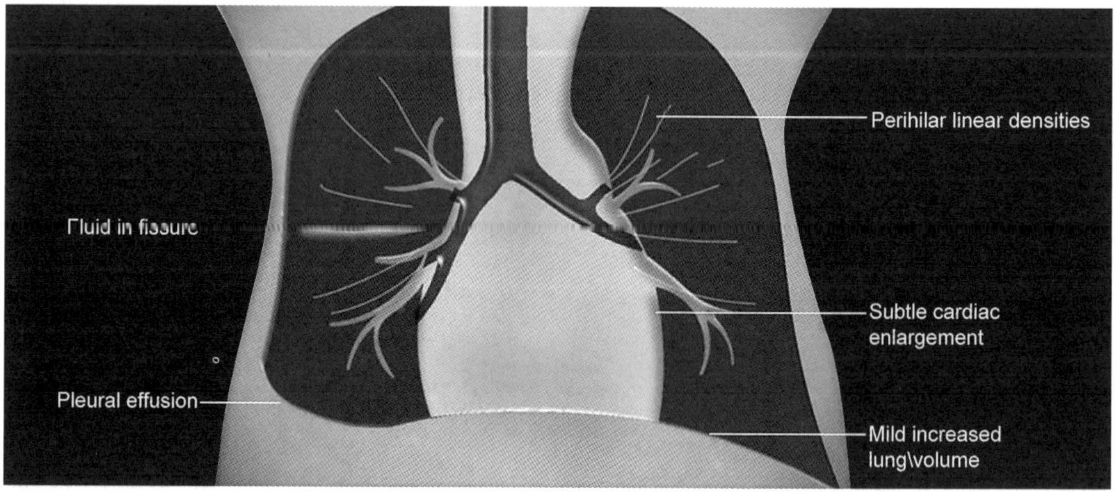

FIG. 48: Illustrated imaging features of TTN.

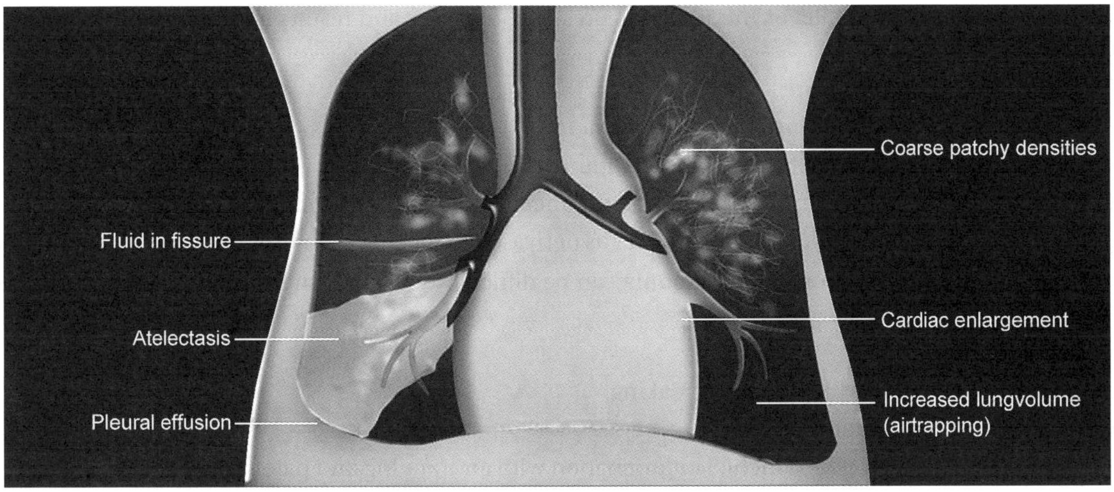

FIG. 49: Illustrated imaging features of MAS.

4. **Bronchopulmonary dysplasia (BPD)**:

   Chronic pulmonary disorder of prematurity.

   Results from the use of high positive-pressure mechanical ventilation and high concentration oxygen in neonates.

   Chest X-ray findings:
   - Areas of air trapping with hyperinflated lung fields.
   - Ill-defined reticular markings with rounded lucent areas diffusely involving hyperinflated lungs.
   - Cardiomegaly may be present resulting in development of pulmonary hypertension
   - Areas of atelectasis may be seen.
   - Interstitial thickening, fibrosis.
   - Four stages of radiographic changes of BPD have been described:

   Stage I (first week): Typical granular opacity of RDS seen.

   Stage II (second week): Includes generalized haziness and plethora.

   Stage III (third week): Involves cystic changes alternating irregular opacities.

   Stage IV (fourth week): Characterized by hyperinflation, extensive stranding, and an enlarged heart in the giving rise to bubbly appearance.

   HRCT findings:

   Stage 1: Show changes of respiratory distress syndrome, pneumothorax, and pulmonary interstitial emphysema.

   Stage 2: Interlobular septal thickening is the most common finding.

   Stage 3: Characterized by linear atelectasis and fibrotic changes.

5. **Pulmonary interstitial emphysema**:
   - Primarily occurred in premature infants but can also manifest in adults.
   - Abnormal location of gas in pulmonary interstitium and lymphatics. Most often due to positive pressure ventilation.
   - The increased air pressure within the alveoli and alveolar airspaces disrupts the adjacent lung interstitial tissue, damaging the lung structure.

   Chest X-ray findings:
   - Spherical cystic or linear, oval radiolucencies in the interstitium radiating from the hilum.
   - Affected segment is often hyperexpanded and static in volume on multiple radiographs.
   - Overall lung volume is increased.
   - Complications occurred as pneumothorax, pneumomediastinum, or pneumopericardium.

- The heart tends to get smaller as intrathoracic pressure increases and results in diminished venous return into the chest.

HRCT is confirmatory, findings are:

- Cystic/linear radiolucencies in the affected segment.
- Typically show a line and dot pattern in interstitium of lung lined by air.
- Better visualization of a pneumothorax or pneumomediastinum or pneumopericardium.
- If incidentally detected in adults, it may appear as perivascular lucent or low- attenuating haloes and small cysts.

6. **Pneumonia**: Congenital or neonatal pneumonia can be difficult to distinguish from other entities such as RDS or bronchopulmonary dysplasia.

   Imaging features:

   - Increased lung volume with perihilar streaking.
   - Diffuse or focal consolidation.
   - Viral pneumonia shows peribronchial inflammation with air trapping and patchy atelectasis.
   - Pleural effusions can be seen.

7. **Pneumothorax**:

   - Air in the pleural space leads to lung collapse.
   - Chest X-ray reveals the absence of lung markings on the affected side.
   - Show shift of mediastinal structures.

8. **Congenital diaphragmatic hernia (CDH)**:

   A defect in the diaphragm allows abdominal contents into the chest, causing lung compression.

   Imaging findings:

   - Indistinct diaphragm or defect in diaphragmatic outline with opacification of part of or all the hemithorax.
   - Cystic lucencies in thorax.
   - Paucity of bowel in abdomen and continuity of bowel between abdomen and chest.
   - Shift of mediastinum to contralateral side.
   - Antenatal USG help for diagnosis of CDH.

9. **Congenital lobar overinflation (CLO)**:

   It is also known as congenital lobar overinflation, or congenital lobar emphysema or congenital alveolar overdistension.

   It is a condition in which there is hyperexpansion of a lobe of the lungs. Imaging findings:

   - Immediate postpartum—affected lobe shows homogenously opaque or diffuse reticular pattern.
   - Later—areas of hyperlucency and hyperinflation of the affected lobe.
   - Unilateral opacification of the affected lobe due to fluid retention.
   - Mass effect can be severe with displacement of midline structures and atelectasis of the cpntralateral side.

10. **Pulmonary sequestration**:

    Spectrum of broncho pulmonary foregut malformation.

    Aberrant formation of segmental lung tissue that has no connection with the bronchial tree or pulmonary arteries.

    Imaging features:

    - Triangular soft tissue density mass with smooth/lobulated contour in the lung base.
    - May show cystic spaces if intralobar variety/infected.
    - CT demonstrates the arterial supply by the descending aorta, venous drainage.

11. **Congenital pulmonary airway malformation (CPAM)**:

    It is a spectrum of bronchopulmonary foregut malformations. Multicystic masses of lung tissue with abnormal bronchial proliferations.

    CPAM is divided into 5 types (0–4) according to the recent classification.

    Type 1 (75% of cases) is composed of variable sized cysts, with at least one dominant cyst larger than 2 cm in diameter.

    Type 2 (10–15% of cases) is composed of smaller multiple cysts of the same size, less than 1 cm in diameter.

Type 3 solid mass composed of microcysts.

Type 0 consists of small cysts, similar to type 3 in appearance.

Type 4 (a few %) large cysts, similar to types 1 and 2 in appearance. *Imaging features*:

- In type I and II, multiple thin-walled cysts containing air and varying in size are seen.
- Type III lesions appear solid.
- Infection of the cysts causes air-fluid levels.
- Large lesions may cause a mass effect with resultant mediastinal shift, depression, and even inversion of the diaphragm.

2. Enumerate causes of neonatal respiratory distress. Describe in detail pathophysiology and imaging findings in hyaline membrane disease. [2+(2+6)][DNB Dec 20, AIIMS May 24]

Causes of respiratory distress in newborn:

1. **Intrathoracic**:
   a. Medical causes:
      - Respiratory distress syndrome (RDS)
      - Transient tachypnoea of the newborn (TTN)
      - Meconium aspiration syndrome
      - Bronchopulmonary dysplasia (BPD)
      - Pulmonary interstitial emphysema (PIE) and complications
      - Pulmonary hemorrhage.
      - Pulmonary underdevelopment
      - Patent ductus arteriosus (PDA)
      - Pulmonary lymphangiectasia
      - Persistent pulmonary hypoplasia of the newborn
      - Leaky lung syndrome
      - Neonatal pulmonary infection/neonatal pneumonia
      - Thyroid transcription factor-1 deficiency
      - Pulmonary interstitial glycogenosis

   b. Surgical causes:
      - Esophageal atresia and tracheoesophageal fistula.
      - Congenital diaphragmatic hernia (CDH)
      - Diaphragmatic eventration
      - Congenital pulmonary airway malformation (CPAM)
      - Pulmonary sequestration
      - Congenital lobar overinflation (CLO)
      - Enteric duplication cyst
      - Bronchogenic cyst
2. **Extra thoracic**:
   a. Central nervous system
      - Hemorrhage
      - Vein of Galen malformation
      - Increased pressure including hydrocephalus

   b. Neuro-muscular and MSK
      - Werdnig-Hoffman disease
      - Skeletal abnormality:
        - Osteogenesis imperfecta
        - Thanatophoric dwarfism
        - Asphyxiating thoracic dystrophy of Jeune.

   c. Tumor
   d. Trauma
   e. Extrathoracic airway obstruction
   f. Abdominal:
      - Perforation
      - Necrotising enterocolitis
      - Obstruction
      - Mass/visceromegaly
      - Ascites
3. **Systamic causes**:
   a. Sepsis
   b. Profound anemia
   c. Hypothermia
   d. Hypovolemic shock
   e. Electrolyte imbalance
   f. Adrenal insufficiency
   g. Severe acidosis

Hyaline Membrane Disease

It is also known as surfactant deficiency disorder/lung disease of prematurity.

It is a result from insufficient production of surfactant in preterm neonates.

Surfactant is crucial for reducing surface tension in the alveoli and preventing their collapse during exhalation.

Risk Factors

- **Prematurity**: GA <36 weeks
- **Low birth weight**: <2 kg
- Maternal diabetes
- Multiple gestation
- Perinatal asphyxia

Pathophysiology (Flowchart 12)

Insufficient production of surfactant resulting in increased surface tension of alveoli causes alveolar collapse (atelectasis)

↓

Reducing the surface area available for gas exchange, leading to hypoxemia and increased work of breathing

↓

Reduced gas exchange causes low oxygen (hypoxemia) and increased carbon dioxide (hypercapnia) levels, resulting in respiratory acidosis, causes pulmonary vasoconstriction, worsening oxygen delivery

↓

The collapsed alveoli and damaged epithelial cells lead to the leakage of proteinaceous material into the alveoli, forming the characteristic hyaline membranes. These membranes further impair gas exchange.

FLOWCHART 12: Pathophysiology of hyaline membrane disease.

Imaging Findings (Fig. 50)

1. **Chest X-ray**:
   - Low lung volumes.
   - Diffuse, bilateral and symmetrical granular opacities in early stages.
   - Air bronchograms may be seen.

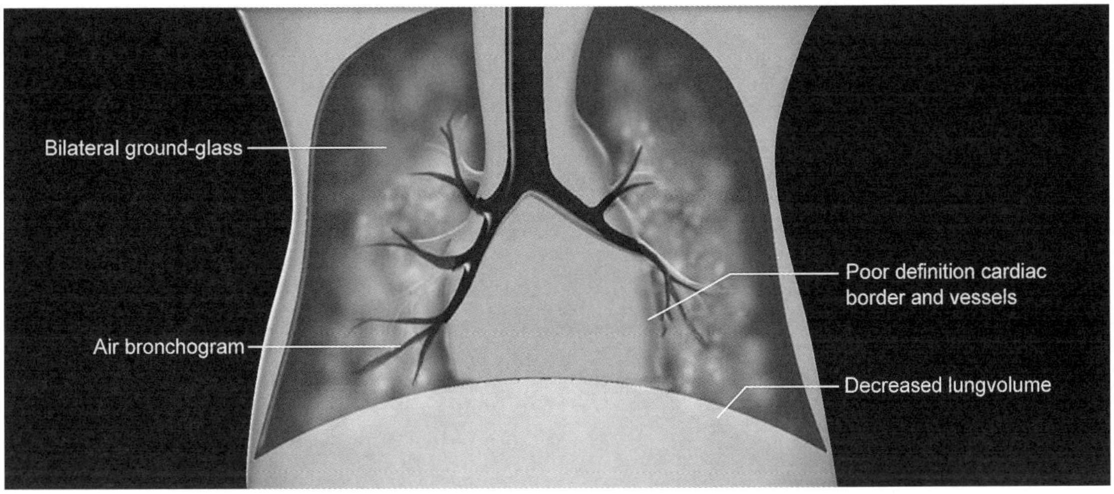

FIG. 50: Illustrated imaging features of RDS.

- Consolidation/alveolar opacity-silhouetting cardiomediastinal and diaphragmatic contours (advanced stages).
- Complete white out lungs due to extensive consolidation.
- Bell-shaped thorax.

USG findings:

- “Solid capping” lung due to coalescent of B lines.
- Retrodiaphragmatic hyperechogenicity seen.

Diagnosis of RDS excluded if:

- Normal CXR at 6 hours after birth.
- Hyperinflated lung in nonventilated patient.

3. The role of imaging in a newborn with respiratory distress. [10] [MD (WBUHS) 19]

The role of Imaging in a Newborn with respiratory distress:

The imaging modality used for evaluation of respiratory distress in newborn babies are

1. **Chest X-ray (CXR)**:
   - First-line imaging in a newborn with respiratory distress.
   - Provides a rapid assessment of the lungs, airways, heart, diaphragm and any structural abnormalities.
   - Identify common causes of respiratory distress in newborn.
2. **Ultrasound (US)**:
   - Used for its portability and lack of radiation.
   - Useful for assessing lung consolidation, pleural effusions, and detecting pneumothorax.
   - Cardiac ultrasound (echocardiography)is used for structural heart defects.
   - Abdominal ultrasound can help identify congenital anomalies like diaphragmatic hernias or abdominal masses affecting respiratory function.
3. **CT Scan**:
   - Not commonly used due to high radiation exposure.
   - Used in complex cases.
4. **MRI**:
   - Less commonly used.
   - Fetal MRI may be done in some cases before birth to identify structural abnormalities which leads to respiratory distress in after birth.

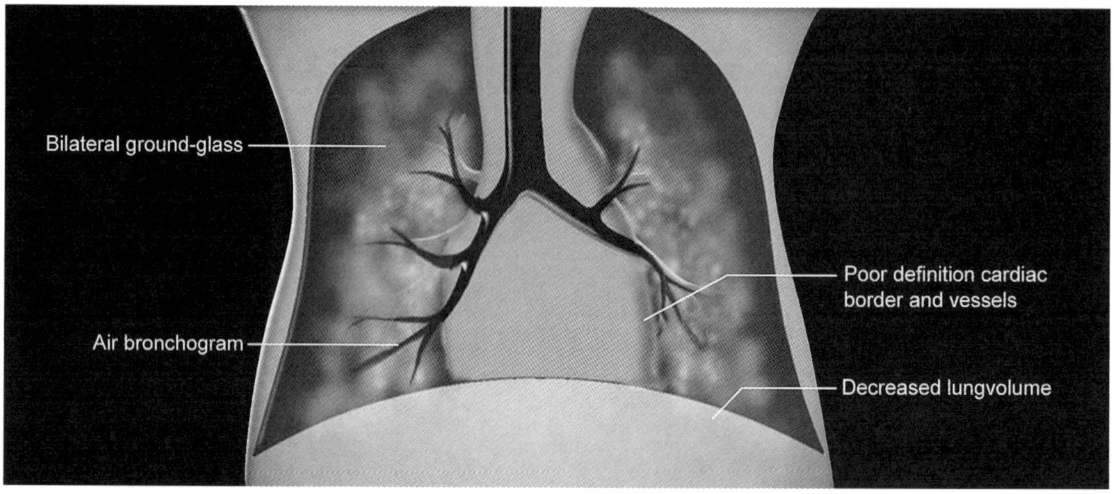

FIG. 51: Imaging features of RDS.

5. **Fluoroscopy**:
   - May be used conditions like tracheoesophageal fistula or esophageal atresia.

Causes of respiratory distress diagnosed with imaging in newborns are radiographic features of respiratory distress in newborn:

1. **Respiratory distress syndrome (RDS) (Fig. 51)**:
   Insufficient production of surfactant (type 2) in preterm. Also called hyaline membrane disease/lungs of prematurity.
   Chest X-ray:
   - Low lung volumes.
   - Diffuse, bilateral and symmetrical granular opacities in early stages.
   - Air bronchograms may be seen.
   - Consolidation/alveolar opacity–silhouetting cardiomediastinal and diaphragmatic contours (advanced stages).
   - Complete white out lungs due to extensive consolidations.
   - Bell-shaped thorax.

   USG findings:
   - "Solid capping" lung due to coalescent of B-lines.
   - Retrodiaphragmatic hyperechogenicity seen.
2. **Transient tachypnoea of the newborn (TTN) (Fig. 52)**:
   Retained fetal fluid or delayed clearance of fetal lung fluids. Also called wet lung diseases.
   Full term neonates by caesarean section/precipitous labor.
   Chest X-ray findings:
   - Diffuse interstitial edema predominantly perihilar seen as perihilar streakiness
   - Small pleural effusions—fluid in fissures.
   - Lung volume may be normal or increased.
   - Perihilar alveolar opacities in severe cases.
   - Normal chest radiograph by 48–72 hours postpartum.

   USG findings: "Double lung point sign"—a sharp boundary between aerated superior lung fields and coalescent "B-lines" (representing interstitial edema) in the basal lung fields.
3. **Meconium aspiration syndrome (MAS) (Fig. 53)**:
   Occurs in full term/post-term neonates.
   Due to inhalation of meconium-stained amniotic fluid. *Chest X-ray findings*:
   - Increased lung volumes due to hyperinflated lungs with flattened hemidiaphragms.
   - Asymmetric patchy pulmonary opacities.

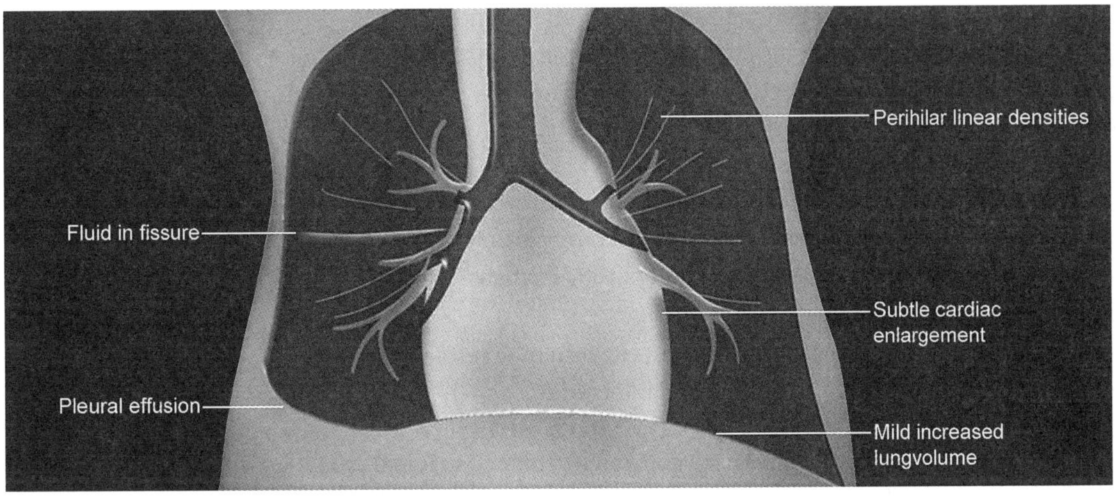

FIG. 52: Imaging features of TTN.

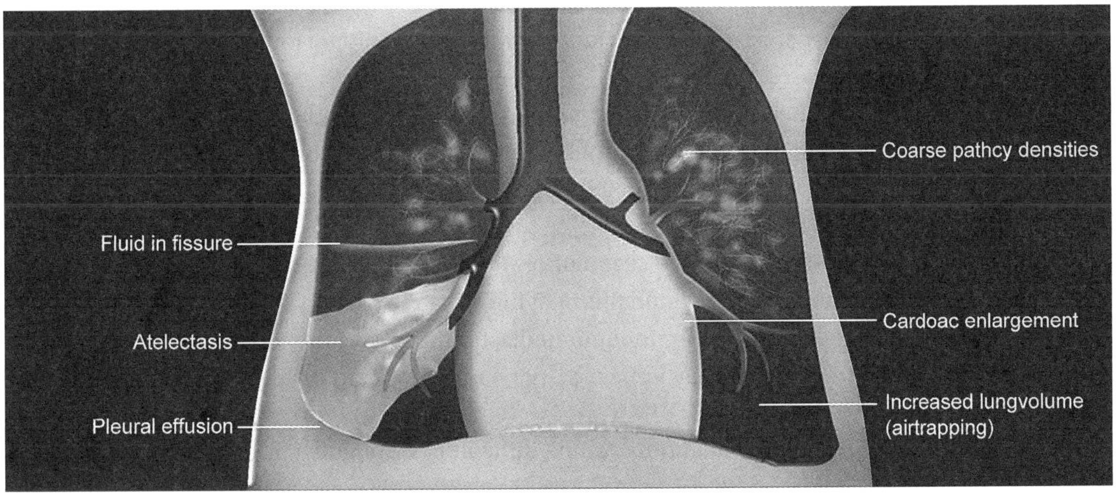

FIG. 53: Imaging features of MAS.

- Areas of air trapping (due to small airway obstruction).
- Pleural effusions can be seen.
- Pneumothorax or pneumomediastinum seen in 20–40% of cases.
- Multifocal consolidation due to chemical pneumonitis.
- Pulmonary interstitial emphysema.

4. **Bronchopulmonary dysplasia (BPD)**:

   Chronic pulmonary disorder of prematurity.

   Results from the use of high positive-pressure mechanical ventilation and high concentration oxygen in neonates.

   Chest X-ray findings:

   - Areas of air trapping with hyperinflated lung fields.
   - Ill-defined reticular markings with rounded lucent areas diffusely involving hyperinflated lungs.
   - Cardiomegaly may be present resulting in development of pulmonary hypertension
   - Areas of atelectasis may be seen.
   - Interstitial thickening, fibrosis.
   - Four stages of radiographic changes of BPD have been described:

     Stage I (first week): Typical granular opacity of RDS seen.

Stage II (second week): Includes generalized haziness and plethora.

Stage III (third week): Involves cystic changes alternating irregular opacities.

Stage IV (fourth week): Characterized by hyperinflation, extensive stranding, and an enlarged heart in the giving rise to bubbly appearance.

HRCT Findings

Stage 1: Shows changes of respiratory distress syndrome, pneumothorax, and pulmonary interstitial emphysema.

Stage 2: Interlobular septal thickening is the most common finding.

Stage 3: Characterized by linear atelectasis and fibrotic changes.

5. **Pulmonary interstitial emphysema**:
   - Primarily occurred in premature infants but can also manifest in adults.
   - Abnormal location of gas in pulmonary interstitium and lymphatics. Most often due to positive pressure ventilation.
   - The increased air pressure within the alveoli and alveolar airspaces disrupts the adjacent lung interstitial tissue, damaging the lung structure.

   Chest X-ray findings:
   - Spherical cystic or linear, oval radiolucencies in the interstitium radiating from the hilum.
   - Affected segment is often hyperexpanded and static in volume on multiple radiographs.
   - Overall lung volume is increased.
   - Complications occurred as pneumothorax, pneumomediastinum, or pneumopericardium.
   - The heart tends to get smaller as intrathoracic pressure increases and results in diminished venous return into the chest.

   HRCT is confirmatory and findings are:
   - Cystic/linear radiolucencies in the affected segment.
   - Typically show a line and dot pattern in interstitium of lung lined by air.
   - Better visualization of a pneumothorax or pneumomediastinum or pneumopericardium.
   - If incidentally detected in adults, it may appear as perivascular lucent or low- attenuating haloes and small cysts.
6. **Pneumonia**: Congenital or neonatal pneumonia can be difficult to distinguish from other entities such as RDS or bronchopulmonary dysplasia.

   Imaging features:
   - Increased lung volume with perihilar streaking.
   - Diffuse or focal consolidation.
   - Viral pneumonia shows peribronchial inflammation with air trapping and patchy atelectasis.
   - Pleural effusions can be seen.
7. **Pneumothorax**:
   - Air in the pleural space leads to lung collapse.
   - Chest X-ray reveals the absence of lung markings on the affected side.
   - Show shift of mediastinal structures.
8. **Congenital diaphragmatic hernia (CDH)**: A defect in the diaphragm allows abdominal contents into the chest, causing lung compression.

   Imaging findings:
   - Indistinct diaphragm or defect in diaphragmatic outline with opacification of part of or all the hemithorax.
   - Cystic lucencies in thorax.
   - Paucity of bowel in abdomen and continuity of bowel between abdomen and chest.
   - Shift of mediastinum to contralateral side.
   - Antenatal USG help for diagnosis of CDH.

9. **Congenital Lobar Overinflation (CLO)**: Also known as congenital lobar overinflation, or *congenital lobar emphysema or congenital alveolar overdistension.*

   It is a condition in which there is hyperexpansion of a lobe of the lungs.

   Imaging findings:

   - Immediate postpartum-affected lobe shows homogenously opaque or diffuse reticular pattern.
   - Later—areas of hyperlucency and hyperinflation of the affected lobe.
   - Unilateral opacification of the affected lobe due to fluid retention.
   - Mass effect can be severe with displacement of midline structures and atelectasis of the cpntralateral side.

10. **Pulmonary sequestration**: Spectrum of broncho pulmonary foregut malformation.

    Aberrant formation of segmental lung tissue that has no connection with the bronchial tree or pulmonary arteries.

    Imaging features:

    - Triangular soft tissue density mass with smooth/lobulated contour in the lung base.
    - May show cystic spaces if intralobar variety/infected.
    - CT demonstrates the arterial supply by the descending aorta, venous drainage.

11. **Congenital pulmonary airway malformation (CPAM)**:

    It is a spectrum of bronchopulmonary foregut malformations. Multicystic masses of lung tissue with abnormal bronchial proliferations.

    CPAM is divided into 5 types (0–4) according to the recent classification.

    Type 1 (75% of cases) is composed of variable sized cysts, with at least one dominant cyst larger than 2 cm in diameter.

    Type 2 (10–15% of cases) is composed of smaller multiple cysts of the same size, less than 1 cm in diameter.

    Type 3 solid mass composed of microcysts.

    Type 0, small cysts, similar to type 3 in appearance.

    Type 4 (a few %) large cysts, similar to types 1 and 2 in appearance. Imaging features:

    - Type I and II, multiple thin-walled cysts containing air and varying in size are seen.
    - Type III lesions appear solid.
    - Infection of the cysts causes air-fluid levels.
    - Large lesions may cause a mass effect with resultant mediastinal shift, depression, and even inversion of the diaphragm.

4. Describe the congenital anomalies of the lung. [10][MD (WBUHS) 20] Congenital anomalies of the lung (Flowchart 13).

1. **Underdevelopment anomalies**: Classified into three types as agenesis, aplasia, and hypoplasia.
   - Pulmonary agenesis, and aplasia:
     - Nearly same term.
     - Occur on either side.
     - Associated with congenital anomalies and poor prognosis.
     - Agenesis: absence of pulmonary parenchyma, its bronchus and vascular structures.
     - Aplasia: absence of pulmonary parenchyma , its bronchus and vascular structures,
     - A short rudimentary bronchus is present.
     - *Imaging findings*:
       1. Opacified hemithorax with and marked ipsilateral mediastinal shift.
       2. Hyperlucency in the anterior chest due to herniation of contralateral hyperinflated lung on lateral film radiography.
       3. Pulmonary aplasia—differentiated from pulmonary agenesis by presence rudimentary blind-ending bronchus on CT.
       4. The heart is displaced into posterior hemithorax on the side of agenesis or aplasia.

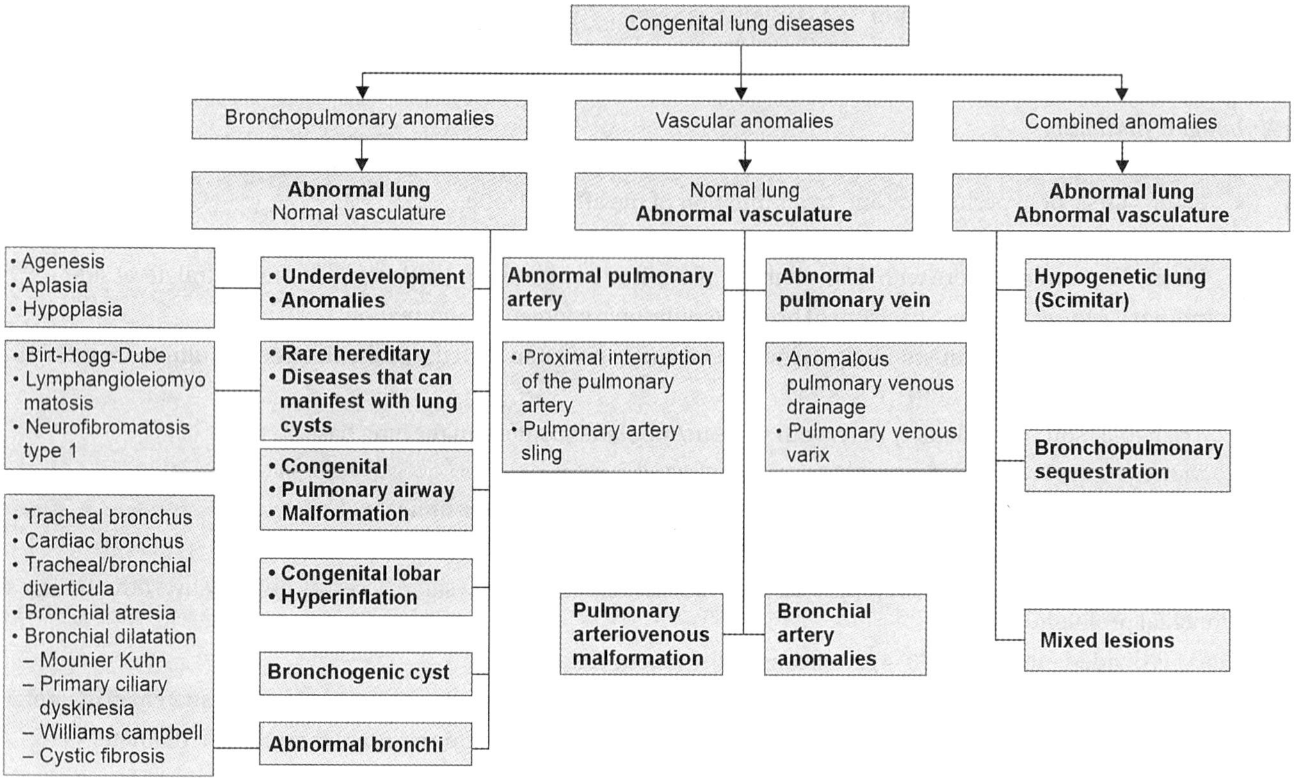

FLOWCHART 13: Types of congenital lung diseases.

- Pulmonary hypoplasia:
  - Abnormal lung development associated with a reduction in lung volume and decrease in number of alveoli and bronchial divisions.
  - Deficient lobes or segments may be present.
  - Associated with:
    i. Hypogenetic lung (scimitar) syndrome,
    ii. Proximal interruption of pulmonary artery,
    iii. Lung compression during development (congenital diaphragmatic hernia, space occupying lesions, CPAM, sequestration, thoracic deformity, or oligohydramnios).
  - *Imaging features* (X-ray + CT): Decrease in ipsilateral lung volume and pulmonary artery, narrowing of intercostal spaces, compensatory hyperinflation, and mediastinal shift.

2. **Congenital pulmonary airway malformation (CPAM)**:
   - It is a spectrum of bronchopulmonary foregut malformations
   - CPAM also known as congenital cystic adenomatoid malformation (CCAM)
   - It is an intralobar mass of disorganized lung tissue, derived primarily from bronchioles, and cystic or multicystic.
   - Most common in lower lobe.
   - CPAM is divided into 5 types (0–4) according to the recent classification.
   - *Imaging findings*:

   Type 1 (65%):
   i. One or more cysts, >2 cm in diameter
   ii. Large air-filled multicystic lesion.
   iii. Sometimes with air-fluid levels (when infection superimposed).

   Type 2 (20–25%):
   i. Multiple cysts <2 cm in diameter
   ii. Air-filled multicystic mass with focal consolidation.

Type 3 (10%):

i. Microscopic (<3–5 mm) cysts.

ii. Appears as solid mass.

Type 4:

i. Small cysts.

ii. Similar to type 3 in appearance.

Type 5:

i. Large cysts.

ii. Similar to types 1 and 2 in appearance.

3. **Congenital lobar hyperinflation (CLH):**
   - Known as congenital lobar emphysema.
   - Associated with partial or complete bronchial obstruction due to deficient cartilage, external compression, anomalous vessel or bronchogenic cyst or luminal abnormalities such as mucosal folds.
   - Hyperinflation of one or multiple lobes.
   - The left upper and right middle lobes are most commonly affected.
   - Imaging features (X-ray + CT):
     - Overinflation and air trapping in the affected lobe.
     - Hyperlucency of the affected lung.
     - Mass effect on adjacent structures including compressive atelectasis, mediastinal shift to the contralateral hemithorax, separated ribs, and flattened diaphragm on the ipsilateral side.
4. **Bronchogenic cysts**: Foregut duplication cysts and due to abnormal development of the lung bud.
   - Bronchogenic cysts are filled with fluid (serous, hemorrhagic, or highly viscous and gelatinous).
   - Most common in the medial lung and the lower lobes.

   Imaging findings:
   - *Chest X-ray*: May appear as a solitary, round to oval, well-defined mass.
   - *CT scan*: Shows a fluid-filled round to oval cyst (low attenuation), thin walled occasionally calcified, well-circumscribed, may contain any air-fluid level when infected.
5. **Abnormal bronchi**:
   - Tracheal bronchus:
     - Known as pig bronchus.
     - Originates from the right wall of the trachea, usually within 2 cm of the carina.
     - Usually supply the apical segment of right upper lobe.
     - Axial CT, coronal reconstruction and 3D reconstruction images can depict abnormal bronchus.
     - Recurrent pneumonia and bronchiectasis can be seen, observed in adults
   - Cardiac bronchus:
     - Originates from the inferomedial of the right main or intermediate bronchus.
     - It may end blindly or be accompanied by rudimentary lung tissue.
     - May terminate into mediastinum.
     - Can cause repeated infection and hemoptysis.
   - Tracheal/bronchial diverticula:
     - Congenital and acquired.
     - The congenital diverticula are located in the posteromedial border of the right main bronchus or posterolateral border of the right trachea.
     - Acquired tracheal diverticula occur due to the increased intraluminal pressure and weakened tracheal wall.
     - CT demonstrated both paratracheal cyst and communication to the tracheal lumen.
   - Bronchial atresia:
     - Congenital bronchial atresia is characterized by developmental defect of focal obstruction or narrowing of a lobar, segmental or subsegmental bronchus with a normal distal airway.

- The most commonly affected lobe is the left upper lobe followed by the right upper and right middle lobes;
- Imaging findings (X-ray+CT):
  1. Air trapping seen in distal lungdue to decreased perfusion.
  2. Affected lung is hyperlucent, hypovascular and increased volume resulting in mediastinal shift.
  3. Mucus accumulates within dilated bronchi distal to the obstruction, resulting in central mass-like opacity show tubular configuration and finger-in-glove appearance or a rounded shape with or without air-fluid level.

6. **Scimitar Syndrome**:
   - Also known as hypogenetic lung syndrome or congenital pulmonary venolobar syndrome or scimitar.
   - Rare congenital anomaly that almost always affects the right lung.
   - Characterized by:
     - Hypoplasia of the lung with abnormal segmental or lobar anatomy.
     - Hypoplasia of the ipsilateral pulmonary artery.
     - Anomalous pulmonary venous return to the inferior vena cava (scimitar vein)
     - Anomalous systemic arterial supply to a portion of the hypoplastic lung.
   - Imaging findings(X-ray+CT):
     - Small, hyperlucent hypoplastic right lung.
     - Associated with dextroversion of the heart
     - Mediastinal shift to the right.
     - Hyperinflation of the contralateral side, and a curvilinear anomalous vein with a scimitar-like appearance.
7. **Pulmonary sequestration**:
   - Pulmonary sequestration congenital malformation resulting from abnormal budding of the foregut.
   - Presenting with dysplastic nonfunctional pulmonary tissue that is not related to the normal tracheobronchial tree and without normal pulmonary arterial or bronchial communication.
   - Supplied from branches of the thoracic or abdominal aorta.
   - Divided into two types as intralobar and extralobar. Extralobar sequestrations have their own pleura, drain into the systemic venous circulation, association with up to 60% of other congenital anomalies, present in childhood
   - Intralobar sequestrations are anomalies that can be seen in adulthood. They usually drain into the ipsilateral pulmonary venous system and do not have their own pleura, but share pleural investment with adjacent pleura.
   - Findings on imaging:
     1. *Chest X-ray*: Can show an abnormal mass, typically in the lower lobes.
     2. *CT or MRI*: Demonstrates a solid or cystic mass, and contrast-enhanced CT shows an anomalous artery arising from the aorta, confirming the diagnosis.
8. **Pulmonary arteriovenous malformation (PAVM)**:
   - Direct communication between the pulmonary artery and vein.
   - 35–67% of cases are associated with Osler-Weber-Rendu syndrome (hereditary hemorrhagic telangiectasia)
   - Most commonly found in the lower lobes, although they can occur in any lobe. They can be seen as single or multiple lesions involving one or both lungs.
   - *Imaging findings*:
     - Contrast-enhanced CT and 3D reconstructions help in diagnosis of PAVM in detail.
     - A large single sac, a mass of enlarged vascular structures, and direct communication between artery and vein seen.
     - Mural thrombi or calcifications may also occasionally be seen.
     - PAVM with a single feeding artery and a single draining vein is defined as simple, while PAVM with two or more feeding arteries or draining veins is defined as complex PAVM.

5. Describe the classification of developmental lung anomalies. Discuss CT findings in any three common developmental lung anomalies. [4+6]

Classification of developmental lung anomalies **(Flowchart 14)**:
CT findings for the three common developmental lung anomalies are as follows:

1. **Pulmonary hypoplasia**:
   - Volume reduction in affected side with compensatory overinflation of opposite side.
   - Mediastinum shifted toward the affected side due to a reduction in lung volume.
   - Absent or rudimentary bronchus with collapsed lung on the same side
   - Reduced/rudimentary/absent underlying peripheral pulmonary vascular markings.
   - Associated with rib crowding and rib abnormalities.
   - Hypoplastic airways may be seen in affected side.
2. **Congenital Pulmonary Airway Malformation (CPAM)**:
   - It is a spectrum of bronchopulmonary foregut malformations
   - CPAM also known as congenital cystic adenomatoid malformation (CCAM)
   - It is an intralobar mass of disorganized lung tissue, derived primarily from bronchioles, and cystic or multicystic.
   - Most common in lower lobe.
   - *CPAM is divided into 5 types (0–4) according to the recent classification.*
   - *Imaging findings*:
     - Type 1 (65%):
       - One or more cysts, >2 cm in diameter
       - Large air-filled multicystic lesion.
       - Sometimes with air-fluid levels (when infection superimposed).

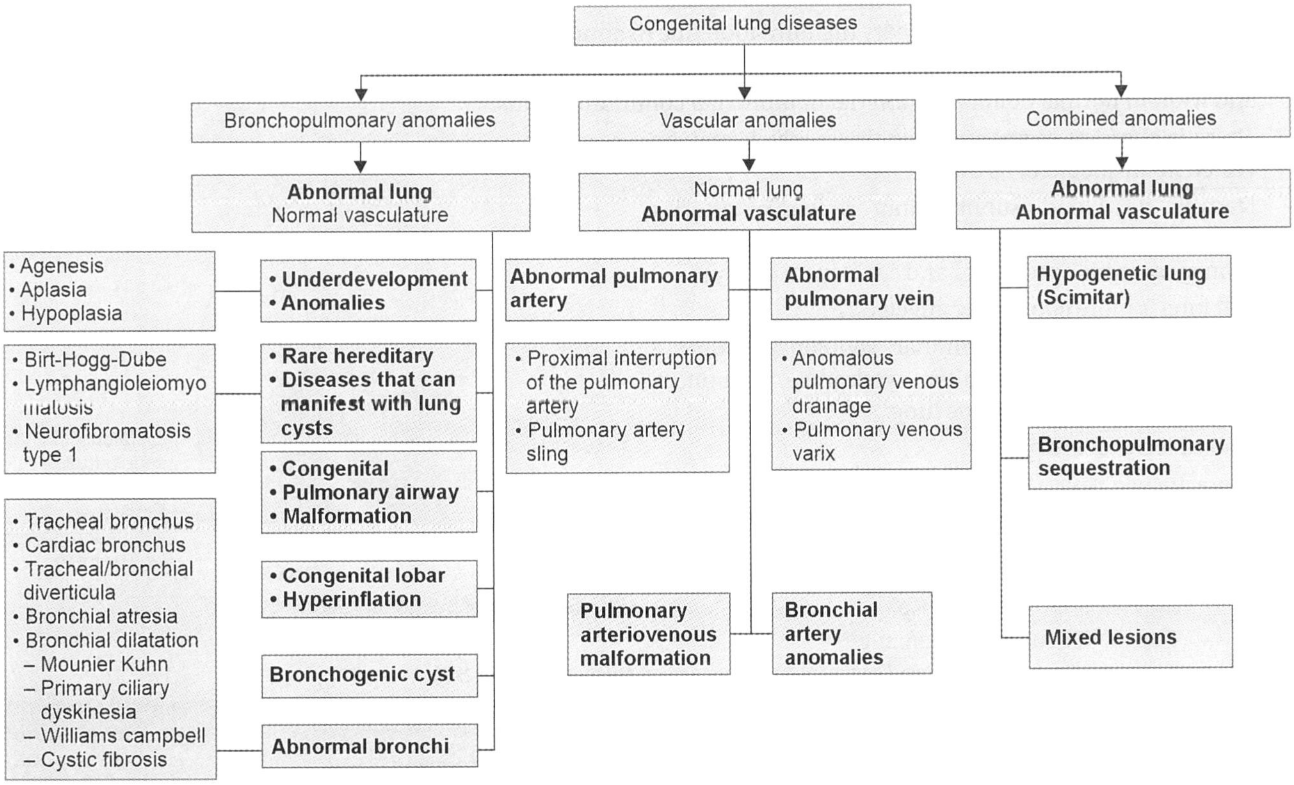

FLOWCHART 14: Types of congenital lung diseases.

- Type 2 (20–25%):
  - Multiple cysts <2 cm in diameter
  - Air-filled multicystic mass with focal consolidation.
- Type 3 (10%):
  - Microscopic (<3–5 mm) cysts.
  - Appears as solid mass.
- Type 0 (a few %)
  - Small cysts.
  - Similar to type 3 in appearance.
- Type 4 (a few %)
  - Large cysts.
  - Similar to types 1 and 2 in appearance.

3. **Bronchogenic cysts**:
   - Foregut duplication cysts and due to abnormal development of the lung bud.
   - Bronchogenic cysts are filled with fluid (serous, haemorrhagic, or highly viscous and gelatinous).
   - Most common in the medial lung and the lower lobes.

   Imaging findings:
   - *Chest X-ray*: May appear as a solitary, round to oval, well-defined mass.
   - *CT Scan*: Shows a fluid-filled round to oval cyst (low attenuation), thin walled occasionally calcified, well-circumscribed, may contain any air-fluid level when infected.

6. Write a short note on: Pulmonary sequestration. [5] [MD (WBUHS) 20]

Introduction

- It is a congenital bronchopulmonary malformation due to abnormal budding of the foregut.
- Presenting with dysplastic non-functional pulmonary tissue that is not related to the normal tracheobronchial tree and without normal pulmonary arterial or bronchial communications.
- There is aberrant segmental lung tissue which may be vested in the pleura of its own.
- Derives its blood supply from systemic arteries (classically from descending thoracic aorta, but also from mesenteric, intercostal and subclavian artery).
- Left lung is more commonly affected.
- It is a part of congenital pulmonary venolobar syndrome which consists of Schimitar syndrome, pulmonary sequestration and horseshoe lung.
- Also called **accessory lung.**
- There are two types **(Fig. 54)**:
  1. Intralobar sequestration (ILS)
  2. Extralobar sequestration (ELS)
     - Extralobar intrathoracic
     - Extralobar subdiaphragmatic

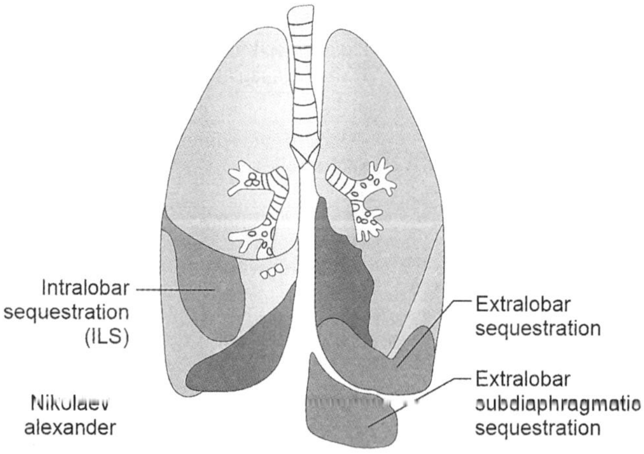

FIG. 54: Types of pulmonary sequestration.

Difference between intralobar and extralobar types are as follows **(Table 35)**.

TABLE 35: Difference between intralobar and extralobar sequestration.

Incidence	*More common (75%)*	*Less common (25%)*
Gender predisposition	Equal	Men 4:1
Laterality	Left > right	Left > right

Continued...

Continued...

Incidence	*More common (75%)*	*Less common (25%)*
Pleural investment	Shares visceral pleura of parent lobe	Separate visceral pleura
Bronchial communication	Yes	No
Location	Posterior basal segments (Approx. 60% on left)	Above, below or within diaphragm (Approx. 90% on left)
Arterial supply	Systemic	Systemic: rare pulmonary
Venous drainage	Pulmonary venous	Systemic venous (azygos. IVC, portal)
Associated anomalies	Rare	>50%
Presentation	Early adulthood with a history of pulmonary infection, chronic cough, or asthma. Asymptomatic mass (15%)	Mostly present during first 6 months of life due to respiratory or feeding problems
Radiographic features	Homogeneous consolidation with irregular margins or uniformly dense mass with smooth or lobulated contours.	Single well defined, homogeneous, triangular shaped opacity in the lower thorax. May present ease where in the thoracic cavity.

Imaging Features

Modality of choice: Contrast enhanced CT. Radiographic feaures:

1. **Chest X-ray**:
   - A homogenous well defined opacity or cystic mass in the lower lobes (especially the left side).
   - Air-fluid levels may be seen in cases of infected sequestrations.
   - *Barium studies*: To see whether communication with gastrointestinal tract is present or not.
2. **CE CT**:
   - Sequestered tissue appears as a well-defined solid mass, cystic lesion, or both.
   - Air-filled cysts or areas of consolidation may be seen, when there is infection or recurrent pneumonia.
   - Detects the anomalous arterial supply from the aorta, concurrent anomalous veins.
   - Differentiating between intralobar and extralobar sequestrations
3. **CT angiography**: Gold standard for identifying the abnormal systemic blood supply from the aorta and venous drainage, helping differentiate between ILS and ELS.
4. **MRI**:
   - *T1*: The sequestrated segment tends to be of comparatively high signal to normal lung tissue[14]
   - *T2*: Also tends to be of comparatively high signal[14]
   - *MRA*: Can be helpful in demonstrating anomalous arterial supply.

Associated Anomalies

- Congenital pulmonary airway malformation–*hybrid lesion* (concurrent presence of congenital pulmonary airway malformation and sequestration)
- Scimitar syndrome
- Congenital heart disease
- Congenital diaphragmatic hernia

Differential Diagnosis

- Congenital pulmonary airway malformation
- Scimitar syndrome
- Pneumonia
- Lung abscess
- Bronchogenic cyst
- Arteriovenous malformation

Management

Intralobar sequestration-surgery-segmental lobectomy. Extralobar-conservative treatment.

7. Write a short note on Scimitar Syndrome. [5] [MD (WBUHS) 20, MD (WBUHS) 19]

Introduction

It is a rare congenital syndrome in which there is partial or complete lung hypoplasia in the ipsilateral side which is drained by anomalous pulmonary vein into the systemic veins.

Right Lung is Affected

Characterized by

- Hypoplasia of the lung with abnormal segmental or lobar anatomy.
- Hypoplasia of the ipsilateral pulmonary artery.
- Anomalous pulmonary venous return to the inferior vena cava (scimitar vein)
- Anomalous systemic arterial supply to a portion of the hypoplastic lung.

It is a part of congenital pulmonary venolobar syndrome which consists of schimitar syndrome, pulmonary sequestration and horseshoe lung.

Also known as hypogenetic lung syndrome.

Pathophysiology

An anomalous pulmonary vein drains the affected lung into suprahepatic IVC or other systemic arteries like portal vein, azygous vein or right atrium or coronary sinus.

This anomalous vein looks like Scimitar (Turkish sword).

Imaging Features

- **Modality of choice**: Contrast enhanced CT
- **Radiographic features**:
  1. *Abnormal venous drainage (scimitar vein)*: An anomalous pulmonary vein draining from the right lung into the inferior vena cava (IVC).This vein has a curvilinear course resembling a scimitar sword and is most visible on the right side.
  2. *Hypoplastic right lung*: Hypoplastic right lung with Hyperinflation of the contralateral side. There is reduction in the number of bronchopulmonary segments in right lung.
  3. *Cardiac dextroposition*: The heart displaced toward the right side due to the smaller size of the right lung.
  4. *Mediastinal Shift*: Toward the right side due to hypoplastic lung with right diaphragmatic elevation.
  5. Abnormal systemic arterial supply may originate from the aorta or its branches, providing blood to the right lower lobe.

Associated Anomalies

- Lung sequestration.
- Lung segmentation anomalies—horseshoe lung.
- Congenital heart disease—ASD, VSD, PDA, and TOF.
- Vertebral anomalies—hemivertebra.
- Ipsilateral diaphragmatic anomalies: hernia or accessory diaphragm.
- Bronchial branching anomalies.

Differential Diagnosis

- Right middle lobe collapse (on frontal chest radiograph).
- Pulmonary sequestration.
- Swyer-James syndrome.
- Unilateral absence of pulmonary artery.

Pleura and Diaphragm

1. Classify pleural tumors. Briefly discuss chest radiographic and CT findings of malignant mesothelioma. [3+3+4] [MD (WBUHS) 23]

Classification of Pleural Tumors

- **Primary pleural tumors**:
  - Mesothelial tumors
    - Pleural malignant mesothelioma
    - Well-differentiated papillary mesothelioma
    - Adenomatoid tumor of pleura
  - Mesenchymal tumors
    - Solitary fibrous tumor (pleural fibroma)
    - Pleural angiosarcoma
    - Pleural synovial sarcoma
    - Desmoid-type fibromatosis of pleura
    - Calcifying fibrous tumor of pleura
    - Desmoplastic round cell tumor of pleura
  - Lymphoproliferative disorders
    - Primary pleural lymphoma
    - Pyothorax-associated lymphoma
    - Primary effusion lymphoma
- **Secondary lesions that can involve the pleura**:
  - Metastases:
    - Lung cancer
    - Breast carcinoma
    - Ovarian cancer
    - Lymphoma
    - Gastric carcinoma
    - Thymic epithelial tumors (thymoma)
  - Invasive tumors to the pleura
    - Thymic epithelial tumors (thymoma) with pleural invasion
    - Pericardial tumors with pleural invasion
    - Invasive chest wall tumors
    - Ewing sarcoma family of tumors with pleural invasion

Radiographic findings of malignant mesothelioma **(Fig. 55)**:

Chest X-ray

- A unilateral pleural effusion with diffuse pleural thickening is common finding.
- Diffuse pleural thickening or extensive lobular pleural-based masses are seen in about half of cases.
- The pleural thickening and masses are seen along the fissures and may simulate an intraparenchymal mass.
- Tumor growth leads to nodular thickening of interlobar fissures and lung encasement with a rind-like appearance.
- Volume loss of affected hemithorax leads to tracheomediastinal shift, elevated hilum, elevated diaphragm, and reduced intercostal spaces.
- When mediastinal or diaphragmatic pleura is involved, there may be shaggy mediastinal/heart or diaphragmatic contours.
- Punctate calcifications may be seen due to osseous and cartilaginous differentiation.

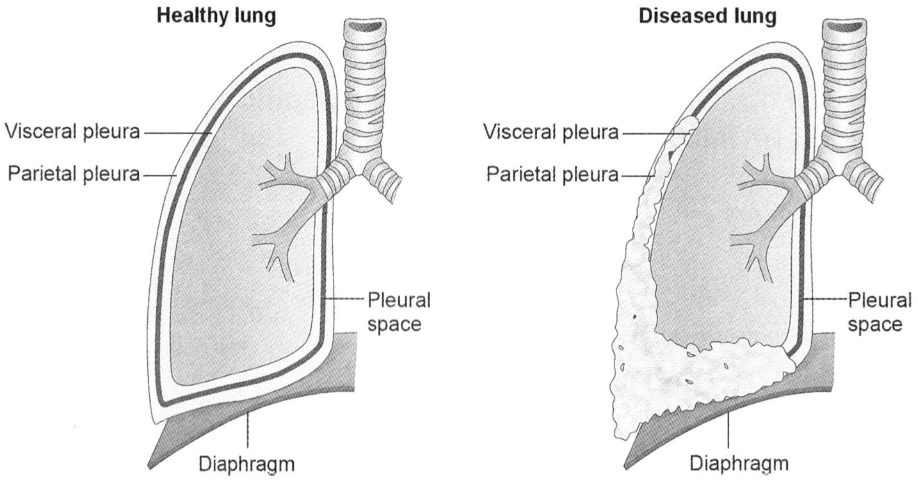

FIG. 55: Involvement of pleura and lung in malignant mesothelioma.

- Rib destruction or extension can be seen.
- Mediastinal or hilar lymphadenopathy may be seen.

CT findings: Imaging modality of choice for the extent of primary disease and locoregional extension of disease.
- Nodular or lobular or diffuse pleural thickening is the most common manifestation.
- Pleural thickening >1 cm suggestive of malignant disease.
- Pleural effusion, mediastinal pleural involvement, and interlobar pleural involvement are seen.
- Circumferential pleural thickening with rind-like encasement of the lung and ipsilateral volume loss is seen.
- Involvement of pleural fissure is seen.
- Calcified pleural plaque may be present if there is asbestos exposure.
- Local invasion includes:
  - *Mediastinal invasion*: Loss of the interface with the mediastinal fat, or greater than 50% circumferential invasion of the trachea or esophagus.
  - *Pericardial invasion*: Results in pericardial thickening, effusion, nodularity, or soft tissue.
  - *Chest wall involvement*: Loss of normal extrapleural fat or invasion of the intercostal muscles or bony destruction.
  - *Diaphragmatic extension*: It is less reliably diagnosed on CT; however, loss of fat plane with diaphragm and subdiaphragmatic structures may suggest invasion.
  - *Pulmonary metastasis*: Seen in the form of parenchymal nodules, masses or lymphangitis carcinomatosis.

CT parameters of unresectability of the disease are:
- Multifocal or diffuse invasion of the chest wall.
- Invasion of the mediastinal structures or spine.
- Transmural invasion of the pericardium.
- Involvement of the contralateral pleura.
- Transdiaphragmatic extension.
- Metastatic disease.

2. Discuss various imaging signs of diaphragmatic injury. Describe the differences between blunt and penetrating diaphragmatic injury. Discuss signs to differentiate diaphragmatic hernia from eventration and paralysis. [5+2+3] [DNB June 20]

Various imaging signs of diaphragmatic injuries are:

Chest X-ray (CXR) signs: Not specific for diagnosis; however, the following signs help in the diagnosis.

- **Elevation of the hemidiaphragm**: This is a common but nonspecific sign. The diaphragm on the injured side may appear higher.
- **Absent diaphragmatic outline**: A disruption of the smooth contour of the diaphragm may indicate a tear.
- **Collar sign**: Herniation of a hollow viscus (stomach, colon, small bowel) into the chest with or without focal constriction of the viscus at the site of the tear.
- **Crescent sign**: Visualization of the stomach or bowel loops in the thorax, especially on the left side, as air-filled loops.
- **Contralateral mediastinal shift**: If the injury causes a large hernia or diaphragmatic rupture, the mediastinum may shift towards the unaffected side.
- Basal atelectasis may be seen.
- **Pleural effusion/hydrothorax/hemothorax**: Associated with rib fracture.

CT Scan Signs

CT is the most sensitive modality for detecting diaphragmatic injuries, especially in trauma cases.

1. **Direct signs**:
    - Direct discontinuity of the diaphragm
    - Dangling diaphragm sign
2. **Indirect signs**:
    - Collar sign
    - Intrathoracic herniation of viscera
    - Dependent viscera sign
    - Contiguous injury on either side of the diaphragm
    - Sinus cutoff sign
3. **Signs of uncertain origin**:
    - Thickening of the diaphragm
    - Hypoattenuated diaphragm
    - Fractured rib
    - Diaphragmatic/peridiaphragmatic contrast extravasation
4. **Discontinuous diaphragm sign**: Visualization of direct discontinuity of the diaphragm along with segmental non-visualization of the diaphragm.
5. **Dangling diaphragm sign**: It is characterized by the free edge of the torn diaphragm curling inward, instead of remaining parallel to the body wall.
6. **Collar sign or Hourglass sign**: Visualization of a focal, waist-like constriction of the herniating abdominal viscus at the level of the torn diaphragm.
7. **Dependent viscera sign**: The abnormal positioning of abdominal organs like the liver or stomach or bowel, where they lie directly against the posterior ribs without the intervening diaphragm.
8. **Organ herniation**: Visualization of an intra-abdominal organ within the thoracic cavity through a defect in the diaphragm.
9. **Associated injuries**: Rib fractures, hemothorax (blood in the chest), pneumothorax (air in the chest), or injuries to adjacent organs.

Ultrasound Signs

- **Diaphragmatic motion abnormalities**: Demonstrate paradoxical movement of the diaphragm.
- Absent or reduced diaphragmatic excursion.

Differences between blunt and penetrating diaphragmatic injury **(Table 36)**:

TABLE 36: Difference between blunt and penetrating diaphragmatic injury.

Features	*Blunt diaphragmatic injury*	*Penetrating diaphragmatic injury*
Cause	High energy trauma like-car accident, falls from height. Sudden increase in intrabdominal /intrathoracic pressure	Direct trauma like–stab wounds, gunshot.
Mechanism	Torn due to sudden increase pressure or compression.	Puncture the diaphragm creating immediate defects.
Injury size	Larger often measuring 5–15 cm, irregular defect, left >right	Small <1 cm defect, clean tears at the site of puncture.
Symptoms	Subtle or delayed with respiratory distress, pain.	Immediate with pain and difficulty in breathing or sign of organ damage.

Differentiating sign of diaphragmatic hernia from eventration and paralysis are given in **(Table 37).**

TABLE 37: Differentiating sign of diaphragmatic hernia from eventration and paralysis.

Eventration vs. Hernia vs. Palsy			
	Eventration	*Phrenic nerve palsy*	*Hernia*
cXR	Unbroken continuity	Smooth convex	Broken outline
	Elevation of diaphragm or focal bulge	High hemidiaphragm	Focal elevation of high hemidiaphragm
	No basal atelectasis	Basal atelectasis	Pleural effusion, basal atelectasis
Fluoroscopy	Paradoxical movement	More marked Paradoxical Movement	Paradoxical movement
+ Inspiration	Some degree of downward movement	No downward movement	
Shift of mediastinum			Present

3. Draw a schematic diagram describing anatomy of diaphragm and imaging features of diaphragmatic injury on chest X-ray, ultrasound, CT and MRI. [2+2+2+2+2][DNB Dec 20]

Schematic diagram of diaphragm anatomy is given in **Figure 56.**

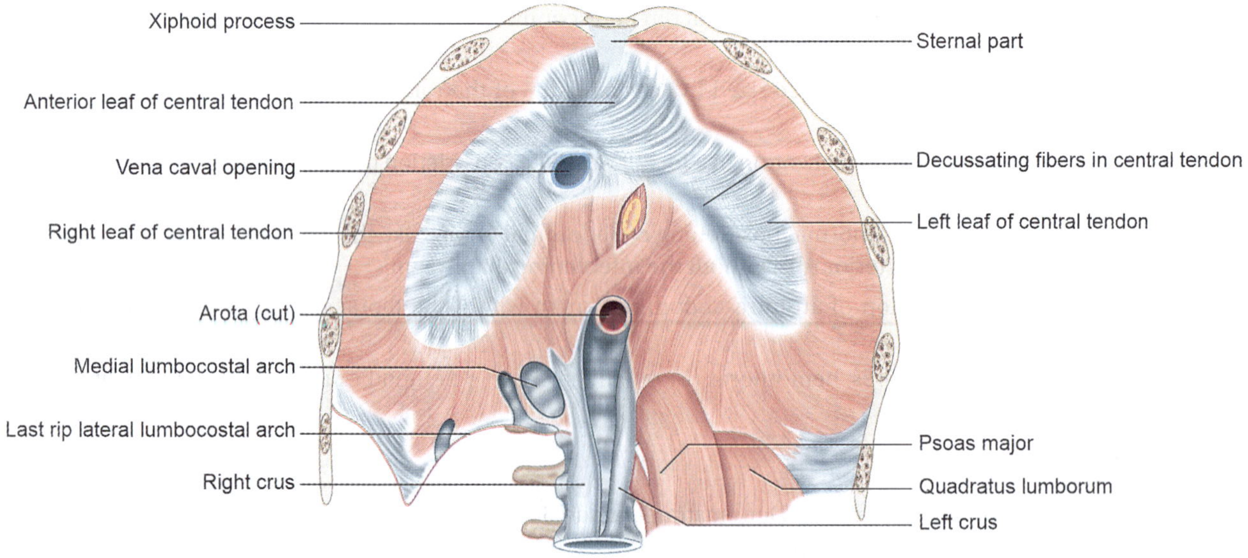

FIG. 56: Normal anatomy of diaphragm.

Imaging features of diaphragmatic injury:[27]

1. **Chest X-ray**:
   a. Elevation of the hemidiaphragm: This is a common but nonspecific sign. The diaphragm on the injured side may appear higher.
   b. Absent diaphragmatic outline: A disruption of the smooth contour of the diaphragm may indicate a tear.
   c. Collar sign: Herniation of a hollow viscus (stomach, colon, small bowel) into the chest with or without focal constriction of the viscus at the site of the tear.
   d. Crescent sign: Visualization of the stomach or bowel loops in the thorax, especially on the left side, as air-filled loops.
   e. Contralateral mediastinal shift: Shift towards the unaffected side in case of large injury.
   f. Basal atelectasis may be seen.
   g. Pleural Effusion/hydrothorax/hemothorax: Associated with rib fracture.
2. **Computed tomography**:
   a. *Diaphragmatic discontinuity*: Visualization of direct discontinuity of the diaphragm alongwith segmental nonvisualization of the diaphragm.
   b. *Dangling diaphragm sign*: It is characterized by the free edge of the torn diaphragm curling inward, instead of remaining parallel to the body wall.
   c. *Collar sign or Hourglass sign*: Visualization of a focal, waist-like constriction of the herniating abdominal viscus at the level of the torn diaphragm.
   d. *Dependent viscera sign*: The abnormal positioning of abdominal organs like the liver or stomach or bowel, where they lie directly against the posterior ribs without the intervening diaphragm.
   e. *Organ herniation*: Visualization of an intra-abdominal organ within the thoracic cavity through a defect in the diaphragm.
   f. *Associated Injuries*: Rib fractures, hemothorax (blood in the chest), pneumothorax (air in the chest), or injuries to adjacent organs.
3. **Magnetic resonance imaging (MRI)**:
   a. Diaphragmatic discontinuity seen as disruption of T1 hypointense line.
   b. Herniation of abdominal contents seen through disruption of hypointense line into thoracic cavity.
   c. Diaphragmatic elevation or inversion seen at the side of injured due to loss of muscle tone.

4. What role radiologist plays in the diagnosis of patient who has pleural effusion. [10] [MD (WBUHS) 19]

Role of radiologists in the diagnosis of pleural effusion:

Pleural effusion: Characterized by the abnormal accumulation of fluid in the pleural space surrounding the lungs **(Flowchart 15)**.

1. **Imaging modalities**:
   a. *X-ray*:
      - Costo-phrenic (CP) angle blunting—1st recognizable findings in PA view of chest-indicates ~175 mL of pleural fluid present.
      - On lateral radiograph ~75 mL of fluid.
      - Lateral decubitus ~10 ml of fluid.
      - Fluid extending into the lateral aspect of the minor fissure and slightly separating the lobes often results in an opacity resembling a rose thorn (the "thorn sign")
      - With increasing effusion-fluid seen lateral to lower ribs-lung is fixed medially by hilum and inferior pulmonary ligaments; medial fluid collections are usually smaller.

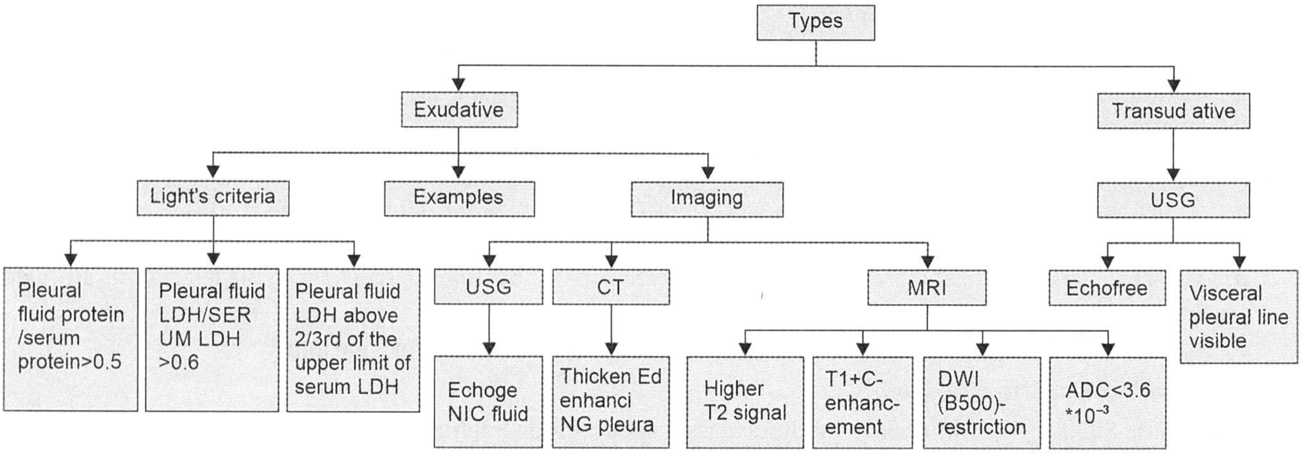

FLOWCHART 15: Types of pleural effusion.

- Meniscus sign: In case of large effusion there is homogenous opacification of lower chest with obliteration of CP angle and hemidiaphragm with concave superior margin and higher in lateral side.
- In larger effusion there is significant or complete lung atelectasis and results in a mediastinal shift to the opposite side and diaphragmatic inversion.

Effusion on supine radiograph

- Hazy veil like opacity affecting the whole or lower part of hemithorax due to layering of the effusion posteriorly with preserved vascular opacities in the overlying lung.
- Obscuration or poor definition of the hemidiaphragm.
- Blunting of the costophrenic angle.
- Thickening of the minor fissure
- Widening of the paraspinal interface.
- With large effusions, an apical cap may be seen

Subpulmonic effusion

- On PA and lateral CXR- high hemidiaphragm with an unusual contour that peaks more laterally than usual, straight medial segment and falls away rapidly to the CP angle laterally which may or may not be blunted.
- On left side, separation of more than 2 cm of stomach bubble from the lung.

Lamellar effusion

Vertical band of soft tissue density between the lung and chest wall with blunting of the right costophrenic angle-mimicking the appearance of pleural thickening.

Loculated pleural fluid

- Fluid collection between the visceral and parietal pleura and in fissures
- Loculated pleural fluid collections are limited in extent by pleural adhesions.
- Often exudative and results from adhesions.
- Transudates may cause loculation without adhesions, particularly within fissures mimicking masses—pseudotumours/phantom tumour, most common in patients with congestive heart failure.
- Typically, fluid collections in a fissure are rounded or lenticular and may show a tapering triangular opacity or "beak" at the point atwhich they merge with the fissure itself.
- Loculated collection appears sharply marginated when its surface is parallel to the X-ray beam and ill-defined when viewed en face.
- On frontal radiograph—appear sharply marginated, and the lateral radiograph—ill defined.

Empyema:

- Caused by anaerobic organisms/TB.
- *CXR findings*: Lenticular in shape with smooth margins
  - Does not respect fissural boundaries.
  - Altered shape in AP and lateral views
  - Segmental disregard.
  - Produce obtuse angle with the pleura.

b. *USG*:

- Ultrasound (US) is noninvasive, portable, radiation free bedside tool for diagnosing and managing pleural effusions, especially in ICU patients.
- Detects small amounts of pleural fluid, as small as 3–5 mL.
- US can determine the size and location of the effusion.
- Help in guiding thoracentesis and chest tube drainage with real time imaging, ensures accurate and safe placement of the needle.
- US can help diagnose co-existing lung diseases.
- US can categorize pleural effusions as simple or complex based on their appearance
- Simple pleural effusions: Anechoic and usually transudative.
- Complex pleural effusions: Can be homogeneously echogenic, heterogeneously echogenic, or have septations. Complex effusions are often exudative.
- Exudative effusions often demonstrate punctate, hyperechoic floating foci within the effusion, called plankton sign. Septations may be seen in the pleural fluid, and may indicate underlying infection but can be seen in chylothorax or hemothorax
- Effusions with heterogeneous echogenicity with swirling echoes suggest high cellular content that is often associated with malignancy.
- Fibrinous stranding, septations, and loculations also suggest an exudative effusion.

c. *CT*:

- Pleural effusion appears lower in attenuation than pleural thickening or consolidated or collapsed lung on non-contrast CT.
- On contrast CT, both airless lung and thickened pleura enhance.
- Detects small amounts of fluid and is also often able to identify the underlying intrathoracic causes (e.g., malignant pleural deposits or primary lung neoplasms) and subdiaphragmatic diseases (e.g., subdiaphragmatic abscess).
- Free pleural effusion appears as crescent shaped.
- Large effusions often extend into the major fissures, displacing the lower lobes medially and posteriorly.
- Atelectasis is common in patients with large effusions, and atelectatic lung may be seen floating within the fluid.
- Presence of thickened parietal pleura in association with a pleural effusion suggests that the fluid collection is an exudate.
- CT shows air within the fluid collection and multiple air bubbles or multiple air-fluid levels.

On axial CT images, a number of CT signs are helpful in differentiating ascites from pleural effusion **(Table 38)**:

Loculated pleural fluid:

- A localized collection
- An elliptical or lenticular shape (rather than crescentic).
- A nondependent location.
- If air is present within a loculated effusion, multiple septations may be seen, resulting in multiple air bubbles, localized air collections, or air-fluid levels.

- Loculated effusions are often associated with pleural thickening, best seen with contrast enhancement.

If both visceral and parietal pleural surfaces are thickened—split pleura sign.

2. **Guidance for procedures**: Radiologists often use ultrasound to guide thoracentesis/ drain fluid for both therapeutic relief and diagnostic testing with real-time imaging.
3. **Monitoring**: Radiologists help in monitoring the progression or resolution of pleural effusions, detect complications, or guide further interventions.

TABLE 38: Difference between ascites and pleural effusion on the basis of CT signs.

Differences between ascites and pleural effusion on the basis of CT signs		
Feature	***Ascites***	***Pleural effusion***
Diaphragmatic circle	Center	Outside
Displaced crus sign	Posteromedial	Anterolateral
Bare area sign	Seen	Not seen
Interface (abdominal viscera)	Sharp	Hazy
Lung	Anterior	Surrounds
Caudally	Increases	Deceases
Cranially	Decreases	Increases

Miscellaneous

1. Enumerate causes of unilateral opaque hemithorax. Describe the role of imaging in the evaluation of unilateral opaque hemithorax in an adult. [3+7]

Causes of unilateral opaque hemithorax:

- No mediastinal shift
  - Consolidation
  - Pleural effusion
  - Malignant pleural mesothelioma
- With mediastinal shift away from the opaque hemithorax
  - Massive pleural effusion
  - Large intrathoracic tumor
  - Diaphragmatic hernia
- With mediastinal shift towards the opaque hemithorax
  - Lung collapse
  - Post pneumonectomy
  - Lymphangitis carcinomatosis
  - Pulmonary aplasia, hypoplasia, and agenesis
  - Malignant pleural mesothelioma

Role of imaging in the evaluation of unilateral opaque hemithorax:

- **Chest X-ray (CXR)**:
  - First-line imaging modality for identifying gross abnormalities.
  - Deviation of trachea and mediastinum can help differentiate between causes (e.g., mediastinal shift toward the opacity in lung collapse and shift away in pleural effusion).
  - Air bronchograms seen in alveolar consolidation (pneumonia or lung collapse).
  - Silhouette sign localize lesions based on which borders (e.g., heart, diaphragm) are obscured.
- **Ultrasound (US)**:
  - Ultrasound (US) is easily available portable bedside tool for diagnosing and managing pleural effusions and other lung pathology like-consolidation, ARDS especially in ICU patients.
  - It can distinguish between transudates, exudates, and empyema.
  - Help in guiding thoracentesis and chest tube drainage with real time imaging, ensures accurate and safe placement of the needle

- **Computed Tomography**:
  - Gold standard for detailed anatomical assessment of lung parenchyma, pleura, and mediastinal structures in case of opaque hemithorax.
  - CT pulmonary angiography (CTPA) imaging-used in case pulmonary embolism is suspected as a cause of lung collapse or effusion.
- **Magnetic Resonance Imaging (MRI)**:
  - Less commonly used.
  - Mainly used for differentiating soft tissue masses (e.g., tumors) or in cases of chest wall involvement in case of opaque hemithorax.
- **Fluoroscopy**:
  - Dynamic imaging used to help to identify diaphragmatic paralysis or hernias.
- **Positron Emission Tomography (PET)**:
  - Rarely used.
  - Used in opacified hemithorax due to malignancy for metabolic activity of masses or lymph nodes.
- **Bronchoscopy with Imaging Guidance**:
  - Used in airway obstruction that led to lung collapse or atelectasis.

Imaging findings in differential diagnosis of unilateral opaque hemithorax **(Fig. 57)**:

- **Consolidation**:
  - Homogenous increase in opacity in the lungs that obscure the blood vessels and airway.
  - Air bronchograms/air-filled bronchi visible running through the consolidated area.
  - Silhouette sign seen when there is loss of normal borders between heart, diaphragm, or vessels, with adjacent consolidation area.
  - Lung volume generally preserved.
- **Pleural effusion**:
  - Blunting of the costophrenic angle-earliest signs of pleural effusion.
  - Meniscus sign: in case of large effusion there is—homogenous opacification of lower chest with obliteration of CP angle and hemidiaphragm with concave superior margin and higher in lateral side
  - A large effusion may cause a uniform opacity.
  - In massive pleural effusion, there is shift of the mediastinum away from the side of the effusion.
  - Loss of diaphragmatic outline noted in affected side.

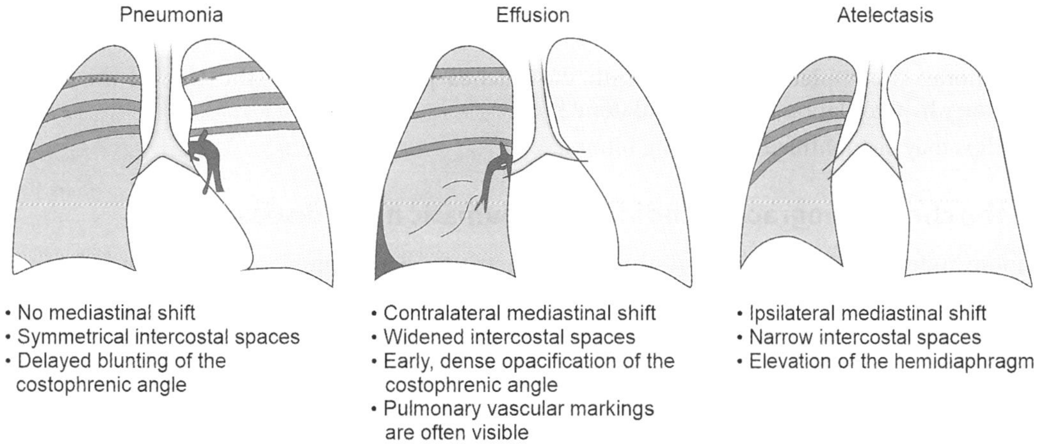

FIG. 57: Causes of opaque hemithorax and their imaging findings.

  - Pleural effusion appears lower in attenuation than pleural thickening or consolidated or collapsed lung on noncontrast CT.
  - Presence of thickened parietal pleura in association with a pleural effusion suggests that the fluid collection is an exudate on CT.
  - CT shows air within the fluid collection and multiple air bubbles or multiple air-fluid levels.
- **Malignant pleural mesothelioma**:
  - Unilateral pleural effusion with diffuse pleural thickening is common finding.
  - Nodular or lobular or diffuse pleural thickening is the most common manifestation.
  - Pleural thickening >1 cm suggestive of malignant disease.
  - Volume loss of affected hemithorax leads to tracheomediastinal shift, elevated hilum, elevated diaphragm, and reduced intercostal spaces.
- **Pulmonary aplasia, and agenesis**:
  - Opacified hemithorax with and marked ipsilateral mediastinal shift.
  - Hyperlucency in the anterior chest due to herniation of contralateral hyperinflated lung on lateral film radiography.
  - Pulmonary aplasia differentiated from pulmonary agenesis by presence rudimentary blind-ending bronchus on CT.
  - The heart is displaced into posterior hemithorax on the side of agenesis or aplasia.
- **Diaphragmatic hernia**:
  - Indistinct diaphragm or defect in diaphragmatic outline with opacification of part of or all the hemithorax.
  - Cystic lucencies in thorax.
  - Paucity of bowel in abdomen and continuity of bowel between abdomen and chest.
  - Shift of mediastinum to contralateral side.
- **Lung collapse**:
  - Direct signs
    - Displacement of fissures
    - Crowding of pulmonary vessels
  - Indirect signs
    - Elevation of the ipsilateral hemidiaphragm
    - Crowding of the ipsilateral ribs
    - Shift of the mediastinum towards the side of atelectasis
    - Compensatory hyperinflation of normal lobes
    - Hilar displacement towards the collapse
    - Shifting granuloma sign
- **Postpneumonectomy**:
  - The hemithorax is completely opacified with the trachea pulled towards the side of the abnormality and compensatory hyperinflation of the contralateral lung.
  - Surgical clips may be identified at the lung hilum.

2. Describe the chest radiographic findings in rheumatic heart disease. [5]

Chest radiographic findings in rheumatic heart disease is due structural and functional of the valves (mainly mitral and aortic valve), findings are:

- **Cardiomegaly**: The heart may appear globally enlarged due to chronic valvular disease like-left atrial and left ventricular enlargement with combined mitral and aortic valve disease.
- **Left atrial enlargement**: A common finding in mitral stenosis, which is frequently seen in RHD.
  - *Double density sign*: An overlapping contour of the left atrium over the right heart border.

  - *Splaying of the carina*: Widening of the angle (normally <90°) between the mainstem bronchi due to an enlarged left atrium.
  - *Straightening of the left heart border*: The left atrium enlarges and pushes against the adjacent structures.
- **Pulmonary edema**: Due to increased pressure in the pulmonary circulation from left-sided heart failure. Findings are:
  - Prominent pulmonary vessels in the upper lobes (cephalization).
  - Kerley B lines (horizontal lines at the lung bases due to interstitial edema).
  - Alveolar edema or "bat-wing" appearance in severe cases.
- **Aortic root dilatation**: If the aortic valve is involved (aortic stenosis or regurgitation), there may be enlargement of the ascending aorta.
- **Pulmonary hypertension**: In advanced cases, secondary pulmonary hypertension may occur.
  - Enlargement of the main pulmonary artery.
  - Prominent pulmonary artery branches.
- **Mitral valve calcification**: X-ray as dense linear opacities at the level of the mitral annulus.
- **Right ventricular hypertrophy**: In cases of advanced pulmonary hypertension, there may be enlargement of the right heart, specifically the right ventricle.

3. USG in pleural and parenchymal pathology. [10] [DNB June 22]

USG in pleural pathology: It is used in diagnosis and management of pleural pathology.
It is noninvasive, portable, radiation-free, and used in bedside, especially for ICU patients. Common pathologies that are diagnosed using ultrasound are:

- **Pleural effusion**:
  Highly sensitive: Ultrasound can detect small amounts of pleural fluid (3–5 mL). *Characterization of fluid*:
  - *Simple pleural effusions*: Anechoic and usually transudative (e.g., in heart failure).
  - *Complex pleural effusions*: Can be homogeneously echogenic, heterogeneously echogenic, or have septations. Complex effusions are often exudative.
  - Exudative effusions often demonstrate punctate, hyperechoic floating foci within the effusion, called plankton sign. Septations may be seen in the pleural fluid, and may indicate underlying infection but can be seen in chylothorax or hemothorax.
  - Effusions with heterogeneous echogenicity with swirling echoes suggest high cellular content that is often associated with malignancy.
  - Fibrinous stranding, septations, and loculations also suggest an exudative effusion.
  - *Empyema*: Appears as a complex, echogenic fluid with possible septations, suggesting pus in the pleural space.
- **Guidance for procedures and biopsy**:
  - Help in guiding thoracentesis and chest tube drainage with real time imaging, ensures accurate and safe placement of the needle.
  - Pleural biopsy: Ultrasound can guide pleural biopsies, particularly in suspected malignancy or TB.
- **Pleural thickening**:
  - Pleural thickening is a focal lesion arising from the visceral or parietal pleura >3 mm in width with or without an irregular margin.
  - Pleural thickening neither displays movement relative to the chest wall during respiration nor contains movable strands or echo densities.
  - In a pleural effusion, transmitted motion during respiratory or cardiac cycles causes a color signal known as the fluid color sign.
  - In case of pleural thickening no colored signals are detected as pleural thickening has no movable part.

- **Pleural masses**: USG can visualize pleural-based tumors, differentiating them from chest wall masses or lung parenchymal lesions and help in guided biopsy or FNAC.
- **Pneumothorax**:
  - Absence of lung sliding: Normally, on USG pleura slide against each other during respiration, which is called lung sliding. The absence of this sign suggests pneumothorax.
  - Barcode/Stratosphere Sign: In M-mode, a pneumothorax can present as a "barcode" or "stratosphere" pattern, in contrast to the normal "seashore" appearance in a healthy lung.
  - Lung point: The point where the pneumothorax ends and normal lung sliding begins, which helps estimate the size of the pneumothorax.
- **Diaphragmatic paralysis**: USG can evaluate diaphragmatic movement, detecting diaphragmatic paralysis or paresis.

USG in Parenchymal Pathology (Flowchart 16)

Lung pathology that are diagnosed in USG are:

- **Pulmonary edema**:
  - Presence of multiple B-lines (which are vertical, hyperechoic lines, comet-tail artifacts that arise from the pleural line and extend downwards and move with respiration).
- **Pneumonia and consolidation**:
  - Consolidation or hepatization of the lung—hypoechoic regions of lung with a tissue-like echotexture, often compared to the liver (hepatization of the lung).
  - Shred sign: Consolidated lung tissue appears as a subpleural hypoechoic region that has an irregular deep border which abuts normally aerated lung, which has echogenic artifacts.
  - Unilateral B-lines or bilateral B-lines
  - Possible small pleural effusion
  - Reduced lung sliding due to thickened pleura in severe cases–dynamic air bronchograms (atelectasis has static bronchograms)

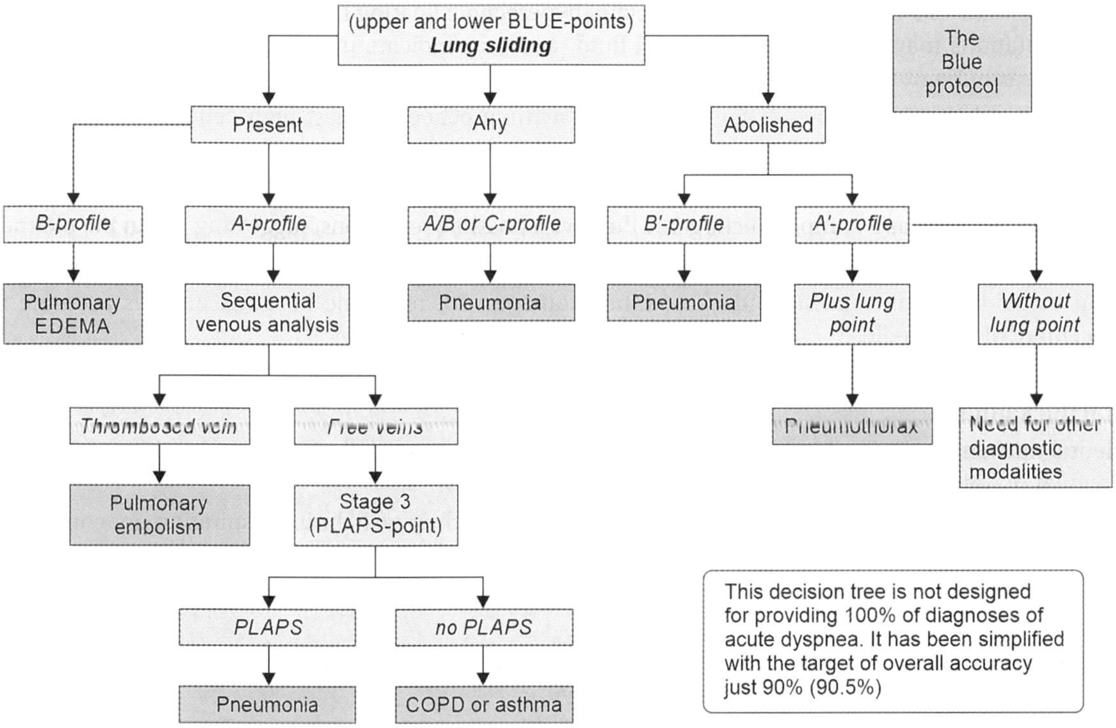

FLOWCHART 16: The blue protocol of USG in lung emergency.

- **Acute Respiratory Distress Syndrome (ARDS)**:
  - Normal lung sliding.
  - Multiple and bilateral B-lines indicating alveolar and interstitial involvement, consolidations, pleural thickening, and small subpleural consolidations.
- **Pulmonary fibrosis**:
  - Multiple, irregular B-lines, which are typically more widely spaced compared to pulmonary edema.
  - Pleural line may appear irregular and thickened due to fibrosis.
- **Lung contusion (trauma)**:
  - Show consolidation areas that resemble pneumonia but are more localized to the area of trauma.
  - These areas are hypoechoic with tissue-like echotexture, similar to the liver

Advantages

- Rapid diagnosis.
- *Portable and repeatable*: Ideal for critically ill patients in ICU settings
- No radiation exposure.
- *Guides procedures*: Useful for guiding thoracentesis or chest tube placement in cases of pleural effusion or pneumothorax.

Limitations

- **Operator dependent**: The accuracy of diagnosis depends on the skill and experience of the operator.
- **Limited in certain conditions**: Air in the lungs (as seen in emphysema) can limit the visualization of deeper structures.

4. Differentials of calcifications on Chest X-ray. [5] [DNB Dec 21]

Differential of calcifications on a chest X-ray are:[28]

1. **Lung parenchyma**:
   a. Calcified granuloma:
      - A variety of infections can produce a granulomatous tissue response and result in intrathoracic dystrophic calcifications.
      - Typically, small nodular calcifications scattered throughout the lung fields.
      - Tuberculosis (TB) is a common cause of intrathoracic calcifications and present as parenchymal granulomas, mediastinal lymph nodes, and fibronodular areas, diffuse nodular calcification of the lungs may be the result of a hematogenous infection.
      - *Histoplasma capsulatum* infections give rise to calcified intrathoracic deposits like-calcified mediastinal lymph nodes, broncholithiasis, mediastinal granuloma and solitary or multiple intrapulmonary calcified histoplasmomas.
      - *Coccidioides immitis* infection is a rare occurrence of dystrophic calcification. may occur in healing coccidioidal granulomas.
      - Sarcoidosis may produce multiple micronodular calcifications, which is radiographically similar to pulmonary alveolar microlithiasis.
      - Hypercalcemia secondary to granulomatous infections or supplemental vitamin D is a rare occurrence but may contribute to calcification of intrathoracic granulomas.

   b. *Pneumoconiosis*:
      - Silicosis, Coal Worker's pneumoconiosis.
      - Calcifications in upper lung zones, may coalesce, with eggshell calcification of lymph nodes.

   c. *Hamartoma*:
      - Shows popcorn-like calcifications which is pathognomonic for hamartoma. d)Metastatic Disease (e.g., Osteosarcoma, Mucinous Adenocarcinoma):
      - Predominantly in upper lobe.

- Multiple calcified nodules in the lung parenchyma.
- Most calcified pulmonary metastases are from primary sarcomas such as osteogenic, chondrosarcoma, synovial sarcomas, giant cell tumor, malignant mesenchymoma and fibrosarcoma of the breast, mucinous adenocarcinomas

2. **Lymph Node Calcifications**:
   a. Granulomatous disease:
      - Seen in tuberculosis, sarcoidosis.
      - Dense calcified lymph nodes, often in the hilar or mediastinal regions.

   b. Pneumoconiosis:
      - Seen in silicosis, coal Worker's pneumoconiosis:
      - Eggshell calcification of hilar lymph nodes.

   c. Postirradiation or chemotherapy: Lymph nodes may show heterogeneous calcifications post-therapy seen in lymphoma.

3. **Pleural calcifications**:
   a. Old empyema or hemothorax: Localized pleural calcifications, especially where infection or bleeding occurred.
   b. Asbestosis (Pleural Plaques): Plaque-like calcifications on the diaphragm and parietal pleura adjacent to anterior ribs, usually bilateral.
   c. Mesothelioma: Rarely can show calcifications.

4. **Cardiac and great vessel**:
   a. Pericardial calcifications: Seen in chronic pericarditis, appears as a dense ring-like calcification around the heart.
   b. Aortic arch calcification: Due to atherosclerosis, seen in older patients, linear calcifications along the aortic arch.
   c. Mitral or aortic valve calcifications: Seen in degenerative or rheumatic valve disease as nodular calcifications.

5. **Mediastinal and other causes**:
   a. Thymoma or teratoma: Focal areas of calcifications seen in anterior mediastinal masses.
   b. Aortic aneurysm: Calcifications may be seen outlining the aneurysm wall.
   c. Rib Fractures: Healing rib fractures can develop calcified calluses.
   d. Breast tissue calcifications: These can be sometimes be seen on a chest X-ray.

5. Differentials of cavitary pulmonary lesions. [5] [DNB Dec 21]

Introduction: Gas filled space within nodule, mass or consolidation is called cavity.[29] Differentials of pulmonary cavitary lesions:

1. **Infective**:
   - Organisms such as: *Staphylococcus aureus*, *Klebsiella pneumoniae*, *Mycobacterium tuberculosis,* fungal (Aspergillosis, Histoplasmosis, Coccidioidomycosis).
   - Septic emboli
   - Aspiration

   Infection in pre-existing bulla, sequestration, bronchogenic cyst

2. **Neoplastic**:
   - Lung carcinoma
   - Metastasis
   - Lymphoma
   - Tracheobronchial papillomatosis

3. **Vascular**: Infarction

4. **Inflammatory**:
    - Granulomatosis with polyangiitis
    - Rheumatoid nodules
    - Progressive massive fibrosis
    - Sarcoidosis
5. **Traumatic**:
    - Hematoma
    - Traumatic lung cyst
6. **Congenital(rare etiologies)**:
    - Congenital pulmonary airway malformation
    - Bronchogenic cyst
    - Pulmonary sequestration

Imaging findings of cavitary pulmonary lesions:

1. **Infectious causes**
    a. *Tuberculosis*:
        - A cavitary lesion with total air content (may have an air–fluid level), and with a thick irregular wall, often associated with consolidations.
        - Most frequently seen in the apical and posterior segments of upper lobes, and the superior segments of lower lobes.

    b. *Lung abscess*:
        - Cavity filled with pus developed in a pneumonia site
        - Caused by *Klebsiella Pneumoniae, Pseudomonas Aeruginosa*, or anaerobic organisms.
        - On CT – a cavity with thick irregular wall and inner margin, enhanced after contrast, often surrounded by consolidation causing poorly defined outer margins.

    c. *Fungal Infections*: *Aspergillosis*: Seen in the immunocompromised patients.

        On CT it manifests as a cavity in an upper lobe or, containing a well-defined oval or round mass (called fungus ball), dense, and mobile when the patient changes position.

        Histoplasmosis, Coccidioidomycosis: Can form cavitary lesions, usually in chronic cases.

    d. *Septic Emboli*:
        - Associated with intravenous drug use or endocarditis.
        - Bilateral asymmetrical alveolar cavitary nodules, that can excavate and converge
        - Located in the periphery and lung bases.
        - Often have a feeding vessel.
        - Wedge-shaped peripheral opacitics arc also a common manifestation

    e. Pneumatocele: Formed after infections like *Staphylococcus aureus* pneumonia, these are thin-walled cavities.

2. **Neoplastic causes**
    a. *Primary lung cancer*: Squamous cell carcinoma often cavitates. These lesions typically have thick, irregular walls, and are often solitary.

    b. *Metastatic disease*:
        - Appear as multiple sharp spherical nodules with cavitations.
        - A feeding artery can be seen in small metastases.
        - Seen in squamous cell carcinoma from head and neck, adenocarcinoma.

3. **Autoimmune/inflammatory causes**:
    a. Granulomatosis with polyangiitis (Wegener's): Multiple, bilateral and scattered cavitary lesions commonly range from 2 to 4 cm in size with variable wall thickness.

b. *Rheumatoid nodules*:
   - Multiple nodules (≥4 nodules) that are peripherally located with smooth borders, and surrounded by small satellite nodules.
   - Usually seen in patients with long-standing disease.
4. **Traumatic lung cyst**: *Pulmonary contusion*: Can lead to cavitary lesions following trauma.
5. **Vascular causes**
   a. *Pulmonary infarction*:
      - Cavitation can occur after a pulmonary embolism.
      - These are irregular in shape and are often peripheral.
6. **Congenital causes**
   a. *Bronchogenic cyst*: Although usually noncavitating, but after infection or ruptures cavitary lesions may formed.

Interventions in Chest

1. Role of intervention radiology in massive hemoptysis. [5] [MD (WBUHS) 20]

Massive or Life-threatening hemoptysis generally refers to either of the following criteria:

- Hemoptysis >300 mL/day.
- Any volume hemoptysis leading to >1 g/dL drop in hemoglobin or >5% drop in hematocrit OR
- Any volume hemoptysis leading to respiratory failure (SpaO2 <60%) OR
- Any volume hemoptysis leading to hypotension (systolic blood pressure <90 mm Hg).
  Role of interventional radiology in case of massive hemoptysis are: Bronchial artery embolization (BAE):[30]

Indications

- Massive or recurrent hemoptysis not controlled by medical management.
- Bleeding from identifiable bronchial or nonbronchial systemic arteries.
- Unstable patients unsuitable for surgery.
- **Preprocedural imaging and diagnosis**:
  - Diagnostic angiography helps in localizing the source of bleeding in case of massive hemoptysis.
  - Preprocedurally localize the site of bleeding and assess the vascular anatomy.
  - And also detect abnormal vascular structures such as dilated bronchial arteries or non-bronchial systemic arteries involved in the bleeding.
- **Procedure**:
  - Primary, most effective and commonly procedure used for massive hemoptysis.
  - >90% of massive hemoptysis is due to bronchial circulation.
  - In angiography at first, we identify the bronchial arteries or other vessels.
  - Then a small catheter is inserted through the femoral artery, guided toward the bronchial arteries, which are source of the bleeding.
  - Embolic agents (such as coils, particles, or liquid embolics) are injected to block the arteries which are responsible for bleeding.
- **Nonbronchial systemic embolization**: In cases of bleeding from nonbronchial arteries like intercostal or internal mammary arteries, IR can also perform for embolization to stop bleeding.
- **Advantages over surgery**:
  - BAE provides a life-saving, minimally invasive alternative to surgical interventions like lobectomy or pneumonectomy.
  - Surgery is usually reserved for patients who fail embolization or have recurrent hemoptysis.
- **Postprocedure monitoring and follow-up**: After embolization, follow-up imaging and clinical evaluation are necessary to ensure no re-bleeding occurs. Recurrent hemoptysis can occur in up to 30% of cases, often requiring repeat IR interventions.

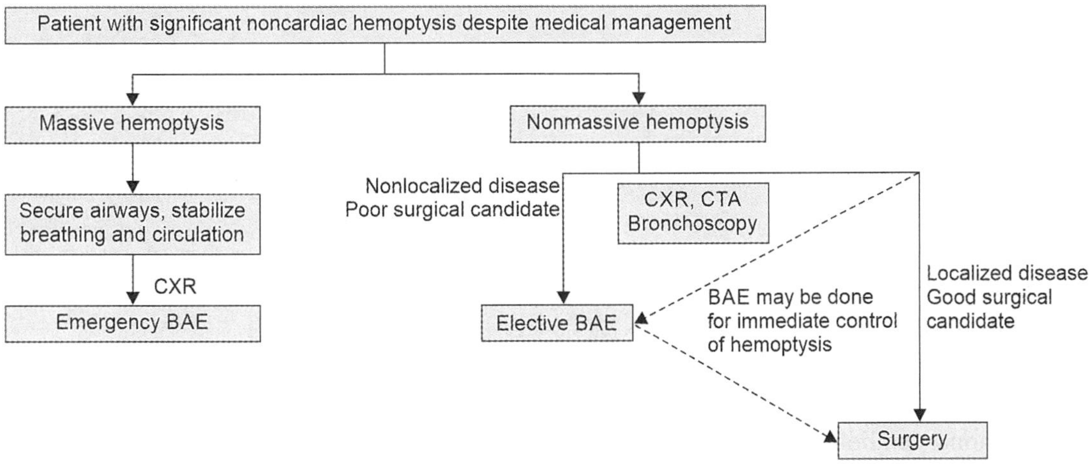

FLOWCHART 17: Stepwise approach of patients with hemoptysis.

Advantages

- Minimally invasive with high success rates (70–90% immediate control).
- Can be repeated if re-bleeding occurs.
- Avoids the risks of surgery.

Limitations

- Not effective in case bleeding from pulmonary arteries or other sources such as pulmonary vein.
- Embolization carries risks such as spinal cord ischemia (rarely due to collateral damage to the artery of Adamkiewicz).

Approach to a patient with hemoptysis is given in **Flowchart 17.**

2. What are the causes of massive hemoptysis? Describe the process of Bronchial artery embolization in case of intractable hemoptysis. [10] [MD (WBUHS) 24, MD (WBUHS) 19, AIIMS May 23]

Causes of massive hemoptysis:

1. **Infective**:
   - Active tuberculosis (most common cause worldwide)
   - Aspergillosis
   - Bacterial pneumonia
   - Bronchitis
   - Lung abscess
2. **Tracheobronchial**:
   - Bronchiectasis
   - Cystic fibrosis
   - Foreign body
   - Tumor - bronchogenic carcinoma, metatstasis
   - Bronchial telengiectasia
3. **Cardiovascular**:
   - Congenital heart disease—mitral stenosis
   - Aortic aneurysm
   - Left ventricular failure
4. **Vasculitis**: Granulomatosis with polyangiitis, Goodpasture's syndrome

5. **Iatrogenic**:
   - Pulmonary artery catheterization
   - Trauma due to bronchoscopy
6. **Blunt trauma**:
   - Pulmonary contusion
   - Tracheobronchial injury
7. **Miscellaneous**:
   - Bleeding diathesis
   - Anticoagulation therapy
   - Pulmonary infarction due to thromboembolism
   - AV malformation
   - Septic pulmonary emboli
   - Pulmonary endometriosis

Process of Bronchial artery embolization in case of intractable hemoptysis:

Bronchial artery embolization is an interventional radiology (IR) procedure that is used in control intractable hemoptysis (severe, recurrent bleeding from the lungs) that does not respond to conventional treatments.

Steps involved in bronchial artery embolization are:

- **Preprocedure evaluation**:
  - Before procedure patient is assessed with clinical and imaging modalities.
  - Multidetector CT is the modality of choice for evaluation of hemoptysis.
  - Contrast-enhanced CT and CT angiography detect airway, parenchymal as well as vascular causes of hemoptysis.
  - Fiberoptic bronchoscopy is more accurate in localizing the site of active bleed and useful if there is multifocal/bilateral lung disease.
  - Local anesthesia (for sedation) or general anesthesia used—depending on the patient's condition.
- **Route of catheter placement**:
  - Transfemoral arterial access is most commonly used for bronchial circulation. Transbrachial/transaxillary access may be used in case of increased aortic tortuosity and to selectively catheterize branches of subclavian artery.
  - Under real-time X-ray guidance (fluoroscopy), the catheter is navigated through the arterial system to reach the bronchial arteries, which supply blood to the lungs and are often the source of the bleeding.
- **Thoracic aortogram**:
  - Securing a vascular sheath in the femoral artery, then take flush aortogram using 5F angiographic pigtail catheter (having multiple side holes).
  - The loop of the pigtail catheter is formed in the proximal DTA.
  - 25–30 mL of ~80% diluted contrast (concentration≥300 mg iodine/mL) is injected at flow rate of 18 mL/s.
  - The contrast run is acquired in digital subtraction angiography (DSA).
  - Identify abnormal bronchial and nonbronchial systemic collaterals from DTA for facilitation of selective catheterization.
- **Superselective catheterization**:
  - The bronchial arteries are hooked using angiographic catheters like renal double curve (RDC)/cobra catheter.
  - Reverse seeking catheter (like Simmons) may also be used.
  - Once the artery is hooked, then check contrast injected, making them visible on fluoroscopic imaging.
- **Embolization**:
  - Embolic agents, such as polyvinyl alcohol (PVA) particles, gel foam, micro-coils, microspheres, glue are used.
  - Polyvinyl alcohol (PVA) particles most commonly used.
  - Embolic agents are carefully introduced through the catheter to block the targeted bronchial arteries. Advantages of PVA over gel foam include permanency of embolization (since gelatin sponge gets resorbed).

- The embolic agents cause a temporary or permanent obstruction in the abnormal blood vessels, cutting off the blood flow to the affected area and reducing or stopping the hemorrhage.

- **Confirmation and catheter removal**:
  - After embolization, an additional angiogram is performed to confirm the effectiveness of the procedure and ensure that there is no further blood flow to the bleeding vessels.
  - The catheter is then removed, and pressure is applied to the puncture site to prevent bleeding.
- **Postprocedure monitoring**: Patients are monitored closely for a few hours to ensure stability and check for any immediate complications, such as mild chest pain, fever, or signs of infection.
- **Outcome and follow up**:
  - BAE is effective IR procedure in stopping hemoptysis in about 85–90% of cases.
  - Recurrence may occur, especially in patients with chronic conditions
  - Long-term follow-up is necessary, particularly for patients with underlying lung diseases.
  - Repeat embolization may be required if bleeding recurs.

Basic steps in the procedure of bronchial artery embolization **(Flowchart 18)**.

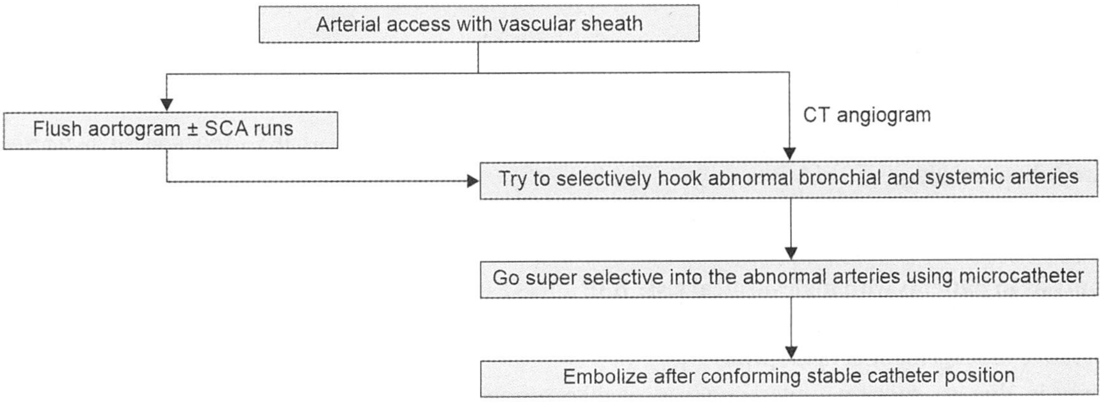

FLOWCHART 18: Basic steps of bronchial artery embolization.

3. Enumerate the causes of hemoptysis in adult patient. Briefly discuss indications, techniques and complications of radiological interventions in them. [2+2+4+2] [DNB Dec 20]

Causes of hemoptysis in adult patient:

1. **Infective**:
   - Active tuberculosis (most common cause worldwide)
   - Aspergillosis
   - Bacterial pneumonia
   - Bronchitis
   - Lung abscess
2. **Tracheobronchial**
   - Bronchiectasis
   - Cystic fibrosis
   - Foreign body
   - *Tumor*: Bronchogenic carcinoma, metastasis
   - Bronchial telengiectasia
3. **Cardiovascular**:
   - Congenital heart disease—mitral stenosis
   - Aortic aneurysm
   - Left ventricular failure

4. **Vasculitis**: Granulomatosis with polyangiitis and Goodpasture's syndrome
5. **Iatrogenic**:
   - Pulmonary artery catheterization
   - Trauma due to bronchoscopy
6. **Blunt trauma**:
   - Pulmonary contusion
   - Tracheobronchial injury
7. **Miscellaneous**:
   - Bleeding diathesis
   - Anticoagulation therapy
   - Pulmonary infarction due to thromboembolism
   - AV malformation
   - Septic pulmonary emboli
   - Pulmonary endometriosis

Indications of radiological interventions in the causes of hemoptysis:

Bronchial artery embolization is commonly used IR to control hemoptysis, particularly when it is recurrent or life-threatening.[31] The indications for performing BAE:

- **Massive or life-threatening hemoptysis**: Loss of large volumes of blood (more than 100–600 mL in 24 hours) leads to airway obstruction.
- Recurrent episode of hemoptysis (three or more episodes per week with ≥100 mL of blood).
- Hemoptysis not controlled by endoscopic or pharmacologic interventions.
- **Hemoptysis in patients with high surgical risk**: BAE offers a less invasive alternative to surgery and is the preferred choice for managing hemoptysis in high-risk surgical patients.
- Preoperative management of hemoptysis
- Hemoptysis due to specific underlying causes like–bronchiectasis, tuberculosis and fungal infections, lung malignancy.

Technique of bronchial artery embolization:
The steps BAE are:

- Transfemoral arterial access is routinely used.
- A catheter is guided to the bronchial arteries using fluoroscopy.
- Five or six French sheaths are used for the insertion of selective catheters like reverse- curved catheters (Mikaelson, Simmons I, SOS Omni) or forward-looking catheters (such as Cobra, HIH, and RC).
- Left mainstem bronchus is a convenient fluoroscopic landmark for location of bronchial arteries.
- To start embolization procedure, it is necessary to look at bronchial arteriogram for location.
- Abnormal angiographic findings that suggest the site of bleeding include tortuosity, hypervascularity, hypertrophy, extravasation, aneurysms, and bronchial artery to the pulmonary artery or vein shunting.
- If the site of hemorrhage is known, all abnormal bronchial arteries supplying that region should be embolized.
- Embolic agents that used are-polyvinyl alcohol (PVA) particles ranging in size from 300 to 500 μm, other microspheres gelatin sponge, thrombin, coils and glue.
- Postprocedure After embolization, follow-up imaging may be done to ensure the bleeding is controlled.

Basic steps in the procedure of bronchial artery embolization **(Flowchart 19)**.

Complications of radiological interventions:

1. **Chest pain**: Most common.
2. **Spinal cord ischemia**: Most dangerous complication.
   - Can lead to spinal cord infarction and transverse myelitis.
   - Use of ionic contrast agents.
   - Embolization of *Artery of Adamkeiwicz* or any dominant radicular branch of anterior spinal artery

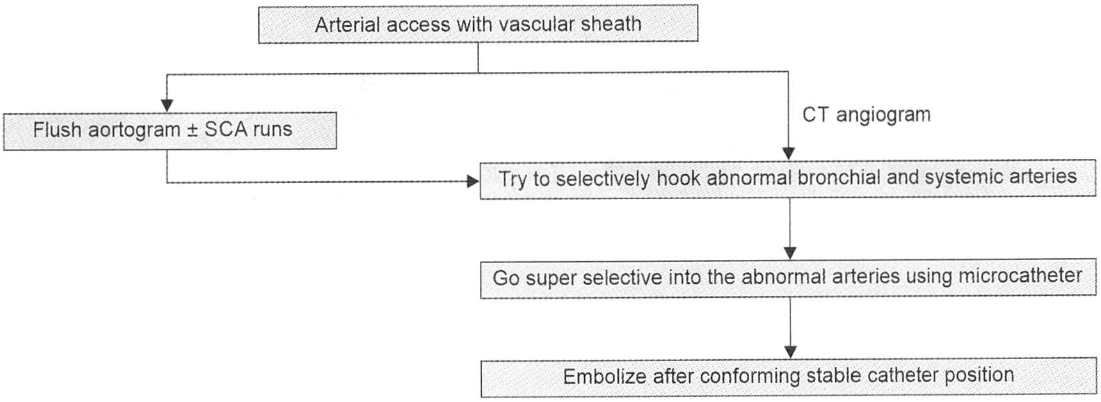

FLOWCHART 19: Basic steps of bronchial artery embolization.

Artery of Adamkeiwicz:
- It is the largest anterior medullary branch arising from T5–L5 levels
- Most common: T8–L1 level
- The right intercostobronchial artery contributes or originates with the artery of Adamkeiwicz
- Accidental embolization of this artery leads to spinal ischemia and infarction.
- So, preembolization angiography is done to identify the course of this artery which resembles a hair pin loop.

3. **Transient dysphagia**: Occurs if the esophageal arteries are affected but regresses spontaneously.
4. Aortic or bronchial artery dissection
5. Bronchial infarction
6. Bronchoesophageal fistula
7. **Nontarget embolization**:
   - Pulmonary infarction
   - Ischemic colitis
   - Transient cortical blindness
   - Referred pain to head and neck region
8. **Recurrent bleeding**:
   - *Bleeding from nonembolized*: Aberrant or non-aberrant bronchial artery
   - Recanalization of embolized bronchial artery
   - Non bronchial systemic collaterals

4. Anatomy of bronchial artery. b) Indications, technique and complications of bronchial artery embolization. [4+(2+2+2)] [DNB Dec 20]

Bronchial Artery Anatomy

- Bronchial arteries arise from the descending thoracic aorta at T3–T8 level.
- **Most common**: T5–T6 level.
- The right bronchial or intercostobronchial artery arises from right lateral or anterolateral surface of the descending thoracic aorta. It often has common origin with the posterior intercostal artery.
- The left bronchial artery arises from the anterior surface of aorta or concavity of the arch. It can arise superior or inferior to the left main bronchus.
- They go along the bronchi to the respiratory bronchiole and anastomose with the pulmonary circulation.
- They supply the trachea, bronchi, vagus nerve, lymph nodes, posterior mediastinum, vasa vasorum of aorta, pulmonary artery and vein and middle third of esophagus.
- There are variations in bronchial artery anatomy **(Fig. 58)**.

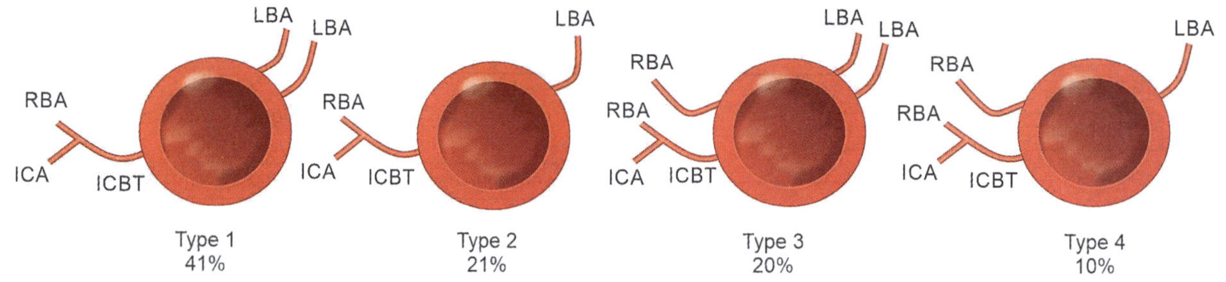

FIG. 58: Anatomical variations of bronchial artery.

(ICA: intercostal artery; ICBT: intercostal-bronchial trunk; LBA, left bronchial artery; RBA, right bronchial artery)

According to Cauldwell Classification

Type 1: Two left and one right bronchial arteries

Type 2: One bronchial arteries on each side

Type 3: Two bronchial arteries on each side

Type 4: Two right and one left bronchial arteries (opposite of type 1)

Prevalence: Type 1>type 2>type 3>type 4

Normal diameter if bronchial artery:

- At origin <1.5 mm
- *At entry into bronchopulmonary segment*: 0.5 mm

Aberrant origins of bronchial arteries:

- Abdominal aorta
- Subclavian arteries
- Thyrocervical arteries
- Internal mammary arteries
- Superior intercostal artery
- Innominate artery
- Coronary arteries
- Pericardiophrenic artery
- Inferior phrenic artery

Indications of radiological interventions in the causes of hemoptysis:

Bronchial artery embolization is commonly used IR to control hemoptysis, particularly when it is recurrent or life-threatening. The indications for performing BAE:

- **Massive or life-threatening hemoptysis**: Loss of large volumes of blood (more than 100–600 mL in 24 hours) leads to airway obstruction.
- Recurrent episode of hemoptysis (three or more episodes per week with ≥100 mL of blood).
- Hemoptysis not controlled by endoscopic or pharmacologic interventions.
- **Hemoptysis in patients with high surgical risk**: BAE offers a less invasive alternative to surgery and is the preferred choice for managing hemoptysis in high-risk surgical patients.
- Preoperative management of hemoptysis
- Hemoptysis due to specific underlying causes like-bronchiectasis, tuberculosis and fungal infections, lung malignancy.

Technique of bronchial artery embolization

The steps BAE are:

- Transfemoral arterial access is routinely used.
- A catheter is guided to the bronchial arteries using fluoroscopy.

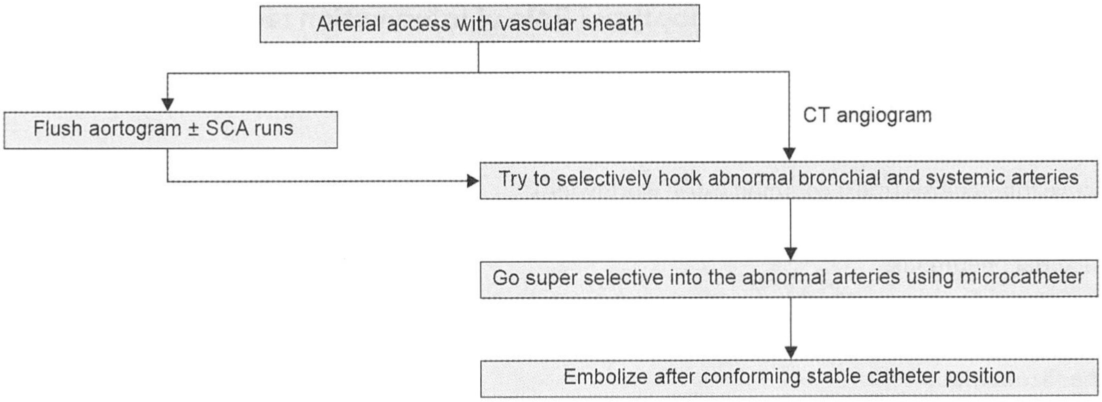

FLOWCHART 20: Basic steps of bronchial artery embolization.

- Five or six French sheaths are used for the insertion of selective catheters like reverse- curved catheters (Mikaelson, Simmons I, SOS Omni) or forward-looking catheters (such as Cobra, HIH, and RC).
- Left mainstem bronchus is a convenient fluoroscopic landmark for location of bronchial arteries.
- To start embolization procedure, it is necessary to look at bronchial arteriogram for location.
- Abnormal angiographic findings that suggest the site of bleeding include tortuosity, hypervascularity, hypertrophy, extravasation, aneurysms, and bronchial artery to the pulmonary artery or vein shunting.
- If the site of hemorrhage is known, all abnormal bronchial arteries supplying that region should be embolized.
- Embolic agents that used are -polyvinyl alcohol (PVA) particles ranging in size from 300 to 500 μm, other microspheres gelatin sponge, thrombin, coils and glue.
- Postprocedure: After embolization, follow-up imaging may be done to ensure the bleeding is controlled.

  Basic steps in the procedure of bronchial artery embolization **(Flowchart 20)**.

Complications of radiological interventions:

1. **Chest pain**: Most common.
2. **Spinal cord ischemia**: Most dangerous complication
   - Can lead to spinal cord infarction and transverse myelitis.
   - Use of ionic contrast agents.
   - Embolization of *Artery of Adamkeiwicz* or any dominant radicular branch of anterior spinal artery

   Artery of Adamkeiwicz:
   - It is the largest anterior medullary branch arising from T5–L5 level.
   - Most common: T8–L1 level
   - The right intercostobronchial artery contributes or originates with the artery of Adamkeiwicz.
   - Accidental embolization of this artery leads to spinal ischemia and infarction.
   - So, pre-embolization angiography is done to identify the course of this artery which resembles a hair pin loop.
3. **Transient dysphagia**: Occurs if the esophageal arteries are affected but regresses spontaneously.
4. Aortic or bronchial artery dissection.
5. Bronchial infarction.
6. Bronchoesophageal fistula.
7. **Nontarget embolization**:
   - Pulmonary infarction
   - Ischemic colitis
   - Transient cortical blindness
   - Referred pain to head and neck region
8. **Recurrent bleeding**:

- Bleeding from nonembolized—aberrant or nonaberrant bronchial artery
- Recanalization of embolized bronchial artery
- Nonbronchial systemic collaterals

5. Enumerate causes of massive hemoptysis? Role of intervention radiology in management of hemoptysis. [2+8] [MD (WBUHS) 22]

Causes of hemoptysis in adult patient:

1. **Infective**:
   - Active tuberculosis (most common cause worldwide)
   - Aspergillosis
   - Bacterial pneumonia
   - Bronchitis
   - Lung abscess
2. **Tracheobronchial**:
   - Bronchiectasis
   - Cystic fibrosis
   - Foreign body
   - Tumor—bronchogenic carcinoma, metastasis
   - Bronchial telengiectasia
3. **Cardiovascular**:
   - Congenital heart disease—-mitral stenosis
   - Aortic aneurysm
   - Left ventricular failure
4. **Vasculitis**: Granulomatosis with polyangiitis, Goodpasture's syndrome
5. **Iatrogenic**:
   - Pulmonary artery catheterization
   - Trauma due to bronchoscopy
6. **Blunt trauma**:
   - Pulmonary contusion
   - Tracheobronchial injury
7. **Miscellaneous**:
   - Bleeding diathesis
   - Anticoagulation therapy
   - Pulmonary infarction due to thromboembolism
   - AV malformation
   - Septic pulmonary emboli
   - Pulmonary endometriosis

Role of intervention radiology in management of hemoptysis:

1. **Bronchial artery embolization**:
   a. Primary, most effective and commonly procedure used for massive hemoptysis.
   b. >90% of massive hemoptysis is due tbronchial circulation.
   c. Advantages:
      i. Minimally invasive with high success rates (70–90% immediate control).
      ii. Can be repeated if re-bleeding occurs.
      iii. Avoids the risks of surgery.

   Steps involved in bronchial artery embolization are:
   - *Preprocedure evaluation*:
     - Before procedure patient is assessed with clinical and imaging modalities.
     - Multidetector CT is the modality of choice for evaluation of hemoptysis.

  - Contrast-enhanced CT and CT angiography detect airway, parenchymal as well as vascular causes of hemoptysis.
  - Fiberoptic bronchoscopy is more accurate in localizing the site of active bleed and useful if there is multifocal/bilateral lung disease.
  - Local anesthesia (for sedation) or general anesthesia - used depending on the patient's condition.
- *Route of catheter placement*:
  - Transfemoral arterial access is most commonly used for bronchial circulation. Transbrachial/transaxillary access may be used in case of increased aortic tortuosity and to selectively catheterize branches of subclavian artery.
  - Under real-time X-ray guidance (fluoroscopy), the catheter is navigated through the arterial system to reach the bronchial arteries, which supply blood to the lungs and are often the source of the bleeding.
- *Thoracic aortogram*:
  - Securing a vascular sheath in the femoral artery, then take flush aortogram using 5F angiographic pigtail catheter (having multiple side holes).
  - The loop of the pigtail catheter is formed in the proximal DTA.
  - 25–30 mL of ~80% diluted contrast (concentration ≥300 mg iodine/mL) is injected at flow rate of 18 mL/s.
  - The contrast run is acquired in digital subtraction angiography (DSA).
  - Identify abnormal bronchial and non-bronchial systemic collaterals from DTA for facilitation of selective catheterization.
- *Super selective catheterization*:
  - The bronchial arteries are hooked using angiographic catheters like RDC (renal double curve)/cobra catheter.
  - Reverse seeking catheter (like Simmons) may also be used.
  - Once the artery is hooked, then check contrast injected, making them visible on fluoroscopic imaging.
- *Embolization*:
  - Embolic agents, such as polyvinyl alcohol (PVA) particles, gel foam, micro-coils, microspheres, glue are used.
  - Polyvinyl alcohol (PVA) particles most commonly used.
  - Embolic agents are carefully introduced through the catheter to block the targeted bronchial arteries. Advantages of PVA over gelfoam include permanency of embolization (since gelatin sponge gets resorbed).
  - The embolic agents cause a temporary or permanent obstruction in the abnormal blood vessels, cutting off the blood flow to the affected area and reducing or stopping the hemorrhage.
- *Confirmation and catheter removal*:
  - After embolization, an additional angiogram is performed to confirm the effectiveness of the procedure and ensure that there is no further blood flow to the bleeding vessels.
  - The catheter is then removed, and pressure is applied to the puncture site to prevent bleeding.
- *Postprocedure monitoring*: Patients are monitored closely for a few hours to ensure stability and check for any immediate complications, such as mild chest pain, fever, or signs of infection.
- *Outcome and follow up*:
  - BAE is effective IR procedure in stopping hemoptysis in about 85–90% of cases.
  - Recurrence may occur, especially in patients with chronic conditions
  - Long-term follow-up is necessary, particularly for patients with underlying lung diseases.
  - Repeat embolization may be required if bleeding recurs.

2. **Preprocedural imaging and diagnosis**:
   a. Diagnostic angiography helps in localizing the source of bleeding in case of massive hemoptysis.
   b. Preprocedurally localize the site of bleeding and assess the vascular anatomy.
   c. And also detects abnormal vascular structures such as dilated bronchial arteries or nonbronchial systemic arteries involved in the bleeding.
3. **Nonbronchial systemic embolization**: In cases of bleeding from nonbronchial arteries like intercostal or internal mammary arteries, IR can also perform for embolization to stop bleeding.

4. **Advantages over surgery**:
   a. BAE provides a life-saving, minimally invasive alternative to surgical interventions like lobectomy or pneumonectomy.
   b. Surgery is usually reserved for patients who fail embolization or have recurrent hemoptysis.
5. **Postprocedure monitoring and follow-up**: After embolization, follow-up imaging and clinical evaluation are necessary to ensure no rebleeding occurs. Recurrent hemoptysis can occur in up to 30% of cases, often requiring repeat IR interventions.

6. Hemoptysis—role of radiology and intervention. [10] [DNB June 22]

Role of radiology in hemoptysis:

Radiology is essential in the evaluation and management of hemoptysis, identifies bleeding source, underlying causes, and help in therapeutic interventions. Different radiological imaging modalities are:

- **Chest X-ray**:
  - Initial imaging screening for evaluation of hemoptysis. It detects common causes, such as infections, lung masses, bronchiectasis, and infiltrates.
  - *Limitations*: X-rays may miss small lesions or bleeding sources in early or minor cases, requiring further imaging.
- **Computed tomography**:

  CT protocol for evaluation of hemoptysis **(Table 39)**:

TABLE 39: CT protocol for evaluation of hemoptysis.

Imaging parameter	***Details***
contrast material (mL)	110–125
Contrast material injection rate (mL/sec)	4–5
No. of acquisitions	1
Tuning of bolus tracking	Middle descending aorta
Coverage	Lower neck through the celiac axis
Reconstructions	
Vascular and soft tissue	
Planes of imaging	Axial, coronal, sagittal
Section thickness (mm)	1
Kernel	Standard
Lungs	
Section interval thickness (mm)	3/2
Kernel	Dedicated lung
Postprocessing	Performed as needed with dedicated software
Double-oblique reconstruction	–
Curved reconstruction	–
Maximum intensity projection	–
Three-dimensional volumetric reconstruction	–
Optional sequences	
Noncontrast sequence	Consider in patients with penetrating trauma, prior surgery, or a history of anaphylaxis after iodinated contrast enhanced sequence
Portal venous phase, with fixed 70-sccond delay	Consider in patients with tumors or pneumonia, because parenchymal and tumor enhancement are optimized in this phase

- *CT angiography (CTA)*: Provides detailed anatomy of the bronchial arteries and pulmonary vasculature, locating the exact source of bleeding. CT bronchial angiography (CTBA) delineating the hypertrophied bronchial and nonbronchial systemic arteries which are the causes of hemoptysis **(Fig. 59)**.[32]
- *Localization and etiology*: Detect variety of underlying causes, such as bronchiectasis, tuberculosis, aspergilloma, arteriovenous malformations, malignancies, and other vascular abnormalities.

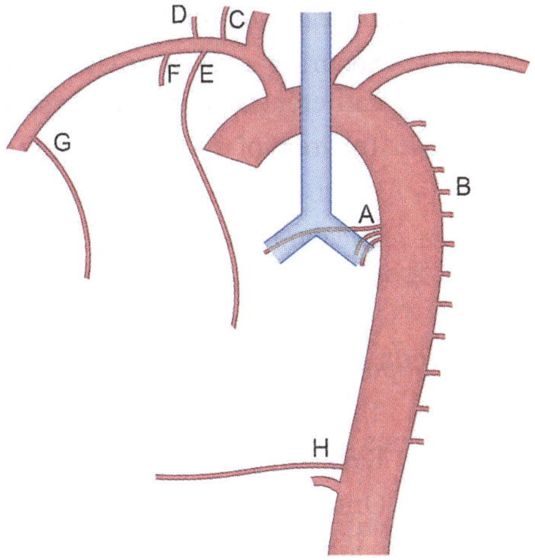

FIG. 59: Diagram shows common bronchial and nonbronchial systemic arterial sources of hemoptysis, which are highly variable among patients. A, The most common branching pattern for orthotopic bronchial arteries, with one right and two left bronchial arteries arising at the T5-T6 level, is shown. An ectopic bronchial artery (dashed red line) arises from the undersurface of the aortic arch. These variants may also arise from other systemic arteries. B, Posterior intercostal arteries arise at each level and course through the intercostal spaces to anastomose with anterior intercostal arteries (not shown). Several branches of the proximal or midsubclavian artery may give rise to transpleural collateral vessels including, C, the vertebral artery; D, the thyrocervical trunk; E, the internal mammary artery; and, F, the costocervical trunk. G, The lateral thoracic artery traverses the lateral chest wall and may also produce transpleural collateral vessels. H, Inferior phrenic arteries may arise directly from the abdominal aorta or as branches from the celiac axis and can occasionally be a source of hemoptysis, primarily in collateral vessels through the inferior pulmonary ligament.

- **Bronchoscopy**: Not a radiological procedure, but often combined with CTA. CT is more useful to identify the cause while bronchoscopy is more accurate in localizing the site of active bleed.
- **Role in preinterventional planning**:
  - *Embolization planning*: CTA is essential in planning for bronchial artery embolization or other interventional procedures, as they help the vascular anatomy and determine the catheterization approach.
  - Surgical planning.
- **Follow-up and post-treatment evaluation**:
  - Post-procedure CT evaluate the success of embolization or surgical interventions, ensuring no residual bleeding or other complications.
  - Detecting recurrence: Follow-up is important in patients with chronic or recurrent hemoptysis.

Role of intervention radiology in management of hemoptysis:

1. **Bronchial artery embolization**:
   a. Primary, most effective and commonly procedure used for massive hemoptysis.
   b. >90% of massive hemoptysis is due tbronchial circulation.
   c. Advantages:
      i. Minimally invasive with high success rates (70–90% immediate control).
      ii. Can be repeated if re-bleeding occurs.
      iii. Avoids the risks of surgery.

   Steps involved in bronchial artery embolization are:
   - *Preprocedure evaluation*:
     - Before procedure patient is assessed with clinical and imaging modalities.
     - Multidetector CT is the modality of choice for evaluation of hemoptysis.
     - Contrast-enhanced CT and CT angiography detect airway, parenchymal as well as vascular causes of hemoptysis.
     - Fiberoptic bronchoscopy is more accurate in localizing the site of active bleed and useful if there is multifocal/bilateral lung disease.
     - Local anesthesia (for sedation) or general anesthesia—used depending on the patient's condition.
   - *Route of catheter placement*:
     - Transfemoral arterial access is most commonly used for bronchial circulation. Transbrachial/transaxillary access may be used in case of increased aortic tortuosity and to selectively catheterize branches of subclavian artery.
     - Under real-time X-ray guidance (fluoroscopy), the catheter is navigated through the arterial system to reach the bronchial arteries, which supply blood to the lungs and are often the source of the bleeding.

- *Thoracic aortogram*:
  - Securing a vascular sheath in the femoral artery, then take flush aortogram using 5F angiographic pigtail catheter (having multiple side holes).
  - The loop of the pigtail catheter is formed in the proximal DTA.
  - 25–30 mL of ~80% diluted contrast (concentration≥300 mg iodine/mL) is injected at flow rate of 18 mL/s.
  - The contrast run is acquired in digital subtraction angiography (DSA).
  - Identify abnormal bronchial and nonbronchial systemic collaterals from DTA for facilitation of selective catheterization.
- *Super selective catheterization*:
  - The bronchial arteries are hooked using angiographic catheters like RDC (renal double curve)/cobra catheter.
  - Reverse seeking catheter (like Simmons) may also be used.
  - Once the artery is hooked, then check contrast injected, making them visible on fluoroscopic imaging.
- *Embolization*:
  - Embolic agents, such as polyvinyl alcohol (PVA) particles, gel foam, micro-coils, microspheres, glue are used.
  - Polyvinyl alcohol (PVA) particles most commonly used.
  - Embolic agents are carefully introduced through the catheter to block the targeted bronchial arteries. Advantages of PVA over gelfoam include permanency of embolization (since gelatin sponge gets resorbed).
  - The embolic agents cause a temporary or permanent obstruction in the abnormal blood vessels, cutting off the blood flow to the affected area and reducing or stopping the hemorrhage.
- *Confirmation and catheter removal*:
  - After embolization, an additional angiogram is performed to confirm the effectiveness of the procedure and ensure that there is no further blood flow to the bleeding vessels.
  - The catheter is then removed, and pressure is applied to the puncture site to prevent bleeding.
- *Postprocedure monitoring*: Patients are monitored closely for a few hours to ensure stability and check for any immediate complications, such as mild chest pain, fever, or signs of infection.
- *Outcome and follow up*:
  - BAE is effective IR procedure in stopping hemoptysis in about 85–90% of cases.
  - Recurrence may occur, especially in patients with chronic conditions
  - Long-term follow-up is necessary, particularly for patients with underlying lung diseases.
  - Repeat embolization may be required if bleeding recurs.

2. **Preprocedural imaging and diagnosis**:
   a. Diagnostic angiography helps in localizing the source of bleeding in case of massive hemoptysis.
   b. Preprocedurally localize the site of bleeding and assess the vascular anatomy.
   c. And also detects abnormal vascular structures such as dilated bronchial arteries or nonbronchial systemic arteries involved in the bleeding.
3. **Nonbronchial systemic embolization**:
   a. In cases of bleeding from nonbronchial arteries like intercostal or internal mammary arteries, IR can also perform for embolization to stop bleeding.
4. **Advantages over surgery**:
   a. BAE provides a life-saving, minimally invasive alternative to surgical interventions like lobectomy or pneumonectomy.
   b. Surgery is usually reserved for patients who fail embolization or have recurrent hemoptysis.
5. **Postprocedure monitoring and follow-up**: After embolization, follow-up imaging and clinical evaluation are necessary to ensure no rebleeding occurs. Recurrent hemoptysis can occur in up to 30% of cases, often requiring repeat IR interventions.

CARDIOVASCULAR IMAGING

Cardiac Imaging

1. Discuss the radiological anatomy of coronary arteries. Describe the technique of CT coronary angiography. Discuss the recent advances in assessment of coronary artery stenosis by CT angiography. [3+3+4] [MD (WBUHS) 23, [MD (WBUHS) 18, MD (WBUHS) 17, DNB June 20]

The coronary arteries supply blood to the heart muscle and branch from the ascending aorta **(Fig. 60)**. There are two main coronary arteries:

a. **Left Main or left coronary artery (LCA)**
   i. Left anterior descending (LAD)
      – Diagonal branches (D1 and D2)
      – Septal branches
   ii. Circumflex (Cx): Obtuse marginal branches (M1 and M2)

b. **Right coronary artery (RCA)**
   i. Acute marginal branch (AM)
   ii. AV node branch
   iii. Posterior descending artery (PDA)

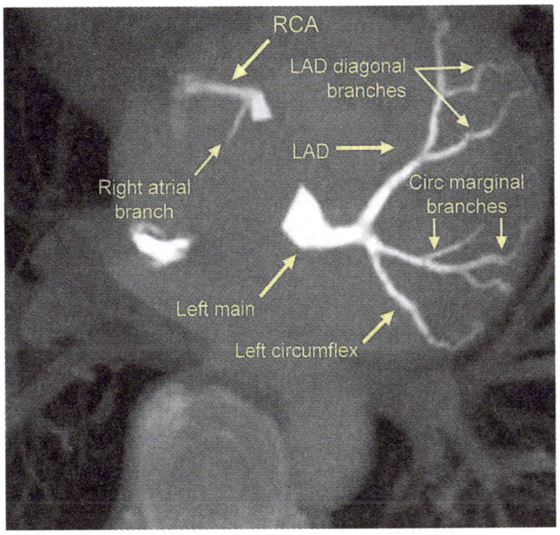

FIG. 60: Radiological anatomy of coronary arteries.

Right Coronary Artery (RCA)

- **Origin**: Arises from the right aortic sinus.
- **Course**: Travels in the right atrioventricular groove (coronary sulcus) toward the inferior aspect of the heart.
- **Branches**:
  - **AV nodal branch**: Supplying the atrioventricular septal area and the atrioventricular node.
  - **Acute marginal artery**: Supplies the right ventricle.
  - **Posterior descending artery (PDA)**: Supplies the inferior wall of the left ventricle and part of the interventricular septum.

Left Coronary Artery (LCA)

- **Origin**: Arises from the left aortic sinus.
- **Divisions**:
- **Left main coronary artery (LMCA)**: Short segment that bifurcates into:
  - **Left anterior descending artery (LAD)**:
    - **Course**: Runs down the anterior interventricular groove toward the apex of the heart.
    - **Branches**: Diagonal branches supply the anterior wall and the septum.
  - **Left circumflex artery (LCX)**:
    - **Course**: Runs in the left atrioventricular groove, supplying the lateral and posterior walls of the left ventricle.
    - **Branches**: Obtuse marginal branches that supply the lateral wall.

Dominance

- **Right Dominant**: PDA arises from RCA
- **Left Dominant**: PDA arises from LCX
- **Codominant**: Both RCA and LCX supply the PDA

CT coronary angiography (CTCA) is a noninvasive imaging modality used to visualize the coronary arteries and assess for coronary artery disease.[33]

Here's a detailed overview of the technique:

- **Preparation**:
  - *Patient assessment*: Evaluate medical history, including any allergies to iodinated contrast, renal function, and contraindications to the procedure.
  - *Informed consent*: Explain the procedure and obtain consent.
  - *Hydration*: Ensure the patient is well-hydrated to promote kidney function postcontrast.
  - *Medication review*: Consider premedication with beta-blockers to control heart rate if necessary.
- **Equipment**:
  - *CT scanner*: Use a multi-detector CT (MDCT) scanner, ideally with dual-source or 256-slice capability for high-resolution images.
  - *IV access*: Establish intravenous access for contrast injection.
- **Scanning Protocol**:
  - *Patient positioning*: Position the patient supine with arms raised above the head to minimize motion artifacts.
  - *Electrocardiogram (ECG) Monitoring*: Continuous ECG monitoring is performed to synchronize imaging with the cardiac cycle.
  - *Contrast administration*: Inject iodinated contrast agent (60–100 mL) via a power injector at a rate of 4–5 mL/s, typically followed by a saline flush.
- **Timing of the scan**: *Bolus tracking*: Use bolus tracking software to determine the optimal timing for image acquisition. The scan is triggered when the contrast reaches a predefined threshold in the ascending aorta.
- **Image acquisition**:
  - *Scan duration*: The actual imaging is typically performed during a single breath-hold (10–20 seconds) to minimize motion artifacts.
  - *Phase selection*: Images are acquired in multiple phases of the cardiac cycle, usually during diastole, when the coronary arteries are best visualized.
- **Postprocessing**: *Image reconstruction*: Use advanced algorithms to reconstruct the images in various planes (axial, coronal, sagittal) and create 3D models of the coronary arteries.

Recent Advances in Assessment of Coronary Artery Stenosis by CT Angiography

Over the last 5 years, there has been rapid advancement in CT technology, with increasing number of detectors and gantry rotation time. These have led to application of functional MDCT techniques for better evaluation of coronary artery disease. Two of these techniques are myocardial stress CT perfusion and CT-derived fractional flow reserve (CT-FFR). Both CT perfusion and FFRCT are complementary to CTCA and offer greater specificity and positive predictive value for detecting hemodynamically significant coronary artery disease (CAD) compared with anatomic imaging alone. The two strategies are particularly valuable in guiding clinical management for patients with moderate stenosis (50–70%) detected on CTCA and in special circumstances when the accuracy of CTCA is compromised, such as in patients with coronary stents and heavily calcified arteries offers an opportunity for comprehensive non-invasive evaluation of coronary anatomy and function within a single imaging session, leveraging both the strong negative predictive value of CTCA in low to-intermediate-risk patients and the higher specificity and positive predictive value of CT perfusion and FFRCT in intermediate- to high-risk patients.

2. Write short note on Ebstein anomaly. [5] [MD (WBUHS) 23]

Definition: Ebstein anomaly is a rare congenital heart defect characterized by an abnormal tricuspid valve and its positioning within the heart. The tricuspid valve is malformed and positioned lower than normal in the right ventricle, leading to functional impairments and complications.[34]

Pathophysiology

- **Malformation of the tricuspid valve**: In Ebstein anomaly, the tricuspid valve leaflets are malformed, often causing them to be elongated or dysplastic. The valve is displaced downward into the right ventricle, which can lead to varying degrees of right ventricular dysfunction.

- **Dilated atria**: The abnormal positioning and function of the tricuspid valve can cause enlargement of the right atrium, leading to atrial arrhythmias, such as atrial fibrillation.
- **Potential for right heart failure**: Depending on the severity, the right ventricle may become compromised, contributing to heart failure symptoms.

Clinical Presentation

- Symptoms can vary widely, ranging from asymptomatic individuals to those presenting with severe cyanosis, heart failure, or arrhythmias. Common symptoms include:
- Fatigue
- Shortness of breath
- Palpitations
- Cyanosis (in severe cases)

Diagnosis

Echocardiography: This is the primary diagnostic tool, revealing:

- Malpositioned tricuspid valve
- Enlarged right atrium
- Right ventricular dilation
- Possible interatrial shunt (e.g., patent foramen ovale or atrial septal defect)

Electrocardiogram (ECG): May show signs of right atrial enlargement or arrhythmias.

- CXR- right-sided cardiomegaly due to an elongated and enlarged right atrium which may result in an elevated apex. Classically, the heart is described as having a "box shape".

Management

- **Medical management**: Initially focuses on managing symptoms, including:
  - Heart rate control for arrhythmias
  - Diuretics for fluid overload
- **Surgical options**: In cases of severe dysfunction or symptoms, surgical intervention may be necessary, which can include:
  - Tricuspid valve repair or replacement
  - Palliative procedures to improve right heart function

Prognosis

Early diagnosis and appropriate management can significantly improve outcomes. Long-term follow-up is essential due to the risk of arrhythmias and heart failure.

3. Classify congenital heart disease. Discuss PDA. [10] [MD (WBUHS) 20]

Congenital heart disease (CHD) can be classified based on several criteria, including the nature of the defect, hemodynamic consequences, and clinical presentation. The most common classifications are:

1. **By hemodynamic characteristics**
   - *Cyanotic heart defects*: Conditions that result in low oxygen levels in the blood, leading to cyanosis (bluish discoloration). Examples include:
     - Tetralogy of Fallot
     - Transposition of the great arteries
     - Tricuspid atresia
     - Total anomalous pulmonary venous return

- *Acyanotic heart defects*: Conditions that do not cause cyanosis, often due to left-to- right shunting of blood. Examples include:
  - Atrial septal defect (ASD)
  - Ventricular septal defect (VSD)
  - Patent ductus arteriosus (PDA)
  - Coarctation of the aorta

2. **By anatomical location**:
   - *Left-to-right shunts*: Conditions where blood flows from the left side of the heart to the right side, leading to volume overload. Examples include:
     - ASD
     - VSD
     - PDA
   - *Right-to-left shunts*: Conditions where blood flows from the right side of the heart to the left side, bypassing the lungs. Examples include:
     - Tetralogy of Fallot
     - Transposition of the great arteries
3. **By timing of presentation**:
   - *Early-onset defects*: Presenting symptoms in infancy or early childhood.
   - *Late-onset defects*: Symptoms may not manifest until later in childhood or adulthood.

Patent Ductus Arteriosus (PDA)

Definition: Patent ductus arteriosus (PDA) is a congenital heart defect characterized by the failure of the ductus arteriosus, a fetal blood vessel connecting the pulmonary artery to the aorta, to close after birth. This results in an abnormal communication between the aorta and pulmonary artery.

Pathophysiology

- **Shunting of blood**: In PDA, blood flows from the aorta (higher pressure) to the pulmonary artery (lower pressure) during systole, leading to increased blood flow to the lungs.
- **Volume overload**: The left atrium and left ventricle may become volume overloaded over time, potentially leading to heart failure if left untreated.

Clinical Presentation

- **Symptoms in infants**: May present with:
  - Tachypnea (rapid breathing)
  - Poor feeding or growth failure
  - Sweating with feeding
  - Signs of heart failure (e.g., lethargy, respiratory distress)
- **Symptoms in older children/adults**: May be asymptomatic or present with:
  - Exercise intolerance
  - Palpitations
  - Fatigue Diagnosis
- **Physical Examination**:
  - Continuous "machinery" murmur heard best at the left infraclavicular area.
  - Wide pulse pressure and bounding pulses may be noted.
- **Echocardiography**: The primary diagnostic tool, revealing:
  - Visualization of the PDA and assessment of shunt direction and volume.
  - Evaluation of associated structural heart defects.
- **Chest X-ray**: May show cardiomegaly and increased pulmonary vascular markings.

Management

- **Medical management**:
    - *Indomethacin*: In preterm infants, this nonsteroidal anti-inflammatory drug can promote closure of the PDA.
    - *Diuretics*: For managing heart failure symptoms.
- **Surgical or interventional closure**:
    - *Percutaneous closure*: Using coils or devices to occlude the PDA, often performed in older children and adults.
    - *Surgical ligation*: Indicated in cases where percutaneous closure is not feasible or in larger PDAs.

Prognosis

Excellent outcomes: With timely intervention, the prognosis for PDA is generally good, particularly when diagnosed and treated early. Long-term follow-up is essential to monitor for any residual effects or complications.

4. Describe advantages and pitfalls of cardiac MRI. [10] [MD (WBUHS) 19, AIIMS Dec 23]

Cardiac MRI (magnetic resonance imaging) is a valuable imaging modality for assessing various cardiac conditions.35 Here are the key advantages and pitfalls of cardiac MRI:

Advantages

- **High soft-tissue contrast**: Provides excellent visualization of cardiac structures, allowing for detailed assessment of myocardium, valves, and surrounding tissues.
- **No ionizing radiation**: Unlike CT scans and traditional angiography, MRI does not use ionizing radiation, making it safer for repeated use.
- **Functional assessment**: Accurately measures cardiac volumes, ejection fraction, and wall motion, enabling evaluation of cardiac function and performance.
- **Tissue characterization**: Can differentiate between types of myocardial tissue (e.g., ischemic vs. non-ischemic) and identify conditions like fibrosis, edema, and inflammation.
- **Multiplanar imaging**: Allows for imaging in multiple planes (axial, coronal, sagittal) without repositioning the patient, facilitating comprehensive evaluation.
- **Evaluation of congenital heart disease**: Provides detailed anatomical information and functional assessment in patients with congenital heart defects.
- **Assessment of cardiomyopathies**: Excellent for diagnosing and characterizing various cardiomyopathies, including hypertrophic and dilated cardiomyopathy.

Pitfalls

- **Longer scan times**: MRI scans can take longer than other modalities, which may be challenging for patients who cannot hold their breath or remain still.
- **Patient claustrophobia**: The enclosed nature of MRI machines can cause discomfort or anxiety for some patients.
- **Limited availability**: MRI is not as widely available as other imaging modalities, and access may be limited in certain settings.
- **Contraindications**: Patients with certain implants (e.g., pacemakers, defibrillators) or severe renal impairment (risk of nephrogenic systemic fibrosis from gadolinium) may not be suitable candidates.
- **Artifacts**: Motion artifacts from respiratory or cardiac motion can affect image quality. Strategies like breath-holding or cardiac gating are often used to mitigate this.
- **Gadolinium-based contrast risks**: While rare, there is a risk of adverse reactions to gadolinium contrast agents, including allergic reactions and nephrogenic systemic fibrosis in patients with severe kidney dysfunction.
- **Cost and time**: MRI can be more expensive than other imaging modalities, and the longer acquisition times can lead to longer wait times for patients.

5. Mitral stenosis, etiology, and radiographic findings. [10] [MD (WBUHS) 19]

Definition: Mitral stenosis is a narrowing of the mitral valve opening, which obstructs blood flow from the left atrium to the left ventricle during diastole. This condition can lead to increased pressure in the left atrium, pulmonary circulation, and ultimately heart failure.[36]

Etiology

- **Rheumatic fever**: The most common cause in developing countries, often following untreated streptococcal throat infections. It leads to scarring and deformity of the mitral valve.
- **Congenital heart disease**: Some individuals are born with a malformed mitral valve, which can lead to stenosis.
- **Calcific degeneration**: In older adults, calcification of the mitral valve may occur, leading to stenosis.
- **Infective endocarditis**: Infection of the valve can cause vegetations that may impair valve function.
- **Other conditions**: Conditions such as systemic lupus erythematosus or other connective tissue disorders may also contribute to mitral stenosis.

Radiographic Findings

Radiographic imaging plays a key role in the evaluation of mitral stenosis, particularly in identifying complications and assessing heart size and pulmonary vascular changes.

- **Chest X-ray**:
  - *Left atrial enlargement*:
    - A prominent feature due to the increased pressure in the left atrium.
    - This can manifest as a double-contoured silhouette on the right heart border.
  - *Pulmonary congestion*:
    - Increased vascular markings, indicative of pulmonary venous hypertension.
    - Possible presence of pulmonary edema, which may appear as fluffy opacities or Kerley B lines.
  - *Cardiomegaly*: Enlargement of the heart shadow, particularly affecting the left atrium and possibly the right heart due to volume overload.
- **Echocardiography**: Essential for evaluating the degree of stenosis and assessing the structure of the mitral valve. Findings may include
  - Thickened mitral valve leaflets.
  - Reduced mitral valve area.
  - Impaired diastolic filling of the left ventricle.
- **Cardiac MRI**: Can provide additional information about left atrial size, function, and the presence of any thrombus formation in the left atrium.

6. Discuss the plain radiographic findings in congenital heart diseases. [10]

Plain radiography can provide valuable information in the assessment of congenital heart diseases (CHDs). Here are some common findings associated with various types of congenital heart defects:

- **Atrial septal defect (ASD)**:
  - Cardiomegaly: Enlargement of the right atrium and ventricle may be noted due to volume overload
  - Pulmonary Vascularity: Increased pulmonary vascular markings may be observed due to increased blood flow to the lungs.
- **Ventricular septal defect (VSD)**:
  - Cardiomegaly: Similar to ASD, there may be right and left ventricular enlargement.
  - Pulmonary Vascularity: Increased pulmonary vascular markings due to left-to-right shunting.
- **Patent ductus arteriosus (PDA)**:
  - Cardiomegaly: Often mild to moderate enlargement of the heart, particularly the left atrium and left ventricle.
  - Pulmonary Vascularity: Prominent pulmonary vascular markings due to increased blood flow.
  - Aortic Arch: A "figure of 3" sign may be seen on lateral views due to a dilated aortic arch.

- **Tetralogy of Fallot**:
  - Boot-shaped Heart: Characteristic appearance due to right ventricular hypertrophy and upturned cardiac apex.
  - Cardiomegaly: Right ventricular enlargement can lead to overall heart enlargement.
  - Pulmonary Vascularity: Decreased pulmonary vascular markings may be seen due to right-to-left shunting.
- **Transposition of the great arteries (TGA)**:
  - Cardiomegaly: The heart may appear enlarged.
  - Pulmonary Vascularity: Typically, pulmonary vascular markings may be decreased due to the lack of adequate pulmonary blood flow.
  - Aortic and Pulmonary Arteries: On some views, the aorta may appear to lie anterior and to the right of the pulmonary artery.
- **Coarctation of the aorta**:
  - Figure 3 Sign: On a lateral view, the aorta may show a characteristic "figure of 3" appearance due to the coarctation.
  - Cardiomegaly: May be present in severe cases.
  - Collateral Circulation: Prominent collateral vessels may be visible, particularly in the intercostal areas.
- **Pulmonary stenosis**:
  - *Right ventricular hypertrophy*: The heart may appear enlarged due to right ventricular hypertrophy.
  - Pulmonary vascularity: May be normal or decreased depending on the severity of the stenosis.
- **Hypoplastic left heart syndrome**:
  - *Cardiomegaly*: Often shows significant cardiomegaly, especially of the right heart structures.
  - *Pulmonary vascularity*: Pulmonary vascular markings may be increased if there is significant pulmonary blood flow.

7. Triple rule out CT coronary angiography: Technique, its principle and protocol. [10] [DNB June 22]

Triple Rule Out (TRO) CT Coronary Angiography is a comprehensive imaging technique used to assess three critical conditions that can cause acute chest pain: coronary artery disease (CAD), pulmonary embolism (PE), and aortic dissection (AD).[37] Here's an overview of its technique, principle, and protocol.

Technique

1. **Preparation**:
   - *Patient Assessment*: Review medical history for contraindications (e.g., allergies to contrast, renal impairment).
   - *Informed Consent*: Explain the procedure and obtain consent.
   - *Hydration*: Ensure the patient is well-hydrated.
   - *Medication Review*: Premedicate with beta-blockers if necessary to control heart rate.
2. **Equipment**: *CT Scanner*: Use a multidetector computed tomography (MDCT) scanner, ideally with high-speed capabilities (e.g., 256-slice or dual-source CT) to minimize motion artifacts.

Principle

The principle of Triple Rule Out CTCA is to simultaneously evaluate the coronary arteries, the pulmonary vasculature, and the aorta, allowing for a comprehensive assessment of chest pain. By using advanced imaging techniques, it captures the three vascular systems in a single acquisition, enabling quick and accurate diagnosis.

Protocol

- **Patient positioning**: Position the patient supine with arms above the head to reduce motion artifacts.
- **ECG monitoring**: Continuous ECG monitoring is essential to synchronize imaging with the cardiac cycle.
- **Contrast administration**: Administer an iodinated contrast agent (typically 60–100 mL) via a power injector at a rate of 4–5 mL/s, followed by a saline flush.

- **Scan timing**: *Bolus Tracking*: Use bolus tracking to determine the optimal timing for image acquisition. The scan is triggered when contrast reaches a predefined threshold in the aorta.
- **Image acquisition**:
  - *Breath-hold Scanning*: Perform the scan during a single breath-hold, typically lasting 10–20 seconds.
  - *Acquisition Phases*: Obtain images during various phases of the cardiac cycle, focusing on diastole for optimal coronary artery visualization.
- **Postprocessing**:
  - Image Reconstruction: Use advanced algorithms to reconstruct images in multiple planes (axial, coronal, and sagittal) and create 3D models.
  - Evaluation: Assess coronary arteries for stenosis, the pulmonary vasculature for emboli, and the aorta for dissection or aneurysm.
- **Interpretation**: A radiologist interprets the images, evaluating the presence of CAD, PE, or AD, providing a comprehensive report for clinical decision-making.

8. Cardiac tumors and imaging. [10] [DNB June 22, RG 18]

Cardiac tumors, though rare, can be primary (originating in the heart) or secondary (metastatic). Imaging plays a crucial role in their diagnosis, characterization, and management.[38] Here's an overview of common types of cardiac tumors and the imaging modalities used to assess them:

Types of Cardiac Tumors

- **Primary tumors**:
  - *Myxoma*: The most common primary cardiac tumor, often located in the left atrium.
  - *Fibroma*: Usually found in the ventricular myocardium; often associated with arrhythmias.
  - *Rhabdomyoma*: Commonly seen in children and associated with tuberous sclerosis.
  - *Sarcoma*: Aggressive tumors, often arising from the heart wall; includes angiosarcoma and leiomyosarcoma.
- **Secondary tumors**: *Metastatic disease*: More common than primary tumors, often from lung, breast, or melanoma.

Imaging Modalities

- **Echocardiography**:
  - *Technique*: Often the first-line imaging modality, using transthoracic (TTE) or transesophageal (TEE) approaches.
  - *Findings*: Tumors may appear as masses attached to cardiac walls or valves, with echogenicity varying based on the tumor type. Myxomas typically have a "pedunculated" appearance.
- **Cardiac MRI**:
  - *Technique*: Provides detailed images of cardiac structures and is useful for characterizing tumors based on tissue composition.
  - *Findings*: Offers high soft tissue contrast; myxomas appear as hyperintense masses on T2-weighted images. MRI can assess tumor involvement with surrounding structures and evaluate for infiltration in cases of sarcomas.
- **CT Angiography**:
  - *Technique*: Useful for assessing larger tumors, their extent, and any associated vascular involvement.
  - *Findings*: Can show the relationship of the tumor with surrounding structures and provide information on coronary artery involvement.
- **Positron Emission Tomography (PET)**:
  - *Technique*: Can be used in conjunction with CT for metabolic activity assessment of suspected tumors.
  - *Findings*: Helps differentiate between benign and malignant tumors based on metabolic activity, particularly useful for sarcomas.

Differential Diagnosis

When evaluating cardiac masses, it's essential to consider differential diagnoses, including:

- Thrombus (especially in the context of atrial fibrillation).
- Pericardial cysts or effusions.
- Abscesses or infectious masses.

9. Imaging protocol in 50-year-old with acute chest pain. Likely causes and Imaging findings. [10] [DNB Dec 21]

When evaluating a 50-year-old patient with acute chest pain, a systematic imaging protocol is essential to diagnose the underlying cause. Here's an overview of the likely causes of acute chest pain, the recommended imaging protocol, and expected imaging findings.

Likely Causes of Acute Chest Pain

- **Cardiovascular Causes**:
  - *Myocardial Infarction (MI)*: STEMI or NSTEMI.
  - *Angina*: Stable or unstable angina.
  - *Aortic Dissection*: Life-threatening condition requiring immediate evaluation.
  - *Pulmonary Embolism (PE)*: Can present with sudden chest pain and dyspnea.
- **Pulmonary Causes**:
  - *Pneumothorax*: Collapsed lung.
  - *Pneumonia*: Infection leading to chest pain and respiratory symptoms.
  - *Pleural Effusion*: Accumulation of fluid in the pleural space.
- **Gastrointestinal Causes**:
  - *Esophageal Spasm*: Can mimic cardiac pain.
  - *Gastroesophageal Reflux Disease (GERD)*: Common cause of noncardiac chest pain.
- **Musculoskeletal Causes**:
  - *Costochondritis*: Inflammation of the cartilage connecting ribs to the sternum.
  - *Rib Fractures*: Trauma-related pain.

Assessment

- **Initial Assessment**:
  - *Electrocardiogram (ECG)*: First-line assessment to rule out acute coronary events.
  - *Chest X-ray (CXR)*: Quick and useful for initial evaluation of thoracic structures.
- **Further Imaging Based on Findings**: CT Angiography (CTA) of the Chest:
  Indicated if aortic dissection or pulmonary embolism is suspected. Provides detailed evaluation of the aorta and pulmonary vasculature.
  - Echocardiography: Useful for assessing cardiac function and detecting wall motion abnormalities in cases of suspected MI.
  - MRI or Additional CT Scans: If there's a suspicion of other causes, such as cardiac tumors or complex anatomical issues.

Imaging Findings

- **Chest X-ray**:
  - *Normal*: May appear normal in cases of MI or angina.
  - *Cardiomegaly*: Signs of heart failure or structural abnormalities.

- *Pleural Effusion*: Blunting of the costophrenic angles.
- *Pneumothorax*: Visible pleural line and absence of vascular markings in the affected lung.

- **CT Angiography**:
  - *Aortic Dissection*: Intimal flap separating the true and false lumen; may show "double-barrel" aorta.
  - *Pulmonary Embolism*: Filling defects in pulmonary arteries; "saddle embolus" may appear at the bifurcation.
  - *Coronary Artery Disease*: Stenosis or occlusion in coronary arteries.
- **Echocardiography**:
  - *Myocardial Infarction*: Regional wall motion abnormalities.
  - *Aortic Dissection*: Pericardial effusion or abnormal aortic movement.
  - *Valvular Issues*: Abnormalities in valve function may be identified.

10. MRI in ischemic heart disease. [5]

Magnetic Resonance Imaging (MRI) plays a crucial role in the assessment and management of ischemic heart disease (IHD).[39] It provides detailed information about cardiac structure, function, and perfusion, which is essential for diagnosing and guiding treatment decisions. Here's an overview of the use of MRI in ischemic heart disease:

1. **Types of MRI Techniques in IHD**:
   a. Cardiac MRI (CMR):
      i. *T1 and T2-weighted Imaging*: Useful for assessing myocardial structure and detecting abnormalities.
      ii. *Late Gadolinium Enhancement (LGE)*: Highlights areas of myocardial scarring or fibrosis, indicative of previous ischemia or infarction.
      iii. *Functional Imaging*: Measures left ventricular (LV) volumes, ejection fraction (EF), and wall motion abnormalities.
   b. Stress MRI:
      i. *Pharmacological Stress*: Using agents like dobutamine to simulate exercise and assess myocardial perfusion and function under stress.
      ii. *Perfusion Imaging*: Can evaluate blood flow to the myocardium during rest and stress conditions.
2. **Indications for MRI in Ischemic Heart Disease**:
   - *Assessment of Myocardial Viability*: Distinguishing between viable myocardium and scarred tissue, which can guide revascularization strategies.
   - *Evaluation of Cardiac Function*: Providing detailed measurements of LV function, including EF and volume changes.
   - *Identification of Ischemic Areas*: Localizing regions of ischemia and assessing their significance.
   - *Characterization of Myocardial Tissue*: Differentiating between acute and chronic ischemic changes through LGE imaging.
3. **Advantages of MRI in IHD**:
   - *No Ionizing Radiation*: MRI is safe for repeated use, making it ideal for monitoring chronic conditions.
   - *High Soft Tissue Contrast*: Provides excellent visualization of cardiac structures, helping to detect subtle changes.
   - *Comprehensive Assessment*: Simultaneously evaluates morphology, function, and perfusion, offering a complete picture of cardiac health.
4. **Limitations**:
   - *Availability and Cost*: MRI may not be as readily available as other imaging modalities and can be more expensive.
   - *Patient Claustrophobia*: Some patients may experience anxiety in the MRI machine.
   - *Contraindications*: Patients with certain implanted devices (e.g., pacemakers) or severe renal impairment may not be suitable candidates for MRI.
5. **Imaging Findings in IHD**:
   - *Myocardial Infarction*: Areas of LGE indicate necrotic tissue; the extent correlates with the severity of the infarction.

- *Myocardial Ischemia*: Regional wall motion abnormalities may be observed during stress testing.
- *Viable Myocardium*: Presence of hyperenhanced areas on LGE imaging may indicate hibernating myocardium, which could benefit from revascularization.

11. Radiographic findings in congenital cyanotic heart disease. [5] [DNB Dec 21]

Congenital cyanotic heart diseases are a group of structural heart defects that lead to low oxygen levels in the blood, resulting in cyanosis.
Radiographic imaging plays a critical role in diagnosing and assessing these conditions. Here are the common types of congenital cyanotic heart diseases and their associated radiographic findings:

- **Tetralogy of Fallot (ToF)**:
  - *Boot-shaped Heart*: The cardiac silhouette may appear "boot-shaped" due to right ventricular hypertrophy and an upturned cardiac apex.
  - *Right Atrial Enlargement*: Often seen due to right ventricular overload.
  - *Decreased Pulmonary Vascularity*: Reduced blood flow to the lungs may result in decreased pulmonary vascular markings on X-ray.
- **Transposition of the Great Arteries (TGA)**:
  - *Cardiomegaly*: May be present, particularly in older infants or children.
  - *Pulmonary Vascularity*: Typically decreased due to inadequate pulmonary blood flow; the main pulmonary artery may appear prominent.
  - *Aortic and Pulmonary Arteries*: The aorta may lie anterior and to the right of the pulmonary artery.
- **Tricuspid Atresia**:
  - *Cardiomegaly*: Enlarged heart, especially the right atrium.
  - *Increased Pulmonary Vascularity*: Often seen in patients with associated VSD or shunts (e.g., PDA).
  - *Hypoplastic Right Ventricle*: The right ventricle may be underdeveloped, which can be inferred from the shape and size of the heart.
- **Total Anomalous Pulmonary Venous Return (TAPVR)**:
  - *Snowman or Figure-of-8 Appearance*: This characteristic shape is due to the configuration of the cardiac silhouette and pulmonary venous structures.
  - *Cardiomegaly*: Often present due to volume overload.
  - *Increased Pulmonary Vascularity*: Particularly in supracardiac type where pulmonary veins drain into the left innominate vein.
- **Pulmonary Atresia with VSD**:
  - *Cardiomegaly*: Enlarged heart due to right ventricular hypertrophy.
  - *Decreased Pulmonary Vascularity*: May be observed if blood flow to the lungs is significantly compromised.
  - *Increased Right Atrial Pressure*: This can result in right atrial enlargement.
- **Hypoplastic Left Heart Syndrome (HLHS)**:
  - *Cardiomegaly*: Significant enlargement of the heart, especially of the right structures.
  - *Increased Pulmonary Vascularity*: May be noted depending on the presence of shunts.
  - *Diminished Left Heart Structures*: The aorta may appear small, and there may be a lack of normal left ventricular silhouette.

12. Imaging findings mitral stenosis. [5] [DNB Dec 21]

Mitral stenosis (MS) is a narrowing of the mitral valve opening, leading to impaired blood flow from the left atrium to the left ventricle. Various imaging modalities can be used to assess mitral stenosis, with specific findings noted in each. Here are the typical imaging findings across different modalities:

- **Chest X-ray**:
  - *Left Atrial Enlargement*: The most common finding; the left atrium may appear enlarged, leading to a "double contour" on the right heart border.

- *Pulmonary Venous Congestion*: Increased vascular markings may indicate congestion in the pulmonary circulation.
- *Cardiomegaly*: Overall enlargement of the heart may be noted, primarily due to left atrial enlargement.
- *Pulmonary Edema*: In advanced cases, there may be signs of pulmonary edema, such as Kerley B lines.

- **Echocardiography**:
  - *Mitral Valve Appearance*: The mitral valve may appear thickened and calcified, with restricted leaflet motion.
  - *Left Atrial Enlargement*: Significant enlargement of the left atrium is often observed.
  - *Doppler Studies*: Continuous wave Doppler shows elevated transmitral gradient and may quantify the severity of stenosis (with mean gradients typically >5 mmHg indicating significant stenosis).
  - *Left Ventricular Function*: Normal or mildly reduced left ventricular systolic function, depending on the chronicity of the condition.
- **Transesophageal Echocardiography (TEE)**:
  - *Detailed Visualization*: Provides a clearer view of the mitral valve morphology, allowing better assessment of calcification and subvalvular structures.
  - *Thrombus Detection*: TEE is particularly useful for detecting left atrial thrombus, which can occur due to stasis in the enlarged left atrium.
- **Cardiac MRI**:
  - *Assessment of Valve Structure*: Can provide detailed information about the mitral valve morphology and surrounding structures.
  - *Functional Assessment*: Evaluates left atrial and left ventricular volumes and function.
  - *Tissue Characterization*: Allows for the assessment of myocardial fibrosis, which can occur in chronic MS.
  - Cardiac Catheterization (less common for initial diagnosis but may be used):
  - *Hemodynamic Assessment*: Measures pressures in the left atrium, left ventricle, and pulmonary artery, helping quantify the severity of stenosis.
  - *Gradient Measurement*: Can directly measure the pressure gradient across the mitral valve.

13. Dark and white blood cardiac MRI. Viability scans in IHD. [10] [DNB June 21]

Cardiac MRI (CMR) is a powerful imaging tool for assessing myocardial viability, particularly in ischemic heart disease (IHD). It can provide critical information regarding the presence of viable myocardium and help guide treatment decisions.

Dark and White Blood Imaging

- **Dark Blood Imaging**:
  - *Technique*: Involves using inversion recovery techniques to nullify the signal from blood, allowing for clearer visualization of myocardial structures.
  - *Applications*: Useful for assessing myocardial morphology, detecting edema (e.g., in cases of acute myocardial infarction), and evaluating the extent of scarring.
- **White Blood Imaging**:
  - *Technique*: In this method, the blood is not nulled, allowing for better visualization of the blood pool and cardiac chambers.
  - *Applications*: Important for evaluating cardiac function, chamber sizes, and flow dynamics. It provides comprehensive information about the heart's anatomy and function.

Viability Scans in IHD

- **Assessment of Myocardial Viability**:
  - CMR can differentiate between viable and nonviable myocardial tissue. Areas of infarction that are not viable will typically show no functional recovery after revascularization.
  - *Late Gadolinium Enhancement (LGE)*: A key CMR technique that identifies scar tissue. Viable myocardium typically shows little to no enhancement, while infarcted areas exhibit pronounced enhancement.

- **Clinical Implications**:
  - Viability assessment helps in determining candidacy for revascularization procedures (e.g., PCI or CABG).
  - Identifying hibernating myocardium (viable but underperfused) can guide therapeutic strategies and improve patient outcomes.

14. Constrictive Pericarditis–CT Imaging. Radiographic Imaging of mitral valve diseases. [10] [DNB June 21]

Overview: Constrictive pericarditis is a condition where the pericardium becomes thickened and fibrotic, leading to impaired diastolic filling of the heart.[40] CT imaging is particularly useful in diagnosing this condition.

CT Imaging Characteristics

- **Pericardial Thickness**: Increased thickness (>3 mm) of the pericardium is a hallmark sign.
- **Calcification**: Presence of calcified pericardium is often observed, especially in chronic cases.
- **Pericardial Effusion**: May be present, though typically limited in size due to the constrictive nature.
- **Heart Shape**: The heart may appear "flattened" or have a characteristic "box-like" shape due to external compression.
- **Atrial and Ventricular Morphology**: Right atrial enlargement and signs of diastolic dysfunction may be noted.
- **Pulmonary Vein and Superior Vena Cava**: Assessment of venous structures may show compression or displacement due to the thickened pericardium.

CT Advantages

- Provides high-resolution images of the pericardium.
- Noninvasive assessment, allowing for a clear evaluation of both the pericardium and adjacent structures.

Radiographic Imaging of Mitral Valve Diseases

Overview: Mitral valve diseases, including mitral regurgitation and stenosis, can be evaluated using various imaging modalities. Radiographic imaging plays a crucial role in the initial assessment and ongoing monitoring.

Imaging Techniques

- **Chest X-ray**:
  - Findings:
    - *Cardiomegaly*: Enlargement of the heart silhouette in cases of severe mitral regurgitation.
    - *Pulmonary Congestion*: Kerley B lines, pulmonary edema, and pleural effusions can indicate heart failure secondary to mitral valve disease.
    - *Mitral Annular Calcification*: May be seen as calcifications around the mitral valve area.
- **Echocardiography**:
  - Role:
    - First-line imaging modality for evaluating mitral valve structure and function.
    - Provides information on valve morphology, severity of regurgitation or stenosis, and associated left atrial and ventricular changes.
- **Cardiac MRI**:
  - Advantages:
    - Excellent for assessing the extent of left atrial enlargement and left ventricular function.
    - Can visualize the mitral valve in detail and assess for associated pathologies (e.g., chordae tendineae rupture).
- **CT Angiography**:
  - Utility:
    - Sometimes used to assess for mitral valve anatomy and related structures, particularly in planning for surgical interventions.

15. Describe the Imaging Protocol and Role of MRI in Evaluation of Ischemic Heart Disease. [5+5] [DNB June 20, DNB June 18]

Overview: Cardiac MRI (CMR) is a noninvasive imaging modality that plays a crucial role in the evaluation of ischemic heart disease (IHD). It provides detailed anatomical and functional information, helping to assess myocardial viability, perfusion, and the extent of ischemic damage.

Imaging Protocol

- **Preparation**:
  - *Patient Preparation*: Ensure the patient is comfortable and inform them about the procedure. Assess for contraindications (e.g., pacemakers, certain implants).
  - *Monitoring*: Continuous monitoring of vital signs during the exam.
- **Sequence Selection**:
  - Standard Protocols:
    - *Localizer Sequence*: To position the heart accurately.
    - *Cine Imaging*: Typically performed using steady-state free precession (SSFP) sequences to evaluate cardiac function and wall motion.
    - *Late Gadolinium Enhancement (LGE)*: Administer gadolinium contrast and perform imaging to identify scarred or infarcted myocardium.
    - *T1 and T2 Mapping*: Assess myocardial edema and fibrosis, especially in acute settings.
    - *Perfusion Imaging*: Use stress perfusion imaging (typically with adenosine or regadenoson) to evaluate myocardial perfusion.
- **Image Acquisition**:
  - *Slice Orientation*: Acquire images in standard views (short axis, long axis, and apical views) to cover the entire left ventricle.
  - *Timing*: Perform LGE imaging at least 10–15 minutes after gadolinium administration to allow optimal contrast between viable and non-viable myocardium.
- **Postprocessing**: Analyze the images using dedicated software to assess wall motion, volume measurements, and LGE patterns.

Role of MRI in Evaluation of Ischemic Heart Disease

- **Assessment of Myocardial Viability**:
  - *LGE Imaging*: Differentiates between viable myocardium and scar tissue, guiding decisions for revascularization.
  - *Identifying hibernating myocardium*: Areas that are underperfused but still viable can be identified, helping in planning interventions.
- **Evaluation of Cardiac Function**: *Cine MRI*: Provides quantitative data on left ventricular ejection fraction (LVEF), volumes, and wall motion abnormalities, crucial for assessing the impact of ischemia on cardiac function.
- **Assessment of Myocardial Ischemia**: *Perfusion Studies*: Can identify areas of ischemia by evaluating blood flow during rest and stress, helping to pinpoint regions at risk.
- **Characterization of Cardiac Structures**: Detailed assessment of the mitral valve, coronary arteries (when combined with angiography), and other cardiac structures.
- **Monitoring Disease Progression**: Useful for longitudinal studies to monitor changes in myocardial viability and function over time, especially postintervention.

16. Role of Nuclear Imaging, Cardiac MRI, and MDCT in Evaluating Ischemic Heart Disease [2+4+4] [MD (WBUHS) 17, DNB Dec 20]

Ischemic heart disease (IHD) can be evaluated using several advanced imaging modalities, each providing unique insights into myocardial structure and function.[41] Here's a comparison of nuclear imaging, cardiac MRI (CMR), and multi-detector computed tomography (MDCT).

1. **Nuclear Imaging**

   Overview: Nuclear imaging techniques, such as Single Photon Emission Computed Tomography (SPECT) and Positron Emission Tomography (PET), are valuable for assessing myocardial perfusion and viability.

   Key roles:

   - Myocardial Perfusion Imaging: SPECT/PET can evaluate regional blood flow, helping to identify areas of ischemia and myocardial infarction.
   - Viability Assessment: Can differentiate between viable and nonviable myocardium, guiding decisions regarding revascularization.
   - Risk Stratification: Provides prognostic information regarding the risk of future cardiac events based on perfusion patterns.
   - Quantitative Analysis: Offers quantitative data on perfusion defects, aiding in clinical decision-making.

   Advantages:

   - Widely available and relatively easy to perform.
   - Can be combined with exercise or pharmacological stress tests.

2. **Cardiac MRI (CMR)**

   Overview: CMR is a noninvasive imaging modality that provides high-resolution images of cardiac structures and detailed functional assessment.

   Key Roles:

   - Assessment of Cardiac Function: Cine MRI allows for accurate measurement of left ventricular ejection fraction (LVEF) and wall motion abnormalities.
   - Viability Assessment: Late gadolinium enhancement (LGE) identifies myocardial scar and viable tissue, crucial for treatment planning.
   - Characterization of Myocardial Tissue: T1 and T2 mapping can assess myocardial edema and fibrosis.
   - Detailed Anatomical Imaging: Offers comprehensive views of cardiac structures, including valves and chambers.

   Advantages:

   - No radiation exposure.
   - Provides both functional and anatomical information in a single study.

3. **Multi-detector Computed Tomography (MDCT)**

   Overview: MDCT is primarily used for coronary artery imaging and can assess coronary artery disease (CAD) and myocardial perfusion.

   Key Roles:

   - Coronary Artery Imaging: Excellent for noninvasive coronary angiography to evaluate the presence and severity of CAD.
   - Assessment of Coronary Anatomy: Provides detailed anatomical information about the coronary vessels, including stenosis and plaque characterization.
   - Perfusion Imaging: CT perfusion studies can evaluate myocardial blood flow, though less common than nuclear methods.

   Advantages:

   - Rapid acquisition, often leading to shorter exam times.
   - High spatial resolution for coronary artery visualization.

In clinical practice, the choice of imaging modality often depends on patient factors, availability, and the specific information required for diagnosis and management of ischemic heart disease. Each modality has its strengths and can complement one another to provide a comprehensive evaluation.

17. Define pulmonary edema and describe its pathophysiology. Enumerate causes and imaging features in pulmonary edema. [2+2+(2+4)] [DNB Dec 20, RG 18]

Definition: Pulmonary edema is a condition characterized by the accumulation of excess fluid in the lungs' interstitial spaces and alveoli. This leads to impaired gas exchange and can result in respiratory distress and hypoxemia.

Pathophysiology

- **Increased Hydrostatic Pressure**: Commonly due to left-sided heart failure, which elevates pressure in the pulmonary circulation, leading to fluid leakage into the alveoli.
- **Increased Permeability**: Conditions such as pneumonia, acute respiratory distress syndrome (ARDS), and sepsis can cause inflammation and increased permeability of the alveolar-capillary membrane, allowing fluid to enter the lungs.
- **Decreased Oncotic Pressure**: Hypoproteinemia (low protein levels in the blood) can reduce the oncotic pressure, causing fluid to move from the vascular space to the interstitial space.
- **Lymphatic Obstruction**: Conditions affecting the lymphatic system (e.g., tumors, infections) can impair fluid drainage from the lungs.

Causes of Pulmonary Edema

- **Cardiogenic Causes**:
  - *Congestive heart failure (CHF)*: Left-sided heart failure is the most common cause.
  - *Myocardial infarction*: Can lead to acute heart failure.
  - *Arrhythmias*: Such as atrial fibrillation.
- **Noncardiogenic Causes**:
  - *Acute respiratory distress syndrome (ARDS)*: Often due to sepsis, trauma, or pneumonia.
  - *Pulmonary infections*: Such as pneumonia.
  - *Toxic inhalation*: Exposure to harmful substances (e.g., smoke, chemicals).
  - *Neurologic causes*: Such as seizures or high-altitude pulmonary edema (HAPE).
  - *Medications*: Certain drugs can cause pulmonary edema, including some chemotherapeutics and nonsteroidal anti-inflammatory drugs (NSAIDs).
- **Other Causes**:
  - *Hypoalbuminemia*: Due to liver disease or nephrotic syndrome.
  - *Pulmonary embolism*: Can lead to right-sided heart strain and subsequent pulmonary edema.

Imaging Features of Pulmonary Edema

- **Chest X-ray**:
  - *Bilateral Opacities*: Often described as "bat-wing" or "butterfly" distribution, indicating alveolar fluid.
  - *Kerley B-Lines*: Short horizontal lines seen at the lung bases, indicating interstitial edema.
  - *Cardiomegaly*: In cardiogenic pulmonary edema, the heart may appear enlarged.
  - *Pleural Effusions*: May be present, particularly in chronic cases.
- **CT Imaging**:
  - *Ground-glass Opacities*: Indicate fluid in the interstitial space and alveoli.
  - *Consolidation*: In cases of pneumonia leading to pulmonary edema.
  - *Septal Thickening*: Can indicate interstitial edema.
  - *Pleural Effusions*: As with X-ray, CT is better at characterizing the volume and extent of effusions.
- **Ultrasound**:
  - *B-lines (Lung Rocket Signs)*: Vertical lines originating from the pleural line, indicating interstitial edema.
  - *Pleural Effusions*: Can be evaluated and measured.

Nuclear Medicine

1. Scintigraphy in cardiac imaging. [5] [DNB Dec 21]

Definition: Nuclear medicine is a specialized branch of medical imaging that uses small amounts of radioactive materials (radiopharmaceuticals) to diagnose and treat various diseases, including cancer, heart disease, and certain neurological disorders.

Key Components of Nuclear Medicine

- **Radiopharmaceuticals**: These are compounds that combine a radioactive isotope with a biologically active molecule. They can be injected, ingested, or inhaled, allowing for targeted imaging of specific organs or tissues.
- **Imaging Techniques**: Single Photon Emission Computed Tomography (SPECT): A type of nuclear imaging that provides 3D images of the distribution of radiopharmaceuticals in the body. Commonly used for cardiac imaging, bone scans, and evaluating brain disorders.
- **Positron Emission Tomography (PET)**: Utilizes positron-emitting radiopharmaceuticals to visualize metabolic activity in tissues. Often combined with CT (PET/CT) for anatomical localization. Widely used in oncology to assess tumor metabolism and response to therapy.
- **Therapeutic Applications**: Certain radiopharmaceuticals can also be used for treatment, such as:

Radioiodine Therapy: Used for hyperthyroidism and thyroid cancer. Radium-223: For metastatic prostate cancer.

Peptide Receptor Radionuclide Therapy (PRRT): For neuroendocrine tumors. Applications of Nuclear Medicine

- **Cardiology**:
  - Myocardial perfusion imaging to assess blood flow and detect coronary artery disease.
  - Evaluation of cardiac function and viability.
- **Oncology**:
  - Tumor localization, staging, and monitoring response to treatment.
  - Detection of metastases.
- **Neurology**:
  - Evaluation of conditions such as Alzheimer's disease, epilepsy, and movement disorders.
  - Functional imaging of brain metabolism.
- **Endocrinology**:
  - Assessment of thyroid function and abnormalities.
  - Localization of neuroendocrine tumors.
- **Bone Scintigraphy**:
  - Detection of bone metastases, fractures, infections, and other bone disorders.

Advantages and Limitations Advantages

- Provides functional imaging that can reveal metabolic activity and physiological processes.
- Minimally invasive and can often be performed on an outpatient basis.
- Can provide information that may not be available through other imaging modalities.

Limitations

- Exposure to radiation, though typically low and considered safe.
- Availability of radiopharmaceuticals and specialized equipment.
- Limited resolution compared to some other imaging techniques (e.g., CT or MRI).

Scintigraphy in Cardiac Imaging and Vascular Imaging

Definition: Scintigraphy, or nuclear imaging, involves the use of radioactive isotopes to evaluate the function and perfusion of the heart.[42] It is primarily utilized for diagnosing and managing various cardiac conditions.

Key Components of Cardiac Scintigraphy

- **Radiopharmaceuticals**:
  - Common agents include:
    - *Technetium-99m (Tc-99m) Sestamibi*: Used for myocardial perfusion imaging.
    - *Thallium-201*: Less frequently used but still applicable for assessing perfusion.
    - *Gallium-67*: Sometimes utilized for evaluating cardiac inflammation or infection.

- **Imaging Techniques**: Single Photon Emission Computed Tomography (SPECT): Provides 3D images of myocardial perfusion, capturing blood flow to the heart muscle during stress and rest.
- **Positron Emission Tomography (PET)**: Offers enhanced resolution and is used for assessing myocardial perfusion and viability.

Applications

- **Myocardial Perfusion Imaging**:
  - Stress testing (exercise or pharmacological) to evaluate blood flow during increased heart workload.
  - Resting studies to identify ischemic areas and infarcts.
- **Assessment of Cardiac Function**: Measures left ventricular ejection fraction (LVEF) and wall motion abnormalities.
- **Viability Assessment**: Helps determine if damaged myocardium can recover, influencing decisions about revascularization.
- **Detection of Cardiac Events**: Identifies complications from coronary artery disease, such as myocardial infarction.

Advantages and Limitations

- **Advantages**:
  - Noninvasive with functional insights.
  - High sensitivity for ischemic heart disease.
- **Limitations**:
  - Radiation exposure, albeit low.
  - Potential for false positives or negatives.

Vascular Imaging

Definition: Vascular imaging encompasses various techniques used to visualize the vascular system (arteries and veins) for diagnosing diseases like atherosclerosis, aneurysms, and vascular blockages.

Key Techniques in Vascular Imaging

- **Ultrasound**: **Doppler ultrasound**: Evaluates blood flow and detects abnormalities such as stenosis or occlusion. It's commonly used for carotid arteries, venous insufficiency, and peripheral artery disease.
- **Computed Tomography Angiography (CTA)**: Provides detailed 3D images of blood vessels using contrast material. It is effective in assessing conditions like aneurysms, arterial stenosis, and vascular malformations.
- **Magnetic Resonance Angiography (MRA)**: Uses magnetic resonance imaging to visualize blood vessels. It can assess vascular conditions without ionizing radiation and is particularly useful for renal and cerebral arteries.
- **Digital Subtraction Angiography (DSA)**: An invasive procedure that uses contrast and fluoroscopy to visualize blood vessels. It is the gold standard for diagnosing vascular diseases but involves a higher risk due to the invasive nature.

Applications of Vascular Imaging

- **Detection of Aneurysms**: Identifies dilations in blood vessels that could lead to rupture.
- **Assessment of Atherosclerosis**: Evaluates the presence and extent of plaque buildup in arteries, helping to guide treatment decisions.
- **Evaluation of Vascular Malformations**: Identifies congenital or acquired vascular anomalies.
- **Guidance for Interventions**: Assists in planning for surgical or endovascular interventions.

Advantages and Limitations

- **Advantages**:
  - Noninvasive and can provide real-time assessment (especially with ultrasound).
  - CTA and MRA offer detailed imaging without radiation exposure.

- **Limitations**:
  - Some techniques involve contrast agents that may have risks (e.g., nephrotoxicity).
  - Invasive procedures like DSA carry inherent risks.

Vascular Imaging

1. Discuss various types of aortic aneurysms and their radiological evaluation. [10] [MD (WBUHS) 20]

Aortic aneurysms are localized dilations of the aorta, classified primarily by their location and morphology.[43] The most common types are:

Types of Aortic Aneurysms

- **Abdominal Aortic Aneurysm (AAA)**:
  - *Location*: Typically occurs below the renal arteries, in the abdominal portion of the aorta.
  - *Morphology*: Most commonly fusiform (spindle-shaped) but can also be saccular (localized bulge).
- **Thoracic Aortic Aneurysm (TAA)**: *Location*: Found in the thoracic region of the aorta, often between the aortic arch and the diaphragm.
- **Types**:
  - *Ascendant aneurysm*: Involves the ascending aorta. Aortic Arch Aneurysm: Involves the arch of the aorta.
  - *Descending aneurysm*: Located in the descending thoracic aorta.
- **Thoracoabdominal Aortic Aneurysm**:
  - *Location*: Extends from the thoracic aorta into the abdominal aorta.
  - *Clinical Importance*: Often requires complex surgical management due to involvement of both thoracic and abdominal sections.
- **Peripheral Aneurysms**: **Location**: While not strictly aortic, aneurysms can occur in the branches of the aorta, such as the femoral or popliteal arteries.

Radiological Evaluation

Radiological imaging plays a crucial role in the diagnosis, assessment of size, and management of aortic aneurysms. Common modalities include:

- **Ultrasound**:
  - *Use*: First-line imaging for suspected AAA, especially in emergency settings.
  - *Findings*: Can visualize the aneurysm, assess size, and detect thrombus or rupture. It is non-invasive and does not involve radiation.
- **Computed Tomography (CT) Angiography**:
  - *Use*: Gold standard for evaluating the size, extent, and morphology of aortic aneurysms.
  - Findings: Provides detailed anatomical information about the aneurysm and surrounding structures.
  - Can identify complications like dissection or rupture. Offers 3D reconstructions for surgical planning.
  - Contrast Agent: Requires intravenous contrast, which can pose risks in patients with renal impairment.
- **Magnetic Resonance Angiography (MRA)**:
  - *Use*: Useful for patients who cannot receive iodinated contrast or for assessing aortic arch aneurysms.
  - *Findings*: Provides excellent soft tissue contrast and can visualize the aorta without radiation.
  - *Limitations*: Longer acquisition times and may be less available in emergency settings.
- **Chest X-ray**:
  - *Use*: Initial imaging in cases of thoracic aneurysms.
  - *Findings*: May show a widened mediastinum or abnormal aortic contour, but is not definitive.

- **Digital Subtraction Angiography (DSA)**:
  - *Use*: Primarily for therapeutic purposes rather than initial diagnosis.
  - *Findings*: Offers high-resolution images of blood vessels but is invasive.

2. Describe briefly the imaging of aortic aneurysm, rupture, and dissection. [10] [MD (WBUHS) 19, MD (WBUHS) 17]

Aortic conditions such as aneurysms, ruptures, and dissections require precise imaging for diagnosis, management, and surgical planning.[2] Here's a brief overview of the imaging modalities and their findings for each condition.

- **Aortic Aneurysm Imaging Modalities**:
  - Ultrasound:
    - *Use*: Often the first-line imaging for suspected abdominal aortic aneurysms (AAA).
    - *Findings*: Visualizes the aneurysm, measures its size, and assesses the presence of thrombus or complications.
  - Computed Tomography (CT) Angiography:
    - *Use*: Gold standard for diagnosing and evaluating aortic aneurysms.
    - *Findings*: Detailed visualization of the aneurysm, including size, morphology (fusiform or saccular), and involvement of branches.
    - 3D reconstructions aid in surgical planning.
  - Magnetic Resonance Angiography (MRA):
    - *Use*: Useful for patients who cannot receive contrast or for assessing the thoracic aorta.
    - *Findings*: Good soft tissue contrast and visualization of the aorta and surrounding structures.
- **Aortic Rupture Imaging Modalities**:
  - CT Angiography:
    - *Use*: Most effective in diagnosing aortic rupture.
    - *Findings*: Extravasation of contrast material indicates active bleeding. Hemoperitoneum or hematoma in the mediastinum may be noted.

  Visualization of the aneurysm and its relationship to surrounding structures is critical.
  - Ultrasound:
    - *Use*: Rapid assessment in emergency settings, especially for AAA.
    - *Findings*: May show free fluid (hemoperitoneum) or hematoma around the aorta.
  - X-ray: *Use*: Limited role; may show indirect signs such as a widened mediastinum but is not definitive.
- **Aortic Dissection Imaging Modalities**:
  - CT Angiography:
    - *Use*: Preferred method for diagnosing aortic dissection.
    - *Findings*: Double lumen appearance indicating true and false lumens. Intimal flap visualized separating the two lumens.

  Assessment of the extent of dissection and involvement of branches.
  - Magnetic Resonance Angiography (MRA):
    - *Use*: Noninvasive option, particularly in cases where radiation exposure should be minimized.
    - *Findings*: Similar to CT, showing intimal flap and double lumen; provides excellent soft tissue detail.
  - Transesophageal Echocardiography (TEE):
    - *Use*: Useful for bedside evaluation, particularly in unstable patients.
    - *Findings*: Can visualize the intimal flap and assess cardiac involvement; highly sensitive for diagnosing aortic dissection.

3. Imaging in Patent Ductus Arteriosus (PDA). [10] [MD (WBUHS) 19]

Patent ductus arteriosus (PDA) is a congenital heart defect characterized by the failure of the ductus arteriosus, a fetal blood vessel, to close after birth. This condition can lead to increased blood flow to the lungs and heart, resulting in heart failure and pulmonary hypertension if left untreated. Imaging plays a critical role in the diagnosis and management of PDA. Imaging Modalities for PDA:

- **Echocardiography**:
  - *Use*: The first-line imaging modality for diagnosing PDA, especially in infants and children.
  - *Findings*: Color Doppler: Demonstrates the left-to-right shunt across the PDA, visualizing the flow from the aorta to the pulmonary artery.

  M-mode and 2D Imaging: Can show the size of the ductus and assess its hemodynamic significance.

  Assessment of Associated Heart Defects: Echocardiography can evaluate for other congenital heart defects that may coexist with PDA.
- **Chest X-ray**:
  - *Use*: Often part of the initial evaluation.
  - *Findings*:
    - May show cardiomegaly due to volume overload.
    - Increased pulmonary vascular markings indicating elevated pulmonary blood flow.
    - Possible left atrial and ventricular enlargement.
- **Computed Tomography (CT) Angiography**:
  - *Use*: Helpful in cases where echocardiography is inconclusive or when surgical intervention is planned.
  - *Findings*:
    - Can provide detailed anatomical information about the PDA and surrounding structures.
    - Visualizes collateral circulation if present and assesses the size of the ductus.
- **Magnetic Resonance Imaging (MRI)**:
  - *Use*: Useful in certain cases, particularly for detailed anatomical assessment or in patients with contraindications to CT.
  - *Findings*:
    - Provides excellent soft tissue contrast and can visualize the ductus, as well as any associated structural abnormalities.
    - May be used to assess pulmonary vascularity and cardiac function.
- **Angiography**:
  - *Use*: Generally reserved for cases where interventional treatment is planned.
  - *Findings*: Direct visualization of the PDA and measurement of shunt size. Assessment of collateral circulation.

4. Enumerate the causes of superior vena cava obstruction (SVCO) and their imaging features. [10] [MD (WBUHS) 19]

Superior vena cava obstruction (SVCO) is a condition where blood flow through the superior vena cava (SVC) is impeded, leading to a range of clinical symptoms.[44]

Common Causes of SVCO

Malignancy

- **Lung Cancer**:
  - Imaging features: CT may show a mass in the right lung apex (Pancoast tumor) or mediastinal lymphadenopathy compressing the SVC.
- **Lymphoma**:
  - Imaging features: Enlarged lymph nodes in the mediastinum, often seen on CT or PET scans.
- **Metastatic Disease**:
  - Imaging features: Presence of metastatic lesions in the mediastinum or lung, causing compression.

- **Thrombosis:**
  - Primary thrombosis: Rare but can occur, particularly in patients with hypercoagulable states.
  - Secondary thrombosis: Often occurs in association with central venous catheters or pacemakers.
  - Imaging features: CT or ultrasound may show a thrombus within the SVC. Dilated collateral veins may also be observed.
- **Fibrosing Mediastinitis**
  - Imaging features: CT shows thickening of the mediastinal structures and possible mass effect on the SVC.
- **Aortic Aneurysm**:
  - Imaging features: CT may reveal an aneurysm compressing the SVC, often with associated dilation of the aorta.
- **Congenital Anomalies**:
  - Example: Congenital absence of the SVC or aberrant veins.
  - Imaging features: MRI or CT can demonstrate abnormal venous anatomy.
- **Trauma**:
  - Imaging features: CT may show direct injury to the SVC, hematoma, or associated thoracic injuries.
- **Infection**:
  - Example: Tuberculosis or other granulomatous infections can cause lymphadenopathy compressing the SVC.
  - Imaging features: CT may reveal lymph node enlargement and associated pulmonary findings.

Imaging Modalities

- **Computed Tomography (CT)**:
  - The primary imaging modality for assessing SVCO. It can provide detailed information about the cause and extent of obstruction.
  - CT venography can visualize the SVC and any associated thrombosis.
- **Magnetic Resonance Imaging (MRI)**: Useful for assessing soft tissue structures and identifying vascular involvement without radiation exposure.
- **Ultrasound**: Helpful in evaluating thrombosis, especially in cases of catheter-related SVCO.
- **Chest X-ray**: Can show indirect signs of SVCO, such as mediastinal widening or prominent collateral veins, but is not specific.

5. Classify aortic dissection. Enumerate the salient radiological findings to differentiate true lumen and false lumen. [4+6] [MD (WBUHS) 22]

Aortic dissection can be classified based on various criteria, including the location of the dissection and the involvement of the aortic arch. The most commonly used classification systems are:

- **Stanford Classification**:
  - *Type A*: Involves the ascending aorta, regardless of whether the descending aorta is involved. This type is more critical and often requires surgical intervention.
  - *Type B*: Involves only the descending aorta, typically starting after the left subclavian artery. It is usually managed medically unless complications arise.
- **DeBakey classification**:
  - *Type I*: Involves the ascending aorta, arch, and descending aorta.
  - *Type II*: Involves only the ascending aorta.
  - *Type III*: Involves the descending aorta, starting distal to the left subclavian artery. It can be further divided into IIIa (extending to the diaphragm) and IIIb (distal to the diaphragm).

  Radiological imaging is critical for diagnosing and characterizing aortic dissection. Key findings to differentiate between the true lumen and false lumen include:
- **Computed Tomography (CT) Angiography**:
  - *Double lumen appearance*: The most characteristic sign, showing two distinct lumens: the true lumen (usually smaller) and the false lumen (wider).

  - *Intimal flap*: A linear, hyperdense structure seen between the true and false lumens, indicating the separation of the aortic wall layers.
  - *Lumen size*: The true lumen typically appears smaller compared to the false lumen, which may have a larger diameter and may contain thrombus.
  - *Branch vessel involvement*: Evaluate whether branches of the aorta are perfused via the true lumen or false lumen. The false lumen may compress or obstruct branch vessels.
  - *Blood flow direction*: The flow in the true lumen typically shows antegrade flow towards the distal aorta, whereas the false lumen may exhibit variable flow patterns.
- **Magnetic Resonance Imaging (MRI)**:
  - *High-resolution images*: Similar findings as CT, with the ability to evaluate the aortic wall and detect complications such as rupture or hematoma.
  - *True versus false lumen*: MRI provides excellent soft tissue contrast, allowing differentiation between the two lumens based on their signal characteristics.
- **Transesophageal Echocardiography (TEE)**:
  - *Intimal flap visualization*: Can directly visualize the intimal flap and assess the relationship between the true and false lumen.
  - *Lumen size*: TEE can measure the diameters of both lumens, aiding in assessing the hemodynamic significance.

6. Imaging in Varicose Veins. [5] [DNB Dec 21]

Varicose veins are dilated, tortuous veins that occur in the legs due to valve incompetence, leading to venous insufficiency.

Proper imaging is essential for diagnosis, assessment of severity, and planning treatment. Here are the key imaging modalities used in evaluating varicose veins:

- **Ultrasound**:
  - *Type*: Duplex ultrasound (combination of B-mode and Doppler ultrasound).
  - *Use*: First-line imaging modality for evaluating varicose veins.
  - *Findings*:
    - *Anatomical Assessment*: Visualizes the superficial and deep venous systems, identifying incompetent valves and areas of reflux.
    - *Venous Flow*: Doppler imaging shows the direction and velocity of blood flow. Reflux (backward flow) during the Valsalva maneuver indicates valve incompetence.
    - *Thrombosis*: Detects any associated thrombus in the veins.
- **Magnetic Resonance Imaging (MRI)**:
  - *Use*: Less common for routine evaluation but useful in complex cases or when other soft-tissue pathologies are suspected.
  - *Findings*:
    - Provides detailed images of soft tissues, allowing assessment of venous anatomy and any related complications (e.g., deep vein thrombosis).
    - Can visualize the entire venous system without ionizing radiation.
- **Computed Tomography (CT) Venography**:
  - *Use*: Primarily used when ultrasound findings are inconclusive or in surgical planning.
  - *Findings*:
    - Detailed anatomical depiction of the venous system, including the superficial and deep veins.
    - Can show the extent of varicosities and any associated abnormalities.
- **Sclerotherapy and Endovenous Laser Therapy (EVLT)**:
  - *Use*: While not imaging techniques per se, ultrasound guidance is often used during these minimally invasive treatments.
  - *Findings*:
    - Real-time imaging allows precise targeting of varicose veins for injection or laser treatment.

7. Imaging in chronic pulmonary thromboembolism (PTE). [5] [DNB Dec 21]

Chronic pulmonary thromboembolism, often resulting from unresolved acute pulmonary embolism, leads to persistent obstruction of the pulmonary arteries. This condition can cause pulmonary hypertension and right heart strain.[45] Accurate imaging is essential for diagnosis and management. Here are the key imaging modalities used in evaluating chronic PTE:

- **Computed Tomography Pulmonary Angiography (CTPA)**
  - *Use*: The primary imaging modality for evaluating pulmonary embolism, including chronic changes.
  - *Findings*:
    - *Acute Emboli*: Filling defects in the pulmonary arteries.
    - *Chronic Changes*:
      - Vessel narrowing or occlusion, often with recanalization.
      - Mosaic perfusion pattern due to variable perfusion of lung segments.
      - Signs of pulmonary hypertension, such as dilated pulmonary arteries and right heart strain.
- **Magnetic Resonance Imaging (MRI)**
  - *Use*: Less common but valuable for patients with renal impairment or allergies to iodinated contrast.
  - *Findings*:
    - Can assess vascular anatomy and detect filling defects.
    - Provides information about right heart function and pulmonary artery pressures.
    - Useful in visualizing associated cardiac changes (e.g., right ventricular hypertrophy).
- **Ventilation-perfusion (V/Q) Scan**
  - *Use*: Particularly useful in cases of suspected chronic PTE when other imaging modalities are contraindicated.
  - *Findings*:
    - *Mismatched Defects*: Areas of decreased perfusion without corresponding ventilation abnormalities indicate chronic emboli.
    - Patterns of chronic embolization may reveal areas of lung that are persistently under-perfused.
- **Chest X-ray**
  - *Use*: Initial imaging may reveal indirect signs of chronic PTE.
  - *Findings*:
    - Often normal in chronic cases but may show: Enlarged right heart silhouette.
    - Signs of pulmonary hypertension (e.g., increased vascular markings).
    - Effusions or other complications.
- **Echocardiography**
  - *Use*: Provides functional assessment of the right heart and pulmonary artery pressures.
  - *Findings*:
    - Right ventricular enlargement or hypertrophy.
    - D-shaped left ventricle during diastole indicating pressure overload.
    - Possible thrombus visualization in the right heart.

8. Peripheral arterial disease—imaging with advantages and disadvantages. [10] [DNB June 21]

Peripheral arterial disease (PAD) is a common condition resulting from atherosclerosis, leading to reduced blood flow to the limbs. Various imaging modalities are employed to diagnose and assess PAD, each with its own advantages and disadvantages.

- **Ultrasound (Doppler Ultrasound)**
  - *Use*: Noninvasive assessment of blood flow and arterial anatomy.
  - Advantages:
    - No radiation exposure.
    - Real-time imaging and functional assessment of blood flow (Doppler).

    - Cost-effective and widely available.
    - Can detect stenosis and occlusions.
  - Disadvantages:
    - Operator-dependent; quality may vary.
    - Limited visualization of deeper vessels.
    - May not provide detailed anatomical information compared to other modalities.
- **Ankle-Brachial Index (ABI)**
  - *Use*: A simple, non-invasive test comparing blood pressure in the ankle with that in the arm.
  - Advantages:
    - Quick and easy to perform.
    - No specialized equipment required.
    - Provides a quantitative measure of arterial occlusion.
  - Disadvantages:
    - May be inaccurate in patients with calcified arteries (e.g., diabetes).
    - Cannot localize the specific site of obstruction.
- **Computed Tomography Angiography (CTA)**
  - *Use*: Detailed imaging of peripheral arteries, particularly for surgical planning.
  - Advantages:
    - High-resolution images and 3D reconstructions of the vascular anatomy.
    - Can assess the extent of arterial disease and collateral circulation.
    - Non-invasive compared to traditional angiography.
  - Disadvantages:
    - Requires iodinated contrast, which poses risks (e.g., nephrotoxicity).
    - Radiation exposure.
    - May miss small vessel disease.
- **Magnetic Resonance Angiography (MRA)**
  - Use: Imaging of peripheral arteries, especially useful for patients allergic to contrast agents.
  - Advantages:
    - No ionizing radiation.
    - Excellent soft tissue contrast and visualization of vascular structures.
    - Can assess the arterial tree and surrounding tissues.
  - Disadvantages:
    - Longer acquisition times; less available in emergency settings.
    - May require gadolinium-based contrast, which carries a risk for patients with renal impairment.
    - Expensive compared to other modalities.
- **Digital Subtraction Angiography (DSA)**
  - Use: Invasive imaging used for definitive diagnosis and treatment of PAD.
  - Advantages:
    - Gold standard for visualizing vascular anatomy and lesions.
    - Allows for simultaneous therapeutic interventions (e.g., angioplasty).
    - High-resolution images of blood vessels.
  - Disadvantages:
    - Invasive procedure with associated risks (e.g., bleeding, infection).
    - Requires contrast media, with risks similar to those in CTA.
    - Not suitable for all patients due to comorbidities.

9. Describe various types of aortic dissection. Discuss the role of imaging in evaluation of aortic dissection. [5+5] [DNB June 20, MD (WBUHS) 24]

Aortic dissection is a serious condition characterized by a tear in the aortic intima, allowing blood to flow between the layers of the aortic wall. It can be classified primarily by the location of the dissection and the involvement of the aortic arch.

- **Stanford Classification**
  - *Type A*: Involves the ascending aorta, regardless of whether the descending aorta is involved. This type is more critical and often requires surgical intervention.
  - *Type B*: Involves only the descending aorta, typically starting distal to the left subclavian artery. This type is usually managed medically unless complications arise.
- **DeBakey Classification**
  - *Type I*: Involves the ascending aorta, arch, and descending aorta.
  - *Type II*: Involves only the ascending aorta.
  - *Type III*: Involves the descending aorta, starting distal to the left subclavian artery. It can be further divided into:
    - *IIIa*: Extending to the diaphragm.
    - *IIIb*: Distal to the diaphragm.

Role of Imaging in Evaluation of Aortic Dissection

Imaging is crucial in diagnosing and managing aortic dissection.

- **Computed Tomography (CT) Angiography**
  - *Use*: Gold standard for diagnosing aortic dissection.
  - *Findings*:
    - Visualization of the intimal flap separating the true and false lumens.
    - Measurement of the size of the true and false lumens.
    - Assessment of branch vessel involvement.
    - Identification of complications such as pericardial effusion or aortic rupture.
  - *Advantages*: Rapid acquisition, high resolution, and the ability to visualize the entire aorta.
- **Magnetic Resonance Imaging (MRI)**
  - *Use*: Useful for detailed assessment, particularly in patients with renal impairment who cannot receive contrast.
  - *Findings*:
    - Similar to CT, showing the intimal flap and dual lumen appearance.
    - Provides excellent soft tissue contrast and can assess surrounding structures.
  - *Advantages*: No radiation exposure; useful for evaluating complex cases or chronic dissections.
- **Transesophageal Echocardiography (TEE)**
  - *Use*: Often used in unstable patients or during surgical procedures.
  - *Findings*:
    - Direct visualization of the aorta, including the intimal flap.
    - Assessment of hemodynamic status and right heart involvement.
  - Advantages: Provides real-time imaging and can be performed at the bedside.
- **Chest X-ray**
  - *Use*: Initial imaging that may show indirect signs of aortic dissection.
  - *Findings*:
    - Possible widening of the mediastinum or abnormal aortic contour.
    - Indirect signs of complications (e.g., pleural effusion).
  - *Advantages*: Quick and widely available but not diagnostic.

- **Digital Subtraction Angiography (DSA)**
  - *Use*: Primarily for therapeutic purposes or when non-invasive imaging is inconclusive.
  - *Findings*:
    - Direct visualization of the aorta and any associated vascular lesions.
  - *Advantages*: High-resolution images and ability to perform interventions, such as stenting or balloon angioplasty.

10. Discuss the imaging approach to acute limb ischemia. Discuss the interventional radiological treatment options for it. [5+5] [DNB June 20]

Acute limb ischemia (ALI) is a critical condition characterized by a sudden decrease in blood flow to the extremities, often requiring prompt diagnosis and intervention.[46] The imaging approach plays a crucial role in determining the extent of ischemia, identifying the underlying cause, and guiding treatment.

- **Initial Assessment**:
  - Clinical Evaluation:
    - Assessment of symptoms (pain, pallor, pulselessness, paresthesia, paralysis, and poikilothermia).
    - Risk factors (e.g., history of peripheral arterial disease, recent surgery, embolic events).
- **Imaging Modalities**:
- **Doppler Ultrasound**:
  - *Use*: First-line imaging modality for assessing blood flow in the affected limb.
  - *Findings*:
    - Detects the presence of arterial occlusion or significant stenosis. Provides information about collateral circulation and perfusion status.
  - Advantages: Noninvasive, widely available, and provides real-time assessment.
- **Computed Tomography Angiography (CTA)**:
  - *Use*: Gold standard for detailed anatomical evaluation of arterial occlusions.
  - *Findings*:
    - Visualizes the extent of arterial blockage and identifies the location of thrombus or embolus.
    - Can assess collateral circulation and any anatomical abnormalities.
  - Advantages: Quick, high-resolution images; allows for 3D reconstructions.
- **Magnetic Resonance Angiography (MRA)**:
  - *Use*: Alternative to CTA, especially in patients with renal impairment.
  - *Findings*:
    - Similar to CTA in identifying vascular occlusions and collateral pathways.
  - Advantages: No ionizing radiation; excellent soft tissue contrast.
- **Digital Subtraction Angiography (DSA)**:
  - *Use*: Considered the gold standard for intra-arterial imaging, often performed when intervention is planned.
  - *Findings*: Provides real-time imaging of blood flow and vascular anatomy. Can identify and characterize lesions during intervention.
  - *Advantages*: High-resolution images and the ability to treat identified lesions during the same procedure.

Interventional Radiological Treatment Options

Interventional radiology offers various treatment options for acute limb ischemia, particularly when the underlying cause is identified and can be addressed.

- **Catheter-directed Thrombolysis**:
  - *Procedure*: Administration of thrombolytic agents (e.g., tPA) directly into the thrombus via a catheter.
  - *Indications*: Suitable for patients with significant thrombus and limb salvage potential.
  - *Advantages*: Minimally invasive and can restore blood flow while preserving the limb.

- **Mechanical Thrombectomy**:
  - *Procedure*: Involves the use of devices (e.g., stent retrievers, aspiration devices) to remove thrombus from occluded arteries.
  - *Indications*: Effective in acute thrombotic occlusions and often performed in conjunction with thrombolysis.
  - *Advantages*: Rapid restoration of blood flow; can be used in conjunction with other treatments.
- **Angioplasty and Stenting**:
  - *Procedure*: Balloon angioplasty may be performed to open narrowed or blocked arteries, often followed by stenting to maintain patency.
  - *Indications*: Suitable for chronic stenoses and acute occlusions caused by atherosclerotic disease.
  - *Advantages*: Minimally invasive; can be performed during DSA.
- **Surgical Options**: While not interventional radiology, surgical options (e.g., bypass grafting, embolectomy) may be necessary if the interventional approaches are unsuccessful or not feasible.

11. (a) Enumerate causes of inferior rib notching. (b) Describe X-ray, CT and MRI findings in Coarctation of aorta. (c) Briefly discuss role of interventional radiology in its management. [2+(2+2+2)+2] [DNB Dec 20, MD (WBUHS) 17, AIIMS Dec 23]

a. Causes of Inferior Rib Notching

- **Coarctation of the Aorta**: The most common cause, where collateral circulation erodes the ribs.
- **Aortic Arch Anomalies**: Conditions such as a double aortic arch or a right aortic arch may cause similar notching.
- **Thoracic Outlet Syndrome**: Compression of the neurovascular structures can lead to rib notching due to chronic irritation.
- **Hematologic Disorders**: Conditions such as sickle cell disease, leading to bone changes.
- **Bone Diseases**: Osteogenesis imperfecta or other skeletal dysplasias can contribute to abnormal rib morphology.
- **Tumors**: Localized growths or metastatic disease affecting the ribs.

b. X-ray, CT, and MRI Findings in Coarctation of the Aorta

- **X-ray Findings**:
  - Indirect Signs:
    - *Rib Notching*: Typically seen on the inferior borders of the ribs (most commonly the 3rd to 8th ribs) due to erosion from collateral circulation.
    - *Cardiac Silhouette*: Possible left ventricular hypertrophy (LVH) and changes in the cardiac silhouette.
    - *Widened Mediastinum*: Indicating possible aortic dilation proximal to the coarctation.
- **CT Findings**:
  - Direct Visualization:
    - *Site of Coarctation*: Narrowing of the aorta, typically located just distal to the left subclavian artery.
    - *Collateral Circulation*: Prominent collateral vessels (e.g., intercostal arteries) compensating for the obstruction.
    - *Associated Anomalies*: May reveal additional aortic arch anomalies or vascular malformations.
- **MRI Findings**:
  - Comprehensive Assessment:
    - *Aortic Narrowing*: Clear visualization of the aorta and assessment of the coarctation.
    - *Flow Dynamics*: Evaluation of blood flow before and after the coarctation site.
    - *Heart Structure*: Assessment of cardiac anatomy, function, and any associated abnormalities (e.g., LVH).

c. Role of Interventional Radiology in Management of Coarctation of the Aorta

Interventional radiology plays a significant role in the management of aortic coarctation, particularly in patients who may not be ideal candidates for open surgical repair or in cases of recurrent coarctation.

- **Balloon Angioplasty**:
  - *Procedure*: A balloon catheter is inserted and inflated at the site of coarctation to widen the narrowed segment.
  - *Indications*: Effective in both pediatric and adult patients, especially for those with discrete coarctation.
  - *Advantages*: Minimally invasive with shorter recovery times compared to surgical options.
- **Stenting**:
  - *Procedure*: Following balloon angioplasty, a stent may be deployed to maintain the widened aortic lumen.
  - *Indications*: Often used in cases of recurrent coarctation or in conjunction with angioplasty to provide additional support.
  - *Advantages*: Helps to prevent re-narrowing and can improve long-term outcomes.
- **Management of Complications**:
  - Interventional radiology can also address complications arising from coarctation, such as aneurysm formation or residual stenosis, using minimally invasive techniques.

12. (a) Arterial and Venous Anatomy of the Lower Limb with help of diagram. (b) Imaging features of deep venous thrombosis. [5+5] [DNB Dec 20]

- **Femoral Artery**:
  - Continuation of the external iliac artery, passing through the femoral triangle.
  - Gives off several branches, including the profunda femoris (deep femoral artery).
- **Popliteal Artery**:
  - Continuation of the femoral artery as it passes behind the knee.
  - Branches into the anterior and posterior tibial arteries.
- **Anterior Tibial Artery**:
  - Supplies the anterior compartment of the leg.
  - Continues down to become the dorsalis pedis artery.
- **Posterior Tibial Artery**:
  - Supplies the posterior compartment of the leg.
  - Branches into the medial and lateral plantar arteries at the foot.
- **Peroneal (Fibular) Artery**:
  - Branches off the posterior tibial artery.
  - Supplies the lateral compartment of the leg.

Venous Anatomy (Fig. 61)

- **Superficial Venous System**:
  - *Great saphenous vein*: Begins at the dorsum of the foot, ascends along the medial side of the leg and thigh, draining into the femoral vein.
  - Small saphenous vein: Begins at the lateral side of the foot, ascends along the posterior aspect of the leg, draining into the popliteal vein.
- **Deep venous system**:
  - Femoral vein: Continuation of the popliteal vein as it passes through the adductor canal.
  - Popliteal vein: Formed by the union of the anterior and posterior tibial veins behind the knee.
  - *Tibial veins*: Accompany the respective arteries and drain the muscles of the leg.

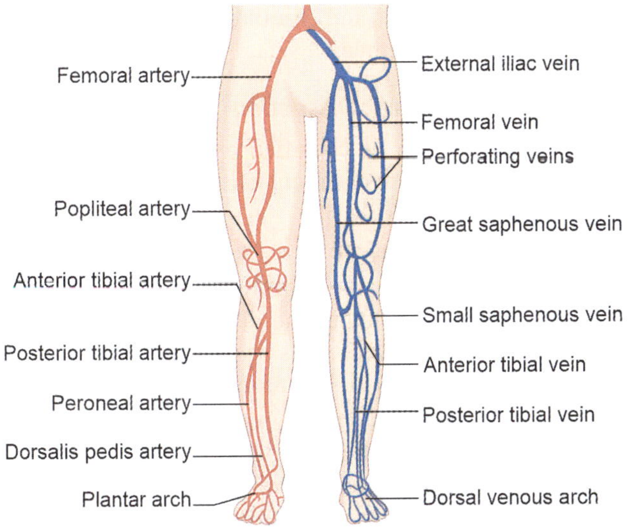

FIG. 61: Arterial and venous anatomy of lower limb arterial anatomy.

Imaging Features of Deep Venous Thrombosis (DVT)

- **Ultrasound:**[47]
  - Compression Ultrasonography: Lack of compressibility of the vein indicates the presence of a thrombus.
  - Doppler Ultrasound: Reduced or absent venous flow in the affected segment.
  - Appearance: Thrombus may appear as an echogenic mass within the vein.
- **CT Venography:**
  - *Use*: High-resolution imaging to evaluate DVT, particularly in complex cases or for planning treatment.
  - *Findings*:
    - Filling defects within the venous lumen indicating thrombus.
    - Visualization of collateral circulation in chronic cases.
- **Magnetic Resonance Imaging (MRI)**:
  - *Use*: Helpful for evaluating DVT in patients with contraindications to CT or ultrasound.
  - *Findings*:
    - Thrombus appears as an area of low signal intensity on T2-weighted images.
    - May show associated muscle edema or signs of post-thrombotic syndrome.
- **Plain Radiography**:
  - *Use*: Limited utility but may show indirect signs such as:
    - Enlargement of the affected limb (swelling).
    - Signs of venous distension.

13. Define Acute Aortic Syndrome. Classify aortic dissection. Describe its imaging features on CT angiography and its management. [1+2+(4+3)] [DNB Dec 20, MD (WBUHS) 24]

Definition: Acute aortic syndrome (AAS) is a term that encompasses a group of life- threatening conditions involving the aorta. It includes:

- Aortic dissection
- Aortic rupture
- Aortic intramural hematoma
- Penetrating aortic ulcer

These conditions can present with similar clinical symptoms, such as sudden severe chest or back pain, and require urgent diagnosis and management.

Classification of Aortic Dissection

Aortic dissection can be classified based on its location and the involvement of different segments of the aorta **(Fig. 62)**:

- **Stanford Classification**:
  - *Type A*: Involves the ascending aorta, regardless of whether the descending aorta is involved. This type often requires surgical intervention.
  - *Type B*: Involves only the descending aorta, typically starting distal to the left subclavian artery. Management is often medical, but intervention may be needed if complications arise.

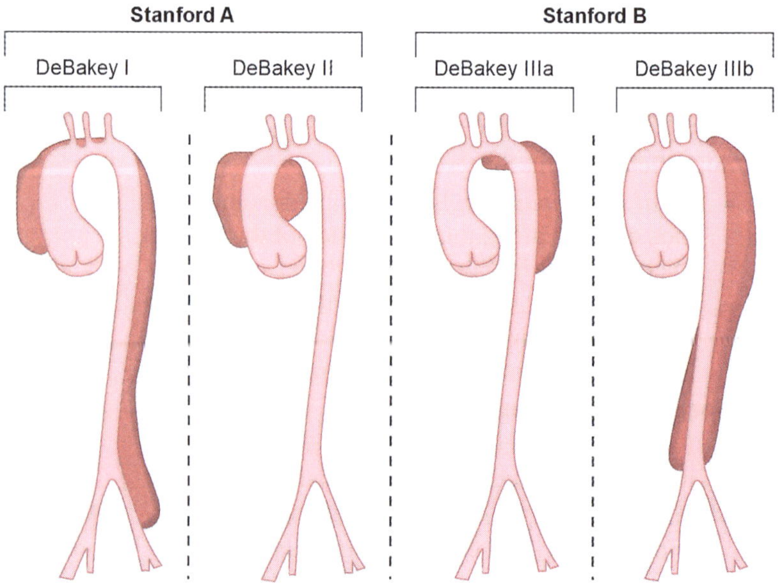

FIG. 62: Classification of aortic dissection.

- **DeBakey Classification**:
  - *Type I*: Involves the ascending aorta, aortic arch, and descending aorta.
  - *Type II*: Involves only the ascending aorta.
  - *Type III*: Involves the descending aorta, starting distal to the left subclavian artery.
    - *IIIa*: Extends to the diaphragm.
    - *IIIb*: Distal to the diaphragm.

Imaging Features on CT Angiography

CT Angiography (CTA) is the gold standard for diagnosing aortic dissection. Key Imaging Features:

- **Intimal Flap**:
  - A prominent feature that separates the true lumen from the false lumen.
  - Visible as a linear structure within the aorta.
- **Dual Lumens**: The presence of two distinct channels within the aorta: the true lumen and the false lumen.
- **Aortic Diameter**: Enlargement of the aorta may be noted, particularly in Type A dissections.
- **Branch Vessel Involvement**: Assessment of any involvement of major branches (e.g., carotid, subclavian) to determine the extent of the dissection.
- **Associated Findings**:
  - Hemopericardium (fluid around the heart) may be seen in cases of aortic rupture.
  - Evidence of ischemia in supplied organs (e.g., renal, mesenteric) if there is compromised blood flow.

Management of Aortic Dissection

Management depends on the type of dissection:

- **Type A Aortic Dissection**:
  - Surgical Intervention:
    - Requires immediate surgical repair, often involving replacement or grafting of the affected aortic segment.
    - Options may include open surgery or endovascular repair, depending on the situation.
- **Type B Aortic Dissection**:
  - Medical Management:
    - Initial management typically includes blood pressure control (using beta-blockers) to reduce the shearing forces on the aorta.
    - Pain management is also critical.
  - Surgical or Endovascular Intervention: Indicated if there are complications such as aneurysm formation, rupture, or significant ischemia.

REFERENCES

1. Whitley AS, Jefferson G, Holmes K, Sloane C, Anderson C, Hoadley G. Clark's Positioning in Radiography, 13th edition. London: CRC Press; 2015.
2. Webb WR, Higgins CB. Thoracic imaging: Pulmonary and Cardiovascular Radiology. Philadelphia: Lippincott Williams and Wilkins; 2011
3. Khandelwal N, Gupta AK, Chowdhury V (Eds). AIIMS-MAMC-PGI's Comprehensive Textbook of Diagnostic Radiology. New Delhi; Jaypee Brothers Medical Publishers (P) Ltd; 2016.
4. Sutton D, Aggarwal B. A Textbook of Radiology and Imaging. Gurgaon, Haryana: Elsevier India; 2023.
5. Adam A, Dixon AK, Gillard JH, Schaefer-Prokop C. Grainger and Allison's diagnostic radiology. Philadelphia: Elsevier Health Sciences; 2020.
6. Godoy MC, Leitman BS, De Groot PM, Vlahos I, Naidich DP. Chest radiography in the ICU: Part 1, Evaluation of airway, enteric, and pleural tubes. AJR Am J Roentgenol. 2012;198(3):563-71.

7. Godoy MC, Leitman BS, De Groot PM, Vlahos I, Naidich DP. Chest radiography in the ICU: Part 2, Evaluation of cardiovascular lines and other devices. AJR Am J J Roentgenol. 2012;198(3):572-81.
8. Silverstone L. (2024). Aspergilloma. [online] Available from https://radiopaedia.org/articles/aspergilloma?lang=gb [Last accessed December, 2024].
9. Yang W, Sirajuddin A, Zhang X, Liu G, Teng Z, Zhao S, et al. The role of imaging in 2019 novel coronavirus pneumonia (COVID-19). Eur Radiol. 2020;30(9):4874-82.
10. Verschakelen JA, De Wever W. Computed Tomography of the Lung: A Pattern Approach. Heidelberg, Berlin: Springer; 2018.
11. Singh S, Jankharia B. Clinico radiological series: Imaging of interstitial lung disease. Lung India. 2017;34(4):403.
12. Hobbs S, Chung JH, Leb J, Kaproth-Joslin K, Lynch DA. Practical imaging interpretation in patients suspected of having idiopathic pulmonary fibrosis: Official recommendations from the Radiology Working Group of the Pulmonary Fibrosis Foundation. Radiol Cardiothoracic Imaging. 2021;3(1):e200279.
13. Revzin MV, Raza S, Warshawsky R, D'agostino C, Srivastava NC, Bader AS, et al. Multisystem Imaging Manifestations of COVID-19, Part 1: Viral Pathogenesis and Pulmonary and Vascular System Complications. Radiographics. 2020;40(6):1574-99.
14. Kanne JP, Bai H, Bernheim A, Chung M, Haramati LB, Kallmes DF, et al. COVID-19 imaging: What we know now and what remains unknown. Radiology. 2021;299(3):E262-79.
15. Durhan G, Tan AA, Düzgün SA, Akkaya S, Arıyürek OM. Radiological manifestations of thoracic hydatid cysts: pulmonary and extrapulmonary findings. Insights Imaging. 2020;11(1):116.
16. Grover SB, Grover H, Antil N, Patra S, Sen MK, Nair D. Imaging approach to pulmonary infections in the immunocompromised patient. Indian J Radiol Imaging. 2022;32(01):81-112.
17. Jeong YJ, Yi CA, Lee KS. Solitary pulmonary nodules: Detection, characterization, and guidance for further diagnostic workup and treatment. AJR Am J Roentgenol. 2007;188(1):57-68.
18. Carter BW, Benveniste MF, Madan R, Godoy MC, De Groot PM, Truong MT, et al. ITMIG classification of mediastinal compartments and multidisciplinary approach to mediastinal masses. Radiographics. 2017;37(2):413-36.
19. Raoof S, Amchentsev A, Vlahos I, Goud A, Naidich DP. Pictorial essay: Multinodular disease: A high-resolution CT scan diagnostic algorithm. Chest. 2006;129(3):805-15.
20. Boitsios G, Bankier AA, Eisenberg RL. Diffuse pulmonary nodules. AJR Am J Roentgenol. 2010;194(5):W354-66.
21. Lee KC, Kang EY, Yong HS, Kim C, Lee KY, Hwang SH, et al. A stepwise diagnostic approach to cystic lung diseases for radiologists. Korean J Radiol. 2019;20(9):1368-80.
22. Biko DM, Lichtenberger III JP, Rapp JB, Khwaja A, Huppmann AR, Chung EM. Mediastinal masses in children: Radiologic-pathologic correlation. Radiographics. 2021;41(4):1186-207.
23. Ranganath SH, Lee EY, Restrepo R, Eisenberg RL. Mediastinal masses in children. AJR Am J Roentgenol. 2012;198(3):W197-216.
24. Rafiee H (Ed). Chapman and Nakielny's Aids to Radiological Differential Diagnosis. Amsterdam: Elsevier; 2019.
25. Wittram C, Kalra MK, Maher MM, Greenfield A, McLoud TC, Shepard JA. Acute and chronic pulmonary emboli: Angiography–CT correlation. AJR Am J Roentgenol. 2006;186 (6_Suppl_2):S421-9.
26. Moore AJE, Wachsmann J, Chamarthy MR, Panjikaran L, Tanabe Y, Rajiah P. Imaging of Acute Pulmonary Embolism: An update. Cardiovasc Diagn Ther. 2018;8(3):225-43.
27. Panda A, Kumar A, Gamanagatti S, Patil A, Kumar S, Gupta A. Traumatic diaphragmatic injury: A review of CT signs and the difference between blunt and penetrating injury. Diagn Interv Radiol. 2014;20(2):121-8.
28. Khan AN, Al-Jahdali HH, Allen CM, Irion KL, Al Ghanem S, Koteyar SS. The calcified lung nodule: What does it mean? Ann Thorac Med. 2010;5(2):67-79.
29. Naggar A, Laasri K, Berrada K, Kabila B, El Aoufir O, Laamrani FZ, et al. Differential diagnoses of cavitary lung lesions on computed tomography: A pictorial essay. Egypt J Radiol Nucl Med. 2023;54(1):149.
30. Fruchter O, Schneer S, Rusanov V, Belenky A, Kramer MR. Bronchial artery embolization for massive hemoptysis: long-term follow-up. Asian Cardiovasc Thorac Ann. 2015;23(1):55-60.
31. Almeida J, Leal C, Figueiredo L. Evaluation of the bronchial arteries: Normal findings, hypertrophy and embolization in patients with hemoptysis. Insights Imaging. 2020;11:1-5.
32. Marquis KM, Raptis CA, Rajput MZ, Steinbrecher KL, Henry TS, Rossi SE, et al. CT for Evaluation of Hemoptysis. Radiographics. 2021;41(3):742-61.
33. Lee SI, Miller JC, Abbara S, Achenbach S, Jang IK, Thrall JH. Coronary CT angiography. J Am Coll Radiol. 2006;3(7):560-4.
34. Allen HD, Driscoll DJ, Shaddy RE, Feltes TF. Moss and Adams' heart disease in infants, children, and adolescents: Including the fetus and young adult. Philadelphia: Lippincott Williams and Wilkins; 2013.
35. Danias PG. Cardiovascular MRI: 150 Multiple-Choice Questions and Answers. Totowa; NJ: Humana Press; 2008.
36. Bonow RO, Otto CM, Bonow RO. Valvular Heart Disease. A Companion to Braunwald's Heart Disease. Amsterdam: Elsevier; 2020.
37. Budoff MJ, Shinbane JS (Eds). Cardiac CT imaging: Diagnosis of Cardiovascular Disease. Berlin, Germany: Springer; 2010.

38. Ho S, Reddy GP. Cardiovascular imaging. Korean J Radiol. 2011;1229(6929):2005-8330.
39. Zoneraich S. Heart Disease: A Textbook of Cardiovascular Medicine. JAMA. 1997;277(15):1247.
40. Mettler FA, Guiberteau MJ. Essentials of Nuclear Medicine and Molecular Imaging. Philadelphia: Elsevier Health Sciences; 2018.
41. Matsuo S (Ed). Clinical Nuclear Cardiology: Practical Applications and Future Directions. Sharjah, United Arab Emirates: Bentham Science Publishers; 2018.
42. Hutchison SJ. Aortic Diseases: Clinical Diagnostic Imaging Atlas. Philadelphia: Elsevier Health Sciences; 2008.
43. Zygmunt Jr JA (Ed). Venous Ultrasound. Boca Raton: CRC Press; 2020.
44. Rosado-de-Christenson ML, Martínez-Jiménez S. Diagnostic Imaging: Chest: Amsterdam: Elsevier Health Sciences; 2022 Feb 15.
45. Kaufman JA, Lee MJ. Vascular and Interventional Radiology: The Requisites. Philadelphia: Elsevier Saunders; 2013.
46. Pellerito JS, Polak JF. Introduction to Vascular Ultrasonography. Philadelphia: Elsevier Saunders; 2019.

CHAPTER

4 Gastrointestinal and Hepatobiliary Imaging

Sayeka Khatun, Priyanka Rathore

QUESTIONS

Imaging Techniques

1. Write a short note on CT enteroclysis. [5] [MD (WBUHS) 23]
2. Discuss the current status of conventional techniques and advances in GI imaging. [10] [MD (WBUHS) 22]
3. Write a short note on: CT enteroclysis and MR enteroclysis. [5] [MD (WBUHS) 22]
4. Discuss techniques, indications, and applications of MR enteroclysis. [10] [MD (WBUHS) 24, MD (WBUHS) 22]
5. MR enteroclysis. [5] [MD (WBUHS) 24, DNB Dec 21]
6. MRCP. [5] [DNB Dec 21]
7. MRI hepatobiliary contrast agent and its use in differentiating liver lesions. [10] [DNB June 21]

The Acute Abdomen

1. Discuss the radiological features of (a) Midgut volvulus and (b) Intussusception. [5+5] [MD (WBUHS) 21]
2. What is intestinal malrotation? Enumerate various types of intestinal malrotation. Describe the radiological findings in a case of midgut volvulus. [2+3+5]
3. (a) Role of plain radiograph in a case of acute abdomen. (b) Role of MRI in acute pancreatitis. [5+5] [DNB June 20]

Infections, Inflammation and Neoplasms

1. Briefly describe the etiopathology and imaging findings of ileocecal tuberculosis. Discuss the features that are useful to differentiate it from Crohn's disease. [3+2+5] [MD (WBUHS) 23, AIIMS May 23]
2. Discuss the common causes of pain in the right iliac fossa and radiological evaluation. [4+6] [MD (WBUHS) 23, MD (WBUHS) 18]
3. Write a short note on: Radiological features of Crohn's disease. [5] [MD (WBUHS) 19]
4. Discuss the role of various imaging modalities in the evaluation of intestinal tuberculosis. [10] [MD (WBUHS) 22]
5. Enumerate the causes of lower gastrointestinal bleeding. Describe briefly the role of imaging and intervention in a case of lower gastrointestinal bleeding. [3+(4+3)]
6. Role of virtual colonoscopy. Technique and contraindications. Imaging findings of colonic polyps on virtual colonoscopy. [10] [DNB Dec 21]
7. Role of CT in initial imaging and follow-up of GIST. [5] [MD (WBUHS) 24, DNB Dec 21, AIIMS Dec 24]

8. (a) Imaging features of intestinal TB on barium meal follow-through and CT (b) difference between intestinal TB and Crohn's disease. [10] [DNB June 21]

Liver and Biliary Tract

1. Write in brief about the technique of triple-phase CT scan for focal hepatic lesions. Describe triple-phase CT scan findings in hepatocellular carcinoma (HCC). [5+5] [MD (WBUHS) 18, AIIMS May 24]
2. List the indications of hepatobiliary scintigraphy in children and adults. Describe briefly the principle, technique, and findings on scintigraphy in a case of neonatal jaundice. [2+2+2+4] [MD (WBUHS) 23]
3. Discuss different imaging modalities in the evaluation of focal hepatic lesions. [10] [MD (WBUHS) 20, AIIMS May 23]
4. Noninvasive evaluation of primary liver tumor. [10] [MD (WBUHS) 20]
5. Role of interventional radiology in hepatic malignancy. [10] [MD (WBUHS) 21]
6. Discuss the imaging protocol for focal liver lesions. What are the differentiating features of hepatic hemangioma, focal hepatocellular carcinoma, and solitary metastatic lesion? [3+7] [MD (WBUHS) 22]
7. Enumerate various interventions in the biliary tract. Briefly discuss the indications, contraindications, procedure and complications of Percutaneous Transhepatic Biliary Drainage (PTBD). [2+8]
8. Role of imaging in chronic liver disease. [10] [DNB June 22]
9. Hyperenhancing tumors of liver and imaging. [10] [DNB June 22]
10. Caroli's disease. [5] [DNB Dec 21]
11. (a) LIRAD, its main features, and categories (b) use of LIRAD in liver lesion management. [10] [DNB June 21]
12. Role of ultrasound, MRI, and scintigraphy in assessment of biliary atresia. [3+4+3] [MD (WBUHS) 17]
13. Describe briefly segmental anatomy of liver with a line diagram. Describe imaging (CT and MRI) features in hepatocellular carcinoma. [4+(3+3)] [DNB June 20, AIIMS May 23]

Pancreas

1. Discuss in brief the pancreatic masses and its imaging features in brief. [5+5] [MD (WBUHS) 23]
2. Briefly state the anatomical variations of pancreaticobiliary tree with suitable diagrams. [10] [MD (WBUHS) 19]
3. Describe the embryology and development of the pancreas. Describe the imaging features of any one important congenital anomaly of the pancreas. [7+3] [MD (WBUHS) 24, MD (WBUHS) 22]
4. Cystic pancreatic tumors and imaging. [10] [DNB June 22]
5. X-ray findings in acute pancreatitis. [5] [DNB Dec 21, MD (WBUHS) 18]
6. (a) CT imaging in pancreatitis. (b) What is groove pancreatitis? (c) Radiological difference between focal mass forming pancreatitis and pancreatic adenocarcinoma. [10] [DNB June 21]
7. Define pancreatic divisum. Briefly discuss the embryological basis with the help of a diagram. Describe imaging findings on MDCT, MRCP, and ERCP. [2+2+(2+2+2)]
8. Discuss the classification and imaging features of cystic neoplasms of pancreas. [3+7] [DNB June 20, AIIMS May 24]

Vascular Diseases

1. Imaging in mesenteric ischemia. [10] [DNB June 22]
2. (a) Radiographic, ultrasound and MDCT findings in acute mesenteric ischemia. (b) Role of intervention in this condition. [(2+2+2) +4]
3. Discuss the causes and radiological features of Budd-Chiari Syndrome. Discuss the role of interventional radiology in treatment of Budd-Chiari Syndrome. [7+3] [DNB June 20, MD (WBUHS) 24]
4. What are the various causes of acute mesenteric ischemia? Discuss the role of radiology in its diagnosis and management. [3+(5+2)] [DNB June 20]

Miscellaneous

1. Enumerate the common causes of Epigastric disorder in a young adult mentioning the various imaging procedures to come to a diagnosis. [10] [MD (WBUHS) 19]
2. What are the causes of abdominal mass in children below the age of 5 years? Discuss in brief the imaging modalities to investigate the case. [3+7] [MD (WBUHS) 22]
3. Imaging of necrotizing enterocolitis. [10] [DNB June 22]
4. Causes of dysphagia. Role of barium swallow. [5] [DNB Dec 21]
5. Abdominal trauma-imaging approach. Splenic injury imaging. [10] [DNB June 21]
6. Draw a schematic diagram of anorectal junction on coronal plane, depicting internal and external sphincters. Describe the types of anorectal fistula with the help of a diagram and briefly discuss MR imaging protocol in their evaluation. [3+(3+4)]
7. Name various motility disorders of esophagus. Discuss pathophysiology and imaging findings of cardia achalasia. [3+(2+5)]
8. Enumerate various internal hernias. Discuss in detail imaging features of any two internal hernias. [2+8] [DNB June 20, AIIMS Dec 24]
9. Enumerate types of perianal Fistula with their imaging findings. [10] [MD (WBUHS) 19]

Interventions

1. Write a short note on transjugular liver biopsy. [5] [MD (WBUHS) 23]
2. Write a short note on PAIR therapy. [5] [MD (WBUHS) 23]
3. Write a short note on ablative interventional techniques in focal liver lesions. [5] [MD (WBUHS) 23]
4. Role of interventional radiology in obstructive jaundice. [10] [MD (WBUHS) 20, RG 18, AIIMS Dec 24]
5. Write a short note on: Transjugular intrahepatic portosystemic shunt (TIPS). [5] [MD (WBUHS) 24, MD (WBUHS) 22]
6. Techniques and role of interventional management in malignant liver tumors. [10] [DNB Dec 21]

ANSWERS

Imaging Techniques

1. Write a short note on CT enteroclysis. [5] [MD (WBUHS) 23]

Definition

Computed tomographic (CT) enteroclysis is a hybrid technique that combines fluoroscopic small bowel examination with CT abdomen. In this method, luminal contrast is introduced with the help of a nasojejunal tube placed fluoroscopically prior to CT examination.

Indication

a. In inflammatory bowel disease (IBD) to look for bowel wall and mucosal enhancement and extraluminal abnormalities, such as mesenteric adenitis and abscess.
b. As a complementary investigation with capsule endoscopy.
c. Unexplained Gastrointestinal (GI) bleeding or anemia.
d. Staging of known Crohn's disease.
e. Unexplained pain abdomen with no evidence of significant small bowel distension on plain X-ray.
f. Low-grade small bowel obstruction.
g. Diagnosis of small bowel neoplasm.

Technical Requirements

1. Sixteen slices or more CT scanner.
2. WW- 360HU, WL- 40HU.

Patient Preparation

- Low residue diet with ample fluids.
- NPO for 8 hours.
- Laxative a day prior to the examination.

Premedication

a. **Metoclopramide (10 mg)**:
    - Given orally 60 min before the CT examination.
    - Help in gastric emptying.
b. **Glucagon (1 mg) or Buscopan (20 mg)**:
    - Given intravenously prior to scanning.
    - It decreases bowel peristalsis.

There are two methods:

1. With positive contrast use 4–15% water soluble contrast or dilute 6% barium.
2. With neutral contrast using .5% methylcellulose, water, low density barium (most commonly used).

Sinus tract and fistula study are done with the help of positive contrast and mural enhancement pattern abnormality is done with the help of neutral contrast.

Technique

1. CT enteroclysis with neutral luminal contrast and intravenous contrast material:
   - *Fluoroscopic phase*:
     - 13F enteroclysis catheter is used. The balloon is positioned to the left of the spine in the descending part of the duodenum.
     - 0.3 mg of Glucagon is injected intravenously.
     - 1.5 L of water is introduced at a rate of 130–150 mL/min and transferred patient to the CT.
   - *CT Phase:*
     - 0.3 mg of glucagon is injected intravenously.
     - 1.5 L of water/oral contrast is infused at 100–150 mL/min.
     - 150 mL of intravenous contrast is injected. CT images are obtained at a delay of 50 seconds, i.e., in the late arterial/early postal venous phase.
2. CT enteroclysis with positive luminal contrast and no IV contrast:
   - *Fluoroscopic Phase*:
     - 13F catheter is used. The balloon of the catheter is placed in the descending part of the duodenum.
     - 2 L 12% water soluble contrast material/6% barium contrast is infused at the rate of 50–150 mL/min.
     - Fluoroscopy and radiography till contrast material reaches the cecum.
   - *CT Phase*:
     - 500–1,000 mL of water-soluble contrast is infused at rate of 60–160 mL/min before and during the CT examination.

Advantage

1. It gives information about luminal and extraluminal abnormality.
2. Neutral contrast agent gives information about mural enhancement pattern-target, homogenous, heterogenous, diminished, length of involvement, degree of thickening, location, and associated abnormalities.
3. Positive contrast agent gives information about the sinus tract and fistula and about the site of bowel obstruction.

Comparison with Other Methods

1. **CT Enterography**:
   - Intravenous contrast material enhanced abdominopelvic CT following ingestion of large volume (1.5–2 L) of neutral/positive contrast agent is called CT enterography.
   - It is an alternative for CT enteroclysis when expertise in enteroclysis catheter placement is not available.
   - The disadvantage of this technique is that there is inadequate bowel loop distension.
2. **MR Enteroclysis**: It has no radiation exposure and safe contrast agents however it is not accurate as compared to CT enteroclysis.
3. **Capsule Endoscopy**: Capsule endoscopy is superior to CT enteroclysis for mucosal evaluation but the disadvantage of this technique includes retention of the capsule and poor localization of the mucosal lesion.

2. Discuss the current status of conventional techniques and advances in GI imaging. [10] [MD (WBUHS) 22]

A plain radiograph of the abdomen has been limited to bedside evaluation and for initial evaluation of bowel distension and free intra-abdominal air.[1]

CT is done as an initial technique replacing X-ray for evaluation of acute abdomen, such as acute appendicitis, peritonitis, bowel obstruction, and blunt trauma.

For evaluation of the esophagus, barium study has a role limited to motility disorders and is largely replaced by endoscopy which is the first line of investigation.

For stomach, and duodenum barium meal study is superior to endoscopy in functional abnormalities like reflux, delayed emptying, and infiltrative process.

For other conditions like dyspepsia and abdominal pain it is only complimentary to endoscopy.

For evaluation of small bowel CT enteroclysis/enterography is a technique of choice rather than barium small bowel follow-through examination.

Evaluation of colorectal diseases has been taken over by colonoscopy as the initial technique. In the evaluation of colonic pathology also CT examination has superseded the barium enema.

Advances in GI Imaging

Following are newer techniques in the evaluation of GI tract:

a. Ultrasonography
b. CT enteroclysis
c. CT enterography
d. MR enteroclysis
e. PET CT enteroclysis and PET CT colonography
f. Nuclear scintigraphy
g. Capsule endoscopy

a. **Ultrasonography**:
   - USG is considered of limited value for the evaluation of the gastrointestinal tract due to inherent bowel gases. However high-frequency transducers can be used for the evaluation of bowel wall and appendicitis especially in lean patients and children.
   - Using endoscopic US can help in the evaluation of the upper GI tract. Also, by incorporating a biopsy instrument we can obtain a biopsy sample from the bowel wall.
   - Endosonography can also help in staging the bowel wall tumor. Similarly, transrectal USG can help in staging colorectal carcinoma.
   - Anal endosonography can help in the evaluation of traumatic defects in anal sphincter in patients with fecal incontinence.
   - The use of color Doppler and power Doppler imaging can help in the differentiation of active (increased blood flow) bowel thickening and chronic (no increased blood flow) bowel wall thickening.

b. **CT enteroclysis**: This is a hybrid technique that combines small bowel fluoroscopy with CECT abdomen. There are two methods: (1) With positive oral contrast and no IV contrast. (2) With neutral oral contrast and IV contrast. Positive oral contrast is used for the evaluation of low-grade bowel obstruction and fistula and sinuses. And neutral contrast is used for the evaluation of inflammatory bowel diseases, obscured GI bleeding, and neoplasms. Patient preparation is done with laxative a day prior to examination and nil per oral for 8 hours.

   There are two phases:

   1. Fluoroscopic phase: During this phase enteroclysis catheter is placed in the descending duodenum and contrast material is introduced.
   2. CT phase: The fluoroscopic phase is followed by the CT phase during which an additional 1.5–2 L of contrast is introduced followed by obtaining images in the late arterial/early portal venous phase.

   Advantages:
   - CT enteroclysis helps in the evaluation of the bowel wall as well as mesentery.
   - Better bowel distension.

c. **CT enterography**:
   - Similar to CT enteroclysis except that contrast is given orally.
   - It can be done in places where expertise for fluoroscopic enteroclysis tube placement is not available.
   - Advantages: It is more compliant to patients.
   - Disadvantages: Inadequate bowel loop distension.

d. **MR enteroclysis**:

   Advantages:
   - Functional information.
   - Excellent soft tissue contrast.
   - Multiplanar imaging capabilities.

- Imaging technique and patient preparation are the same as CT enteroclysis Methylcellulose is used as a luminal contrast agent.
- Gadopentetate dimeglumine is used as IV contrast agent.

e. **PET CT enteroclysis and PET CT colonography**:
- CT and MR enteroclysis provide excellent anatomical information but they fail to show the metabolic status of the disease activity. PET CT enteroclysis and PET CT colonography are a fusion of a metabolic imaging technique, i.e., PET and an anatomical imaging technique i.e., CT enteroclysis. This fusion helps in the localization of active disease focus.
- MOA PET imaging exploits the property of malignant cells and inflammatory conditions which have higher uptake of glucose and metabolism of glucose.
- Method:
  - Patient preparation is the same as CT enteroclysis.
  - Two liter of Methylcellulose is introduced via nasojejunal tube followed by injection of 10 mCi of IV 18 fluoro-deoxyglucose. Followed by obtaining images 60 min after FDG injection.
- Limitation:
  - Physiological uptake of FDG in various abdominal/pelvic organs.
  - Poor image resolution.
- Advantage: Detect significantly higher number of lesions in Crohn's disease, ileocecal TB, and ulcerative colitis.

f. **Nuclear scintigraphy**:
- In this technique, radionuclide labeled white blood cell scintigraphy is used for evaluation of actively inflamed bowel.
- Radionuclide used-Gallium 67, Indium, Technetium.
- Method: Blood is removed from the patient, white blood cells are separated and labeled, and reinjected. Radionuclides accumulate at the site of active inflammation.
- Advantage: Help to differentiate between active and inactive disease.

3. Write a short notes on: CT enteroclysis and MR enteroclysis. [5] [MD (WBUHS) 22]

The following comparative table **(Table 1)** depicts the salient features of CT and MR enteroclysis.

TABLE 1: Showing the salient features of CT and MR enteroclysis.

CT enteroclysis	*MR enteroclysis*
Definition: It is a hybrid technique that combines fluoroscopy with CECT abdomen for evaluation of various GI pathologies like IBD, bowel neoplasm, bowel obstruction, sinuses, and fistula.	Definition: It is an invasive method of MRI for evaluation of small bowel especially Crohn's disease.
Indication: • Obscured GI bleeding • Inflammatory bowel disease. • As complementary investigation with capsule endoscopy • Staging Crohn's disease. • Low-grade small bowel obstruction.	Indication: • Assessment of Crohn's disease and its complications. • Adhesions. • Radiation enteritis. • Scleroderma. • Bowel malignancy.
Patient preparation: • Nil per oral for 8 hrs. • The laxative day prior to the examination. • Low residue diet.	
Method: 1. With positive contrast agent ex-barium sulfate solution and water-soluble contrast agent. 2. With neutral contrast agent ex-water, methylcellulose, and dilute barium solution.	Method: Methylcellulose/water is used as a luminal contrast agent.

Continued...

Continued...

CT enteroclysis	***MR enteroclysis***
Technique: • Fluoroscopic phase: 13fr enteroclysis catheter placed in descending part of duodenum and 1.5 L of contrast agent introduced. • CT phase: Injection glucagon/buscopan followed by the introduction of 1.5 L of contrast and obtaining images after 50 second delay, i.e., in late arterial and early portal venous phase.	Technique: • Fluoroscopy phase: – Nasoduodenal tube is placed in descending duodenal segment. – 1–3 L of .5% methylcellulose/water solution introduced through an electric infusion pump at a rate of 80–200 mL/min. • MRI phase: The following sequences are used- – HASTE, FISP, FLASH, and VIBE with postcontrast images.
Advantages: • It helps in the evaluation of both luminal and extraluminal abnormalities. • By different patterns of abnormality in CT enteroclysis, i.e., 1. Mural enhancement-target, homogenous, heterogenous, diminished 2. Length of involvement 3. Degree of wall thickening 4. Symmetric vs asymmetric thickening 5. Location, i.e., proximal versus distal. 6. Associated abnormality, i.e., mesenteric changes we can differentiate between diseases.	Advantages: • No radiation exposure • Better soft tissue resolution • Multiplanar imaging.
Disadvantage: • It needs the expertise to insert an enteroclysis tube. • Long study time.	Disadvantage: • Long scanning time as compared to CT enteroclysis. • Susceptible to motion and breathing artifacts. • Less sensitive as compared to CT enteroclysis. • MR incompatible implants and devices preclude the scan.

4. Discuss techniques, indications, and applications of MR enteroclysis. [10] [MD (WBUHS) 24, MD (WBUHS) 22]

Definition

It is an invasive method of MRI for the evaluation of small bowel diseases especially Crohn's disease.

The main disadvantage of conventional imaging is that it does not give information about extraluminal disease and radiation exposure at a younger age. MR enteroclysis can be used for the evaluation of small bowel disease with its excellent soft tissue contrast, lack of radiation exposure, and multiplanar imaging.

Patient preparation:

- Nil per oral for 8 hours.
- The laxative day before the study.

MR enteroclysis technique and pulse sequences:

- Patient position- Prone position. By exerting mild pressure on the anterior abdominal wall, it helps in separating small bowel loops.
- With a nasojenunal tube 1.5–2 L of water solution/methylcellulose is introduced using MR compatible MR pump at the rate of 80–150 mL/min till it reaches the terminal ileum.

Followed by obtaining MR images. The following sequences can be used:

- HASTE
- FISP
- T1W FLASH with gadopentate dimeglumine in .1 mmol/kg.

Indication

- Assessment of Crohn's disease and its complications.
- Adhesions.
- Radiation enteritis.
- Scleroderma.
- Bowel malignancy

Technique

- **Fluoroscopy phase**:
  - Nasoduodenal tube is placed in descending duodenal segment.
  - 1–3 L of .5% methylcellulose/water solution introduced through an electric infusion pump at a rate of 80–200 mL/min.
- **MRI Phase**: The following sequences are used: HASTE, FISP, FLASH, AND VIBE with postcontrast images.

Advantages

- No radiation exposure
- Better soft tissue resolution
- Multiplanar imaging

Disadvantage

- Long scanning time as compared to CT enteroclysis.
- Susceptible to motion and breathing artifacts.
- Less sensitive as compared to CT enteroclysis.
- MR incompatible implant and devices preclude the scan.

5. MR enteroclysis. [5] [MD (WBUHS) 24, DNB Dec 21]

Definition

It is an invasive method of MRI for evaluation of small bowel especially Crohn's disease.

Indication

- Assessment of Crohn's disease and its complications.
- Adhesions.
- Radiation enteritis.
- Scleroderma.
- Bowel malignancy.

Technique

- **Fluoroscopy phase**:
  - Nasoduodenal tube is placed in descending duodenal segment.
  - 1–3 L of .5% methylcellulose/water solution introduced through electric infusion pump at rate of 80–200 mL/min.
- **MRI Phase: Following sequences are used**: HASTE, FISP, FLASH AND VIBE with postcontrast images.

Advantages

- No radiation exposure
- Better soft tissue resolution
- Multiplanar imaging.

Disadvantage

- Long scanning time as compared to CT enteroclysis.
- Susceptible to motion and breathing artifacts.
- Less sensitive as compared to CT enteroclysis.
- MR incompatible implant and devices preclude the scan.

6. MRCP. [5] [DNB Dec 21]

Magnetic resonance cholangiopancreatography (MRCP) is a noninvasive imaging technique used to visualize the bile ducts, gallbladder, and pancreatic ducts. It is a specialized application of magnetic resonance imaging (MRI) focusing on the biliary and pancreatic ductal systems.[2]

Principle: High water content in the biliary and pancreatic duct fluid and its static nature is used to aid in visualization in all MRCP sequences.

MRCP protocol:

- **Patient preparation**:
  - At least 4 hours of fasting prior to the examination to reduce fluid secretions in the stomach.
  - Administration of antiperistaltic agent.
  - Oral administration of iron oxide contrast or blueberry juice to reduce overlapping signals from stomach fluid.
- **Technical Requirement**- ≥ 1.5T MRI scanner.
  - **Technique**:
    - T2W Breathhold HASTE Sequence, 3D T2W FSE Sequence
    - Additional T1W sequence can be obtained to look for parenchymal abnormality.
    - MRCP uses magnetic fields and radio waves to create detailed images of the bile ducts and surrounding structures without the need for contrast dye or invasive procedures.
  - **Indications**: It is commonly used to diagnose conditions, such as:
    - Bile duct obstructions,
    - Gallstones,
    - Acute cholecystitis
    - Acute pancreatitis
    - Benign biliary stricture
    - Malignant biliary stricture ex-cholangiocarcinoma, pancreatic adenocarcinoma.
    - Tumors
    - Congenital anomalies in the biliary tree.
    - Postsurgical anatomy and complications.
  - **Advantages**:
    - MRCP is noninvasive.
    - Does not involve ionizing radiation.
    - Provides high-resolution images that can guide further treatment or interventions.
    - As compared to ERCP it gives both protectional and cross-sectional images of bile trees.
    - It gives information on the bile tree both proximal and distal to the lesion.
    - When combined with T1 and T2WI it gives information about extraductal abnormalities as well.
  - **Comparison with ERCP**: Unlike endoscopic retrograde cholangiopancreatography (ERCP), which is both diagnostic and therapeutic, MRCP is purely diagnostic.

7. MRI hepatobiliary contrast agent and its use in differentiating liver lesions. [10] [DNB June 21]

Magnetic resonance imaging with hepatobiliary contrast agents plays a crucial role in the evaluation and characterization of liver lesions. These agents are specifically designed to enhance imaging of the liver and biliary system, offering significant advantages in differentiating benign from malignant lesions.[3]

Type of Hepatobiliary Contrast Agent

Hepatobiliary contrast agents, also known as liver-specific or targeted agents, are gadolinium-based compounds that are selectively taken up by hepatocytes (liver cells) and excreted into the bile.

The most commonly used agents include:

1. **Gadoxetate disodium (Gd-EOB-DTPA):** It has both extracellular and hepatocyte-specific phases, allowing dynamic imaging followed by delayed hepatobiliary phase imaging.
2. **Gadobenate dimeglumine (Gd-BOPTA/MultiHance):** It has partial hepatocyte uptake, making it useful for both vascular and hepatobiliary phase imaging.

Mechanism of Action

After intravenous administration, these agents distribute into the extracellular fluid space during the initial dynamic phases (arterial, portal venous, and delayed phases). Subsequently, during the hepatobiliary phase (typically 20 minutes for gadoxetate and 60 minutes for multiphase postinjection), they are taken up by functioning hepatocytes and excreted into the biliary system. Lesions without functioning hepatocytes (e.g., most malignant tumors) appear hypointense (darker) relative to the surrounding liver parenchyma during this phase, while lesions with functioning hepatocytes (e.g., some benign lesions) appear hyperintense (brighter).

Used in differentiating liver lesions – the main differentiating points among the different liver lesions are presented in a tabular form **(Tables 2 and 3)** as follows:

1. Benign Lesions

TABLE 2: Showing the main differentiating points among the different benign liver lesions.

Focal nodular hyperplasia (FNH)	*Hepatocellular adenoma*	*Regenerative nodules*
FNH typically shows hyperintensity during the hepatobiliary phase due to its high content of functioning hepatocytes.	Depending on the subtype, some adenomas may take-up the contrast agent, but generally, they appear isointense or slightly hyperintense.	Often seen in cirrhotic livers, these nodules can uptake the contrast, appearing hyperintense.

2. Malignant Lesions

TABLE 3: Shows the main differentiating points among the different malignant liver lesions.

Hepatocellular carcinoma	*Metastases*	*Cholangiocarcinoma*
Most HCCs appear hypointense in the hepatobiliary phase, as they generally lack normal hepatocyte function. However, well-differentiated HCCs might show some uptake.	Metastatic liver lesions do not contain functioning hepatocytes, and thus appear hypointense during the hepatobiliary phase, aiding in differentiation from benign lesions.	Typically, hypointense is due to the lack of hepatocytes in these malignant tumors.

Clinical Advantages

The use of hepatobiliary contrast agents enhances the accuracy of MRI in characterizing liver lesions, particularly in distinguishing between benign and malignant tumors.

The Acute Abdomen

1. Discuss the radiological features of (a) Midgut volvulus and (b) Intussusception. [5+5] [MD (WBUHS) 21]

Midgut Volvulus

Midgut volvulus is a life-threatening condition where the intestine twists around the superior mesenteric artery, leading to bowel obstruction and potential ischemia. Prompt diagnosis is crucial, and imaging plays a key role. Here are the key imaging findings:

1. **Upper Gastrointestinal (UGI) Series**:
   a. Corkscrew Appearance: The most classic finding is a "corkscrew" or "spiral" configuration of the twisted bowel loops, particularly seen in the duodenum and proximal jejunum.
   b. Malpositioned Duodenojejunal Junction: Normally located to the left of the spine at the level of the duodenal bulb, in midgut volvulus, this junction is displaced or not visualized in the correct location.
2. **Abdominal X-ray**:
   - Double Bubble Sign: This can be seen in neonates, indicating a proximal obstruction.
   - Distended Bowel Loops: There may be evidence of distended bowel loops with air-fluid levels, though this finding is nonspecific.
3. **Ultrasound (US)**:
   - Whirlpool Sign: This is a key finding where the superior mesenteric vein and surrounding mesentery are seen twisting around the superior mesenteric artery, resembling a whirlpool.
   - Doppler Ultrasound: May show reduced or absent blood flow in the twisted mesenteric vessels, indicating compromised blood supply.
4. **CT Scan**:
   - Whirlpool Sign: Similar to ultrasound, CT can clearly depict the twisted bowel and mesentery around the superior mesenteric artery.
   - Malpositioned SMV: Normally superior mesenteric vein is on the right side of the superior mesenteric artery. The superior mesenteric vein (SMV) may be positioned abnormally relative to the superior mesenteric artery (SMA) in the midgut volvulus.

Intussusception

Intussusception occurs when a segment of the intestine telescopes into an adjacent segment, leading to obstruction and potential ischemia.

Imaging is critical for diagnosis, particularly in pediatric patients. Here are the key imaging findings:

1. **Ultrasound**:
   - Target Sign: The most characteristic finding on ultrasound, appearing as concentric rings of alternating echogenicity, resembling a "bull's-eye" or "donut." This sign is seen in the transverse view.
   - Pseudo-kidney Sign: In the longitudinal view, the intussuscepted bowel appears as an elongated mass with layers that resemble the structure of a kidney.
2. **Abdominal X-ray**:
   - Soft Tissue Mass: An abdominal X-ray may show a soft tissue mass in the right upper quadrant or other locations, often with signs of bowel obstruction such as distended loops of bowel with air-fluid levels.
   - Absence of Gas in the Distal Bowel: There may be a lack of gas beyond the point of obstruction.
3. **Air or Contrast Enema: Coiled Spring Sign**: During a contrast or air enema, the intussusception appears as a coiled spring pattern due to the trapped bowel folds. This technique is both diagnostic and therapeutic, as it can often reduce intussusception.

2. What is intestinal malrotation? Enumerate various types of intestinal malrotation. Describe the radiological findings in a case of midgut volvulus. [2+3+5]

Intestinal malrotation is a congenital condition resulting from abnormal rotation and fixation of the midgut during fetal development. This condition affects the positioning and attachment of the bowel loops within the abdominal cavity.

Embryology

During normal fetal development, the intestines undergo a series of rotations as they return to the abdominal cavity from the umbilical cord. In malrotation, this process is incomplete or abnormal, leading to improper positioning of the intestines, usually with the cecum and duodenojejunal junction in abnormal locations.

Clinical Presentation

Intestinal malrotation often presents in neonates and infants with bilious vomiting, abdominal distension, and signs of bowel obstruction. It can also present later in life with chronic abdominal pain or failure to thrive. The most serious complication is midgut volvulus, where the intestines twist around the superior mesenteric artery, leading to bowel ischemia and necrosis.

Intestinal malrotation refers to a spectrum of congenital anomalies resulting from improper rotation and fixation of the bowel loop during embryonic development. The types of malrotation are classified based on the stage at which the developmental process is interrupted.

The main types:

1. **Nonrotation**:
   - In nonrotation, the midgut fails to undergo its normal 270° rotation. As a result, the small intestine remains predominantly on the right side of the abdomen, while the colon is on the left side.
   - Clinical Implications: Although it may be asymptomatic, nonrotation increases the risk of volvulus due to the abnormal positioning of the bowel.
2. **Incomplete Rotation**:
   - In this type, the rotation is incomplete, typically leaving the duodenojejunal junction abnormally positioned to the right of the midline, and the cecum and appendix are often located in the upper abdomen or near the midline.
   - Clinical Implications: This form of malrotation is associated with a high risk of midgut volvulus and intestinal obstruction.
3. **Reversed Rotation**:
   - Description: In reversed rotation, the midgut undergoes an abnormal counterclockwise rotation, leading to the transverse colon lying posterior to the superior mesenteric artery and the duodenum anterior to it.
   - Clinical Implications: This can cause the transverse colon to become compressed by the superior mesenteric artery, leading to symptoms of bowel obstruction.
4. **Mixed Rotation**:
   - This type involves a combination of nonrotation and incomplete rotation patterns, leading to complex and unpredictable bowel positioning.
   - Mixed rotation poses a significant risk of volvulus, bowel obstruction, and other complications.

Radiological Findings in Midgut Volvulus

Midgut volvulus is a surgical emergency where the intestine twists around the superior mesenteric artery, leading to obstruction and potential ischemia. Radiological imaging is crucial for diagnosis.

Key radiological findings include:

1. **Upper Gastrointestinal (UGI) Series**:
   - Corkscrew Appearance: This is the classic finding, where the twisted bowel loops create a spiral or corkscrew pattern, particularly in the duodenum and proximal jejunum.
   - Malpositioned duodenojejunal junction: In a normal UGI series, the duodenojejunal junction is located to the left of the spine. In midgut volvulus, this junction is displaced, usually to the right of the midline or lower than usual.
2. **Abdominal X-ray**:
   - Double Bubble Sign: This sign can be seen in neonates, indicating proximal bowel obstruction with dilated stomach and proximal duodenum.
   - Distended Bowel Loops: There may be generalized distention of bowel loops with air-fluid levels, indicative of obstruction, though this finding is nonspecific.
3. **Ultrasound**:
   - Whirlpool Sign: This is a key diagnostic feature where the superior mesenteric vein (SMV) and surrounding mesentery are seen twisting around the superior mesenteric artery (SMA), resembling a whirlpool.
   - Abnormal SMV Positioning: The SMV may be seen anterior to or on the left side of the SMA, which is abnormal.

4. **CT Scan**:
   - Whirlpool Sign: Similar to ultrasound, CT can show the twisted bowel and mesentery around the SMA, confirming volvulus.
   - Malpositioned SMV and SMA: The relationship between the SMV and SMA is reversed or abnormal, which is characteristic of malrotation and volvulus.
5. **Absence of Bowel Gas: Bowel Ischemia**: In severe cases, there may be a paucity of bowel gas distal to the volvulus site, indicating possible bowel ischemia or necrosis.

3. (a) Role of plain radiograph in a case of acute abdomen. (b) Role of MRI in acute pancreatitis. [5+5] [DNB June 20]

a. Role of Radiograph in a Case of Acute Abdomen

Plain radiographs (X-rays) being cheap and easily available are a valuable initial imaging tool in the evaluation of patients with acute abdomen, helping to guide further management. Key roles of radiographs include:

1. **Detection of Bowel Obstruction: Air-fluid Levels and Distended Bowel Loops**: Radiographs can reveal dilated loops of the bowel with air-fluid levels, which are suggestive of bowel obstruction.
2. **Identification of Free Air (Pneumoperitoneum): Air Under the Diaphragm**: On an upright chest X-ray, free air under the diaphragm indicates pneumoperitoneum, a sign of gastrointestinal perforation, which is a surgical emergency.
3. **Detection of Calcifications: Gallstones, kidney stones, and pancreatic calcifications**: Radiographs can identify radiopaque calcifications, such as gallstones, kidney stones, or calcifications in the pancreas, which can be associated with acute cholecystitis, renal colic, or chronic pancreatitis, respectively.
4. **Evaluation of Intestinal Gas Patterns: Abnormal Gas Distribution**: Radiographs can show abnormal gas patterns, such as generalized ileus (with diffuse bowel distension).
5. **Assessment of Foreign Bodies: Radiopaque Foreign Bodies**: In cases of ingestion or insertion of foreign objects, radiographs can help locate radiopaque foreign bodies in the gastrointestinal tract, aiding in their further management.

b. Role of MRI in Acute Pancreatitis

Although CECT is the imaging investigation of choice for acute pancreatitis, MRI plays a crucial role in the assessment and management of acute pancreatitis, offering detailed imaging of the pancreas and surrounding structures. Here are a few points:

1. **Detailed Pancreatic Imaging: High-resolution Images**: MRI provides superior soft tissue contrast, which helps in assessing the extent of pancreatic inflammation and necrosis. Contrast-enhanced MRI can further aid in giving information about the extent of necrosis.
2. **Detection of Complications**:
   - Pancreatic Necrosis: MRI is highly sensitive in detecting areas of necrosis within the pancreas, which is crucial for prognosis and management.
   - Peripancreatic Fluid Collections: MRI is effective in identifying and characterizing fluid collections, including acute peripancreatic fluid collections, pseudocysts, and walled-off necrosis, which can guide therapeutic interventions. Also, an MRI can help in identifying communication between the main pancreatic duct and the collection which is very important for further management.
3. **Assessment of Biliary and Ductal Systems: MR cholangiopancreatography (MRCP)**: MRI can be combined with MRCP to noninvasively visualize the biliary and pancreatic ducts. This is particularly useful in identifying gallstones, MPD calcifications, strictures, or other ductal anomalies that may cause or complicate acute pancreatitis.
4. **Evaluation of severity: Severity Assessment**: MRI can assess the severity of acute pancreatitis by evaluating the extent of pancreatic inflammation, necrosis, and involvement of surrounding tissues. This helps in predicting the clinical course and planning management.
5. **Avoiding Radiation Exposure: Safe Imaging Modality**: Unlike CT, MRI does not use ionizing radiation, making it a safer option for repeated imaging for patients requiring regular follow-up.

Infections, Inflammation and Neoplasms

1. Briefly describe the etiopathology and imaging findings of ileocecal tuberculosis. Discuss the features that are useful to differentiate it from Crohn's disease. [3+2+5] [MD (WBUHS) 23, AIIMS May 23]

Etiopathogenesis

1. **Causative Agent**: Ileocecal tuberculosis (TB) is caused by Mycobacterium tuberculosis.
2. **Pathways of Infection**:
   - Hematogenous Spread: TB bacteria can spread to the gastrointestinal tract through the bloodstream from a primary site, such as the lungs.
   - Ingestion of Infected Material: Ingestion of sputum containing TB bacilli or infected food can directly infect the intestines.
   - Contiguous Spread: TB can spread directly from adjacent infected organs like the peritoneum.
3. The most common site of infection is the ileocecal region because of abundant lymphoid tissue, prolonged stasis, increased rate of absorption in the region, and closer contact of the bacilli with the mucosa of the region.
4. **Pathology**: The disease typically causes chronic inflammation, leading to thickening of the bowel wall, fibrosis, and formation of caseating granulomas. This can result in strictures, obstruction, or fistulas. The lesion may be:
   1. Hyperplastic with long segment narrowing, rigidity, and loss of distensibility.
   2. Ulcerative.
   3. Ulcero-hyperplastic
   4. Carcinoma type with short annular defect and overhanging edges.

Imaging Findings

1. **Barium studies (BMFT)**: The salient features of ileocecal tuberculosis on barium meal follow-through studies are presented **(Table 4)** as follows:

TABLE 4: Showing the main findings of ileocecal tuberculosis on barium meal follow-through examination.

Early involvement	*Advanced disease*
Thickening of the ileocecal valve and wide gaping of the valve with narrowing of terminal ileum - called an inverted umbrella sign/fleisher sign.	• Symmetric, annular, "napkin ring" stenosis of the ileocecal valve. • Shrunken and retracted cecum. • Narrowing of terminal ileum. • Dilated proximal ileum. • "Gooseneck deformity"- Loss of ileocecal angle with dilated ileum hanging from contracted and retracted cecum.

2. **CT scan**:
   - Ileocecal Mass: CT often reveals circumferential thickening of the cecum and terminal ileum with irregular thickening of the ileocecal valve.
   - Lymphadenopathy: Enlarged mesenteric lymph nodes with central caseation (necrosis) are seen.
   - Fibrosis and Strictures: CT may also show strictures and localized bowel wall thickening, which can lead to obstruction.
3. **Ultrasound**:
   - Bowel Wall Thickening: Ultrasound can demonstrate circumferential thickening of the wall of the terminal ileum and cecum along with adjacent lymphadenopathy.
4. **MRI**:
   - MRI provides detailed images of the bowel wall and surrounding structures, showing thickening, strictures, and peritoneal involvement. It is particularly useful in assessing the extent of the disease.

Differentiating Ileocecal Tuberculosis from Crohn's Disease

Ileocecal tuberculosis and Crohn's disease are both chronic inflammatory conditions that primarily affect the ileocecal region, making their differentiation challenging. However, specific clinical features and imaging findings can help distinguish between the two **(Table 5)**.

TABLE 5: Showing the main differentiating points between ileocecal tuberculosis and Crohn's disease.

Findings	*TB*	*Crohn's disease*
Patient history	Patients often present with a history of tuberculosis exposure, positive tuberculin test, residing in TB-endemic areas, etc.	• Patient's symptoms are relapsing remitting type. • Family history of inflammatory disease may be present.
Symptom onset	• Subacute to chronic onset of fever, night sweats, weight loss, etc. • Diarrhea is less frequent.	• Chronic symptoms of diarrhea, weight loss and recurrent abdominal pain. • May be associated with perianal fissures and fistula. • Extraintestinal manifestations may be present like arthritis and skin involvement. • Diarrhea is more frequent.
Imaging findings		
Site	Cecum more common	Terminal ileum is more common
Length of involvement	Short segment	Long segment
Multiple site involvement	Uncommon (<4)	Common
Skip lesions		
Type of enhancement	Homogenous	Stratified
Mural stratification	Rarely seen	Common
Perianal fistula	Uncommon	Common
Mesenteric abscesses	Uncommon	Common
Interbowel fistula	Rare	Common
Stricture	Concentric	Eccentric with sacculation
Enterolith	More common	Less common
Increased Mesenteric vascularity	Uncommon	Common
Fibrofatty proliferation	Uncommon	Common
Mesenteric Nodes	Larger, Necrotic	Small homogenous
Omental involvement	Often present	Rare
Ascites	Present	Absent
Solid organ involvement	May be present	Very rare
Endoscopic		
Mucosal changes	Transverse ulcers, pseudopolyps	Deep longitudinal ulcers, aphthous ulcers
Skip lesions	Uncommon	More common
Fistulae	Uncommon	Common
Patulous ileocecal valve	Common	Rare
Anorectal disease	Uncommon	Common
Histology		
Granuloma	Multiple, confluent, caseating, submucosal	Microgranuloma, single, nonconfluent, noncaseating
Disproportionate submucosal inflammation	Common	Rare

2. Discuss the common causes of pain in the right iliac fossa and radiological evaluation. [4+6] [MD (WBUHS) 23, MD (WBUHS) 18]

Common Causes of Pain in the Right Iliac Fossa

1. **Acute Appendicitis**: The **most common** cause of right iliac fossa pain, especially in children and young adults. It presents with acute onset sharp pain that typically starts around the umbilicus and later localizes to the right iliac fossa, often accompanied by nausea, vomiting, and fever.
2. **Ileocecal Tuberculosis**: A chronic infection caused by Mycobacterium tuberculosis affecting the ileocecal region. Patients may experience chronic pain, weight loss, fever, and a lump in the right iliac fossa.
3. **Crohn's Disease**: An inflammatory bowel disease that often affects the terminal ileum. It causes chronic, crampy pain in the right iliac fossa, often associated with diarrhea and weight loss.
4. **Ovarian or Adnexal Pathology**: Conditions like ovarian cysts, torsion, or ectopic pregnancy can cause right iliac fossa pain in women. The pain is typically sharp and sudden in onset, often associated with vomiting and menstrual irregularity.
    1. Intussusception
    2. Acute Gastroenteritis/infective colitis
    3. Epiploic appendagitis
    4. Endometriosis
    5. Ureteric Stone
    6. Pelvic inflammatory disease
    7. Diverticulitis.

Radiological Evaluation of Pain in the Right Iliac Fossa

Radiological imaging plays a crucial role in the diagnosis and management of right iliac fossa pain, helping to identify the underlying cause and guide appropriate treatment:

The common causes of pain in the right iliac fossa along with their corresponding imaging findings are presented in the following table **(Table 6)**.

TABLE 6: Showing the common causes of pain in the right iliac fossa along with their corresponding imaging findings.

	USG	*CT*	*X-ray*	*MRI*
Acute appendicitis	• First-line investigation, • Advantages easily available, lack of ionizing radiation • Noncompressible dilated (>6mm) appendix. With periappendiceal fluid ± appendicolith.	• CECT is done when USG findings are inconclusive and also when abscess formation or perforation is suspected. • Dilated appendix with periappendiceal fat stranding and fluid with/without appendicolith.	Limited role. May show appendicolith. Perforation.	Same as CT
Ileocecal tuberculosis	• First-line investigation. • Shows thickening of terminal ileum and cecum with multiple lymph nodes showing central necrosis.	Thickening of ileocecal valve, wall of the terminal ileum and cecum with multiple necrotic lymph nodes.	Limited role. May show perforation or bowel obstruction.	Same as CT
Crohn's disease	First-line investigation. Shows thickening of terminal ileum and cecum with small lymph nodes in right iliac fossa.	Mural stratification and thickening of the wall of terminal ileum and caecum, skip lesions. Small homogenous lymph nodes in the right iliac fossa.	Limited role. May show bowel perforation.	Bowel wall thickening and mural stratification.

Continued...

Continued...

	USG	CT	X-ray	MRI
Pelvic inflammatory disease	• Investigation of choice to rule out gynecological conditions. • May show ovarian cysts/ adnexal lesions like ectopic pregnancy.	May help in confirming the finding on USG.		With better soft tissue resolution. It helps in confirming the ovarian cysts and adnexal lesions.
Ureteric calculus	Shows additional findings like hydronephrosis.	NCCT KUB is an investigation of choice for detecting ureteric calculus.	May shows a calculus along the course of the ureter.	

1. **Ultrasound**:
   - First-line Imaging modality: Ultrasound is often the initial imaging modality due to its accessibility, lack of radiation, and ability to provide real-time images. It is particularly useful in evaluating appendicitis, gynecological conditions, and bowel-related issues.
   - Appendicitis: The classic findings include a noncompressible, dilated appendix (>6 mm in diameter), wall thickening, and increased vascularity (hyperemia) on Doppler imaging. The presence of an appendicolith or periappendiceal fluid collection may also be seen.
   - Gynecological Pathologies: Ultrasound is essential for identifying ovarian cysts, ovarian torsion, or ectopic pregnancy, which may present with right iliac fossa pain. Features like ovarian enlargement, lack of blood flow (in torsion), and free fluid in the pelvis can be indicative.
2. **CT Scan**:
   - Comprehensive Evaluation: A contrast-enhanced CT scan of the abdomen and pelvis is often performed if the diagnosis remains uncertain after ultrasound or if there are signs of complications. CT provides excellent anatomical detail and can identify a wide range of conditions.
   - Appendicitis: CT findings include an enlarged appendix (>6 mm), periappendiceal fat stranding, appendicoliths, and complications like abscess or perforation.
   - Crohn's Disease: CT can show segmental bowel wall thickening, skip lesions, mesenteric fat stranding, and complications such as fistulas or abscesses.
   - Ileocecal Tuberculosis: Characteristic findings include ileocecal wall thickening, mesenteric lymphadenopathy with central necrosis, and the "cecal mass" appearance.
3. **MRI**:
   - Specialized Imaging: MRI is particularly useful in evaluating gynecological conditions, bowel pathology, and in cases where radiation exposure is a concern (e.g., in young patients or pregnant women). It offers superior soft-tissue contrast.
   - Crohn's Disease: MRI enterography can show bowel wall thickening, stratification, and the presence of fistulas or abscesses, which are characteristic of Crohn's disease.
   - Gynecological conditions: MRI can provide detailed images of ovarian cysts, torsion, and pelvic inflammatory disease, helping to confirm the diagnosis when ultrasound findings are inconclusive.
4. **Plain Abdominal X-ray**:
   - Limited Role: While less commonly used as the first line for right iliac fossa pain, an abdominal X-ray can be helpful in specific situations, such as detecting bowel obstruction (air-fluid levels), perforation (free air under the diaphragm), or foreign bodies.
   - Appendicitis: Occasionally, an appendicolith may be visible on an X-ray, suggesting appendicitis.
5. **Barium Studies**:
   - Selective Use: Barium studies, like a barium enema, are rarely used in acute settings but can be helpful in chronic cases to evaluate conditions like Crohn's disease or ileocecal tuberculosis. They can show strictures, fistulas, or mass lesions in the bowel.

3. Write a short note on: Radiological features of Crohn's disease. [5] [MD (WBUHS) 19]

Radiological Features of Crohn's Disease

Crohn's disease is a chronic inflammatory bowel disease that can affect any part of gastrointestinal tract from mouth to anal canal. About two third of the cases however affect small bowel either in isolation or with colonic involvement. Small intestinal involvement can be assessed either endoscopically or radiologically. Advantage of endoscopy is direct visualization of mucosa and the ability to take a biopsy. Advantage of radiology is noninvasive and visualization of entire small bowel. Also, assessment of wall and extraintestinal changes.

Small bowel follow through and enteroclysis were investigation of choice earlier but now a day CT enterography/enteroclysis and MR enterography/enteroclysis are investigation of choice for evaluation of Crohn's disease.

Radiological Classification of Crohn's Disease (Table 7)

TABLE 7: Radiological classification of Crohn's disease.

Active inflammatory subtype	Fibrostenotic subtype	Fistulizing/perforating subtype	Reparative/regenerative subtype
Minimal changes-superficial ulcers	Minimal stenosis	Deep fissuring ulcers sinus tracts	Regenerative polyp
Severe changes-deep ulcers/ Cobblestone mucosa Wall thickening	Severe stenosis	Fistula with other organs	

Barium Studies

Once considered investigation of choice for Crohn's disease. Following are imaging findings on double contrast barium study:

- **Aphthous Ulcers**:
  - Earliest radiologically appreciable findings. They are superficial mucosal erosions well appreciated on double contrast barium meal follow through.
  - Deep fissuring ulcers and cobblestone—as a result of deep transverse and longitudinal ulcers separated by residual edematous mucosa.
- **Stricture**:
  - Stenosis of the bowel with or without prestenotic dilatation
  - Sinus tract or fistula
  - Radiological imaging is crucial for diagnosing and assessment of Crohn's disease.
- **USG**:
  - Thickening of the wall of terminal ileum and cecum with mesenteric lymph nodes.
  - Color Doppler may show increased vascularity and hyperemia in active disease.

Hydrogen peroxide-enhanced ultrasonography can be done by injecting a solution of 30% hydrogen peroxide and 70% povidone-iodine mixture into the skin orifice of the enterocutaneous fistula which enhances visualization of the tract.

CTE/MRE

1. **Bowel Wall Thickening: Segmental Thickening**: The bowel wall is often thickened and shows mural stratification, typically in a segmental or patchy manner. This thickening can be asymmetric and involves both the small intestine and the colon, with the terminal ileum being the most commonly affected area.
2. **Skip Lesions**: Discontinuous Involvement One of the hallmark features of Crohn's disease is the presence of "skiplesions," where segments of the diseased bowel are interspersed with normal, healthy bowel. This pattern helps differentiate Crohn's from other inflammatory bowel diseases like ulcerative colitis.
3. **Strictures**: Narrowing of the lumen chronic inflammation can lead to fibrotic strictures, which cause narrowing of the bowel lumen. These strictures may be seen as areas of narrowed bowel on imaging, often leading to obstruction.

4. **Fistulas and Abscesses: Transmural Inflammation**: Crohn's disease can cause deep, transmural inflammation that may result in the formation of fistulas (abnormal connections between the bowel and other organs or skin) and abscesses. These can be identified in imaging studies like CT or MRI.
5. **Fat Stranding and Mesenteric Changes**:
   - Creeping Fat: Increased fat deposition around the affected bowel loops, known as "creeping fat," is a common finding. This may be accompanied by mesenteric fat stranding and enlarged lymph nodes, reflecting ongoing inflammation.
   - "Comb sign": Prominent vasa recta of mesenteric vessels representing pericentric inflammation and bowel wall inflammation.
6. In addition, MRE can help in differentiating fibrostenotic wall thickening from active inflammatory. Fibrostenotic thickening will be hypointense on both T1W and T2WI.

4. Discuss the role of various imaging modalities in the evaluation of intestinal tuberculosis. [10] [MD (WBUHS) 22]

Intestinal tuberculosis is a challenging condition to diagnose due to its nonspecific clinical presentation, which often mimics other gastrointestinal diseases like Crohn's disease, lymphoma, or malignancies. Imaging plays a critical role in the evaluation, diagnosis, and management of intestinal TB. Here is an overview of the role of imaging in this context:

1. **Detection of the lesion**: Imaging, particularly through modalities like CT scans and MRI, helps in identifying characteristic features of intestinal TB. The presence of asymmetric wall thickening in the ileocecal region, strictures, and enlarged mesenteric lymph nodes with central necrosis are hallmark signs that suggest intestinal TB.
2. **Differentiation from Other Diseases**: One of the major roles of imaging is to differentiate intestinal TB from other conditions like Crohn's disease, bowel malignancies, gastroenteritis, etc. While both conditions can present with bowel wall thickening and strictures, TB often involves shorter segments of the intestine and shows more pronounced lymphadenopathy with central necrosis.
3. **Guidance for Biopsy**: Imaging can be used to guide percutaneous biopsies, especially in cases where the diagnosis is uncertain. Identifying the most affected areas via imaging can increase the diagnostic yield of biopsies.
4. **Assessment of Complication**: Complications such as bowel perforation, abscess formation, and fistulas are not uncommon in intestinal TB. Imaging modalities, including CT and MRI, are essential in assessing these complications. CT, in particular, is invaluable in emergency settings for the quick assessment of perforation or the presence of abscesses, which may require surgical intervention.
5. **Monitoring of Treatment Response**: Imaging is also critical in monitoring the response to antitubercular therapy (ATT). Serial imaging studies can show the resolution of bowel wall thickening, reduction in lymph node size, and healing of strictures. Persistent or worsening findings on imaging may suggest treatment failure, drug resistance, or complications, necessitating a change in the therapeutic approach.

5. Enumerate the causes of lower gastrointestinal bleeding. Describe briefly the role of imaging and intervention in a case of lower gastrointestinal bleeding. [3+(4+3)]

Lower GI bleeding refers to bleeding originating from a source distal to the ligament of Treitz, typically from the small intestine, colon, rectum, or anus. Common causes include:

1. **Diverticular Disease**: Diverticulosis is the most common cause of lower GI bleeding in adults, particularly in older individuals.

   They are most commonly in the descending colon. Bleeding is abrupt, massive, and painless. Meckel's diverticulum is a congenital anomaly of the distal ileum. It is the cause of acute hemorrhage in children and young adults. Meckel's diverticulum is identified with a Tc-99m-pertechnetate scan.
2. **Angiodysplasia**: They are mucosal telangiectasia in the colon, usually in the cecum and ascending colon, which can lead to bleeding. On angiography they appear as vascular tuft with early opacification of draining veins.
3. **Colorectal Cancer**: Malignancies in the colon or rectum can cause bleeding, often presenting as occult blood or overt hematochezia.

4. **Inflammatory Bowel Disease**: Includes Crohn's disease and ulcerative colitis, which can cause bleeding due to ulceration of the intestinal mucosa.
5. **Hemorrhoids**: Dilated veins in the rectum or anus that can cause bright red bleeding, typically painless.
6. **Ischemic Colitis**:
   - It can be occlusive like in embolization, thrombosis, and aneurysm or nonocclusive like in hypovolemia and cardiac dysfunction. Reduced blood flow to the colon, often presenting with sudden onset of pain and bloody diarrhea.
   - The hallmark on the barium enema is a thumb-printing sign due to submucosal hemorrhage and edema.
7. **Infectious Colitis**: It can cause bloody diarrhea.
8. **Radiation Proctitis**: Bleeding caused by damage to the rectal mucosa following radiation therapy for pelvic malignancies.
9. **Aortoenteric Fistula**: Due to rupture of an arteriosclerotic aortic aneurysm into the small intestine. It occurs due to arterial reconstructive surgery with fistula formation between the synthetic graft and bowel lumen.

Role of Imaging and Intervention in Lower GI Bleeding

1. Diagnostic Imaging

1. **CT Angiography (CTA)**: CTA (Arterial phase) is often the first imaging modality used in the evaluation of acute lower GI bleeding. It is highly sensitive and specific for detecting active bleeding by identifying contrast extravasation within the bowel lumen. It also provides anatomical details that can help localize the bleeding source and guide further intervention.
2. **Colonoscopy**: Colonoscopy is both a diagnostic and therapeutic tool. It allows direct visualization of the lower GI tract and can often identify the bleeding source. Additionally, therapeutic interventions such as clipping, coagulation, or injection therapy can be performed during the procedure.
3. **Radionuclide Scintigraphy (Sulphur Colloid and Tagged Red Blood Cell Scan)**:
   - It can detect bleeding as low as .1 mL/min. Half-life of sulfur colloid scan is 2.5–3 min. If active bleeding is occurring during this short time the tracer would extravasate in the bowel. Sulphur colloid can detect bleeding rates as low as .1 mL/min. Tc-99m labelled RBC has a half-life of 2 hours and hence it is useful for evaluating intermittent GI bleeding.
   - This imaging modality is more sensitive than CTA for detecting slow bleeding rates but lacks precise localization. It is used in cases where other imaging is inconclusive or if the bleeding is intermittent.

2. Interventional Radiology

- **Angiography and Embolization**: Angiography plays a significant role in the diagnosis and management of patients with gastrointestinal hemorrhage. Angiography is diagnostic if the rate of bleeding exceeds .5 mL/min. In case of intermittent bleeding, less invasive examinations can be used, and emergency angiography may not be required.
- If CTA or colonoscopy identifies an active bleeding source, angiography can be performed to confirm the location and provide catheter-directed therapeutic embolization. This is particularly useful in patients who are not candidates for surgery. Angiography finding of active GI hemorrhage is active extravasation with puddling of contrast which persists in the venous phase. Delayed phase may show contrast in the intestinal lumen.

6. Role of virtual colonoscopy. Technique and contraindications. Imaging findings of colonic polyps on virtual colonoscopy. [10] [DNB Dec 21]

Virtual colonoscopy, also known as CT colonography, is a noninvasive imaging technique used to screen for colorectal polyps and cancer. It has emerged as an alternative to traditional optical colonoscopy, particularly in patients who cannot undergo the conventional procedure (the gold standard investigation for screening of colorectal cancer is optical colonoscopy and occult blood).

CT colonography may represent a reasonable alternative screening method in patients who cannot undergo or refuse colonoscopy and would otherwise remain unscreened; in fact, the benefits of CT colonography employment in CRC mass screening are actually under evaluation and its potential role as a first-line screening modality is emerging.

Role of Virtual Colonoscopy

1. **Screening for Colorectal Cancer**: Virtual colonoscopy is primarily used for screening asymptomatic individuals for colorectal cancer and precancerous polyps. It is especially useful in patients who are at average risk or who cannot undergo traditional colonoscopy due to sedation risks, anticoagulation therapy, or other medical conditions.
2. **Alternative to Optical Colonoscopy**: It serves as an alternative for patients who refuse or are unable to tolerate a conventional colonoscopy. Virtual colonoscopy can visualize the entire colon, including areas that might be inaccessible during a traditional colonoscopy due to strictures or tortuosity.
3. **Detection of Extracolonic Pathologies**: Apart from identifying polyps and cancers within the colon, virtual colonoscopy can also detect extracolonic findings, such as abdominal aortic aneurysms, renal masses, or liver lesions, which may warrant further investigation.
4. **Follow-up Postpolypectomy**: Virtual colonoscopy can be used as a follow-up tool in patients who have had polyps removed, to ensure there is no recurrence or new polyp formation.
5. **Assessing Incomplete Colonoscopies**: In cases where traditional colonoscopy is incomplete (e.g., due to obstructive lesions or patient discomfort), virtual colonoscopy can be used to evaluate the remaining colon.

Technique of Virtual Colonoscopy

1. **Bowel Preparation**: Similar to traditional colonoscopy, a thorough bowel cleansing is required to remove stool and fluids from the colon. This typically involves a clear liquid diet/low residue diet and the use of laxatives or purgatives 24 hours before the procedure. Laxatives like magnesium citrate, sodium phosphate, and polyethylene glycol can be used.
2. **Colon Distention**: To obtain clear images, the colon is gently distended with air or carbon dioxide, which is insufflated through a small tube inserted into the rectum. This step is crucial as it expands the colon walls, allowing better visualization of the mucosal surface.
3. Spasmolytic like buscopan are agent of choice especially in the case of stricture, stenosing carcinoma, and diverticula. If contraindicated or not available glucagon(1mg) may be used.
4. **CT Imaging**: The patient is then positioned on the CT table. The scan should be done on MDCT (>4 rows) , and a low-dose CT scan(120KVp) and mAs 50 of the abdomen and pelvis is performed.1mm thin sections obtained with 50–70% overlapping of slices. IV contrast is not mandatory and is only used if the patient has symptoms of colorectal cancer, for staging known colorectal cancer, metachronous disease, or metastases. The scan is usually done twice: once with the patient lying on their supine and once on the prone position to ensure full visualization of the colon. Automatic exposure control and iterative reconstruction are used for dose reduction.
5. **Image Reconstruction and Analysis**: The CT data are processed to create two-dimensional and three-dimensional images of the colon.
6. **Interpretation**: Radiologists analyze the images for the presence of polyps, masses, or other abnormalities. Lesions larger than 6 mm typically warrant further evaluation, which may include a traditional colonoscopy for biopsy or removal.

"Polyp" is defined as a structure with homogeneous soft-tissue attenuation that arises from the colonic mucosa, characterized by a fixed point of attachment to the bowel wall and projecting into the colonic lumen.

A "mass" is defined as any colonic lesion with soft-tissue attenuation, greater than 3 cm in its largest dimension.

1. **Polypoid Lesions**: Polyps appear as well-defined, round, or ovoid protuberances arising from the colonic mucosa. They typically project into the lumen of the colon and can vary in size from a few millimeters to several centimeters.
2. **Surface Characteristics**: The surface of a polyp on virtual colonoscopy is usually smooth, but larger polyps may have an irregular or lobulated surface. The detailed 3D reconstructions enable visualization of these surface features, aiding in the differentiation between benign and potentially malignant polyps.
3. **Soft Tissue Density**: Polyps typically exhibit soft tissue density on CT images, which distinguishes them from other intraluminal contents, such as residual stool or air bubbles. The soft tissue density helps in confirming the presence of a true polyp rather than a pseudolesion.

4. **Stalked (Pedunculated) vs. Sessile Polyps**: Polyps can be classified based on their attachment to the colonic wall. Pedunculated polyps are attached to the mucosa by a narrow stalk, appearing as a mushroom-like structure, while sessile polyps have a broad base and are flatter against the mucosa. Virtual colonoscopy effectively differentiates these types based on their appearance.
5. **Contrast Enhancement and 3D Views**: Contrast enhancement in virtual colonoscopy is not typically required, but the 3D views and "fly-through" navigation allow radiologists to assess the polyp's size, shape, and relation to surrounding structures. These views help in determining the clinical significance of the polyp and the need for further intervention, such as traditional colonoscopy or polypectomy.

Contraindications of Virtual Colonoscopy

1. **Acute Colonic Conditions**: Patients with active inflammatory bowel disease, diverticulitis, or suspected bowel perforation should not undergo CT colonography due to the risk of bowel perforation and exacerbation of these conditions.
2. **Recent Colonic Surgery**:
3. **Severe Cardiopulmonary Conditions**: Patients with severe cardiopulmonary conditions, such as uncontrolled heart failure or severe chronic obstructive pulmonary disease (COPD), may not tolerate bowel insufflation.
4. **Pregnancy**: Although the radiation dose used in virtual colonoscopy is low, it is generally contraindicated in pregnant women due to potential risks to the fetus.
5. Inability to undergo bowel preparation.

7. Role of CT in initial imaging and follow-up of GIST. [5] [MD (WBUHS) 24, DNB Dec 21, AIIMS Dec 24]

Gastrointestinal stromal tumors are mesenchymal neoplasms of the gastrointestinal tract. Immunohistochemically they are C KIT (CD 117) and CD 34 positive.

Most GIST are benign with variable malignant potential. Malignant potential is assessed with size and mitotic figure rate on pathology. Tumors <2 cm are usually benign and >5cm are aggressive.

Role of CT in Imaging and Follow-up of Gastrointestinal Stromal Tumors (GIST)

Computed Tomography (CT) plays a critical role in the initial imaging, diagnosis, and follow-up of GISTs:

1. **Initial Detection and Characterization**: CT is the primary imaging modality for detecting GISTs. GIST may be submucosal, intramural or subserosal in location. Imaging cannot differentiate between benign and malignant lesions. On CT, GISTs typically appear as well-defined, heterogeneous masses, often with areas of necrosis, hemorrhage, or cystic degeneration. Calcifications may be seen. Tumors may exhibit an exophytic/endophytic or combined growth pattern and can be located anywhere along the gastrointestinal tract, most commonly in the stomach and small intestine. Ascites, lymph nodes, and metastatic deposits indicate malignancy.
2. **Tumor Staging**: CT is essential in staging GISTs by assessing tumor size, local invasion, and the presence of metastases. Common sites of metastasis include the liver and peritoneum. CT accurately delineates the extent of the disease, which is crucial for surgical planning and determining prognosis.
3. **Evaluation of Treatment Response**: For patients receiving targeted therapy, such as imatinib, CT is used to monitor the tumor's response. A decrease in tumor size and density on CT, along with reduced enhancement, indicates a positive response to treatment. The modified response evaluation criteria in solid tumors (mRECIST) guidelines are often used to assess treatment response.
4. **Detection of Recurrence**: During follow-up, CT scans are performed regularly to detect any signs of tumor recurrence. Recurrence can manifest as a new mass, an increase in the size of residual lesions, or new metastatic lesions. Regular CT imaging allows for early detection and prompt management of recurrences.
5. **Surgical Planning and Postoperative Follow-up**: CT aids in preoperative planning by providing detailed anatomical information about the tumor's relationship with surrounding structures. Postoperatively, CT is used to monitor the surgical site for any residual disease, complications, or recurrence.

8. (a) Imaging features of intestinal TB on barium meal follow-through and CT (b) difference between intestinal TB and Crohn's disease. [10] [DNB June 21]

Imaging Features of intestinal TB on Barium Meal Follow-through and CT

Barium Studies (BMFT) **(Table 8)**:

TABLE 8: Representing features of ileocecal tuberculosis on barium meal follow-through.

Early involvement	*Advanced disease*
Thickening of the ileocecal valve and wide gaping of the valve with narrowing of terminal ileum - called an inverted umbrella sign/Fleisher sign.	Symmetric, annular, "napkin ring" stenosis of the ileocecal valve. Shrunken and retracted cecum. Narrowing of terminal ileum. Dilated proximal ileum. "Goose-neck deformity"- Loss of ileocecal angle with Dilated ileum hanging from contracted and retracted cecum. • String Sign: Narrowing of the terminal ileum or other affected segments may produce a "string sign," where the lumen appears narrowed and irregular, resembling a string. This is due to the thickening and fibrosis of the bowel wall. • Pseudopolyps and Mucosal Nodularity: Mucosal irregularity with the appearance of pseudopolyps and nodules can be seen, especially in the terminal ileum, reflecting granulomatous inflammation. • Fistulae and Sinuses: Although less common, barium studies may reveal the presence of fistulae or sinus tracts, which can develop due to the chronic inflammatory process in TB.

CT Imaging Features: CT enterography (CTE) is an investigation of choice for the evaluation of ileocecal TB.

1. **Concentric Bowel Wall Thickening**: CT enterography typically shows asymmetric, concentric thickening of the bowel wall, particularly in the ileocecal region. This thickening is often associated with the narrowing of the lumen.
2. **Lymphadenopathy**: Mesenteric lymph nodes are commonly enlarged, with a characteristic central area of low attenuation due to caseous necrosis. The presence of these "necrotic" lymph nodes is a key feature of TB on CTE.
3. **Adhered Bowel Loops**: Thickened bowel loops may appear adhered together due to the presence of fibrosis, and inflammatory exudates.
4. **Complications**: Complications such as perforation, abscess formation, and fistulas may also be visualized on CT, providing a comprehensive evaluation of the extent of the disease.

Differences Between CT Features of Intestinal Tuberculosis and Crohn's Disease

The main differences between CT Features of Intestinal Tuberculosis and Crohn's disease are represented in the following table **(Table 9)**:

TABLE 9: Shows the main differences between CT features of intestinal tuberculosis and Crohn's disease.

Findings	*Tb*	*Crohn's disease*
Patient history	Patients often present with H/o tuberculosis exposure, positive tuberculin test, reside in TB endemic areas, etc.	• The patient's symptoms are relapsing-remitting type. • A family history of inflammatory disease may be present.
Symptom onset	• Subacute to the chronic onset of fever, night sweats, weight loss, etc. • Diarrhea is less frequent.	• Chronic symptoms of diarrhea, weight loss, and recurrent abdominal pain. • May be associated with perianal fissures and fistula. • Extraintestinal manifestations may be present like arthritis and skin involvement. • Diarrhea is more frequent.
Imaging findings		
Site	Cecum more common	Terminal ileum is more common

Continued...

Continued...

Findings	***Tb***	***Crohn's disease***
Length of involvement	Short segment	Long segment
Multiple site involvement	Uncommon (<4)	Common
Skip lesions		
Type of enhancement	Homogenous	Stratified
Mural stratification	Rarely seen	Common
Perianal fistula	Uncommon	Common
Mesenteric abscesses	Uncommon	Common
Interbowel fistula	Rare	Common
Stricture	Concentric	Eccentric with sacculation
Enterolith	More common	Less common
Increased mesenteric vascularity	Uncommon	Common
Fibrofatty proliferation	Uncommon	Common
Mesenteric nodes	Larger, Necrotic	Small homogenous
Omental involvement	Often present	Rare
Ascites	Present	Absent
Solid organ involvement	May be present	Very rare
Endoscopic		
Mucosal changes	Transverse ulcers, pseudopolyps	Deep longitudinal ulcers, aphthous ulcers
Skip lesions	Uncommon	More common
Fistulae	Uncommon	Common
Patulous ileocecal valve	Common	Rare
Anorectal disease	Uncommon	Common
Histology		
Granuloma	Multiple, confluent, caseating, submucosal	Microgranuloma, single, nonconfluent, noncaseating
Disproportionate submucosal inflammation	Common	Rare

Liver and Biliary Tract

1. Write in brief about the technique of triple-phase CT scan for focal hepatic lesions. Describe triple-phase CT scan findings in hepatocellular carcinoma (HCC). [5+5] [MD (WBUHS) 18, AIIMS May 24]

The Technique of Triple-phase CT Scan for Focal Hepatic Lesions

A triple-phase CT scan is a useful examination for the assessment of focal hepatic lesions. It involves acquiring images during three different phases i.e., arterial, portal venous, and delayed phase of contrast enhancement to assess the vascular characteristics of liver lesions:

1. **Patient Preparation: Fasting**: Fasting for at least 4–6 hours before the scan to reduce the risk of adverse reactions to contrast and to minimize the presence of gastric contents that could obscure the liver.

2. **Administration of Contrast: Contrast Injection**: Iodinated contrast material is administered intravenously at a rate of 3–5 mL/second using a power injector. The total amount of contrast usually ranges from 100 to 150 mL, depending on the patient's body weight and renal function.
3. **Imaging Phases**:
   - Arterial Phase (Late Arterial Phase): This phase is typically acquired 15–25 seconds after the start of the contrast injection. During this phase, the hepatic arteries enhance, allowing for the detection of hypervascular lesions, such as hepatocellular carcinoma, which appear more conspicuous due to their early uptake of contrast.
   - Portal Venous Phase: Acquired approximately 60–70 seconds after the start of the contrast injection, this phase allows for optimal enhancement of the liver parenchyma and portal vein. It is crucial for identifying hypovascular lesions, such as metastases or cholangiocarcinoma, which may be more conspicuous in this phase due to the relative lack of enhancement compared to the surrounding liver.
   - Delayed Phase (Equilibrium Phase): This phase is typically captured 3–5 minutes after contrast injection. During this phase, the contrast begins to wash out from the liver parenchyma, and certain lesions, like HCC, may exhibit a characteristic washout, becoming hypoattenuating relative to the enhanced liver tissue. Fibrotic or scar tissue within lesions may retain contrast longer, aiding in characterization.
4. **Image Acquisition and Reconstruction**:
   - Thin-slice Imaging: Images are usually acquired with thin slices (1–3 mm) to provide detailed anatomy and to allow for multiplanar reconstructions (MPR), which are helpful in lesion localization and assessment.
   - Post-processing: After image acquisition, the data are reconstructed to create axial, coronal, and sagittal images, and sometimes 3D reconstructions, which can be valuable for surgical planning or further characterization of the lesion.
5. **Interpretation**: Radiologists evaluate the images across all three phases, comparing the enhancement patterns of the focal lesion with that of the surrounding liver parenchyma. Key features such as arterial phase hyperenhancement, portal venous phase hypodensity, and delayed washout are analyzed to characterize the lesion and differentiate between benign and malignant entities.

Triple-phase CT Scan Findings in Hepatocellular Carcinoma

Hepatocellular carcinoma is the most common primary liver cancer, and triple-phase CT scanning is an essential imaging modality for its diagnosis and characterization. The technique involves imaging the liver in three phases after the administration of intravenous contrast: arterial, portal venous, and delayed phases. Here are the typical findings in HCC during these phases:

1. **Arterial Phase Hyperenhancement**:
   - Finding: HCC typically shows early, intense enhancement during the arterial phase (15–25 seconds postcontrast administration). This hyperenhancement is due to the tumor's predominantly arterial blood supply, distinguishing it from the surrounding liver parenchyma, which is mainly supplied by the portal vein.
   - Significance: The arterial phase hyperenhancement is a hallmark of HCC, helping differentiate it from benign liver lesions such as hemangiomas, which do not enhance in this pattern.
2. **Portal Venous Phase Washout**:
   - Finding: In the portal venous phase (60–70 seconds postcontrast), HCC often shows "washout," appearing hypodense (darker) compared to the surrounding liver tissue, which enhances uniformly. This occurs because the tumor washes out the contrast faster than the normal liver parenchyma.
   - Significance: Washout is a key feature that suggests malignancy, particularly HCC, and is critical in differentiating it from benign lesions that maintain contrast enhancement.
3. **Delayed Phase Hypoattenuation**:
   - Finding: During the delayed phase (3–5 minutes postcontrast), HCC lesions typically continue to appear hypoattenuating relative to the surrounding liver. The delayed washout further confirms the presence of the tumor.
   - Significance: Persistent hypoattenuation in the delayed phase is a characteristic finding in HCC, distinguishing it from other hypervascular lesions that may retain contrast longer, such as fibrolamellar HCC or certain metastases.

4. **Capsule Appearance**:
   - Finding: A fibrous capsule may be visible around the tumor, particularly in the delayed phase, appearing as a hyperdense rim. This capsule is associated with well-differentiated HCC and can help in confirming the diagnosis.
   - Significance: The presence of a capsule suggests a slower-growing, more indolent form of HCC, which can influence management decisions.
5. **Intratumoral Heterogeneity**:
   - Finding: HCCs often show internal heterogeneity due to necrosis, hemorrhage, or fat content, leading to areas of differing enhancement within the tumor. Some regions may not enhance at all, while others may enhance unevenly.
   - Significance: This heterogeneity can help distinguish HCC from other liver tumors, such as metastases, which tend to have more uniform enhancement patterns.

2. List the indications of hepatobiliary scintigraphy in children and adults. Describe briefly the principle, technique, and findings on scintigraphy in a case of neonatal jaundice. [2+2+2+4] [MD (WBUHS) 23]

Indications of Hepatobiliary Scintigraphy in Children and Adults

Hepatobiliary scintigraphy, also known as a HIDA scan (hepatobiliary iminodiacetic acid scan), is a nuclear medicine imaging technique used to evaluate the function of the liver, gallbladder, and bile ducts. The indications for this procedure can vary between children and adults due to differences in common disease presentations in these populations.

Indications in Children

1. **Neonatal Cholestasis**: To differentiate between extrahepatic biliary atresia (EHBA) and neonatal hepatitis. Hepatobiliary scintigraphy is crucial in determining whether there is a patent bile duct system.
2. **Biliary Atresia**: To confirm or exclude the diagnosis of biliary atresia, a condition where the bile ducts are blocked or absent, preventing bile from draining from the liver to the intestine.
3. **Congenital Biliary Disorders**: For the evaluation of congenital anomalies of the bile ducts, such as choledochal cysts or Caroli disease.
4. **Postsurgical Assessment**: To assess the patency and function of the bile ducts after surgical procedures, such as the Kasai portoenterostomy in infants with biliary atresia.
5. **Acute Cholecystitis**: Although less common in children, hepatobiliary scintigraphy can be used to diagnose acute cholecystitis when ultrasound findings are inconclusive.

Indications in Adults

1. **Acute and Chronic Cholecystitis**: To diagnose acute cholecystitis, especially when ultrasound findings are equivocal. The test is useful for identifying cystic duct obstruction, a key feature of acute cholecystitis. It is also used in the evaluation of chronic cholecystitis to assess gallbladder function.
2. **Biliary Dyskinesia**: To assess gallbladder ejection fraction in patients with suspected biliary dyskinesia, where symptoms such as biliary colic occur without evidence of gallstones.
3. **Bile Leak Detection**: To detect bile leaks following trauma, surgery (e.g., cholecystectomy), or liver transplantation. Hepatobiliary scintigraphy can pinpoint the site of the leak.
4. **Evaluation of Jaundice**: In the workup of jaundice, particularly when the cause is unclear, hepatobiliary scintigraphy can help assess the functional integrity of the biliary system.
5. **Postliver Transplantation**: To assess biliary drainage and detect complications such as biliary obstruction or leaks following liver transplantation.
6. **Assessment of Biliary Obstruction**: To determine the presence and level of biliary obstruction, especially when other imaging modalities (like ultrasound or MRCP) provide inconclusive results.

7. **Postoperative Complications**: To evaluate for complications following biliary surgery, such as bile duct injuries or strictures that might lead to impaired bile flow.

Scintigraphy in Neonatal Jaundice: Principle, Technique, and Findings

Principle

Hepatobiliary scintigraphy, commonly known as a HIDA scan, is a nuclear medicine imaging technique that evaluates the function of the liver, gallbladder, bile ducts, and small intestine. The principle behind the test involves the intravenous administration of a radiopharmaceutical agent, usually a technetium-99m-labeled iminodiacetic acid (Tc-99m IDA) derivative. This radiotracer is selectively taken up by hepatocytes and excreted into the bile, mimicking the physiological process of bile formation and flow. The gamma camera detects the radiation emitted by the radiotracer, providing real-time images of the hepatobiliary system.

In the context of neonatal jaundice, hepatobiliary scintigraphy is primarily used to differentiate between extrahepatic biliary atresia (EHBA) and other causes of neonatal cholestasis, such as neonatal hepatitis. The ability of the radiotracer to pass from the liver into the bowel is key to determining whether the biliary system is obstructed or not.

Technique

1. **Preparation**:
   - Patient Preparation: The neonate should be adequately hydrated, and oral feeding may need to be withheld for a few hours before the scan to reduce gastrointestinal motility that could obscure imaging.
   - Phenobarbital Pretreatment: In some cases, phenobarbital is administered for 3–5 days prior to the scan to enhance biliary excretion by stimulating hepatic enzyme activity. This helps in distinguishing EHBA from hepatocellular dysfunction.
2. **Radiopharmaceutical Administration**: The radiopharmaceutical, typically Tc-99m mebrofenin or Tc-99m DISIDA (diisopropyl iminodiacetic acid), is injected intravenously. The usual dose is adjusted for the neonate's weight.
3. **Imaging Protocol**:
   - Initial Imaging: Immediately after the injection, dynamic imaging is performed to capture the uptake of the tracer by the liver. This is usually done over a period of 60 minutes.
   - Delayed Imaging: If the initial images do not show tracer activity in the bowel, delayed images are taken at intervals (usually 4–24 hours later) to allow sufficient time for the tracer to pass through the biliary system if it is patent.
4. **Interpretation**: The images are interpreted by analyzing the time-activity curves, the pattern of tracer uptake by the liver, and its subsequent excretion into the bile ducts and small intestine.

Findings

1. **Normal Findings**: In a healthy neonate, the radiotracer is rapidly taken up by the liver, with clear visualization of the biliary tree and gallbladder within 30–60 minutes. The tracer should then pass into the small intestine, indicating a patent biliary system. This pattern effectively rules out biliary atresia.
2. **Biliary Atresia (EHBA)**:
   - Absence of Bowel Excretion: In EHBA, the radiotracer is taken up by the liver but fails to enter the small intestine, even on delayed imaging. The tracer may accumulate in the liver and gallbladder (if present), but there is no visualization of the bowel.
   - Persistent Liver Uptake: The liver continues to show persistent uptake of the tracer, indicating an obstructed bile flow due to atresia of the extrahepatic bile ducts. The gallbladder may not be visible if it is underdeveloped or absent.
3. **Neonatal Hepatitis: Delayed but Present Bowel Excretion**: In cases of neonatal hepatitis, the radiotracer shows delayed excretion into the bowel. There is often a prolonged retention of the tracer in the liver, and the biliary ducts and gallbladder may be visualized, but with delayed or reduced intensity. The key finding is that bowel excretion, although delayed, is eventually seen, distinguishing it from biliary atresia.
4. **Other Conditions**:
   - Alagille Syndrome: In this genetic disorder, the scintigraphy may show poor tracer excretion similar to neonatal hepatitis but associated clinical findings and genetic tests help in the diagnosis.

- Choledochal Cyst: If a choledochal cyst is present, the radiotracer may accumulate in the cyst, showing a dilated biliary tree with delayed emptying.

3. Discuss different imaging modalities in the evaluation of focal hepatic lesions. [10] [MD (WBUHS) 20, AIIMS May 23]

Liver lesions, due to their varied etiology and clinical significance, require accurate imaging to differentiate between benign and malignant conditions. Here is a breakdown of liver lesions, classifications, and how imaging modalities contribute to their diagnosis:

Categories of Liver Lesions

A. **Focal Liver Lesions**:
   - **Benign lesions that are usually asymptomatic**: These do not require treatment unless symptomatic like hepatic hemangiomas, focal nodular hyperplasia (FNH), and benign liver cysts.
   - **Benign lesions that often require treatment**: Lesions that have potential complications, such as bleeding or infection. For example, Hepatic adenoma (risk of hemorrhage or malignant transformation), hepatic abscess (requires drainage), and symptomatic hepatic adenomas.
   - **Malignant lesions**: Primary or secondary (metastatic) tumors of the liver. For example, Hepatocellular carcinoma, cholangiocarcinoma, hepatic angiosarcoma, and metastatic liver lesions from primary cancers (e.g., colorectal cancer).

B. **Diffuse Liver Lesions**:
   - Vascular Diseases: Conditions affecting liver blood flow, such as Budd-Chiari syndrome or hepatic venous congestion.
   - Inflammatory Conditions: Liver diseases like hepatitis and cirrhosis.
   - Storage Disorders: Diseases like hepatic steatosis (fatty liver), hemochromatosis (iron overload), and Wilson's disease (copper accumulation).

Imaging Modalities in Focal Hepatic Lesions

1. **Ultrasound (US)**:
   - **Role**: First-line imaging for liver lesions, valuable for screening and differentiating simple cysts, solid lesions, and fatty liver changes.
   - **Lesion Characteristics**:
     - **Hemangioma**: Typically appears as a well-defined, hyperechoic lesion; occasionally heterogeneous in larger hemangiomas.
     - **Hepatocellular Carcinoma**: Variable appearance; can be hypoechoic or hyperechoic. Doppler US may reveal hypervascularity.
     - **Liver Metastases**: Often hypoechoic with a halo or "target" appearance, although this varies with the primary tumor type.
     - **Fatty Liver Disease**: Diffuse hyperechogenicity compared to the renal cortex, indicating hepatic steatosis.
   - **Contrast-enhanced Ultrasound (CEUS)**: Used to differentiate benign from malignant lesions based on real-time contrast dynamics.
     - **HCC**: Shows rapid arterial phase enhancement followed by washout in the portal venous phase.
     - **Hemangiomas**: Show peripheral nodular enhancement with gradual centripetal filling over time, consistent with benign vascular lesions.
     - **Metastases**: Generally, show rapid washout after early arterial enhancement, a pattern suggesting malignancy.

2. **Computed Tomography**
   - **Protocols**:
     - **Noncontrast CT**: Detects hepatic steatosis, iron/calcium deposition, and baseline densities of liver lesions.
     - **Single-phase (portal venous phase)**: Conducted 70 seconds postcontrast injection, captures maximum liver enhancement. Useful for evaluating hypovascular lesions and diffuse liver diseases like cirrhosis and hypovascular metastases (e.g., colorectal metastasis).

- **Dual-phase (arterial and portal venous phases)**: Captures liver images in both arterial (35 seconds postcontrast) and portal venous phases, better identifying hypervascular lesions like HCC, metastatic renal cell carcinoma, and breast cancer metastasis.
- **Triphasic (arterial, portal venous, and delayed phases)**: Provides nonenhanced, arterial, and portal phases; often essential for hypervascular lesions, particularly in cirrhotic patients.

- **Lesion Characteristics**:
  - **Hepatocellular Carcinoma**: Enhances in the arterial phase (due to hypervascularity) with washout in the portal venous phase, often showing a rim of hypointensity on delayed phases.
  - **Hemangioma**: Appears as a hypodense lesion with peripheral nodular enhancement in the arterial phase, followed by centripetal filling over time, a hallmark of this benign vascular lesion.
  - **Cholangiocarcinoma**: Shows delayed enhancement due to its fibrous stroma. The triphasic CT is particularly useful, as the delayed phase better highlights the fibrous composition.
  - **Fatty Liver Disease**: On noncontrast CT, hepatic attenuation appears at least 10 Hounsfield units (HU) lower than the spleen. In the portal venous phase, 25 HU less than the spleen suggests steatosis.

3. **Magnetic Resonance Imaging**:
   - **Sequences**:
     - **T1-Weighted Imaging**: Fatty lesions (e.g., hepatic adenoma with fat) appear hyperintense, while most other liver lesions are hypointense.
     - **T2-Weighted Imaging**: Cystic and vascular lesions like hemangiomas appear hyperintense; malignancies (e.g., HCC) typically show mild hyperintensity.
     - **In-phase and Out-of-phase Gradient Echo**: Identifies hepatic steatosis by showing signal drop on out-of-phase images.
     - **Dynamic Contrast Phases**: Arterial, portal venous, and delayed phases help evaluate vascularity and enhancement patterns.
     - **Hepatobiliary-specific Contrast Agents**: Gadoxetic acid (Gd-EOB-DTPA) and similar agents can enhance liver imaging in the hepatobiliary phase, distinguishing lesions based on hepatocyte uptake.
   - **Lesion Characteristics**:
     - **HCC**: Shows arterial enhancement with portal venous washout. Differs from other lesions due to high signal in T2 and hyperintense rim in delayed phase.
     - **Focal Nodular Hyperplasia (FNH)**: Iso- or hyperintense in hepatobiliary phase due to contrast retention by hepatocytes. Often has a central scar visible on T2-weighted imaging, enhancing in delayed phases.
     - **Hepatic Adenoma**: Appears hypointense in the hepatobiliary phase, distinguishing it from FNH. Often shows early arterial enhancement with rapid washout.
     - **Hemangiomas**: T1 hypointense, T2 hyperintense, with peripheral nodular enhancement that fills centrally over time.
4. **Positron Emission Tomography-computed Tomography (PET-CT)**:
   - **Role**: Primarily for evaluating metastatic disease, recurrence, and treatment response, as PET-CT detects metabolic activity in malignancies.
   - **Lesion Characteristics**:
     - **Metastatic Lesions**: Hypermetabolic metastases (e.g., from colorectal cancer) appear as FDG-avid foci. These lesions generally show increased FDG uptake, making PET useful for identifying and staging metastatic disease.
     - **Hepatocellular Carcinoma**: Has variable FDG uptake; FDG-PET is not routinely used in HCC diagnosis but may be helpful in specific cases.
   - **Limitations**: PET has limited sensitivity for lesions under 1 cm, which may be challenging in cases of small metastases or early HCC.
5. **Nuclear Medicine (SPECT and PET)**:
   - **Role**: Useful for staging malignancy, assessing metastatic spread, and response to therapies.

- **Lesion Characteristics**: **Hypermetabolic Liver Metastases**: These lesions are often visible on FDG-PET scans and are particularly relevant for patients with known cancers (e.g., colorectal carcinoma).
- **Treatment and Therapeutics**: Used in TARE (trans-arterial radioembolization) or radio-labeled therapies to target hepatic lesions directly.

6. **Angiography**:
   - **Role**: Primarily an interventional tool; used in procedures like trans-arterial chemoembolization (TACE) and radioembolization for HCC.
   - **Lesion Characteristics**:
     - **HCC**: Detailed arterial anatomy and tumor vascularity are mapped out before procedures such as TACE.
     - **FNH and Hypervascular Metastases**: Angiography helps characterize the vascular supply, providing essential details for surgical or interventional planning.

4. Noninvasive evaluation of primary liver tumor. [10] [MD (WBUHS) 20]

Primary liver tumors are tumors that originate within the liver, and they can be either benign or malignant. Here is a list of the main primary liver tumors:

Benign Primary Liver Tumor

- **Hepatic Hemangioma**: Most common benign liver tumor; typically, asymptomatic.
- **Focal Nodular Hyperplasia (FNH)**: Hypervascular with a central scar; second most common.
- **Hepatic Adenoma**: Risk of bleeding and rare malignant transformation.
- **Biliary Cystadenoma**: Rare, cystic, potential for malignancy.

Malignant

- **Hepatocellular Carcinoma**: Most common malignant tumor; linked to cirrhosis.
- **Cholangiocarcinoma**: Bile duct cancer, poor prognosis, often diagnosed late.
- **Hepatoblastoma**: Common in young children, rare in adults.
- **Angiosarcoma**: Rare, aggressive, linked to chemical exposures.
- **Fibrolamellar Carcinoma**: Affects young adults with, a better prognosis than HCC.

Each of these tumors has unique imaging characteristics, aiding in their diagnosis and differentiation from other liver lesions.

Evaluation of These Tumors

1. **Hepatic Hemangioma (Benign)**:
   - **Ultrasound (US)**:
     - Typically appears as a well-defined, hyperechoic lesion.
     - Larger hemangiomas may show heterogeneous echotexture.
   - **Contrast-Enhanced Ultrasound (CEUS)**:
     - Shows peripheral nodular enhancement in the arterial phase.
     - Gradual centripetal filling, with complete filling in the delayed phase.
   - **CT**:
     - **Noncontrast**: Hypodense lesion.
     - **Arterial phase**: Peripheral nodular enhancement.
     - **Delayed phase**: Progressive centripetal filling; often fully filled in delayed phases.
   - **MRI**:
     - **T1-weighted**: Hypointense.
     - **T2-weighted**: Hyperintense (characteristic "light bulb" sign on T2).
     - **Postcontrast (Gadolinium)**: Peripheral nodular enhancement with centripetal filling over time.

2. **Focal Nodular Hyperplasia (FNH) (Benign)**:
   - **Ultrasound**:
     - Iso- or hypoechoic lesion with a central scar in larger lesions.
     - Color Doppler may show central vascularity.
   - **CEUS**:
     - Early arterial phase enhancement with centrifugal filling.
     - Iso enhancement to liver parenchyma in the portal and delayed phases.
   - **CT**:
     - **Noncontrast**: Often iso- or hypodense.
     - **Arterial phase**: Homogeneous, intense enhancement.
     - **Delayed phase**: Central scar may enhance.
   - **MRI**:
     - **T1-weighted**: Iso- or hypointense.
     - **T2-weighted**: Central scar appears hyperintense.
     - **Hepatobiliary phase (e.g., with gadoxetic acid)**: Retains contrast and appears hyperintense relative to surrounding liver tissue.
3. **Hepatic Adenoma (Benign but Risk of Malignancy)**:
   - **Ultrasound**: Hyperechoic or iso-echoic, sometimes heterogeneous due to fat or hemorrhage.
   - **CEUS**:
     - Arterial phase hyperenhancement with early, marked washout in the portal phase.
     - Can show heterogeneous enhancement due to internal hemorrhage or fat.
   - **CT**:
     - **Noncontrast**: May appear hypodense or show fat content.
     - **Arterial phase**: Rapid enhancement due to vascularity.
     - **Portal venous and delayed phases**: Washout is typical.
   - **MRI**:
     - **T1-weighted**: Hyperintense if fat is present.
     - **T2-weighted**: Variable; hyperintense if hemorrhage or fat is present.
     - **Postcontrast**: Arterial enhancement with rapid washout.
     - **Hepatobiliary phase**: Typically appears hypointense, distinguishing it from FNH.
4. **Biliary Cystadenoma (Benign but Malignant Potential)**:
   - **Ultrasound**:
     - Multiloculated cystic structure with thin septations.
     - Often shows internal septations or solid nodules.
   - **CT**:
     - **Noncontrast**: Hypodense, cystic lesion.
     - **Postcontrast**: Septal and mural enhancement.
   - **MRI**:
     - **T1-weighted**: Hypointense, but proteinaceous content may increase intensity.
     - **T2-weighted**: Hyperintense with septal enhancement on postcontrast images.
5. **Hepatocellular Carcinoma (Malignant)**:
   - **Ultrasound**:
     - Variable; may be hypoechoic, hyperechoic, or mixed echogenicity.
     - Color Doppler shows hypervascularity.
   - **CEUS**:
     - Rapid arterial phase hyperenhancement.
     - Washout in the portal and delayed phases.

- **CT**:
  - Noncontrast: Often hypo- or iso-dense.
  - Arterial phase: Enhances due to arterial supply.
  - Portal venous phase: Washout appearance.
  - Delayed phase: Capsule enhancement may be visible.
- **MRI**:
  - T1-weighted: Hypointense.
  - T2-weighted: Mildly hyperintense.
  - Postcontrast: Arterial enhancement with washout in portal venous and delayed phases.
  - Hepatobiliary phase (with gadoxetic acid): Typically, hypointense due to lack of functional hepatocytes.

6. **Cholangiocarcinoma (Malignant)**:
   - **Ultrasound**: Hypoechoic, irregular mass; may show biliary ductal dilation.
   - **CT**:
     - Noncontrast: Hypodense or isodense.
     - Arterial phase: Peripheral enhancement.
     - Portal venous and delayed phases: Progressive, delayed enhancement due to fibrous stroma.
   - **MRI**:
     - T1-weighted: Hypointense.
     - T2-weighted: Hyperintense due to fibrous content.
     - Postcontrast: Progressive enhancement in delayed phases due to fibrotic tissue.

   Magnetic Resonance Cholangiopancreatography (MRCP): May show bile duct dilation and obstruction.
7. **Hepatoblastoma (Pediatric Malignant Tumor)**:
   - **Ultrasound**:
     - Heterogeneous mass, often with calcifications.
     - Color Doppler can show hypervascularity.
   - **CT**:
     - Noncontrast: Heterogeneous with calcifications.
     - Arterial phase: Hypervascular enhancement.
     - Portal venous phase: May show washout.
   - **MRI**:
     - T1-weighted: Variable; can be hypointense.
     - T2-weighted: Hyperintense with heterogeneous appearance.
     - Postcontrast: Arterial enhancement with possible washout.
8. **Angiosarcoma (Aggressive Malignant Tumor)**:
   - **Ultrasound**:
     - Heterogeneous, often complex echotexture.
     - May show hypervascularity on Doppler imaging.
   - **CT**:
     - Noncontrast: Hypodense, heterogeneous.
     - Arterial phase: Irregular, heterogeneous enhancement.
     - Delayed phase: Persistent enhancement in some areas.
   - **MRI**:
     - T1-weighted: Hypointense or heterogeneous.
     - T2-weighted: Hyperintense with hemorrhagic areas.
     - Postcontrast: Irregular, heterogeneous enhancement due to vascular nature.

9. **Fibrolamellar Carcinoma (Subtype of HCC, Malignant)**:
   - **Ultrasound**: Large, heterogeneous mass; may show central scar.
   - **CT**:
     - Noncontrast: Heterogeneous, often hypodense.
     - Arterial phase: Hyperenhancement with possible central scar.
     - Delayed phase: Central scar may show delayed enhancement.
   - **MRI**:
     - T1-weighted: Hypointense with hyperintense central scar.
     - T2-weighted: Central scar is hyperintense.
     - Postcontrast: Arterial enhancement with delayed central scar enhancement.

5. Role of interventional radiology in hepatic malignancy. [10] [MD (WBUHS) 21]

Interventional radiology is essential in managing liver tumors, particularly hepatocellular carcinoma. It helps in the following aspects described below:

- **Diagnosis**: Image-guided biopsies (needle core and fine-needle aspiration) help confirm HCC and assess tumor grade.
- **Treatment**: Transarterial therapies (e.g., TACE and TARE) and percutaneous ablations (e.g., RFA and MWA) target tumors directly, sparing healthy liver tissue, especially for nonsurgical candidates.
- **Advanced Disease**: For advanced HCC, these interventions aim to control symptoms, slow progression, and improve quality of life, with TARE beneficial in cases with portal vein thrombosis.
  Interventional radiology thus supports diagnosis, localized treatment, and palliation in HCC.

Interventional Procedures in Treatment Aspects

1. Transarterial Therapies

Rationale: These therapies take advantage of the liver's dual blood supply. While the liver receives 75% of its blood flow from the portal vein, tumors such as HCC are supplied predominantly by the hepatic artery. By targeting the hepatic artery, these treatments can deliver agents directly to the tumor while sparing healthy liver tissue.

1.1. **Bland Embolization**:
   - **Mechanism**: Small particles (40–50 μm) are injected to block the tumor's arterial blood supply, leading to ischemia and tumor necrosis.
   - **Indications**: Occasionally used in centers where TACE is not preferred or as an alternative to chemotherapy. Bland embolization may offer similar outcomes to TACE for some patients.
   - **Procedure**: Performed under fluoroscopic guidance; selective cannulation of the feeding hepatic artery branches is achieved, followed by injection of embolic particles until complete stasis is reached.

1.2. **Transarterial Chemoembolization (TACE)**:
   - **Mechanism**: Combines localized chemotherapy with embolization to enhance tumor necrosis. Chemotherapeutic agents (e.g., doxorubicin, cisplatin) are mixed with lipiodol, a radiopaque oil that stays within the tumor, acting as a carrier and microembolic agent. Lipiodol accumulates in the tumor, allowing prolonged drug exposure.
   - **Indications**: Ideal for intermediate-stage HCC with preserved liver function; contraindicated in cases of portal vein thrombosis or severely impaired liver function.

   Procedure:
   - A catheter is advanced into the hepatic artery, and a microcatheter is used to selectively deliver the chemoembolic mixture to the tumor.
   - After the chemotherapeutic agent and lipiodol are administered, additional embolic particles (polyvinyl alcohol or gel foam) are used to block blood flow.
   - Completion angiography confirms tumor ischemia.

   Preparation and Postcare:
   - Patients are well hydrated to reduce nephrotoxicity risk, and preprocedure antibiotics are administered to prevent infection.

- Postprocedure, patients may experience postembolization syndrome (pain, fever, nausea), which is managed with antiemetics and NSAIDs.

1.3. **Drug-eluting Beads (DEB-TACE)**:
- **Mechanism**: Polyvinyl alcohol beads loaded with chemotherapeutic agents are delivered to the tumor. These beads release the drug slowly over time, extending tumor exposure and reducing systemic side effects.
- **Advantages**: Compared to conventional TACE, DEB-TACE maintains a lower systemic drug concentration, reducing toxic effects and improving response rates.
- **Procedure**: Similar to conventional TACE, with beads delivered directly to the tumor's arterial supply using a microcatheter.

1.4. **Transarterial Radioembolization (TARE)**:
- **Mechanism**: Yttrium-90 (Y-90) radioactive microspheres are injected into the hepatic artery to deliver localized radiation to the tumor. These beta-emitting spheres have a short range (1–2 mm), minimizing exposure to surrounding liver tissue.
- **Indications**: Used for larger or unresectable tumors; effective in cases of portal vein thrombosis, as the minimal embolic effect allows continued blood flow.
- **Procedure**:
  - A detailed angiogram maps the tumor's arterial supply, and any gastrointestinal branches are embolized to prevent off-target effects.
  - A test dose of 99mTc MAA (macroaggregated albumin) is used to assess lung shunt fraction.
  - After dose calculation, the Y-90 microspheres are delivered intra-arterially under real-time imaging guidance.
- **Postprocedure**: Follow-up imaging (CT or MRI) at 6 weeks assesses necrosis and treatment response. Common side effects include fatigue, mild liver toxicity, and, rarely, radiation-induced complications.

2. Percutaneous Ablative Therapies

Rationale: These therapies destroy tumor tissue directly and are best suited for small, localized tumors. These techniques are minimally invasive and use imaging guidance for precise targeting.

2.1. **Radiofrequency Ablation (RFA)**:
- **Mechanism**: RFA uses high-frequency electrical currents to generate heat within the tumor, causing coagulative necrosis.
- **Indications**: Best for tumors <3 cm, located away from large blood vessels (to avoid the "heat sink" effect).
- **Procedure**:
  - Under ultrasound or CT guidance, a needle electrode is inserted into the tumor. The electrode generates an alternating current, heating the tissue to 50–100°C for 4–6 minutes.
  - Expandable electrodes allow larger areas to be treated, and cooling mechanisms can control heat distribution.
- **Postprocedure**: CT imaging at 1 week shows a nonenhancing area of necrosis. Follow-up imaging every 3–4 months assesses for residual disease.
- **Complications**: Risks include hepatic abscess, bleeding, bile duct injury, and tumor seeding along the needle tract. For tumors near critical structures, 5% dextrose can be injected as a buffer.

2.2. **Microwave Ablation (MWA)**:
- **Mechanism**: Uses microwave energy to generate heat and achieve higher intratumoral temperatures than RFA.
- **Advantages**: MWA heats tissue faster, treats larger tumors, and is less affected by the heat sink effect. It also allows multiple applicators to be used simultaneously.
- **Procedure**: Similar to RFA, but MWA is quicker, making it suitable for larger or difficult-to-treat tumors.

2.3. **Cryoablation**:
- **Mechanism**: Uses cycles of freezing and thawing to destroy tumor cells. Ice crystals form within the cells during freezing, causing cell death.
- **Advantages**: Reduced procedural pain and clear visualization of the "ice ball" on imaging, allowing precision treatment. Cryoablation preserves the structure of nearby blood vessels and visceral lining.
- **Procedure**: Performed under imaging guidance; ideal for tumors close to sensitive structures (e.g., gallbladder, bowel).

2.4. **Chemical Ablation**:
- **Types**: Percutaneous Ethanol Injection (PEI) or Acetic Acid Injection.
- **Mechanism**: Injected chemicals cause dehydration and necrosis of tumor cells.
- **Application**: Primarily used for small tumors (<3 cm) or when thermal ablation is contraindicated. PEI is most effective in small, well-defined HCCs.

3. Post-treatment and Response Evaluation

- **Postprocedure Care**: Patients typically receive IV fluids, antibiotics, antiemetics, and pain control. Post-embolization syndrome (fever, pain, nausea) is common but self-limited.
- **Response Evaluation**: At 6 weeks, CT or MRI assesses necrosis. The lack of contrast enhancement within the tumor indicates a complete response. Residual disease may appear as enhancing areas, requiring further treatment.
- **Repeat Treatments**: For TACE, additional cycles are performed until complete necrosis is achieved. If there is no response after two cycles, TACE may be discontinued.

6. Discuss the imaging protocol for focal liver lesions. What are the differentiating features of hepatic hemangioma, focal hepatocellular carcinoma, and solitary metastatic lesion? [3+7] [MD (WBUHS) 22]

Imaging Protocol for Focal Liver Lesions

1. **Computed Tomography**:
   - **Unenhanced CT**: Useful for detecting fat, and calcifications, and assessing hepatic steatosis.
   - **Single-phase CT**: Portal venous phase (70 seconds postcontrast) is standard for evaluating diffuse liver conditions and hypovascular lesions.
   - **Dual-phase CT**: Late arterial and portal phases enhance visualization of hypervascular lesions (e.g., HCC and metastases).
   - **Triphasic CT**: Combines noncontrast, arterial, portal venous, and sometimes delayed phases, essential for hypervascular lesions like HCC and cholangiocarcinoma.
2. **Magnetic Resonance Imaging (MRI)**:
   - **Multi-phase Protocol**: Includes arterial, portal, equilibrium, and hepatobiliary phases with hepatocyte-specific contrast agents for detailed characterization.
   - Sequences:
     - **T1-Weighted**: Identifies fat or hemorrhage.
     - **T2-Weighted**: Highlights cystic or vascular lesions (e.g., hemangiomas).
   - **Diffusion-weighted Imaging**: Useful for detecting malignancies.
   - **Applications**: Differentiate lesions like FNH, hepatic adenoma, and HCC based on contrast uptake patterns.
3. **Ultrasound**:
   - **Gray-scale and Color Doppler US**: First-line for lesion detection and assessing vascularity.
   - **Contrast-enhanced US (CEUS)**: Real-time contrast dynamics for characterizing vascular patterns:
     - HCC: Arterial phase enhancement with rapid washout.
     - Hemangioma: Peripheral nodular enhancement with gradual filling.

The differentiating imaging features for hepatic hemangioma, focal hepatocellular carcinoma, and solitary metastatic lesions:

1. **Hepatic Hemangioma**:
   - **Ultrasound**: Typically appears as a well-defined, hyperechoic lesion with posterior acoustic enhancement. Large hemangiomas may appear heterogeneous.
   - **CT**:
     - **Noncontrast**: Generally hypodense.
     - **Arterial Phase**: Shows peripheral, nodular enhancement.

  - **Portal and Delayed Phases**: Progressive centripetal fill-in, leading to complete or near-complete filling of the lesion over time.
- **MRI**:
  - **T1-Weighted**: Hypointense.
  - **T2-Weighted**: Strongly hyperintense ("light bulb sign").
  - **Postcontrast**: Peripheral nodular enhancement with gradual centripetal filling on delayed images.

2. **Focal Hepatocellular Carcinoma**:
   - **Ultrasound**: Variable appearance; maybe hypoechoic, hyperechoic, or heterogeneous. Color Doppler often shows hypervascularity.
   - **CT**:
     - **Noncontrast**: Iso- or hypodense.
     - **Arterial Phase**: Intense enhancement due to hypervascularity.
     - **Portal Phase**: Rapid washout, often with a hypodense appearance.
   - **MRI**:
     - **T1-Weighted**: Hypointense.
     - **T2-Weighted**: Mildly hyperintense.
     - **Postcontrast**: Arterial phase enhancement with washout in the portal or delayed phase. Often hypointense in the hepatobiliary phase (with liver-specific contrast).
3. **Solitary Metastatic Lesions**:
   - **Ultrasound**: Typically, hypoechoic but may vary depending on the primary cancer.
   - **CT**:
     - **Noncontrast**: Hypodense.
     - **Arterial Phase**: Hypervascular metastases (e.g., from renal cell carcinoma or melanoma) show arterial enhancement; hypovascular metastases may not enhance significantly.
     - **Portal Phase**: Washout of hypervascular metastases; hypovascular metastases appear hypodense.
   - **MRI**:
     - **T1-Weighted**: Generally hypointense.
     - **T2-Weighted**: Hyperintense.
     - **Postcontrast**: Variable enhancement depending on vascularity. Hypervascular metastases enhance in the arterial phase with washout in the portal phase, while hypovascular lesions may enhance minimally.

7. Enumerate various interventions in the biliary tract. Briefly discuss the indications, contraindications, procedure and complications of percutaneous transhepatic biliary drainage (PTBD). [2+8]

Interventions in the Biliary Tract

- Percutaneous transhepatic biliary drainage (PTBD)
- Endoscopic retrograde cholangiopancreatography (ERCP)
- Percutaneous transhepatic cholangiography (PTC)
- Biliary stenting (endoscopic or percutaneous)
- Biliary stone extraction (ERCP)
- Biliary balloon dilation
- Biliary brush cytology and biopsy
- Choledocholithotomy (removal of bile duct stones)
- Biliary radiofrequency ablation
- Photodynamic therapy (PDT) in malignant biliary obstruction

Indications, Contraindications, Procedure and Complications of Percutaneous Transhepatic Biliary Drainage

Indications

1. **Biliary Obstruction**:
   - Patients with biliary-enteric anastomosis.
   - When endoscopic approach fails to provide adequate drainage.
   - In obstructions above the insertion of cystic duct (high level obstruction).
   - In order to decrease bilirubin to allow patients to get chemotherapy.
2. **Biliary Leak**:
   - Iatrogenic
   - Post-traumatic.
3. **Cholangitis**:
   - Intrasegmental cholangitis.
   - Patients with altered anatomy (Roux-en-Y anatomy).
   - Failure of ERCP to provide appropriate drainage.
   - Cholangitis should be diagnosed using clinical presentation (RUQ pain and fever) and jaundice (hyperbilirubinemia).
   - Recurrent cholangitis due to intrahepatic choledocholithiasis. PTBD can be utilized to facilitate transhepatic and lithotripsy.
4. **Biliary Drainage in Patients with Hilar/Perihilar Malignancy.**

Contraindications

- **Uncorrectable Coagulopathy**: PTBD is contraindicated in patients with severe bleeding disorders.
- **Massive Ascites**: Increases the risk of leakage and infection.
- **Severe Hepatic Encephalopathy**: PTBD may worsen encephalopathy by disrupting bile flow.
- **Inaccessible Biliary Tree**: Anatomical variations or dense fibrosis that prevent safe access to the biliary system.

Procedure

1. **Preprocedural Preparation**: Coagulation parameters are checked and corrected if needed. Broad-spectrum antibiotics are administered to prevent infection.
2. **Patient Positioning**: The patient is positioned supine or in a slightly oblique position for optimal liver and bile duct visualization.
3. **Imaging Guidance**: Ultrasound and fluoroscopy are used to guide the needle into a peripheral intrahepatic bile duct.
4. **Needle Insertion**: A thin needle is advanced into the liver and bile duct system, confirmed by bile aspiration.
5. **Contrast Injection**: Contrast is injected to opacify the biliary system, identifying the site and extent of obstruction.
6. **Catheter Placement**: A guidewire is advanced into the bile duct, followed by a catheter for external drainage or an internal-external stent for bile flow into the duodenum.

Postprocedure Care

1. Closely monitor vital signs and patient's condition (every 15–30 minutes for 2 hours and then every 4 hours) for 24 hours for any signs/symptoms of sepsis and hemorrhage.
2. Check wound dressing for evidence of bile leak.
3. Skin around the catheter should be evaluate every 24 hours.
4. Flush the catheter daily with 10 mL saline.
5. Catheter outputs should be recorded daily.

Complications

- **Infection and Sepsis**: Cholangitis or sepsis may occur, especially if bile leaks into the peritoneum.
- **Bleeding**: Hemorrhage can result from liver puncture, especially in patients with coagulopathy.
- **Bile Leak and Peritonitis**: Leakage of bile into the peritoneum can lead to chemical peritonitis.
- **Pneumothorax or Hemothorax**: Accidental puncture of the pleura or blood vessels during needle insertion.
- **Catheter Occlusion or Displacement**: The catheter may become blocked or dislodged, requiring repositioning.
- **Subcapsular Hematoma**: A localized collection of blood under the liver capsule can occur due to needle injury.

8. Role of imaging in chronic liver disease. [10] [DNB June 22]

Imaging plays a pivotal role in the diagnosis, management, and monitoring of chronic liver disease (CLD), providing essential insights into liver structure, function, and complications.[4] It's role:

A. **Diagnosis**: Ultrasound is the first-line imaging modality for initial liver assessment, detecting early changes like fatty infiltration and fibrosis.

B. **Staging of Fibrosis**: MRI and transient elastography (fibroscan) measure liver stiffness, allowing noninvasive staging from fibrosis to cirrhosis.

C. **Progression**: Serial imaging with US or MRI tracks liver changes over time, enabling assessment of disease progression.

D. **Portal Hypertension Evaluation**: Doppler US assesses portal vein flow and detects signs of portal hypertension, such as splenomegaly, varices, and ascites.

E. **Hepatocellular Carcinoma Detection**: MRI and contrast-enhanced CT identify and characterize liver nodules, crucial for HCC surveillance in cirrhotic patients.

F. **Vascular Assessment**: CT and MRI angiography evaluate the hepatic and portal veins, detecting complications like thrombosis and collateral formation.

G. **Guiding Interventions**: Imaging guides liver biopsies, trans-jugular intrahepatic portosystemic shunt (TIPS) placements, and other interventional procedures.

H. **Fat Quantification**: MRI allows noninvasive measurement of hepatic steatosis, important for assessing fatty liver disease in CLD patients.

I. **Liver Volume and Regeneration Potential**: CT and MRI assess liver volume, aiding in planning for liver resection or transplant.

J. **Detection of Extrahepatic Manifestations**: Imaging identifies complications like splenomegaly, ascites, and varices, showing systemic effects of advanced CLD.

Imaging findings in chronic liver disease (CLD): It may vary by modality and disease stage, with distinct features for diagnosing, staging, and evaluating complications. Here is a summary of key imaging findings:

1. **Ultrasound**:
   - **Surface Nodularity**: Commonly seen in cirrhosis (88% sensitivity, 82–95% specificity).
   - **Coarse and Heterogeneous Echotexture**: Reflects the overall changes in liver parenchyma.
   - **Segmental Hypertrophy/Atrophy**: Hypertrophy of the caudate and lateral left lobe, with atrophy in posterior right lobe.
   - **Caudate Width**: Measurement >0.65 indicates cirrhosis (43–84% sensitivity, 100% specificity).

   Signs of Portal Hypertension:
   - **Enlarged Portal Vein**: >13 mm (95–100% specificity).
   - **Slow Portal Flow**: <15 cm/s.
   - **Reversal/to-and-fro Flow**: Indicates portal hypertension.
   - **Portal Venous Thrombosis**: Can show cavernous transformation.
   - **Enlarged Mesenteric and Splenic Veins**: >10 mm.
   - **Doppler Flow Changes**: Loss of respiratory variation, and "corkscrew" hepatic arteries indicating compensatory changes.

- Splenomegaly, Ascites, Fatty Change: May be observed in advanced disease.
- **Sonoelastography**: Helps assess fibrosis (values >7 kPa indicate advanced fibrosis; 12.5–15 kPa suggest cirrhosis).

2. **CT**:
   - **Early Cirrhosis**: Generally insensitive.
   - **Established Findings**:
     - Surface and Parenchymal Nodularity: Suggestive of cirrhosis.
     - Regenerative Nodules: Isodense/hyperdense to liver parenchyma.
     - Siderotic Nodules: Hyperdense due to iron accumulation.
   - **Fatty Change**: Variable presentation.
   - **Parenchymal Heterogeneity**: Seen pre and postcontrast.
   - **Portal Venous Supply to Dysplastic Nodules**: Important for distinguishing from HCC.
   - **Signs of Portal Hypertension**: Enlargement of portal vein, thrombosis, splenomegaly, and portosystemic collaterals.
   - **Upper Abdominal Lymphadenopathy**: Seen in end-stage disease.
3. **MRI**:
   - **Early Cirrhosis**: MRI is also insensitive in early stages.
   - **Established Findings**:
     - **Regenerative Nodules**: Typically, isointense on T1 and T2; no early enhancement as they have portal venous supply.
     - **Siderotic Nodules**: Hypointense on T2 due to iron deposition.
     - **Dysplastic Nodules**: Variable appearance; low-grade resemble regenerative nodules, high-grade may resemble HCC.
     - **Small Hepatocellular Carcinoma:**
       - T1 C^+ (Gadolinium): Early arterial enhancement, washout, and possible late capsule enhancement.
       - T2: Typically, mildly or moderately hyperintense.
     - **MR Angiography**: Used to assess portal vein patency and portosystemic collaterals.

Nuclear Medicine (Hepatobiliary Scintigraphy) Findings

- **Functional Assessment**: Detects hepatocyte dysfunction and biliary obstruction in advanced disease.
- **Liver-spleen Scintigraphy**: Used less frequently, but may show altered liver uptake in cirrhosis.

FibroScan (Transient Elastography) Findings

Liver Stiffness Measurement: Used to noninvasively assess and quantify the degree of fibrosis, especially useful in early staging.

9. Hyperenhancing tumors of liver and imaging. [10] [DNB June 22]

Hyperenhancing liver tumors are characterized by their increased contrast enhancement during the arterial phase of imaging, typically appearing brighter than surrounding liver parenchyma. This enhancement pattern helps differentiate them from other liver lesions and is crucial in narrowing down potential diagnoses.

Types of Hyperenhancing Liver Tumors and Their Imaging Features

1. **Hepatocellular Carcinoma:**[5]
   - **US**: May appear hypoechoic or heterogeneous. Color Doppler may show increased vascularity, and larger lesions may display a mosaic pattern or a peripheral halo.
   - **CEUS**: Shows arterial hyperenhancement followed by washout in the portal venous phase, characteristic of malignancy.
   - **CT**: Demonstrates arterial-phase hyperenhancement with washout in portal or delayed phases. A capsule appearance may also be seen in delayed phases.
   - **MRI**: Typically, hyperintense on T1-weighted images with arterial-phase enhancement and washout on delayed images. Restricted diffusion is also a key feature on diffusion-weighted imaging (DWI).

2. **Focal Nodular Hyperplasia (FNH)**:
   - **US**: Usually iso- or hypoechoic compared to surrounding liver tissue; a central scar may appear hyperechoic.
   - **CEUS**: Exhibits strong, homogeneous arterial-phase enhancement with no washout in delayed phases, helping to differentiate it from malignant lesions.
   - **CT**: Arterial-phase enhancement and isodense in portal phases. A central scar, if present, may show delayed enhancement.
   - **MRI**: Iso- or hyperintense on T2-weighted images, with central scar showing delayed enhancement on T1 postcontrast sequences. The lesion remains isointense or slightly hyperintense in delayed phases without washout.
3. **Hepatic Adenoma**:
   - **US**: Often appears as a well-defined, slightly hyperechoic mass. Large lesions may show heterogeneity due to hemorrhage or necrosis.
   - **CEUS**: Shows homogeneous arterial-phase enhancement without washout, remaining iso- or hyperechoic in delayed phases.
   - **CT**: Homogeneous arterial enhancement, no washout. Fat components appear as hypodense regions on noncontrast CT. Hemorrhage or necrotic areas can make the lesion heterogeneous.
   - **MRI**: Typically, hyperintense on T1 with fatty or hemorrhagic areas. Homogeneous enhancement in the arterial phase, remaining isointense or slightly hyperintense without washout.
4. **Hemangioma**:
   - **US**: Generally hyperechoic with sharp margins. Larger lesions may appear more heterogeneous due to thrombosis or fibrosis.
   - **CEUS**: Peripheral nodular enhancement with centripetal fill-in over time, a pattern distinctive for hemangioma.
   - **CT**: Peripheral nodular enhancement with progressive, centripetal fill-in, which becomes hyperdense in delayed phases.
   - **MRI**: Very hyperintense on T2-weighted images with gradual centripetal fill-in on dynamic sequences, matching blood pool intensity in delayed phases.
5. **Hypervascular Metastases**:
   - **US**: Echogenicity varies based on the primary tumor; lesions may appear hypo- or hyperechoic and are often multiple.
   - **CEUS**: Rapid arterial enhancement with washout in delayed phases, similar to HCC.
   - **CT**: Typically shows arterial-phase hyperenhancement with washout. Often presents as multiple lesions scattered throughout the liver.
   - **MRI**: Lesions are hypointense on T1 and variable on T2, with arterial enhancement and washout. High signal on DWI also aids in diagnosis.
6. **Fibrolamellar Hepatocellular Carcinoma (FL-HCC)**:
   - **Imaging**: FL-HCC shows arterial phase hyperenhancement with heterogeneity due to the fibrotic stroma, which may enhance in delayed phases.
   - **Other Features**: Central scar may be seen but lacks delayed enhancement, unlike FNH.
   - **Associated Factors**: Seen in younger patients without chronic liver disease.
7. **Angiosarcoma**:
   - **Imaging**: Typically presents with early peripheral arterial enhancement and heterogeneity, often showing rapid washout and areas of necrosis.
   - **Other Features**: May show large, irregular, and infiltrative growth with vascular invasion.
   - **Associated Factors**: Rare, associated with exposure to vinyl chloride, thorium dioxide, or arsenic.

10. Caroli's disease. [5] [DNB Dec 21]

Caroli disease is a rare congenital disorder characterized by segmental, nonobstructive dilation of the intrahepatic bile ducts. It is part of the spectrum of fibropolycystic liver diseases and can present as isolated bile duct dilation or as part of Caroli syndrome, which also involves congenital hepatic fibrosis.

Types of Caroli Disease

- **Simple Caroli Disease**: Involves focal or segmental saccular dilation of intrahepatic bile ducts without fibrosis.
- **Caroli Syndrome**: Associated with congenital hepatic fibrosis, which leads to portal hypertension and liver dysfunction.

Clinical Presentation

- **Symptoms**: Patients may present with recurrent episodes of cholangitis (biliary infections), abdominal pain, and jaundice.
- **Complications**: Increased risk of cholangiocarcinoma, liver abscesses, and secondary biliary cirrhosis.

Imaging Findings

Imaging plays a critical role in diagnosing Caroli disease, helping to visualize the characteristic features of bile duct dilation and complications.

1. **Ultrasound**:
   - **Intrahepatic Ductal Dilatation**: Shows "cystic" or "saccular" dilations in the liver, often described as a "string of beads" appearance due to alternating dilated and nondilated segments.
   - **Central Dot Sign**: Dilated bile ducts around a fibrovascular bundle seen as echogenic "dots" in the center of cystic areas.
   - **Hepatomegaly and Splenomegaly**: Common in Caroli syndrome due to portal hypertension.
2. **Computed Tomography**:
   - **Dilated Intrahepatic Bile Ducts**: Appear as cystic structures, often distributed throughout the liver.
   - **Central Dot Sign**: Small enhancing dots within the dilated ducts on contrast-enhanced CT, representing portal vein radicles surrounded by dilated bile ducts.
   - **Liver Fibrosis**: Seen in Caroli syndrome, with atrophic or nodular liver contour.
   - **Biliary Stones and Sludge**: CT may show stones or biliary sludge, common due to bile stasis.
3. **Magnetic Resonance Imaging (MRI) and Magnetic Resonance Cholangiopancreatography (MRCP)**:
   - **MRCP**: Noninvasive, best modality for visualizing the "string of beads" appearance of segmental ductal dilations.
   - **Central Dot Sign**: Also visible on T2-weighted MRI and MRCP, showing high signal intensity in the dilated bile ducts surrounding a low-signal portal vein branch.
   - **Fibrosis and Portal Hypertension**: MRCP and MRI also reveal signs of portal hypertension, such as splenomegaly and varices in Caroli syndrome.
4. **Cholangiography (ERCP or Percutaneous)**: Rarely used today due to the availability of MRCP, but historically performed to confirm diagnosis, showing cystic dilations in intrahepatic ducts.

Management

- **Antibiotics**: For treating and preventing recurrent cholangitis.
- **Endoscopic and Surgical Interventions**: ERCP for stone removal; partial liver resection may be considered in localized disease.
- **Liver Transplantation**: May be considered in diffuse disease with complications like severe portal hypertension or biliary cirrhosis.

Prognosis

The prognosis depends on the extent of liver involvement and presence of complications. Caroli syndrome has a more severe course due to portal hypertension and associated complications. Regular follow-up is essential due to the increased risk of cholangiocarcinoma.

11. (a) LIRAD, its main features and categories (b) use of LIRAD in liver lesion management. [10] [DNB June 21]

Liver imaging reporting and data system (LI-RADS) is a standardized system developed by the American College of Radiology (ACR) to help radiologists assess and categorize liver lesions, particularly in patients at risk for hepatocellular carcinoma. It ensures consistency in reporting, improves diagnostic accuracy, and guides management.

Major Features of LI-RADS

- **Arterial Phase Hyperenhancement (APHE)**: **Nonrim APHE**: This feature involves a lesion that shows greater enhancement than the surrounding liver tissue during the arterial phase without a rim-like enhancement pattern. Rim enhancement is not characteristic of HCC.
- **Nonperipheral Washout**: **Washout Appearance**: A decrease in lesion enhancement on the portal venous or delayed phases, leading to hypo-enhancement. It suggests malignancy, particularly HCC.
- **Capsule**: **Enhancing Capsule**: A smooth, uniform border that surrounds the lesion, observed in delayed imaging phases. It is an indicator of more developed HCC.
- **Size**: **Larger Lesions**: Lesions over a certain size threshold (e.g., >10 mm) have an increased likelihood of being HCC.
- **Threshold Growth**: Rapid Growth: An increase in lesion size by 50% or more within 6 months is highly suggestive of malignancy, qualifying for LI-RADS category adjustment to LR-5 if accompanied by APHE.
- Example: For a lesion >10 mm with APHE, capsule, and washout, these combined features would classify it as LR-5 (definitely HCC).

LI-RADS Categories

LI-RADS categories **(Table 10)** range from LR-1 (definitely benign) to LR-5 (definitely HCC), with intermediate categories like LR-3 (indeterminate probability) and LR-4 (probable HCC) helping guide diagnosis and management.

TABLE 10: LI-RADS categories of hepatic lesions.

LI-RADS	*Description*	*Management*
Negative	No observations detected	Return to surveillance in 6 months
LR-NC	Not categorizable due to image degradation or omission	Repeat or alternative imaging in <3 months
LR-1	Definitely benign observation	Return to surveillance in 6 months
LR-2	Probably benign	Consider repeat diagnostic imaging in 6 months.
LR-3	Intermediate probability of malignancy	Repeat or alternative imaging in 3–6 months
LR-4	Probably HCC	Multidisciplinary discussion for further work-up
LR-5	Definitely HCC	Multidisciplinary discussion for management consensus
LR-M	Probably/definite malignancy not HCC-specific	Multidisciplinary discussion. Consider biopsy
LR-TIV	Definite tumor in the vein	Multidisciplinary discussion, may include biopsy

LI-RADS Category Details

- **LR-1 (Definitely Benign)**: Observations with nonenhancing features like cysts, hemangiomas, or benign perfusion changes.
- **LR-2 (Probably Benign)**: Likely benign but not definitive; could include cysts or benign pseudolesions without malignant features.
- **LR-3 (Intermediate Probability)**: Lesions with a mix of benign and malignant characteristics, often requiring further follow-up or imaging. Examples include nodules <20 mm without major malignant indicators
- **LR-4 (Probably HCC)**: Lesions with nonrim APHE and additional HCC features such as capsule or washout, indicating high suspicion for HCC.
- **LR-5 (Definitely HCC)**: Lesions over 10 mm with nonrim APHE, washout, and/or growth meeting all diagnostic criteria for HCC.

Additional LI-RADS Categories

- **LR-TIV (Tumor in Vein)**: Indicates vascular invasion by tumor, typically from HCC, and is associated with advanced disease.

- **LR-M (Malignant, not HCC)**: Used for lesions with malignancy features but atypical for HCC, such as those with rim APHE, peripheral washout, or delayed central enhancement—often seen in intrahepatic cholangiocarcinoma (iCCA).
- **LR-TR (Treated HCC)**: Classification for post-treatment lesions, assisting in the monitoring and assessment of recurrence.
- **LR-NC (Noncategorizable)**: Observations in cases where technical limitations prevent reliable imaging interpretation.

Use of LI-RADS in Liver Lesion Management

LI-RADS plays a critical role in the management of liver lesions by:

- **Guiding Surveillance and Follow-Up**: Categories such as LR-1 and LR-2 lesions typically do not require aggressive follow-up, while LR-3 lesions often prompt closer monitoring or repeat imaging.
- **Providing Diagnostic Confidence for HCC**: LR-4 and LR-5 categories help determine lesions with high probability of HCC, supporting decisions regarding interventions such as biopsy, surgical resection, or liver transplantation listing.
- **Differentiating HCC from Other Malignancies**: LR-M lesions highlight potential malignancies that are not HCC, allowing clinicians to consider alternative diagnoses, which may lead to different treatment pathways (e.g., chemotherapy for metastatic disease).
- **Guiding Treatment Decisions**:
  - **LR-5**: When lesions are categorized as LR-5 (definitive for HCC), they can be treated as HCC without biopsy, streamlining treatment planning for therapies like ablation or liver transplantation.
  - **LR-TIV**: Identification of vascular invasion (LR-TIV) in liver tumors indicates advanced disease, directing treatment away from surgical options towards systemic or palliative care.
- **Improving Multidisciplinary Communication**: By providing a clear and standardized classification, LI-RADS facilitates communication between radiologists, hepatologists, surgeons, and oncologists, enhancing team-based management and treatment planning.

12. Role of ultrasound, MRI, and scintigraphy in assessment of biliary atresia. [3+4+3] [MD (WBUHS) 17]

Biliary atresia **(Fig. 1)** is a congenital biliary disorder that is characterized by an absence or severe deficiency of the extrahepatic biliary tree. It is one of the most common causes of neonatal cholestasis, often causing cirrhosis immediately and leading to death and accounts for over half of children who undergo liver transplantation.[6]

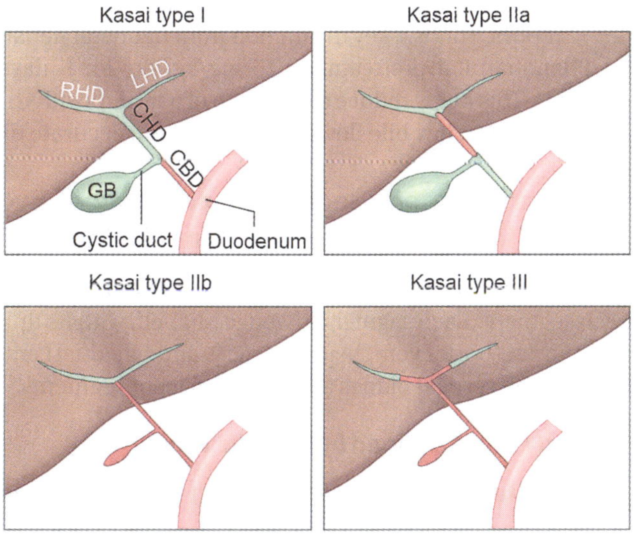

FIG. 1: Biliary atresia.

Ultrasound Findings in Biliary Atresia

- **Triangular Cord Sign**:
  - Seen as echogenic fibrous tissue located anterior to the portal vein.
  - Significance: Indicates the fibrotic ductal remnant of the extrahepatic bile duct and is considered a characteristic sign of biliary atresia.
- **Hepatic Artery Changes**:
  - **Increased Hepatic Arterial Caliber**: Enlargement of the hepatic artery may be noted as a response to the impaired biliary system.
  - **Subcapsular Hepatic Arterial Flow on Doppler**: Abnormal Doppler findings, including increased blood flow to the liver capsule, indicate compensatory changes.

- **Specific Measurements**:
  - Right proximal hepatic artery diameter often exceeds 1.5 mm.
  - Hepatic artery to portal vein diameter ratio is typically >0.45, which can help in differentiating biliary atresia from other causes of neonatal jaundice.
- **Gallbladder Ghost Triad**: Features of the "ghost" gallbladder on ultrasound can provide additional clues:
  - **Atretic Gallbladder**: The gallbladder is often shortened, measuring less than 19 mm in length.
  - **Irregular or Lobular Contour**: The shape and structure of the gallbladder may be altered, showing irregularity or a lobulated appearance.
  - **Indistinct Wall and Lack of Smooth Mucosal Lining**: The mucosal lining is often incomplete, and the wall is not sharply delineated.
- **Gallbladder Contraction Index**: In biliary atresia, contraction of the gallbladder is often reduced, with a length-to-width ratio >5.2, indicating a decreased contraction index for the patient's age.

Magnetic Resonance Imaging (MRI)

MRI, particularly MR cholangiopancreatography (MRCP), provides detailed anatomical information and is valuable in confirming findings from ultrasound:

- **Ductal System Visualization**: MRCP is instrumental in visualizing the biliary tree. In biliary atresia, the extrahepatic biliary tree is often not visualized, while intrahepatic biliary ducts are typically of smaller caliber.
- **Fibrosis Assessment**: MRI can evaluate hepatic fibrosis, which may be evident as biliary atresia progresses.
- **Hepatobiliary Phase Imaging**: With hepatobiliary contrast agents (such as Gd-EOB-DTPA), biliary excretion can be indirectly assessed. Lack of excretion into the duodenum may suggest atresia.
- **Complementary Role**: MRI can aid in differential diagnosis by excluding other causes of neonatal cholestasis, such as choledochal cysts or Alagille syndrome.

Nuclear Medicine Findings (Hepatobiliary Scintigraphy or HIDA Scan)

- **Hepatobiliary Tracers**: Tc-99m DISIDA (diosgenin) and BRIDA (mebrofenin): These radiotracers are preferred because of their high hepatic extraction rates and short transit times.
- **Imaging Findings**:
  - In cases of biliary atresia, the tracer typically demonstrates good hepatic uptake (indicating functional hepatic cells).
  - No Excretion into Small Bowel: A lack of biliary excretion is typically observed, even on delayed images at 24 hours. This is a key distinction from neonatal hepatitis, in which delayed excretion into the bowel may still occur.

Phenobarbital pretreatment (5 mg/kg/day for 5 days) is often used to boost bile secretion by stimulating liver enzymes. This helps reduce the chance of a false-positive result on a hepatobiliary scan in patients with a functional bile duct system but low bile flow, ensuring a more accurate diagnosis.

13. Describe briefly segmental anatomy of liver with a line diagram. Describe imaging (CT and MRI) features in hepatocellular carcinoma. [4+(3+3)] [DNB June 20, AIIMS May 23]

The liver's segmental anatomy (**Fig. 2**) is organized based on independent vascular, biliary, and lymphatic systems for each segment. Each segment is wedge-shaped, with its tip pointing toward the porta hepatis, where its own branch of the portal triad (portal vein, hepatic artery, and bile duct) enters. Segment boundaries are defined by hepatic veins, which run in three vertical planes and drain adjacent segments.[7]

Vertical Planes Defined by Hepatic Veins

- **Right Hepatic Vein**: Divides the right lobe into right lateral (posterior) and right medial (anterior) sections.
- **Middle Hepatic Vein**: Lies along Cantlie's line (from the IVC to the gallbladder fossa) and divides the liver into right and left lobes.
- **Left Hepatic Vein**: Divides the left lobe into left medial and left lateral sections.

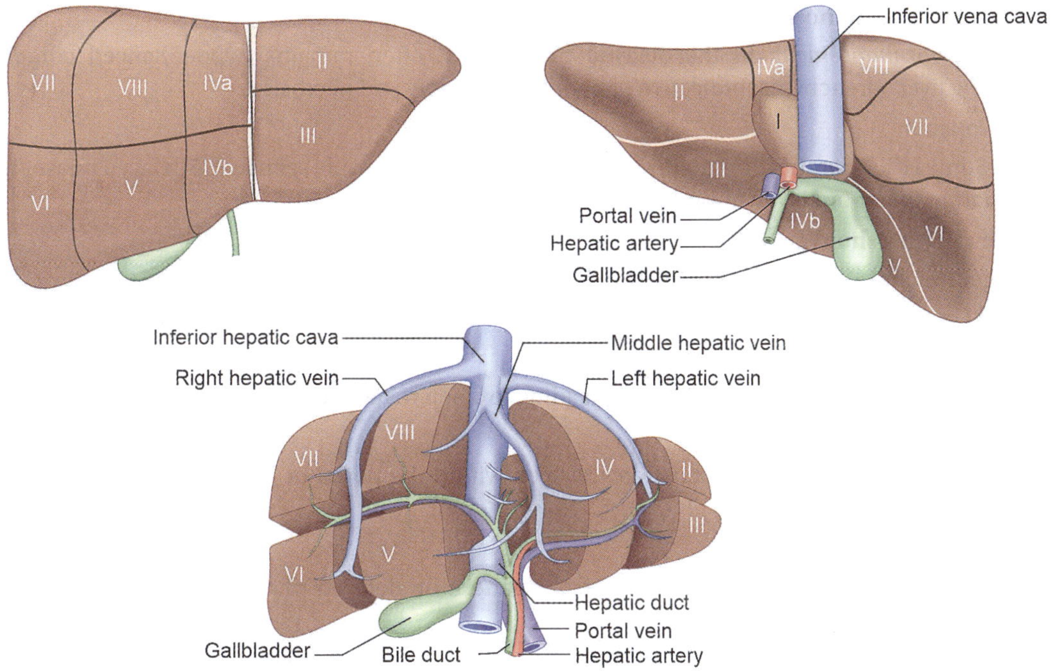

FIG. 2: Segmental anatomy of liver.

Horizontal Division by Portal Plane

Each section is further divided by the portal vein into superior and inferior segments:

- **Left Lateral**: Segment II (superior) and III (inferior)
- **Left Medial**: Segment IVa (superior) and IVb (inferior)
- **Right Medial**: Segment VIII (superior) and V (inferior)
- **Right Lateral**: Segment VII (superior) and VI (inferior)

Caudate Lobe (Segment I)

Located posteriorly, bounded by the IVC, ligamentum venosum, and porta hepatis, with dual blood supply from both right and left portal veins. It drains directly into the IVC.

Segment Arrangement

The segments are numbered in a clockwise fashion from segment II to VIII, starting superiorly on the left lobe:

- **Left Lobe**: Segments II (superior) and III (inferior), separated by the left hepatic vein.
- **Quadrate Lobe (Segment IV)**: Located between left and middle hepatic veins, divided into IVa (above portal plane) and IVb (below portal plane).
- **Right Lobe**: Segments V to VIII, with V and VIII between the middle and right hepatic veins. Each hepatic vein drains multiple segments adjacent to it, forming the boundaries of each section, and enhancing understanding of liver anatomy for surgical and radiological procedures.

CT Features of Hepatocellular Carcinoma

1. **Arterial Phase Hyperenhancement (APHE)**:
   - Key Feature: HCC typically shows hyperenhancement during the arterial phase, meaning the tumor enhances more than the surrounding liver tissue.
   - Nonrim enhancement: HCC lacks peripheral rim enhancement, unlike other lesions like metastases.
2. **Portal Venous Phase Washout**:
   - Washout: HCC often demonstrates hypoenhancement in the portal venous phase, indicating washout due to the tumor's high arterial supply and poor venous drainage.

3. **Delayed Phase Hypoenhancement**:
   - *Persistent hypoenhancement*: In the delayed phase, HCC often remains hypoenhanced compared to the surrounding liver parenchyma, indicative of poor blood supply and necrosis.
4. **Enhancing Capsule**:
   - Capsule: Some HCCs may have a smooth or irregular enhancing capsule seen in the delayed phase. This suggests a more mature tumor but is not always present.
5. **Size and Growth (threshold growth)**:
   - Size: Larger lesions (>2 cm) are more likely to be HCC.
   - Threshold Growth: If the lesion grows by more than 50% in 6 months, it is highly suspicious for HCC.
6. **Intratumoral Necrosis**:
   - Necrosis: HCC often shows areas of necrosis, leading to a heterogeneous enhancement pattern on CT.
7. **Vascular Invasion**:
   - Portal Vein Invasion: Tumor thrombus may be seen within the portal or hepatic veins, appearing as a filling defect.
8. **Mosaic Pattern**:
   - Mosaic Architecture: Rarely, HCC shows a mosaic pattern on delayed-phase CT due to areas of necrosis and fibrosis.

LI-RADS and CT Imaging

- **LR-5**: Definitely HCC, with arterial hyperenhancement, washout, and enhancing capsule.
- **LR-4**: Likely HCC, with arterial hyperenhancement and at least one additional feature.
- **LR-3**: Intermediate probability of HCC.
- **LR-1**: Definitely benign (e.g., cysts, hemangiomas).

CT plays a critical role in diagnosing, staging, and managing HCC, especially in cirrhotic livers.

MRI Features of Hepatocellular Carcinoma

1. **T1-Weighted Imaging**:
   - Signal: HCC appears iso- or hypointense compared to surrounding liver tissue.
   - Intratumoral Fat: Some HCCs may appear hyperintense on T1 due to fat content.
   - Enhancement after Contrast:
   - T1 C^+ (Gadolinium): Typically shows arterial-phase hyperenhancement (APHE) due to its arterial blood supply.
   - Washout: After the arterial phase, HCC demonstrates rapid washout, becoming hypointense in the portal venous or delayed phases.
   - Rim Enhancement: Some HCCs show rim enhancement, which is suggestive of an enhancing capsule.
2. **T2-Weighted Imaging**:
   - Signal: The tumor may appear moderately hyperintense on T2-weighted images, though this can vary.
3. **Hepatobiliary Phase (with Eovist/Primovist)**:
   - APHE and Washout: Well-differentiated HCCs may lack typical APHE and can appear hypointense in the hepatobiliary phase.
   - Retained Contrast: In some cases, well-differentiated HCCs with functional hepatocytes may retain contrast in the hepatobiliary phase (10–15%).
4. **Diffusion-weighted Imaging (DWI)**:
   - High Signal: HCC typically shows high signal intensity on DWI due to the presence of cellularity and restricted diffusion, which enhances sensitivity and specificity.
5. **Superparamagnetic Iron Oxide (SPIO) Enhancement**:
   - Increased Sensitivity: Use of SPIO contrast agents can improve the detection of small HCCs by making the tumor more conspicuous against the surrounding liver tissue.

Pancreas

1. Discuss in brief the pancreatic masses and its imaging features in brief. [5+5] [MD (WBUHS) 23]

Pancreatic Tumors: Classification

Primary (95%)

A. **Solid Tumors:**
   i. Pancreatic adenocarcinoma (85–95%)
   ii. Pancreatic neuroendocrine tumor
   iii. Solid pseudopapillary tumor
   iv. Pancreatoblastoma
   v. Pancreatic lymphoma

B. **Cystic Tumors:**
   i. Serous cystadenoma
   ii. Mucinous cystic neoplasm
   iii. Intraductal papillary mucinous tumor of the pancreas

Metastatic Lesions (5%)

Brief description and imaging features of pancreatic masses:

1. **Pancreatic Ductal Adenocarcinoma (PDAC):**
   - **Incidence and Presenting Features:** The most common pancreatic malignancy, representing 85–90% of pancreatic tumors. Commonly presents with painless jaundice due to bile duct obstruction, especially when in the pancreatic head. Other symptoms include weight loss, abdominal or back pain, and new-onset diabetes in some cases. It has a poor prognosis, with a 5-year survival rate of less than 10%.
   - **Location:** Predominantly in the pancreatic head.
   - **Imaging Features:**
     - **CT:** Hypoattenuating mass on contrast-enhanced scans with irregular margins; common findings include pancreatic ductal dilation (double duct sign), vascular invasion, and encasement of adjacent vessels.
       MRI: Hypointense on T1-weighted images and moderately hyperintense on T2. Diffusion restriction is common, indicating cellularity.
     - **Endoscopic Ultrasound (EUS):** Hypoechoic mass with irregular borders; facilitates biopsy for confirmation.
     - **PET/CT:** Often shows increased FDG uptake but not typically first-line for diagnosis.

2. **Pancreatic Neuroendocrine Tumors (PNETs):**
   - **Incidence:** Comprise 1–2% of pancreatic tumors; can be functional (insulinoma, gastrinoma) or nonfunctional.
   - **Imaging Features:**
     - **CT:** Typically, hypervascular on arterial phase imaging due to rich blood supply, appearing as well-defined, enhancing masses.
     - **MRI:** Iso- or hyperintense on T2-weighted images, showing avid arterial enhancement.
     - Somatostatin Receptor Imaging (SRI): Gallium-68 DOTATATE PET/CT has high sensitivity for detecting primary lesions and metastases.
     - **EUS:** Useful for detecting small lesions and performing biopsies.

3. **Cystic Neoplasms of the Pancreas:**
   A. **Serous Cystadenoma:** It is a typically benign pancreatic tumor, most commonly seen in older women. Types:
     - **Microcystic/Honeycomb Pattern:** Comprises multiple small cysts with a central scar (30%) and sometimes calcifications.
     - **Macrocystic:** Contains larger cysts, challenging to distinguish from mucinous cystic neoplasms or pseudocysts.
     - **Mixed and Solid:** Less common presentations.

Imaging Features:

- **Ultrasound**: Lobulated, cystic mass with a honeycombed pattern in microcystic cases.
- **CT/MRI**: Well-defined, lobulated mass without ductal communication. Microcystic lesions have a central scar with possible calcifications, while macrocystic forms show fewer, larger cysts.
- **Enhancement**: Hypervascular enhancement can sometimes mimic cystic neuroendocrine tumors.
- **Growth**: Larger tumors (>4 cm) may grow up to 20 mm per year, potentially causing symptoms.

B. **Mucinous Cystic Neoplasm (MCN)**: It is a premalignant pancreatic cystic tumor predominantly affecting women, with a potential to transform into mucinous cystadenocarcinoma.

Characteristics:

- Seen exclusively in women, typically aged 40–50 ("Mother" demographic). Located mostly in the body and tail of the pancreas (95%).
- Often symptomatic, presenting with vague abdominal pain.

Imaging Features:

- **Ultrasound**: Appears as a well-defined, macrocystic mass with thick internal septations.
- **CT**:
  - Shows a well-defined, multilocular cystic lesion with thick wall septations.
  - Peripheral calcifications are seen in about 25% of cases, which is a distinguishing feature.
- **MRI**:
  - T1: Low signal intensity.
  - T2: High signal intensity in the cystic components.
  - Clear definition of thickened septations and absence of communication with the pancreatic duct.

C. **Intraductal Papillary Mucinous Neoplasm (IPMN)**:

Feature: Communication with the main pancreatic duct or its branches, distinguishing it from other cystic pancreatic lesions.

Imaging features:

- **Ultrasound**: Shows small, thin-walled cysts or dilated ducts (>5 mm for main duct type). Mural nodules may appear hyperechoic.
- **CT**: Appears as cystic hypodense lesions. Main duct dilation >5 mm is characteristic of main duct IPMN. Calcifications are rare.
- **MRI/MRCP**:
  - **Main Duct Type**: Dilation >5 mm, with mucin-filled ducts and possible thinning of pancreatic parenchyma. Enhancing mural nodules may indicate malignancy.
  - **Branch Duct Type**: Multiple dilated side branches, often resembling a "bunch of grapes."
  - **Mixed Type**: Shows branch duct dilation with additional main duct involvement.

4. **Solid Pseudopapillary Tumor (SPT)**:
   - **Incidence**: Rare, affecting predominantly young women.
   - **Imaging Features**:
     - **CT**: Well-defined encapsulated lesion with mixed solid and cystic components.
     - **MRI**: Shows heterogeneous enhancement due to hemorrhage within the tumor; distinctive appearance due to hemorrhagic degeneration.
5. **Acinar Cell Carcinoma**:
   - **Incidence**: Rare, accounts for less than 1% of pancreatic cancers.
   - **Imaging Features**:
     - **CT/MRI**: Appears as a large, well-circumscribed, and often hypervascular mass. Tends to be more aggressive than adenocarcinoma and may present with metastasis.
6. **Pancreatoblastoma**:
   - **Incidence**: Rare pediatric pancreatic tumor, mainly in children but can occasionally occur in adults.

- **Imaging Features**:
  - **Ultrasound**: Large, well-defined, heterogeneous mass with solid and multilocular cystic areas, containing hyperechoic septae. Biliary duct dilatation is uncommon.
  - **CT**: Well-defined, heterogeneous mass with solid and cystic components, enhancing septae, and sometimes fine calcifications. Commonly located in the pancreatic head and presents as a large solitary mass; hypodense hepatic metastases may occur.
  - **MRI**:
    - **T1**: Low to intermediate signal intensity.
    - **T2**: Heterogeneously hyperintense.

7. **Lymphoma (Primary Pancreatic or Secondary Involvement)**:
   - **Incidence**: Rare as a primary tumor; pancreas may be involved secondarily by nonHodgkin lymphoma.
   - **Imaging Features**:
     - **CT**: Homogeneous mass, generally without pancreatic duct dilation; minimal contrast enhancement.
     - **MRI**: Iso- to hypointense on T1 and hyperintense on T2; minimal enhancement on postcontrast images.
     - **PET/CT**: FDG avidity is high, aiding in differentiation from PDAC.
8. **Metastatic Lesions to the Pancreas**:
   - **Primary Sources**: Commonly from renal cell carcinoma, melanoma, lung, and breast cancer.
   - **Imaging Features**:
     - **CT**: Typically hypervascular, well-defined lesions; can appear as multiple masses.
     - **MRI**: Hyperintense on T2-weighted images; shows early arterial phase enhancement similar to PNETs

2. Briefly state the anatomical variations of pancreaticobiliary tree with suitable diagrams. [10] [MD (WBUHS) 19]

Developmental anatomy of pancreas: The pancreas forms from two buds, dorsal and ventral, which appear as foregut outgrowths in the fifth gestational week **(Fig. 3A)**. By the seventh week, the ventral bud rotates behind the duodenum to fuse with the dorsal bud **(Figs. 3B and C)**. The ventral bud develops into the posterior head and uncinate process, while the dorsal bud forms the anterior head, body, and tail. After fusion, the ductal systems connect: the ventral duct (duct of Wirsung) drains into the major papilla, while the dorsal duct (main pancreatic duct and duct of Santorini) drains into the minor papilla **(Fig. 3D)**.

Anatomical Variations

A. **The Pancreatic Duct Varies in Shape (Figs. 4A to D)**:
   - Descending (50%): Gentle downward path.

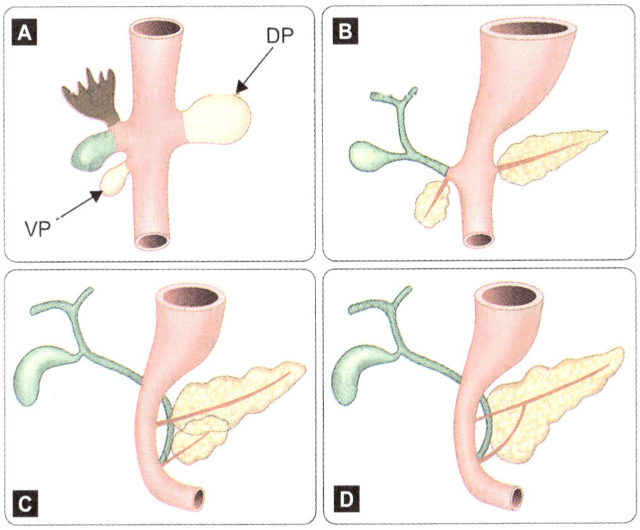

FIGS. 3A to D: Developmental anatomy of pancreaticobiliary tree.

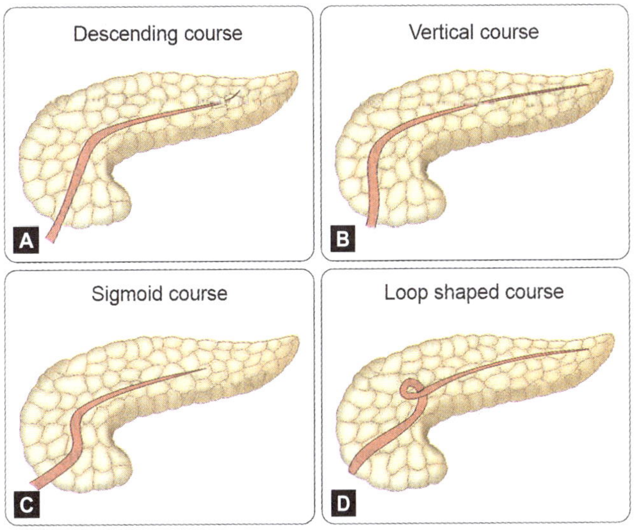

FIGS. 4A TO D: Various shapes of pancreatic duct.

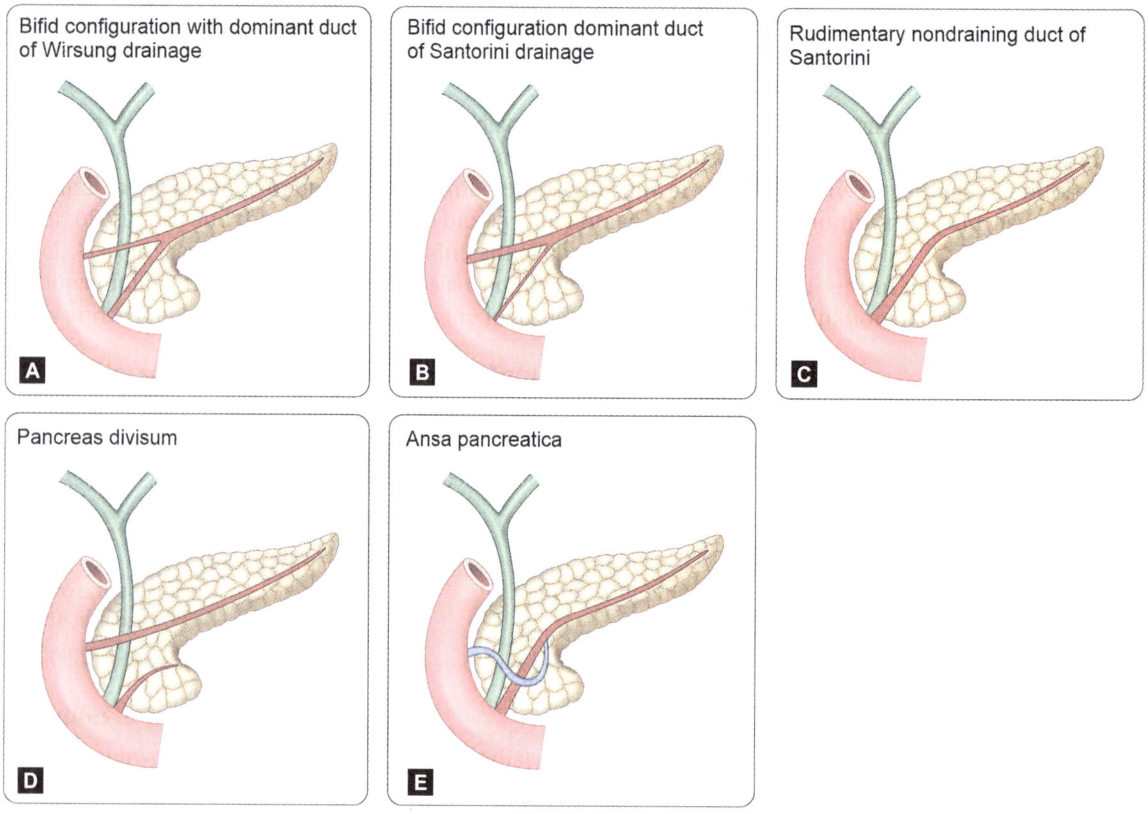

FIGS. 5A to E: Different types of pancreatic duct configurations.

- Sigmoid: S-shaped curve.
- Vertical: Straight down.
- Loop: Rare, looped shape in the head.

B. **The Pancreatic Duct Configurations are as Follows (Figs. 5A to E)**:
- Bifid Configuration (60%): Dominant duct of Wirsung with a bifurcation.
- Absent Duct of Santorini (30%): Only the duct of Wirsung is present.
- Dominant Duct of Santorini without Divisum (1%): Santorini is the primary duct.
- Ansa Pancreatica: The duct of Santorini forms a reversed-S shape, connecting to a side branch of the duct of Wirsung.

C. **Anomalous Pancreaticobiliary Ductal Junction**: It involves the fusion of the pancreatic duct and CBD outside the duodenal wall, creating a long common channel (>15 mm). This condition is often linked to choledochal cysts and an increased risk of biliary tract carcinoma.

D. **Pancreas Divisum**: It occurs in 4–14% of people due to failed fusion of dorsal and ventral ducts. There are three types:
1. Type 1 (Classical): Total fusion failure.
2. Type 2: Dominant dorsal drainage with no duct of Wirsung.
3. Type 3 (Incomplete): Small communication between ducts.

Most pancreatic drainage occurs via the minor papilla, while the head drains through the major papilla. Though often asymptomatic, it can cause recurrent acute pancreatitis due to inadequate drainage. MRCP is the preferred noninvasive diagnostic tool, with MDCT also useful in visualizing the ducts. Rarely, a Santorinicele (cystic dilation) can form in the duct of Santorini.

E. **Annular Pancreas**: It occurs in about 1 in 20,000 people due to the ventral bud's failure to rotate with the duodenum, resulting in a band of pancreatic tissue encircling the duodenum, either partially or completely.

- **Presentation**:
  - **Neonates**: Severe vomiting from duodenal obstruction.
  - **Adults**: May be asymptomatic or present with abdominal pain, postprandial fullness, vomiting, pancreatitis, or jaundice.
- **Diagnosis**:
  - MRCP/ERCP: Identifies the annular pancreatic duct encircling the duodenum.
  - CT/MRI: Shows pancreatic tissue ring around the duodenum, though a full ring is not required for diagnosis.
  - Special Imaging: Secretin-enhanced MRCP helps evaluate ductal anatomy if standard MRCP is unclear.

F. **Ectopic Pancreas**:
- Definition: Pancreatic tissue outside the normal location.
- Location: Mostly in the gastric antrum, duodenum, jejunum.
- Size: 0.5–2 cm (up to 5 cm).
- Symptoms: Often asymptomatic; can cause bleeding, obstruction, or rarely adenocarcinoma.
- Imaging: Seen as a submucosal lesion on barium studies with central umbilication; no specific CT features.

G. **Pancreatic Agenesis/Hypoplasia**:
- Total Agenesis: Rare, not compatible with life.
- Partial Agenesis
- Complete Dorsal Agenesis: Missing anterior head, neck, body, tail.
- Partial Dorsal Agenesis: Some dorsal pancreas tissue remains.
- Risk: Higher diabetes risk due to loss of islet cells.

Anatomic Variations of Biliary Tree

1. **Aberrant Biliary Ducts**:
   - **Types**: Crossover anomaly (right duct drains to left) and accessory right duct (drains into common hepatic or cystic duct).
   - **Risk**: Can cause duct injury or leaks if unnoticed in surgery.
   - **Imaging**: Detected by MRCP, CT cholangiography, or ERCP.
2. **Aberrant Cystic Duct Insertion**:
   - **Low Insertion**: Cystic duct joins the distal CBD, seen in 9% of people.
   - **Insertion into RHD**: Rare variant where cystic duct connects to the right hepatic duct.
   - **Risk**: Unrecognized variants can cause misidentification and accidental injury to CBD or RHD during laparoscopic cholecystectomy.
   - **Imaging**: MRCP is effective for identifying these variations presurgery.
3. **Bile Duct Cysts (Todani Classification) (Fig. 6)**:
   - **Type 1 (Choledochal Cyst)**: Fusiform dilation of the extrahepatic bile duct (80–90% of cases).
     - Associated with reflux of pancreatic secretions; requires resection due to risk of complications.
   - **Type 2 (Diverticulum)**: Saccular outpouching from the extrahepatic bile duct, seen in 3% of cases.
   - **Type 3 (Choledochocele)**: Bulging of the distal bile duct into the duodenum, often incidental but may cause abdominal symptoms.
   - **Type 4**:
     - **4A**: Multiple cysts in intra- and extrahepatic ducts.
     - **4B**: Multiple cysts only in the extrahepatic duct.

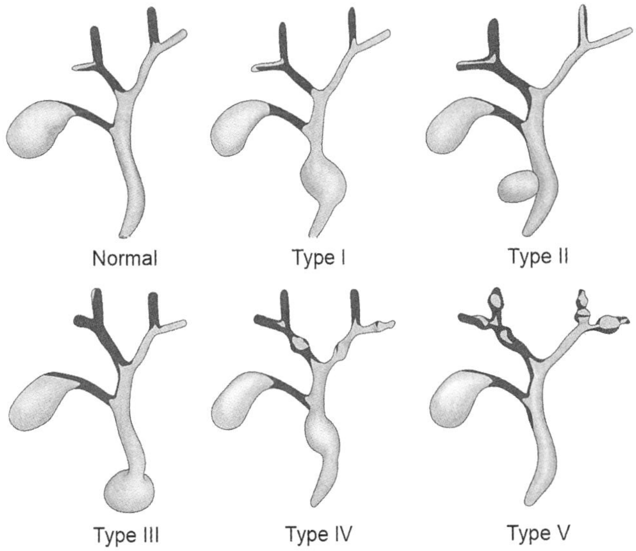

FIG. 6: Different types of bile duct cysts.

- **Type 5 (Caroli's Disease)**: Cystic dilation of intrahepatic bile ducts, associated with renal cystic disease and increased risk of liver complications.
- **Imaging**: Primarily diagnosed using MRCP and ERCP for detailed visualization.

4. **Biliary Abnormalities with Situs Anomalies**:
   - **Situs Inversus**: Bile ducts and abdominal organs are reversed in a mirror-image configuration.
   - **Situs Ambiguous with Polysplenia**: Stomach and multiple small spleens are in the right upper quadrant, with the liver and gallbladder near the midline.

3. Describe the embryology and development of the pancreas. Describe the imaging features of any one important congenital anomaly of the pancreas. [7+3] [MD (WBUHS) 24, MD (WBUHS) 22]

Embryologic Development of the Pancreas

- **Four Weeks Gestation**: The pancreas originates from the endodermal lining of the duodenum.
  - **Buds Formation**: Two outpouchings develop at the foregut-midgut junction **(Fig. 7A)**:
  - **Ventral Bud (caudal)**: This bud eventually forms the posterior portion of the pancreatic head and the uncinate process.
  - **Dorsal Bud (cranial)**: This bud gives rise to the anterior portion of the head, body, and tail of the pancreas.
- **Six Weeks Gestation**:
  - As the foregut elongates, the ventral pancreas rotates clockwise behind the duodenum, along with the gallbladder and bile duct **(Fig. 7B)**.
  - This rotation positions the ventral pancreatic bud posteroinferiorly to the dorsal bud, allowing for their future fusion.

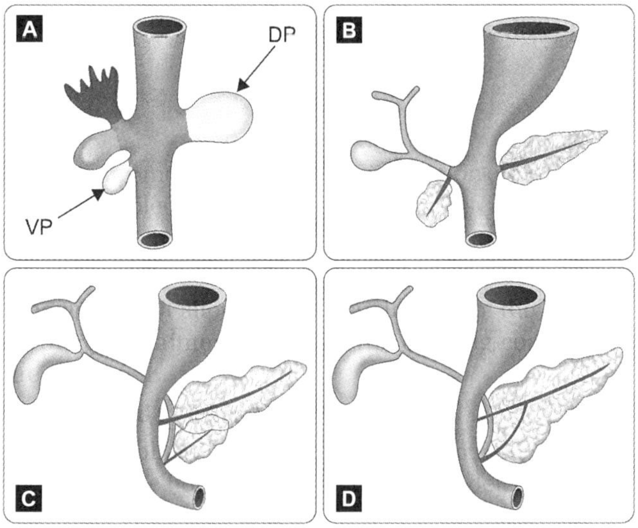

FIGS. 7A to D: Above figures show normal embryologic development of pancreas.

- **Seven Weeks Gestation**:
  - **Fusion**: The dorsal and ventral buds fuse, forming a single pancreatic organ **(Fig. 7C)**.
  - **Duct Formation**: Main Pancreatic Duct (Wirsung): Formed from the ventral pancreatic duct and the distal portion of the dorsal duct.
  - **Accessory Duct (Santorini)**: May persist if the proximal part of the dorsal pancreatic duct remains, providing an additional drainage pathway.
  - **Major Papilla Formation**: The ventral pancreatic duct joins with the common bile duct (CBD), resulting in the shared exit into the duodenum at the major papilla.
  - This fusion and rotation establish the adult configuration of the pancreas and its ducts, allowing coordinated drainage into the duodenum **(Fig. 7D)**.

Congenital Anomalies of Pancreas

- Pancreas Divisum
- Annular Pancreas
- Ectopic (Heterotopic) Pancreas
- Accessory Pancreatic Lobe
- Pancreatic Agenesis
- Dorsal Pancreatic Agenesis
- Hypoplasia of the Dorsal Pancreas
- Anomalous Pancreaticobiliary Junction

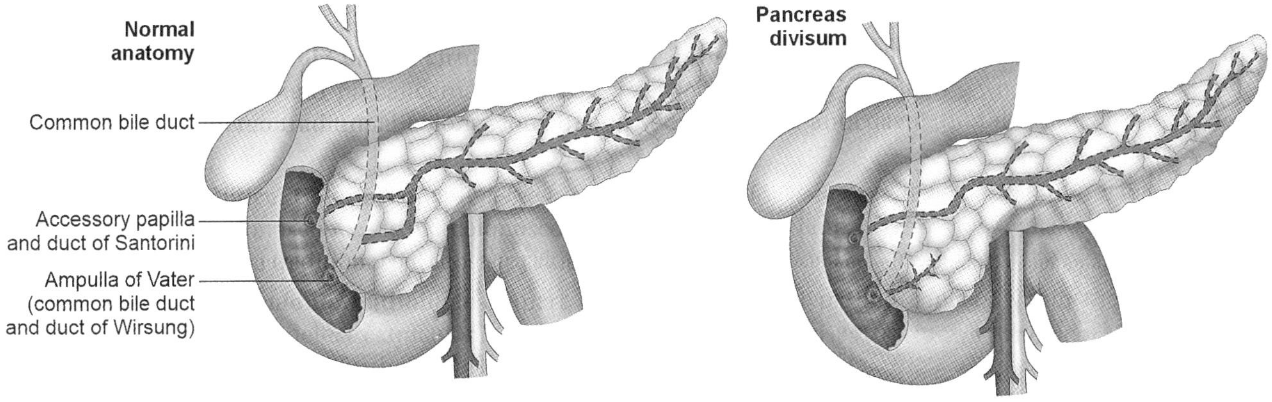

FIG. 8: Pancreatic divisum.

Imaging Features of Pancreatic Divisum (Fig. 8)

- **ERCP**:
  - Ventral Duct: Appears short and tapered, ends abruptly without crossing the midline.
  - Acinarization: Noted in the head after filling attempt, indicating obstruction.
  - Importance: A truncated ventral duct in adults may indicate malignancy; further imaging correlation recommended.
- **MRCP**:
  - Dorsal Duct: Drains into the minor papilla via the duct of Santorini; appears prominent and continuous.
  - Ventral Duct: Short, noncommunicating with the dorsal duct; joins distal bile duct, draining into the major papilla.
  - Pancreatic Head: May have an elongated appearance.
  - Secretin-Enhanced MRCP: Improves visualization and sensitivity of ductal anatomy.
- **CECT**:
  - Duct of Santorini: Prominent, runs parallel to the duct of Wirsung, without connection between them.
  - Chronic Pancreatitis Findings (if present): Beaded, dilated dorsal duct, sometimes with calcifications in chronic cases.

These imaging features assist in confirming pancreatic divisum, with MRCP preferred for its noninvasive nature.

4. Cystic pancreatic tumors and imaging. [10] [DNB June 22]

Common Cystic Neoplasms

- IPMN: Intraductal papillary mucinous neoplasm
- SCN: Serous cystic neoplasm
- MCN: Mucinous cystic neoplasm

Uncommon Cystic Neoplasms

- SPEN (solid pseudopapillary epithelial neoplasm)
- Tumors with cystic degeneration: adenocarcinoma—neuroendocrine tumor

Diagnostic Features of Pancreatic Cystic Neoplasms

- **Consideration**: Suspect if no history of pancreatitis or trauma.
- **Morphological Indicators**:
  - Thick, irregular rim
  - Septations

  - Presence of solid components
  - Dilated pancreatic duct (>3 mm)
  - Calcifications
- **Serous Cystic Neoplasm**: Important to identify, as it has no malignant potential; symptoms typically arise only from size increase.
- **Diagnostic Challenge**: Small cysts may limit definitive diagnosis.

Imaging Features of Serous Cystic Neoplasm

1. **Plain Radiograph**:
   - Usually nonspecific and normal.
   - May show amorphous central calcification over the pancreas.
2. **Ultrasound**:
   - Appears as a nonspecific hypoechoic mass in the pancreatic head.
   - Internal echoes may indicate microcysts; oligocystic subtype may show identifiable cysts.
3. **CT**:
   - Multicystic, lobulated mass in the pancreatic head, resembling a "bunch of grapes."
   - Individual cysts are typically <20 mm and greater than six in number (except oligocystic type).
   - Enhancing central scar with possible stellate calcification (~20% of cases).
4. **MRI**:
   - Appears as a cluster of small cysts with no communication with the pancreatic duct.
   - **T1**: Low signal intensity.
   - **T2**: High signal in cystic components; central fibrous scar (if present) appears low signal.
   - **T1 with Contrast (Gd)**: Fibrous septa may enhance on delayed images.

Imaging Features of Intraductal Papillary Mucinous Neoplasm (IPMN)

1. **General Features**:
   - **Ductal Communication**: IPMNs communicate with the main pancreatic duct or its branches, unlike mucinous cystadenomas.
   - **Calcifications**: Rare (~13% in resected IPMNs).
2. **Fluoroscopy (ERCP)**:
   - Shows dilated pancreatic ducts (segmental, diffuse, or branch type).
   - May reveal polypoid mural tumors or mucinous filling defects.
   - Mucin may be seen at the ampulla of Vater.
3. **Ultrasound**:
   - **Main Duct Type**: Shows thin-walled cysts or dilated hypoechoic ducts (>5 mm).
   - **Mural Nodules and Mucin**: Hyperechoic; may be difficult to differentiate from pancreatic tissue.
4. **CT**:
   - Hypodense, cystic lesions; main duct dilated (>5 mm) in main duct IPMN.
   - Communication with pancreatic ducts can be challenging to detect.
   - Calcifications uncommon in IPMN.
5. **MRI/MRCP**:
   - **Main Duct Type**: Dilated pancreatic duct (>5 mm) filled with low-density mucin; parenchyma may be thinned.
   - **Mucin Bulging**: Mucinous material may bulge from ampulla of Vater (uncommon but pathognomonic).
   - **Branch Duct Type**: Dilated side branches with a "bunch of grapes" appearance, mimicking cystic tumors.
   - **Mixed Type**: Features of both main duct and branch duct types with main duct dilatation (>5 mm).
   - **Mural Nodules**: Concerning for malignancy, especially if they enhance after contrast.

Imaging Features of Mucinous Cystadenoma (MCN)

1. **Demographics**:
   - Exclusively seen in women, typically aged 40–50.
   - Often located in the pancreatic **body and tail** (95%).
2. **Morphology**:
   - Large, macrocystic lesion with **thick-walled septations**.
   - **Peripheral calcifications** in 25% of cases, aiding in specific diagnosis.
   - No communication with the main pancreatic duct.
3. **CT Findings**:
   - Large cystic lesion with **peripheral calcification**.
   - **Internal septations** and **thick walls**.
   - Nonlobulated, smooth capsule.
4. **MRI Findings**:
   - Better depiction of **internal septations** on T1-weighted images postgadolinium.
   - Absence of ductal communication.
5. **Clinical Presentation**:
   - Typically, symptomatic with vague abdominal pain.
   - May present with sudden pain due to rapid cyst enlargement or complications.

Imaging Features of Solid Pseudopapillary Neoplasm (SPMN)

1. **Demographics**: Rare, primarily affects young women aged 20–30.
2. **Morphology**:
   - Solid and cystic mass with a well-defined **capsule**.
   - **Early "hemangioma-like" enhancement** in solid portions on imaging.
3. **CT Findings**:
   - Large, encapsulated mass, typically in the **pancreatic head**.
   - **Mixed solid and cystic components** due to cystic or necrotic degeneration.
   - **Central nonenhancing areas** indicating cystic or necrotic regions.
   - May show **intratumoral hemorrhage**, adding to mixed appearance.
4. **MRI Findings**:
   - Solid portions enhance early, while cystic/necrotic areas lack enhancement.
   - Hemorrhagic components may appear hyperintense on T1-weighted images.

Imaging Features of Neuroendocrine Tumor with Cystic Degeneration

1. **Type**: Nonfunctioning, also known as an islet cell tumor.
2. **Appearance**: Large mass, often with cystic or necrotic areas.
3. **Enhancement**: Hypervascular with peripheral (ring) enhancement, unlike serous cystic neoplasms which enhance centrally.
4. **CT Findings**: Hypervascular mass with central necrosis, giving a cystic-like appearance.

5. X-ray findings in acute pancreatitis. [5] [DNB Dec 21, MD (WBUHS) 18]

Acute pancreatitis is a sudden inflammation of the pancreas that can range from mild to severe and potentially life-threatening. It results from the premature activation of pancreatic enzymes, leading to autodigestion of the pancreas and surrounding tissues.

X-ray Findings in Acute Pancreatitis: Radiographs are indeed limited in diagnosing acute pancreatitis, as they are often insensitive and lack specificity. Many patients with acute pancreatitis have normal radiographic findings, and the signs seen on X-rays are not specific enough to confirm the condition.

Abdominal X-ray:

1. **Sentinel Loop Sign**: A localized ileus or isolated dilated loop of small bowel, often in the left upper quadrant, indicating inflammation near the pancreas.
2. **Colon Cut-off Sign**: Gas in the transverse colon that abruptly stops near the splenic flexure, suggesting inflammation spreading from the pancreas.
3. **Generalized Ileus**: Diffuse gaseous distension throughout the small and large bowel may occur in severe cases.
4. **Other Signs**: Rarely, you may see pancreatic calcifications in cases of chronic pancreatitis superimposed on acute exacerbations.

Chest X-ray:

1. **Pleural Effusion**: Most commonly left-sided but may be bilateral, reflecting inflammatory changes near the diaphragm.
2. **Basilar Atelectasis**: Due to diaphragmatic irritation or decreased lung expansion from abdominal pain.
3. **Acute Respiratory Distress Syndrome (ARDS)**: In severe cases, diffuse pulmonary infiltrates can be seen if ARDS develops.

6. (a) CT imaging in pancreatitis. (b) What is groove pancreatitis? (c) Radiological difference between focal mass forming pancreatitis and pancreatic adenocarcinoma. [10] [DNB June 21]

a. CT Findings in Acute Pancreatitis

Typical Pancreatic Findings

- **Parenchymal Enlargement**: Focal or diffuse enlargement due to inflammation.
- **Edema**: Changes in density within the pancreas, creating a swollen appearance.
- **Indistinct Margins**: Blurred pancreatic edges from surrounding inflammation.
- **Retroperitoneal Fat Stranding**: Inflammatory changes in the peripancreatic fat.
- **Necrosis**:
    - **Liquefactive Necrosis**: Nonenhancing areas within the pancreas, typically visible about a week after onset to differentiate from edema.
    - **Infected Necrosis**: Challenging to distinguish from aseptic necrosis, but the presence of gas (emphysematous pancreatitis) suggests infection.
    - **Abscess Formation**: Circumscribed fluid collection with little necrotic tissue, distinct from infected necrosis.
- **Hemorrhage**:
    - High-attenuation Fluid: Seen in the retroperitoneum or around the pancreas, indicating bleeding.
- **Calcifications**: Indicates underlying chronic pancreatitis in some cases.
- **Retroperitoneal Fat Necrosis**: Low-density areas with minimal heterogeneity, sometimes resembling carcinomatosis.

Dual-Energy CT

- Differentiates necrotic debris, hematomas, and viable tissue in necrotizing pancreatitis.
- Virtual noncontrast images help identify hematoma in hemorrhagic pancreatitis and distinguish it from parenchymal enhancement.
- Improves detection of noncalcified gallstones or isoattenuating cholesterol stones as potential causes.

b. Groove Pancreatitis

Groove Pancreatitis is a rare type of chronic pancreatitis that affects the "groove" between the pancreatic head, duodenum, and common bile duct (CBD). It primarily occurs in middle-aged men with a history of heavy alcohol use, and it has no association with autoimmune disease or gallstones.

Causes and Pathophysiology

The exact cause is unclear, but contributing factors may include:

- Alcohol abuse (strongest association)
- Functional obstruction of the duct of Santorini
- Brunner gland hyperplasia
- Increased pancreatic secretion viscosity from smoking or alcohol use.

Groove pancreatitis is often divided into:

- **Pure form**: Limited to the pancreaticoduodenal groove.
- **Segmental form**: Extends from the groove into the pancreatic head, sometimes causing secondary changes in the entire pancreas.

Clinical Presentation

Patients present variably with either acute or chronic symptoms:

- **Acute**: Severe abdominal pain, nausea, vomiting, and sometimes gastric outlet obstruction.
- **Chronic**: Jaundice (due to CBD narrowing), chronic weight loss, and pain that may mimic malignancy.

Imaging Features

On CT and MRI:

- Ill-defined soft tissue density or cystic changes in the pancreaticoduodenal groove.
- Thickened duodenal wall and possible small cysts in the groove or duodenal wall.
- Minimal to no pancreatic duct dilation and no lymphadenopathy, differentiating it from malignancy.

c. Radiological Difference between Focal Mass Forming Pancreatitis and Pancreatic Adenocarcinoma

Ultrasound

- **Mass Forming Pancreatitis**:
  - Location in the pancreatic head.
  - Ill-defined, often lobulated mass.
  - Common calcifications.
  - Dilated but unobstructed duct.
- **Adenocarcinoma**:
  - Located in the head and uncinate process.
  - Ill-defined, infiltrative mass.
  - Rare calcifications.
  - Abrupt ductal cutoff with dilation.

Computed Tomography

- **Mass Forming Pancreatitis**:
  - Enlarged/atrophic areas, calcifications.
  - Dilated duct without abrupt truncation.
  - Possible cystic areas (pseudocysts).
- **Adenocarcinoma**:
  - Hypoattenuating, infiltrative mass.
  - Abrupt ductal cutoff (double duct sign).
  - Vascular invasion and enlarged lymph nodes.
  - Potential distant metastasis.

MRI/MRCP

- **Mass Forming Pancreatitis**:
  - T1 iso- or hypointense, T2 hyperintense (cystic areas).
  - Dilated duct without abrupt termination.
  - Cystic changes; minimal vascular encasement.
- **Adenocarcinoma**:
  - T1 hypointense, mildly T2 hyperintense, restricted diffusion.
  - Abrupt duct cutoff, double duct sign.
  - Vascular invasion and lymphadenopathy.

PET/CT

- **Mass forming Pancreatitis**: Mild FDG uptake (inflammation).
- **Adenocarcinoma**: High FDG uptake (malignancy).

7. Define pancreatic divisum. Briefly discuss the embryological basis with the help of a diagram. Describe imaging findings on MDCT, MRCP, and ERCP. [2+2+(2+2+2)]

Pancreas Divisum: It is a congenital anatomical variant of the pancreatic ductal system where the dorsal pancreatic duct (which includes the main pancreatic duct and duct of Santorini) drains into the minor papilla without connecting to the ventral duct (duct of Wirsung), which drains into the major papilla **(Fig. 9)**. This separation results in two distinct drainage pathways:

- Dorsal duct drains the majority of the pancreas (body and tail) through the minor papilla.
- Ventral duct drains a smaller portion of the pancreas (head and uncinate process) through the major papilla.

Because the minor papilla is narrower, the pancreas divisum can lead to impaired drainage, causing increased pressure and a predisposition to abdominal pain and idiopathic pancreatitis in some individuals.

Embryology: Embryology of Pancreas Divisum

Pancreas divisum arises due to an incomplete fusion of the dorsal and ventral pancreatic buds during embryonic development, a process that normally culminates in the seventh week of gestation.

Normal Embryologic Development of the Pancreas

- **Four Weeks Gestation**:
  - The pancreas originates from the endodermal lining of the duodenum.
  - **Buds Formation**: Two outpouchings develop at the foregut-midgut junction **(Fig. 10A)**:

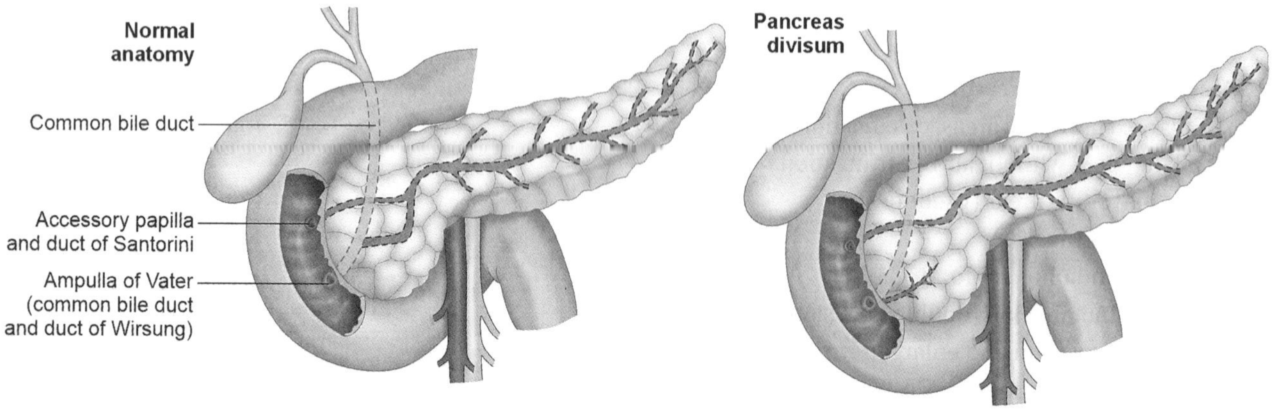

FIG. 9: Pancreatic divisum.

- **Ventral Bud (caudal)**: This bud eventually forms the posterior portion of the pancreatic head and the uncinate process.
- **Dorsal Bud (cranial)**: This bud gives rise to the anterior portion of the head, body, and tail of the pancreas.

- **Six Weeks Gestation**:
  - As the foregut elongates, the ventral pancreas rotates clockwise behind the duodenum, along with the gallbladder and bile duct **(Fig. 10B)**.
  - This rotation positions the ventral pancreatic bud posteroinferiorly to the dorsal bud, allowing for their future fusion.
- **Seven Weeks Gestation**:
  - **Fusion**: The dorsal and ventral buds fuse, forming a single pancreatic organ **(Fig. 10C)**.
  - **Duct Formation**: Main pancreatic duct (Wirsung): Formed from the ventral pancreatic duct and the distal portion of the dorsal duct.
  - **Accessory Duct (Santorini)**: May persist if the proximal part of the dorsal pancreatic duct remains, providing an additional drainage pathway.
  - **Major Papilla Formation**: The ventral pancreatic duct joins with the common bile duct (CBD), resulting in the shared exit into the duodenum at the major papilla.
  - This fusion and rotation establish the adult configuration of the pancreas and its ducts, allowing coordinated drainage into the duodenum **(Fig. 10D)**.

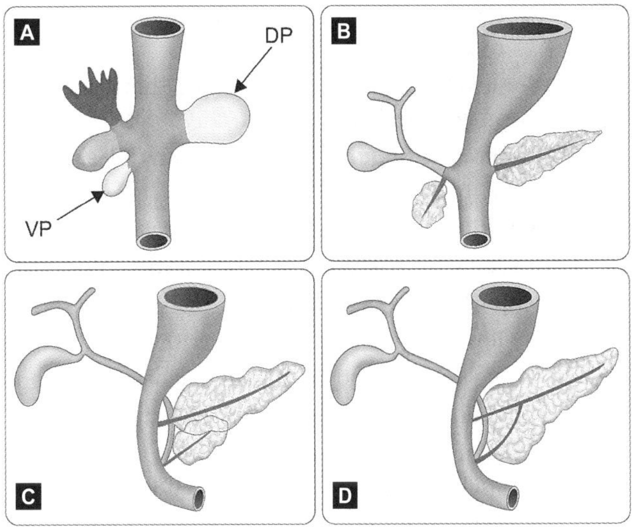

FIGS. 10A to D: Figures show normal embryologic development of pancreas.

Formation of Pancreas Divisum

In pancreas divisum, fusion of the dorsal and ventral ducts fails:

- The dorsal duct remains as the primary drainage pathway, connecting to the minor papilla and draining the body and tail.
- The ventral duct drains only the head and uncinate process through the major papilla.

Imaging Features

A. **MDCT**:
  - **Anatomy Visualization**: Less sensitive than MRCP, but sensitivity/specificity >90% in some studies.
  - **Dorsal Duct**: May appear dilated and can be traced from the pancreatic tail to the minor papilla.
  - **Ventral Duct**: Typically, smaller and harder to visualize, draining only the posterior head and uncinate.
  - **Pancreatic Morphology**: Abnormal contour of head and neck, large pancreatic head, or two distinct lobes separated by a fat cleft.
  - **Associated Pancreatitis Findings**: Acute/Chronic Pancreatitis: Enlargement, fat stranding, cysts, atrophy, calcifications, and fluid collections.

B. **Magnetic Resonance Cholangiopancreatography (MRCP)**:
  - Best noninvasive modality for visualizing the pancreatic ductal anatomy, especially the drainage patterns of the dorsal and ventral pancreatic ducts.
  - **Lack of Communication**: No connection between the dorsal and ventral ducts.
  - **Dorsal Duct (Duct of Santorini)**:
    - Dominant drainage pathway, appears long and narrow, draining most of the pancreas into the minor papilla.
    - May show constant, mildly dilated caliber without normal tapering toward the tail.
    - Santorinicele: Focal cystic dilation of the duct of Santorini visible on MRCP.

    - Crossing Ducts Sign: Anatomic crossing of the dorsal duct and common bile duct on MRCP MIP reconstructions.
  - **Ventral Duct (Duct of Wirsung)**: Shorter and drains the posterior pancreatic head and uncinate process into the major papilla.
  - **Pancreatic Signal**: High T2 and low T1 signal intensity in cases of superimposed pancreatitis, with possible peripancreatic fluid.
  - **Secretin-Enhanced MRCP**: Improves visualization by distending pancreatic ducts, aiding in diagnosis.

C. **Endoscopic Retrograde Cholangiopancreatography (ERCP)**: Most accurate but invasive:
  - **Major Papilla Cannulation**:
    - Reveals the short, tapered ventral duct.
    - No flow beyond the pancreatic head with contrast injection.
    - Guidewire does not extend past the head.
  - **Minor Papilla Cannulation**: Shows the long, possibly dilated dorsal duct, draining nearly the entire pancreas except for the posterior head and uncinate.
    - No communication observed between the dorsal and ventral ducts.
    - Cannulation of the minor papilla can be technically challenging due to its small size.

8. Discuss the classification and imaging features of cystic neoplasms of pancreas. [3+7] [DNB June 20, AIIMS May 24]

Common Cystic Neoplasms

- IPMN: Intraductal papillary mucinous neoplasm
- SCN: Serous cystic neoplasm
- MCN: Mucinous cystic neoplasm

Uncommon Cystic Neoplasms

- Solid pseudopapillary epithelial neoplasm (SPEN)
- Tumors with cystic degeneration: adenocarcinoma—neuroendocrine tumor

Diagnostic Features of Pancreatic Cystic Neoplasms

- **Consideration**: Suspect if no history of pancreatitis or trauma.
- **Morphological Indicators**:
  - Thick, irregular rim
  - Septations
  - Presence of solid components
  - Dilated pancreatic duct (>3 mm)
  - Calcifications
- **Serous Cystic Neoplasm**: Important to identify, as it has no malignant potential; symptoms typically arise only from size increase.
- **Diagnostic Challenge**: Small cysts may limit definitive diagnosis.

Imaging Features of Serous Cystic Neoplasm

1. **Plain Radiograph**:
   - Usually nonspecific and normal.
   - May show amorphous central calcification over the pancreas.
2. **Ultrasound**:
   - Appears as a nonspecific hypoechoic mass in the pancreatic head.
   - Internal echoes may indicate microcysts; oligocystic subtypes may show identifiable cysts.

3. **CT**:
   - Multicystic, lobulated mass in the pancreatic head, resembling a "bunch of grapes."
   - Individual cysts are typically <20 mm and greater than six in number (except oligocystic type).
   - Enhancing central scar with possible stellate calcification (~20% of cases).
4. **MRI**:
   - Appears as a cluster of small cysts with no communication with the pancreatic duct.
   - **T1**: Low signal intensity.
   - **T2**: High signal in cystic components; central fibrous scar (if present) appears low signal.
   - **T1 with Contrast (Gd)**: Fibrous septa may enhance on delayed images.

Imaging Features of Intraductal Papillary Mucinous Neoplasm (IPMN)

1. **General Features**:
   - **Ductal Communication**: IPMNs communicate with the main pancreatic duct or its branches, unlike mucinous cystadenomas.
   - **Calcifications**: Rare (~13% in resected IPMNs).
2. **Fluoroscopy (ERCP)**:
   - Shows dilated pancreatic ducts (segmental, diffuse, or branch type).
   - May reveal polypoid mural tumors or mucinous filling defects.
   - Mucin may be seen at the ampulla of Vater.
3. **Ultrasound**:
   - **Main Duct Type**: Shows thin-walled cysts or dilated hypoechoic ducts (>5 mm).
   - **Mural Nodules and Mucin**: Hyperechoic; may be difficult to differentiate from pancreatic tissue.
4. **CT**:
   - Hypodense, cystic lesions; main duct dilated (>5 mm) in main duct IPMN.
   - Communication with pancreatic ducts can be challenging to detect.
   - Calcifications uncommon in IPMN.
5. **MRI/MRCP**:
   - **Main Duct Type**: Dilated pancreatic duct (>5 mm) filled with low-density mucin; parenchyma may be thinned.
   - **Mucin Bulging**: Mucinous material may bulge from ampulla of Vater (uncommon but pathognomonic).
   - **Branch Duct Type**: Dilated side branches with a "bunch of grapes" appearance, mimicking cystic tumors.
   - **Mixed Type**: Features of both main duct and branch duct types with main duct dilatation (>5 mm).
   - **Mural Nodules**: Concerning for malignancy, especially if they enhance after contrast.

Imaging Features of Mucinous Cystadenoma (MCN)

1. **Demographics**:
   - Exclusively seen in women, typically aged 40–50.
   - Often located in the pancreatic **body and tail** (95%).
2. **Morphology**:
   - Large, macrocystic lesion with **thick-walled septations**.
   - **Peripheral calcifications** in 25% of cases, aiding in specific diagnosis.
   - No communication with the main pancreatic duct.
3. **CT Findings**:
   - Large cystic lesion with **peripheral calcification**.
   - **Internal septations** and **thick walls**.
   - Nonlobulated, smooth capsule.

4. **MRI Findings**:
   - Better depiction of **internal septations** on T1-weighted images postgadolinium.
   - Absence of ductal communication.
5. **Clinical Presentation**:
   - Typically, symptomatic with vague abdominal pain.
   - May present with sudden pain due to rapid cyst enlargement or complications.

Imaging Features of Solid Pseudopapillary Neoplasm (SPMN)

1. **Demographics**: Rare, primarily affects young women aged 20–30.
2. **Morphology**:
   - Solid and cystic mass with a well-defined **capsule**.
   - **Early "hemangioma-like" enhancement** in solid portions on imaging.
3. **CT Findings**:
   - Large, encapsulated mass, typically in the **pancreatic head**.
   - **Mixed solid and cystic components** due to cystic or necrotic degeneration.
   - **Central nonenhancing areas** indicating cystic or necrotic regions.
   - May show **intratumoral hemorrhage**, adding to mixed appearance.
4. **MRI Findings**:
   - Solid portions enhance early, while cystic/necrotic areas lack enhancement.
   - Hemorrhagic components may appear hyperintense on T1-weighted images.

Imaging Features of Neuroendocrine Tumor with Cystic Degeneration

1. **Type**: Nonfunctioning, also known as an islet cell tumor.
2. **Appearance**: Large mass, often with cystic or necrotic areas.
3. **Enhancement**: Hypervascular with peripheral (ring) enhancement, unlike serous cystic neoplasms which enhance centrally.
4. **CT Findings**: Hypervascular mass with central necrosis, giving a cystic-like appearance.

Vascular Diseases

1. Imaging in mesenteric ischemia. [10] [DNB June 22]

Mesenteric ischemia is a potentially life-threatening condition that results from insufficient blood flow to the intestines. Imaging plays a critical role in the diagnosis and management of this condition.

Classification and Types

- **Acute MI (AMI)**: Sudden reduction in blood flow, presenting as severe, disproportionate abdominal pain, nausea, vomiting, and diarrhea. Peritonitis suggests irreversible ischemia.
- **Chronic MI (CMI)**: Develops gradually, characterized by postprandial pain, weight loss, and food aversion, often due to atherosclerotic narrowing of the mesenteric vessels.
- **Acute-on-Chronic MI**: Acute ischemic episodes superimposed on chronic ischemic conditions.

AMI is further divided into:

- Occlusive MI (embolism, thrombosis, venous thromboembolism).
- Nonocclusive MI (NOMI), typically in critically ill patients without clear arterial or venous blockage.

Imaging Modalities for Mesenteric Ischemia

1. **Plain Radiography**:
   - **Role**: Often an initial imaging tool, but limited specificity and sensitivity for diagnosing mesenteric ischemia.

- **Findings**: May show signs of bowel ischemia such as pneumatosis intestinalis, portal venous gas, or bowel distension, although these are typically late findings.
- **Limitations**: Nonspecific, as these findings may appear in other conditions as well.

2. **Ultrasound (US) with Doppler**:
   - **Role**: Useful for visualizing mesenteric vessels, particularly the superior mesenteric artery (SMA) and coeliac artery.
   - **Findings**:
     - **Early-phase AMI**: Doppler can show SMA occlusion and bowel spasm.
     - **Intermediate-phase**: Limited by bowel gas accumulation, which causes acoustic impedance.
     - **Late-stage**: Fluid-filled loops, decreased peristalsis, bowel wall thinning, and peritoneal free fluid. In venous occlusion, findings may include portal thrombus, decreased peristalsis, intraluminal secretions, and mural thickening.
3. **Computed Tomography Angiography (CTA)**:
   - Primary imaging modality with high sensitivity (90–100%) and specificity.
   - **Protocol**: Thin-section imaging in arterial and venous phases, with bolus tracking for timing. Split-bolus protocol can reduce radiation and contrast dose.
   - **Key Findings**:
     - **Arterial Thromboembolism**: Low-attenuation filling defects within mesenteric arteries, absent bowel wall enhancement, or "paper-thin" bowel wall. Severe cases may show pneumatosis intestinalis and porto-mesenteric venous gas.
     - **Mesenteric Venous Thrombosis (MVT)**: Filling defects in mesenteric veins, mural thickening, and a "halo" or "target" sign due to submucosal edema.
     - **Nonocclusive Mesenteric Ischemia (NOMI)**: Narrowing of mesenteric vessels with the "string-of-sausages" appearance, subtle signs of bowel wall hyperenhancement, and perienteric stranding.
4. **Catheter Angiography**: Now primarily for therapeutic interventions (e.g., thrombolysis, stenting) rather than diagnostic use.
5. **Dual-energy CT (DECT)**:
   - Enhanced bowel wall contrast with virtual noncontrast (VNC) and iodine maps.
   - Low-energy monochromatic images (40–60 keV) highlight subtle enhancement differences in ischemic bowel segments.
6. **CT Findings in Specific Mesenteric Ischemia Types**:
   - **Chronic Mesenteric Ischemia (CMI)**: Visualizes arterial stenosis at mesenteric vessel origins and collateral vessels.
   - **Colonic Ischemia**: Bowel wall thickening, hypoenhancement, and, in severe cases, pneumatosis intestinalis or perforation.
7. **Magnetic Resonance Angiography (MRA)**:
   - **Role**: High sensitivity and specificity for evaluating occlusions or stenoses, especially in chronic mesenteric ischemia.
   - **Findings**: Effective for identifying proximal vessel occlusions or high-grade stenoses, particularly of the coeliac trunk or SMA.

2. (a) Radiographic, ultrasound and MDCT findings in acute mesenteric ischemia. (b) Role of intervention in this condition. [(2+2+2)+4]

Radiographic Features

Often an initial imaging tool, but limited specificity and sensitivity for diagnosing mesenteric ischemia.

- **Nonspecific Findings**: Plain radiographs may not be diagnostic but can show:
  a. Dilated bowel loops

b. Gasless abdomen
c. Pneumatosis intestinalis (late-stage finding)
d. Portal venous gas (advanced ischemia)

Ultrasound Features in AMI

1. **Mesenteric Artery and Vein Assessment (Doppler Ultrasound)**
   - **Reduced or Absent Flow**: Lack of Doppler flow in the superior mesenteric artery (SMA) or superior mesenteric vein (SMV) can indicate arterial or venous occlusion.
   - **Increased Resistive Index (RI)**: A high RI in the SMA may suggest vasospasm or impaired blood flow.
   - **Visible Thrombus**: Direct visualization of a thrombus in the SMA or SMV is rare but possible. Thrombi may appear as echogenic structures within the vessel lumen.
2. **Bowel Wall Findings**:
   - **Bowel Wall Thickening**: Hypoechoic or "target" appearance due to edema or hemorrhage within the bowel wall layers.
   - **Loss of Normal Stratification**: Disrupted bowel wall layers, indicating severe ischemia or impending necrosis.
   - **Diminished or Absent Peristalsis**: Reduced or absent bowel motility can indicate severe ischemia and may suggest nonviable bowel.
3. **Intramural and Portal Venous Gas**:
   - **Pneumatosis Intestinalis**: Small gas bubbles within the bowel wall can sometimes be visualized as hyperechoic foci with ring-down artifacts.
   - **Portal Venous Gas**: Hyperechoic foci within the portal vein and its branches, often associated with poor prognosis, seen as moving bright spots on real-time imaging.
4. **Mesenteric and Peritoneal Findings**:
   - **Mesenteric Fat Stranding**: Increased echogenicity of the mesenteric fat, suggesting inflammation.
   - **Free Fluid (Ascites)**: The presence of free fluid around bowel loops can indicate advanced ischemia or bowel infarction, particularly if it appears complex or echogenic.

MDCT

Imaging Protocol

1. **Phases**: A triple-phase protocol (noncontrast, arterial, and venous phases) is typically used.
   - **Noncontrast Phase**: Helps detect bowel wall hemorrhage and intramural gas.
   - **Arterial Phase**: Critical for evaluating the mesenteric arteries, identifying thrombus or emboli, and assessing arterial flow.
   - **Venous Phase**: Essential for detecting mesenteric venous thrombosis and for evaluating bowel wall enhancement and surrounding mesenteric structures.
2. **Key MDCT Findings in AMI**:
   - **Vascular Findings**:
     - **Arterial Occlusion**: Seen as a filling defect within the superior mesenteric artery (SMA) or other mesenteric vessels.
     - **Venous Thrombosis**: Filling defects in the mesenteric veins, commonly in the superior mesenteric vein (SMV).
     - **Nonocclusive Mesenteric Ischemia (NOMI)**: Reduced vessel caliber, with narrowed SMA due to vasospasm or low-flow states, often related to systemic hypoperfusion.
   - **Bowel Wall Findings**:
     - **Bowel Wall Thickening**: Due to edema or inflammation, with "target" or "halo" appearance.
     - **Abnormal Enhancement**: In early AMI, hyperenhancement of the bowel wall due to vascular congestion; in advanced ischemia, hypoenhancement indicates necrosis.
     - **Intramural Gas (Pneumatosis)**: Indicates severe ischemia and impending or ongoing bowel infarction.

   - **Portal Venous Gas**: Seen as small air bubbles in the portal vein branches, indicating severe ischemic injury and poor prognosis.
- **Mesenteric Findings**:
   - **Mesenteric Fat Stranding**: Inflammatory changes in the surrounding mesentery.
   - **Engorgement of Mesenteric Veins**: Due to venous congestion in venous AMI.
   - **Ascites**: Small amounts of fluid around the affected bowel loops, often associated with advanced ischemia.

Intervention

In acute mesenteric ischemia (AMI), rapid intervention is essential to restore blood flow and prevent bowel necrosis. Here is a summary of key interventions:

- **Catheter-directed Thrombolysis**:
  - Indication: Used in thrombotic or embolic AMI, especially in frail patients with early-stage ischemia.
  - Procedure: Thrombolytic agents are delivered directly into the thrombus via catheter through a femoral arterial approach. Often combined with heparin for better clot dissolution.
  - Advantages: Minimally invasive, reduces need for open surgery.
- **Angioplasty and Stenting**:
  - Indication: Employed when vascular stenosis underlies AMI, commonly in mesenteric arterial thrombosis (MAT).
  - Procedure: A balloon-expandable stent is placed after angioplasty to widen the stenotic segment. Thrombo-aspiration or thrombolysis may be combined to prevent distal embolization.
  - Advantages: Effective for restoring blood flow in cases without bowel necrosis.
- **Intra-arterial Vasodilator Therapy for nonocclusive Mesenteric Ischemia (NOMI)**:
  - Indication: NOMI cases where vasoconstriction causes reduced mesenteric blood flow.
  - Procedure: Vasodilators (e.g., papaverine) are infused via catheter in the SMA to relieve vasospasm, improving blood flow.
  - Advantages: Reduces mortality by restoring perfusion without surgery.
- **Surgical Intervention**:
  - Indication: For irreversible ischemia, bowel necrosis, or failed endovascular attempts.
  - Procedure: Options include embolectomy, bypass grafting, or bowel resection depending on the extent of ischemia.
  - Advantages: Direct visualization allows assessment of bowel viability.
- **Management of Mesenteric Venous Thrombosis (MVT)**:
  - Indication: AMI due to venous occlusion.
  - Procedure: Initial management is anticoagulation with heparin. Severe cases may require thrombolysis and thromboaspiration via TIPS or transhepatic routes.
  - Advantages: Restores venous drainage, preventing long-term complications.

Each intervention targets different AMI causes, aiming to restore blood flow while minimizing risks and preventing bowel damage.

3. Discuss the causes and radiological features of Budd-Chiari Syndrome. Discuss the role of interventional radiology in treatment of Budd-Chiari Syndrome. [7+3] [DNB June 20, MD (WBUHS) 24]

Budd-Chiari Syndrome (BCS), or hepatic venous outflow obstruction, occurs when hepatic veins are partially or completely blocked, impairing liver blood drainage. Clinical symptoms typically arise when at least two hepatic veins are obstructed, causing liver congestion, ascites, and abdominal pain. Diagnosis is confirmed via imaging (Doppler US, CT, MRI) that shows vein occlusion and collateral circulation.

Causes of Budd-Chiari Syndrome

- **Thrombotic Causes**:
  - **Polycythemia Vera**: Increases blood viscosity, leading to clots.
  - **Thrombocytosis**: Excess platelets promote clotting.

  - **Antiphospholipid Syndrome, PNH**: Autoimmune disorders causing recurrent clotting.
  - **Pregnancy/Postpartum, Oral Contraceptives**: Hormonal changes increase clot risk.
  - **Sickle Cell Disease**: Abnormal blood cells cause blockages.
  - **Dehydration, Sepsis**: Contribute to clot formation.
- **External Compression (25%)**:
  - **Congenital**: Hepatic vein/IVC web, diaphragm interruptions.
  - **Tumor Invasion**: Cancers like renal or liver carcinoma, leiomyosarcoma can compress veins.
- **Autoimmune and Inflammatory**:
  - **Phlebitis**: Inflammation due to conditions like bone marrow transplant or chemoradiotherapy.
  - **Behçet's Disease**: Autoimmune vasculitis causing clotting.
- **Idiopathic**: One-third of cases have no clear cause.

Imaging Features

A. **Sonographic Findings in Budd-Chiari Syndrome**:
  - **Gray-scale Sonography**:
    - **Caudate Lobe Enlargement**: Hypertrophy of the caudate lobe.
    - **Ascites**: Presence of free fluid in the abdomen.
    - **Splenomegaly**: Enlargement of the spleen.
    - **Hepatic Vein Abnormalities**: Narrowing, lack of visualization, or thrombosis of hepatic veins.
    - **Caudate Vein Diameter**: Caudate vein ≥3 mm on grayscale suggests Budd-Chiari syndrome.
  - **Color Doppler Sonography**:
    - **Absent or Flat Hepatic Vein Flow**: Reduced or absent blood flow in hepatic veins.
    - **Reversed Flow**: Reverse flow in the hepatic veins, inferior vena cava (IVC), or both.
    - **Intrahepatic Collateral Pathways**: Formation of collateral vessels within the liver.
    - **Portal Vein Flow**: Slow hepatofugal flow (<11 cm/s), indicating reversed or slowed portal blood flow.

B. **CT Imaging in Budd-Chiari Syndrome**:
  - **Acute BCS**:
    - Patchy liver enhancement: Central liver shows strong enhancement, while peripheral areas are hypoattenuating.
    - Hepatic vein thrombosis: Hypoattenuating hepatic veins and IVC compression due to enlarged caudate lobe.
    - Ascites and splenomegaly are common.
  - **Subacute/Chronic BCS**:
    - Intrahepatic collaterals and hypoperfused liver areas visible.
    - Enlarged hepatic artery and possible IVC calcification.
    - Portal vein thrombosis may develop.
  - **Regenerative Nodules**: Seen in chronic cases, hyperattenuating in arterial phase, differentiable from hepatocellular carcinoma.
  - **Advanced MDCT**: Multiplanar reformation aids in detailed evaluation of venous structures and liver changes.

C. **MRI Features in Budd-Chiari Syndrome**:
  - **T2-weighted Images**:
    - Peripheral liver changes: Heterogeneous increased signal intensity in the peripheral liver.
    - Lack of hepatic vein and IVC visualization: T2-weighted sequences don't show these vessels.
  - **T2-weighted Gradient-Recalled Echo***: Useful for detecting absence of flow in the hepatic veins and IVC.
  - **T1-weighted Images with Contrast**:
    - **Hepatic vein and IVC occlusion**: Clear visualization of occluded veins.
    - **In acute BCS**: Normal or increased enhancement of the caudate lobe, with decreased peripheral liver enhancement.
    - **In chronic BCS**: Enhancement may be more variable and subtle.

- **Regenerative Nodules**:
  - **T1-weighted images**: Nodules are bright and hypervascular postcontrast.
  - **T2-weighted images**: Nodules are typically isointense or hypointense compared to liver.
  - Distinguish from hepatocellular carcinoma based on signal characteristics.

D. **Angiographic Findings in Budd-Chiari Syndrome**:
- **Spiderweb Pattern**: A pathognomonic "spiderweb" pattern of collateral vessels in the IVC or hepatic venography.
- **Thrombosis**: Thrombus within the hepatic veins or inferior vena cava.
- **IVC Compression**: Long segmental compression of the IVC due to caudate lobe hypertrophy.
- **Hepatic Artery Changes**: Dilated hepatic arteries and arterioportal shunts due to reduced venous outflow.

Role of Interventional Radiology in Budd-Chiari Syndrome Treatment

Interventional radiology (IR) is central in managing BCS, especially for patients with refractory symptoms or progressive liver dysfunction.

- **Percutaneous Transhepatic Angioplasty (PTA) and Stenting**:
  - **Indications**: Primarily used in patients with stenosis or short-segment occlusions of hepatic veins or IVC.
  - **Procedure**: Balloon angioplasty dilates the stenosed hepatic vein or IVC segment, followed by stent placement if needed to maintain vessel patency.
  - **Outcome**: PTA and stenting effectively restore venous outflow and reduce portal hypertension in select cases.
- **Transjugular Intrahepatic Portosystemic Shunt (TIPS)**:
  - **Indications**: TIPS is used when angioplasty or stenting is not feasible, or in cases with severe portal hypertension.
  - **Procedure**: Creates a shunt between the portal vein and hepatic vein, reducing portal hypertension and decompressing the liver.
  - **Outcome**: TIPS provides effective symptomatic relief, improves venous outflow, and can prevent variceal bleeding and ascites.
- **Thrombolysis and Thrombectomy**:
  - **Indications**: Acute BCS with recent thrombus formation in hepatic veins or IVC.
  - **Procedure**: Catheter-directed thrombolysis administers thrombolytic agents directly into the clot, while thrombectomy mechanically removes the clot.
  - **Outcome**: Thrombolysis/thrombectomy can restore venous patency but carries a higher risk of bleeding complications.
- **Surgical Shunts and Liver Transplantation**: For advanced or refractory cases where IR options are insufficient or in cases of fulminant liver failure, surgical shunts or liver transplantation may be considered.

4. What are the various causes of acute mesenteric ischemia? Discuss the role of radiology in its diagnosis and management. [3+(5+2)] [DNB June 20]

Causes of Acute Mesenteric Ischemia (AMI)

- **Arterial Thrombosis (50% of cases)**: Primary cause is a thrombus in the superior mesenteric artery (SMA) or celiac artery, often associated with atherosclerosis.
- **Arterial Embolism (25–40%)**: Embolism from the heart (due to atrial fibrillation, valvular disease, or myocardial infarction) or other embolic sources can occlude the mesenteric arteries.
- **Nonocclusive Mesenteric Ischemia (NOMI)**: Mesenteric vasospasm often due to systemic hypotension, heart failure, or vasoconstrictor drugs.
- **Venous Thrombosis (5–15%)**: Thrombosis in the mesenteric veins (e.g., superior mesenteric vein (SMV)) or portal vein, often seen in patients with hypercoagulable states like polycythemia, antiphospholipid syndrome, or oral contraceptive use.
- **External Compression**: Compression due to tumors, retroperitoneal fibrosis, or abdominal aortic aneurysm (AAA).

Radiographic Features

Often an initial imaging tool, but limited specificity and sensitivity for diagnosing mesenteric ischemia.

Nonspecific findings: Plain radiographs may not be diagnostic but can show:

a. Dilated bowel loops
b. Gasless abdomen
c. Pneumatosis intestinalis (late-stage finding)
d. Portal venous gas (advanced ischemia)

Ultrasound Features in AMI

1. **Mesenteric Artery and Vein Assessment (Doppler Ultrasound)**:
   - **Reduced or Absent Flow**: Lack of Doppler flow in the superior mesenteric artery (SMA) or superior mesenteric vein (SMV) can indicate arterial or venous occlusion.
   - **Increased Resistive Index (RI)**: A high RI in the SMA may suggest vasospasm or impaired blood flow.
   - **Visible Thrombus**: Direct visualization of a thrombus in the SMA or SMV is rare but possible. Thrombi may appear as echogenic structures within the vessel lumen.
2. **Bowel Wall Findings**:
   - **Bowel Wall Thickening**: Hypoechoic or "target" appearance due to edema or hemorrhage within the bowel wall layers.
   - **Loss of Normal Stratification**: Disrupted bowel wall layers, indicating severe ischemia or impending necrosis.
   - **Diminished or Absent Peristalsis**: Reduced or absent bowel motility can indicate severe ischemia and may suggest nonviable bowel.
3. **Intramural and Portal Venous Gas**:
   - **Pneumatosis Intestinalis**: Small gas bubbles within the bowel wall can sometimes be visualized as hyperechoic foci with ring-down artifacts.
   - **Portal Venous Gas**: Hyperechoic foci within the portal vein and its branches, often associated with poor prognosis, seen as moving bright spots on real-time imaging.
4. **Mesenteric and Peritoneal Findings**:
   - **Mesenteric Fat Stranding**: Increased echogenicity of the mesenteric fat, suggesting inflammation.
   - **Free Fluid (Ascites)**: The presence of free fluid around bowel loops can indicate advanced ischemia or bowel infarction, particularly if it appears complex or echogenic.

MDCT

Imaging Protocol

1. **Phases**: A triple-phase protocol (noncontrast, arterial, and venous phases) is typically used.
   - **Noncontrast Phase**: Helps detect bowel wall hemorrhage and intramural gas.
   - **Arterial Phase**: Critical for evaluating the mesenteric arteries, identifying thrombus or emboli, and assessing arterial flow.
   - **Venous Phase**: Essential for detecting mesenteric venous thrombosis and for evaluating bowel wall enhancement and surrounding mesenteric structures.
2. **Key MDCT Findings in AMI**:
   - **Vascular Findings**:
     - **Arterial Occlusion**: Seen as a filling defect within the superior mesenteric artery (SMA) or other mesenteric vessels.
     - **Venous Thrombosis**: Filling defects in the mesenteric veins, commonly in the superior mesenteric vein (SMV).
     - **Nonocclusive Mesenteric Ischemia (NOMI)**: Reduced vessel caliber, with narrowed SMA due to vasospasm or low-flow states, often related to systemic hypoperfusion.
   - **Bowel Wall Findings**:
     - **Bowel Wall Thickening**: Due to edema or inflammation, with "target" or "halo" appearance.
     - **Abnormal Enhancement**: In early AMI, hyperenhancement of the bowel wall due to vascular congestion; in advanced ischemia, hypoenhancement indicates necrosis.

  - **Intramural Gas (Pneumatosis)**: Indicates severe ischemia and impending or ongoing bowel infarction.
  - **Portal Venous Gas**: Seen as small air bubbles in the portal vein branches, indicating severe ischemic injury and poor prognosis.
- **Mesenteric Findings**:
  - **Mesenteric Fat Stranding**: Inflammatory changes in the surrounding mesentery.
  - **Engorgement of Mesenteric Veins**: Due to venous congestion in venous AMI.
  - **Ascites**: Small amounts of fluid around the affected bowel loops, often associated with advanced ischemia.

Intervention

In acute mesenteric ischemia (AMI), rapid intervention is essential to restore blood flow and prevent bowel necrosis. Here is a summary of key interventions:

- **Catheter-directed Thrombolysis**:
  - Indication: Used in thrombotic or embolic AMI, especially in frail patients with early-stage ischemia.
  - Procedure: Thrombolytic agents are delivered directly into the thrombus via catheter through a femoral arterial approach. Often combined with heparin for better clot dissolution.
  - Advantages: Minimally invasive, reduces need for open surgery.
- **Angioplasty and Stenting**:
  - Indication: Employed when vascular stenosis underlies AMI, commonly in mesenteric arterial thrombosis (MAT).
  - Procedure: A balloon-expandable stent is placed after angioplasty to widen the stenotic segment. Thromboaspiration or thrombolysis may be combined to prevent distal embolization.
  - Advantages: Effective for restoring blood flow in cases without bowel necrosis.
- **Intra-arterial Vasodilator Therapy for Nonocclusive Mesenteric Ischemia:**
  - Indication: NOMI cases where vasoconstriction causes reduced mesenteric blood flow.
  - Procedure: Vasodilators (e.g., papaverine) are infused via a catheter in the SMA to relieve vasospasm, improving blood flow.
  - Advantages: Reduces mortality by restoring perfusion without surgery.
- **Surgical Intervention**:
  - Indication: For irreversible ischemia, bowel necrosis, or failed endovascular attempts.
  - Procedure: Options include embolectomy, bypass grafting, or bowel resection depending on the extent of ischemia.
  - Advantages: Direct visualization allows assessment of bowel viability.
- **Management of Mesenteric Venous Thrombosis (MVT)**:
  - Indication: AMI due to venous occlusion.
  - Procedure: Initial management is anticoagulation with heparin. Severe cases may require thrombolysis and thromboaspiration via TIPS or transhepatic routes.
  - Advantages: Restores venous drainage, preventing long-term complications.

Each intervention targets different AMI causes, aiming to restore blood flow while minimizing risks and preventing bowel damage.

Miscellaneous

1. Enumerate the common causes of epigastric disorder in a young adult mentioning the various imaging procedures to come to a diagnosis. [10] [MD (WBUHS) 19]

A. Gastroesophageal Reflux Disease

- **Fluoroscopy**:
  - Reflux: Demonstration of contrast material moving from the stomach into the esophagus during dynamic imaging.
  - Hiatus Hernia: Visualization of the stomach pushing through the diaphragm into the thoracic cavity.

- **Endoscopy**:
  - Reflux Esophagitis: Erythema, erosions, and ulcerations in the esophageal lining.
  - Barrett's Esophagus: Presence of columnar cells replacing the normal squamous cells, indicating potential precancerous changes.
- **24-hour pH Monitoring**: Measurement of acid levels in the esophagus to assess the frequency and duration of acid reflux episodes.

B. Gastric Ulcer

Radiographic Features

Although historically barium studies were the mainstay of investigation for suspect peptic ulceration, endoscopy has in most centers, largely replaced the barium meal. Many younger radiologists/training radiologists have rarely if ever performed a full diagnostic barium meal, and the 'art' of this examination is gradually being lost.

In the acute setting CT is the modality of choice for assessing a patient with acute abdominal pain, and in some settings may be able to identify the site of bleeding prior to endoscopy.

Plain Radiograph

Abdominal films have little role in the setting of vague/chronic upper abdominal pain and have a very low yield. In the acute setting, an erect chest x-ray is invaluable as it not only often allows the diagnosis of pneumoperitoneum to be made with confidence, but also gives treating clinicians' important information of the patients' general health (e.g., cardiomegaly, aspiration pneumonia, pulmonary metastases).

Barium meals are performed with liquid barium and an effervescent to distend the stomach with gas and allow a 'double-contrast' image.

Features of ulceration include:

- Pocket of barium filling the ulcer crater
- 85% round; 15% linear
- 10–15% of ulcers are multiple
- Postbulbar ulcers should raise the possibility of Zollinger-Ellison syndrome especially if ulcers are multiple and gastric folds are thickened
- Edematous collar of swollen mucosa (to be distinguished from the rolled edges of a malignant ulcer)
- Radiating folds of mucosa away from the ulcer

CT

Ideal technique and findings depend on the presentation. Perforation is usually a straightforward diagnosis, often with abundant pneumoperitoneum visible. The site of perforation is sometimes visible as a region of discontinuity in the stomach or duodenal wall.

Hemorrhage can be challenging to identify and requires a multi-phase scan without positive oral contrast (typically noncontrast, arterial and delayed phase scans are obtained) and the presence of active bleeding. Extravasation and pooling/accumulation of contrast into the lumen of the bowel may be seen.

C. Gastritis

Gastritis, the inflammation of the stomach lining, can present with various radiological features depending on the underlying cause and severity. Here are some common imaging modalities and their associated findings:

1. **X-ray**:
   - Air Fluid Levels: In cases of severe gastritis with possible gastric outlet obstruction.
   - Dilated Stomach: May indicate a functional obstruction or severe inflammation.
2. **Ultrasound**:
   - Thickened Gastric Wall: Wall thickness greater than 5 mm can suggest inflammation.
   - Increased Echogenicity: Suggests edema in the gastric wall.
   - Peritoneal Fluid: Possible presence in cases of erosive gastritis or complications.

3. **CT Scan**:
   - Gastric Wall Thickening: More pronounced than in ultrasound, indicating inflammation.
   - Enhancement of the Gastric Wall: Seen with contrast enhancement, indicating active inflammation.
   - Mucosal Edema: Appears as low attenuation areas within the wall.
   - Lymphadenopathy: Enlarged regional lymph nodes may be seen, especially in cases of chronic or infectious gastritis.
4. **Endoscopic Findings**: While not strictly radiological, endoscopy can provide critical visual information:
   - Erythema and Edema: Visual signs of inflammation.
   - Erosions or Ulcers: Indicates more severe forms of gastritis.
   - Mucosal Atrophy: Seen in chronic gastritis.

D. Acute Pancreatitis

Acute pancreatitis is characterized by inflammation of the pancreas, and various radiological imaging techniques can help diagnose and assess its severity. Here are some key imaging features associated with acute pancreatitis:

1. **Ultrasound**:
   - Peritoneal Fluid: Presence of fluid collections in the peritoneal cavity.
   - Pancreatic Edema: Increased echogenicity or enlargement of the pancreas.
   - Gallstones: Identification of gallstones, which are a common cause of acute pancreatitis.
   - Fluid Collections: Detection of fluid collections around the pancreas (e.g., peripancreatic fluid).
2. **Computed Tomography**:
   - Pancreatic Enlargement: Swelling of the pancreas due to inflammation.
   - Peripancreatic Fat Stranding: Increased attenuation in the surrounding fat indicating inflammation.
   - Fluid Collections: Formation of pseudocysts or necrotic collections.
   - Necrosis: Areas of nonenhancement within the pancreas indicating necrotizing pancreatitis.
   - Complications: Potential complications like abscess formation, vascular complications, or portal vein thrombosis.
3. **Magnetic Resonance Imaging (MRI)**:
   - Pancreatic Edema: Similar to CT, showing increased signal intensity in T2-weighted images.
   - Fluid Collections: Well-defined fluid collections can be visualized.
   - Necrotic Tissue: Differentiation of necrotic versus viable pancreatic tissue.
   - Biliary Tract Evaluation: Better visualization of the biliary tree to assess for obstructions.
4. **Endoscopic Ultrasound (EUS)**:
   - Early Diagnosis: Useful for early detection of pancreatitis and complications.
   - Pseudocysts: Can assess and characterize pancreatic pseudocysts.
   - Biliary Causes: Allows direct visualization of the bile ducts and can help identify obstructions.
5. **Radiographic Features**:
   - Calcifications: In chronic cases or severe acute pancreatitis, calcifications may develop.
   - Vascular Complications: Signs of thrombosis or hemorrhage can be assessed via CT angiography if necessary.

2. What are the causes of abdominal mass in children below the age of 5 years? Discuss in brief the imaging modalities to investigate the case. [3+7] [MD (WBUHS) 22]

Common Causes of Abdominal Mass in Children Below the Age of 5 Years

- **Malignant Hepatic Neoplasm**:
  1. Hepatoblastoma
  2. Hepatocellular Carcinoma

- **Benign Hepatic Neoplasm**:
  1. Hemangioma
- **Renal Mass**:
  1. Wilm's tumor
  2. Neuroblastoma

Malignant Hepatic Neoplasm

1. **Hepatoblastoma**:
   - **Ultrasound**:
     - Hypoechoic Mass: The tumor typically appears as a solid, hypoechoic mass relative to normal liver tissue.
     - Vascularity: Increased vascularity can be noted on Doppler ultrasound.
     - Calcifications: Focal calcifications may be present but are not always seen.
   - **Computed Tomography**:
     - Mass Appearance: Hepatoblastoma often presents as a large, heterogeneous mass that can be well-defined or infiltrative.
     - Enhancement Patterns: On contrast-enhanced CT, the tumor typically shows heterogeneous enhancement, with areas of necrosis.
     - Vascular Invasion: The presence of portal vein invasion or hepatic vein involvement can be evaluated.
     - Lymphadenopathy: Regional lymphadenopathy may be present.
   - **Magnetic Resonance Imaging (MRI)**:
     - T1-weighted Imaging: Hepatoblastoma usually appears hypointense to the surrounding liver on T1-weighted images.
     - T2-weighted Imaging: It is often hyperintense on T2-weighted images due to its high-water content.
     - Enhancement Characteristics: Postcontrast, the tumor may show variable enhancement depending on the degree of necrosis and the presence of fibrous tissue.
     - Capsule: An incomplete capsule may be observed, and surrounding edema can be noted.
2. **Hepatocellular Carcinoma**:
   - **Ultrasound**:
     - Heterogeneous echogenicity: The tumor may appear hypoechoic or isoechoic relative to normal liver tissue.
     - Mass effect: Presence of a solid mass, often with irregular margins.
     - Vascular invasion: Possible Doppler signal showing increased blood flow.
   - **CT Scan**:
     - Well-defined or irregular mass: Often appears as a hypervascular lesion, especially during the arterial phase.
     - Heterogeneous enhancement: May show central necrosis or calcifications.
     - Portal vein invasion: Thrombosis or invasion can be seen.
   - **MRI**:
     - High signal intensity on T2-weighted images: Depending on the degree of necrosis and fat content.
     - Arterial phase enhancement: Similar to CT, with washout in the portal venous phase.
     - Capsule formation: Some tumors may demonstrate a surrounding capsule.

Benign Hepatic Neoplasm

1. **Hemangiomas**:
   - **Ultrasound**:
     - Typically, well-defined hyperechoic lesions, a small proportion (10%) are hypoechoic, which may be due to a background of hepatic steatosis, where the liver parenchyma itself is of increased echogenicity.
     - Color Doppler: May show peripheral feeding vessels.

  - Contrast-enhanced ultrasound:
    - Arterial phase: Peripheral nodular discontinuous enhancement
    - Portal venous and delayed phases: continued "filling-in" of the lesion, until the entire hemangioma is hyperechoic relative to background liver
    - Central hemorrhagic portions of cavernous hemangiomas remain nonenhancing
- **CT**: Most hemangiomas are relatively well-defined. The dynamic enhancement pattern is related to the size of its vascular space. Features of typical lesions include:
  - Noncontrast: Often homogeneous hypoattenuating (<20 hounsfield units) relative to liver parenchyma.
  - Late arterial phase: Typically show discontinuous, nodular, peripheral enhancement (small lesions may show uniform enhancement)
  - Portal venous phase: Progressive peripheral enhancement with more centripetal fill-in
  - Delayed phase: Further irregular fill-in and therefore iso or hyper-attenuating to liver parenchyma.
- **MRI**: Typical features include:
  - T1: hypointense relative to liver parenchyma
  - T2: hyperintense relative to liver parenchyma, but less than the intensity of CSF or of a hepatic cyst
  - T1C +(Gd): Often shows peripheral nodular discontinuous enhancement which progresses centripetally (inward) on delayed images
  - Hemangiomas tend to retain contrast on delayed (>5 minutes) contrast-enhanced images
  - Atypical hemangiomas may demonstrate slightly altered enhancement patterns
  - T1 C + (hepatobiliary contrast, Eovist):
    - Hemangiomas show a wide range of appearances on delayed imaging so this is less useful
    - High-flow hemangiomas may show "pseudo washout'—this is thought to be due to increased contrast uptake from the adjacent liver parenchyma and should not be confused with true washout.

Renal Mass

1. **Wilms Tumor**:
   - **Plain radiograph**: Abdominal x-ray typically reveals a large soft tissue opacity displacing bowel. This is only relevant if found incidentally since a radiograph should never be used for the assessment of an abdominal mass. The only exception would be a resource-poor setting where an abdominal radiograph is the only imaging modality available.
   - **Ultrasound**: Ultrasound is a very useful examination and in almost every situation will be the primary investigation of choice. It is helpful to localize the mass to the kidney and also distinguish from other causes of renal masses (e.g., hydronephrosis). Although many of the features seen on CT/MRI can also be identified on US, the former are required to adequately stage the disease and is established in protocols for Wilms tumor staging in North America and Europe.
     - Wilms tumor appears as solid mass on ultrasound that may have vascular invasion with smooth margins. Cystic or necrotic areas may be anechoic and hypoechoic respectively while hemorrhage/fat/calcification appear as hyperechoic.
     - Doppler examination can be performed to examine the renal vein and IVC to assess for the presence of tumor thrombus.
   - **CT**: There is no value of CT multiphase abdomen and pelvis in characterizing renal tumors in children. CT scan done in portal venous phase is sufficient to characterize Wilms tumor.

     Wilms tumors are heterogeneous soft-tissue density masses with infrequent areas of calcification (~15%) and fat density regions. Enhancement is also patchy and allows for better delineation of the relationship between the mass and kidney. 10–20% of cases have lung metastases at the time of diagnosis.
   - **MRI**: Where MRI is available it is the investigation of choice for staging since it does not involve ionizing radiation. It is also the most accurate modality in assessing for IVC involvement where protocols have been optimized. These tumors appear heterogeneous on all sequences and frequently contain blood products.
     - T1: Hypointense

- T1C+ (Gd): Heterogeneous enhancement
- T2: Hyperintense

2. **Neuroblastoma**:
   - **Ultrasound**: Neuroblastoma on ultrasound demonstrates a heterogeneous mass with internal vascularity. Often there are areas of necrosis that appear as regions of low echogenicity. Calcification may or may not be evident on ultrasound.
   - **CT**: On CT, the tumor typically is heterogeneous with calcifications seen in 80–90% of cases. Areas of necrosis are of low attenuation. The tumor morphology is often helpful, with the mass seen insinuating itself beneath the aorta and lifting it off the vertebral column. It tends to encase vessels and may lead to compression. Adjacent organs are usually displaced, although in more aggressive tumors direct invasion of the psoas muscle or kidney can be seen. The latter can make distinguishing neuroblastoma from Wilms tumor difficult. Lymph node enlargement is often present.
   - **MRI**:
     - MRI is superior to all other modalities in assessing:
       - The organ of origin
       - Intracranial or intraspinal disease
       - Bone marrow disease
     - On MRI:
       - T1: heterogeneous and iso to hypointense
       - T2: heterogeneous and hyperintense
       - Cystic/necrotic areas have very high intensity
       - Signal voids may be evident
       - T1 C+ (Gd): Variable and heterogeneous enhancement

3. Imaging of necrotizing enterocolitis. [10] [DNB June 22]

Necrotizing enterocolitis (NEC) is a serious gastrointestinal condition primarily affecting premature infants. Radiological imaging plays a crucial role in diagnosing and managing NEC. Here are some key imaging features associated with the condition:

1. **Abdominal X-ray**:
   - Dilated bowel loops: Increased air in the intestines, especially in the proximal segments.
   - Pneumatosis intestinalis: Presence of air within the bowel wall, appearing as linear streaks or bubbles on X-ray.
   - Portal venous gas: Air within the portal venous system, indicating severe disease.
   - Free air: Signs of perforation, such as free air under the diaphragm.
2. **Ultrasound**:
   - Bowel wall thickening: Increased thickness of the bowel wall, often greater than 3 mm.
   - Increased peristalsis: Hyperactive bowel sounds may be noted.
   - Pneumatosis: Similar to X-ray findings, with visualized gas within the bowel wall.
   - Fluid collections: Possible presence of intra-abdominal fluid or abscesses.

   CT scan:
   - Severe bowel wall edema: Marked thickening and enhancement of the bowel wall.
   - Bowel ischemia: Reduced perfusion can be observed in advanced cases.
   - Gas patterns: Similar findings to X-ray, with more detailed visualization of pneumatosis and portal venous gas.
   - Complications: Identification of perforations, strictures, or fistulas.

   MRI:
   - Bowel wall features: Can provide detailed imaging of the bowel wall structure and adjacent tissues.
   - Soft tissue evaluation: Useful for assessing complications such as abscess formation or necrotic changes.

4. Causes of dysphagia. Role of barium swallow. [5] [DNB Dec 21]

Causes of Dysphagia

A. **Mechanical Oropharyngeal Dysphagia**:
- Zenker's diverticulum
- Cricopharyngeal bar or stenosis
- Cervical (mucosal) Web-Plummer-Vinson syndrome
- Retropharyngeal abscess
- Oropharyngeal tumor
- Head and neck surgery
- Stricture-caustic, post-radiation

B. **Motor Oropharyngeal Dysphagia**:
1. *Central nervous system*:
   - Stroke
   - Parkinson's disease
   - Brainstem tumors
   - Alzheimer's disease
2. *Degenerative diseases*:
   - Drugs (Phenothiazines, benzodiazepines)
   - Amyotrophic lateral sclerosis
   - Huntington's chorea
   - Multiple sclerosis
3. *Peripheral nervous system*:
   - Spinal muscular atrophy
   - Guillain-Barré syndrome
   - Post-polio syndrome
   - Drugs (Botulinum toxin and cytotoxics)
   - Myasthenia gravis
4. *Myogenic*:
   - Dermatomyositis, polymyositis
   - Thyrotoxic myopathy
   - Drugs (amiodarone, alcohol, cholesterol lowering drug)

C. **Mechanical Esophageal Dysphagia**:
1. *Intrinsic narrowing*:
   i. Inflammatory/infective esophagitis
   ii. Webs and rings
   iii. Benign strictures
   iv. Malignant stricture
   v. Foreign body
2. *Extrinsic narrowing*

D. **Motor Esophageal Dysphagia**:
1. *Diseases of smooth muscles*:
   i. Weak muscle contraction or LES tone
   ii. Enhanced muscle contraction

2. *Disorders of inhibitory innervation*:
   i. Diffuse esophageal spasm (DES)
   ii. Achalasia
   iii. Contractile (muscular/lower esophageal ring)

Dysphagia Lusoria

The esophagus may be compressed by a congenitally aberrant right subclavian artery. In the rare case that this is symptomatic, a diagnosis of dysphagia lusoria is made. At CT the diagnosis is straightforward. Fluoroscopically, an oblique tubular extrinsic impression is seen in the upper esophagus. Treatment is generally nonoperative with PPIs unless symptoms are severe.

Dysphagia Aortica

The acquired equivalent of dysphagia lusoria is compression of the posterior wall of the lower esophagus by a tortuous or dilated aorta: hence the term dysphagia aortica. Older women of short stature are predisposed.

Role of Barium Swallow in Dysphagia

A barium swallow, also known as a barium esophagram, is a radiographic imaging study used to evaluate swallowing difficulties (dysphagia). Here is how it plays a role in the assessment and management of dysphagia:

1. **Diagnosis of Structural Abnormalities**:
   - Identifies Obstructions: The test can reveal structural issues such as strictures, tumors, or foreign bodies that may be obstructing the esophagus.
   - Detects Anatomical Anomalies: It can also show congenital abnormalities or anatomical variations that could contribute to swallowing difficulties.
2. **Assessment of Motility Disorders**:
   - Evaluates Esophageal Function: A barium swallow assesses how well the esophagus moves and can help identify motility disorders like achalasia or esophageal spasms.
   - Swallowing Dynamics: It provides insight into the timing and coordination of swallowing phases, which can be disrupted in certain conditions.
3. **Functional Evaluation**:
   - Swallowing Phases: The test allows for visualization of the oral, pharyngeal, and esophageal phases of swallowing, helping to pinpoint where the dysfunction occurs.
   - Visualizes Contrast Passage: The movement of barium through the esophagus can highlight issues like delayed transit or reflux.
4. **Guiding Further Management**:
   - Treatment Planning: Results can inform treatment options, such as dietary modifications, swallowing therapy, or surgical interventions if necessary.
   - Follow-Up: It can be used to monitor changes over time, especially after treatment interventions.
5. **Noninvasive Nature**:
   - Safe and Accessible: The procedure is generally safe and noninvasive, making it a common first step in the evaluation of dysphagia.

5. Abdominal trauma-imaging approach. Splenic injury imaging. [10] [DNB June 21]

Radiological imaging plays a crucial role in the evaluation of abdominal trauma. The common imaging modalities include X-rays, ultrasound, and CT scans, each offering unique insights into the nature and extent of injuries. Here are some key features observed in various imaging techniques:

1. **X-ray Imaging**:
   - Free Air: Presence of pneumoperitoneum suggests perforation of hollow viscera.
   - Fractures: Rib and pelvic fractures may indicate potential intra-abdominal injuries.
   - Hemoperitoneum: Indirect signs such as fluid levels can indicate blood accumulation.

2. **Ultrasound**:
   - Focused Assessment with Sonography for Trauma (FAST): Rapid assessment for free fluid or organ injuries.
   - Free Fluid: Anechoic areas in the abdomen suggest blood or other fluids.
   - Organ Lacerations: Hypoechoic or complex lesions in solid organs (liver, spleen).
   - Pneumoperitoneum: Visualization of air under the diaphragm.
3. **CT Imaging**:
   - Solid Organ Injuries: Lacerations or contusions in the liver, spleen, or kidneys can be characterized by:
     - Liver: Hematoma or laceration patterns (grade I–V based on severity).
     - Spleen: Subcapsular hematomas, lacerations.
     - Kidneys: Perirenal hematoma, lacerations, and vascular injuries.
   - Bowel Injuries: Signs of perforation include:
     - Extravasation of contrast: Indicates bowel wall disruption.
     - Bowel wall thickening: May suggest contusion or ischemia.
   - Vascular Injuries: Contrast-enhanced CT can reveal:
     - Vascular hematomas: Aneurysms or lacerations of major vessels (e.g., aorta, mesenteric vessels).
   - Fluid Collections: Identification of hemoperitoneum or other fluid collections.
4. **MRI**: Generally, not first-line for acute trauma but can provide detailed information on soft tissue injuries and is useful for evaluating certain chronic or subtle injuries.

Splenic Injury Imaging

Imaging plays a crucial role in diagnosing and assessing splenic injuries. Here are the primary imaging modalities used:

- **Ultrasound**:
  - Often the first-line imaging modality, especially in unstable patients.
  - Can quickly assess for free fluid (hemoperitoneum) and splenic lacerations.
  - Limited in assessing the extent of injury in some cases.
- **Computed Tomography**:
  - The gold standard for evaluating splenic injuries, particularly in stable patients.
  - Provides detailed images of the spleen and surrounding structures.
  - Can classify injuries into grades based on the American Association for the Surgery of Trauma (AAST) scale:
    - Grade I: Hematoma <10% of spleen volume or laceration <lcm
    - Grade II: Hematoma 10–50% or laceration 1–3 cm
    - Grade Ill: Hematoma >50% or laceration >3 cm
    - Grade IV: Laceration involving segmental or entire spleen
    - Grade V: Vascular injury or splenic pedicle injury
- **Magnetic Resonance Imaging (MRI)**: Not commonly used for acute trauma but can be helpful in chronic cases or for assessing splenic pathology when CT or US findings are inconclusive.
- **Plain X-rays**: Limited use; can occasionally show indirect signs of splenic injury, such as free air or rib fractures, but not specific for splenic injuries.

6. Draw a schematic diagram of anorectal junction on coronal plane, depicting internal and external sphincters. Describe the types of anorectal fistula with the help of a diagram and briefly discuss MR imaging protocol in their evaluation. [3+(3+4)]

Anorectal fistulas are abnormal connections between the anal canal or rectum and the skin surrounding the anus. They are often the result of an infection in the anal glands that leads to the formation of an abscess. Here are the main types of anorectal fistulas:

1. **Intersphincteric Fistula**:
   - The most common type.

- Located between the internal and external anal sphincters.
- Often associated with an abscess that drains into the skin.

2. **Transsphincteric Fistula**:
    - Passes through both the internal and external sphincter muscles.
    - Can be more complex and may require surgical intervention.
3. **Suprasphincteric Fistula**:
    - Starts above the sphincter muscles and curves around them to reach the skin.
    - Typically, more challenging to treat due to its location.
4. **Extrasphincteric Fistula**:
    - Arises above the sphincter complex, often from conditions like Crohn's disease or trauma.
    - Can involve significant tissue and may be associated with other diseases.
5. **Complex Fistulas**:
    - These can involve multiple tracts or branches and are often associated with inflammatory bowel disease, previous surgeries, or other conditions.
    - They require a more individualized treatment approach.

MRI is a crucial imaging modality for assessing anorectal fistulas, providing detailed information about their anatomy and any associated complications. Here is a general outline of MRI protocols for evaluating anorectal fistulas:

Patient Preparation

- **Informed Consent**: Explain the procedure and obtain consent.
- **Fasting**: Patients may be instructed to fast for a few hours prior to the exam.
- **Bowel Preparation**: Some protocols suggest a mild laxative or enema to clear the rectum.

MRI Technique

1. **Patient Positioning**: Typically, the patient is positioned supine on the MRI table. Use of a coil designed for pelvic imaging may be beneficial.
2. **Sequences**:
    - T1-weighted Imaging:
        - Spin-echo or turbo spin-echo sequences.
        - Helps identify the fistulous tract and any associated abscess.
    - T2-weighted Imaging:
        - Spin-echo or turbo spin-echo sequences.
        - Provides excellent contrast between soft tissues; helpful for assessing the anatomy and surrounding structures.
    - Fat-Saturation Techniques: Use of fat-saturated sequences, especially in T2-weighted images, enhances visualization of the fistula.
3. **Protocol Details**:
    - Field strength: 1.5 T or 3.0 T MRI machines are typically used.
    - Slice Thickness: 3–5 mm with a gap of 1 mm, depending on the specific system and coils used.
    - Field of View (FOV): Adjust based on the size of the region being imaged, typically around 20–30 cm.
    - Number of Axial/Coronal/Sagittal Sequences: Usually include multiple planes (axial, coronal, and sagittal) for comprehensive assessment.
    - Additional Sequences:
        - Dynamic MRI: Sometimes used for functional assessment, though not standard in all protocols.
        - Contrast-enhanced Imaging: May be utilized in specific cases to evaluate more complex anatomy or to identify associated conditions.

7. Name various motility disorders of esophagus. Discuss pathophysiology and imaging findings of cardia achalasia. [3+(2+5)]

Esophageal Motility Disorders

These disorders are those which are attributable to esophageal neuromuscular function and are commonly associated with dysphagia, chest pain or heart burn. The dysphagia is slowly progressive and occurs to both liquid and solid foods. The esophageal motility can be easily assessed at fluoroscopy with the patient in the prone right anterior oblique (RAO) position. Two to five individual swallows should be observed at fluoroscopy as the bolus passes. It is important to remember that in patients suspected of having an esophageal motility disorder, individual swallow should be evaluated, as a second or double swallow would interfere with primary peristalsis and limit evaluation of esophageal motility. Specific motility disorders consist of diffuse esophageal spasm (DES), achalasia and scleroderma. However, the motility disorders may not fall into any of these categories and may occur in association with GERD.

- **Primary Motility Disorder**:
  - Nonspecific esophageal motility disorder
  - Diffuse esophageal spasm
  - Achalasia
- **Secondary Motility Disorder**:
  - Scleroderma
  - Achalasia

Pathophysiology

Achalasia is an uncommon motility disorder of the esophagus characterized by a loss of primary esophageal peristalsis, incomplete relaxation of the lower esophageal sphincter in response to deglutition, increased resting LES pressure, and increased intraesophageal pressure. All these lead to esophageal dilatation or megaesophagus. Of all the conditions associated with esophageal dilatation like achalasia, inflammatory narrowing, progressive systemic sclerosis (PSS), and carcinoma; achalasia causes the most severe generalized dilatation.

Imaging Features

- **Barium Swallow Study**:
  - Dilated Esophagus: A significant dilation of the esophagus is often observed.
  - Bird-beak Appearance: The tapering of the esophagus at the gastroesophageal junction, resembling a bird's beak.
  - Stasis of Barium: Retention of barium in the esophagus due to impaired peristalsis.
  - Endoscopy:
  - Esophageal Dilation: The esophagus may appear enlarged and have a smooth, thickened appearance.
  - Incomplete Closure of Lower Esophageal Sphincter:
  - Visible during endoscopy, indicating failure to relax.
- **CT Scan**:
  - Esophageal Distension: Enlargement of the esophagus, particularly in the distal part.
  - Thickened Esophageal Wall: Often seen in chronic cases.
- **Manometry**: Although not an imaging technique, esophageal manometry shows increased resting lower esophageal sphincter pressure and absent peristalsis.

8. Enumerate various internal hernias. Discuss in detail imaging features of any two internal hernias. [2+8] [DNB June 20, AIIMS Dec 24]

Types of Internal Hernias

- Left paraduodenal
- Right paraduodenal
- Pericecal

- Foramen of Winslow
- Intersigmoid
- Transmessenteric

Foramen of Winslow Hernia

A hernia through the foramen of Winslow is a type of internal hernia in which abdominal contents herniate into the lesser sac through a natural opening between the greater and lesser peritoneal cavities. These hernias are uncommon, accounting for about 8% of all internal hernias, and most commonly involve the small bowel.

Key Imaging Characteristics

1. **CT Findings**:
   - Gas filled Loops in the Lesser Sac: CT shows cluster of gas filled small bowel loops within the lesser sac, positioned posterior to liver hilum, anterior to Inferior Vena cava and between the stomach and pancreas.
   - Narrowing at the Foramen of Winslow: Herniated bowel loops taper as they pass through the Foramen of Winslow, located beneath the free edge of the lesser omentum.
   - Mesenteric Vessel Stretching: The mesenteric vessels stretch through the foramen, sometimes causing vascular engorgement if there's compression or obstruction.
   - Anterior and Lateral Displacement of Stomach: There is often anterior and lateral displacement of stomach due to mass effect from herniated bowel loops.
   - Signs of Small Bowel Obstruction: Findings such as dilated bowel loops and air fluid level may indicate small bowel obstruction.
2. **Conventional Radiographs**: Gas-filled bowel cluster: Radiographs can show localized, circumscribed collection of gas-filled loops in upper abdomen typically located medial and posterior to stomach, potentially extending to a position anterior to hepatic flexure.
3. **Barium Studies**:
   - Shift in Position of Stomach and Duodenum: On barium studies the stomach and the first and second parts of Duodenum may appear anteriorly and laterally displaced.
   - Mass Effect and Bowel Displacement: Barium studies reveal mass effect causing displacement of stomach and duodenum.
   - Appearance of Cecal Volvulus: If the herniated sac contains the cecum, it may resemble a cecal volvulus.
   - Obstruction Transition Zone Near Hepatic Flexure: The zone where obstruction occur is often found near the hepatic flexure.
4. **Additional Features and Complications**:
   - Gallbladder Distention or Jaundice: Rare cause may show a distended Gallbladder or Jaundice due to pressure on the common bile ducts.
   - Reentry into Greater Peritoneal Cavity: If defects exist in the gastrocolic or gastrohepatic omentum, herniated loops may re-enter the greater peritoneal cavity.

Imaging Features of Right Paraduodenal Hernia

Right paraduodenal hernias are congenital internal hernia involving bowel herniation through Waldeyer's fossa.

Imaging specially CT and barium studies play a crucial role in diagnosing this rare condition. Key imaging features are as follows:

1. **Location and Encapsulation**:
   - The herniated small bowel loops are typically found inferior and lateral to the descending duodenum, within the right half of transverse mesocolon or behind the ascending mesocolon.
   - The hernia forms a fixed, encapsulated, ovoid cluster of small bowel loops in the right mid-abdomen, often seen on both CT and barium studies.
2. **Relationship with Superior Mesenteric Vessels**:
   - The herniated bowel loops can loop behind the superior mesenteric artery and superior mesenteric vein, often near the root of mesentery.

- On CT jejunal branches of SMA and SMV may course posteriorly and to the right of parent vessels to supply the herniated loops.
- The SMA, ileocolic artery and the right colic vein may be displaced anteriorly due to the mass effect from the herniated bowel, with vessels engorgement visible in case of obstruction.

3. **Afferent and Efferent Loops**: Unlike left paraduodenal hernias, right paraduodenal hernias shows closely opposed and narrowed afferent and efferent loops on imaging.
4. **Small Bowel, Obstruction (SBO)**: Signs of small bowel obstruction may be present, with dilated bowel loops proximal to the hernia sac and air fluid level often seen on CT.
5. **Nonrotation and Midgut Malrotation**:
   - A more ventral and left ward position of SMV relative to SMA.
   - Absence of normal horizontal duodenum.
   - However, the cecum typically remains in its normal location.
6. **Barium Study Findings**:
   - A barium gastrointestinal study shows an ovoid encapsulated cluster of bowel loops situated lateral and inferior to the descending duodenum.
   - The encapsulated loops appear fixed, with narrowing of both afferent and efferent bowel segments.

9. Enumerate types of perianal fistula with their imaging findings. [10] [MD (WBUHS) 19]

Perianal fistulae **(Fig. 11)** can be classified into several types based on their anatomy and associated imaging features.

1. **Intersphincteric Fistula**:
   Imaging Features:
   - Located between the internal and external anal sphincter.
   - Seen on MRI as a low-signal tract extending from the anal canal to the inter-sphincteric space.
   - May show fluid or abscess formation.
2. **Trans-sphincteric Fistula**:
   Imaging Features:
   - Passes through both the internal and external sphincter muscles.
   - Appears as a tract that crosses the sphincter complex on MR, often with a higher signal intensity compared to surrounding tissues.
   - Can show associated abscesses.
3. **Suprasphincteric Fistula**:
   Imaging Features:
   - Starts above the sphincter complex and may extend superiorly or laterally.
   - MRI may show a tract that ascends above the sphincter and may be associated with perianal or pelvic abscesses.
4. **Extrasphincteric Fistula**:
   Imaging Features:
   - Originates from the rectum or sigmoid colon and bypasses the anal sphincters.
   - Typically identified on MRI or CT as a tract that does not follow the typical path of anal sphincters and may have an external opening away from the anal region.

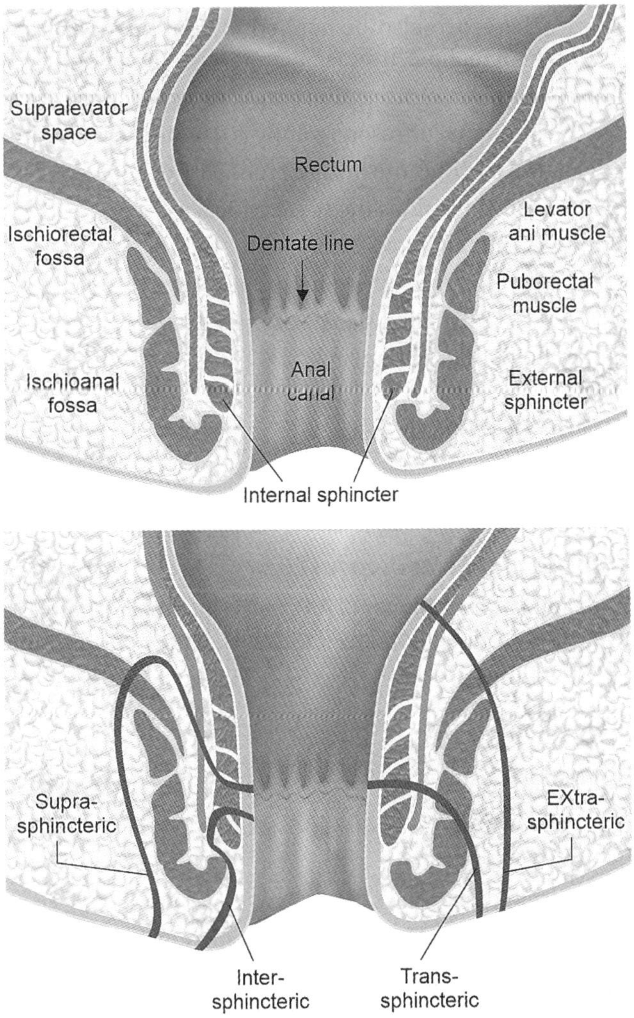

FIG. 11: Different types of fistulae are shown in the above diagram.

5. **Horseshoe Fistula**:

   Imaging Features:

   - A variation of trans-sphincteric fistula that has bilateral extensions around the anal sphincter.
   - MRI may show a horseshoe-shaped tract connecting two external openings.

   Radiographic Features:

   - **Fistulography**:
     - Fistulography is a traditional radiological technique used to define the anatomy of fistulas, yet it is an unreliable technique and is difficult to interpret.
     - In fistulography, the external opening is catheterized with a fine cannula, and a water-soluble contrast agent is injected to define the fistulous tract.
     - It has two major drawbacks:
       - Difficult to assess secondary extensions secondary to lack of proper filling with contrast material.
       - Inability to visualize the anal sphincters and to determine their relationship to the fistula.
   - **Ultrasound**: The benefits of ultrasonography over MRI are the former's ubiquity and lower operating costs. There are three ultrasonography methods for the evaluation of perianal fistulae, whether cryptoglandular or Crohn disease associated:
     - Endoanal ultrasound (EAUS)
     - Transvaginal ultrasound (TVUS)
     - Transperineal ultrasound (TPUS)

     These can also be applied in combination. Infusion of hydrogen peroxide into the fistulous tract renders it hyperechoic, thus facilitating its delineation.

     Doppler interrogation can show hyperemia in active Crohn's disease.

     Endoanal ultrasonography is deemed less sensitive than endoanal MR for deep supralevator disease.
   - **MRI**: MRI is the imaging modality of choice.

     Active fistulous tracts are typically:
     - T1: isointense to muscle
     - T2: high signal compared to fat
     - T2-FS: high signal compared to fat
     - T1 C+: enhancing

Interventions

1. Write a short note on transjugular liver biopsy. [5] [MD (WBUHS) 23]

Transjugular Liver Biopsy (TJLB)

Transjugular liver biopsy (TJLB)[8] serves as an alternative to percutaneous liver biopsy, especially for patients with diffuse liver disease, coagulopathy, or ascites. It may be combined with transjugular intrahepatic portosystemic shunt (TIPSS) or venography.

Indications

i. Massive ascites
ii. Coagulopathy
iii. Hepatic peliosis
iv. Morbid obesity
v. Failed or contraindicated percutaneous liver biopsy

Contraindications

Few, but ideally correct coagulopathy (INR >1.7, platelets <40). Not suitable for focal liver lesions.

Procedure

- **Equipment**: TJLB set, 18 G puncture needle, 9 F sheath, guidewires, catheters.
- **Positioning**: Patient supine; local anesthesia, or general anesthesia if uncooperative.
- **Technique**:
  A. **Puncture**: Under ultrasound, puncturing the right internal jugular vein, advancing a .035" guide wire to the superior vena cava.
  B. **Sheath Placement**: Inserting a 9 F sheath over the guidewire. 21–22 G micropuncture set is required for children or coagulopathy cases.
  C. **Guide Access**: Navigating the wire and catheter through the vena cava and right atrium to the right hepatic vein, with ECG monitoring.
  D. **Venogram**: Confirmation was made by placing a catheter in the right hepatic vein with a venogram.
  E. **Biopsy**: Inserting a 7 F TJLB sheath, positioning it, and with a trucut needle 2–3 liver tissue cores are obtained.

Complications

a. Hemorrhage: Often venous but may occasionally be arterial, necessitating angiography/embolization.
b. Capsular Rupture/Hemoperitoneum: Ensure adequate liver parenchyma anterior to the right hepatic vein or use the left lobe/middle hepatic vein if necessary.
c. Pneumothorax
d. Hemobilia
e. Hepatic artery-portal vein/biliary duct fistulation
f. Hepatic artery pseudoaneurysm

2. Write a short note on PAIR therapy. [5] [MD (WBUHS) 23]

PAIR Therapy (Puncture, Aspiration, Injection, Re-aspiration) is a minimally invasive, image-guided treatment used primarily for hepatic hydatid cysts caused by *Echinococcus granulosus.*[9] This procedure is an alternative to surgery, especially in patients with cysts that are not suitable for surgical removal.

Indications

- Uncomplicated, active hydatid cysts (WHO classification CE1 and CE3a)
- Cysts that are superficial or pose a risk of rupture
- Patients who are poor surgical candidates or refuse surgery

Contraindications

- Cysts communicating with the biliary tree (risk of bile leak)
- Inactive, calcified cysts (as they usually do not require intervention)
- Pregnancy (due to the use of scolicidal agents)
- Cysts located in areas that are inaccessible for safe puncture

Procedure

- **Puncture (P)**:
  - Under ultrasound or CT guidance, the cyst is punctured using a fine needle. This step is done with utmost care to prevent spillage and minimize the risk of anaphylaxis.
  - Local anesthesia is administered.
- **Aspiration (A)**: The cyst contents were rapidly aspirated, detaching the endocyst. The aspirated fluid was tested for bilirubin (dipstick), scolex viability, and cultured. A yellow fluid or positive bilirubin test led to the procedure being halted.
- **Injection (I)**: The team injected 20% hypertonic saline into the cyst, leaving it for 20 minutes. Ultrasound showed a "snowflake appearance," confirming proper instillation.

- **Re-aspiration (R)**: The saline was re-aspirated, and the laminated membrane detachment was confirmed by ultrasound. The scolex viability test was repeated, and if viable scolices were found, the PAIR process was repeated.
- **Follow-Up**: An ultrasound was performed within 24 hours to check for leaks. If no complications were found, the patient was discharged. Monthly follow-ups continued until the cyst resolved, with three-monthly checks afterward.

Advantages

- Minimally invasive with fewer complications compared to open surgery
- Shorter hospital stay and faster recovery
- Suitable for patients with contraindications for surgery
- Effective for reducing cyst size and managing symptoms

Complications

- **Anaphylaxis**: Due to spillage of cyst fluid; preprocedure preparation should include anti-anaphylactic measures.
- **Biliary Fistula**: May occur if the cyst is in communication with the biliary system.
- **Infection**: Rare, but can be managed with antibiotics.

3. Write a short note on ablative interventional techniques in focal liver lesions. [5] [MD (WBUHS) 23]

Ablative interventional techniques are minimally invasive procedures used to treat focal liver lesions, especially in patients who are not candidates for surgical resection due to poor liver function, advanced disease, or tumor location. These techniques aim to destroy or shrink tumors by applying thermal or chemical energy directly to the lesion under imaging guidance (ultrasound, CT, or MRI). These procedures are commonly used for hepatocellular carcinoma (HCC), liver metastases, and other benign lesions.

1. **Radiofrequency Ablation (RFA)**:
   - **Mechanism**: Uses high-frequency electrical currents to generate heat within tumors, causing necrosis.
   - **Indications**: Best for tumors <3 cm and away from large blood vessels.
   - **Procedure**: A needle electrode is inserted under imaging guidance (ultrasound/CT) to heat the tumor.
   - **Complications**: Includes hepatic abscess, bleeding, bile duct injury, and tumor seeding.
2. **Microwave Ablation (MWA)**:
   - **Mechanism**: Uses microwave energy to heat tumors, achieving higher temperatures than RFA.
   - **Advantages**: Faster heating, suitable for larger tumors, and less affected by the "heat sink" effect.
   - **Procedure**: Similar to RFA, but quicker and effective for larger or complex tumors.
3. **Cryoablation**:
   - **Mechanism**: Cycles of freezing and thawing cause cell death by ice crystal formation.
   - **Advantages**: Reduced pain, clear imaging of "ice ball," and preservation of nearby vessels.
   - **Procedure**: Performed under imaging guidance, ideal for tumors near critical structures.
4. **Chemical Ablation**:
   - **Mechanism**: Direct injection of substances (e.g., ethanol) into tumors to cause necrosis.
   - **Indications**: Used for small tumors or adjunct to other treatments.
   - **Procedure**: Chemical agent is injected directly into the tumor under imaging guidance.

These techniques offer nonsurgical treatment options for liver lesions, with the choice of method depending on tumor size, location, and surrounding anatomy.

4. Role of interventional radiology in obstructive jaundice. [10] [MD (WBUHS) 20, RG 18, AIIMS Dec 24]

Interventional radiology (IR) plays a crucial role in the diagnosis and management of obstructive jaundice, which occurs when there is a blockage in the bile ducts that impedes the flow of bile, leading to jaundice. Obstructive jaundice can result from a variety of causes such as tumors, strictures, or stones in the bile ducts. IR offers minimally invasive solutions for both diagnostic evaluation and therapeutic interventions.

Diagnostic Role

- **Percutaneous Transhepatic Cholangiography (PTC)**:
  - Indication: Used when noninvasive imaging (such as ultrasound or CT) is inconclusive or when a definitive diagnosis is needed.
  - Procedure: A needle is inserted through the skin into the liver, and a contrast agent is injected into the bile ducts under fluoroscopic guidance to visualize blockages, strictures, and ductal anatomy.
  - Benefit: Provides detailed images of bile duct obstructions, aiding in diagnosis and planning of treatment.
- **Endoscopic Retrograde Cholangiopancreatography (ERCP)**:
  - Indication: Primarily used to visualize the biliary and pancreatic ducts. Can be diagnostic and therapeutic.
  - Procedure: A flexible endoscope is passed through the duodenum, and a contrast agent is injected into the bile duct to detect blockages or other abnormalities.
  - Benefit: Allows direct visualization and offers the ability to perform interventions like stenting or stone removal during the procedure.

Therapeutic Role

- **Percutaneous Transhepatic Biliary Drainage (PTBD)**: Percutaneous Transhepatic Biliary Drainage (PTBD) is a key interventional radiology procedure for managing obstructive jaundice, which occurs when there is a blockage in the bile ducts, leading to a buildup of bile in the liver. PTBD provides a direct way to drain bile and relieve symptoms, especially in patients who cannot undergo endoscopic or surgical intervention.
  - **Role of PTBD in Obstructive Jaundice**:
    - **Symptom Relief**: PTBD provides immediate relief from jaundice symptoms, such as itching and skin discoloration, by diverting bile externally, thereby reducing serum bilirubin levels.
    - **Infection Management**: In cases of cholangitis (bile duct infection), PTBD relieves obstruction, reducing the infection source and allowing effective biliary drainage to prevent septic complications.
    - **Preoperative Stabilization**: PTBD is often used to reduce bilirubin levels before surgical procedures, especially in patients with malignant jaundice, improving the safety of surgery and postsurgical outcomes.
    - **Palliative Care**: For patients with inoperable malignancies causing biliary obstruction (e.g., pancreatic or cholangiocarcinoma), PTBD helps manage symptoms and improve quality of life by enabling bile drainage and reducing pain from biliary distention.
  - **Procedure Steps**:
    - **Access**: A needle is introduced percutaneously through the liver into the obstructed bile duct under ultrasound or fluoroscopic guidance.
    - **Contrast Injection**: After confirmation of the obstruction location, contrast dye is injected to visualize the biliary anatomy.
    - **Catheter Insertion**: A drainage catheter is inserted over a guidewire, enabling bile to drain either externally or internally (via the duodenum).
  - **Benefits of PTBD in Obstructive Jaundice**:
    - **Minimally Invasive**: PTBD offers a less invasive alternative for patients not suited for surgery or endoscopic retrograde cholangiopancreatography (ERCP).
    - **Immediate Relief**: It provides rapid reduction of bilirubin and symptom relief.
    - **Diagnostic Advantage**: PTBD can also help assess the nature and extent of the biliary obstruction, guiding further treatment options.
  - Complications of PTBD include bleeding, bile leakage, infection, and catheter dislodgement.
- **Biliary Stenting**:
  - Indication: Used for patients with malignant biliary obstruction (e.g., pancreatic cancer, cholangiocarcinoma) or benign strictures.

  - Procedure: A stent (either metal or plastic) is placed within the bile duct to open up the obstruction, allowing bile to flow freely into the intestine.
  - Benefit: Offers long-term relief from obstructive jaundice symptoms, especially in malignant cases where surgery is not an option.
- **Stone Extraction**:
  - Indication: Used for patients with choledocholithiasis (stones in the common bile duct) causing obstruction.
  - Procedure: Stones can be removed through ERCP or, in some cases, percutaneously under fluoroscopic guidance.
  - Benefit: Relieves obstruction and improves bile flow, reducing the need for surgery in many cases.
- **Endoscopic Stent Placement**:
  - Indication: Used in cases of malignant obstruction (e.g., pancreatic or biliary cancer) to relieve symptoms.
  - Procedure: A stent is inserted through the duodenum during ERCP to maintain bile duct patency.
  - Benefit: Less invasive than surgery and can significantly improve the quality of life in patients with advanced cancer.
- **Percutaneous Cholangioscopy**:
  - Indication: Used in complex cases where the anatomy is difficult to assess via conventional imaging or when a precise diagnosis is required.
  - Procedure: A flexible cholangioscope is inserted through the skin to directly visualize the bile ducts and collect biopsies.
  - Benefit: Allows for accurate diagnosis and targeted therapy (e.g., stenting or biopsy).

Role in Palliation

- **Indication**: In patients with inoperable cancer or advanced disease, IR interventions like biliary stenting provide palliation by alleviating jaundice, pruritus, and improving the quality of life.
- **Benefit**: Minimally invasive approach with faster recovery and reduced risk compared to surgery.

Postoperative Biliary Obstruction

- **Indication**: After gallbladder surgery or liver transplant, bile duct obstruction may occur.
- **Procedure**: IR techniques like stenting or percutaneous drainage can be used to manage postoperative biliary obstruction.
- **Benefit**: Reduces the need for reoperation and helps in managing complications like bile leaks or strictures.

5. Write a short note on: Transjugular intrahepatic portosystemic shunt (TIPS). [5] [MD (WBUHS) 24, MD (WBUHS) 22]

Transjugular Intrahepatic Portosystemic Shunt (TIPS/TIPSS)

TIPS is a procedure for treating portal hypertension by creating a direct connection between a hepatic vein and a portal vein branch, allowing blood to bypass the liver and reduce portal pressure.[10] The target portosystemic gradient is <12 mm Hg.

Indications

- Acute variceal bleeding unresponsive to medication or endoscopic treatment
- Recurrent variceal bleeding (preventative)
- Refractory ascites requiring frequent drainage
- Hepatic hydrothorax not managed by diet and diuretics
- Portal hypertensive gastropathy
- Hepatorenal syndrome
- Lower GI or stomal varices
- Malignant compression of hepatic or portal veins
- Moderate Budd-Chiari syndrome not responsive to anticoagulation

Contraindications

- **Absolute**:
  - Severe chronic liver disease or acute liver failure
  - Resistant severe encephalopathy
  - Severe right heart failure
  - Uncontrolled sepsis.
- **Relative**:
  - Right heart failure
  - Cavernous transformation of the portal vein
  - Cystic hepatic disease
  - Occlusive portal vein thrombus
  - Polycystic kidney disease
  - Hepatic malignancy or hemangioma.
- **Procedure Details**:
  - **Access**: Ultrasound-guided vascular access via the right internal jugular vein; vascular sheath inserted into the right atrium.
  - **Venography**: Angiographic catheter advanced to a hepatic vein for venography.
  - **Needle Puncture**: TIPS needle is rotated and advanced to connect the hepatic and portal veins.
  - **Portal Venogram and Guidewire**: Contrast confirms portal vein access. Guidewire inserted to ensure stability.
  - **Pressure Measurement and Stenting**: Portal pressure is measured. A balloon catheter dilates the track, and a stent is placed. Poststent portal pressure confirms adequate gradient reduction.
  - **Verification**: Venography checks cessation of variceal bleeding.

Complications

- **Acute**:
  - Hemorrhage (hemoperitoneum, intrahepatic hematoma)
  - Hepatic infarction
  - Gallbladder puncture
  - Sepsis
  - Vascular site hematoma
  - Unintentional arterial access
  - Acute kidney injury
- **Long-term**:
  - Uncontrollable encephalopathy
  - Recurrence of portal hypertension
  - Stent occlusion or migration
  - Hepatic venous stenosis
  - Stent infection (rare with PTFE stents)

Methods to Assess Patency

- Color Doppler ultrasound
- CT angiography
- Portography with portal manometry

TIPS remains a key intervention in managing complex cases of portal hypertension, offering an effective bridge to liver transplantation or a long-term solution for various complications.

6. Techniques and role of interventional management in malignant liver tumors. [10] [DNB Dec 21]

1. **Radiofrequency Ablation (RFA) Technical Aspects:**
   - **Equipment:** A generator produces radiofrequency energy, which is delivered to the tumor via a specially designed electrode needle.
   - **Guidance:** The needle is inserted into the tumor under **image guidance**—typically ultrasound, CT, or MRI—to precisely target the lesion.
   - **Procedure:**
     - The electrode is deployed into the tumor, and high-frequency alternating current flows from the needle, creating frictional heating.
     - Temperatures of 60–100°C are generated around the electrode, causing **coagulative necrosis** of the tumor cells.
     - Tumors up to **3–5 cm** in size can be effectively treated.
   - **Ablation Zone:** A margin of 0.5–1 cm beyond the tumor is ablated to ensure complete destruction.
   - **Duration:** Depends on the tumor size, but it usually takes **10–30 minutes** per lesion.

   Key Points:
   - Thermal energy can dissipate near large blood vessels due to the **heat sink effect**, reducing efficacy for tumors located close to vascular structures.
   - Multiple ablation sessions may be required for larger or recurrent tumors.
2. **Microwave Ablation (MWA) Technical Aspects:**
   - **Equipment:** A microwave generator produces microwaves, which are transmitted via an antenna probe inserted into the tumor.
   - **Guidance:** Similar to RFA, the probe is positioned under real-time imaging guidance (CT, ultrasound, or MRI).
   - **Procedure:**
     - The probe emits microwaves that cause the rapid rotation of water molecules within the tissue, generating intense heat (up to 150°C) and destroying cancer cells.
     - MWA heats the tissue **faster and over a larger area** than RFA, making it suitable for larger tumors (up to **5–7 cm**).
     - **Ablation Zone:** The ablation zone is typically more homogenous and extends further from the probe, leading to fewer treatment sessions.

   Key Points:
   - MWA is less affected by the **heat sink effect**, meaning it works well near blood vessels.
   - Microwave ablation is generally faster than RFA (procedure times of **5–15 minutes** per lesion), and fewer probes may be needed to treat large tumors.
3. **Transarterial Chemoembolization (TACE) Technical Aspects:**
   - **Equipment:**
     - A **microcatheter** is used to deliver chemotherapy and embolic agents. The catheter is inserted through the **femoral artery** or **radial artery** and advanced to the hepatic artery.
     - **Fluoroscopy** (X-ray guidance) is used to position the catheter precisely in the artery supplying the tumor.
   - **Procedure:**
     - **Selective catheterization** is performed to isolate the branch of the hepatic artery feeding the tumor (segmental or lobar).
     - Chemotherapeutic drugs (e.g., **doxorubicin** or **cisplatin**) are injected directly into the artery.
     - Embolic agents (gelatin sponges, microspheres, or polyvinyl alcohol particles) are then injected to occlude the artery, cutting off blood flow to the tumor.
     - This dual approach (chemo + ischemia) leads to **tumor cell death.**
   - **Repeat Sessions:** TACE is often repeated every few months depending on tumor response and progression.

Key Points:

- TACE is generally performed in **nonsurgical candidates** and can be used as a **bridging therapy** for patients awaiting liver transplantation.
- It is typically contraindicated in patients with **portal vein thrombosis** due to the risk of ischemic liver damage.

4. **Drug-eluting Beads TACE (DEB-TACE) Technical Aspects**:
   - **Equipment**: Similar to conventional TACE, a catheter is used to deliver the drug-eluting beads. These beads are loaded with chemotherapy drugs (e.g., **doxorubicin**).

   Key Points:
   - The beads are injected into the hepatic artery under **fluoroscopic guidance**.
   - Once in place, the beads gradually release the chemotherapy drug over time, providing **sustained exposure** to the tumor.
   - The embolic nature of the beads also restricts blood flow to the tumor, enhancing tumor necrosis.
   - The extended-release of the drug improves local efficacy and minimizes systemic toxicity.
     - **Advantages**: More controlled release of the chemotherapeutic agent, leading to fewer side effects compared to conventional TACE. Useful in treating **unresectable HCC** or liver metastases.
     - Typically performed in **outpatient settings** and repeated as necessary based on tumor response.

5. **Transarterial Radioembolization (TARE)/Selective Internal Radiation Therapy (SIRT) Technical Aspects**:
   - **Equipment**: Uses **Yttrium-90 (Y-90)** radioisotope-laden microspheres delivered through a microcatheter placed in the hepatic artery.
   - **Procedure**:
     - A catheter is inserted via the femoral or radial artery, and under **fluoroscopic guidance**, it is advanced into the **branch of the hepatic artery** feeding the tumor.
     - The **radioactive microspheres** (Y-90) are infused into the tumor vasculature.
     - These microspheres lodge in the small blood vessels surrounding the tumor and emit **beta radiation** directly to the cancer cells, causing radiation-induced damage while sparing much of the surrounding healthy liver tissue.
   - **Radiation Dose**: Y-90 emits radiation over **14 days**, with limited exposure to surrounding healthy tissues.
   - **Single Session**: Typically, only one session of TARE is needed due to the sustained radiation effect.

   Key Points:
   - **Advantages**: Particularly effective for treating **portal vein invasion** and advanced tumors.
   - **Limitations**: Requires careful patient selection, as radiation-induced liver injury can occur.

6. **Percutaneous Ethanol Injection (PEI) Technical Aspects**:
   - **Equipment**: A **fine needle** is inserted percutaneously into the tumor under **ultrasound guidance**.
   - **Procedure**:
     - Absolute **ethanol (95–100%)** is injected directly into the tumor through the needle.
     - The ethanol causes **tumor cell dehydration**, coagulative necrosis, and destruction of tumor blood vessels.
     - Multiple injections may be needed, especially for larger tumors.
   - **Repeat Sessions**: Often requires several sessions, particularly for tumors larger than 3 cm.

   Key Points:
   - **Advantages**: Simple and cost-effective, particularly useful for small HCC tumors in patients with **poor liver function** or significant comorbidities.
   - **Limitations**: Less effective for large tumors or tumors with irregular borders.

7. **Cryoablation Technical Aspects**:
   - **Equipment**: A **cryoprobe** (hollow needle) is inserted into the tumor under **image guidance** (CT or ultrasound).
   - **Procedure**:
     - The cryoprobe is placed into the tumor and cooled to **–20°C to –40°C** using liquid nitrogen or argon gas, causing ice formation inside the tumor.

- Multiple **freeze-thaw cycles** are performed, which result in tumor cell death due to the formation of ice crystals within the cells and disruption of the cell membrane.
- The ice ball can be monitored in real-time using imaging to ensure complete coverage of the tumor.

▪ **Advantages**: Effective for **larger or irregularly shaped tumors**, and the procedure can be performed in challenging locations near blood vessels and bile ducts.

Key Points:

▪ Cryoablation causes **less collateral damage** to surrounding tissues compared to heat-based ablation methods.
▪ **Limitations**: Risk of **cryoshock** (a systemic inflammatory response) and potential damage to surrounding structures if not carefully monitored.

8. **Irreversible Electroporation (IRE) Technical Aspects**:

▪ **Equipment**: Two or more needle electrodes are placed around the tumor using image guidance (CT or ultrasound).
▪ **Procedure**:
  - High-voltage electrical pulses are delivered between the electrodes to create permanent **nanopores** in the cell membrane.
  - This process disrupts the cell's homeostasis and induces **apoptosis** (programmed cell death) without generating heat.
  - The nonthermal nature of IRE allows it to treat tumors near critical structures like blood vessels or bile ducts.
▪ **Ablation Zone**: The area of cell death extends 0.5–1 cm beyond the electrode placement, ensuring adequate tumor destruction.

Key Points:

▪ **Advantages**: Preserves critical structures that would otherwise be damaged by thermal ablation techniques.
▪ **Limitations**: Requires highly specialized equipment and operator expertise.

REFERENCES

1. In: Sutton D (Ed). A Textbook of Radiology and Imaging, 7th edition. New Delhi: Elsevier; 2022.
2. In: Adam A, Dixon AK, Gillard JH, Schaefer-Prokop C, editors. Grainger and Allison's Diagnostic Radiology. 7th edition. New Delhi: Elsevier Health Sciences; 2020.
3. In: Khandelwal N, Gupta AK, Chowdhury V (Eds). AIIMS-MAMC-PGI's Comprehensive Textbook of Diagnostic Radiology. New Delhi: Jaypee Brothers Medical Publishers Pvt Ltd; 2016.
4. Gaillard F, Walizai T, Hacking C. Cirrhosis. [Online]. Available from: https://radiopaedia.org/articles/cirrhosis?lang=us. [Last accessed December 2024].
5. Gaillard F, Sharma R, Feger J. Hepatocellular carcinoma. Radiopaedia. Available from: https://radiopaedia.org/articles/hepatocellular-carcinoma?lang=us. [Last accessed December, 2024].
6. Singh G, Walizai T, Knipe H. Biliary atresia. [Online] Available from: https://radiopaedia.org/articles/biliary-atresia?lang=us [Last accessed December 2024].
7. Jones J, Campos A, Hirano Y. Couinaud classification of hepatic segments. [Online] Available from: https://radiopaedia.org/articles/biliary-atresia?lang=us [Last accessed December 2024].
8. Desai P, Murphy A, Alhusseiny K. Liver biopsy (transjugular). Available from: https://radiopaedia.org/articles/liver-biopsy-transjugular. [Accessed December, 2024].
9. Khuroo MS. Percutaneous drainage in hepatic hydatidosis—the PAIR technique: concept, technique, and results. J Clin Exp Hepatol. 2021,11(3).592-602.
10. Gaillard F, Murphy A, Lukies M. Transjugular intrahepatic portosystemic shunt. [Online]. Available from: https://doi.org/10.53347/rID-8046. [Last accessed December 2024].

CHAPTER

5 Genitourinary Imaging

Kasturi Rakshit

QUESTIONS

Imaging Techniques

1. Write short note on: CT urography and MR urography. [5] [MD (WBUHS) 24, MD (WBUHS) 22, [MD (WBUHS) 18, DNB Dec 18]
2. MR urography, technique, application, advantages and disadvantages. [10] [DNB June 22]
3. Technique, imaging sequences and clinical application of MR urography. [3+3+4] [MD (WBUHS) 18, DNB Dec 20]

Renal Infections

1. Describe the imaging findings in nontubercular renal infections. [10] [MD (WBUHS) 19]
2. Write short notes on: (a) Emphysematous pyelonephritis. (b) Horseshoe kidney. [5+5] [MD (WBUHS) 22]
3. Pathophysiology, X-ray, USG and CT in genitourinary TB. [10] [DNB June 22, AIIMS May 23, AIIMS Dec 24]

Tumors of the Urogenital Tract

1. Imaging modalities of renal neoplasm with special reference to PET scan. [10] [MD (WBUHS) 19]
2. Various benign and malignant solid renal masses. Imaging features of malignant solid renal masses. [10] [DNB Dec 21, AIIMS Dec 23]
3. Draw and discuss—T-staging of bladder tumors. [5] [DNB Dec 21]

Lower Urinary Tract

1. Discuss role of IVU, CT urography, MR urography in obstructive uropathy. [10] [MD (WBUHS) 20]
2. IVU in the diagnosis of posterior urethral value. [10] [MD (WBUHS) 19]
3. Discuss the types of urinary bladder trauma and role of imaging in diagnosis and management of such cases. [4+6]
4. A 74-year-old with urinary incontinence-approach and role of imaging. [10] [DNB June 22]
5. Draw and discuss—male urethral injury. [5] [DNB Dec 21]
6. Describe TNM staging of bladder cancer. Draw a schematic diagram of T-staging of bladder tumor. Enumerate the role of ultrasound, computed tomography and MRI in the diagnosis and staging of the bladder carcinoma. [2+2+(2+2+2)] [DNB June 20, MD (WBUHS) 18]

Miscellaneous Urinary Tract Lesions

1. Write short note on nephrocalcinosis. [5] [MD (WBUHS) 20]
2. Discuss briefly the role of imaging in a 40-year-old female presenting with hematuria. [10] [MD (WBUHS) 24]

3. Causes of nephrocalcinosis and imaging. [10] [DNB June 22]
4. (a) Bosniak classification of renal cyst 2019 (b) syndromic association of renal cyst in adult. [10] [DNB June 21]
5. Describe approach to a patient in renal trauma with a flowchart and discuss the role of imaging with grades of renal injury. [4+6] [MD (WBUHS) 18, AIIMS May 24]

Retroperitoneum

1. Discuss the retroperitoneal anatomy with suitable diagram. Discuss the common retroperitoneal tumors and appropriate radiological modalities to evaluate them. [4+3+3] [MD (WBUHS) 23, RG 18, AIIMS May 24]
2. Describe retroperitoneal compartments and their contents in reference to medical imaging. [10] [MD (WBUHS) 20]
3. Classify adrenal tumors with their radiological features. [10] [MD (WBUHS) 19]
4. Discuss in brief the imaging modalities in the diagnosis of adrenal lesion. [10] [MD (WBUHS) 22, RG 18]
5. Enumerate the imaging modalities used for adrenal lesions. Describe in brief the CT scan protocol and systematic approach to evaluate adrenal lesions. [2+(3+5)] [MD (WBUHS) 21, MD (WBUHS) 18]
6. (a) Radiological anatomy of retroperitoneum. (b) Cross-sectional imaging in retroperitoneal liposarcoma. [10] [DNB June 21]
7. (a) Imaging evaluation of a patient with Cushing's syndrome. (b) Role of imaging in differentiating adrenal adenoma from adrenal metastasis. [5+5] [DNB Dec 20]

Interventions

1. Discuss the indications and procedure of percutaneous nephrostomy. [3+7] [MD (WBUHS) 23, MD (WBUHS) 17]
2. Classify renal injuries, imaging features and intervention in them. [3+4+3] [MD (WBUHS) 21]
3. What are the indications of embolization in genitourinary tract? Describe the technique of renal artery angioplasty and stenting. [5+5] [MD (WBUHS) 22]

Diseases of Female Pelvis

1. Classify morbid adhesions of placenta. Write down USG findings in ectopic pregnancy. [5+5] [MD (WBUHS) 23]
2. Describe the role of USG and Doppler studies in IUGR. [5+5] [MD (WBUHS) 23, AIIMS Dec 23]
3. Discuss the indications and the procedure of uterine artery embolization. [3+7] [MD (WBUHS) 23, AIIMS Dec 23]
4. Briefly describe development of uterus in reference to different uterine malformations. [10] [MD (WBUHS) 20, AIIMS Dec 23]
5. Write short note on imaging of placenta previa. [5] [MD (WBUHS) 20]
6. Discuss USG in IUGR. [10] [MD (WBUHS) 20]
7. Discuss role of imaging in a suspected case of ectopic pregnancy. [10] [MD (WBUHS) 20]
8. Write short note on: (a) PNDT ACT. (b) Role of Doppler in IUGR. [5+5] [MD (WBUHS) 19]
9. List various causes of female infertility. Discuss the role of HSG and MRI in their evaluation. [2+4+4] [MD (WBUHS) 21]
10. Classify the cystic pelvic lesions in middle-aged female patient. Discuss the imaging features of common cystic lesions. [4+6] [MD (WBUHS) 22, MD (WBUHS) 18]
11. Discuss the role of various imaging modalities in detection of congenital anomalies of the fetus with their advantages and disadvantages. [10] [MD (WBUHS) 22]
12. What are the indications of 1st trimester ultrasound? Briefly discuss the assessment of fetal congenital anomalies by first trimester ultrasound. [4+6] [AIIMS May 24]
13. Discuss the imaging evaluation and differential diagnosis in a 60-year-old woman with postmenopausal bleeding. [4+6]
14. What is fetal growth restriction? Discuss the role of ultrasound and Doppler in its diagnosis and management. [2+8]

15. Uterine artery Doppler in pregnant female. [5]
16. Right pelvic pain in a woman—causes and imaging. [10] [DNB June 22]
17. USG in ectopic pregnancy. [10] [DNB June 22]
18. Role of USG, CT and MRI in endometrial carcinoma. [10] [DNB Dec 21, DNB Dec 18]
19. Role on USG and MRI in morbidly adherent placenta. [10] [DNB Dec 21, AIIMS May 23]
20. Bleeding PV at 18 weeks. Causes and imaging findings. [5] [DNB Dec 21]
21. Oligohydramnios. [5] [DNB Dec 21]
22. MRI in Ca cervix. [5] [DNB Dec 21, AIIMS May 24]
23. Antenatal MRI—indications, safety and protocols. [5] [DNB Dec 21]
24. Different variety of gestational trophoblastic disease and role of imaging. [10] [DNB June 21]
25. (a) Imaging evaluation of female presented with infertility. (b) MRI imaging feature of uterine adenomyosis. [10] [DNB June 21, AIIMS May 23]
26. (a) MRI evaluation method in ovarian mass. (b) Differentiating features of benign and malignant ovarian mass on USG and MRI. [10] [DNB June 21]
27. (a) Enumerate the causes of acute pelvic pain in a young female patient. (b) Role of imaging in ovarian torsion. [4+6]
28. Enumerate various causes of postmenopausal bleeding in a 60-year-old female. Discuss the role of imaging in evaluation of endometrial carcinoma and its management based on staging. [2+(5+3)] [MD (WBUHS) 24]
29. Describe imaging algorithm in a suspected case of ectopic pregnancy. Describe role of imaging in differentiating three common clinical mimics of ectopic pregnancy. [5+5] [MD (WBUHS) 24, DNB June 20]
30. Describe various indications, protocol, advantages, and disadvantages of fetal MRI. [2+3+3+2] [DNB June 20]

Prostrate

1. Imaging of prostate cancer with regards to TRUS and MRI. [5+5] [MD (WBUHS) 23]
2. Describe the protocols and MR imaging features in prostatic carcinoma. [3+7] [MD (WBUHS) 21]
3. Discuss multiparametric MR imaging of the prostate. [10] [MD (WBUHS) 21]
4. Discuss in brief about radiological anatomy of prostrate with its radiological implications. [5+5] [MD (WBUHS) 22]
5. Draw cross-sectional anatomy of prostate. Discuss briefly the role of MRI in prostate pathologies. [2+5] Discuss PIRADS. [3] [MD (WBUHS) 24]

Scrotum and Male Sexual Dysfunction

1. Discuss the role of sonogram in various scrotal pathologies. [10] [MD (WBUHS) 19]
2. What are the common causes of a young adult presenting with acute unilateral scrotal pain and swelling? Discuss the ultrasound/Doppler evaluation of such cases. [5+5] [MD (WBUHS) 22, MD (WBUHS) 17, AIIMS May 24]
3. Color Doppler in testicular torsion. [5]
4. Role of radiology in erectile dysfunction. [10] [DNB June 22]
5. (a) Describe various causes and role of imaging modalities in male infertility. (b) Role of sonography in erectile dysfunction. [(3+3)+4] [AIIMS Dec 24, AIIMS Dec 23]

Vascular Diseases

1. What are the common types of renal artery dysplasia with its clinical features? What are the angiographic features of FMD? [10] [MD (WBUHS) 19]
2. Imaging in renal artery stenosis. [5] [DNB Dec 21, MD (WBUHS) 24]
3. Discuss imaging features of renal artery stenosis on ultrasonography and MR angiography and briefly the role of interventions in its management. [3+3+4] [MD (WBUHS) 24, AIIMS Dec 24]

Recent Advances

1. Discuss radiological evaluation of renal transplant donor. [10] [MD (WBUHS) 20]
2. How would you evaluate donor kidney for renal transplant. Discuss role of ultrasonography and scintigraphy in various types of renal graft dysfunction. [4+3+3] [MD (WBUHS) 21]
3. Briefly discuss USG features of renal transplant. [10] [MD (WBUHS) 19]
4. Briefly discuss the role of ultrasound Doppler in postoperative evaluation of AV fistula for dialysis. [5]
5. Role of imaging in management of renal transplant patient. [10] [DNB June 22]
6. (a) Imaging workup of a potential renal donor. (b) Imaging evaluation of vascular complications of a transplant kidney. [5+5] [DNB June 20]

ANSWERS

Imaging Techniques

1. Write short note on: CT urography and MR urography. [5] [MD (WBUHS) 24, MD (WBUHS) 22, [MD (WBUHS) 18, DNB Dec 18]

CT Urography

Introduction

It is an examination to evaluate the genitourinary tract. Renal parenchyma and urothelium both can be evaluated.[1]

Indications

- Hematuria
- Urolithiasis
- Urothelial thickening
- Renal neoplasm
- Ureteric lesions
- Pelviureteric junction obstruction
- Congenital anomalies

Patient Preparation

- Oral administration of 1 L of water for diuresis and better delineation of the ureters.
- Diuretics and saline infusion can be used.

Technique and Protocol

Two approaches to perform CT urography:

1. CT hybrid urography:
   - It combines CT urography and intravenous urography (IVU).
   - Uses projection radiographs (scout image, scanogram).
   - Post-processing of CT images not required.
   - CT urography and IVU performed at different locations (not preferred) or same location (preferred) by ceiling mounted X-ray tube.
   - Bowel preparation required.
2. CT only—CT urography **(Table 1)**
   - Bowel preparation not required.
   - Post-processing of CT images is required.
   - 125 mL IV contrast medium followed by 250 mL saline administration.
   - MPR of excretory—phase images using MIP and volume rendering.

TABLE 1: CT urography protocol.

Phase	*Timing*	*Range*	*Slice thickness*	*What to detect*
Non-enhanced	Pre-contrast	Lung bases to pubic symphysis	5 mm	Calculi. Hemorrhage/hemorrhagic cysts
Nephrogram	100 sec	Lung bases to pubic symphysis	3 mm	Renal tumors, renal vein thrombosis
Excretory	5–8 min	Lung bases to base of bladder	2 or 3 mm	Papillary necrosis, urothelial carcinoma

There are two techniques:

1. Multiphase and
2. Split bolus

Phases of multiphase CT urography

- Non-contrast
- Nephrographic (80–100 seconds)
- Excretory phase (7–12 minutes)

Split Bolus Technique

- At first, nonenhanced scan is obtained.
- 30–50 mL of intravenous contrast given.
- After 8–10 minutes, 80–100 mL of intravenous contrast given.
- Then after 90 seconds, scan is done.
- Images have combined nephrographic and excretory phases.

Applications

- To detect calculi and resultant obstructive changes.
- To detect hemorrhage in collecting system and within cysts.
- To assess renal tumors, their characterization and extent.
- To evaluate renal vein thrombosis, IVC thrombosis and its extent.
- To detect papillary necrosis and assess its cause and urothelial carcinoma.
- Perinephric and periureteral fat stranding can be seen.

Advantages

- High contrast and spatial resolution.
- Detection of pathologies (listed above).

Disadvantages

- Use of ionizing radiation.
- Use of large amount of contrast.
- Detection of small plaque like thickening of bladder and those near the neck, is difficult.

MR Urography

Introduction

MR urography (MRU) is a noninvasive examination for the assessment of abnormalities of the urinary tract. Both anatomical and functional status can be assessed.[2]

Indications

- Congenital anomalies
- Obstructive uropathy
- Pregnant patients and children requiring imaging of the urinary tract.
- Deranged renal function
- Hematuria

Technique and Protocol

- **Magnet**: 1.5 or 3T
- **Coil**: Eight channel phase array body coil.

There are two types of MR urography:

1. Static fluid MRU (based on T2 W imaging)
2. Excretory MRU (based on T1 W imaging)

Sequences

- **Precontrast**:
  - Localizer—axial, sagittal, coronal
  - 2D T2 FSE—axial, coronal
  - 2D T2 FS FSE—coronal
  - 3D SSFSE OR HASTE (post diuretic)—coronal
  - 3D T1 FS GRE (precontrast)—axial
  - CINE (T2 SSFSE)
- **Postcontrast**: 3D T1 FS GRE (20sec, 45 sec and 5 min)—axial
- **Post-processing**:
  - Maximum intensity projection images—with thin and thick slab
  - Volume rendered images

Patient Preparation

- Intake of fluid is restricted for four hours prior to the commencement of the examination.
- Voiding before the examination to avoid discomfort.
- Administration of 250 mL of intravenous normal saline for distension of collecting system.
- Administration of furosemide (0.1 mg/kg) may be considered.
- Excretory MRU—administration of 0.1 mmol/kg of gadolinium followed by 15-20 mL saline push.

Advantages

- No ionizing radiation is used.
- Ureteral peristalsis can be seen by CINE images as intermittent distention and collapse.
- The level of complete or partial obstruction is determined.
- It can provide anatomical and structural details and details of anomaly if any.
- Assessment of function can also be done as normal renal parenchyma and bladder wall enhance showing the different phases.
- Minimal ascites, perirenal and periureteral edema can also be seen in static fluid MR urography since it is heavily T2 weighted.
- Static fluid MR urography does not use contrast, so it can be used in patients with deranged renal function as well as in pediatric and pregnant patients.

Disadvantages

- Less spatial resolution than CT urography.
- Presence of fluid in the bowel and metal artifacts may interfere with interpretation of the images.
- Bowel and ureteral peristalsis can create artifacts.
- Time-consuming process and requires expertise.
- Difficult for pregnant patients to lie down so long in the machine.
- Air introduced due to any intervention is difficult to differentiate from calculi.
- Small calculi can be missed.

Static MRU: Cannot assess the excretory function.

Excretory MRU: Cannot be used in patients having derangement in excretory function, such as anuric patients.

Applications

- Anomalies of urinary tract—duplex kidney, horseshoe or ectopic kidney.
- For assessment of urinary tract obstruction—its cause, extent and level.
- For assessment of hematuria and determine its cause.
- Imaging modality of choice in children and pregnant patients.
- Imaging modality of choice in case of deranged renal function and allergy to iodinated contrast.
- Preoperative and postoperative assessment.

2. MR urography, technique, application, advantages and disadvantages. [10] [DNB June 22]

Introduction

MR urography (MRU) is a noninvasive examination for the assessment of abnormalities of the urinary tract. Both anatomical and functional status can be assessed.

Indications

- Congenital anomalies
- Obstructive uropathy
- Pregnant patients and children requiring imaging of the urinary tract.
- Deranged renal function
- Hematuria

Technique and Protocol

- **Magnet**: 1.5 or 3T
- **Coil**: Eight channel phase array body coil.

There are two types of MR urography:

1. Static fluid MRU (based on T2 W imaging)
2. Excretory MRU (based on T1 W imaging)

Sequences

- **Precontrast**:
  - Localizer—axial, sagittal, coronal
  - 2D T2 FSE—axial, coronal
  - 2D T2 FS FSE—coronal
  - 3D SSFSE OR HASTE (post diuretic)—coronal
  - 3D T1 FS GRE (precontrast)—axial
  - CINE (T2 SSFSE)
- **Postcontrast**: 3D T1 FS GRE (20 sec, 45 sec and 5 min)—axial
- **Post-processing**:
  - Maximum intensity projection images—with thin and thick slab
  - Volume rendered images

Patient Preparation

- Intake of fluid is restricted for four hours prior to the commencement of the examination.
- Voiding before the examination to avoid discomfort.
- Administration of 250 mL of intravenous normal saline for distension of collecting system.
- Administration of furosemide (0.1 mg/kg) may be considered.
- Excretory MRU—administration of 0.1 mmol/kg of gadolinium followed by 15–20 mL saline push.

Advantages

- No ionizing radiation is used.
- Ureteral peristalsis can be seen by CINE images as intermittent distention and collapse.
- The level of complete or partial obstruction is determined.
- It can provide anatomical and structural details and details of anomaly if any.
- Assessment of function can also be done as normal renal parenchyma and bladder wall enhance showing the different phases.
- Minimal ascites, perirenal and periureteral edema can also be seen in static fluid MR urography since it is heavily T2 weighted.
- Static fluid MR urography does not use contrast, so it can be used in patients with deranged renal function as well as in pediatric and pregnant patients.

Disadvantages

- Less spatial resolution than CT urography.
- Presence of fluid in the bowel and metal artifacts may interfere with interpretation of the images.
- Bowel and ureteral peristalsis can create artifacts.
- Time consuming process and requires expertise.
- Difficult for pregnant patients to lie down so long in the machine.
- Air introduced due to any intervention is difficult to differentiate from calculi.
- Small calculi can be missed.

Static MRU: Cannot assess the excretory function.

Excretory MRU: Cannot be used in patients having derangement in excretory function, such as anuric patients.

Applications

- Anomalies of urinary tract—duplex kidney, horseshoe or ectopic kidney.
- For assessment of urinary tract obstruction—its cause, extent and level.
- For assessment of hematuria and determine its cause
- Imaging modality of choice in children and pregnant patients
- Imaging modality of choice in case of deranged renal function and allergy to iodinated contrast
- Preoperative and postoperative assessment.

3. Technique, imaging sequences and clinical application of MR urography. [3+3+4] [MD (WBUHS) 18, DNB Dec 20]

Introduction

MR urography (MRU) is a noninvasive examination for the assessment of abnormalities of the urinary tract. Both anatomical and functional status can be assessed.

Indications

- Congenital anomalies
- Obstructive uropathy
- Pregnant patients and children requiring imaging of the urinary tract.
- Deranged renal function
- Hematuria

Technique and Protocol

- **Magnet**: 1.5 or 3T
- **Coil**: Eight channel phase array body coil.

There are two types of MR urography:

1. Static fluid MRU (based on T2 W imaging)
2. Excretory MRU (based on T1 W imaging)

Sequences

- **Precontrast**:
  - Localizer—axial, sagittal, coronal
  - 2D T2 FSE—axial, coronal
  - 2D T2 FS FSE—coronal
  - 3D SSFSE OR HASTE (post-diuretic)—coronal
  - 3D T1 FS GRE (precontrast)—axial
  - CINE (T2 SSFSE)
- **Postcontrast**: 3D T1 FS GRE (20 sec, 45 sec and 5 min)—axial
- **Post-processing**:
  - Maximum intensity projection images—withthin and thick slab
  - Volume rendered images

Patient Preparation

- Intake of fluid is restricted for four hours prior to the commencement of the examination.
- Voiding before the examination to avoid discomfort.
- Administration of 250 mL of intravenous normal saline for distension of collecting system.
- Administration of furosemide (0.1 mg/kg) may be considered.
- Excretory MRU—administration of 0.1 mmol/kg of gadolinium followed by 15–20 mL saline push.

Advantages

- No ionizing radiation is used.
- Ureteral peristalsis can be seen by CINE images as intermittent distention and collapse.
- The level of complete or partial obstruction is determined.
- It can provide anatomical and structural details and details of anomaly if any.
- Assessment of function can also be done as normal renal parenchyma and bladder wall enhance showing the different phases.
- Minimal ascites, perirenal and periureteral edema can also be seen in static fluid MR urography since it is heavily T2 weighted.
- Static fluid MR urography does not use contrast, so it can be used in patients with deranged renal function as well as in pediatric and pregnant patients.

Disadvantages

- Less spatial resolution than CT urography.
- Presence of fluid in the bowel and metal artifacts may interfere with interpretation of the images.
- Bowel and ureteral peristalsis can create artifacts.
- Time consuming process and requires expertise.
- Difficult for pregnant patients to lie down so long in the machine.
- Air introduced due to any intervention is difficult to differentiate from calculi.
- Small calculi can be missed.

Static MRU: Cannot assess the excretory function.

Excretory MRU: Cannot be used in patients having derangement in excretory function, such as anuric patients.

Applications

- Anomalies of urinary tract—duplex kidney, horseshoe or ectopic kidney.
- For assessment of urinary tract obstruction—its cause, extent and level.
- For assessment of hematuria and determine its cause.
- Imaging modality of choice in children and pregnant patients.
- Imaging modality of choice in case of deranged renal function and allergy to iodinated contrast.
- Preoperative and postoperative assessment.

Renal Infections

1. Describe the imaging findings in nontubercular renal infections. [10] [MD (WBUHS) 19]

Routinely imaging is not done in infections unless there is:

- Obstruction or complications, such as abscesses, emphysematous pyelonephritis
- Immunocompromised patient
- Diabetic patient
- Postrenal transplant patient
- Failure to respond to antibiotics within 72 hours.

Modality of choice for adults: Contrast enhanced CT
Modality of choice for children: Ultrasound

Acute Pyelonephritis

Introduction

- Acute infection of renal pelvis and parenchyma without formation of abscess.[3]
- Focal or diffuse
- Unilateral or bilateral

Sex predilection: Females > males

Causative Organisms

- *E. coli* (most common)
- *Proteus*
- *Klebsiella*
- *Pseudomonas*
- *H. influenzae*
- *Enterobacter*

Ultrasound

- Low sensitivity
- Enlarged kidney
- Echogenic perinephric and renal sinus fat
- Dilated collecting system
- Urothelial thickening
- Bladder wall thickening ≥2 mm in distended bladder and ≥5 mm in nondistended state.
- Significant PVRU

Modality of choice: Contrast enhanced CT

- Anatomical and functional information of kidney
- Intra- and extrarenal pathology

NCCT:

To look for:

- Calculi
- Obstruction
- Gas
- Hemorrhage

CECT-CT urography protocol:

- Renal enlargement may/may not be present.
- Enlarged kidney—right kidney >1.5 cm than left kidney, left kidney >2 cm than right kidney.
- Striated nephrogram—nonenhancing hypodense bands extending from medulla to the cortex alternating with the normally enhancing parenchyma, caused due to adjacently located normal and obstructed tubules.
- Wedge-shaped hypodense areas—renal capsule is not spared.
- Perinephric fat stranding

[To be differentiated from renal infarct:

  - Cortical rim sign—renal capsule is spared because capsular artery branches earlier.
  - Clinical features are different]

- Delayed persistent enhancement
- Focal form—hypodense rounded lesions and abscess
- Diffuse form—diffuse involvement of kidney

MRI

Modality of choice of pregnant and pediatric patients **(Table 2)**.

TABLE 2: Various magnetic resonance imaging sequences that can be used in assessing acute pyelonephritis.

Sequences	*Description*
Non-contrast	Affected regions in the kidney appear hyperintense on T2-weighted imaging and hypointense on the T1 sequence. reflecting edema within the renal parenchyma
Postgadolinium-based contrast	Correctly depicts the regions of involvement. The findings on MRI follow those of CT namely, increased renal size. perinephric fat stranding, and fluid, and striated nephrograms
Gadolinium-enhanced inversion recovery	Because of tubular obstruction and stasis, less amount of gadolinium accumulates in the affected region of the kidney while the rest of the healthy kidney that is normally perfused shows a much higher signal drop, making the affected region stand out against a backdrop of a generalized signal drop
MRU	Used when an obstruction is suspected
Diffusion-weighted imaging	Areas of pyelonephritis show significantly lower apparent diffusion coefficient values than that of in the normal renal parenchyma

Chronic Pyelonephritis

Introduction

- Occurs due to recurrent or chronic infection to kidney, resulting in fibrosis and scarring of renal pelvis and calyces.
- **Most common cause**: Reflux nephropathy.
- Associated with vesicoureteral reflux in childhood.

Imaging Features

- Decreased size of kidney
- Irregular outline of kidney and architectural distortion.
- Focal parenchymal scars with cortical thinning.
- Underlying calyceal clubbing
- Hypertrophy of residual tissue and perinephric fat.

- Perinephric fascia is thickened.
- Decreased function of kidney
- **DMSA scan (dimercaptosuccinic acid)**: Scarring and photopenia in kidney.

Pyonephrosis

Introduction

- Suppurative infection of the obstructed and dilated collecting system resulting in pus formation
- Urologic emergency—immediate drainage needed.

Imaging Features

- **Intravenous urography**:
  - Enlarged renal shadow
  - Poor contrast excretion
- **Ultrasound**:
  - Dilated collecting system filled with mobile echogenic debris—most reliable sign
  - Shifting fluid levels
  - Presence of sludge
  - Dirty shadows from gas

Computed Tomography

- Cause and level of obstruction
- Thick enhancing pelvicalyceal walls >2 mm
- Dilated collecting system and high attenuation fluid causing obstruction.
- Fluid levels
- Debris or sludge
- Delineate the extent of inflammation in kidney and perinephric region.
- Layering of contrast in delayed images
- Poor renal function

MRI-DWI sequence—low ADC value compared with hydronephrosis.

Xanthogranulomatous Pyelonephritis

- Chronic destructive granulomatous process of kidney most commonly occurring due to obstructing renal stone.
- Mostly unilateral
- **Predisposed population**: Middle-aged female with recurrent UTI.

Histopathology

- Xanthoma cells-localized lipid deposits
- Lipid laden foamy macrophages infiltrate the kidney.
- Inflammation spreads from renal pelvis to medulla to cortex.

Imaging Features

Radiograph:

- Staghorn calculi
- Enlarged renal shadow with obscuration of psoas shadow.

Intravenous urography: Marked decrease in renal function

Ultrasonography:

- Enlarged kidney

- Staghorn calculus in renal pelvis
- Multiple hypoechoic lesions replacing the renal parenchyma.
- Loss of normal renal morphology
- Corticomedullary differentiation lost

Contrast enhanced CT-modality of choice:

- Enlarged nonfunctioning kidney
- Large obstructive staghorn calculus in a contracted renal pelvis.
- Hypodense lesions in the periphery of the kidney.
- Thickening of the perirenal fascia
- **Bear's paw sign**: The appearance of contracted renal pelvis with multiple peripheral hypodense lesions in the renal parenchyma.
- Assessment of extent of the disease to perinephric, anterior and posterior pararenal spaces, psoas muscle, abdominal wall and diaphragm.
- Assessment of the perirenal tissue
- Assessment of complications—development of abscess, fistula to skin or colon.

Emphysematous Pyelonephritis

Introduction

It is a life-threatening rare necrotizing infection of the kidney in which there is accumulation of gas within and around the kidney.

Predisposing Factors

Diabetes mellitus, immunocompromised state, urinary tract obstruction, neoplasms.

Organisms Involved

E. coli (most common), *Proteus, Pseudomonas, Klebsiella* species.

Pathophysiology

There is gas formation in and around the kidney due to infection by these organisms.

Clinical Features

Fever, chills, flank pain, nausea, vomiting

Imaging Features

- **Radiograph**: Presence of air and mottled radiolucencies in the renal areas.
- **Ultrasound**:
  - Dirty shadowing of air is seen in the nondependent location.
  - Reverberation artifacts
  - Kidney is enlarged
  - Can be mistaken with calculi (have dense posterior acoustic shadow and is present in dependent location).
- **Contrast enhanced computed tomography: modality of choice for the diagnosis**:
  - Often diagnosed on noncontrast CT due to derangement of renal function test.
  - Presence of air is confirmed.
  - Perinephric fat stranding and thickening of fascia.
  - Destruction of parenchyma is seen.
  - Perinephric collections and collection within the parenchyma can be assessed.
  - Extension into the retroperitoneum or adjacent spaces or abdominal wall is better assessed.
  - Classification of the condition into type 1 or 2 can be done.

  - Type 1 has more mortality, more air, less collection.
  - Type 2 has less mortality, less air, more collection.
- **CT classification of emphysematous pyelonephritis by Huang and Tseng**:
  - Class 1: Gas in collecting system only.
  - Class 2: Gas in renal parenchyma.
  - Class 3: Gas in renal parenchyma with extrarenal extension.
  - Class 3 divided in two subgroups.
  - Class 3A: Extrarenal extension of gas or abscess to perinephric space.
  - Class 3B: Extrarenal extension of gas or abscess to pararenal space.
  - Class 4: Involvement of bilateral or solitary kidney.

2. Write short notes on: (a) Emphysematous pyelonephritis. (b) Horseshoe kidney. [5+5] [MD (WBUHS) 22]

Emphysematous Pyelonephritis

Introduction

It is a life-threatening rare necrotizing infection of the kidney in which there is accumulation of gas within and around the kidney.

Predisposing Factors

Diabetes mellitus, immunocompromised state, urinary tract obstruction, neoplasms.

Organisms Involved

E. coli (most common), *Proteus*, *Pseudomonas*, *Klebsiella* species.

Pathophysiology

There is gas formation in and around the kidney due to infection by these organisms.

Clinical Features

Fever, chills, flank pain, nausea, vomiting

Imaging Features

- **Radiograph**: Presence of air and mottled radiolucencies in the renal areas.
- **Ultrasound**:
  - Dirty shadowing of air is seen in the nondependent location.
  - Reverberation artifacts
  - Kidney is enlarged
  - Can be mistaken with calculi (have dense posterior acoustic shadow and is present in dependent location).
- **Contract enhanced computed tomography: modality of choice for the diagnosis**:
  - Often diagnosed on noncontrast CT due to derangement of renal function test.
  - Presence of air is confirmed.
  - Perinephric fat stranding and thickening of fascia.
  - Destruction of parenchyma is seen.
  - Perinephric collections and collection within the parenchyma can be assessed.
  - Extension into the retroperitoneum or adjacent spaces or abdominal wall is better assessed.
  - Classification of the condition into type 1 or 2 can be done.
  - Type 1 has more mortality, more air, less collection.
  - Type 2 has less mortality, less air, more collection.

- **CT classification of emphysematous pyelonephritis by Huang and Tseng**:
  - Class 1: Gas in collecting system only.
  - Class 2: Gas in renal parenchyma.
  - Class 3: Gas in renal parenchyma with extrarenal extension.
    Class 3 divided in two subgroups.
    - Class 3A: Extrarenal extension of gas or abscess to perinephric space.
    - Class 3B: Extrarenal extension of gas or abscess to pararenal space.
  - Class 4: Involvement of bilateral or solitary kidney.

Horseshoe Kidney

Introduction

It is a congenital abnormality of the developing kidneys in which lower renal poles are medially facing and connected by isthmus causing rotation of the renal axis. The isthmus may have functional renal tissue or fibrous tissue.[4]

Epidemiology

- 1 in 400 live births
- M:F = 2:1

Associated with:

- Mullerian anomalies
- Vertebral anomalies
- Anorectal anomalies
- Cardiovascular anomalies
- VACTERL
- Pelviureteric junction obstruction, ureteropelvic junction obstruction
- Renal dysplasia
- Ureteric duplication
- Medullary sponge kidney
- Trisomy 18 and Turners syndrome
- Fanconi syndrome

Pathophysiology

The lower poles of the bilateral kidneys are fused (metanephric contact) and the ascent and normal rotation of the kidney is hindered by the inferior mesenteric artery arising from the aorta in the midline at the level of L3.

More prone to trauma, nephrolithiasis, infection, VUR, PUJ obstruction and renal tumors including Wilm's tumor.

Imaging Features

- **Radiograph**: Renal shadows are not seen in renal fossa, calculi may be seen in the contacting lower poles.
  - Intravenous urography:
    - U-shaped nephrogram
    - Hand holding calyces: Lower calyces towards the midline at the level of L3.
    - Flower vase appearance: Ureters curve laterally then take a medial course.
  - Micturating cystourethrogram: Associated vesicoureteric reflux is seen.
- **Ultrasound**:
  - Kidney seen crossing the aorta anteriorly and continuing on the other side.
  - Lower poles cannot be well delineated.
- **Contrast enhanced computed tomography/Magnetic resonance imaging**:
  - The upper poles of the kidneys point superolaterally and the lower poles inferomedially.
  - The degree and site of fusion is established.

- Functional assessment of the parenchyma of the isthmus is done.
- Abnormalities of collecting system or associated anomalies assessed.
- Complications are noted if any.

99mTc-DMSA: Functioning renal tissue over the spine in anterior view.

3. Pathophysiology, X-ray, USG and CT in genitourinary TB. [10] [DNB June 22, AIIMS May 23, AIIMS Dec 24]

Introduction

Tubercular infection of the genitourinary system is the second most common location of tuberculosis in the body after lung.[5]

Route of Spread

- **Secondary**: Hematogenous
- **Primary**: BCG vaccine instillation in bladder

Organism

Mycobacterium tuberculosis

Clinical Features

Fever, weight loss, urinary tract infection, hematuria, sterile pyuria.

Pathophysiology (Box 1)

BOX 1: Pathophysiology of genitourinary TB.

Hematogenous spread of *Mycobacterium* to kidney and reactivation

↓

Formation of microscopic granuloma in periglomerular capillaries

↓

Formation of macroscopic granulomas

↓

Spread from cortex to medulla, renal papilla, pelvis, ureter, bladder

Imaging Features (Table 3 and Figs. 1A to B)

- **Radiograph**:
  - Kidney size:
    - Enlarged kidney shadow: Early stage
    - Shrunken kidney shadow: Late stage
    - May remain normal in size also.
  - Calcification:
    - Most common manifestation
    - Punctate or curvilinear renal parenchymal calcification
    - Lobar calcification lining the distorted lobes
    - Caseous pyonephrosis—cloudy appearance in calyceal distribution
    - Putty kidney—seen in end stage renal tuberculosis. Dense homogenous calcified necrotic tissue seen on abdominal radiograph. Also called as tuberculous autonephrectomy.
- **Chest radiograph**: Features of tuberculosis
- **Bones for skeletal TB**: Vertebrae, hip, SI joints
- **Calcified lymph node**: In abdomen and pelvis

- Calcified adrenals
- **Intravenous urography**: Modality of choice of diagnosis of early tuberculosis as calyceal abnormalities are well demonstrated.
- **Calyces**:
    - Loss of outline of minor calyx.
    - Calyceal dilatation
    - Papillary necrosis

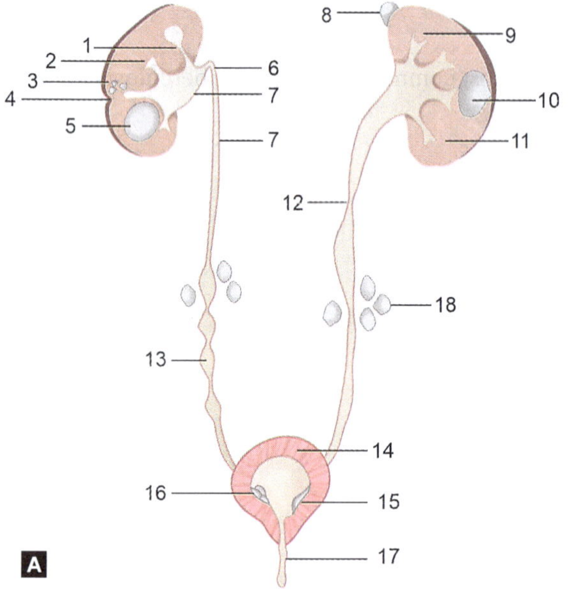

1. Infundibular stenosis with caliectasis
2. Moth-eaten calyx
3. Parenchymal calcification
4. Cortical scarring
5. Caseous mass
6. Hiked-up pelvis
7. Urothelial thickening
8. Adrenal calcification
9. Central papillary necrosis
10. Cortical abscess with rupture into the perinephric space
11. Forniceal papillary necrosis
12. Ureteral stricture
13. Beaded ureter
14. Thickened bladder wall (small capacity bladder)
15. Granulation tissue
16. Intravesical septations
17. Urethral stricture
18. Mesenteric lymph node calcification

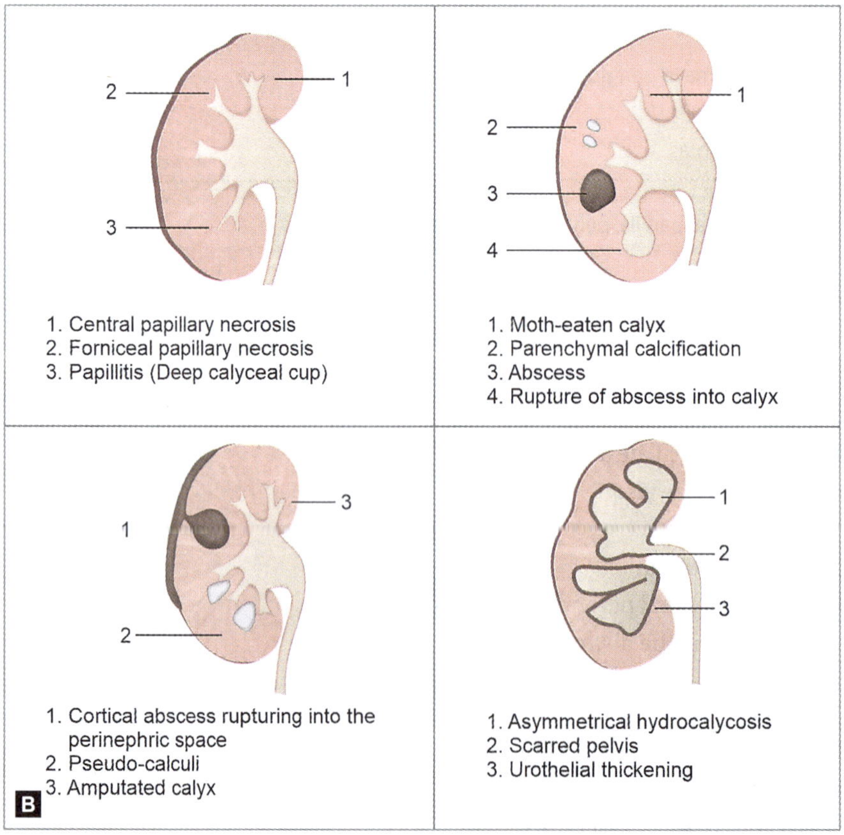

FIGS. 1A and B: Tuberculosis of the urinary tract; (B) Pathological changes of renal tuberculosis.

- **Kidneys**:
  - Moth eaten calyx-irregular and deformation of calyces associated with papillary necrosis.
  - Amputated or phantom calyx-calyceal cutoff due to infundibular stenosis.
  - Hiked up pelvis-stricture at inferior margin of renal pelvis with cephalic retraction.
  - Kerr's kink-infundibular stricture and parenchymal fibrosis produce traction and cause kinking of renal pelvis
  - Abscess-thick irregular peripherally enhancing walls
- **Bladder**:
  - Thimble bladder—fibrosis and contracture of bladder with reduced capacity.
  - Golf hole ureter—wide opening of ureterovesical junction due to fibrosis of trigone resulting in VUR.
- **Ureter**:
  - Beaded or corkscrew ureter—due to fibrosis and stricture.
  - Pipestem ureter—severe thickening with shortening and narrowing.
  - Hydroureteronephrosis
- **Ultrasonography**:
  - Focal caliectasis due to infundibular stenosis
  - Hydroureteronephrosis
  - Urothelial thickening
  - Hyper, hypo or mixed echogenicity masses adjacent to calyces.
  - Renal abscess
  - Echogenic perinephric fat
- **Computed tomography**:
  - Similar features as IVU.
  - Early changes are not seen in CT.
  - Minimally enhancing solid masses.
  - Calcification within masses as mentioned earlier in IVU.
  - Hypodense renal cortex due to hypoperfusion
  - Caliectasis
  - Urothelial thickening in collecting system
  - Stricture ı /

Magnetic Resonance Imaging

- **Sequences**:
  - Static fluid non contrast
  - Heavily T2 weighted
  - Excretory MR urography
- **Imaging features**:
  - Focal hypoperfusion
  - Smaller lesions—hypointense on T1 and T2WI.
  - Larger lesions—centrally hyperintense on T2WI.
  - Contraction of bladder wall-thimble bladder.

TABLE 3: Imaging manifestations and associated classic signs of genitourinary TB.

Affected organ	*Imaging findings*	*Associated imaging signs*
Adrenal glands	• Bilateral involvement • Calcifications in—50% of cases • Mass like gland enlargement in 50%-65% of cases • Peripheral rim enhancement in—50% of cases	

Continued...

Continued...

Affected organ	***Imaging findings***	***Associated imaging signs***
Kidneys	• Parenchyma: • Hypoenhancing granulomas • Striated nephrogram • Abscess and tuberculomas • Autonephrectomy • Pelvicalyceal system: • Papillary necrosis • Focal calyceal blunting and dilatation • Infundibular and/or pelvic stenosis	• "Putty" kidney • "Ball-on-tee" sign • Phantom calyx • "Daisy-flower" kidney
Ureters	• Distal third is most common site • Ureteral thickening with calcifications • Mucosal tuberculomas • Mucosal ulcerations • Sharp angulation at UPJ Strictures and scarring	• "Sawtooth" appearance • Kerr kink • "Pipe stem" ureter • Beaded or "corkscrew ureter
Urinary bladder	• Diffuse or focal wall thickening with calcifications • Mucosal ulcerations and trabeculations • Contracted fibrotic bladder	Thimble-bladder
Urethra	• Affects more men than women • Long-segment strictures • Fistulas to perineum	"Watering can" perineum
Prostate	• Can mimic cancer • Solitary or multiple nodules or masses • Fluid density at CT • Nodular type: Low T2 signal intensity at MRI, with diffusion restriction and DCE • Diffuse type: Low streaky lesions in the peripheral zone at T2-weighted MRI	"Watermelon" prostate
Testis and epididymis	• At US: Diffuse or focal enlargement and heterogeneity with hypoechoic appearance: Rarely miliary pattern of involvement • At MRI: T2-hypointense lesions with variable calcifications	
Vas deferens and/or spermatic-cord	• Enlarged and heterogeneous • Focal or diffuse involvement • Little or no delectable flow at Doppler US	
Seminal vesicles	• Acute phase: Enlarged with or without abscess, wall and septal thickening with calcifications • Chronic phase: Atrophy and calcifications	
Fallopian tubes	• Beaded appearance; interstitial salpingitis can appear like SIN at HSG • Dilated tube with fluid or abscess • Wall thickening with nodular calcifications at CT and MRI	
Uterus and cervix	• At HSG: Asherman syndrome • T-shaped uterus, pseudo-unicornuate appearance, Netter syndrome • At CT and MRI: Thickened endometrium, enlarged heterogeneously enhancing cervix, may show calcifications during chronic stage	"Gloved-finger" uterus
Ovaries	• Tubo-ovarian mass or abscess • May not respect fascial planes	
Vagina and vulva	Enhancing nodule or mass that may mimic malignancy	

(DCE: dynamic contrast enhancement; MSC: hysterosalpingography; SIN: salpingitis isthmica nodosa; UPJ: ureteropelvic junction)

Tumors of the Urogenital Tract

1. Imaging modalities of renal neoplasm with special reference to PET SCAN. [10] [MD (WBUHS) 19]

Following are the imaging appearances of renal masses on different imaging modalities.[3-5]

Abdominal Radiograph

- Loss of psoas margin
- Displacement of retroperitoneal fat
- Central calcification suggests malignancy

Ultrasound

- Often the first modality
- Ideal for pregnant and pediatric patients
- Useful in patients having renal impairment
- Solid or cystic mass
- Hypo- or isoechoic
- Color Doppler–moderate vascularity
- Less accurate for staging RCC

Computed Tomography

Contrast enhanced CT KUB—Modality of choice for evaluation of renal masses **(Flowchart 1)**

- Evaluation of size, shape and extent of tumor.
- Tumor characteristics
- Complications if any, like IVC thrombosis.
- Feasibility of biopsy

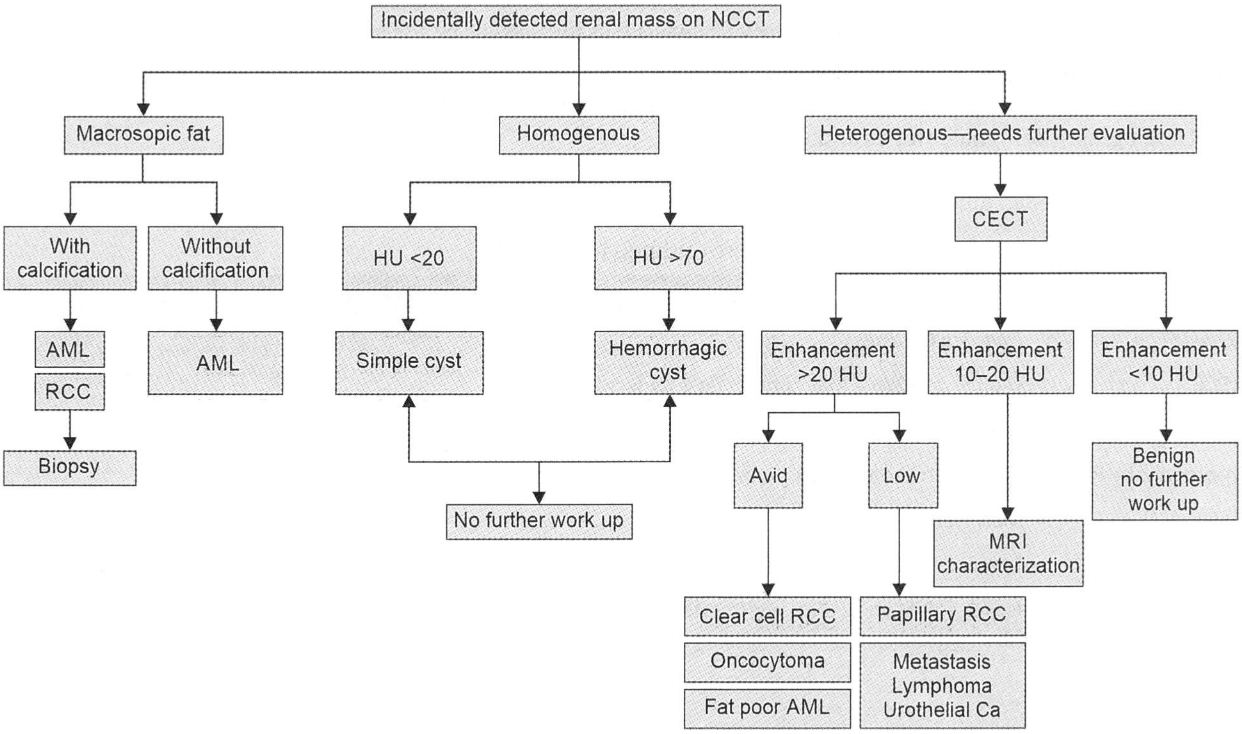

FLOWCHART 1: Algorithmic approach to diagnosis and work up of renal masses on CT scan.

CT Protocol (Table 4)

TABLE 4: CT protocol for renal mass characterization.				
Phases	***Non-contrast***	***Corticomedullary***	***Nephrographic***	***Excretory***
Phase timing	–	40 seconds	90–120 seconds	5–7 minutes
Coverage	Kidneys	Diaphragm through kidneys	Diaphragm through kidneys	Kidneys
Field of view	Whole body	Whole body	Whole body	Whole body
Reconstructions	Axial: 3 mm	• Axial: 3 mm • Coronal: 2 mm • Sagittal: 2 mm	• Axial: 3 mm • Coronal: 2 mm • Sagittal: 2 mm	• Axial: 3 mm • Coronal: 2 mm • Sagittal: 2 mm
*Contrast 100–150 mL low osmolality (LOCM) at 5 mL/s				

Magnetic Resonance

- Useful in patients having genetically increased risk of malignancy like von Hippel-Lindau syndrome.
- Lengthy investigation

MR Protocol (Table 5)

TABLE 5: Multiparametric magnetic resonance protocol for characterization of renal mass.	
Sequences	***Imaging planes***
T1W dual echo gradient (in and opposed phase) T2W	Axial
HASTE	Axial, coronal and sagittal
T2W TSE with fat suppression	Axial
3D fat-saturated TIW SPGR pre-contrast and post-contrast DCE (corticomedullary, nephrographic and excretory)	Axial
Diffusion weighted (b = 50,500, 800), ADC map	Axial
Corticomedullary phase = 40 seconds, nephrographic = 90 seconds, excretory = 3 minutes after IV gadolinium at dose of 0.01 mmoL/kg in patients with GFR >60 mL/min/1.73 m^2 via pressure injector followed by a saline flush.	

- **DWI**: Malignant masses show diffusion restriction.
- **CEMR**: Gadolinium diethylenetriamine penta-acetic acid (Gd-DTPA) used for contrast enhancement of the renal mass.
- MR angiography for renal arteries and veins.
- To look for invasion of renal veins and IVC.
- MRI is superior—can differentiate benign and tumor thrombus.

Imaging features of common solid renal masses are outlined in **Table 6**.

TABLE 6: Imaging features of common solid renal masses.	
Renal lesion	***Imaging features***
ccRCC	High SI on T2WI + may contain fat + hypervascular
Papillary RCC	Low SI on T2WI + may contain hemosiderin + hypovascular
Chromophobe RCC	Iso to high SI on T2 WI + moderate enhancement diagnosis is on histopathology
Classic AML	Macroscopic fat
Minimal fat AML	Low SI on T2WI + may contain microscopic fat + avid early enhancement
Oncocytoma	Iso to high SI on T2 WI + avid/moderate enhancement + may show segmental inversion ⇒ diagnosis on histopathology

Algorithmic approach to diagnosis and work up of renal masses on MRI is presented in **Flowchart 2**.

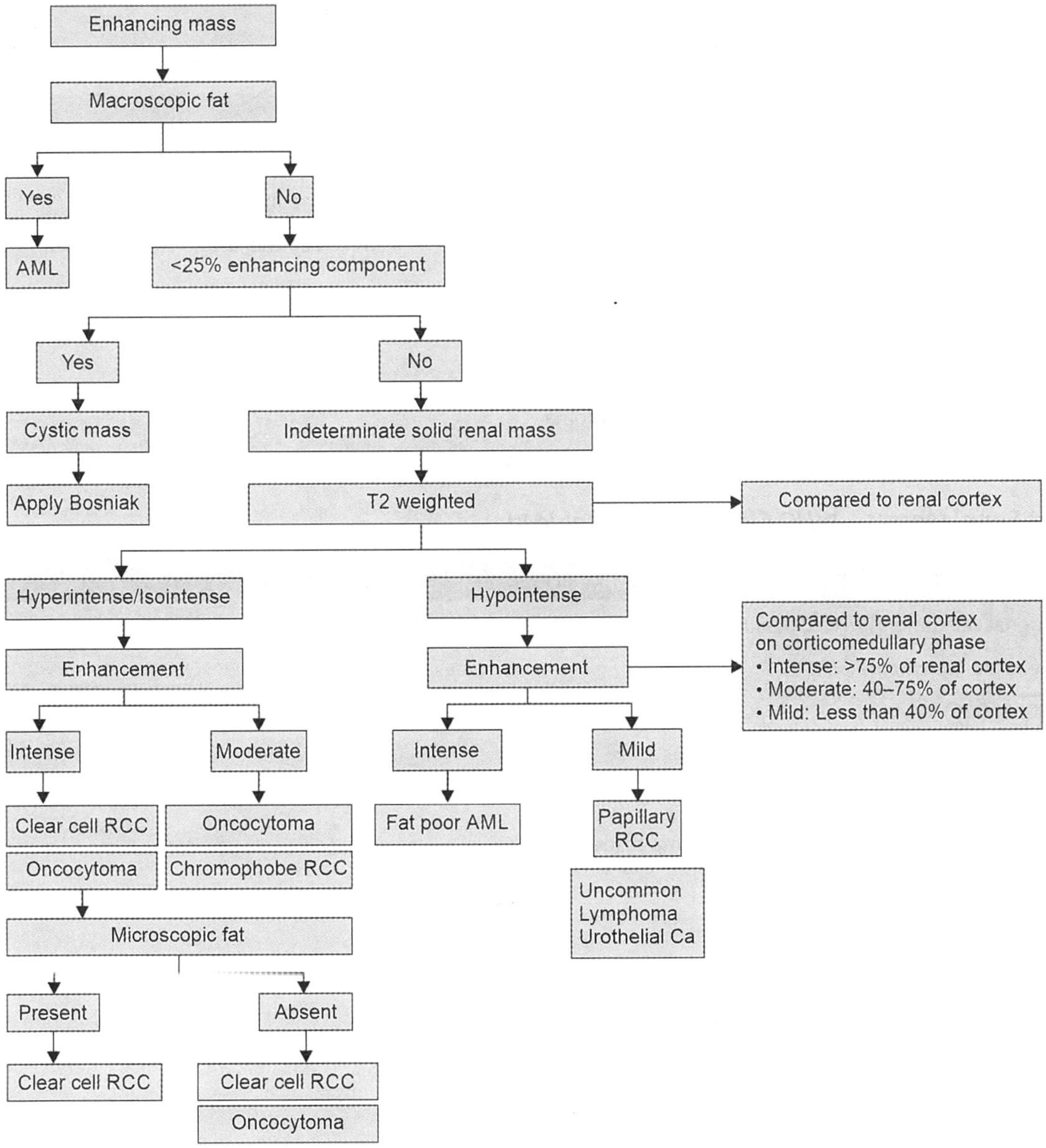

FLOWCHART 2: Algorithmic approach to diagnosis and work up of renal masses on MRI.

PET-CT

- As per NCCN, FDG PET-CT not indicated in RCC.
- Low sensitivity for detecting primary RCC.
- Clear cell RCC has lower FDG uptake.
- **Limitations of PET-CT in RCC**:
- Radiotracers are excreted through kidneys resulting in significant background activity.
- So delineation of RCC from background parenchyma is difficult.

2. Various benign and malignant solid renal masses. Imaging features of malignant solid renal masses. [10] [DNB Dec 21, AIIMS Dec 23]

Benign Renal Masses—WHO Classification (Table 7)

TABLE 7: Benign renal masses–WHO classification.

Renal cell tumors	*Metanephric tumors*	*Mesenchymal tumors*	*Mixed epithelial and mesenchymal tumors*
Oncocytoma	Metanephric adenoma	Angiomyolipoma	Cystic nephroma
Papillary adenoma	Metanephric adenofibroma	Leiomyoma	Mixed epithelial and stromal tumor
	Metanephric stromal tumor	Hemangioma	
		Lymphangioma	
		Reninoma	
		Fibroma	
		Schwannoma	

Malignant Renal Masses—WHO Classification (Table 8)

TABLE 8: Malignant renal masses—WHO Classification.

Malignant renal cell tumors (WHO Classification)
Clear cell renal cell carcinoma (ccRCC)
Papillary RCC (pRCC)
Chromophobe RCC (crRCC)
Multilocular cystic renal cell neoplasm
Hereditary leiomyomatosis and renal cell carcinoma-associated RCC
Collecting duct carcinoma
Renal medullary carcinoma
MIT family translocation RCC
Succinate dehydrogenase—deficient renal carcinoma
Mucinous tubular and spindle cell carcinoma
Tubulocystic RCC
Acquired cystic disease-associated RCC
Clear cell papillary. RCC
Renal cell carcinoma—unclassified

A solid enhancing mass in an adult patient is considered malignant unless proven otherwise.

Two Types of Renal Masses (Table 9 and Fig. 2)

TABLE 9: Main differences between ball- and bean-type renal masses.

Features	*Ball type*	*Bean type*
Renal contour	Deformed	Enlarged but maintained contour
Collecting system	Displaced	Destroyed

Continued...

Continued...

Features	Ball type	Bean type
Examples	Renal cell carcinoma Metastasis Lymphoma Benign: Angiomyolipoma Oncocytoma	Transitional cell carcinoma Infiltrative renal cell carcinoma Medullary duct carcinoma Collecting duct carcinoma Sarcoma Metastasis Lymphoma

Renal Cell Carcinoma (RCC)

Imaging Features

- An arterial hyperenhancing mass is considered RCC, unless proven otherwise.
- Clear cell RCC
- Most common
- **Origin**: Proximal convoluted tubule
- **NCCT**: Hypo to hyperdense lesion

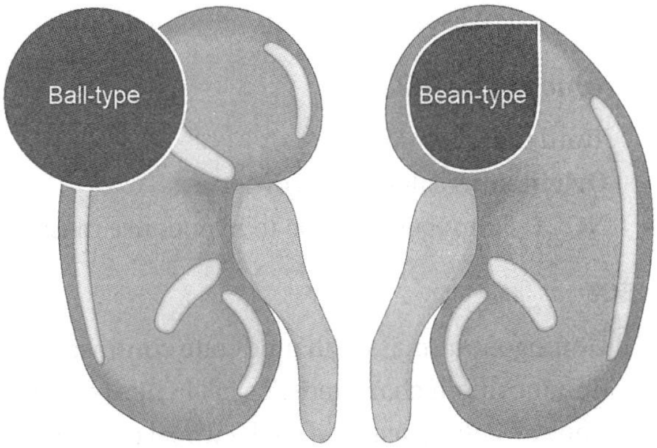

FIG. 2: Ball- and bean-type renal masses.

CECT

- Hypervascular heterogenous mass with moderate to intense enhancement in corticomedullary phase and washout of contrast in nephrographic or delayed phases.
- Hypervascular mass remains hypoattenuating compared with renal parenchyma.
- Hypodense pseudocapsule in corticomedullary phase, hypointense capsule on T1 and T2.
- Can have necrosis, hemorrhage
- Calcification indicates malignancy
- Microscopic fat—common feature
- Cystic degeneration common
- Features of invasion into perirenal and renal sinus fat, renal vein and IVC.
- Metastasis to liver, lung, bone (expansile lytic lesions).

MRI

- T1—Hypo- to isointense lesion
- T2—Heterogeneously hyperintense
- DWI—diffusion restriction. Low ΛDC value correlates with grade.
- Post-contrast—moderate to intense enhancement

Papillary RCC

- Second most common
- **Origin**: Distal convoluted tubule
- **NCCT**: Iso- to hyperdense lesion
- **Small lesions**: Homogenous
- **Large lesions**: Heterogenous

CECT

- Hypovascular heterogenous mass with low enhancement in corticomedullary phase and progressive enhancement in nephrographic or delayed phases.

- Can have necrosis, hemorrhage, calcification.
- **Cystic papillary RCC**: Less common, has papillary projections, mural nodule, and hemorrhagic fluid.
- Tumor to cortex attenuation ratio <0.25—strong predictor.

MRI

- T1—Hypo- to isointense lesion
- T2—hypointense lesion
- DWI—diffusion restriction. Lower ADC value than clear cell RCC.
- **Chemical shift imaging**: Drop in in-phase image due to hemosiderin content.
- **Postcontrast**: Low enhancement in corticomedullary phase and progressive enhancement in nephrographic or delayed phases.

Chromophobe RCC

- Third most common
- **Origin**: Intercalated cells of cortex.
- **NCCT**: Homogenously iso to hypodense mass.

CECT

- Homogenous mass with moderate contrast enhancement in the corticomedullary phase
- Enhancement characteristics fall in between clear cell and papillary RCC.
- Central stellate scar and spoke wheel enhancement may be present.
- **"Segmental enhancement inversion"**: Inversion of pattern of enhancement on excretory phase from that seen on corticomedullary phase.
- Difficult to differentiate from oncocytoma—biopsy is necessary.

MRI

- T1—hypointense lesion
- T2—intermediate to high signal intensity lesion
- DWI—diffusion restriction. Lower ADC value than clear cell RCC.
- Postcontrast—low enhancement in corticomedullary phase and progressive enhancement in nephrographic or delayed phases.

Transitional Cell Carcinoma (TCC)

- Arise from the urothelial lining.
- Arise from pelvicalyceal system or may ascend from bladder TCC via ureter.
- Multiple
- High recurrence
- Congruous or non-congruous involvement—imaging of the entire urinary tract is needed.

Ultrasound

Hyperechoic central mass, difficult to differentiate from sinus fat.

CT

- **Renal TCC**:
  - Smooth or irregular focal hypovascular mass appearing as filling defects.
  - Central mass with loss of sinus fat

- Obstruction of infundibulum causing phantom calyx.
- Fine encrusted calcifications (not renal calculi)
- Infiltrative ill-defined masses which maintain the renal contour.

- **Ureteric TCC**:
  - Irregular eccentric or circumferential wall thickening.
  - Hydronephrosis and hydroureter
  - Goblet sign: Narrowing of ureter with shouldering.
- **Common features**:
  - Absent renal function
  - PUJ obstruction by the mass causing delayed nephrogram.
  - Renal vein and IVC involvement—rare
  - MR urography is done when CT is contraindicated.

The algorithmic approach for characterization of renal masses on CT and MRI are presented in **Flowcharts 3 and 4** as follows:

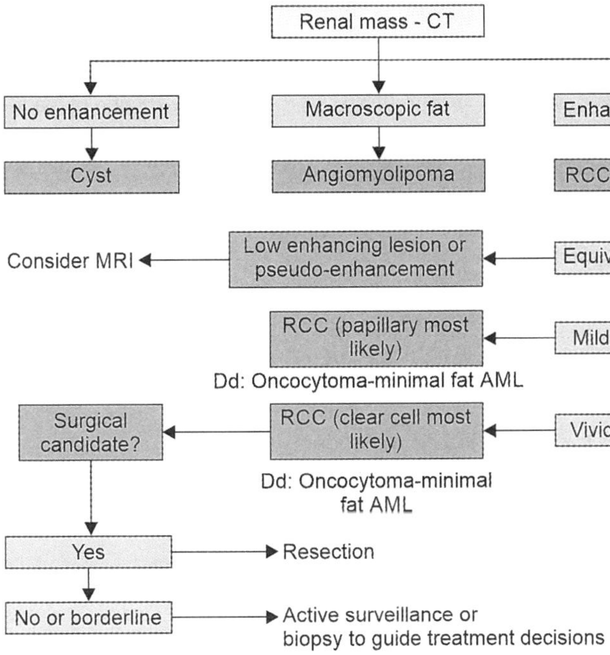

FLOWCHART 3: Algorithmic approach for characterization of renal masses on CT.

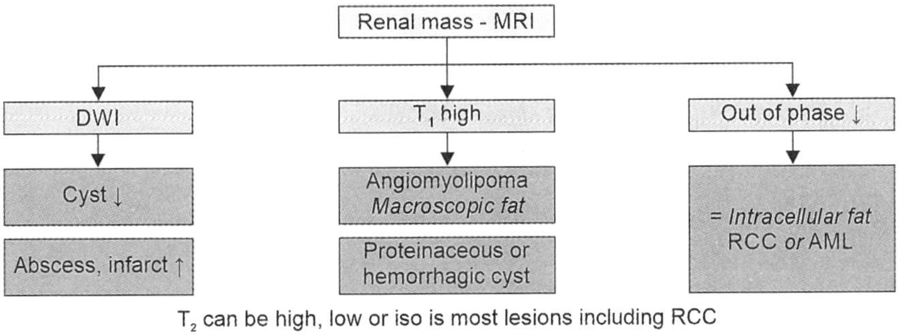

FLOWCHART 4: Algorithmic approach for characterization of renal masses on MRI.

3. Draw and discuss—T-staging of bladder tumors [5] [DNB Dec 21]

TNM Staging of Bladder Cancer (Table 10 and Fig. 3)[6]

TABLE 10: TNM Staging of bladder cancer—8th edition of the American Joint Committee on Cancer (AJCC) Cancer Staging Manual.

Primary Tumor (T)			
TX	Primary tumor cannot be assessed		
TO	No evidence of primary tumor		
Ta	Noninvasive papillary carcinoma		
Tis	Urothelial carcinoma in situ		
TI	Invades lamina propria		
pT2a	Invades superficial muscularis propria		
pT2b	Invades deep muscularis propria		
pT3a	Microscopic perivesical invasion		
pT3b	Macroscopic perivesical invasion		
T4a	Extravesical tumor invades prostatic stroma, uterus, vagina		
T4b	Extravesical tumor invades pelvic wall, abdominal wall		
Lymph Nodes (N)			
NX	Nodes cannot be assessed		
NO	No lymph node metastasis		
NI	Single regional lymph node metastasis in true pelvis		
N2	Multiple regional lymph node metastasis in true pelvis		
N3	Lymph node metastasis to common iliac lymph nodes		
Metastasis (M)			
MO	No distant metastasis		
MIa	Distant metastasis limited to lymph nodes beyond the common iliacs		
MIb	Non-lymph node distant metastasis		
Staging	***T***	***N***	***M***
Stage 0	Ta or Tis	NO	MO
Stage I	TI	NO	MO
Staging	***T***	***N***	***M***
Stage II	T2a or T2b	NO	MO
Stage IIIa	T3a,T3b, or T4a	NO or any NI	MO
Stage IIIb	TI—T4a	N2 or N3	MO
Stage IVa	T4b or any T	Any N	MO or MIa
Stage IVb	Any T	Any N	MIb

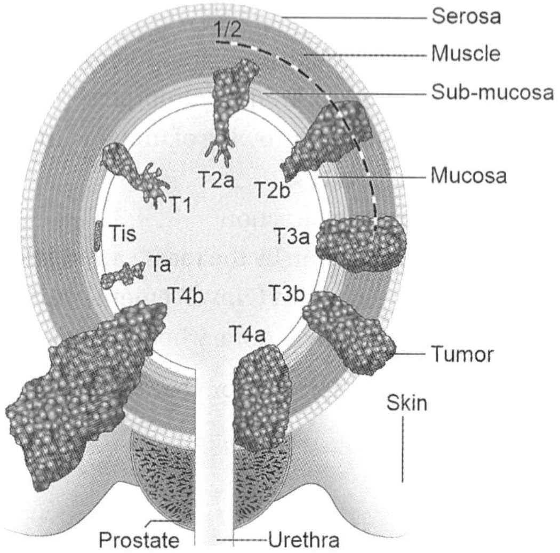

FIG. 3: T-staging of bladder cancer.

- T1–involvement of lamina propria
- T2–involvement of muscularis propria
- T2a–inner half

- T2b–outer half
- T3–involvement of perivesical fat
- T3a–microscopic
- T3b–macroscopic
- T4a–organ involvement
- T4b–pelvic or abdominal wall involvement

Lower Urinary Tract

1. Discuss role of IVU, CT urography, MR urography in obstructive uropathy. [10] [MD (WBUHS) 20]

Introduction

Obstructive uropathy refers to the obstruction of urine flow anywhere along the urinary tract, leading to potential kidney damage. Imaging is essential for diagnosing the location, cause, and severity of the obstruction. It also guides management, such as deciding on surgical intervention, and helps assess the function of the kidneys.

Types of Obstructive Uropathy

1. Acute
2. Chronic

Causes of Obstruction (Table 11, Fig. 4, Box 2, and Flowchart 5)

TABLE 11: Causes of upper urinary tract obstruction

Intrinsic causes	*Extrinsic causes*
intraluminal • Intratubular deposition of crystals (uric acid, drugs) • Stones • Papillary tissue • Blood clots • Fungal ball	**Reproductive system** • Cervix: Carcinoma • Uterus: Pregnancy, tumors, prolapse, endometriosis, pelvic inflammatory disease • Ovary: Tumor, cysts • Prostate: Carcinoma
Intramural • Functional: Pelviureteral or vesicoureteral junction dysfunction • Anatomic: Tumors (benign or malignant) • Infections, granulomas, strictures	**Vascular system** • Aneurysms: Aorta, iliac vessels • Aberrant arteries: Pelviureteral junction • Venous: Ovarian veins, retrocaval ureter
	Gastrointestinal tract • Crohn disease • Pancreatitis • Appendicitis • Diverticulitis • Tumors
	Retroperitoneal space • Lymph nodes • Fibrosis: Idiopathic, drugs, inflammatory or IgG4-related disease • Tumors: Primary or metastatic hematomas • Radiation therapy
	Surgical disruption or ureteral ligation

BOX 2: Causes of lower urinary tract obstruction.

Urethral anatomic causes

Urethral strictures: Trauma, *postinstrumentation*, infections, such as gonococcal urethritis, nongonococcal urethritis, tuberculosis

Posterior urethral valves

- Stones
- Blood clots
- Periurethral abscess
- Phimosis
- Paraphimosis
- Meatal stenosis

Urethral functional causes

Anticholinergic drugs, antidepressants, levodopa

Prostate

- *Benign prostatic hypertrophy*
- *Prostatic carcinoma*

Bladder anatomic causes

- *Bladder cancer*
- *Schistosomiasis* (*Schistosoma haematobium* infection), bladder calculi
- Bladder trauma, pelvic fracture

Bladder functional causes

Neurogenic bladder: Spinal cord defects or trauma, diabetes, multiple sclerosis, Parkinson disease, cerebrovascular accidents

Imaging Features

Intravenous Urography

It is a diagnostic imaging technique used to visualize the urinary tract, including the kidneys, ureters, and bladder, with the aid of intravenous contrast.[7]

Useful in resource-limited environments or when radiation exposure is a concern.

Purpose of IVU in Urinary Tract Obstruction:

- Evaluation of urinary tract anatomy and visualization of any anatomical distortions caused by obstruction.
- Identification of causes of obstruction due to stones, tumors, strictures, or external compression.
- Assessment of kidney function by tracking the excretion of contrast material, giving an indirect measurement of how well the kidneys are working, especially in obstructed systems.

Procedure:

1. Administration of contrast: A radiopaque contrast medium is injected into a vein. This contrast is filtered by the kidneys and excreted into the urine, outlining the renal collecting system, ureters, and bladder on X-ray.
2. Sequential X-rays: X-ray images are taken at various time intervals (typically after 5, 10, and 20 minutes) to track the passage of contrast through the urinary system.
3. Delayed Imaging: In cases of obstruction, delayed images might be necessary to see the contrast material accumulate in dilated areas of the urinary tract (such as in hydronephrosis) or to determine the exact level of obstruction.

Findings in Urinary Tract Obstruction:

- **Hydronephrosis**: IVU can clearly show dilation of the renal pelvis and calyces (hydronephrosis), which is a common result of urinary tract obstruction.
- **Delayed or absent excretion of contrast**: In the presence of a complete or significant obstruction, the contrast material may not be excreted normally, leading to delayed visualization or absence of contrast in the affected kidney or ureter.

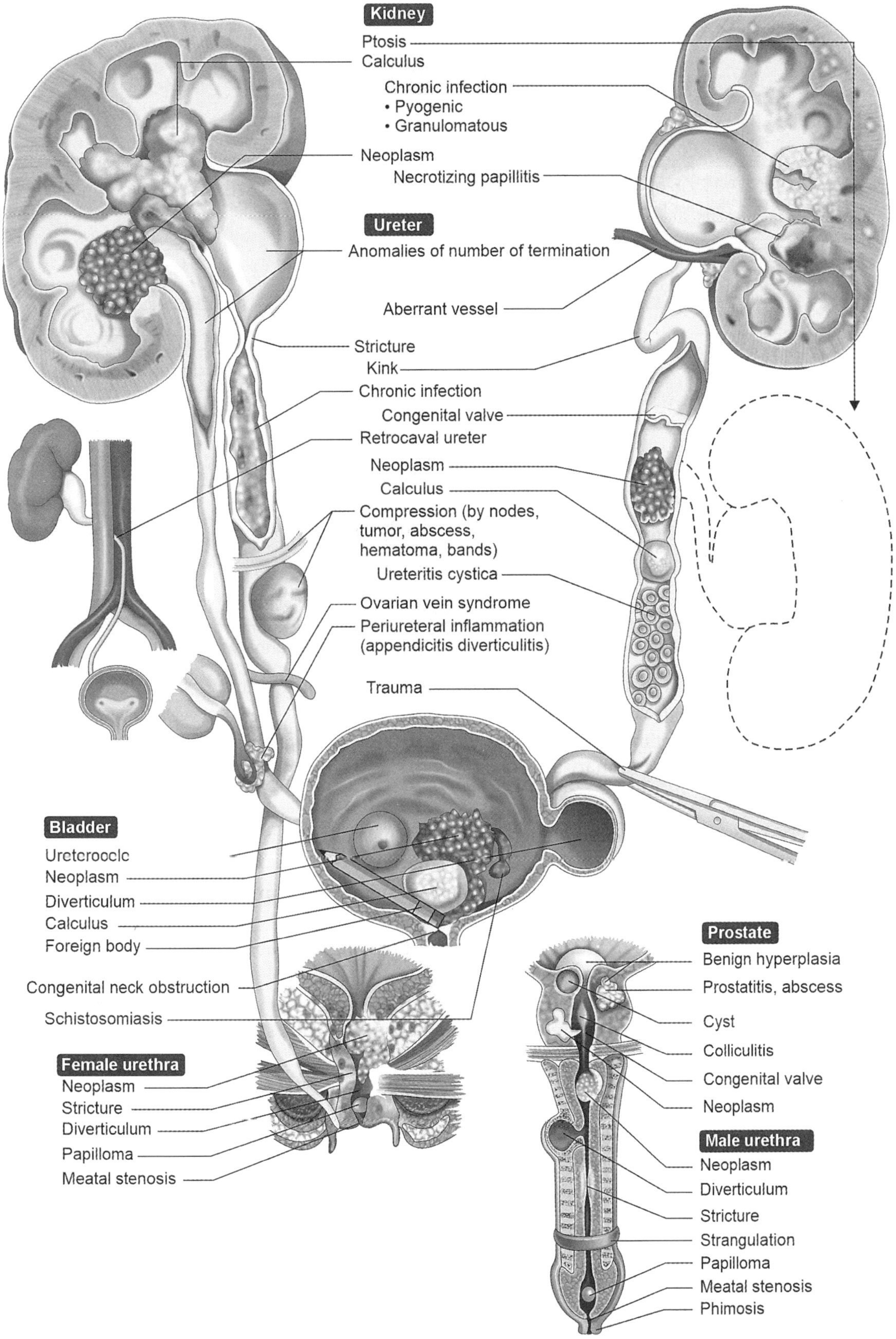

FIG. 4: Causes of obstructive uropathy.

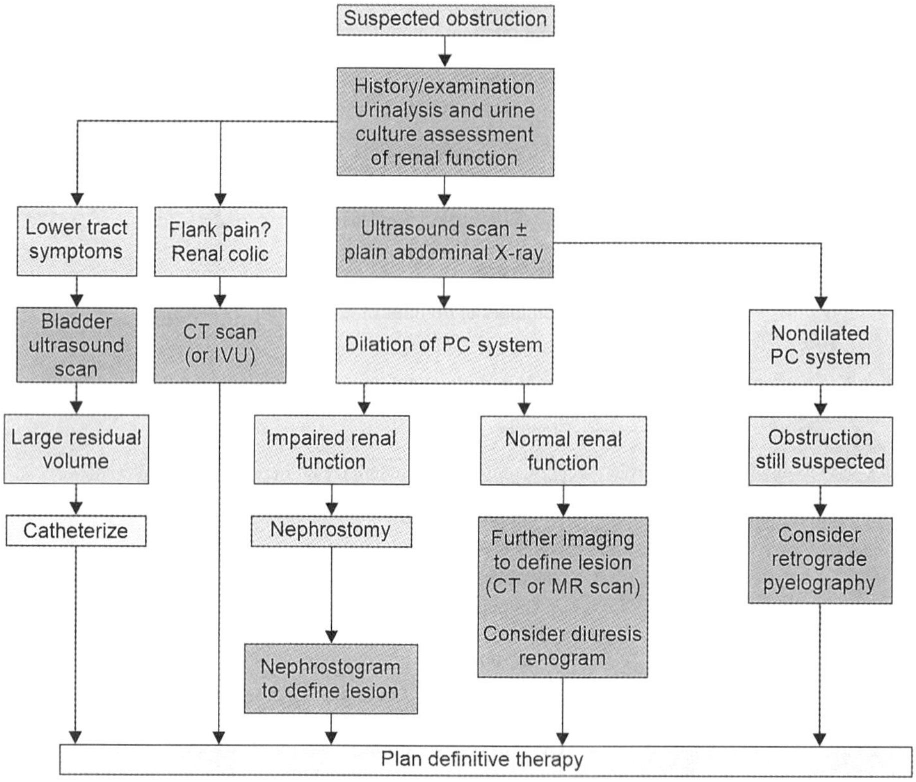

FLOWCHART 5: Algorithmic approach to investigations and management of suspected urinary tract obstruction.

- **Ureteral dilation**: Obstruction in the ureter, due to causes, such as stones or tumors, can lead to dilatation of the ureter upstream of the blockage, visible on IVU.
- **Bladder and urethral obstruction**: In some cases, IVU can show a distended bladder with delayed clearance of contrast material, indicating lower urinary tract obstruction.

Causes of Obstruction:

- **Kidney stones**: IVU can show radiopaque stones within the renal pelvis, calyces, or ureter. The extent of obstruction and the dilatation of the proximal urinary tract can be visualized.
- **Tumors**: Tumors within the kidney or ureter, or even masses external to the urinary tract, can cause obstruction and will manifest as a filling defect or delayed excretion of contrast.
- **Strictures**: Narrowing of the ureter or urethra due to scarring or congenital abnormalities can be seen as a thinning of the contrast-filled lumen, with proximal dilation.
- **External compression**: Masses outside the urinary tract, such as enlarged lymph nodes or tumors, can compress the ureters, leading to obstruction, visible as ureteral dilatation upstream of the site of compression.

Advantages:

- Gives both anatomical and functional information
- Simple and Inexpensive
- Lower radiation dose compared to CT

Disadvantages:

- **Less detailed evaluation than CT**: IVU provides less anatomical detail compared to CT urography, especially in the evaluation of small lesions or subtle causes of obstruction, such as early tumors or mild strictures.
- **Contrast-related risks**: The use of iodinated contrast in IVU poses a risk of allergic reactions or kidney damage, especially in patients with existing renal impairment.
- **Limited use in acute settings**: IVU is generally less useful in acute settings where a rapid diagnosis is needed, as CT urography is faster and more comprehensive.

Comparison with CT Urography:

- CT urography is more commonly used today because it provides detailed cross-sectional images, identifies smaller causes of obstruction, and allows for the diagnosis of a broader range of conditions, including those not related to the urinary system.
- IVU remains useful in settings where radiation dose needs to be minimized, resources are limited, or when the clinical suspicion of a specific condition (e.g., stones or gross hydronephrosis) is high.

MR Urography

Introduction: MR urography (MRU) is a noninvasive examination for the assessment of abnormalities of the urinary tract. Both anatomical and functional status can be assessed.

Indications:

- Congenital anomalies
- Obstructive uropathy
- Pregnant patients and children requiring imaging of the urinary tract
- Deranged renal function
- Hematuria

Technique and protocol:

- **Magnet**: 1.5 or 3T
- **Coil**: Eight channel phase array body coil

There are two types of MR urography:

1. Static fluid MRU (based on T2 W imaging)
2. Excretory MRU (based on T1 W imaging)

Sequences:

- **Precontrast**:
  - Localizer—axial, sagittal, coronal
  - 2D T2 FSE—axial, coronal
  - 2D T2 FS FSE—coronal
  - 3D SSFSE OR HASTE (post diuretic)—coronal
  - 3D T1 FS GRE (precontrast)—axial
  - CINE (T2 SSFSE)
- **Postcontrast**: 3D T1 FS GRE (20 sec, 45 sec and 5 min)—axial
- **Post-processing**:
  - Maximum intensity projection images—withthin and thick slab
  - Volume rendered images

Patient preparation:

- Intake of fluid is restricted for four hours prior to the commencement of the examination.
- Voiding before the examination to avoid discomfort.
- Administration of 250 mL of intravenous normal saline for distension of collecting system.
- Administration of furosemide (0.1 mg/kg) may be considered.
- Excretory MRU—administration of 0.1 mmol/kg of gadolinium followed by 15–20 mL saline push.

Advantages:

- No ionizing radiation is used.
- Ureteral peristalsis can be seen by CINE images as intermittent distention and collapse.
- The level of complete or partial obstruction is determined.
- It can provide anatomical and structural details and details of anomaly if any.

- Assessment of function can also be done as normal renal parenchyma and bladder wall enhance showing the different phases.
- Minimal ascites, perirenal and periureteral edema can also be seen in static fluid MR urography since it is heavily T2 weighted.
- Static fluid MR urography does not use contrast, so it can be used in patients with deranged renal function as well as in pediatric and pregnant patients.

Disadvantages:
- Less spatial resolution than CT urography.
- Presence of fluid in the bowel and metal artifacts may interfere with interpretation of the images.
- Bowel and ureteral peristalsis can create artifacts.
- Time-consuming process and requires expertise.
- Difficult for pregnant patients to lie down so long in the machine.
- Air introduced due to any intervention is difficult to differentiate from calculi.
- Small calculi can be missed.

Static MRU: Cannot assess the excretory function
Excretory MRU: Cannot be used in patients having derangement in excretory function, such as anuric patients.

Applications:
- Anomalies of urinary tract—duplex kidney, horseshoe or ectopic kidney.
- For assessment of urinary tract obstruction—its cause, extent and level.
- For assessment of hematuria and determine its cause.
- Imaging modality of choice in children and pregnant patients.
- Imaging modality of choice in case of deranged renal function and allergy to iodinated contrast.
- Preoperative and postoperative assessment.

CT Urography (Table 1)

Introduction: It is an examination to evaluate the genitourinary tract. Renal parenchyma and urothelium both can be evaluated.

Indications:
- Hematuria
- Urolithiasis
- Urothelial thickening
- Renal neoplasm
- Ureteric lesions
- Pelviureteric junction obstruction
- Congenital anomalies

Patient preparation:
- Oral administration of 1L of water for diuresis and better delineation of the ureters.
- Diuretics and saline infusion can be used.

Technique and protocol:
Two approaches to perform CT urography:

1. CT hybrid urography:
   - It combines CT urography and intravenous urography (IVU).
   - Uses projection radiographs (scout image, scanogram).
   - Post-processing of CT images not required.
   - CT urography and IVU performed at different locations (not preferred) or same location (preferred) by ceiling mounted X-ray tube.
   - Bowel preparation required.

2. CT only—CT urography
    - Bowel preparation not required.
    - Post-processing of CT Images is required.

There are two techniques:

1. Multiphase and
2. Split bolus

Phases of multiphase CT urography

- Non-contrast
- Nephrographic (80–100 sec)
- Excretory phase (7–12 min)

Split bolus technique:

- At first, non-enhanced scan is obtained.
- 30–50 mL of intravenous contrast given
- After 8–10 min, 80–100 mL of intravenous contrast given
- Then after 90 sec, scan is done.
- Images have combined nephrographic and excretory phases

Applications:

- To detect calculi and resultant obstructive changes.
- To detect hemorrhage in collecting system and within cysts.
- To assess renal tumors, their characterization and extent.
- To evaluate renal vein thrombosis, IVC thrombosis and its extent.
- To detect papillary necrosis and assess its cause and urothelial carcinoma.
- Perinephric and periureteral fat stranding can be seen.

Advantages:

- High contrast and spatial resolution.
- Detection of pathologies (listed above).

Disadvantages:

- Use of ionizing radiation
- Use of large amount of contrast
- Detection of small plaque like thickening of bladder and those near the neck, is difficult.

2. IVU in the diagnosis of posterior urethral value. [10] [MD (WBUHS) 19]

Introduction

It is the most common cause of bladder outlet obstruction in newborns.

Pathophysiology

Remnant of Wolffian duct—raised mucosal fold extending obliquely from verumontanum to the inferior aspect of prostatic urethra.

- **Sex predilection**: Exclusive in male child.
- Diagnosed when there is bilateral hydroureteronephrosis.

Types

Based on YOUNG'S classification **(Figs. 5 and 6)**:

- I - valve located inferior to verumontanum (most common)
- II - valve located at superior urethral crest
- III - valve located at inferior urethral crest

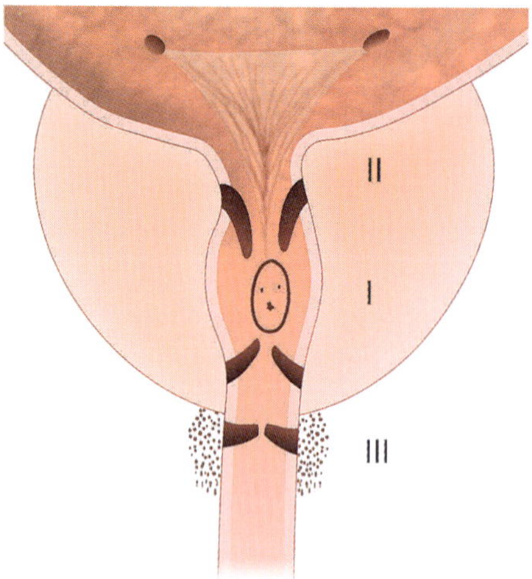

FIG. 5: Young's classification of posterior urethral valves.

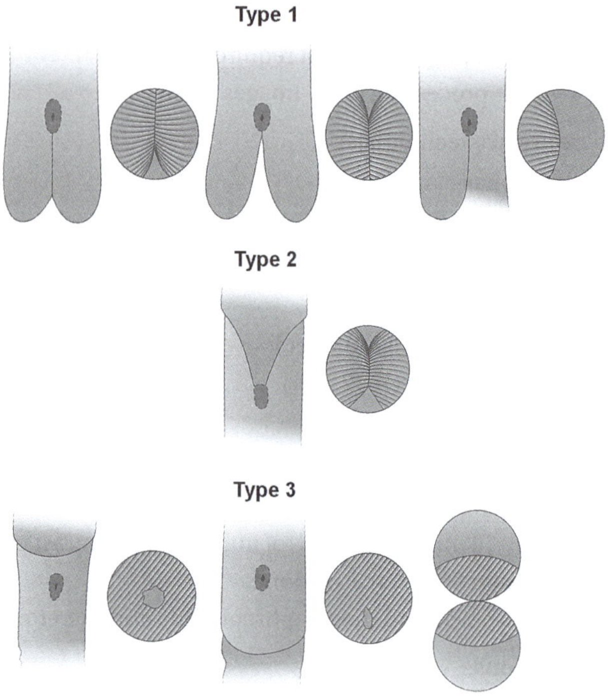

FIG. 6: Types of posterior urethral valves.

Imaging Features in Intravenous Urography

Intravenous Urography

Thin Radiolucent linear filling defect at posterior urethra may be seen.

Micturating urethrography—modality of choice:

- Dilated and elongated posterior urethra.
- Dilatation persisting throughout micturition.
- Vesicoureteral reflux
- Narrow anterior urethra due to obstruction.
- Large volume of residual urine
- Bladder neck hypertrophy, diverticula—due to back pressure changes

Antenatal ultrasound:

- Keyhole appearance of bladder and posterior urethra **(Fig. 7)**.
- Oligohydramnios
- B/L hydronephrosis and hydroureter
- Associated anomalies

Management:
Fulguration of the posterior urethral valve.

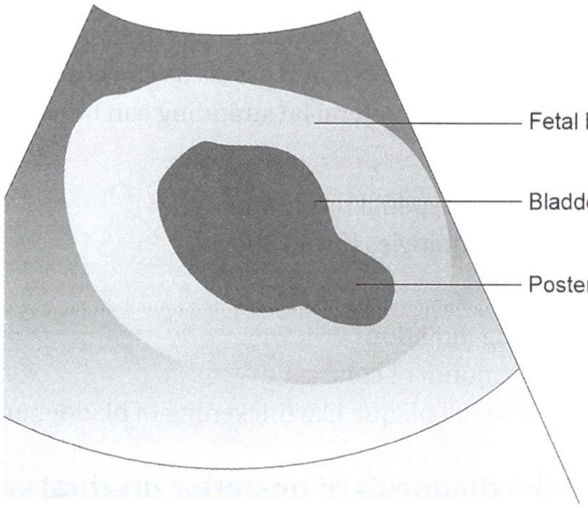

FIG. 7: Keyhole appearance of bladder and posterior urethra in posterior urethral valve.

3. Discuss the types of urinary bladder trauma and role of imaging in diagnosis and management of such cases. [4+6]

Introduction

Urinary bladder is commonly injured organ in blunt trauma. Its evaluation in pelvic bone fracture and RTA is necessary.[8]

Types of Urinary Bladder Trauma

A. Contusion
B. Subserosal bladder rupture

C. Extraperitoneal rupture—more common
D. Intraperitoneal rupture
E. Combined

Mechanism of Injury

- Blunt trauma—most common cause
- Penetrating injuries—gunshot/stab wound
- Motor vehicle accident
- Iatrogenic

Clinical Features

- Hematuria
- Shock
- Hypotension

Modality of choice—CT cystography

Protocol:
- **Machine**: Multidetector CT scanner
- **Position**: Supine
- No anesthesia required.
- Head goes inside the machine.
- **Patient preparation**: Adequate distension of bladder is required.

Sequence:
- Non-contrast—soft tissue and bone window
- Contrast given in bladder via catheter.
- 400 mL of 4% contrast is given by drip set from a reservoir at the maximum height of 100 cm.
- Contrast scan taken.
- After voiding or catheter drainage, another scan taken.

It is performed after ruling out urethral injuries.

Imaging Features

- **Bladder contusion**:
  - Incomplete mucosal tear
  - Formation of hematoma
- **Subserosal bladder rupture**: Subserosal surface tear without extension to the bladder mucosa.
- **Extraperitoneal bladder rupture (Figs. 8A and B)**:
  - Molar tooth or streaky, flame-shaped appearance as contrast leaks into the extraperitoneal spaces.
  - The contrast leaks into prevesical, lateral paravesical spaces, anterior abdominal wall, inguinal regions and upper thigh and presacral space.[9]
  - The contrast can leak into the perineum and scrotum if there is disruption of the urogenital membrane.
  - The contrast can extend retroperitoneally suggesting renal source.
  - Demonstration of the site of bladder rupture rules out renal source.
- **Intraperitoneal bladder rupture (Fig. 9)**:
  - Rent seen at the dome of the bladder.
  - Intraperitoneal spillage of contrast.
  - Contrast fills the peritoneal recesses and surrounds the bowel loops, liver and spleen.
  - Attenuation of contrast is lesser due to dilution by urine in a large space.

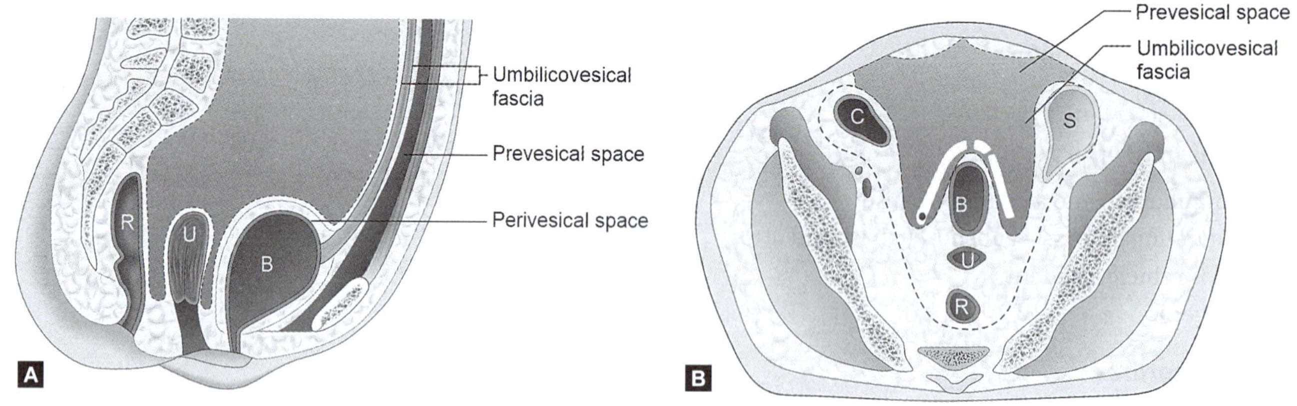

FIGS. 8A and B: Fluid in perivesical space in case of extraperitoneal bladder rupture.

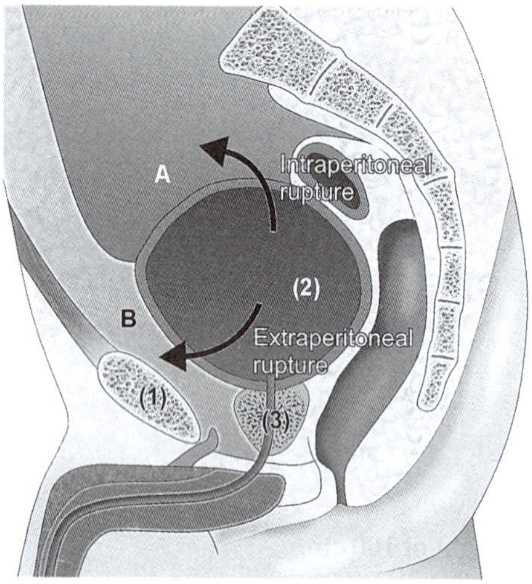

FIG. 9: Intraperitoneal bladder rupture.

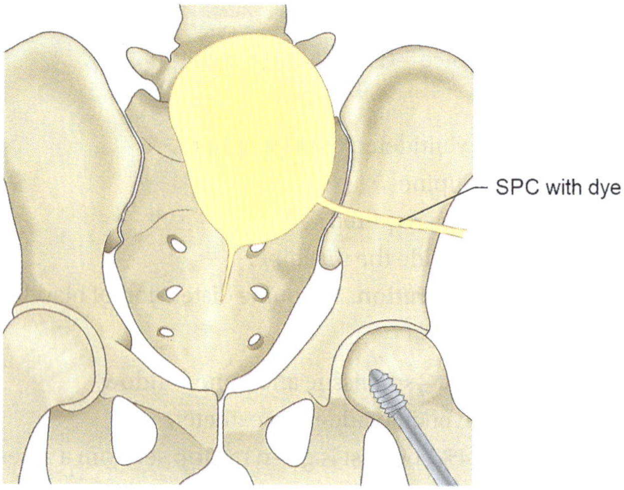

FIG. 10: Pie in the sky bladder in case of pelvic hematoma.

- **Distorted entrapped bladder**—when there is pelvic injury the bladder may get entrapped in the displaced pelvic fracture giving it distorted shape.
- Open reduction and repair of bladder injury is required.

Pie in the Sky Bladder (Fig. 10)

The contrast opacified bladder is lifted high up due to large pelvic hematoma.

Management of Bladder Injuries

Extraperitoneal bladder rupture: It is managed by catheterization of the bladder for 7–10 days. The urinary bladder heals within this time.

Intraperitoneal bladder rupture: Managed surgically.

4. 74-year-old with urinary incontinence-approach and role of imaging. [10] [DNB June 22]

Introduction

Urinary incontinence is involuntary leakage of urine. It is a common condition that can significantly affect quality of life. Most common female health problem.

Causes

- Neurological causes causing bladder dysfunction.

- **Weak pelvic floor muscles**: Pelvic organ prolapse.
- Post-traumatic
- Secondary to obstruction
- Functional causes

History and Examination

- Duration of incontinence
- Any major operation distorting the pelvic floor anatomy, TURP in elderly males.

Imaging Modalities

- **Ultrasound**:
  - Widely available
  - Cost effective
  - No radiation
  - For evaluation of:
    - Hydronephrosis
    - Hydroureter
    - Urinary tract stones
- **Computed tomography**:
  For evaluation of:
  - Nephrolithiasis
  - Pyelonephritis
  - Ectopic insertion of ureter
  - Fistula of urinary tract with uterus, vagina
- **MRI brain and spine**:
  - Spine:
    - Cord compression
    - Cauda equina
    - Spinal epidural abscess
  - Brain: Normal pressure hydrocephalus

Types of Urinary Incontinence and Their Imaging Features

1. **Stress urinary incontinence (SUI)**: The involuntary leakage of urine during activities that increase intra-abdominal pressure (e.g., coughing, sneezing, laughing).
   - Primary cause: Weakness or dysfunction of the pelvic floor muscles or the urethral sphincter.
   - Imaging modalities:
     - Ultrasound (transperineal or transvaginal)
     - Bladder neck descent: During straining or Valsalva, transperineal ultrasound can show abnormal downward movement of the bladder neck and urethra.
     - Angle of urethra: An increase in the urethral-bladder angle during Valsalva suggests loss of urethral support.
   - MRI:
     - Pelvic floor weakness: MRI can show pelvic organ prolapse (e.g., bladder, uterus, or rectum) and loss of integrity of pelvic ligaments or muscles.
     - Urethral hypermobility: MRI during dynamic maneuvers like Valsalva can demonstrate urethral descent.
2. **Urge incontinence (Overactive bladder, OAB)**: Sudden, intense urge to urinate, followed by involuntary leakage.
   - Primary cause: Detrusor muscle overactivity (neurogenic or idiopathic).

- Imaging modalities:
  - Ultrasound:
    - Bladder wall thickness: Ultrasound can show thickening of the bladder wall, which is often seen in overactive bladder conditions. A bladder wall thickness >5 mm is suggestive of bladder outlet obstruction or detrusor overactivity.
    - Post-void residual volume (PVR): Measurement of urine volume after voiding helps assess incomplete bladder emptying, which can be associated with overactivity or outlet obstruction.
  - MRI: Bladder abnormalities: MRI can rule out masses or structural abnormalities, such as diverticula, that may contribute to detrusor overactivity.

3. **Mixed incontinence**: A combination of stress and urge incontinence, which is common in elderly women.
   - Primary cause: Multiple factors, including pelvic floor weakness, bladder overactivity, or obstruction.
   - Imaging modalities:
     - Ultrasound: Features of both SUI (bladder neck descent, urethral hypermobility) and OAB (bladder wall thickening, high post-void residual).
     - MRI: Useful for comprehensive assessment of pelvic anatomy, including both dynamic urethral function and bladder wall characteristics.
4. **Overflow incontinence**: Continuous leakage of urine due to bladder overdistention, often because of an inability to empty the bladder fully.
   - Primary cause: Bladder outlet obstruction or weakened detrusor muscle.
   - Imaging modalities:
     - Ultrasound:
       - Post-void residual (PVR) measurement: Ultrasound is key for detecting high residual volumes, suggesting incomplete bladder emptying. PVR >100 mL is indicative of possible overflow incontinence.
       - Bladder wall thickness: Increased thickness may suggest chronic bladder outlet obstruction or detrusor hypertrophy.
     - MRI: MRI can assess bladder outlet obstruction or neurogenic causes, such as spinal lesions affecting bladder innervation.
5. **Functional incontinence**: Incontinence not due to bladder or urethral dysfunction, but rather due to physical or cognitive impairments that prevent timely voiding.
   - Primary cause: Often linked to mobility issues or dementia in the elderly.
   - Imaging modalities: Ultrasound: Used primarily to rule out other causes of incontinence, such as high PVR or structural abnormalities. Functional incontinence itself usually shows normal bladder and urethral anatomy.
6. **Voiding cystourethrography (VCUG)**: It is less commonly used but can provide detailed dynamic imaging of the bladder and urethra during filling and voiding.
   - Indications:
     - Urethral hyperextension: In cases of stress incontinence, VCUG may show hypermobility of the bladder neck.
     - Bladder diverticula: VCUG may help visualize diverticula or vesicoureteral reflux.
     - Outlet obstruction: In cases of overflow incontinence, VCUG can assess for bladder outlet obstruction, such as in cases of pelvic organ prolapse.
7. **Pelvic organ prolapse**: Descent of pelvic organs, such as the bladder (cystocele), uterus, or rectum, into the vaginal canal, which can contribute to incontinence.
   - Primary cause: Pelvic floor muscle weakness, often due to age-related atrophy, childbirth trauma, or surgery.
   - Imaging modalities:
     - MRI: Dynamic MRI: Provides a detailed assessment of pelvic organ prolapse during straining and rest. It helps evaluate the degree of bladder descent (cystocele) and the involvement of other pelvic organs.
     - Ultrasound (transperineal or transvaginal): Ultrasound can show bladder descent and associated cystocele, which may be contributing to stress or overflow incontinence.

5. Draw and discuss—male urethral injury [5] [DNB Dec 21]

Traumatic urethral injury of male urethra can be divided onto anterior (penile and bulbar) and posterior (membranous and prostatic) injuries **(Fig. 11)**.
Posterior urethral injury is more common.

Causes—blunt trauma, penetrating trauma and iatrogenic

Posterior urethral injury:

- Commonly associated with pelvic fractures.
- Mechanism—motor vehicle accident, fall from height.
- One fifth of the patients also have associated bladder injury.
- Assessed with MCU.

Anterior urethral injury:

- Associated with straddle or shearing injuries and attempted catheterization and instrumentation.
- Fracture is generally not associated.
- Penetrating trauma though rare is associated with anterior urethral injury.
- Assessed with RGU.

Complications:

- Urethral stricture (can occur with urethral contusion also)
- Impotence
- Incontinence
- Mildest injury—type 1
- Commonest injury—type 2

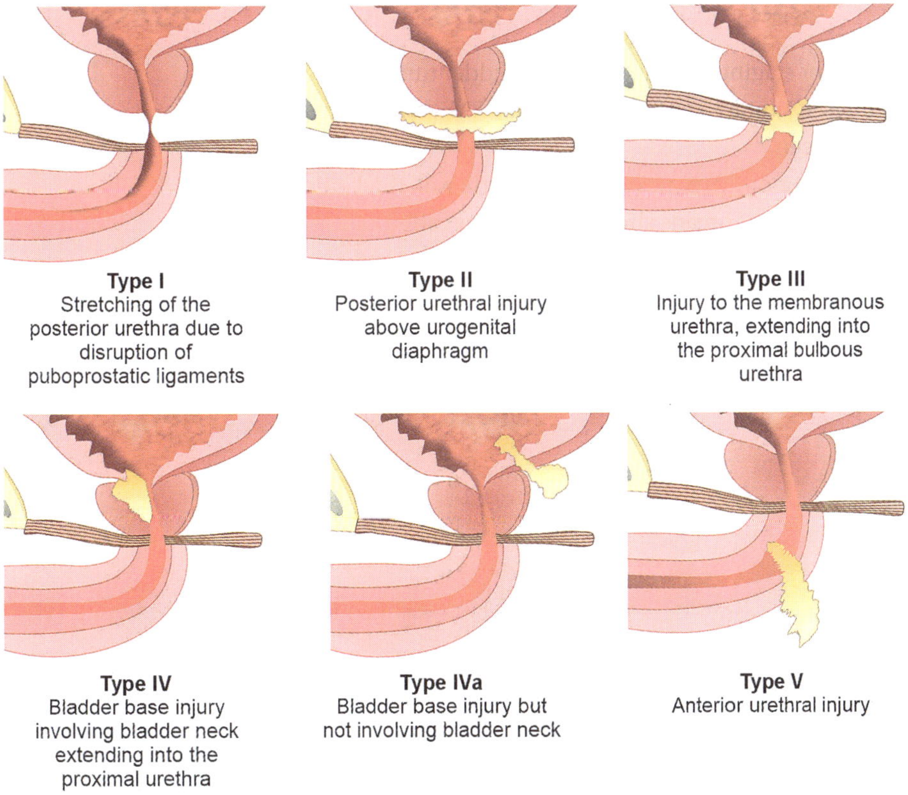

FIG. 11: Types of male urethral injury.

Type two injuries cause partial rupture of urethra mostly and type three cause complete rupture of urethra mostly.

Diagnostic modality of choice:

- Anterior urethral injury—RGU
- Posterior urethral injury—MCU

6. Describe TNM staging of bladder cancer. Draw a schematic diagram of T-staging of bladder tumor. Enumerate the role of ultrasound, computed tomography and MRI in the diagnosis and staging of the bladder carcinoma. [2+2+(2+2+2)] [DNB June 20, MD (WBUHS) 18]

TNM Staging of Bladder Cancer (Table 10 and Fig. 12)

Ultrasound

- Nonmobile sessile/pedunculated variable echogenicity mass with internal vascularity.
- Papillary or focal area of wall thickening
- Mostly hypoechoic
- Color Doppler—internal vascularity
- Involvement of the vesicoureteral junction—hydroureteronephrosis.
- **Advantage of ultrasound is dynamic scanning—to differentiate from clot, change the patient position and application of Doppler shows vascularity in mass, not in clot.**
- **Disadvantage**:
  - Small lesions can be missed.
  - Detection of lesions <5 mm near the bladder neck is difficult.
  - Cannot differentiate layers of bladder wall.
  - Lymph node staging cannot be done.

CT Urography

- Most frequently used for staging and diagnosis of bladder tumors.
- As per ACR guidelines, it should be used along with CEMR abdomen and pelvis.
- Distant spread can be seen.
- Intraluminal polypoidal or nodular mass or asymmetric wall thickening.
- Loss of fat plane with adjacent organs should not be overcalled as invasion.
- **Nephrographic phase**: Variable degree of contrast enhancement.

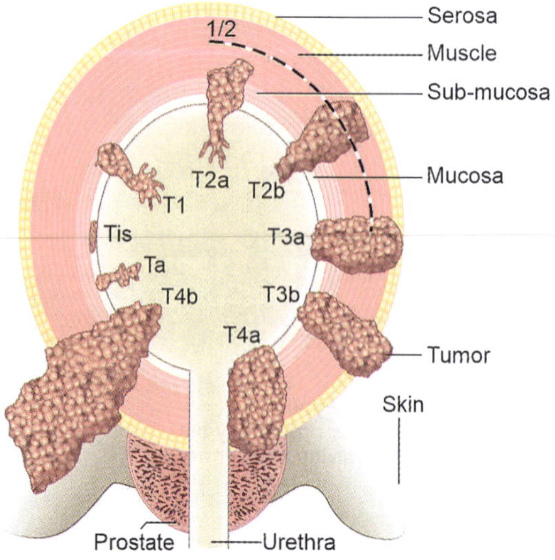

FIG. 12: T-staging of bladder cancer.

- **Delayed phase**: Soft tissue filling defect in the contrast material filled hyperattenuating lumen.
- **Lymph node assessment**:
  - Morphology—round or irregular.
  - Short axis diameter for pelvic (obturator and internal iliac) lymph nodes—8 mm cutoff.
  - Short axis diameter for other lymph nodes—10 mm cutoff.
- Assessment of synchronous lesions (2% chance)
- **Disadvantages**:
  - Fails to detect flat lesions and lesions near the base of the bladder.
  - Cannot accurately assess the degree of invasiveness of the tumor into the wall.
  - Cannot differentiate reliably between recurrence and post-chemotherapy or radiotherapy inflammatory changes.

Magnetic Resonance Imaging

- Multiparametric MRI—modality of choice
- Muscle invasiveness evaluated.
- **Major sequences**: T2W, DWI, DCE (dynamic contrast enhanced) images
- **T2W images**:
  - Tumor is intermediate to hyperintense as compared to hypointense wall.
  - Intact hypointense muscular wall—stage Ta, Tis, T1 (muscle not invaded).
  - Irregular margin at the junction of bladder wall with tumor—stage T2a.
  - Disruption of hypointense muscular wall—stage T2b.
  - Tumor extending into perivesical fat—T3b.
  - Tumor extending into the adjacent organs—T4.
- **DWI images**:
  - Tumor shows restricted diffusion.
  - ADC value correlates with tumor grade (low ADC—high-grade of tumor)
  - Useful sequence to identify tumor in nonmuscle invasive cases.
  - Inchworm sign:
    - Arch-shaped appearance of high signal intensity of tumor with adjacent low signal submucosa.
    - Finding on DWI
    - Stage T1 or below

CEMR

- Dynamic contrast enhanced images—bladder tumors enhance early (45–120s).
- Detrusor muscle is hypoenhancing, so muscle invasion is better evaluated.
- Intact submucosal enhancement—stage T1 or below.
- Irregular inner margin—stage T2a.
- Disruption of hypointense wall and tumor not extending to perivesical fat—stage T2b.
- Enhancing tumor in perivesical fat—stage T3.
- Enhancing tumor extending into the adjacent organs—stage T4.

Assignment of VIRADS Category (Table 12 and Fig. 13)

- Applicable for untreated patients or only diagnostic transurethral resection of bladder tumor.
- The above sequences are considered to give VIRADS score.
- **Dominant sequences**: DWI and DCE.

TABLE 12: VI-RADS categories.

VI-RADS Interpretation
VI-RADS I (muscle invasion is highly unlikely)
VI-RADS 2 (muscle invasion is unlikely to be present)
VI-RADS 3 (the presence of muscle invasion is equivocal
VI-RADS 4 (muscle invasion is likely)
VI-RADS 5 (invasion of muscle and beyond the bladder is very likely)

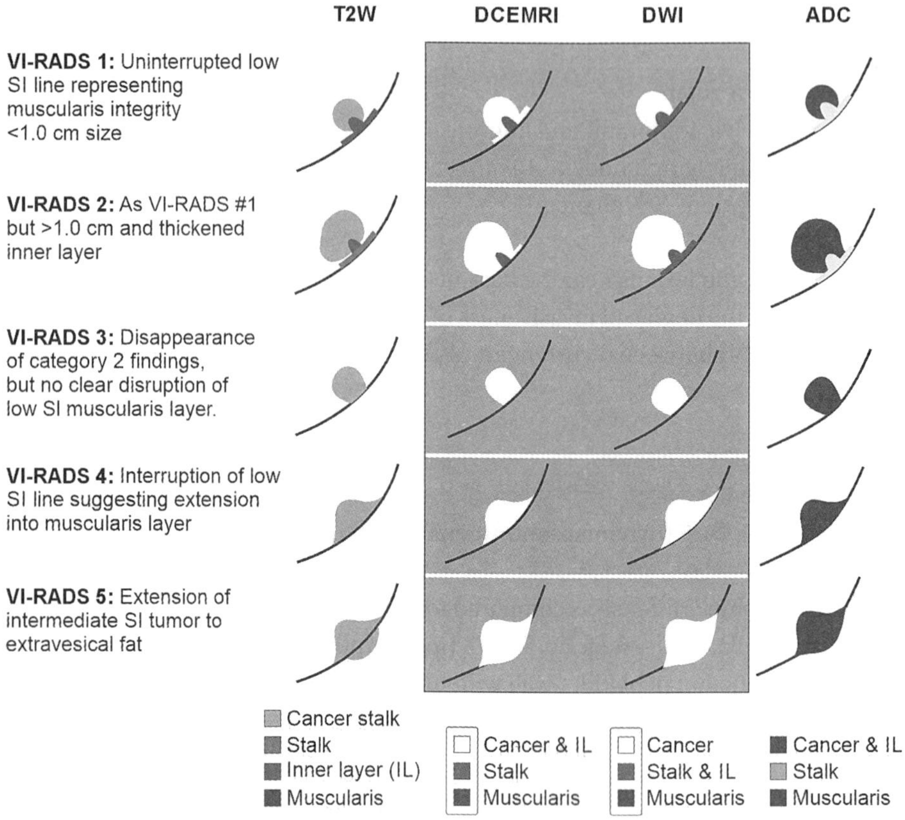

FIG. 13: Schematic illustration of mpMRI appearance of VI-RADS scores.

Miscellaneous Urinary Tract Lesions

1. Write short note on nephrocalcinosis. [5] [MD (WBUHS) 20]

Deposition of calcium in the renal parenchyma (cortex and medulla) is called nephrocalcinosis.
It includes deposition of both calcium phosphate and calcium oxalate.

It is of two types:
- Cortical nephrocalcinosis
- Medullary nephrocalcinosis—more common
- Combined—primary oxalosis

Medullary nephrocalcinosis is caused due to metabolic derangements and cortical nephrocalcinosis is caused due to severe renal cortical disease.

Causes of medullary nephrocalcinosis:
- Hypercalcemia
- Metastatic soft tissue calcification
- Hyperparathyroidism
- Disseminated malignancy causing hypercalcemia
- Sarcoidosis
- Medullary sponge kidney

- Renal tubular acidosis (dense medullary nephrocalcinosis + calculi + renal failure)
- Loop diuretics
- Beta thalassemia
- Inherited tubulopathies
- Oxalosis
- Vitamin D overtreatment, milk alkali syndrome
- Acromegaly, thyrotoxicosis (rare)

Causes of cortical nephrocalcinosis:
- Chronic renal failure
- Hypotensive renal insult (perinatal/septic/hemorrhage)
- Renal cortical necrosis
- Glomerulonephritis
- Renal allograft rejection
- Alport syndrome (sensorineural hearing loss with congenital nephritis)
- Oxalosis
- Ethylene glycol poisoning

Hyperoxaluria causes both cortical and medullary nephrocalcinosis.

Imaging approach to common causes of nephrocalcinosis are presented in **Flowchart 6** as follows:

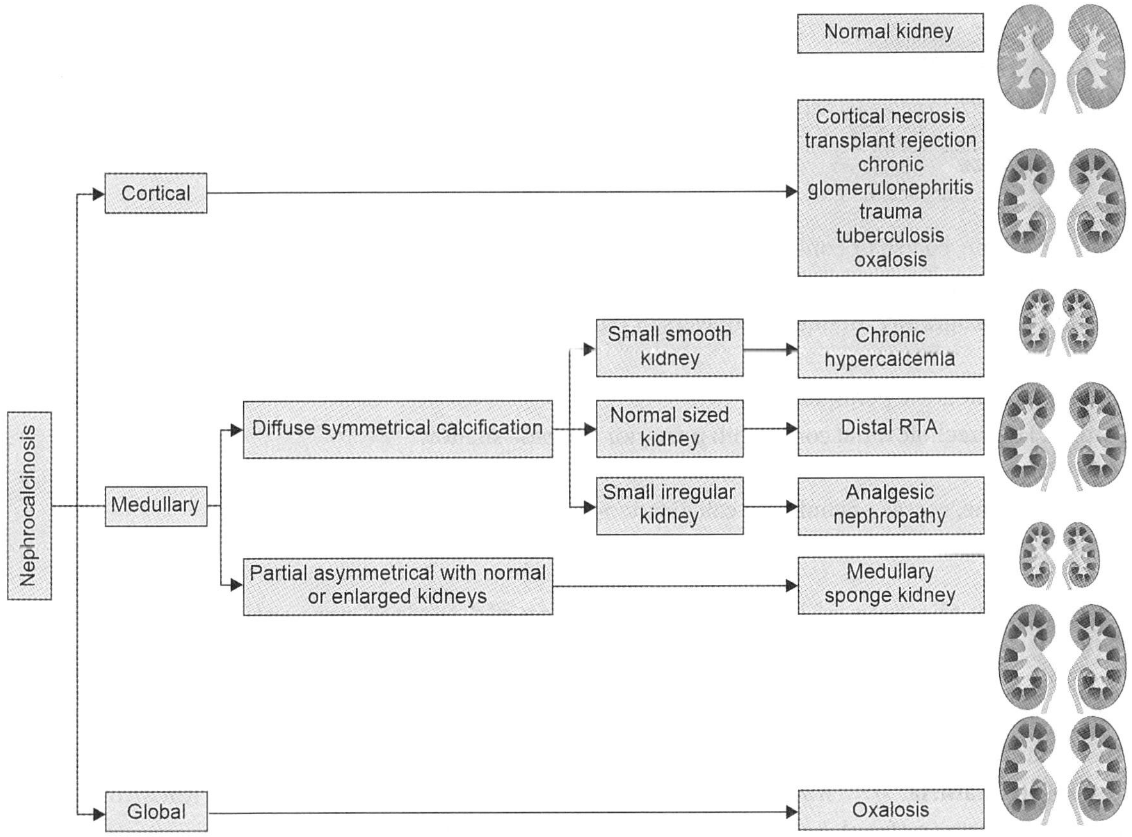

FLOWCHART 6: Imaging approach to common causes of nephrocalcinosis.

Approach to neonatal nephrocalcinosis is presented in **Flowchart 7** as follows:

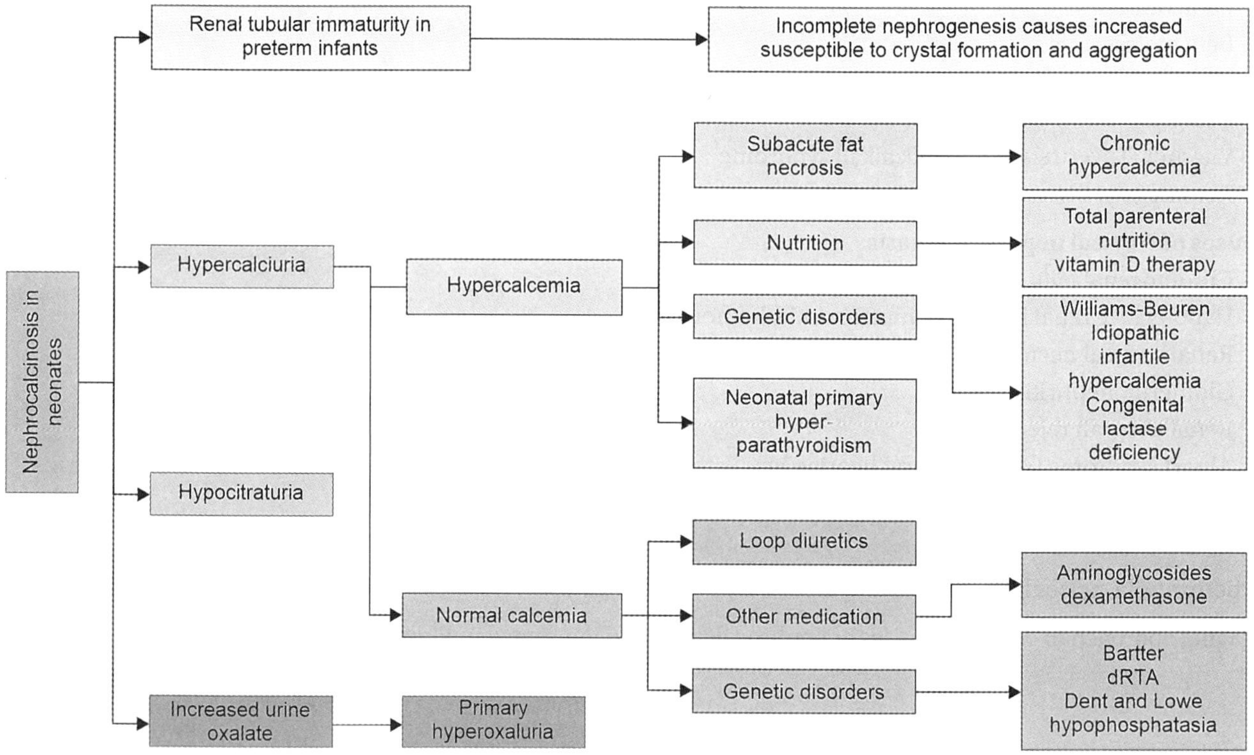

FLOWCHART 7: Approach to neonatal nephrocalcinosis.

Imaging Appearance

- **Radiograph**:
  - Medullary: Fine, coarse or confluent calcifications in renal pyramids.
  - Cortical: Punctate or tram line calcification in the cortex.
  - **IVU and CT urography**: Bouquet of flowers or paint brush appearance in medullary sponge kidney.
- **Ultrasound**:
  - Medullary: Echogenic pyramids
  - Cortical: Hyperechoic renal cortex with posterior acoustic shadow.
- **NCCT KUB**:
  - Medullary: Fine, coarse or confluent calcifications in renal pyramids, dense medulla.
  - Cortical: Increased cortical density and distinct calcifications.

2. Discuss briefly the role of imaging in a 40-year-old female presenting with hematuria. [10] [MD (WBUHS) 24]

Definition

Hematuria means presence of red blood cells in urine.

- **Microscopic hematuria:** >/= 3 RBC/HPF from 2 of 3 properly collected specimens OR >5 RBCs/μL
- **Macroscopic or gross or frank hematuria:** Visible to naked eye OR >2500 RBCs/μL

Etiology

- **Vascular:**
  - Arterial embolism or thrombosis
  - Arteriovenous malformation or fistula

  - Renal vein thrombosis
  - Nutcracker syndrome
- **Glomerular**:
  - IgA nephropathy
  - Alport disease
  - Thin basal membrane nephropathy
  - Other glomerulonephritis
- **Interstitial**:
  - Allergic interstitial nephritis
  - Analgesic nephropathy
  - Renal cystic disease
  - Transplant rejection
  - Pyelonephritis
- **Uroepithelial**:
  - Urothelial carcinoma
  - Renal cell carcinoma
  - Heavy physical exercise
  - Trauma
  - Renal papillary necrosis
  - Cystitis, urethritis, prostatitis
  - Parasitic infections
  - Urolithiasis
  - Radiation
- **Miscellaneous**:
  - Hypercalciuria
  - Hyperuricosuria
  - Sickle cell disease
  - Blood dyscrasias
  - Antiplatelet therapy
  - Connective tissue disorders

Approach to a patient presenting with hematuria is presented in **Flowchart 8** as follows.

Imaging Modalities

1. Abdominal radiograph
2. Ultrasound and color Doppler
3. Intravenous urography, micturating cystourethrography, retrograde urethrography
4. Antegrade pyelography, retrograde pyelography
5. Computed tomography: Nonenhanced, contrast enhanced CT, CT urography, angiography venography, virtual cystoscopy
6. Magnetic resonance imaging: Nonenhanced, contrast enhanced, MR angiography, MR urography
7. Nuclear scan:
   a. Radionuclide scanning
   b. Positron emission tomography

Abdominal Radiograph

- Enlargement of renal shadow in case of obstruction or mass
- Detection of calculi in urinary tract

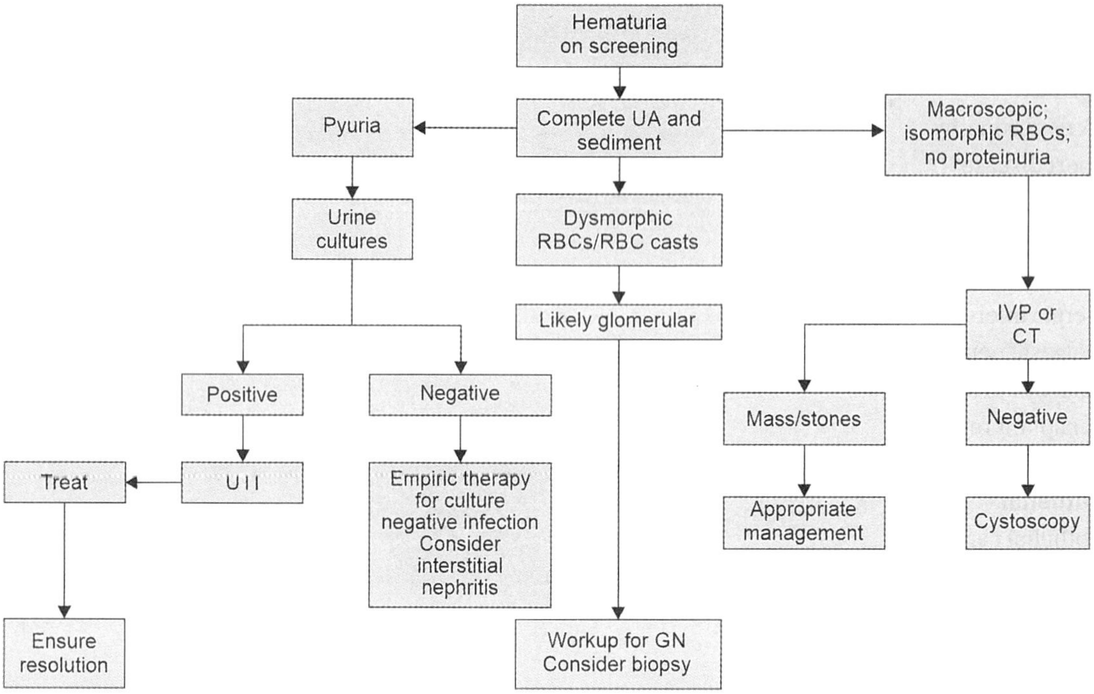

FLOWCHART 8: Approach to a patient presenting with hematuria.

Intravenous Urography

- Filling defects in urinary tract
- Extrinsic compression due to pelvis or retroperitoneal mass
- **Delayed nephrographic phase**: Renal artery stenosis, obstructive uropathy
- **Delayed excretion**: Hydroureteronephrosis
- **Goblet sign**: Shouldering of ureter due to ureteric mass

MCU: Detection of

- Vesicoureteral reflux
- Trauma
- Fistulous communication

RGU: Detection of

- Calculi
- Stricture
- Diverticuli

Ultrasound

- **Advantages**:
  - Accessible, cheap noninvasive painless modality
  - Non-ionizing radiation
  - Sedation not required
- Detection of renal masses, calculi, urothelial thickening
- **Color Doppler**: Minimal to intense color flow within renal masses depending on the histological type
- Assessment of transplant rejection

NCCT

- Detection of small calculi in kidney, ureter and vesicoureteric junction.

- Detection of uric acid and indinavir stones
- Thin collimation CT slices (3–5 mm) are taken from upper pole of kidney to pubic symphysis

CECT

- Corticomedullary phase taken between 25–70 sec
- Cortex enhances more than medulla
- Evaluation of vascular anatomy
- Enhancing hyper/hypovascular mass lesion in kidney—RCC unless proven otherwise
- Transitional cell carcinoma along the ureter—enhancing urothelial thickening, filling defect in excretory phase

CT Urography

There are two techniques:

1. Multiphase and
2. Split bolus

Phases of Multiphase CT urography:

- Non-contrast
- Nephrographic (80–100 sec)
- Excretory phase (7–12 min)

Split bolus technique:

- At first, non-enhanced scan is obtained
- 30–50 mL of intravenous contrast given
- After 8–10 min, 80–100 mL of intravenous contrast given
- Then after 90 sec, scan is done.
- Images have combined nephrographic and excretory phases

Applications:

- To detect calculi and resultant obstructive changes.
- To detect hemorrhage in collecting system and within cysts.
- To assess renal tumors, their characterization and extent.
- To evaluate renal vein thrombosis, IVC thrombosis and its extent.
- To detect papillary necrosis and assess its cause and urothelial carcinoma.
- Perinephric and periureteric fat stranding can be seen.

Advantages:

- High contrast and spatial resolution.
- Detection of pathologies (listed above).

Disadvantages:

- Use of ionizing radiation
- Use of large amount of contrast
- Detection of small plaque like thickening of bladder and those near the neck, is difficult.

MR Urography

There are 2 types of MR urography:

1. Static fluid MRU (based on T2W imaging)
2. Excretory MRU (based on T1W imaging)

Sequences:

- Precontrast
  - Localizer—axial, sagittal, coronal

    - 2D T2 FSE—axial, coronal
    - 2D T2 FS FSE—coronal
    - 3D SSFSE OR HASTE (post diuretic)—coronal
    - 3D T1 FS GRE (precontrast)—axial
    - CINE (T2 SSFSE)
- Postcontrast
    - 3D T1 FS GRE (20sec, 45 sec and 5 min)—axial
- **Post processing**:
    - Maximum intensity projection images—withthin and thick slab
    - Volume rendered images

Patient preparation:

- Intake of fluid is restricted for 4 hours prior to the commencement of the examination.
- Voiding before the examination to avoid discomfort.
- Administration of 250 mL of intravenous normal saline for distension of collecting system.
- Administration of furosemide (0.1 mg/kg) may be considered.
- Excretory MRU- administration of 0.1 mmol/kg of Gadolinium followed by 15–20 mL saline push.

Advantages:

- Non-ionizing radiation is used.
- Ureteral peristalsis can be seen by CINE images as intermittent distention and collapse.
- The level of complete or partial obstruction is determined.
- It can provide anatomical and structural details and details of anomaly if any.
- Assessment of function can also be done as normal renal parenchyma and bladder wall enhance showing the different phases.
- Minimal ascites, perirenal and periureteral edema can also be seen in static fluid MR urography since it is heavily T2 weighted.
- Static fluid MR urography does not use contrast, so it can be used in patients with deranged renal function as well as in pediatric and pregnant patients.

Disadvantages:

- Less spatial resolution than CT urography.
- Presence of fluid in the bowel and metal artifacts may interfere with interpretation of the images.
- Bowel and ureteral peristalsis can create artifacts.
- Time consuming process and requires expertise.
- Difficult for pregnant patients to lie down so long in the machine
- Air introduced due to any intervention is difficult to differentiate from calculi
- Small calculi can be missed.

Static MRU: Cannot assess the excretory function

Excretory MRU: Cannot be used in patients having derangement in excretory function like anuric patients.

Applications:

- Anomalies of urinary tract—duplex kidney, horseshoe or ectopic kidney.
- For assessment of urinary tract obstruction—its cause, extent and level.
- For assessment of hematuria and determine its cause
- Imaging modality of choice in children and pregnant patients
- Imaging modality of choice in case of deranged renal function and allergy to iodinated contrast
- Preoperative and post operative assessment.

Nuclear scan:

- To see renal function
- Radiotracer used- ^{99m}Tc labelled DMSA and DTPA
- Scanned with gamma camera

PET:

- **Radiopharmaceutical used**: 18 fluorodeoxyglucose
- **Avidity present in**:
  - Malignancy
  - Residual or recurrence of tumor
  - Metastasis

3. Causes of nephrocalcinosis and imaging. [10] [DNB June 22]

Deposition of calcium in the renal parenchyma (cortex and medulla) is called nephrocalcinosis.
It includes deposition of both calcium phosphate and calcium oxalate.

It is of two types:

1. Cortical nephrocalcinosis
2. Medullary nephrocalcinosis -more common

Combined – primary oxalosis

Medullary nephrocalcinosis is caused due to metabolic derangements and cortical nephrocalcinosis is caused due to severe renal cortical disease.

Causes of medullary nephrocalcinosis:

- Hypercalcemia
- Metastatic soft tissue calcification
- Hyperparathyroidism
- Disseminated malignancy causing hypercalcemia
- Sarcoidosis
- Medullary sponge kidney
- Renal tubular acidosis (dense medullary nephrocalcinosis + calculi+ renal failure)
- Loop diuretics
- Beta thalassemia
- Inherited tubulopathies
- Oxalosis
- Vitamin D overtreatment, milk alkali syndrome
- Acromegaly, thyrotoxicosis (rare)

Causes of cortical nephrocalcinosis:

- Chronic renal failure
- Hypotensive renal insult (perinatal/septic/hemorrhage)
- Renal cortical necrosis
- Glomerulonephritis
- Renal allograft rejection
- Alport syndrome (sensorineural hearing loss with congenital nephritis)
- Oxalosis
- Ethylene glycol poisoning

Hyperoxaluria causes both cortical and medullary nephrocalcinosis.

Imaging approach to common causes of nephrocalcinosis (*refer* **Flowchart 6**).

Approach to neonatal nephrocalcinosis (*refer* **Flowchart 7**).

Imaging Appearance

- **Radiograph**:
  - Medullary: Fine, coarse or confluent calcifications in renal pyramids
  - Cortical: Punctate or tram line calcification in the cortex
  - **IVU and CT urography**: Bouquet of flowers or paint brush appearance in medullary sponge kidney
- **Ultrasound**:
  - Medullary: Echogenic pyramids
  - Cortical: Hyperechoic renal cortex with posterior acoustic shadow
- **NCCT KUB**:
  - Medullary: Fine, coarse or confluent calcifications in renal pyramids, dense medulla
  - Cortical: Increased cortical density and distinct calcifications

4. (a) Bosniak classification of renal cyst 2019. (b) syndromic association of renal cyst in adult. [10] [DNB June 21]

Bosniak classification of renal cyst 2019 **(Flowchart 9, Tables 13 to 16, and Fig. 14)**

- Incorporated MRI.
- Specific definitions given to the imaging features and all the Bosniak classes.
- Improved inter-rater agreement
- More objective
- Assignment of lower Bosniak class attempted- improved specificity.
- Cyst having less than 25% of solid component is classified as cystic renal mass
- Can be cortical or parapelvic.

Bosniak classification is not applicable to:

- Cysts having more than 25% solid component
- Cysts having thick abundant nodular calcifications
- Hyperattenuating non-enhancing lesions more than 3 cm in size.
- Cysts in renal cell carcinoma syndromes like Von Hippel Lindau syndrome, hereditary leiomyomatosis.

Syndromic association of renal cyst in adult:

1. ADPKD
2. ARPKD
3. VHL
4. Tuberous sclerosis

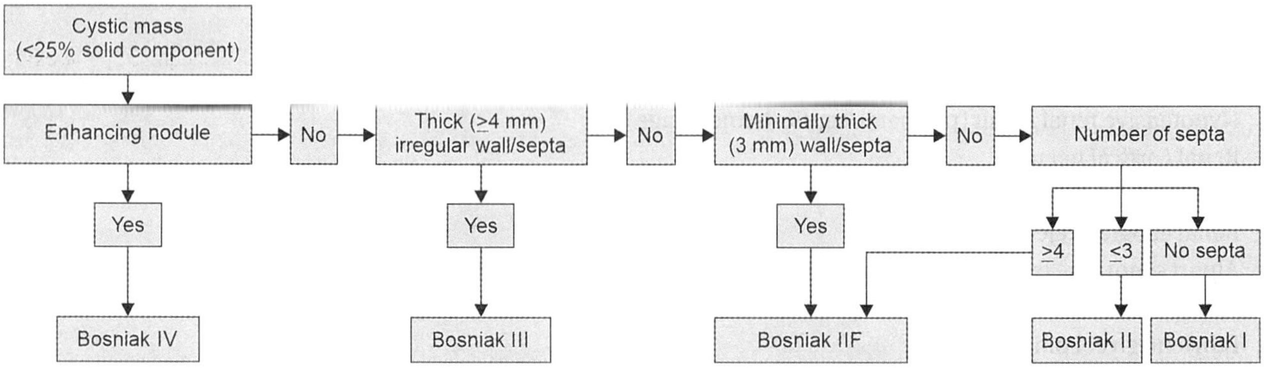

FLOWCHART 9: Algorithmic approach for stratification of cystic renal masses as per Bosniak 2019 version.

TABLE 13: Bosniak classification of renal cyst, version 2019 on CT and MRI.

Class	*CT: Proposed Bosniak Classification, Version 2019*	*MRI: Proposed Bosniak Classification, Version 2019*
I	Well-defined, thin (≤2 mm) smooth wall; homogeneous simple fluid (-9 to 20 HU);no septa or calcifications; the wall may enhance	Well-defined, thin (≤2 mm) smooth wall; homogeneous simple fluid simple fluid (signal intensity similar to CSF); no septa or calcifications; the wall may enhance
II	Six types, all well-defined with thin (≤2 mm) smooth walls: 1. Cystic masses with thin (≤2 mm) and few (1–3) septa; septa and wall may enhance; may have calcification of any type 2. Homogeneous hyperattenuating (≥70 HU) masses at noncontract CT 3. Homogeneous nonenhancing masses >20 HU at renal mass protocol CT (73), may have calcification of any type 4. Homogeneous masses—9 to 20 HU at noncontrast CT 5. Homogeneous masses 21 to 30 HU at portal venous phase CT 6. Homogeneous low-attenuation masses that are too small to characterize	Three types, all well-defined with thin (≤2 mm) smooth walls: 1. Cystic masses with thin (≤2 mm) and few (1–3) enhancing septa; any nonenhancing septa; may have calcification of any type 2. Homogeneous masses markedly hyperintense at T2-weighted imaging (similar to CSF) at noncontrast MRI 3. Homogeneous masses markedly hyperintense at T1-weighted imaging (approximately X2.5 normal parenchymal signal intensity) at noncontract MRI
IIF	Cystic masses with a smooth minimally thickened (3 mm) enhancing wall, or smooth minimal thickening (3 mm) of one or more enhancing septa, or many (≥4) smooth thin (<2 mm) enhancing septa	Two types: 1. Cystic masses with a smooth minimally thickened (3 mm) enhancing wall, or smooth minimal thickening (3 mm) of one or more enhancing septa, or many (≥4) smooth thin (≤2 mm) enhancing septa 2. Cystic masses that are heterogeneously hyperintense at unenhanced fat-saturated T1-weighted imaging
III	One or more enhancing thick (≥4 mm width) or enhancing irregular (displaying ≤3 mm obtusely margined convex protrusion(s) walls or septa	One or more enhancing thick (>4 mm width) or enhancing irregular (displaying ≤3 mm obtusely margined convex protrusion[s]) walls or septa
IV	One or more enhancing nodule(s) (≥4 mm convex protrusion with obtuse margins, or a convex protrusion any size that has acute margins)	One or more enhancing nodule(s) (≥4 mm convex protrusion with obtuse margins, or a convex protrusion any size that has acute margins)

TABLE 14: Suggested terms and phrases to use when reporting cystic renal masses using the Bosniak Classification, version 2019.

Classification	*Suggested term and phrases*
Bosniak I	Benign simple renal cyst requiring no follow-up
Bosniak II	(Option I) Benign Bosniak II renal cyst requiring no follow-up* Option 2) Likely benign Bosniak II renal mass requiring no follow-up**
Bosniak IIF	Bosniak IIF cynic renal mass. The large majority of Bosniak IIF masses are benign. When malignant. nearly all are indolent. Generally, Bosniak IIF masses are followed by imaging at 6 months and 12 months, then annually for a total of 5 years to assess for morphologic change
Bosniak III	Bosniak III cyst is renal mass. Bosniak III masses have an intermediate probability of being malignant. If not already obtained, consider urology consultation
Bosniak IV	Bosniak IV cystic renal mass. The large majority of Bosniak IV masses are malignant. If not already obtained, consider urology consultation

Note: This content is intended for patients in the general population and not those with a renal cell carcinoma syndrome.

*This option is best used for Bosniak II masses that have been confirmed to be cysts (e.g., cysts with few thin septa).

**The Bosniak II category includes some masses that, although they are reliably considered benign, have not been definitively characterized as cysts (e.g., low-attenuation lesions that are too small to characterize).

TABLE 15: Bosniak classification of renal cyst.

Bosniak	*I*	*II*	*IIIF*	*III*	*IV*
Wall thickness	<2 mm	<2 mm	<3 mm	<4 mm	
Septa number	0	1–3	>4		
Smooth enhancing septal thickening	N/A	<2 mm	<3 mm	<4 mm	
Irregular enhancing wall/septal thickening				<3 mm	<4 mm
Enhancing nodule	-	-	-	-	+

TABLE 16: Chances of malignancy with respect to Bosniak classes of renal cyst.

Bosniak classes	*Benign/malignant*
I	Universally benign
II	<1% chances of malignancy
IIF	0–38% chances of malignancy
III	50% chances of malignancy
IV	90% chances of malignancy

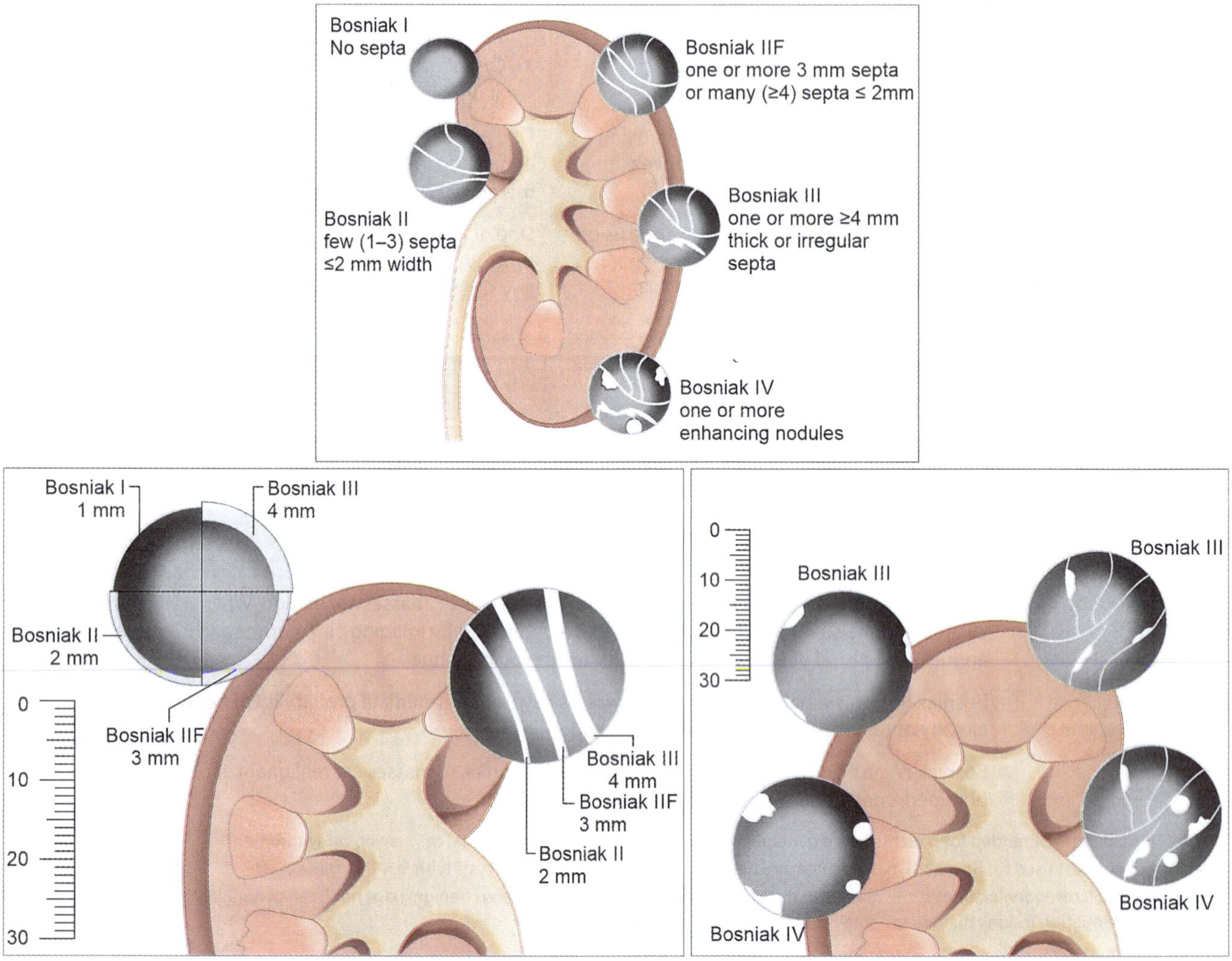

FIG. 14: Bosniak classification of renal cyst.

ARPKD—Autosomal recessive polycystic kidney disease

- Bilateral kidneys are affected.
- Benign etiology.
- Presents in neonate or young adult.
- Kidneys are enlarged, echogenic.
- Corticomedullary differentiation is lost.
- Multiple cystic areas within the kidney, too small too resolve.
- Liver—congenital hepatic fibrosis
- Associated oligohydramnios.

ADPKD—Autosomal dominant polycystic kidney disease

- Bilateral kidneys are affected.
- Benign etiology.
- Familial, 30–50 yrs.
- Kidneys are enlarged.
- multiple varying sized simple and complex cysts within the kidney, pancreas and liver.
- Some cysts may have calcifications.
- Associated—intracranial aneurysm, mitral valve prolapse, aortic aneurysm, bicuspid aortic valve.
- Liver > pancreas > spleen also affected.

VHL—Von Hippel Lindau syndrome

- Bilateral kidneys are affected.
- Cysts are seen in majority of the patients.
- Benign etiology.
- But lifetime risk of RCC is 70%.
- Multiple simple or complex cysts.
- Cystic renal cell carcinoma can be present.

Tuberous sclerosis

- Limited number of small cysts
- One kidney affected
- Benign
- Risk of RCC due to hyperplasia and atypia in the lining cells
- Associated—lymphangioleiomyomatosis, cardiac rhabdomyoma, subependymal hamartomas, cortical tubers

5. Describe approach to a patient in renal trauma with a flowchart and discuss the role of imaging with grades of renal injury. [4+6] [MD (WBUHS) 18, AIIMS May 24]

Genitourinary injuries occur in 10% of blunt trauma patients.

Clinical Features

- Hematuria
- Flank or upper abdomen pain
- Abdominal tenderness
- Palpable mass
- Ecchymosis or abrasion in the abdomen
- Hypotension
- Shock
- Radiograph may reveal rib fracture

Modalities for Evaluation

1. IVU
2. CT
3. Angiography

CT Protocol

- **Mulitidetector CT**: Dual phase or split bolus technique
- **Dual phase**:
  - Arterial phase - 25–30 sec (pseudoaneurysm)
  - Portovenous phase – 65–80 sec (active bleeding and parenchymal disruption)
- **In both techniques**: Delayed images (9 min after porto-venous phase) if required.

Imaging work up in suspected renal trauma is depicted in **Flowchart 10**.

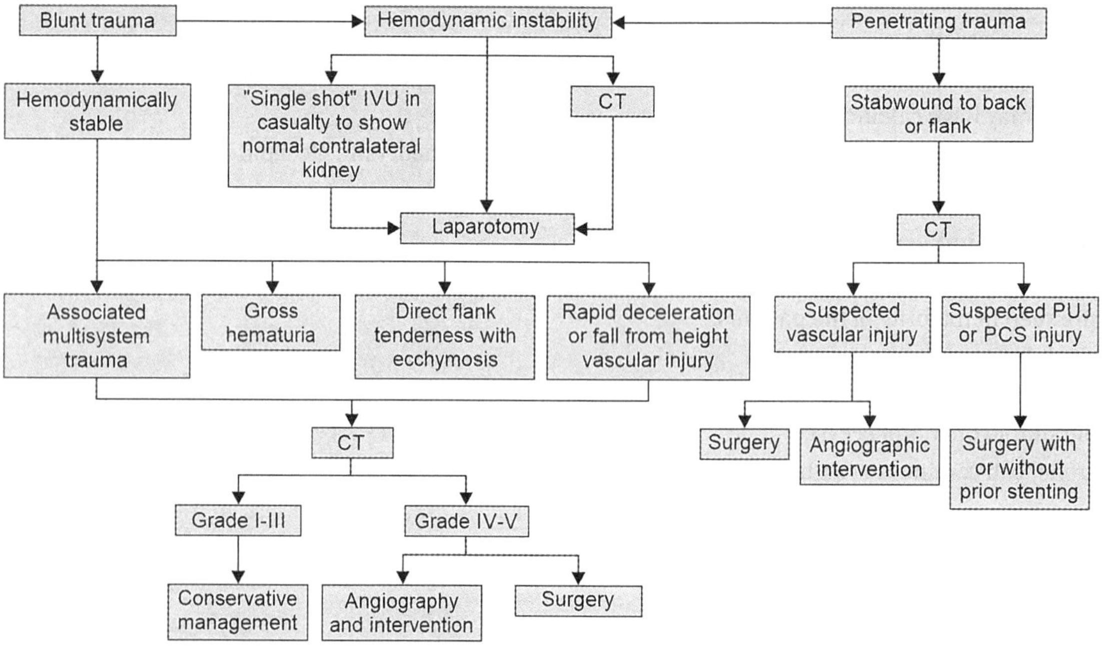

(PUJ: pelviureteric junction; PCS: postconcussion syndrome)

FLOWCHART 10: Imaging work up in suspected renal trauma.

The revised 2018 AAST–OIS grading system for renal injuries is presented as follows (**Table 17 and Fig. 15**).

TABLE 17: Revised 2018 AAST–OIS grading system for renal injuries.

AAST grade	*CT criteria for renal injuries in revised grading system*
I	1. Isolated parenchymal contusions 2. Subcapsular hematoma
II	1. Renal parenchymal laceration ≤10 mm in depth. No involvement of pelvicalyceal system 2. Hematoma in perirenal space limited by anterior renal fascia
III	1. Renal parenchymal laceration >10 mm in depth. No involvement of pelvicalyceal system 2. Any low-grade trauma accompanying injury to vessels or active bleeding limited by anterior renal fascia
IV	1. Renal parenchymal laceration involving pelvicalyceal system 2. Renal pelvis laceration or complete pelviureteric laceration 3. Intimal injury/thrombus of segmental renal artery or vein

Continued...

Continued...

AAST grade	CT criteria for renal injuries in revised grading system
	4. Segmental or complete renal infarction due to renal vessel thrombosis in the absence of active bleeding 5. Active bleeding outside Gerota fascia into the retroperitoneum or peritoneum
V	1. Main renal artery or vein laceration or avulsion from renal hilum 2. Complete devascularization of kidney with active bleeding 3. Shattered kidney

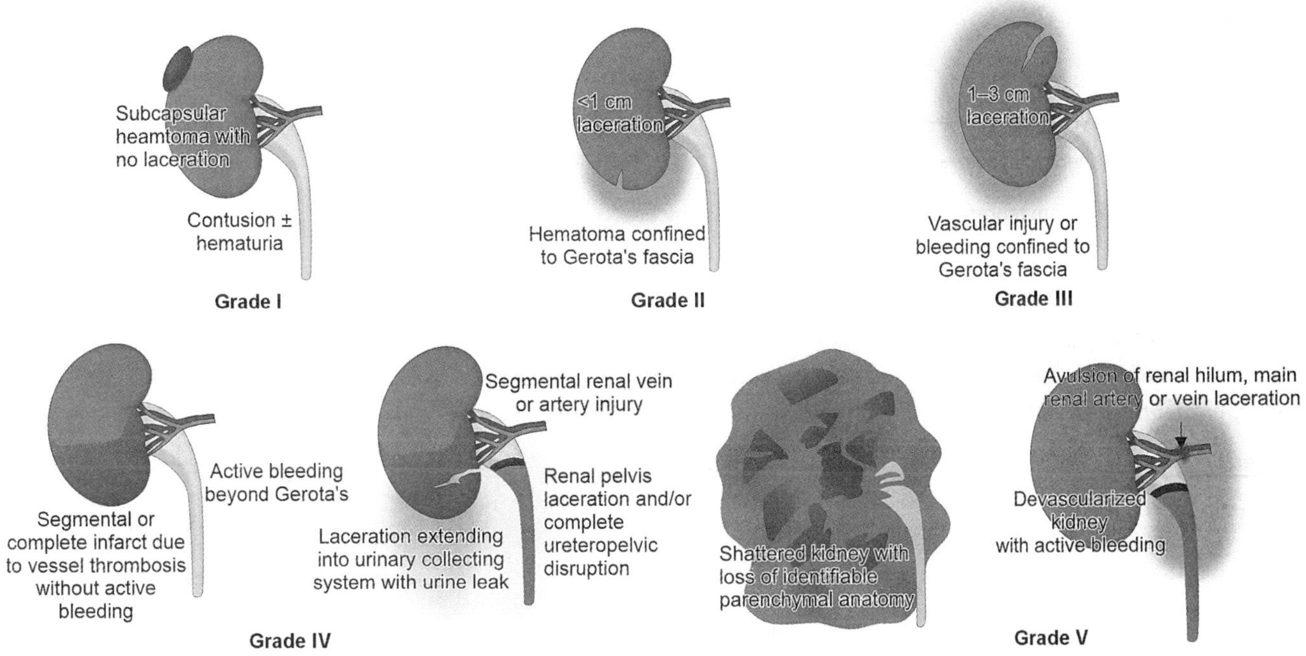

FIG. 15: Revised 2018 AAST–OIS grading system for renal injuries.

According to the revised 2018 AAST–OIS, all renal vascular injuries except thrombosis, are classified as grade V injuries.

Management

- GRADEs I and II—conservative management
- GRADE III—endovascular management in case of active bleeding, pseudoaneurysm and AVM.
- GRADE IV—
  - Segmental vascular injury—low risk (no intervention)
  - Renal pelvis and ureteropelvic junction avulsion-ureteral stenting
  - Perirenal hematoma of size >4 cm and contrast extravasation—arterial embolization
- GRADE V—nephrectomy

Retroperitoneum

1. Discuss the retroperitoneal anatomy with suitable diagram. Discuss the common retroperitoneal tumors and appropriate radiological modalities to evaluate them. [4+3+3] [MD (WBUHS) 23, RG 18, AIIMS May 24]

Introduction

It is the part of the abdomen that lies posterior to the parietal peritoneum and anterior to the transversalis fascia divided by the fascia of Gerota and Zuckerkandl **(Fig. 16)**.

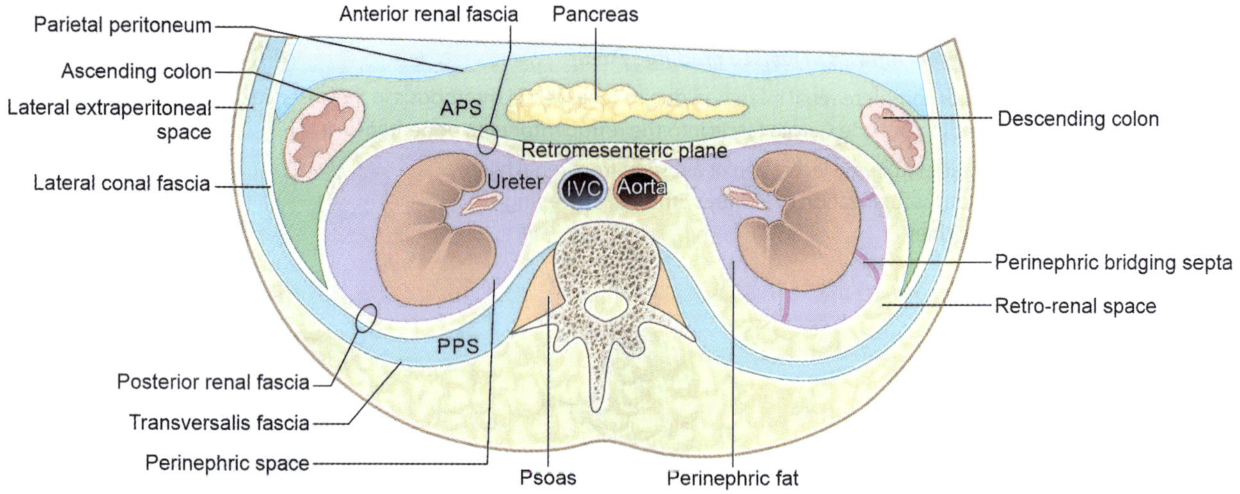

FIG. 16: Schematic diagram representing retroperitoneal anatomy.

Compartments

5 compartments **(Table 18)**

TABLE 18: Retroperitoneal compartments and their contents.

Compartments	*Number*	*Contents*	
Lateral	2	Kidneys on both sides	
Central	1	• Aorta • IVC • Lymphatics	• Located anterior to vertebra • Between the perirenal spaces • Posterior to anterior pararenal space
Posterior	2	Iliopsoas muscles on both sides	Extends from T12 to lesser trochanter, along transversalis fascia

Spaces

3 spaces **(Table 19)**

TABLE 19: Retroperitoneal spaces and their contents.

Spaces	*Contents*	*Relations*
Anterior pararenal space	• Pancreas • D2,3,4 • Ascending and descending colon • Lymph nodes • Fat	• Anteriorly parietal peritoneum • Posteriorly anterior renal fascia (Gerota) • Laterally lateroconal fascia, continuation of Zuckerkandl's fascia
Perirenal space	• Kidney • Adrenal gland • Renal pelvis • Proximal ureter • Renal hilar vessels • Lymph nodes • Fat	• Between anterior and posterior renal fascia • Fluid cannot extend into pelvis from this space
Posterior pararenal space	Fat	Extends from posterior renal fascia to the transversalis fascia, continues anterolaterally as preperitoneal fat

Planes

- These are potentially expansile planes formed by the leaves of fascia **(Table 20)**.
- Visualized in CT only when pathological fluid collections track through them.
- These planes communicate with the pelvis. Hence fluid can be seen tracking through them into the pelvis anterolateral to the psoas muscle.

TABLE 20: Retroperitoneal planes.

Planes	*Between Leaves of*
Retromesenteric plane	Anterior pararenal fascia
Retrorenal plane	Posterior pararenal fascia
Lateroconal plane	Lateroconal fascia

- **Fascia**:
  - Anterior renal fascia - Thinner
  - Posterior renal fascia - Thicker
- **Inferior extension**: Both fasciae meet inferiorly, thus preventing perirenal fluid from going into the pelvis. However, retromesenteric, retrorenal, and lateroconal fascial planes continue downward and extend into the true pelvis. So fluid can track from abdominal retroperitoneum to pelvis anterolateral to psoas muscle.
- **Superior extension**: Both layers fuse with diaphragmatic fascia.

Some common retroperitoneal tumors are:

1. Liposarcoma
2. Undifferentiated pleomorphic sarcoma
3. Leiomyosarcoma
4. Rhabdomyosarcoma
5. Fibrosarcoma
6. Malignant peripheral nerve sheath tumor
7. Extragonadal germ cell tumor
8. Lymphoma
9. Cystadenoma
10. Solitary fibrous tumor
11. Epidermoid cyst

Imaging modalities for evaluation of retroperitoneal masses:

- Abdominal radiograph—obscuration of renal and psoas shadows hints towards the presence of retroperitoneal mass
- Ultrasound—limited visualization of retroperitoneal structures
- Contrast enhanced CT
- Contrast enhanced MRI
- PET CT

Approach to localization of intrabdominal lesions on CECT (Flowchart 11):

- **Beak sign**: Beak like deformation of the edge of the organ
- Phantom organ sign—obscuration of organs by the mass
- Embedded organ sign—part of organ from which the lesion has originated, is embedded in mass with desmoplastic reaction
- Prominent feeding artery sign—the artery feeding the mass originates from the organ of origin
- Floating aorta sign—displacement of the abdominal aorta away from the vertebral column

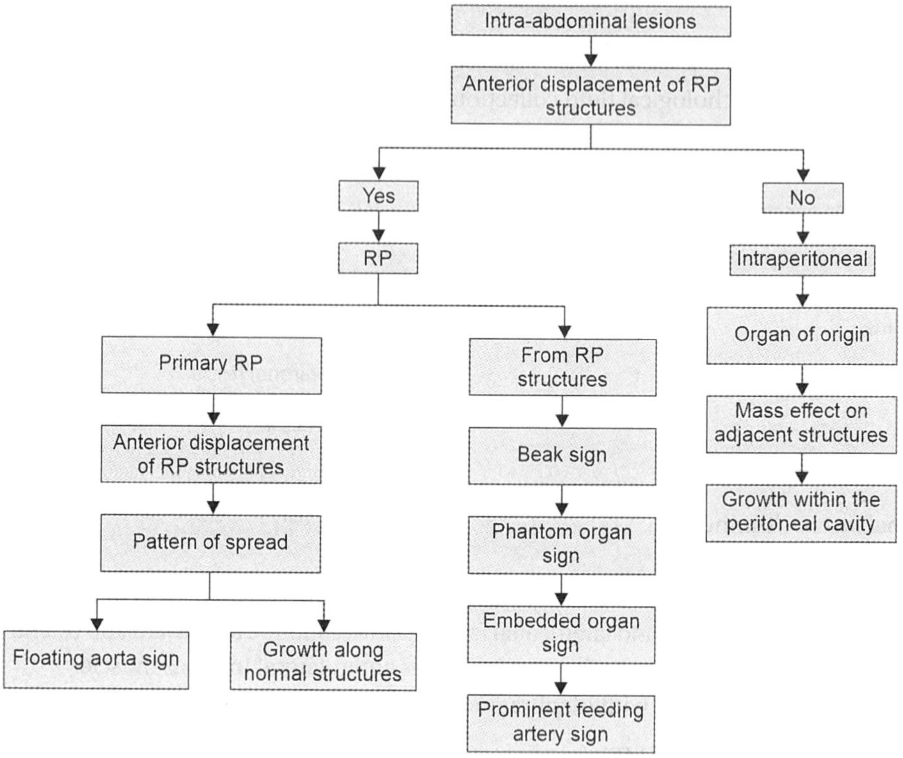

FLOWCHART 11: Approach to localization of intra-abdominal lesions on CECT.

(RP: retroperitoneal)

Diagnostic algorithm of the main retroperitoneal masses in adults is presented as follows is presented in **Flowchart 12** as follows.

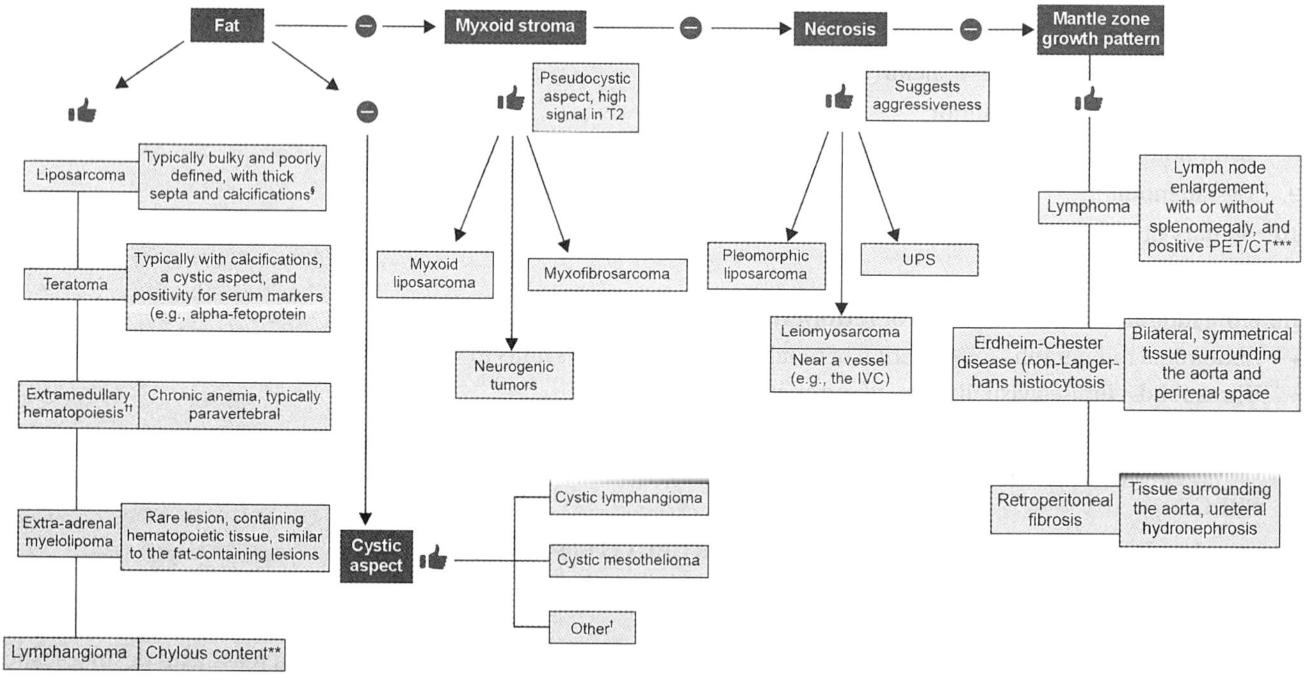

*Most common patterns; **Can result in fat attenuation; *** Strongly positive PET/CT results in some cases; §dedifferentiated liposarcoma (calcification in 30% of cases); †Cystadenoma, cystadeno carcinoma, Müllerian cysts, nonpancreatic pseudocysts, and other cysts; ††Can contain macroscopic fat.

FLOWCHART 12: Diagnostic algorithm of the main retroperitoneal masses in adults.

(UPS: undifferentiated pleomorphic sarcoma; IVC: inferior vena cava)

2. Describe retroperitoneal compartments and their contents in reference to medical imaging. [10] [MD (WBUHS) 20]

Introduction

It is the part of the abdomen that lies posterior to the parietal peritoneum and anterior to the transversalis fascia divided by the fascia of Gerota and Zuckerkandl **(Fig. 16)**.

Compartments

Five compartments **(Table 16)**

Spaces

Three spaces **(Table 17)**

Planes

- These are potentially expansile planes formed by the leaves of fascia **(Table 18)**.
- Visualized in CT only when pathological fluid collections track through them.
- These planes communicate with the pelvis. Hence, fluid can be seen tracking through them into the pelvis anterolateral to the psoas muscle.
- **Fascia**:
  - Anterior renal fascia—thinner
  - Posterior renal fascia—thicker
  - Inferior extension: Both fasciae meet inferiorly, thus preventing perirenal fluid from going into the pelvis.

However, retromesenteric, retrorenal, and lateroconal fascial planes continue downward and extend into the true pelvis.

So fluid can track from abdominal retroperitoneum to pelvis anterolateral to psoas muscle.

Superior extension: Both layers fuse with diaphragmatic fascia.

3. Classify adrenal tumors with their radiological features. [10] [MD (WBUHS) 19]

Classification of Adrenal Tumors (Table 21)

TABLE 21: Classification of adrenal tumors.

Adrenal cortex lesions	• Adenoma (nonfunctioning) • Adenoma (functioning)—cortisol secreting, aldosterone secreting • Hyperplasia (PBMAH—primary bilateral macronodular adrenal hyperplasia) • Adrenocortical carcinoma (secreting or nonsecreting)
Adrenal medulla lesions	• Pheochromocytoma (benign/malignant), Ganglioneuroma • Neuroblastoma, ganglioneuroblastoma
Other stromal lesion	• Hemangioma, angiosarcoma • Myelolipoma—lipoma, teratoma and other mesenchymal lesions
Metastases	More commonly from lung, breast, ovarian, kidney, melanoma, lymphoma, leukemia
Cysts	Endothelial, pseudocyst, epithelial, parasitic, hamartomatous
Adrenal hemorrhage and hematoma	
Infiltrations	Lymphoma, amyloidosis, sarcoidosis
Infections and granulomas	Tuberculosis, histoplasmosis, blastomycosis

Adrenal Adenoma[10]

- Benign tumor of adrenal cortex
- Can be lipid rich and lipid poor

- Can be hyperfunctioning or nonhyperfunctioning
- Can have growth <3 mm/year

Ultrasound

- Well defined, round to oval, homogenous, hypoechoic
- **Color Doppler**: Low vascularity

CT

- **NCCT**: Well defined, round to oval, homogenous
- <3 cm usually
- –2 to 60 HU depending on the amount of fat
- <10 HU high specificity for lipid rich adenoma
- Lipid poor adenoma mimic metastasis on NCCT
- **CECT**: Rapid enhancement and early washout **(Fig. 17)**
  (metastasis also shows rapid enhancement but washout is prolonged)

Contrast washout

$$\text{Absolute contrast washout (APW)} = \frac{\text{Unenhanced CT (HU)} - \text{Delayed CT (HU)}}{\text{Enhanced CT (HU)} - \text{Delayed CT (HU)}} \times 100\%$$

$$\text{Relative contrast washout (RPW)} = \frac{\text{Unenhanced CT (HU)} - \text{Delayed CT (HU)}}{\text{Enhanced CT (HU)}} \times 100\%$$

FIG. 17: Calculation of absolute and relative contrast washout.

APW ≥60%, RPW ≥40%—suggestive of adrenal adenoma.
Dual energy CT: Metastasis and adenoma both can show increased attenuation at 80 kVp but lipid rich adenoma show decrease in attenuation at 140 kVp.

MRI (Fig. 18)

- **T1**: Iso to hypointense
- **T2**: Iso to hypointense
- **Chemical shift imaging**: Signal drop on out of phase image >20%

Adrenal MRI Calculator

$$\text{Adrenal-to-spleen ratio} = \frac{\text{Lesion SI (op)/spleen SI (op)}}{\text{Lesion SI (ip)/spleen SI (ip)}}$$

$$\text{Signal intensity index} = \frac{\text{Lesion SI (ip)/spleen SI (op)}}{\text{Lesion SI (ip)}} \times 100\%$$

FIG. 18: Calculation of signal intensity of adrenal lesion on MRI.

- Adrenal to spleen ratio (ASR) <70%
- Signal intensity index (SI) >5%

Adrenocortical Carcinoma

- Malignancy of the adrenal cortex
- **Can be hyperfunctioning—can present as**:
  - Cushing syndrome
  - Primary hyperaldosteronism
  - Abnormal sexual features

- **Associated with**:
  - Li-Fraumeni syndrome
  - Beckwith-Wiedemann syndrome
  - Familial adenomatous polyposis coli
  - Multiple endocrine neoplasia syndrome (MEN) I
  - Carney's complex
  - Congenital adrenal hyperplasia

Ultrasound

- Large >6 cm, heterogenous mass having necrosis, hemorrhage, cysts and calcifications
- **Color Doppler**: Hypervascular, early enhancement

CT

- NCCT—>43 HU without calcification or hemorrhage—suspicious of malignancy.
- CECT—heterogenous mass with peripheral enhancement.
- <4 cm mass—homogenous, mimics adenoma
- However, APW<60% and RPW <40%
- Presence of calcification indicates adrenocortical carcinoma.
- Invasion of kidney, liver, lymph nodes
- Vascular invasion common

MRI

- **T1**: Hypointense, hyperintense foci indicates hemorrhage.
- **T2**: Hyperintense
- **Chemical shift imaging**: Drop of signal on out of phase images indicating microscopic fat.
- **Post-contrast**: Heterogenous enhancement, delayed washout.

PET CT

Detection of recurrence on follow up.

Pheochromocytoma

- Neural crest cell tumor arising from chromaffin cells of adrenal medulla.
- **10% rule**:
  - Bilateral
  - Extra-adrenal
  - Malignant
  - Children
  - Calcification
  - No hypertension
  - Familial (30%)
- **Associated with**:
  - Von Hippel-Lindau syndrome (VHL)
  - Multiple endocrine neoplasia syndrome (MEN) II
  - familial adenomatous polyposis coli
  - Carney's triad (pheochromocytoma, pulmonary chondroma, gastric GIST)
  - Familial paraganglioma syndrome
  - Neurofibromatosis
  - Sturge weber syndrome
  - Tuberous sclerosis

Ultrasound

- Well defined, large and heterogenous
- Can have calcification
- **Color Doppler**: Hypervascular mass
- **CEUS**: Arterial enhancement

CT

- **Small**: Homogenous
- **Large**: Heterogenous with hemorrhage, necrosis, cystic change.
- **CECT**: Avid enhancement, HU >110 in arterial phase.
- Rapid washout similar to adenoma

MRI

- **T1**: Hypointense
- **T2**: Very hyperintense—**light bulb sign** on T2
- **Chemical shift imaging**: No drop of signal on out of phase images
- **DWI**: Diffusion restriction in malignant pheochromocytoma

MIBG Scan

- When there is biochemical suspicion but routine imaging is inconclusive—to look for extra-adrenal paraganglioma.
- Familial cases

Gallium 68 DOTANOC PET-CT:

- Higher accuracy
- Superior to MIBG scan
- Greater lesion to background tissue contrast.

Adrenal Myelolipoma

- Solitary, <5 cm usually
- Asymptomatic
- Large (>10 cm) lesions cause symptoms
- Can bleed when size >14 cm
- Lesion containing macroscopic fat and hematopoietic tissue.
- Calcification, necrosis, hemorrhage and areas of fibromyxoid degeneration.

CT

- Entirely fatty or solid soft tissue mass containing small areas of fat.
- **Fat attenuation**: –10 to –20 HU
- Capsulated
- May have calcification
- Hemorrhage—high attenuation fluid
- Myeloid component enhances

MRI

- T1 and T2 hyperintense due to fat
- **Hematopoietic marrow**: T1-hypointense, T2-intermediate
- Suppression on T2FS suggests macroscopic fat
- **Chemical shift imaging**: Drop of signal on out of phase images.

D/D

- Retroperitoneal sarcoma
- Exophytic renal angiomyolipoma

Adrenal Cyst

- Rare
- Asymptomatic, incidentally detected
- Unilateral
- F>M
- **Secondary to**:
    - Endothelial or epithelial proliferation
    - Hemorrhage
    - Pseudocyst
    - Parasitic disease (hydatid disease)
    - No enhancement

Radiograph

Laminated, porcelain, such as calcification in case of hydatid cyst.

Ultrasound

- Epithelial cyst—well defined, anechoic, imperceptible wall.
- Hydatid cyst—thick walled, anechoic or having echogenic contents.

CT

- Homogeneous water density lesion
- Non enhancing
- Septations and hyperdense content when infected or associated hemorrhage.
- Wall calcifications may be present.

MRI

- Epithelial cyst—high signal intensity on T2
- **Hydatid cyst**:
    - Cyst within cyst appearance
    - Low intensity pericyst
    - Rim calcification

Metastasis

- Most common malignant adrenal lesion
- Typically bilateral
- Rich blood supply of adrenal gland predisposes to metastasis.
- Metastasis from lung, breast, renal, esophagus, colon, melanoma malignancies.
- No specific imaging features

Ultrasound

Preferred for children

CT

Modality of choice for adults

- Focal soft tissue lesion replacing the gland or diffuse enlargement of the gland.
- **Small**: Homogenous

- **Large**: Heterogenous with calcification, hemorrhage, necrosis
- >10 HU on NCCT
- Enhancement in portovenous phase with delayed washout.
- APW <60% and RPW <40%
- Metastasis from renal cell carcinoma and hepatocellular carcinoma can have fat—early washout in venous phase.
- NCCT—>43 HU without calcification or hemorrhage—suspicious of malignancy.

MRI

- **T1**: Hypointense, hyperintense when metastasis from melanoma
- **T2**: Hyperintense
- **DWI**: No role
- **Chemical shift imaging**: No drop on out of phase images

PET CT

Intense FDG uptake indicating hypermetabolism

Collision Tumor

- Presence of two histologically distinct tumors concurrently in the same adrenal gland.
- Most commonly a metastasis and an adrenal adenoma is present as collision tumor.
- Correlation with previous imaging required.
- Heterogenous signal intensity and rapid enhancement and delayed washout pattern in metastasis.

4. Discuss in brief the imaging modalities in the diagnosis of adrenal lesion. [10] [MD (WBUHS) 22, RG 18]

Imaging Modalities for Adrenal Lesions

- Ultrasound
- Contrast enhanced CT
- Magnetic resonance imaging
- Dual energy CT
- **Nuclear imaging**: MIBG and PET CT

Ultrasound

- Useful only in pediatric patients
- No risk of radiation
- Adrenals can be visualized as Y-shaped structure—a body and two limbs located ventromedially superior to the kidneys.
- Congenital adrenal hyperplasia and adrenal hemorrhage can be ruled out.
- In adults, it is difficult to visualize.
- If there is no adrenal mass seen on ultrasound in an adult patient with/without the visualization of adrenals, the presence of it can be ruled out. **(high negative predictive value)**
- Contrast enhanced ultrasound using microbubbles filled with sulfur hexafluoride—reduction on radiation exposure, safe in patients with renal failure.
- Rapid enhancement and delayed washout in case of malignancies.

CT Scan Adrenal Protocol

- Consent
- Patient in supine position

- Noncontrast scan
- Venous phase—60–70 sec
- Delayed phase—15 minutes
- **Contrast washout calculated (Fig. 19)**:
  - Absolute contrast washout (APW)
  - Relative contrast washout (RPW)

Contrast washout

$$\text{Absolute contrast washout (APW)} = \frac{\text{Unenhanced CT (HU)} - \text{Delayed CT (HU)}}{\text{Enhanced CT (HU)} - \text{Delayed CT (HU)}} \times 100\%$$

$$\text{Relative contrast washout (RPW)} = \frac{\text{Unenhanced CT (HU)} - \text{Delayed CT (HU)}}{\text{Enhanced CT (HU)}} \times 100\%$$

FIG. 19: Calculation of absolute and relative contrast washout.

ROI should occupy 2/3rd of the lesion and away from the edges to prevent volume averaging.

Exclude areas of necrosis calcifications.

APW ≥60%, RPW ≥40%—suggestive of adrenal adenoma.

- Rapid contrast enhancement in adenomas and malignancies.
- Rapid washout in adenoma but delayed washout in malignancies.

MRI (Tables 22 and 23 and Fig. 18)

TABLE 22: MR sequences for adrenal lesion.

MRI protocol	
Chemical shift	Detection of intracellular fat in adenomas
Fat-suppression	Detection macroscopic fat
T2W	Cysts—cystic components Light bulb in pheochromocytomas
Gd-enhanced	Washout enhancement
DWI	No value

- Most important sequence is **Chemical Shift Imaging.**
- Useful when CT is contraindicated or washout values are equivocal.

TABLE 23: Characterization of fat containing lesion on MRI.

Fat content	***Sequence***	***Finding***	***example***
Microscopic fat	Chemical shift imaging	Drop in signal	Adenoma
Macroscopic fat	Fat suppressed	Drop in signal	Myelolipoma

Physics behind:

- The hydrogen ions in fat voxel and water voxel behave differently.
- The hydrogen ions show lower precession frequency in fat voxel in an external magnetic field.
- In T1 GRE images, the signal of the hydrogen ions add up in in-phase images but get cancelled out in out of phase images, in the lesions which have both fat and water content as in adenoma.
- Less sensitive when HU >20 on unenhanced CT.

Adenoma

- **Chemical shift imaging**: Signal drop on out of phase image >20%
- Adrenal to spleen ratio (ASR) <70%
- Signal intensity index (SI) >5%

Dual Energy CT

- **Virtual non-contrast (VNC) images**: VNC images can be derived from contrast enhanced dual energy CT limiting radiation dose.
- **Material decomposition:** By applying voltage at 2 kVp, fat, calcium, water and iodine images are adequately derived by post-processing techniques. Hence, composition of the adrenal mass can be evaluated.

Nuclear medicine:

- **MIBG scan**:
  - Metaiodobenzylguanidine (MIBG) analogue of **nor epinephrine**.
  - Used for detecting lesions of **adrenal medulla.**
  - Detection of any extra-adrenal paraganglioma and metastasis of malignant pheochromocytoma.
- **PET CT (Positron emission tomography)**:
  - 18-fluorodeoxyglucose is injected intravenously after proper preparation of the patient.
  - Areas of high metabolic activity is identified.
  - High negative predictive value.
  - Absence of metabolic activity in a region rules out malignancy or metastasis.

The American College of Radiology algorithm for management of incidental adrenal lesions is shown in **Flowchart 13**.

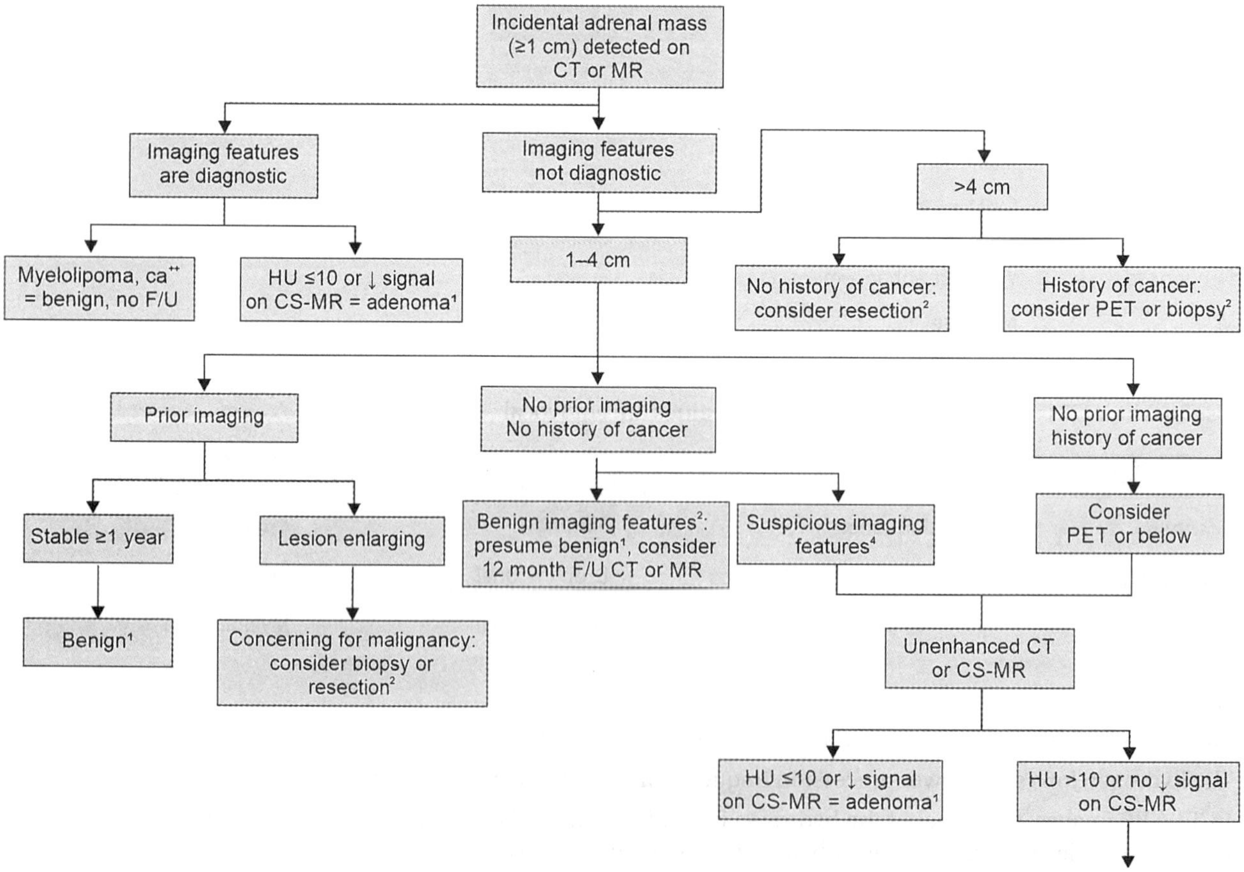

FLOWCHART 13: *Continued...*

Continued...

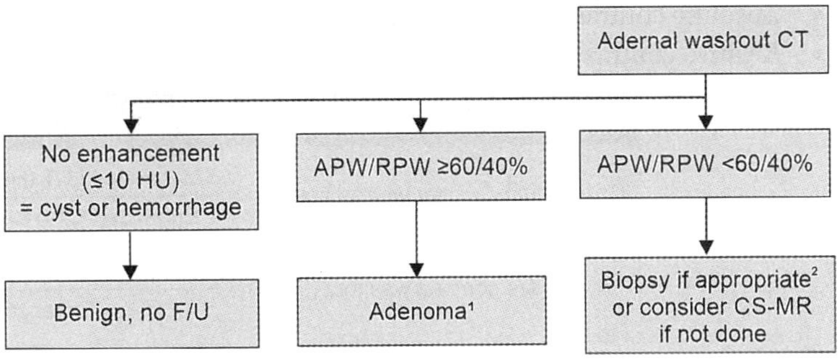

FLOWCHART 13: American College of Radiology—algorithm for management of incidental adrenal lesions.

[1]If patient has clinical signs or symptoms of adenal hyperfunction, consider biochemical evaluation

[2]Consider biochemical testing to exclude pheochromocytoma

[3]Benign imaging features homogeneous, low density, smooth margins

[4]Suspicious imaging feature heterogeneous, necrosis, iregular margins

APW: absolute percentage washout; RPW: relative percentage washout; CS-MR: chemical shift MRI; F/U: follow-up; H/U: hounsfield unit; ↓: decreased

5. Enumerate the imaging modalities used for adrenal lesions. Describe in brief the CT scan protocol and systematic approach to evaluate adrenal lesions. [2+(3+5)] [MD (WBUHS) 24, MD (WBUHS) 18]

Imaging Modalities for Adrenal Lesions

- Ultrasound
- Contrast enhanced CT
- Magnetic resonance imaging
- Dual energy CT
- **Nuclear imaging**: MIBG and PET CT

Ultrasound

- Useful only in pediatric patients
- No risk of radiation
- Adrenals can be visualized as Y-shaped structure—a body and two limbs located ventromedially superior to the kidneys.
- Congenital adrenal hyperplasia and adrenal hemorrhage can be ruled out.
- In adults, it is difficult to visualize.
- If there is no adrenal mass seen on ultrasound in an adult patient with/without the visualization of adrenals, the presence of it can be ruled out. **(high negative predictive value)**
- Contrast enhanced ultrasound using microbubbles filled with sulfur hexafluoride—reduction on radiation exposure, safe in patients with renal failure.
- Rapid enhancement and delayed washout in case of malignancies.

CT Scan Adrenal Protocol

- Consent
- Patient in supine position
- Noncontrast scan
- Venous phase—60–70 sec
- Delayed phase—15 minutes

- **Contrast washout calculated (Fig. 20):**
  - Absolute contrast washout (APW)
  - Relative contrast washout (RPW)

Contrast washout
$$\text{Absolute contrast washout (APW)} = \frac{\text{Unenhanced CT (HU)} - \text{Delayed CT (HU)}}{\text{Enhanced CT (HU)} - \text{Delayed CT (HU)}} \times 100\%$$
$$\text{Relative contrast washout (RPW)} = \frac{\text{Unenhanced CT (HU)} - \text{Delayed CT (HU)}}{\text{Enhanced CT (HU)}} \times 100\%$$

FIG. 20: Calculation of absolute and relative contrast washout.

ROI should occupy 2/3rd of the lesion and away from the edges to prevent volume averaging.
Exclude areas of necrosis calcifications.
APW ≥60%, RPW ≥40%—suggestive of adrenal adenoma.

- Rapid contrast enhancement in adenomas and malignancies.
- Rapid washout in adenoma but delayed washout in malignancies.

MRI (Tables 22 and 23 and Fig. 21)

- Most important sequence is **Chemical Shift Imaging.**
- Useful when CT is contraindicated or washout values are equivocal.

Physics behind:

- The hydrogen ions in fat voxel and water voxel behave differently.
- The hydrogen ions show lower precession frequency in fat voxel in an external magnetic field.
- In T1 GRE images, the signal of the hydrogen ions add up in in-phase images but get cancelled out in out of phase images, in the lesions which have both fat and water content as in adenoma.
- Less sensitive when HU >20 on unenhanced CT.

Adrenal MRI Calculator
$$\text{Adrenal-to-spleen ratio} = \frac{\text{Lesion SI (op)/spleen SI (op)}}{\text{Lesion SI (ip)/spleen SI (ip)}}$$
$$\text{Signal intensity index} = \frac{\text{Lesion SI (ip)/spleen SI (op)}}{\text{Lesion SI (ip)}} \times 100\%$$

FIG. 21: Calculation of signal intensity of adrenal lesion on MRI.

Adenoma

- **Chemical shift imaging**: Signal drop on out of phase image >20%
- Adrenal to spleen ratio (ASR) <70%
- Signal intensity index (SI) >5%

Dual energy CT

- **Virtual non-contrast (VNC) images**: VNC images can be derived from contrast enhanced dual energy CT limiting radiation dose.
- **Material decomposition**: By applying voltage at 2 kVp, fat, calcium, water and iodine images are adequately derived by post-processing techniques. Hence, composition of the adrenal mass can be evaluated.

Nuclear medicine:

- **MIBG scan:**
  - Metaiodobenzylguanidine (MIBG) analogue of **norepinephrine**.
  - Used for detecting lesions of **adrenal medulla**.
  - Detection of any extra-adrenal paraganglioma and metastasis of malignant pheochromocytoma.

- **PET CT (Positron emission tomography)**:
  - 18-Fluorodeoxyglucose is injected intravenously after proper preparation of the patient.
  - Areas of high metabolic activity is identified.
  - High negative predictive value.
  - Absence of metabolic activity in a region rules out malignancy or metastasis.

The American College of Radiology algorithm for management of incidental adrenal lesions is presented in **Flowchart 13**.

6. (a) Radiological anatomy of retroperitoneum. (b) Cross-sectional imaging in retroperitoneal liposarcoma. [10] [DNB June 21]

Introduction

It is the part of the abdomen that lies posterior to the parietal peritoneum and anterior to the transversalis fascia divided by the fascia of Gerota and Zuckerkandl **(Fig. 16)**.

Compartments

Five compartments **(Table 18)**

Spaces

Three spaces **(Table 19)**

Planes

- These are potentially expansile planes formed by the leaves of fascia **(Table 20)**.
- Visualized in CT only when pathological fluid collections track through them.
- These planes communicate with the pelvis. Hence, fluid can be seen tracking through them into the pelvis anterolateral to the psoas muscle.
- **Fascia**:
  - Anterior renal fascia—thinner
  - Posterior renal fascia—thicker
- **Inferior extension**: Both fasciae meet inferiorly, thus preventing perirenal fluid from going into the pelvis.
  However, retromesenteric, retrorenal, and lateroconal fascial planes continue downward and extend into the true pelvis.
  So fluid can track from abdominal retroperitoneum to pelvis anterolateral to psoas muscle.
- **Superior extension**: Both layers fuse with diaphragmatic fascia.

Cross-sectional Imaging in Liposarcoma

Introduction

- Most common primary retroperitoneal malignancy.
- Slow growing tumor of adipose tissue.
- Can arise de novo or from preexisting lipoma.
- Large size at detection
- Can recur

Epidemiology

Male > Female

Types of Liposarcoma

Based on histologic, genetics and biological behavior:

1. Well differentiated—most common, does not metastasis, can dedifferentiate.
2. Dedifferentiated—can metastasis

3. Pleomorphic
4. Myxoid

Imaging Features

Contrast enhanced CT:

- Heterogeneously/homogenously enhancing mass lesion with soft tissue and fat component having septations +/- calcifications
- Can be solid, mixed or pseudocystic
- Usually no prominent vessels.
- Mild or no enhancement.
- Displacement and compression of the adjacent structures, such as kidneys, bowel and bladder.
- Features of invasion may/may not be present.
- Presence of calcification is suggestive of dedifferentiation and poor prognosis.
- Morphologically suspicious lymph nodes—round, heterogenous, enlarged.
- Metastasis occurs to lung and liver—nodules should be sought for.

Magnetic Resonance Imaging

- Useful in iodinated contrast allergy patients.
- Areas of fat, necrosis, hemorrhage as well as solid, cystic and myxoid component can be well characterized.
- Myxoid component is hyperintense on T2, variable signal intensity on T1 and low signal intensity on CT.
- Fat suppressed sequences help delineate amount of fat.
- Similar imaging features as in CT.

FDG–PET

Avid areas indicates high-grade component.

Image-guided Biopsy

- Tumor approached from retroperitoneum.
- 18G needle used.
- 5-6 cores of sample taken from multiple sites.

Differential Diagnosis

- Renal angiomyolipoma
- Adrenal myelolipoma

7. (a) Imaging evaluation of a patient with Cushing's syndrome. (b) Role of imaging in differentiating adrenal adenoma from adrenal metastasis. [5+5] [DNB Dec 20]

Introduction

Cushing's syndrome occurs as a result of excess cortisol (endogenous/exogenous).

Most common cause: Exogenous-steroid administration.

Algorithmic approach for diagnosis and management of Cushing's syndrome is shown in **Flowchart 14.**[11]

Adrenal pathologies that can cause Cushing's syndrome:

- Adrenal adenoma
- Adrenocortical carcinoma

Adrenal Adenoma

- Benign tumor of adrenal cortex

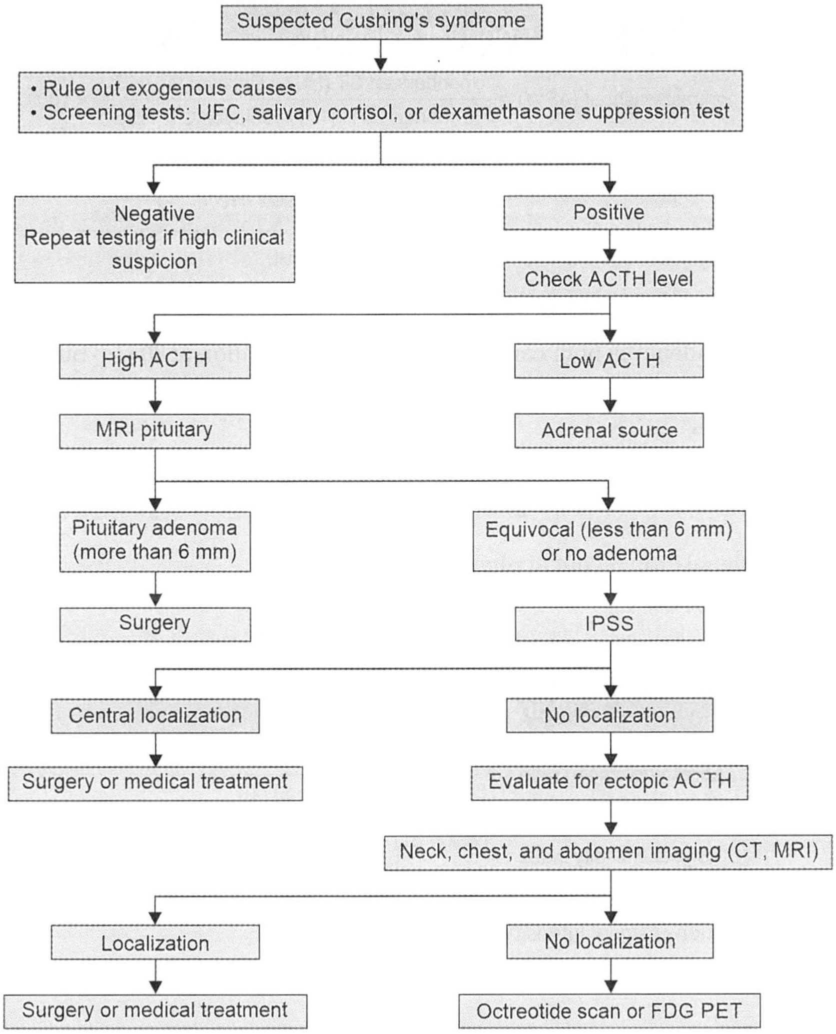

FLOWCHART 14: Algorithm for diagnosis and management of Cushing's syndrome.
(ACTH: adrenocorticotropic hormone; IPSS: inferior petrosal sinus sampling; UFC: urinary free cortisol)

- Can be lipid rich and lipid poor
- Can be hyperfunctioning or nonhyperfunctioning
- Can have growth <3 mm/year

Ultrasound

- Well defined, round to oval, homogenous, hypoechoic.
- **Color Doppler**: Low vascularity.

CT

- **NCCT**: Well defined, round to oval, homogenous.
- <3 cm usually
- –2 to 60 HU depending on the amount of fat
- <10 HU high specificity for lipid rich adenoma
- Lipid poor adenoma mimic metastasis on NCCT
- **CECT**: Rapid enhancement and early washout **(Fig. 22)**

(metastasis also shows rapid enhancement but washout is prolonged)

Contrast washout
Absolute contrast washout (APW) = $\frac{\text{Unenhanced CT (HU)} - \text{Delayed CT (HU)}}{\text{Enhanced CT (HU)} - \text{Delayed CT (HU)}} \times 100\%$
Relative contrast washout (RPW) = $\frac{\text{Unenhanced CT (HU)} - \text{Delayed CT (HU)}}{\text{Enhanced CT (HU)}} \times 100\%$

FIG. 22: Calculation of absolute and relative contrast washout.

APW ≥60%, RPW ≥40%—suggestive of adrenal adenoma.

Dual energy CT: Metastasis and adenoma both can show increased attenuation at 80 kVp but lipid rich adenoma show decrease in attenuation at 140 kVp.

MRI (Fig. 23)

- **T1**: Iso to hypointense
- **T2**: Iso to hypointense
- **Chemical shift imaging**: Signal drop on out of phase image >20%
- Adrenal to spleen ratio (ASR) <70%
- Signal intensity index (SI) >5%

Adrenal MRI Calculator
Adrenal-to-spleen ratio = $\frac{\text{Lesion SI (op)/spleen SI (op)}}{\text{Lesion SI (ip)/spleen SI (ip)}}$
Signal intensity index = $\frac{\text{Lesion SI (ip)/spleen SI (op)}}{\text{Lesion SI (ip)}} \times 100\%$

FIG. 23: Calculation of signal intensity of adrenal lesion on MRI.

Adrenocortical Carcinoma

- Malignancy of the adrenal cortex
- **Can be hyperfunctioning—can present as**:
  - Cushing syndrome
  - Primary hyperaldosteronism
  - Abnormal sexual features
- **Associated with**:
  - Li-Fraumeni syndrome
  - Beckwith-Wiedemann syndrome
  - familial adenomatous polyposis coli
  - Multiple endocrine neoplasia syndrome (MEN) I
  - Carney's complex
  - Congenital adrenal hyperplasia

Ultrasound

- Large >6 cm, heterogenous mass having necrosis, hemorrhage, cysts and calcifications.
- **Color Doppler**: Hypervascular, early enhancement

CT

- NCCT—>43 HU without calcification or hemorrhage—suspicious of malignancy
- CECT—heterogenous mass with peripheral enhancement

- <4 cm mass—homogenous, mimics adenoma
- However, APW<60% and RPW <40%
- Presence of calcification indicates adrenocortical carcinoma
- Invasion of kidney, liver, lymph nodes
- Vascular invasion common

MRI

- T1—hypointense, hyperintense foci indicates hemorrhage.
- T2—hyperintense
- Chemical shift imaging—drop of signal on out of phase images indicating microscopic fat.
- Post-contrast—heterogenous enhancement, delayed washout.

PET CT

Detection of recurrence on follow up.

Differentiating features between adrenal adenoma and adrenal metastasis on imaging (**Table 24**).

TABLE 24: Differentiating features between adrenal adenoma and adrenal metastasis on imaging.

Features	***Adenoma***	***Metastasis***
Vascularity	Hypovascular	Hypervascular
Washout pattern on CECT	Rapid washout	Delayed washout
Chemical shift imaging	Drop of signal on out of phase imaging suggesting microscopic fat	No drop of signal
Laterality	Usually unilateral	Usually bilateral
PET CT	No uptake	Avid uptake of 18-FDG

- Absolute washout of >60% and relative washout of >40 % suggests adenoma.
- HCC and renal metastasis can have fat within them. So, they can show rapid washout making differentiation from adenoma difficult.
- >43 HU on NECT without calcification or hemorrhage—suspicious of malignancy
- Collision tumor—presence of histologically different tumors adjacent to each other in the same gland.
- Metastasis and adenoma can be present concurrently in the same gland.
- Differentiated based on washout pattern and correlation with previous films.

Interventions

1. Discuss the indications and procedure of percutaneous nephrostomy. [3+7] [MD (WBUHS) 23, MD (WBUHS) 17]

The indications of percutaneous nephrostomy shown in **Table 25**.

TABLE 25: Indications of percutaneous nephrostomy.

Indication	***Specific causes***
To relieve obstruction	Urolithiasis, ureteric stricture, malignancy, external compression by various pathologies, retroperitoneal fibrosis
To drain an infected calyceal system	Pyonephrosis
Diversion of urine	Ureteric injury, urine leak, urinary fistula, hemorrhagic cystitis
Access for percutaneous interventions	Ureteric stenting, ureteric balloon dilation percutaneous nephrolithotomy, delivery of chemotherapeutic agents or antifungal drugs

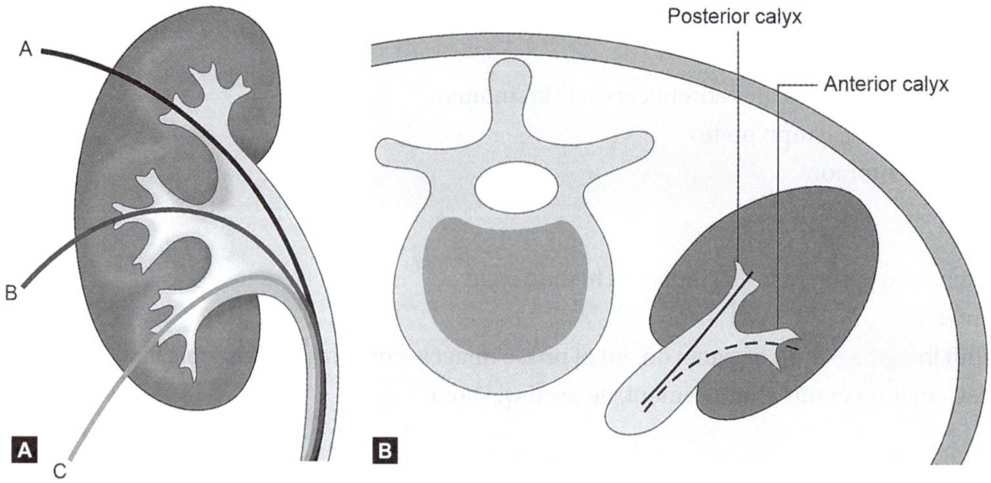

FIGS. 24A and B: Selection of calyx for puncture.

Contraindications: No absolute contraindications

Relative contraindications:

A. Uncorrectable coagulopathy
B. Severe respiratory disorders
C. Uncooperative patients
D. Terminal patients

Preprocedural evaluation: Coagulation parameters to be checked according to the SIR guidelines as nephrostomy is a procedure with significant bleeding risk.

A. INR should be less than 1.5.
B. Platelet should be more than 50,000.
C. APTT should not be more than 1.5 times.

Patient preparation: Antibiotic prophylaxis must be started 1 hour before the procedure.

Procedure:
Patient position:

- Prone position with pillow in the belly to lift it up.
- Right or left lateral decubitus.

Selection of plane: Plane of Brodel **(Figs. 24 and 25)**

Anesthesia: Local infiltration of 5–10 mL of 2% lignocaine given up to the renal capsule.

Steps (Figs. 26A to F):

- Under ultrasound guidance, minor calyx punctured with 18 G (Vygon) needle.
- Tip confirmation done.
- Trocar removed to look for urine flow.
- Sample of urine taken for routine testing and culture and sensitivity testing.
- Diluted iodinated contrast given to opacify pelvicalyceal system.

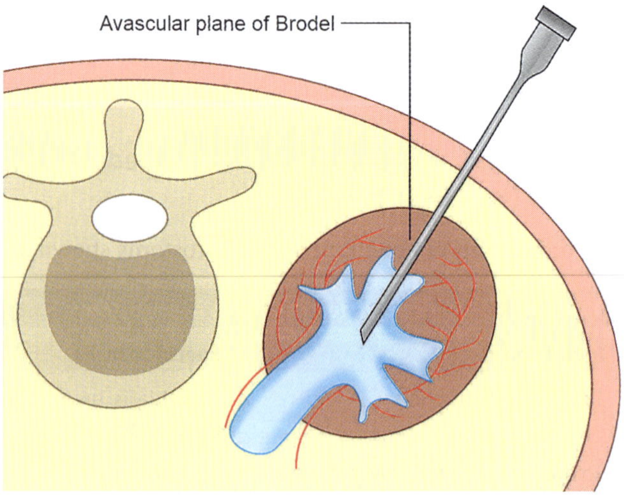

FIG. 25: Avascular plane of Brodel.

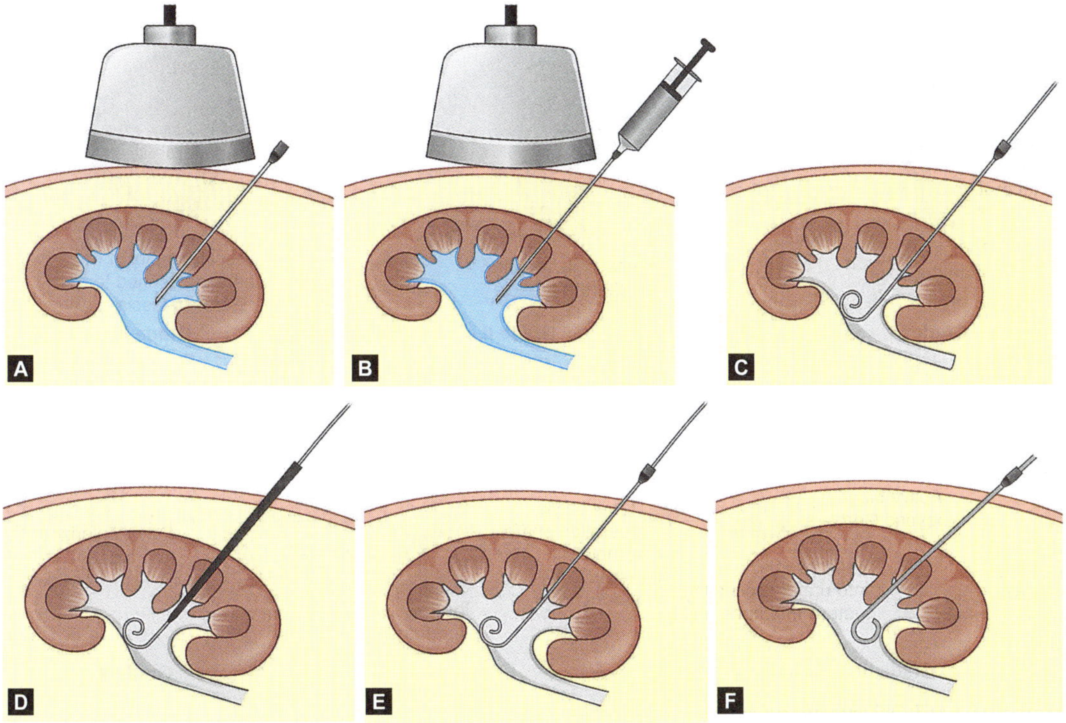

FIGS. 26A to F: Steps of percutaneous nephrostomy.

Under fluoroscopic guidance:

- 0.035 inch guidewire (Amplatz Stiff guidewire) is introduced till ureter.
- 0.035 inch hydrophilic guidewire can also be introduced. If used, it is exchanged by stiff guidewire later.
- In difficult cases, 5 Fr Cobra or Picard catheter is introduced for negotiation of the guidewire.
- Serial dilatation of the tract is done by fascial dilator till the size of the catheter to be introduced.
- 8Fr pigtail catheter is placed over the guidewire and kept in renal pelvis.

Complications:

1. Hemorrhage:
   - Arterial bleed: CT angiogram performed, culprit artery identified, embolization done under fluoroscopy.
   - Venous bleed: Managed conservatively
2. Sepsis: Overdistension of calyces by contrast and excessive manipulation of the guidewire is prevented.

2. Classify renal injuries, imaging features and intervention in them. [3+4+3] [MD (WBUHS) 21]

The revised 2018 AAST-OIS grading system for renal injuries is presented as follows in **Table 17 and Fig. 27**.

According to the revised 2018 AAST-OIS, all renal vascular injuries except thrombosis, are classified as grade V injuries.

Role of Intervention

- Nephrectomy reserved for shattered kidney or vascular pedicle avulsion.
- Endovascular injuries, such as active bleeding, pseudoaneurysm or arteriovenous fistula managed by interventions **(Table 26)**.[12]
- As selectively done as possible.
- Proximal renal artery embolization done in diffuse renal injury with little renal parenchyma left.

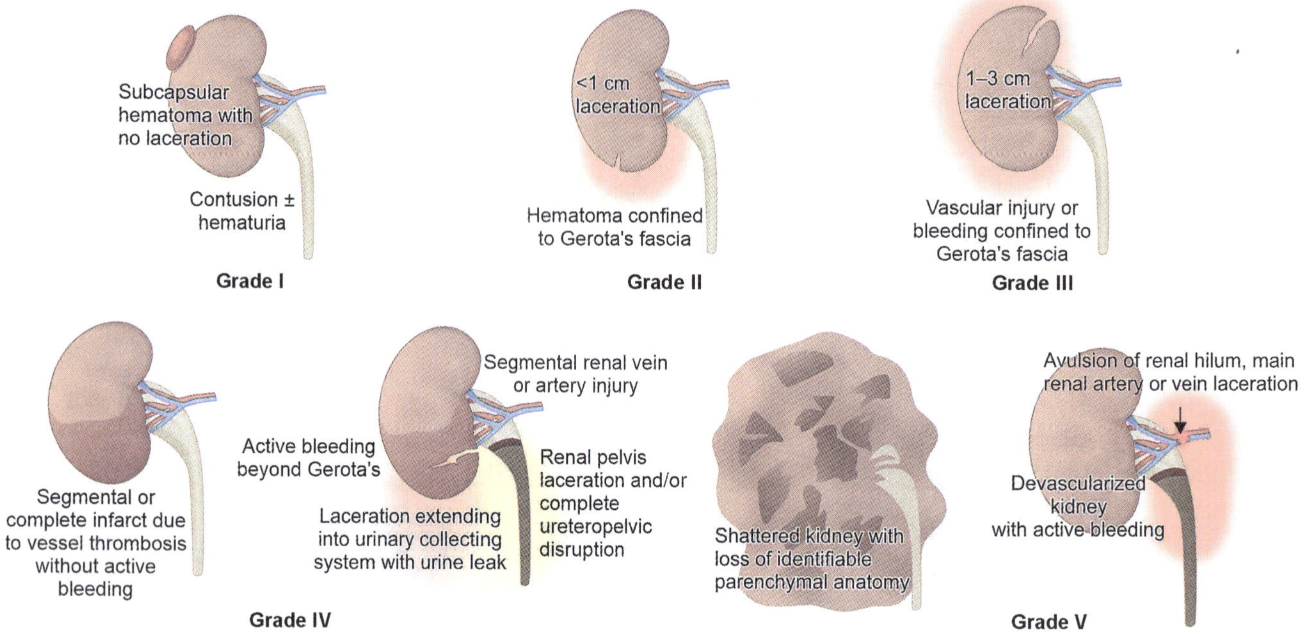

FIG. 27: Revised 2018 AAST-OIS grading system for renal injuries.

TABLE 26: Endovascular interventions in renal artery injury.

Vascular injury ***Site and type of injury***	***Endovascular management***	***Comments***
Main renal artery-dissection, laceration, contrast extravasation	Stent graft	Preserves flow across the site of injury if negotiated safely and successfully
Main renal artery occlusion	Intra-arterial thrombolysis using urokinase or tissue plasminogen activator	Salvages kidney if administered within 6 h of injury
Intrarenal hemorrhage or pseudoaneurysm	Superselective embolization via microcatheter system and microcoils	Targeted embolization: Preserves functioning renal parenchyma
Arteriovenous or arteriocalyceal fistula	Embolization just proximal to fistulous site	Targeted embolization: Preserves functioning renal parenchyma

The recommended protocol for managing nonvascular injuries is presented as follows in **Flowchart 15**.

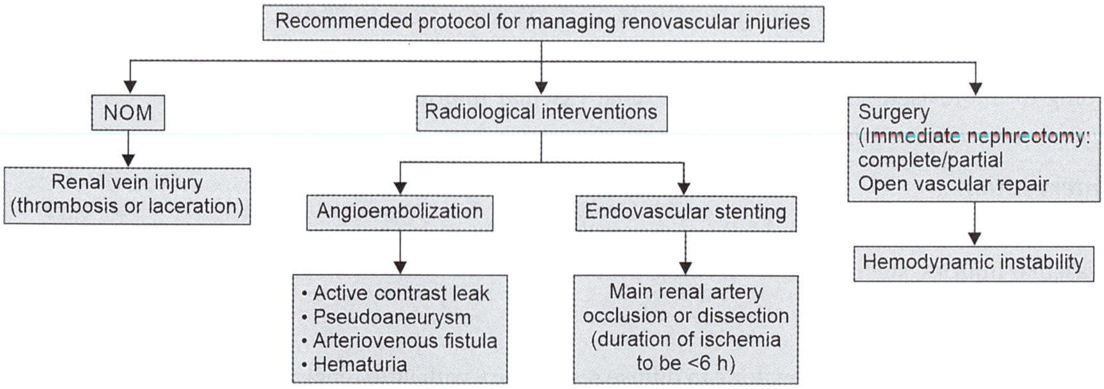

FLOWCHART 15: Recommended protocol for managing non-vascular injuries.

Renal Artery Embolization: *Complication*

- Extremely well tolerated procedure.
- **Complications include**:
    - Renal infarction
    - Renal abscess
    - Hypertension
- Nevertheless, renal function is largely preserved.

Stent Graft

- Renal ischemia is the most critical determinant of the technical success of the endovascular stenting.
- Total duration of ischemia should be <3 hrs in complete and <6 hrs in incomplete arterial occlusion.
- To prevent stent occlusion, anticoagulation should be administered immediately after stent placement.

3. What are the indications of embolization in genitourinary tract? Describe the technique of renal artery angioplasty and stenting. [5+5] [MD (WBUHS) 22]

Indications

Embolization in renal pathologies:

- **Renal tumors**:
    - Angiomyolipoma
    - Renal cell carcinoma—preoperative embolization/palliative therapy
- Nonfunctional kidney/nephrotic syndrome—uncontrollable proteinuria
- End stage PCKD—global embolization
- Renal aneurysms
    - Asymptomatic: >2.0 cm
    - Increase in size
    - Symptomatic: Pain, hypertension, hemorrhage
- Pseudoaneurysm—all are treated regardless of symptoms and size
- Renal AVM—congenital or acquired
- **Renal trauma**:
    - Hemodynamic instability despite resuscitation
    - Grade ≥4 AAST renal injury
    - Fractured kidney
    - Active contrast extravasation

Uterine artery embolization:

- Symptomatic fibroids
- Adenomyosis
- Arteriovenous malformation

Prostatic artery embolization: Benign prostatic hyperplasia

Renal Artery Angioplasty

Introduction

Renal artery angioplasty and stenting is a minimally invasive procedure used to treat renal artery stenosis (narrowing of the renal arteries). The primary goal is to restore adequate blood flow to the kidneys, which can help control hypertension and prevent kidney damage.[13]

Indications of Angioplasty

- Resistant hypertension
- Preserved renal function
- To prevent flash pulmonary edema (CCB related)
- To preserve patency of renal artery

Indications for Stenting

- Failure of angioplasty
- Ostial atherosclerosis
- Repeat angioplasty cannot be done

Criteria of Successful Angioplasty

- Residual stenosis after angioplasty $<30\%$
- $\geq 50\%$ increase in diameter
- Pressure gradient—<20 mm Hg
- ≥ 15 mm Hg decrease in pressure gradient

Complications

- Injury to renal artery
- Perforation
- Dissection
- Thrombosis
- Contrast induced nephropathy
- Restenosis
- Hematoma at puncture site
- **Stent related complications**:
  - Malposition
  - Misdeployment
  - Infection
  - Embolization

Preprocedural Assessment

- **Patient selection**:
  - Size of kidney—8–9 cm
  - Residual function in a solitary kidney.
  - Preservation of glomeruli and tubules—on renal biopsy.
  - Presence of collaterals in arteriography.
- **Medications**: Antiplatelet therapy (e.g., aspirin or clopidogrel) is usually started before the procedure to reduce the risk of thrombus formation. Renal function is assessed to determine contrast agent safety.
- **Informed consent**: Discuss risks (e.g., bleeding, kidney damage, artery rupture) and benefits with the patient.

Procedure

- **Patient position**: Supine
- **Anesthesia**: Local anesthetic
- **Machine used**: Fluoroscopic guidance

Steps

1. Vascular access:
   - The femoral artery is typically the primary access point, although the radial artery may be used.
   - A small incision is made, and a vascular sheath is inserted into the artery to allow the introduction of catheters.
2. Catheter and wire placement:
   - A guidewire is first introduced through the sheath into the femoral artery and advanced into the aorta.
   - A catheter is then guided over the wire into the renal artery using fluoroscopic guidance.
   - Contrast dye injection: Contrast dye is injected through the catheter to visualize the renal arteries and assess the degree of stenosis (narrowing) using real-time fluoroscopy.
3. Balloon angioplasty:
   - Once the stenotic (narrowed) area is identified, a balloon catheter is advanced over the guidewire to the narrowed segment.
   - The balloon is inflated at the site of the stenosis to widen the artery, compressing the plaque against the vessel wall. This is the angioplasty portion of the procedure.
   - The balloon is inflated for several seconds to minutes and then deflated and removed.
4. Stent placement:
   - After angioplasty, a stent (a small mesh-like tube) is typically deployed to keep the artery open. The stent is mounted on a balloon catheter, which is inflated to expand the stent within the artery.
   - The stent remains permanently in the artery, acting as a scaffold to prevent re-narrowing (restenosis).
   - Self-expanding or balloon-expandable stents may be used depending on the patient's anatomy and the degree of stenosis.
   - Post-stenting, another injection of contrast dye is performed to confirm that the artery has been successfully opened and that blood flow to the kidney is restored.
5. Post-dilation (if needed):
   - After stent deployment, balloon post-dilation may be done to further expand the stent and ensure optimal apposition of the stent to the vessel wall.
   - This ensures the stent is properly anchored and the artery is maximally dilated.

Post-Procedural Care

1. Sheath Removal: After the procedure, the femoral sheath is removed, and pressure is applied to the site to prevent bleeding. Alternatively, a closure device may be used to seal the artery.
2. Antiplatelet Therapy: Dual antiplatelet therapy (e.g., aspirin and clopidogrel) is continued to reduce the risk of stent thrombosis.
3. Monitoring: The patient is monitored for signs of complications such as bleeding, hematoma formation, renal function decline, or restenosis.
4. Follow-Up Imaging: After several weeks or months, follow-up imaging (e.g., Doppler ultrasound or CT angiography) is performed to ensure the stent is patent (open) and the artery remains clear.

Outcomes

- Improvement of hypertension
- Improvement of renal function
- **Heart failure**: In patients with "flash" pulmonary edema or recurrent heart failure exacerbations due to renal artery stenosis, stenting can reduce the frequency of these events.

Diseases of Female Pelvis

1. Classify morbid adhesions of placenta. Write down USG findings in ectopic pregnancy. [5+5] [MD (WBUHS) 23]

Introduction

Morbid adhesions of placenta also called Placenta accreta spectrum (PAS), is a term used to describe placenta accreta, increta, and percreta. It results due to trophoblast invasion beyond decidua basalis.[14]

Risk Factors

Most commonly due to previous cesarean section and placenta previa.

The risk factors for morbid adhesions of placenta (MAP) are presented in **Table 27**.

TABLE 27: Risk factors for morbid adhesions of placenta.

- Previous C-section
- Placenta previa
- Other previous uterine surgeries
- Advanced maternal age
- Multiparity
- Uterine irradiation
- Endometrial ablation
- Asherman syndrome
- Uterine leiomyoma
- Uterine anomalies
- Hypertensive disorders of pregnancy
- Smoking

Pathophysiology

Occurs due to placental implantation at an area of abnormal decidualization allowing the chorionic villi to attach and invade into the myometrium.

Classification of morbidly adherent placenta (Fig. 28):

- **Accreta**: Villi attach to the myometrium
- **Increta**: Villi penetrate into the myometrium
- **Percreta**: Villi penetrate through the myometrium to the uterine serosa or adjacent organs.

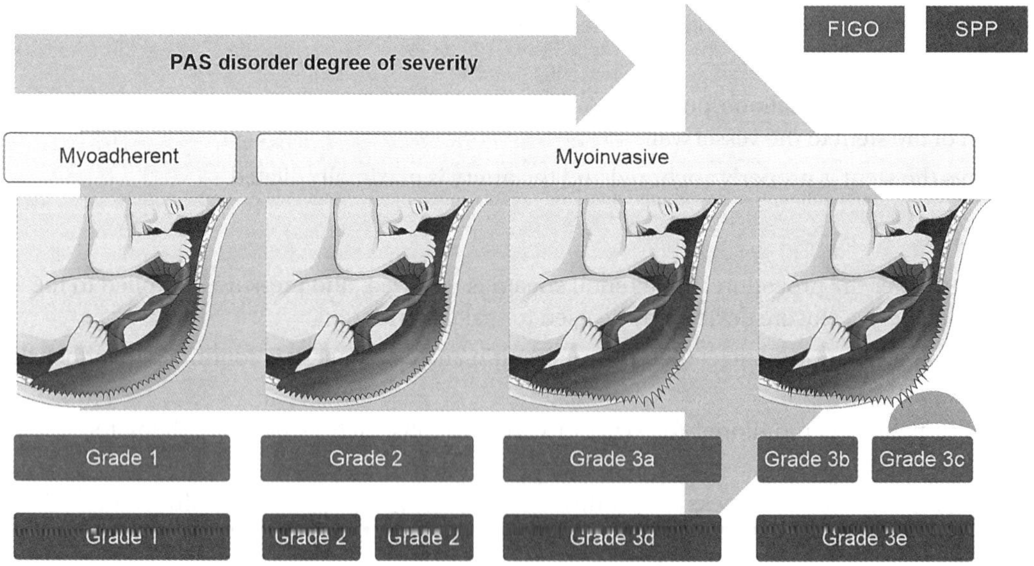

FIG. 28: Placenta accreta spectrum (PAS).

USG Findings in Ectopic Pregnancy (Table 28 and Fig. 29)

TABLE 28: USG findings in ectopic pregnancy.

Type of ectopic gestation	*USG features*
Tubal	• Adnexal mass separate from ovaries • Presence of yolk sac and/or embryo inside the mass is diagnostic

Continued...

Continued...

Type of ectopic gestation	***USG features***
	• The embryo may demonstrate cardiac pulsations • Tubal ring sign – reflective ring surrounding gestational sac • Ring of fire sign – the presence of low impedance vascularity around the lesion on Doppler USG (less specific) • Centrally located fluid collection in the endometrial cavity, known as "pseudogestational sac" can be present with any type of ectopic gestation • Absent intradecidual sac sign
Interstitial	• Eccentrically placed gestational sac with a thin myometrial layer around, less than 5 mm in size • Interstitial line sign—reflective line bordering the intramural gestational sac
Cornual	• Gestational sac surrounded by a thin myometrial layer • 3D coronal reconstruction is helpful in documentation
Ovarian	• Gestational sac with surrounding hyperechoic ring within the ovary
Cervical	• Hourglass appearance of the cervix due to an expanding sac inside the cervical canal • Bimanual sliding sign to rule out an impending abortion sac should not move on bimanual pressure • Vascularity surrounding sac on color Doppler
Scar	• Empty uterus • Gestational sac implanted at or very near the scar line of previous lower segment cesarean section
Intra-abdominal	• Intra-abdominal fetus with an unusual orientation • No defined myometrium • Poorly defined placenta • Bowel loops may be seen around the fetus

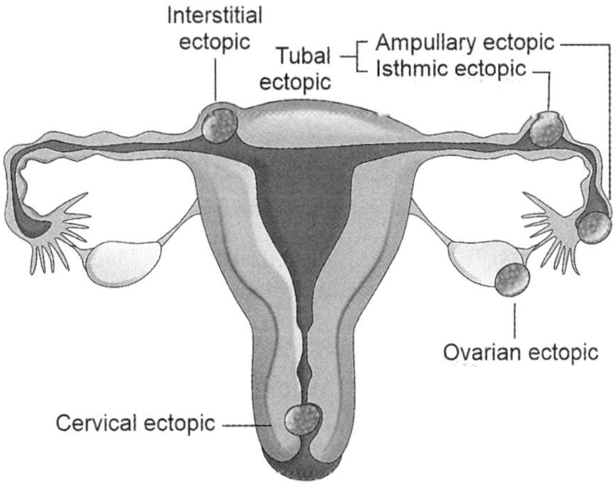

FIG. 29: Schematic diagram showing different locations of ectopic gestation.

Pregnancy of Unknown Location

- A transient stage when no definite intrauterine pregnancy (IUP) is detected on transvaginal ultrasound and no sign of ectopic pregnancy detected.
- **Beta HCG level**: 1000–2000 mIU/mL without an IUP—suspicion of ectopic pregnancy.
- Serial beta HCG monitoring is needed.
- If rise of beta HCG >35% in the next 48 hours—highly suggestive of IUP
- <35% rise—indicates ectopic pregnancy.

2. Describe the role of USG and Doppler studies in IUGR. [5+5] [MD (WBUHS) 23, AIIMS Dec 23]

Intrauterine growth restriction is a condition in which the weight of the fetus is less than <10th percentile without Doppler changes (small for gestational age) and <3rd percentile with Doppler changes.[15]

Small for gestational age (SGA): Between 3rd and 10th percentiles, with normal Doppler studies (umbilical artery, uterine artery, middle cerebral artery)

Fetal growth restriction (FGR):
- <3rd percentile
- <10th percentile with abnormal Doppler studies (umbilical artery, uterine artery, middle cerebral artery)

Role of USG and Doppler in IUGR (Box 3 and Table 29)

BOX 3: Consensus based definitions for early and late fetal growth restriction.

Early-onset FGR (<32 weeks)
- EFW or AC <3rd percentile

  or
- UA with AREDV

  or
- EFW or AC <10th percentile, combined with one or more of the following:
  a. UA PI >95th percentile
  b. UtA PI >95th percentile

Late-onset FGR (≥32 weeks)
- EFW or AC <3rd percentile

  or
- ≥2 of the following 3 criteria:
  a. EFW or AC <10th percentile
  b. EFW or AC crossing percentiles >2 quartiles on growth percentiles
  c. CPR <5th percentile or UA PI >95th percentile

TABLE 29: Main differences between early and late-onset forms of IUGR.

Early-onset FGR (1–2%)	*Late-onset FGR (3–5%)*
Problem: Management	Problem: Diagnosis
Placental disease: Severe (UA Doppler abnormal, high association with preeclampsia)	Placental disease: Mild (UA Doppler normal, low association with preeclampsia)
Hypoxia ++: Systemic cardiovascular adaptation	Hypoxia +/- : Central cardiovascular adaptation
Immature fetus = higher tolerance to hypoxia = natural history	Mature fetus = lower tolerance to hypoxia = no (or very short) natural history
High mortality and morbidity; lower prevalence	Lower mortality (but common cause of late stillbirth); poor long-term outcome; affects large fraction of pregnancies

Sequence of Changes in Doppler Parameters

- Uterine arteries
- Cerebroplacental ratio
- Umbilical artery
- Middle cerebral artery
- Aortic isthmus

- Ductus venosus
- Umbilical vein

Stage based classification and management of FGR is presented as follows (Table 30 and Flowchart 16):

TABLE 30: Stage based classification and management of FGR.

Stage	*Pathophysiological correlate*	*Criteria (any of)*	*Monitoring*	*GA/mode of delivery*
I	Severe smallness or mild placental insufficiency	EFW <3rd centile, CPR <p5 UA PI >p95, MCA PI <p5, UtA PI >p95	Weekly	37 weeks LI
II	Severe placental insufficiency	UA AEDV, reverse AoI	Biweekly	34 weeks CS
III	Low-suspicion fetal acidosis	UA REDV, DV-PI >p95	1–2 days	30 weeks CS
IV	High-suspicion fetal acidosis	DV reverse a flow, cCTG <3 ms, FHR decelerations	12 h	26 weeks CS

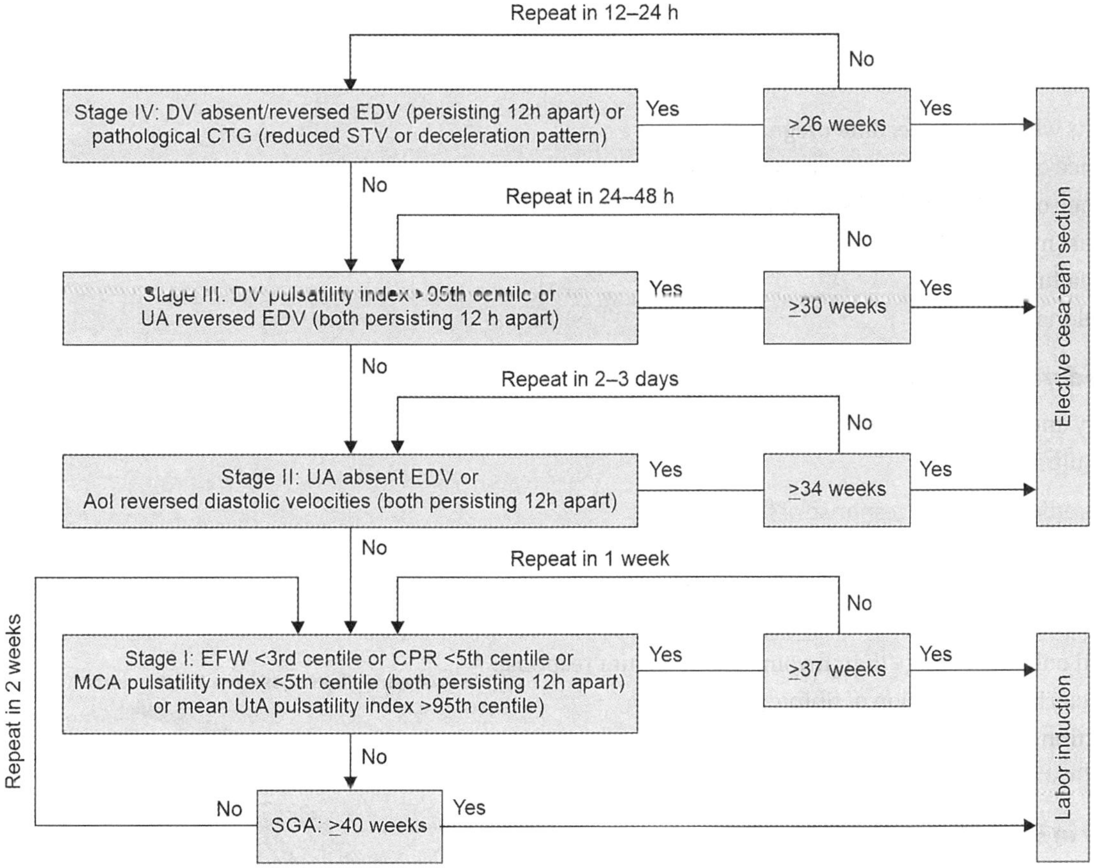

FLOWCHART 16: Stage based decision algorithm for the management of FGR.

(AC: abdominal circumference; AoI: aortic isthmus; AREDV: absent or reversed end-diastolic velocity; CPR: cerebroplacental ratio; CTG: cardiotocography; DV: ductus venosus; EFW: estimated fetal weight; FGR: fetal growth restriction; FHR: fetal heart rate; MCA: middle cerebral artery; PI: pulsatility index; SGA: small for gestational age; UA: umbilical artery; UtA: uterine artery)

Complications of IUGR

- Preeclampsia
- Intrauterine death
- Brain injury
- Fetal distress

3. Discuss the indications and the procedure of uterine artery embolization. [3+7] [MD (WBUHS) 23, AIIMS Dec 23]

Indications

- Symptomatic uterine fibroids (intramural, subserosal, submucosal)
- Adenomyosis
- Dysfunctional uterine bleeding
- Post partum hemorrhage
- Uterine arteriovenous malformation

Absolute Contraindications

- Viable pregnancy
- Active pelvic infection
- Malignancy of uterus and ovaries

Relative Contraindications

- Patients who want to become pregnant
- Presence of intrauterine contraceptive device
- Presence of common blood supply to uterus and ovaries
- Contrast material allergy
- Renal failure
- Coagulopathy

Preprocedural Evaluation

- History and gynaecological examination of the patient
- Pelvic ultrasound

MRI: To predict treatment response of fibroids

- Hyperintensity on T2W indicates hypercellularity—better response
- T1 hyperintense fibroids—poor response due to hemorrhagic necrosis or fat
- Submucosal fibroids—more volume reduction due to radial artery supply
- Fibroid enhancing more than myometrium—better response
- Characterization, location of fibroids
- Prediction of ovarian artery supply of fibroid
- **DWI**: Restriction of malignancies

Anatomy in Brief (Figs. 30 to 32)

- Uterine artery arises from inferior gluteal artery
- U course
- Descending, transverse and ascending parts
- Cervicovaginal arteries arise from transverse part (embolization done distal to this branching to prevent vaginal ischemia)

Anatomical Variations of Uterine Artery (Fig. 31)

Procedure

- Admission
- Informed consent

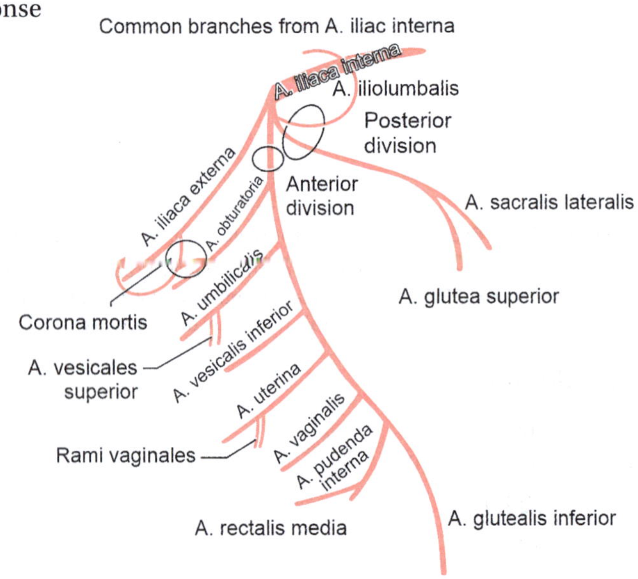

FIG. 30: Uterine artery anatomy.

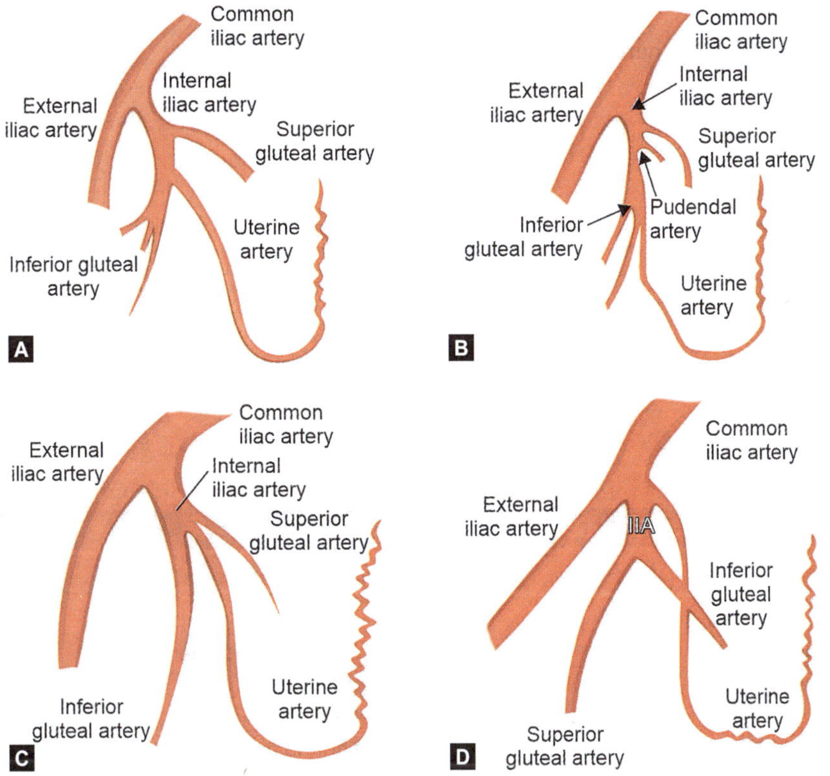

FIGS. 31A to D: Anatomic variations of uterine artery.
A. Uterine artery as 1st branch from inferior gluteal art (type I).
B. Uterine artery as 2nd or 3rd branch from inferior gluteal art (type II)
C. Inferior gluteal, superior gluteal artery, and the uterine artery all arise at the same level (trifurcation) (type III)
D. Uterine artery arises proximal to the origin of the inferior gluteal and superior gluteal arteries (type IV)

- Blood parameters and necessary imaging
- Administration of antibiotics pre and postprocedure.
- Common femoral artery is accessed.
- 5-F Roberts uterine catheter is inserted. Origin of uterine artery is identified. If there is difficulty, cone beam CT is used.
- If not available, cobra catheter is used.
- By microcatheter, selective embolization is done—0.020" micro-catheter is advanced using 0.014" wire
- **Pain management**:
  - Administration of ketorolac and ondansetron 30 mins before the procedure
  - Administration of midazolam and fentanyl during procedure
  - Superior hypogastric nerve block

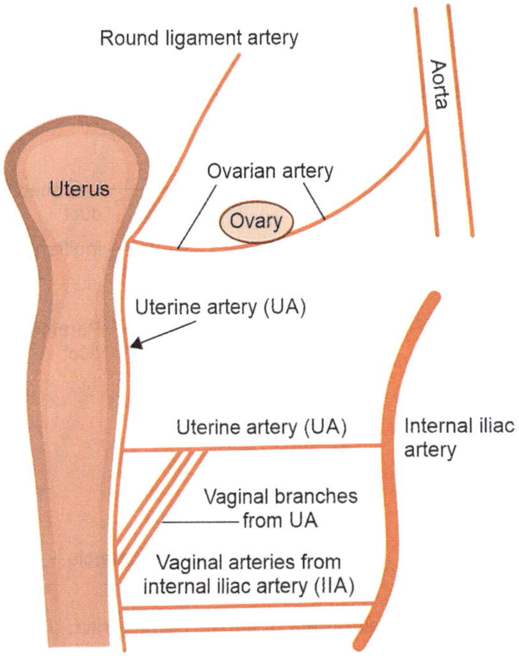

FIG. 32: Arterial anastomotic system–blood supply of uterine artery.

Embolizing Agents

- PVA particles ranging from 350–700
- Embosphere
- NBCA (n-butyl cyanoacrylate)
- Gelfoam
- Vascular coils

Postprocedure

- Hydration antiemetics, NSAIDS, narcotics
- Discharged with antibiotics

Instructions

- Don't use tampons for a week
- Don't have intercourse for a week
- Limit physical activity
- **Visit hospital in case of**:
  - High fever
  - Foul smelling vaginal discharge
  - Severe pelvic pain

Complications (Table 31)

TABLE 31: Complications of uterine artery embolization.

Acute phase	*Subacute and chronic phase*
• Pain • Postembolization syndrome • Sepsis • Bleeding • Groin hematoma • Contrast reaction • Vasovagal response • Pulmonary embolus	• Pain • Transient or permanent amenorrhea • Endometritis • Urinary retention • Passage of fibroid tissue • Delayed contrast reaction • Tubo-ovarian abscess • Uterine necrosis and rupture

4. Briefly describe development of uterus in reference to different uterine malformations. [10] [MD (WBUHS) 20, AIIMS Dec 23]

Development of Uterus (Figs. 33A to C and Flowchart 17)

- Sex determination occurs at the time of conception
- Sex differentiation starts at 6 weeks of gestation

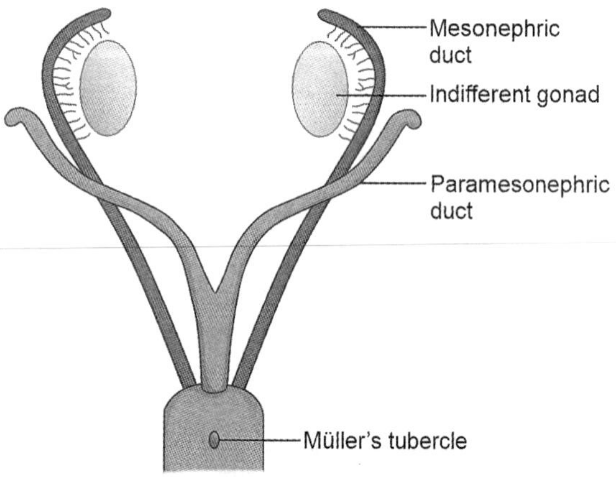

FIG. 33A: Development of female genital tract. Undifferentiated gonad with two pairs of ducts, the Mullerian (paramesonephric) and Wolffian (mesonephric) ducts.

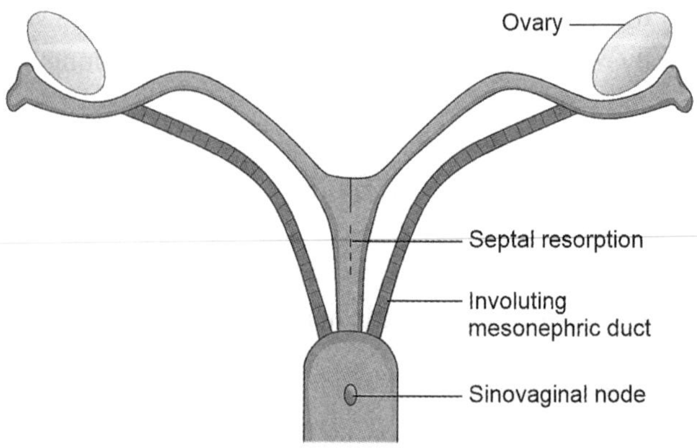

FIG. 33B: Development of female genital tract. Wolffian (mesonephric) ducts involute and the Mullerian (paramesonephric) ducts develop into uterus upper vagina and fallopian tube. The medial portion of the Mullerian ducts fuse in the midline, followed by resorption of the septum.

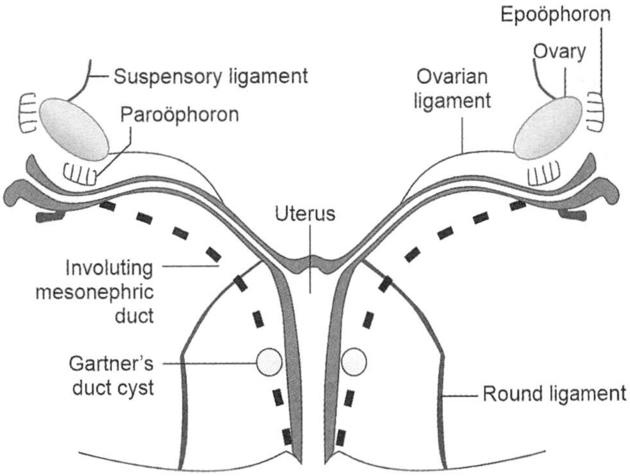

FIG. 33C: Female internal genitalia after its development, at 5 months of embryonic life.

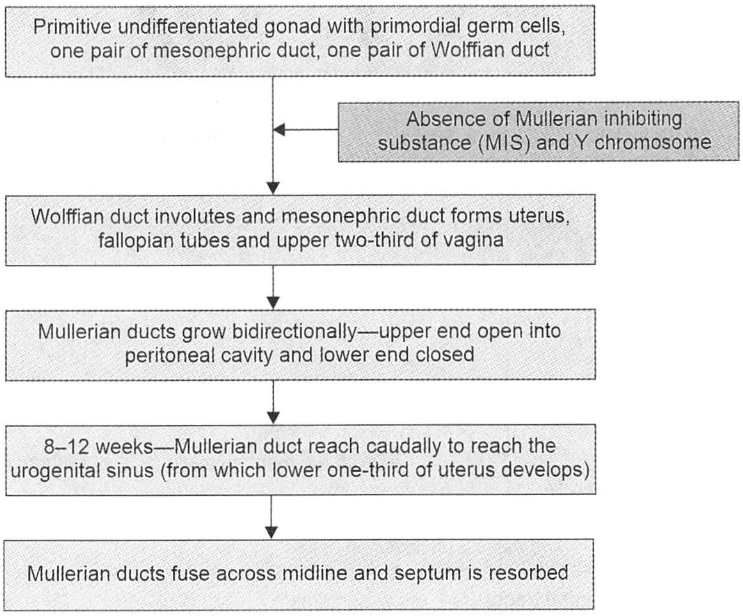

FLOWCHART 17: Steps of development of uterus.

Phases of Mullerian duct development and their defects are outlined as under **(Table 32)**

TABLE 32: Phases of Mullerian duct development and their defects.

Phases of development	*Defect*	*Anomaly*
Organogenesis: Development of Müllerian duct	Failure to develop bilaterally	Aplasia/agenesis (MRKH syndrome)
	Failure to develop unilaterally	Unicornuate uterus
Fusion or unification: Between paired Müllerian ducts	Horizontal fusion defect	Bicornuate uterus, uterus didelphys
Between fused Müllerian duct and urogenital sinus (sinovaginal bulb)	Vertical fusion defect	Transverse vaginal septum, imperforate hymen
Septal resorption or canalization	Defect in resorption or canalization	Septate uterus, arcuate

The different congenital malformations of female genital tract are as follows **(Fig. 34)**

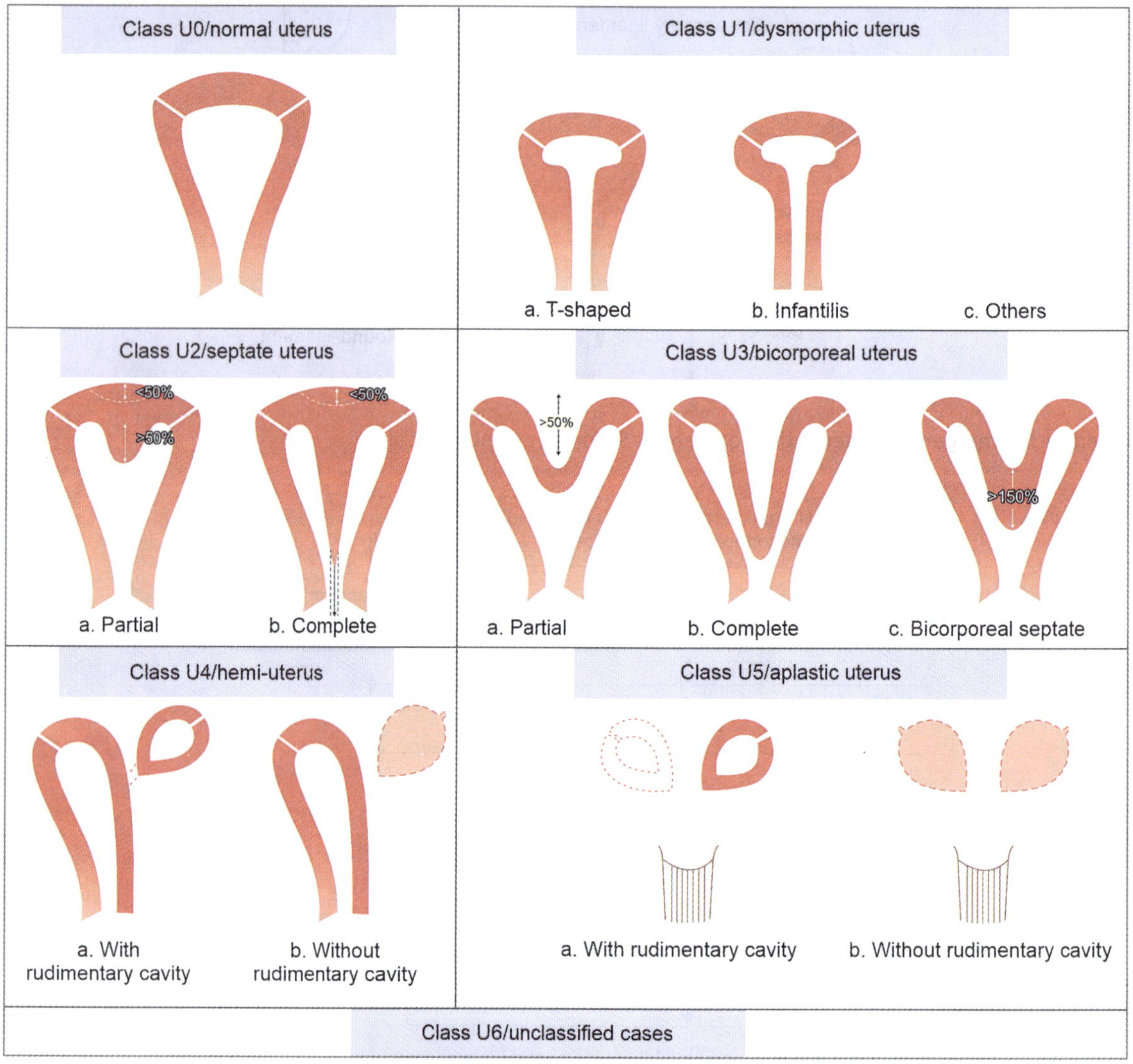

FIG. 34: Congenital malformations of female genital tract.

T shaped uterus-maternal diethylstilbestrol exposure.

The ESHRE-ESGE consensus on the classification of congenital malformations of the female genital tract is presented in **Table 33**.

TABLE 33: ESHRE-ESGE consensus on the classification of congenital malformations of the female genital tract.

ESHRE/ESGE Classification Female Genital Tract Anomalies				
Uterine anomaly			***Cervical/Vaginal anomaly***	
	Main class	***Sub-class***	***Co-existent class***	
u0	Normal uterus		**C0**	Normal cervix
U1	Dysmorphic uterus	a. T-shaped b. Infantilis c. Others	**C1**	Septate cervix
			C2	Double "normal" cervix

Continued...

Continued...

Uterine anomaly		
	Main class	**Sub-class**
U2	Septate uterus	a. Partial b. Complete
U3	Bicorporeal uterus	a. Partial b. Complete c. Bicorporeal septate
U4	Hemi-uterus	a. With rudimentary cavity (communicating or not horn) b. Without rudimentary cavity (horn without cavity/no horn)
U5	Aplastic	a. With rudimentary cavity (bi- or unilateral horn) b. Without rudimentary cavity (bi- or unilateral uterine remnants/aplasia)
U6	Unclassified malformations	
U		
Associated anomalies of non-Müllerian origin		

Cervical/Vaginal anomaly	
Co-existent class	
C3	Unilateral cervical aplasia
C4	Cervical aplasia
V0	Normal vagina
V1	Longitudinal non-obstructing vaginal septum
V2	Longitudinal obstructing vaginal septum
V3	Transverse vaginal septum and/or imperforate hymen
V4	Vaginal aplasia
C	***V***

5. Write short note on imaging of placenta previa. [5] [MD (WBUHS) 20]

Introduction

- Abnormally low-lying placenta that is completely or partially covering the internal os.
- "Previa" in Latin means coming before, in the way. Placenta becomes the presenting part during delivery.
- Important cause of painless vaginal bleeding in the second and third trimesters.

Epidemiology

1/200 pregnancies

Risk Factors

- Previous placenta previa
- Previous cesarean delivery
- Older maternal age
- Multiparity
- Multifetal gestation
- Cigarette smoking
- Assisted conception
- Previous manual removal of placenta

Associated with: Placenta accreta spectrum

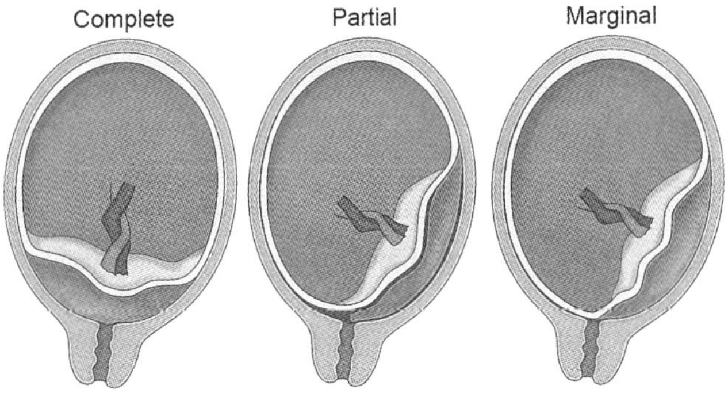

FIG. 35: Types of placenta previa.

Types of Placenta Previa (Fig. 35)

- **Complete**: Placenta covers the internal os completely
- **Partial**: Placenta covers the internal os partially
- **Marginal**: Placenta just reaches the margin of the internal os

Imaging Findings

Transabdominal ultrasound:

- Placenta seen covering the internal os completely or partially.

- If it is touching the margin of the internal os, it is called marginal placenta.
- But the diagnosis of placenta previa is not made before 20 weeks of gestation, as the placenta may migrate upwards later in the gestation.

Transvaginal ultrasound is more accurate in determining the exact distance of the placental margin from the internal os.

Magnetic resonance imaging:

- It is the gold standard imaging for imaging placenta.
- Sagittal images very well demonstrate its relationship to the internal os.

Differential Diagnosis

- **Subchorionic hemorrhage:** It can extend over the cervix mimicking placenta previa.
- **Focal myometrial contraction:** It can give impression that the internal os is close to the placenta.

6. Discuss USG in IUGR. [10] [MD (WBUHS) 20]

Role of USG in IUGR

Intrauterine growth restriction is a condition in which the weight of the fetus is less than <10th percentile without Doppler changes (small for gestational age) and <3rd percentile with Doppler changes.

Role of USG and Doppler in IUGR (refer Box 3 and Table 29)

Sequence of changes in Doppler parameters:

- Uterine arteries
- Cerebroplacental ratio
- Umbilical artery
- Middle cerebral artery
- Aortic isthmus
- Ductus venosus
- Umbilical vein

Stage based classification and management of FGR is presented **(Table 34 and *refer* Flowchart 16)**.

TABLE 34: Stage based classification and management of FGR.

Stage	*Pathophysiological correlate*	*Criteria (any of)*	*Monitoring*	*GA/mode of delivery*
I	Severe smallness or mild placental insufficiency	• EFW <3rd centile • CPR <p5 • UA PI >p95 • MCA PI <p5 • UtA PI >p95	Weekly	37 weeks LI
II	Severe placental insufficiency	• UA AEDV • Reverse AoI	Biweekly	34 weeks CS
III	Low-suspicion fetal acidosis	• UA REDV • DV-PI >p95	1–2 days	30 weeks CS
IV	High-suspicion fetal acidosis	• DV reverse a flow • cCTG <3 ms • FHR decelerations	12 h	26 weeks CS

Complications of IUGR

- Preeclampsia
- Intrauterine death

- Brain injury
- Fetal distress

7. Discuss role of imaging in a suspected case of ectopic pregnancy. [10] [MD (WBUHS) 20]

Introduction

When implantation occurs anywhere other than endometrial cavity, it is called ectopic pregnancy.[16]

Location

- Tubal - ampulla > isthmus > fimbria
- Cervical
- Scar
- Interstitial
- Cornual
- Ovary
- Abdominal

Modalities for Evaluation

Transvaginal Ultrasound: Modality of choice for diagnosing ectopic pregnancy.

USG Findings in Ectopic Pregnancy (Table 28 and Fig. 36)

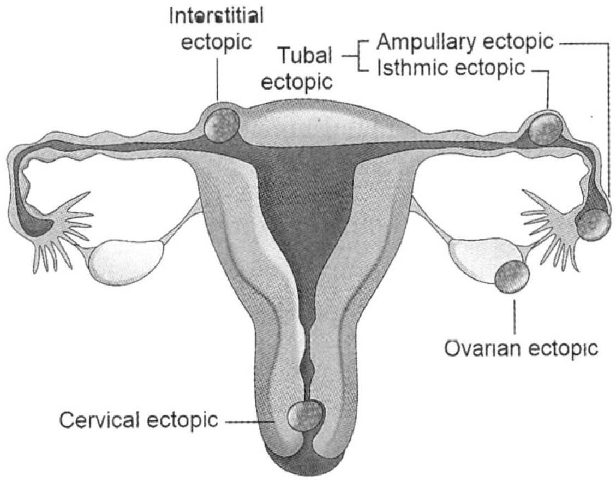

FIG. 36: Schematic diagram showing different locations of ectopic gestation.

Pregnancy of Unknown Location

A transient stage when no definite intrauterine pregnancy (IUP) is detected on transvaginal ultrasound and no sign of ectopic pregnancy detected.

Beta HCG level: 1,000–2,000 mIU/mL without an IUP - suspicion of ectopic pregnancy.

Serial beta HCG monitoring is needed.

If rise of beta HCG >35% in the next 48 hours - highly suggestive of IUP

<35% rise - indicates ectopic pregnancy.

Heterotopic pregnancy: An intrauterine Gestational sac and an ovarian ectopic present concurrently.

Mimics of Ectopic Pregnancy

Corpus luteum:

- Located within ovary
- Can show peripheral vascularity mimicking ring of fire sign of tubal ectopic.
- Thick crenulated wall

- Echogenic contents due to hemorrhage
- Differentiation from ovarian ectopic is important.
- Does not have yolk sac or embryo
- Less echogenic from heterogenous mass type unruptured ovarian ectopic.

8. Write short note on: (a) PNDT ACT. (b) Role of Doppler in IUGR. [5+5] [MD (WBUHS) 19]

The Preconception and Prenatal Diagnostic Techniques Act (Prohibition of Sex Selection Act) 1994

A. Amended in 2003[17]

B. Sex selection and sex determination are prohibited.

C. Sex of the fetus shall not be communicated to the pregnant woman or her relatives by words, signs or any other manner by the person conducting prenatal diagnostic procedure.

D. The clinics conducting ultrasound must be registered.

E. Doctors qualified (listed below) under the act can use diagnostic techniques such as ultrasound.

Any Registered Medical Practitioner with
- Postgraduate degree or diploma or
- Six months of training or
- One year of experience in sonography or image scanning
- Permitted to be registered with a maximum of 2 clinics in a district.
- Gynecologist must have performed at least 20 procedures under the supervision of an experienced gynecologist in this field.

F. The clinics must display the notice- "Disclosure of the sex of the fetus is prohibited under the law" in English as well as in local language.

G. Advertising of sex determination tests is liable for punishment.

Punishments under the act:

1. Offence by any service provider: 3 years imprisonment and/or rupees 10,000 fine.
   Subsequent offence: 5 years imprisonment and/or rupees 50,000 fine.
2. Offence by medical professionals: removal of name from the register for 5 years.
   Subsequent offence: permanent removal.
3. Persons seeking to know the sex of the fetus: up to 3 years imprisonment and/or rupees 50,000 fine.
   Subsequent offence: up to 5 years imprisonment and/or rupees 100,000 fine.
   A woman is presumed to have been compelled by her husband and relatives for undergoing prenatal diagnostic test, so she is not punishable.
4. Advertisement of sex selection tests/procedures: up to 3 years imprisonment and/or rupees 10,000 fine with fine for additional contravention at rupees 500/day.

Forms under the act:

- **FORM A**: For registration or renewal of registration of clinic
- **FORM B**: Certificate of registration
- **FORM C**: Rejection of registration
- **FORM D**: For maintenance of records of the genetic counselling center
- **FORM E**: For maintenance of records of the genetic laboratory
- **FORM F**: For maintenance of records of the genetic clinic/ultrasound clinic/imaging center for prenatal diagnostic test/procedure
- **FORM G**: For taking consent of prenatal diagnostic procedure
- **FORM H**: For maintenance of permanent record for grant/rejection of registration under the Act.

Role of Doppler in IUGR

Intrauterine growth restriction is a condition in which the weight of the fetus is less than <10th percentile without Doppler changes (small for gestational age) and <3rd percentile with Doppler changes.

Role of USG and Doppler in IUGR (Box 3 and Table 29)

Sequence of changes in Doppler parameters:

- Uterine arteries
- Cerebroplacental ratio
- Umbilical artery
- Middle cerebral artery
- Aortic isthmus
- Ductus venosus
- Umbilical vein

Stage based classification and management of FGR is presented as follows **(Table 34 and Flowchart 16)**.

9. List various causes of female infertility. Discuss the role of HSG and MRI in their evaluation. [2+4+4] [MD (WBUHS) 21]

Introduction

Infertility is failure of conception for 12 months or more by a couple having regular unprotected sexual intercourse after ruling out physiological causes such as lactational amenorrhea.

- Primary infertility—infertility in a couple who never had a child.
- Secondary infertility—failure of conception following a previous pregnancy.

The causes of female infertility are listed as follows **(Boxes 4 and 5)**

BOX 4: Genital factors causing female infertility.

Causes of female infertility

Genital factors

- Tubal factors (25–30%) —PID (tubercular and nontubercular), IUD use, Tubal surgery
- Uterine factors - (10%)
  - Congenital—Agenesis, unicornuate, bicornuate didelphys, septate uterus
  - Acquired-fibroid, adenomyosis, synechia, infections
- Ovarian factors (30–40%) – Anovulation, PID, endometriosis
- Cervical factors (5%)—Cervicitis, polyps, Cervical scarring
- Vaginal factors—Vaginitis, Vaginismus, Vaginal atresia, Narrow introitus
- Peritoneal factors (5%)—peritoneal adhesions, Pelvic endometriosis

BOX 5: Systemic factors causing female infertility.

- Age over 35 years, Obesity
- Endocrinopathy- thyroid, hypogonadism, PCOD(10%)
- Psychological
- Immunological:
  - Immunological incompatibility
  - Antiphospholipid antibody syndrome
  - SLE

Tubal occlusion is the most common cause of female infertility-assessed with hysterosalpingography first.

Imaging Evaluation of a Female Patient Presenting with Infertility

- **Modalities available**:
  - Hysterosalpingography (HSG)
  - Ultrasonography (USG)—color Doppler and 3D USG
  - Sonohysterosalpingography (SSG)
  - Hystero-salpingo-contrast sonography (HyCoSy)
- **Ultrasound of thyroid**: To look for causes of hypo/hyperparathyroidism
- **Transabdominal ultrasound**:
  - Position of kidneys
  - Presence or absence of uterus
  - Position of uterus: ante/retroverted
  - Presence of intrauterine contraceptive or other devices
  - Endometrial thickness corresponding to the day of the cycle.
  - Evaluation of fibroid, endometriosis, mullerian anomalies (by using 3D ultrasound), hydrosalpinx
  - Volume of ovaries for polycystic ovarian syndrome (better evaluated on transvaginal scan)
- **Transvaginal ultrasound**: Evaluation of the same structures as transabdominal scan with better detail
- **Hysterosalpingography-evaluation of (Fig. 37)**:
  - Fibroid, polyp
  - Uterine synechiae
  - Mullerian anomalies
  - Infections like tuberculosis
  - Cornual block

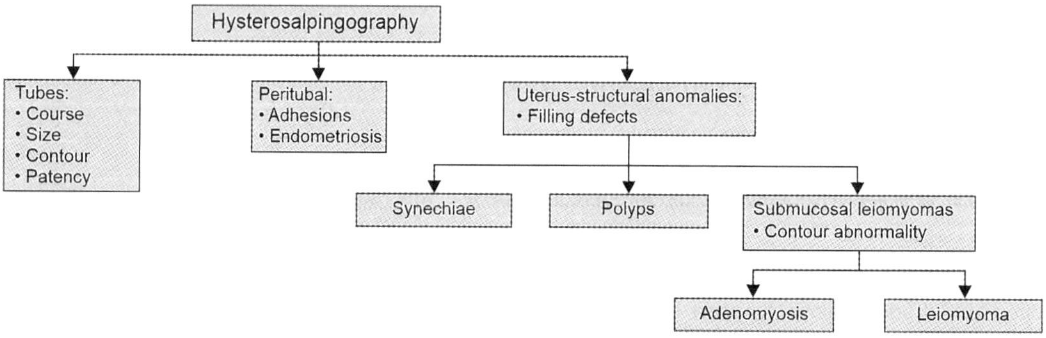

FIG. 37: Role of HSG in female infertility.

Fallopian tube abnormalities are better evaluated on HSG

MRI pelvis and hypothalamic-pituitary axis with dynamic contrast:

1. **MRI pelvis**:

   Protocol:
   - 1.5–3 T magnet
   - Pelvic phased array coil
   - Consent taken
   - Supine position of patient
   - Sequences taken:
     - Axial T1, T2, T2FS, DWI,
     - Sagittal T2
     - Oblique coronal T2
   - Mullerian anomalies-septate, bicornuate uterus most commonly

   The different congenital malformations of female genital tract are as follows **(Fig. 34)**.

The ESHRE-ESGE consensus on the classification of congenital malformations of the female genital tract is presented in the following table **(Table 33)**

- Pelvic masses-fibroid
- Evaluation of endometriosis

2. MRI hypothalamo-pituitary axis with dynamic contrast: to look for pituitary micro or macroadenoma.

Process diagram showing systematic approach to diagnostic imaging for female infertility is presented as follows **(Flowchart 18)**:

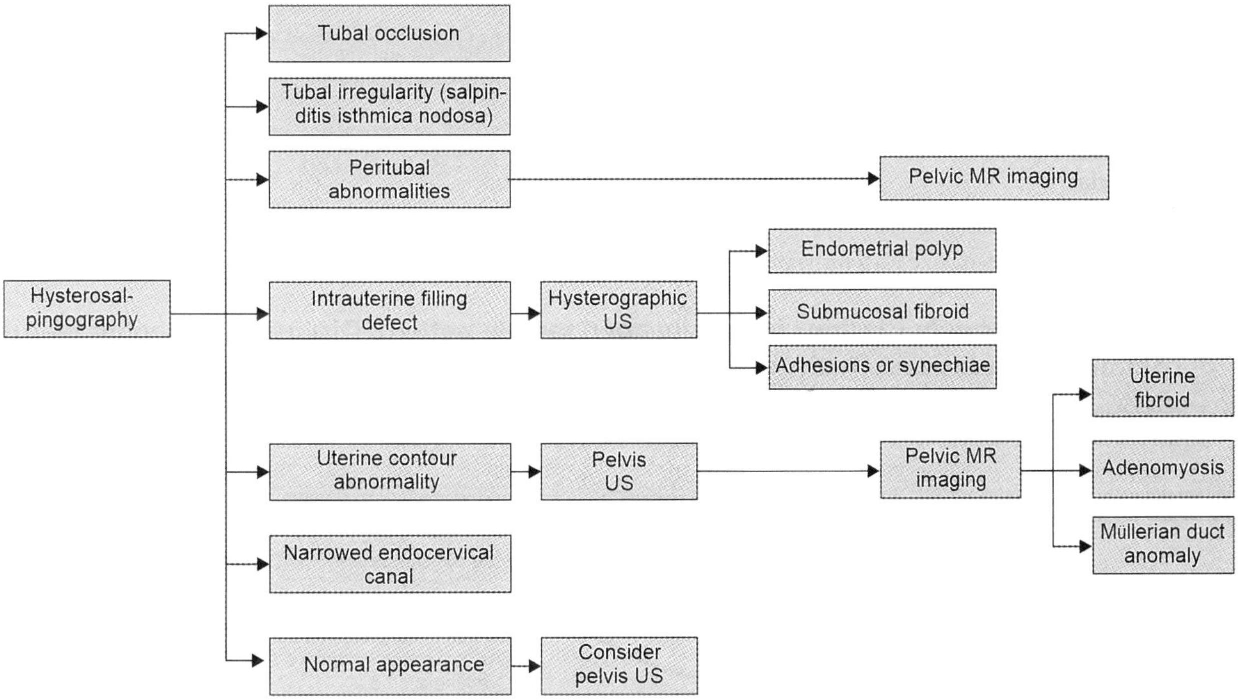

FLOWCHART 18: Process diagram shows a systematic approach to diagnostic imaging for female infertility. Findings from each imaging examination help determine whether further examinations are needed and what modality or modalities would be most useful.

Some common pathologies causing infertility:

Adenomyosis

Definition: The presence of ectopic endometrial tissue within the myometrium.

Types: Diffuse or focal

Modality of choice: MRI

Imaging features in MRI:

- Focal, diffuse or cystic variety
- Thickening of the junctional zone > or equal to 12 mm.
- T1 foci of high signal—presence of hemorrhage
- Ill defined or ovoid focal or diffuse thickening

Fibroid:

- Well circumscribed, homogenously hypointense on T2.
- Subserosal T2 hypointense fibroid may show pedicle
- May have diffusion restriction
- T1 hyperintense areas indicate hemorrhage
- Secondary degeneration common-cystic, hyaline, calcific
- Calcified fibroid is seen in control film of HSG.
- **Cystic degeneration**: High signal on T2, no enhancement in cystic areas

- **Hyaline degeneration**: Cobble stone appearance-postcontrast study
- **Myxoid degeneration**: Very high signal on T2 images and minimal enhancement postcontrast.

Polycystic ovarian disease:
- Common in women of reproductive age
- Infrequent or prolonged menstrual periods-excess male hormone androgen levels
- Multiple small peripherally arrange follicles with echogenic stroma
- Failure of ovulation regularly.

Time of imaging:
- Ideally time days 3–7 of menstruation.
- Irregular cycle any time, or days 3–7 of induced bleeding
- Not applicable at <8 yrs age.

Imaging criteria:
1. >10 cm^3 in volume of one or both ovaries (calculated after exclusion of dominant follicle or luteal cyst if any).
2. ≥20 follicles per ovary of size (2–9 mm) in one or both ovaries.

10. Classify the cystic pelvic lesions in middle aged female patient. Discuss the imaging features of common cystic lesions. [4+6] [MD (WBUHS) 22, MD (WBUHS) 18]

The cystic pelvic lesions are classified as follows **(Fig. 38)**:

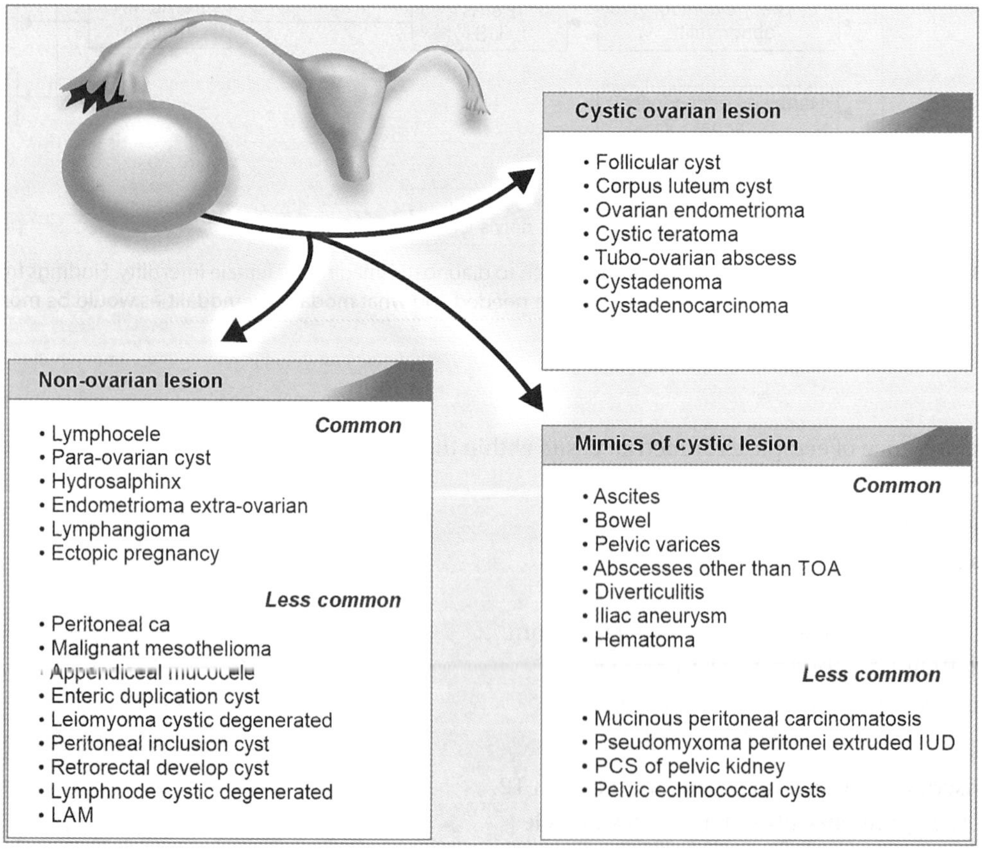

FIG. 38: Classification of cystic pelvic lesions.

Imaging Features of Common Cystic Lesions

Endometrioma (chocolate cyst or endometriotic cyst)

Localized form of endometriosis, usually within the ovary

USG:
- Unilocular cyst with acoustic enhancement
- Diffuse homogenous ground glass echoes
- Less commonly – multiloculated, anechoic cyst, solid-cystic appearance, hyperechoic foci in wall.
- Kissing ovaries
- Anteverted-retroflexed uterus
- Hydrosalpinx – dilated tubular structures with incomplete septations in the adnexa

TVS:
- Helps to assess the soft markers
- Loss of sliding sign indicates obliteration of pouch of Douglas.
- Site specific tenderness

MRI pelvis with contrast:
- Hyperintense on T1 (acute hemorrhage can be hypointense).
- Hyperintense on T1FS
- Hypointense on T2 due to the presence of methemoglobin and deoxyhemoglobin (T2 shading sign)
- Diffusion restriction is variable.
- Postcontrast study-wall may show enhancement (if enhancing mural nodule is present, malignant transformation is to be suspected).
- **T2 dark spot sign**-eccentrically located T2 hypointense and T1 hyperintense nodule, indicate hemosiderin foci due to chronic hemorrhage
- **Kissing ovaries sign**-ovaries are adherent to each other and come in midline posterior to the uterus. Can be associated with bilateral endometriomas.
- **Question mark sign**-anteverted-retroflexed uterus to due adhesions

Difference from hemorrhagic cyst-T2 signal is darker and heterogenous and T1 signal is brighter and more homogenous.

Hemorrhagic Cyst

USG:
- Fine, lacelike, reticular intersecting echoes within the cyst-***cobweb, fishnet, lacy appearance***: specific sign
- An intracystic solid clot
- May have fluid level
- Thin wall
- Clot may adhere to the cyst wall mimicking a nodule
- Retracting clot may have sharp or concave borders
- Posterior acoustic enhancement
- Circumferential blood flow in the cyst wall is typical

Follicular Cyst

- Located within ovary
- Smooth thin walled anechoic cystic structure
- No solid component or septations
- No vascularity
- Can have hemorrhage

Cut off for follow-up imaging (Table 35):

TABLE 35: Cut off for follow up imaging of cysts in premenopausal and postmenopausal women.

	Premenopausal	*Postmenopausal*
Size of cyst	5 cm	3 cm
Follow-up imaging according to ORADS	8–12 weeks	3–5 weeks

Corpus Luteal Cyst

- Located within ovary
- Can show peripheral vascularity mimicking ring of fire sign of tubal ectopic.
- Thick crenulated wall
- Echogenic contents due to hemorrhage
- No solid component
- Smooth thick peripheral enhancement

Hydrosalpinx

Specific signs for diagnosing hydrosalpinx:
- **Waist sign (Fig. 39)**: Indentation along the wall of tortuous tubular cystic structure, causing a waist like narrowing.
- **String of beads sign (Fig. 40)**: Nodular thickening along the cystic tubular structure caused by mucosal folds.

Polycystic Ovarian Syndrome

- Ideally time days 3–7 of menstruation.
- Irregular cycle any time, or days 3–7 of induced bleeding
- Not applicable at <8 yrs age.

Ultrasound criteria:
1. >10 cm^3 in volume of one or both ovaries (calculated after exclusion of dominant follicle or luteal cyst if any).
2. ≥20 follicles per ovary of size (2–9 mm) in one or both ovaries

Dermoid Cyst

Ultrasound:
- Unilocular solid cystic mass
- Septations within cystic component
- Solid component has fat and calcification
- Color Doppler study-twinkling artifact of Rokitansky nodule

CT/MRI:
- Solid cystic lesion containing fat and calcifications/tooth.
- Macroscopic fat identified by fat suppression images or fat density on CT.
- Microscopic fat of fat poor dermoid identified by chemical shift imaging.
- Diffusion restriction in solid areas.
- CEMR - Enhancing solid component with type III curve.
- Capsular penetration - most important sign of malignancy.

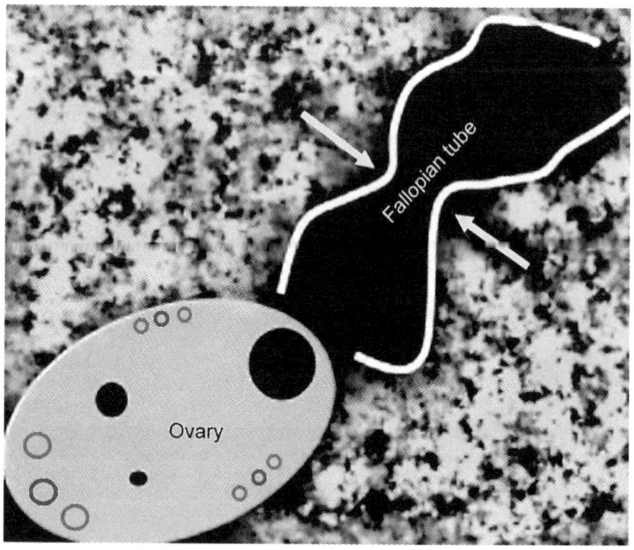

FIG. 39: Schematic diagram of waist sign.

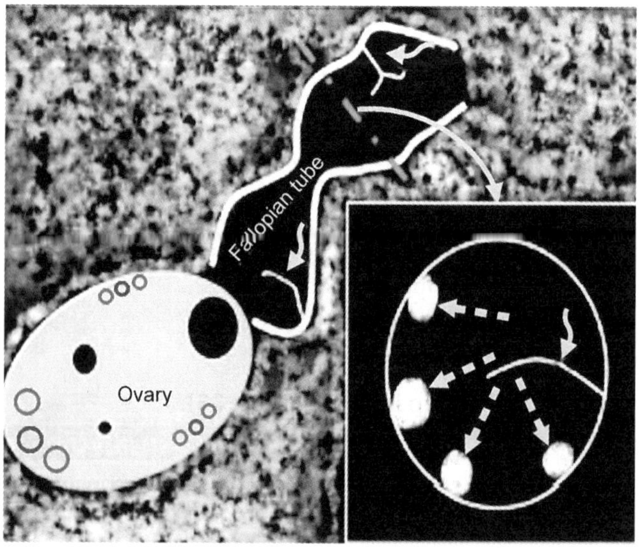

FIG. 40: Schematic diagram of string of beads sign.

11. Discuss the role of various imaging modalities in detection of congenital anomalies of the fetus with their advantages and disadvantages. [10] [MD (WBUHS) 22]

Imaging Modalities for Detection of Congenital Anomalies of the Fetus

Ultrasound

- Modality of choice
- No radiation
- Dynamic scan is possible
- ALARA principle taken care
  - Mechanical index: <1
  - Thermal index: <1
  - Power—as low as possible
  - PRF—low
  - Color gain—high
  - Optimum time gain compensation

Advantages

- Easily available
- Inexpensive
- Noninvasive
- No ionizing radiation
- Painless
- Adequate evaluation of a variety of anomalies

Disadvantages

- Position of the fetus poses a challenge
- Anatomical structures are obscured by the shadow of bony structures

Magnetic Resonance Imaging

- Also called fetal or antenatal MRI
- Done in 1.5-3T
- Supine position
- Sedation may be required
- **Sequence**: HASTE (most important)

Indications of Fetal MRI (Table 36)

Advantages

- Noninvasive
- No ionizing radiation
- Painless
- Position of the fetus does not pose any difficulty for scanning
- Anomalies diagnosed by ultrasound can be confirmed well.
- Scanning in all the three planes and oblique planes is possible.

Disadvantages

- Expensive
- Not easily available

TABLE 36: Indications of fetal MRI.		
Fetal organs	***Indication main category***	***Indication subcategory***
Brain	Congenital anomalies	Ventriculomegaly: corpus callosal dysgenesis: holoprosencephaly; posterior fossa anomalies; malformations of cerebral cortical development
	Screening fetuses with a family risk for brain anomalies	E.g., tuberous sclerosis: corpus callosal dysgenesis: malformations of cerebral cortical development
	Vascular abnormalities	Vascular malformations: hydranencephaly: infarctions; monochorionic twin pregnancy complications
Spine	Congenital anomalies	Neural tube defects: sacrococcygeal teratomas: caudal regression/ sacral agenesis: sirenomelia; vertebral anomalies
Skull, face and neck	Masses of the face and neck	Venolymphatic malformations: hemangiomas: goiter; teratomas; facial clefts
	Airway obstruction	Conditions that may impact parental counseling, prenatal management, delivery planning, and postnatal therapy
Thorax	Masses	Congenital pulmonary airway malformations (congenital cystic adenomatoid malformation, sequestration, and congenital lobar emphysema); congenital diaphragmatic hernia; effusion
	Volumetric assessment of lung	Cases at risk for pulmonary hypoplasia secondary to oligohydramnios, chest mass, or skeletal dysplasias
Abdomen, retroperitoneal and pelvis	Mass	Abdominal-pelvic cyst.: tumors (e.g., hemangiomas, neuroblastomas, sacrococcygeal teratomas, and suprarenal or renal masses), complex genitourinary anomalies (e.g., cloaca), renal anomalies in cases of severe
Abdomen, retroperitoneal and pelvis	Mass	Abdominal-pelvic cyst.: tumors (e.g., hemangiomas, neuroblastomas, sacrococcygeal teratomas, and suprarenal or renal masses), complex genitourinary anomalies (e.g., cloaca), renal anomalies in cases of severe oligohydramnios, and bowel anomalies such as megacystis microcolon
Complications of monochorionic twins		Delineation of vascular anatomy prior to laser treatment of twins: assessment of morbidity after death of a monochorionic co-twin, and improved delineation of anatomy in conjoined twins
Fetal surgery assessment		Meningomyelocele, sacrococcygeal teratomas, processes obstructing the airway (e.g., neck mass or congenital high airway obstruction), complications of monochorionic twins needing surgery, and chest masses.

- Special training of medical personnel required.
- It is a specialized technique that is to be learnt in a dedicated center by the radiologist.
- Uncomfortable for the mother to remain still for so long
- Sedation may be required.

Table 37 showing the fetal congenital anomalies in an organ wise manner:

Postmortem Fetal MRI

- Fetus washed
- MRI is done
- Ideally done before putting the fetus in formalin
- Noninvasive adjuvant to autopsy—which parts to be sent for histopathology can be determined
- Thyroid, meconium and liver appear hyperintense on T1W normally.

TABLE 37: The fetal congenital anomalies in an organ-wise manner.

Organ	*Structure*	*R/S*	*Suggested plane(s)*	*Key features*	*Possible anomalies*
Head and brain	Skull	R	Ax	Oval uninterrupted shape, uniformly hyperechoic	Acrania, cephalocele
	Midline falx	R	Ax	Uninterrupted	Holoprosencephaly
	Lateral ventricles/CP	R	Ax	Symmetric, filled by CP	Ventriculomegaly
	Cranial posterior fossa	R	Sag	Three similar anechoic spaces	Chiari malformation, cystic anomalies
Neck	Nuchal translucency	R	Sag	Thickness <95th centile	Marker for anomalies
Spine	Vertebrae	R	Sag, Co	Uninterrupted vertebral line	Open spina bifida, kyphoscoliosis
	Dorsal skin	R	Sag, Co	Uninterrupted skin	Myelomeningocele
Face	Profile	R	Sag	No flat, no abnormal protrusions, regular chin	Micrognathia, flat face
	Orbits	S	Ax	Anechoic symmetric orbits	An/microphthalmia, hypotelorism
	Anterior palate	S	Co, Ax, Sag	Uninterrupted bone	Cleft
Thorax	Lung fields	R	Ax	Homogeneous structure, shape continuity with abdomen	Pleural effusion, diaphragmatic hernia, lung agenesis, CHAOS, severe skeletal dysplasias
Heart	Heart activity	R	Ax	Regular, 150–170 bpm	Bradycardia, arrhythmias
	Cardiac situs	R	Ax	Apex pointing left, left-sided stomach	Isomerism
	Size and position	R	Ax	Occupies 1/3 of the chest, lies on the midline (2/3 of heart on its left)	Diaphragmatic hernia, hypoplastic RT/LT heart, ectopia cordis
	Four chambers	R	Ax	Four balanced chambers (consider Doppler)	Hypoplastic RT/LT heart, valvular stenosis/atresia, AV septal defect
	Three vessels/arches	S	Ax	V-sign, balanced arches, Doppler suggested	Conotruncal anomalies, valvular stenosis/atresia
GIT and abdominal wall	Stomach	R	Ax, Sag	Round-shaped, anechoic, left-sided	Diaphragmatic hernia, esophageal or duodenal atresia
	Cord insertion	R	Ax, Sag	No bowel protrusion	Exomphalos, gastroschisis, body stalk anomaly
Urinary tract and genitalia	Bladder	R	Ax, Sag	Round-shaped, anechoic, diameter <7 mm	Bladder exstrophy, bilateral renal agenesis, megacystis, LUTO, cloacal anomaly
	Umbilical arteries	R	Ax	Two arteries on bladder sides (Doppler)	Single umbilical artery
	Kidneys	S	Ax, Co	Two symmetric kidneys, homogeneous structure	Renal agenesis, pelvic/horseshoe kidney, cystic/hyperechoic kidneys, hydronephrosis
	Genital tubercle	S	Sag	Flat shape for female, upwards position for males	—
Limbs	Active movements	R	—	Flexion/extension	Neuromuscular anomalies, FADS
	Three segments	R	AX, Sag	Bones present, regular proportions	Limb reduction defects, skeletal dysplasias
	Hands/feet	R	AX, Sag	Present	Limb reduction defects

(R: recommended; S: suggested; Ax: axial; Sag: sagittal; Co: coronal; CP: choroid plexus; CHAOS: congenital high airway obstruction syndrome; bpm: beats per minute; Rt: right; Lt: left; AV: atrioventricular; GIT: gastrointestinal tract; LUTO: lower urinary tract obstruction; FADS: fetal akinesia deformation sequence)

Twin Pregnancy

- Mainly monochorionic diamniotic gestation is assessed because they share the same placenta
- Assessment of complications like TTTS post laser ablation
- Ischemic insult to the donor brain

12. What are the indications of 1st trimester ultrasound? Briefly discuss the assessment of fetal congenital anomalies by first trimester ultrasound. [4+6] [AIIMS May 24]

Indications of First Trimester Ultrasound

- Confirmation of intrauterine pregnancy
- Confirmation of number of gestations
- Confirmation of cardiac activity
- Evaluation of suspected ectopic pregnancy
- Cause of vaginal bleeding
- Assessment of fetal anomalies such as anencephaly
- Measurement of nuchal translucency for aneuploidy screening
- Evaluation of maternal pelvic masses and uterine abnormalities

Assessment of Fetal Congenital Anomalies by First Trimester Ultrasound

Normal ultrasound findings in first trimester pregnancy **(Box 6)**:

BOX 6: Normal ultrasound findings in first trimester pregnancy.

- Nuchal translucency lies within a certain range for a given crown-rump length value
- The nasal bone can be identified as a part of the "equal sign" or the "three-line sign"
- Ductus venosus shows a continuous forward flow on color Doppler
- Fetal cranium shows definite ossification, the falx cerebri is visible, the choroid plexus is seen as a butterfly-shaped symmetric hyperechoic structure, the posterior fossa shows a translucent fourth ventricle, the brain stem is well delineated
- Fetal heart structure and cardiac pulsations can be visualized
- Multiple fetal internal organs such as stomach, kidneys, umbilical arteries, and urinary bladder become visible
- Fetal spine and limb segments can be identified

Table showing the fetal congenital anomalies in an organ wise manner **(Table 37)**.

13. Discuss the imaging evaluation and differential diagnosis in a 60-year-old woman with postmenopausal bleeding. [4+6]

Differential Diagnosis of Post Menopausal Bleeding in a 60-Year-Old Woman

- **Endometrium**:
  - Endometritis
  - Fibroid
  - Endometrial hyperplasia
  - Endometrial polyp
  - Endometrial carcinoma
  - Leiomyosarcoma of uterus
  - Infections: Pyometra
- **Cervix**:
  - Cervicitis
  - Cervical trauma

  - Cervical polyp
  - Cervical carcinoma
- **Vagina**:
  - Atrophic vaginitis
  - Vaginal malignancy
- **Ovary**: Ovarian malignancy (estrogen producing)
- **Vulva**:
  - Trauma
  - Vulvar carcinoma
- **Drugs**:
  - Anticoagulant use
  - Hormone replacement therapy
- **Systemic disease**: Bleeding disorder (thrombocytopenia, leukemia, pancytopenia)
- No cause found

Approach to imaging in a patient presenting with postmenopausal bleeding **(Flowchart 19)**.

Imaging Features of Some Common Pathologies

Endometrial Carcinoma

- **Ultrasound**:
  - Enlarged uterus
  - Thickened heterogenous poorly defined endometrium[18]
  - Large endometrial mass may look polypoidal expanding the endometrial cavity

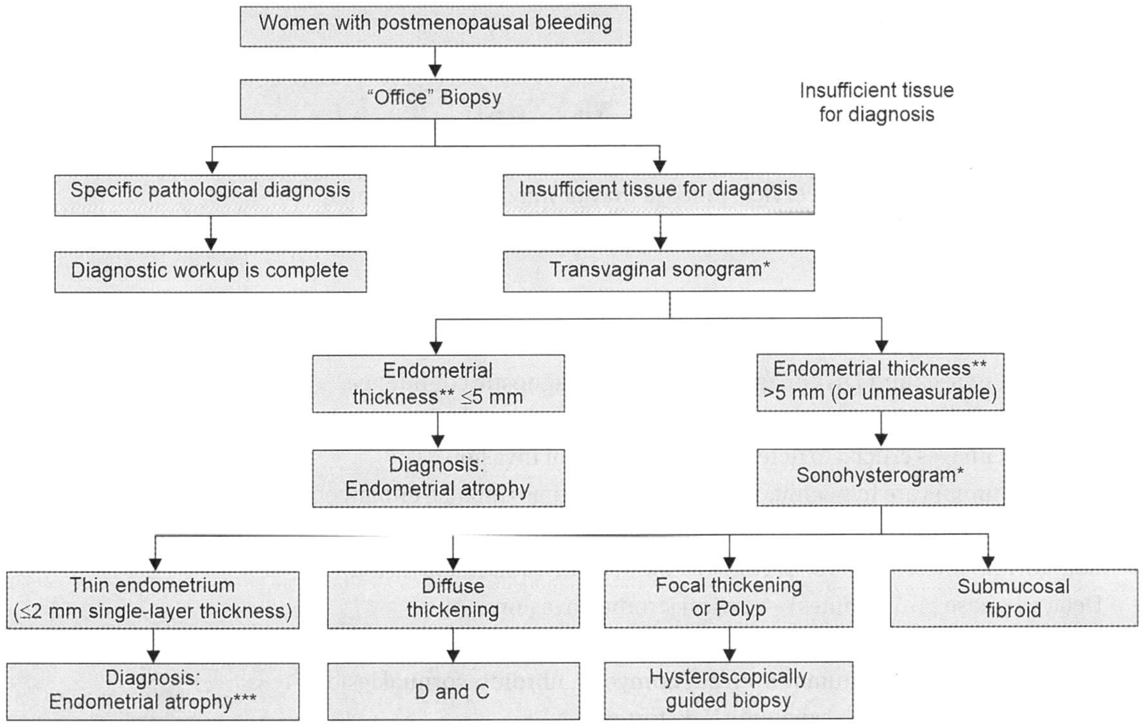

* If the woman has unscheduled bleeding on sequential hormone replacement therapy, sonogram and sonohysterogram should be done shortly after subsequent progesterone withdrawal bleeding
** Double-layer thickness
***Further evaluation may be needed if bleeding persists or patient has risk factors for endometrial carcinoma

FLOWCHART 19: Approach to imaging in a patient presenting with postmenopausal bleeding.

- May be seen as well-defined homogenously echogenic lesion within the endometrial cavity—difficult to differentiate from endometrial hyperplasia or polyp.
- Cystic changes within the lesion.
- Collection within the endometrial cavity due to obstruction
- Interruption of subendometrial halo indicates invasion of myometrium.
- Cannot assess involvement of cervix, parametrium and suspicious lymph nodes

- **Doppler**:
  - Low resistance flow in subendometrial, endometrial and uterine arteries
  - No definite vascular stalk (to differentiate from endometrial polyp.)
- **CT**:
  - Can detect advanced disease (Stage III and above)
  - Important for assessing pelvic lymph nodes and extension to pelvic side walls
  - Cannot accurately evaluate myometrial and cervical invasion and bladder and rectal wall invasion.
- **PET CT**:
  - Useful for assessment of pelvic recurrence and distant metastasis.
  - Metabolically active lesions seen as FDG avid.
- **MR**:
  - Oblique axial and coronal images taken perpendicular to the axis of the endometrium
  - On T1WI, the mass is isointense to normal endometrium and on T2WI the mass is hypointense as compared to normal endometrium but hypointense as compared to the junctional zone.
  - The mass shows less contrast enhancement as compared to myometrium but is more enhancing as compared to the endometrium.
  - Thickened poorly defined endometrium
  - Hematometra or pyometra
  - Enlarged uterus
- **Invasion of cervix**:
  - Tumor may prolapse into the cervix—intactness of the cervical mucosa rules out cervical invasion
  - Invasion of junctional zone and myometrium assessed on T2w images.
  - Extension to the cervix—endocervical mucosa may or may not be disrupted.
  - If myometrium above the cervix is involved, microscopic extension into the cervix cannot be ruled out.
- **Invasion of bladder or rectum**:
  - Interruption of the T2 hypointense muscular wall of bladder and rectum
  - Mass lesion involving the rectal and bladder mucosa
  - Post-contrast images and DWI images increase the diagnostic confidence.
- **Post-contrast study**:
  - Post-contrast images crucial to determine the degree of invasion
  - Endometrial tumors are hypoenhancing except sarcomas (intense enhancement)
    - Early postcontrast (30–60 seconds)—for superficial myometrial invasion
    - Equilibrium phase (120–180 seconds)—for deep myometrial invasion
    - Delayed phase (4–5 minutes)—cervical stromal invasion
- **DWI**:
  - Helps in delineation of the tumor from adenomyosis, fibroids, cornual lesions
  - Useful when junctional zonal anatomy is distorted.
  - Can show vaginal drop metastasis and peritoneal deposits.
  - Invasion into the parametrium:
    - Parametrial soft tissue intensity mass
    - Parametrial fat stranding

- Whickering of the mass into the surrounding parametrium
- Assessed on T2W images.

- **Evaluation of lymph nodes**: Pelvic, paraaortic and common iliac nodes are the drainage sites.
- **Lymph nodes with suspicious features**:
  - More than 10 mm in short axis
  - Round morphology
  - Irregular margin
  - Heterogenous appearance
- **Pitfalls**:
  - Overestimation of the depth of invasion due to the presence of leiomyoma, adenomyosis, cornual tumor.
  - Uterine cornua are thin so overestimation of myometrial invasion is possible.
  - Mimics of endometrial cancer:
    - Secretory or hyperplastic endometrium
    - Retained blood products

These are differentiated by T1 and post-contrast images.

- **Metastasis to ovary**:
  - Bilateral
  - Morphologically similar to endometrial mass
  - Endometrial mass is larger than ovarian mass
- **Primary synchronous tumor of ovary**:
  - Unilateral
  - Presence of lesions like endometriosis
  - Low grade endometrial mass without invasion

Measurement of Myometrial Invasion (Gordon's Method) (Fig. 41)

- A line is drawn over the expected inner edge of the myometrium
- Two lines are drawn perpendicular to the previous line
  - A line measuring the thickness of the tumor (2)
  - Another line measuring the thickness of the whole of the myometrium (3)
  - (2)/(3) gives percentage of myometrial invasion.
  - >50% means deep myometrial invasion upstaging the tumor to IB.

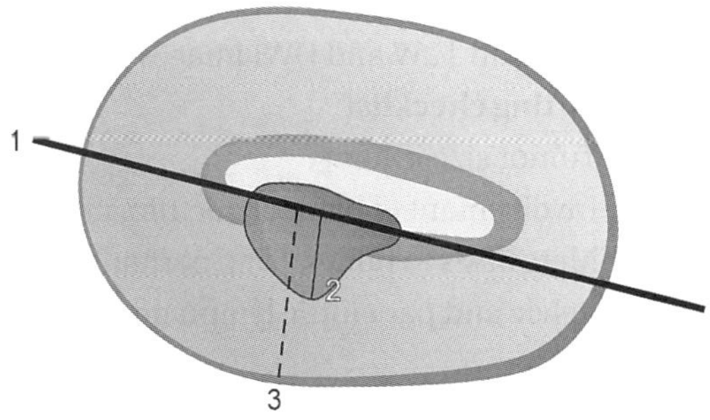

FIG. 41: Measurement of myometrial invasion.

Cervical Carcinoma

- T2W images—cervix is normally hypointense due to dense fibrocollagenous stroma.
- Microscopic disease (stage IA) cannot be visualized.
- Macroscopic disease (stage IB and above) are well visualized on MRI.

Cervical Region

- Ulcerating, infiltrating or exophytic mass lesion
- Loss of normal hypointensity of the cervix on T2w images.
- Mass shows T1W isointense, T2W intermediate to hyperintense signal intensity
- Diffusion restriction in the mass lesion
- Early contrast enhancement
- Hydro/pyometra due to cervical obstruction.

Vaginal Extension

- Loss of normal T2 hypointensity of vaginal wall in case of invasion
- In case of extension, obliteration of the fornices without infiltration of the vaginal wall.

Invasion to Parametrium

- Spiculated extensions from the tumor to the parametrium
- Soft tissue intensity mass in parametrium
- Parametrial fat stranding
- Tumor infiltration into the surrounding vessels and ureter

Extension to Pelvic Wall

- Involvement of obturator internus, piriformis, or levator ani muscles by tumor
- Involvement of ureter may cause hydronephrosis.
- Post-contrast enhancement of the mass and accurate delineation of the extension

Bladder and Rectal Invasion

- Nodular wall thickening
- Interruption of the normal T2 hypointense wall
- Post-contrast enhancement of the mass and accurate delineation of the extension

Lymph Node

- Pelvic and retroperitoneal lymph nodes measuring 10 mm or more in short axis.
- **Suspicious morphological characteristics**:
  - Round shape
  - Irregular margin
  - Central necrosis
  - Nodal group formation
- Assessed on T2W and DWI images—shows DWI restriction
- **Reporting checklist**:
  - Tumor size, extent
  - Involvement of bladder, rectum, ureter, vagina
  - Metastasis to bones, liver, peritoneum if any.
  - Pelvic and paraaortic lymph nodes.

Fibroid

- Well-defined, capsulated
- Subserosal T2 hypointense fibroid may show pedicle
- May have diffusion restriction
- T1 hyperintense areas indicate hemorrhage
- Secondary degeneration common—cystic, hyaline, calcific
- Calcified fibroid is seen in control film of HSG.

Pyometra

- Collection having echogenic debris within the endometrial cavity
- Shows B flow in B mode transabdominal or transvaginal ultrasound
- Uterus is hypervascular on color Doppler
- Associated hydrosalpinx may be seen.

Endometrial Hyperplasia

- Multiple small cysts within the thickened endometrium
- Endometrium is otherwise smooth and has well-defined regular margin.

14. What is fetal growth restriction? Discuss the role of Ultrasound and Doppler in its diagnosis and management. [2+8]

Intrauterine growth restriction is a condition in which the weight of the fetus is <10th percentile without Doppler changes (small for gestational age) and <3rd percentile with Doppler changes.

- Small for gestational age (SGA):
  - Between 3rd and 10th percentiles, with normal Doppler studies (umbilical artery, uterine artery, middle cerebral artery)
- Fetal growth restriction (FGR):
  - <3rd percentile
  - <10th percentile with abnormal Doppler studies (umbilical artery, uterine artery, middle cerebral artery)

Role of USG and Doppler in IUGR (Box 3 and Table 29)

Sequence of Changes in Doppler Parameters

- Uterine arteries
- Cerebroplacental ratio
- Umbilical artery
- Middle cerebral artery
- Aortic isthmus
- Ductus venosus
- Umbilical vein

Stage based classification and management of FGR is presented as follows **(Table 34 and Flowchart 16)**

Complications of IUGR

- Preeclampsia
- Intrauterine death
- Brain injury
- Fetal distress

15. Uterine artery Doppler in pregnant female. [5]

Uterine Artery Doppler in a Pregnant Female

Introduction

- Noninvasive investigation of uteroplacental circulation
- Indicator of uteroplacental resistance
- Screening modality for diagnosing preeclampsia and fetal growth restriction
- Started early in gestation, done at 13 weeks, 18 weeks, 28 weeks, 32 weeks.
- First trimester uterine artery Doppler—prediction of early onset preeclampsia to administer aspirin early
- Diastolic notching—early diastolic notch is common feature in pregnancy.

Technique

- Performed at 11–13 weeks + 6 days
- Maternal bladder emptied

- TAS (preferred) or TVS
- Convex array probe
- Midsagittal section of uterus and cervix
- Lateral movement of transducer to identify aliasing uterine arteries ascending alongside
- **Pulsed Doppler**:
  - Uterine arteries close to internal os
  - 2 mm sample gate
  - Low filter
  - <30-degree angle of insonation
  - PSV should be >60 cm/s—rule out measurement of arcuate arteries
- Both sides reported
- Mean PI calculated
- Conversion to MoM units
- Mean uterine artery PI > 95th percentile- positive screening

Uterine artery Doppler in fetal growth restriction **(Figs. 42 and 43)**:

- **Small for gestational age**: Normal
- **Fetal growth restriction stage 1**: PI > 95 percentile
- **Fetal growth restriction stage 2,3,4**: PI > 99 percentile
- Lesser the better

16. Right pelvic pain in a woman—causes and imaging. [10] [DNB June 22]

Causes of right pelvic pain in a young female patient **(Table 38)**

Approach to a Young Female Patient with Acute Pelvic Pain (Flowchart 20)

Imaging Features of Ovarian Torsion

- **Mode ultrasound**:
  - Enlarged midline ovary
  - Heterogenous echogenicity due to edema and hemorrhage
  - May be hypoechoic or hyperechoic.
  - Follicles displaced towards periphery
  - Central echogenic stroma
- **Follicular ring sign**—echogenicity around the follicles

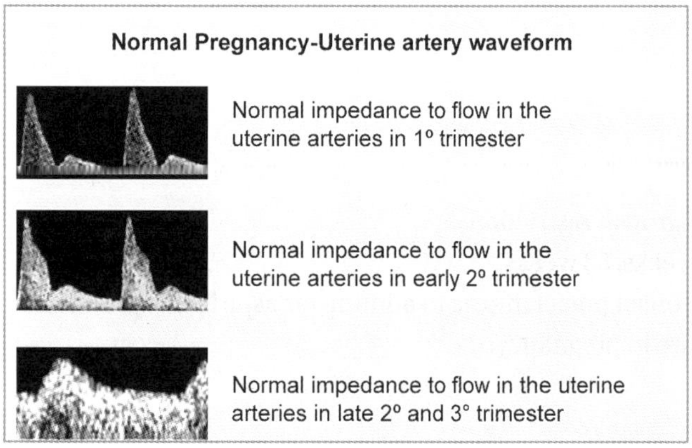

FIG. 42: Normal uterine artery Doppler waveform.

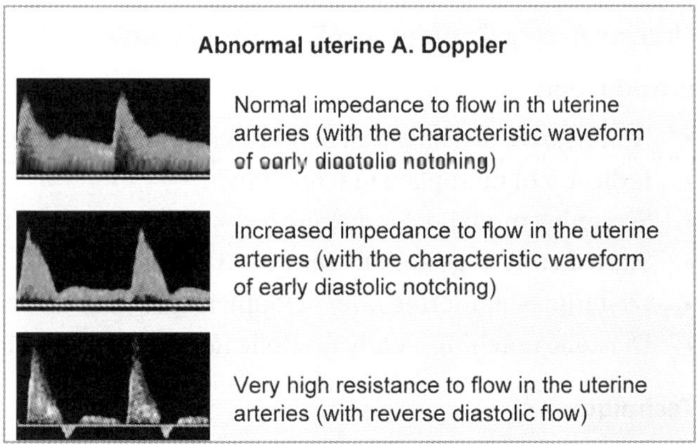

FIG. 43: Abnormal uterine artery Doppler waveform.

TABLE 38: Causes of right pelvic pain in a young female patient.

Gynecologic causes	*Nongynecologic causes*
• Complications of pregnancy – Abortion – Ectopic pregnancy • Ovary – Rupture of a cyst – Torsion of a cyst – Bleeding of corpus luteum – Mittelschmerz – Ovarian hyperstimulation syndrome • Fallopian tubes – Torsion – Infection • Uterus – Degeneration of leiomyomas – Torsion of a fibroid – Pyometra – Endometritis • Acute pelvic inflammatory disease	• Gastrointestinal tract – Appendicitis – Diverticulitis – Mesenteric lymphadenitis – Bowel obstruction • Urinary tract – Cystitis – Pyelonephritis – Nephrolithiasis • Vascular – Mesenteric vascular disease – Aortic aneurysm • Musculoskeletal • Metabolic – Porphyria – Sickle-cell crisis • No evident organic abnormality

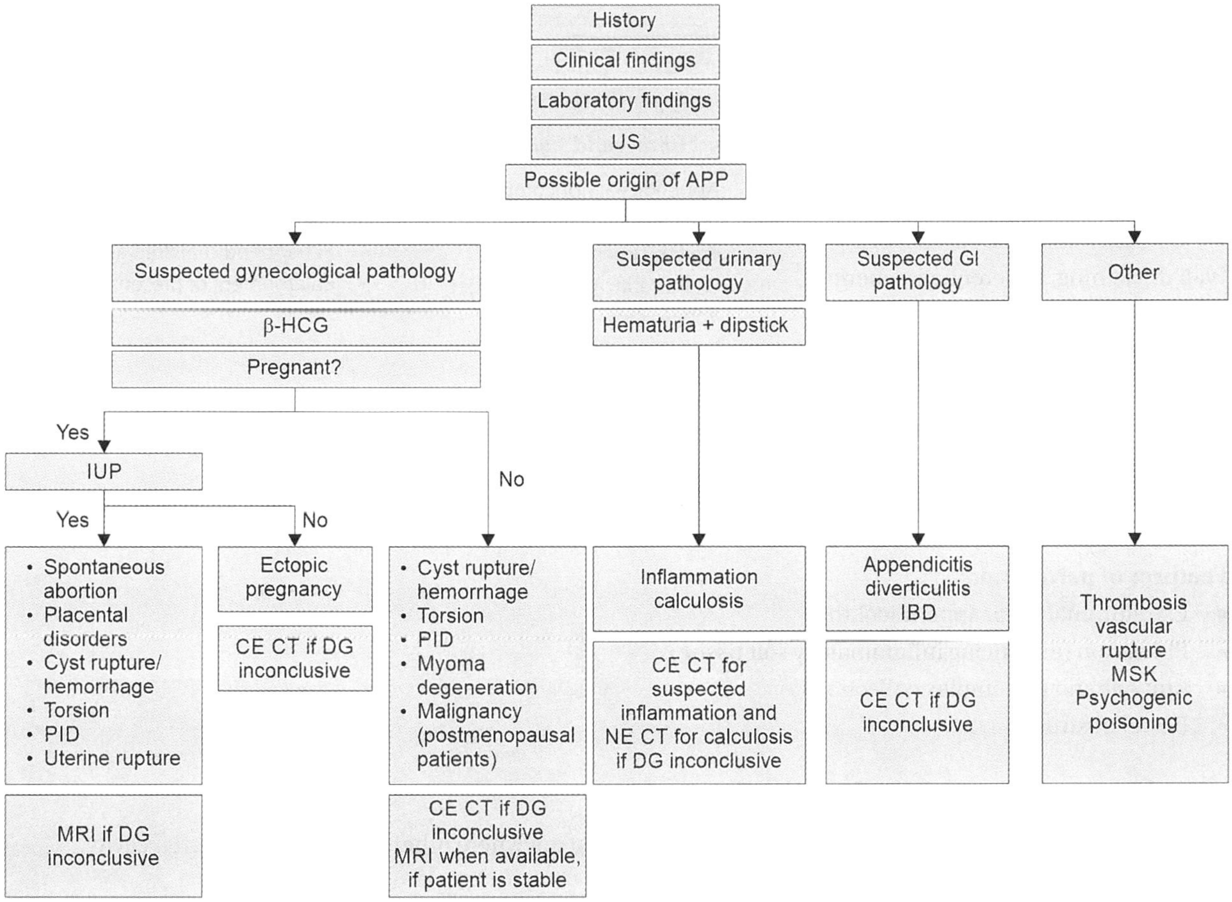

FLOWCHART 20: Approach to a young female patient with acute pelvic pain.

- Adnexal mass identified as the cause of torsion.
- Intraperitoneal free fluid in pelvis.
- Probe tenderness
- **Doppler**:
  - Reduced or absent arterial flow
  - High resistance flow
  - Whirlpool sign: Twisted pedicle giving the appearance of whirlpool
  - Blood flow may be normal if concomitant uterine artery supply is present.
- **Contrast Enhanced CT or MR**:
  - Enlarged midline ovary
  - May be deviated to one side
  - Nonenhancing—if infarcted.
  - Presence of edema, hemorrhage and necrosis
  - Tubal thickening may be present.
- **Management**:
  - Surgical emergency
  - Detorsion and adnexal preservation tried as soon as possible—in young.
  - Salpingo-oophorectomy—if family is complete.

Imaging Features of Appendicitis (Table 39)

CT

- Highly sensitive
- Radiation exposure
- Reserved for patients having
  - Equivocal ultrasound findings
  - Perforation
  - Complications like abscess etc.
- Wall thickening, hyperenhancement
- Appendicolith may be present
- Periappendiceal fat stranding
- Mesenteric lymphadenopathy
- Upper limit of diameter of appendix 10 mm, 6–10 mm equivocal in the absence of other findings.
- Cecal wall thickening
- Arrowhead sign—administration of contrast gives a triangular configuration at the cecum due to wall thickening
- Cecal bar sign—bar like inflammatory tissue between cecum and appendix
- **Features of perforation**:
  - Extraluminal air or appendicolith
  - Phlegmon (enhancing inflammatory soft tissue)
  - Rim enhancing complex collections
  - Bowel obstruction

TABLE 39: Imaging features of acute appendicitis.

Acute Appendicitis: Pearls to Remember	
Direct Ultrasound Signs	***Indirect Ultrasound Signs***
• Appendiceal noncompressibility • Diameter >6 mm • Wall thickness >3 mm • Wall stratification and target appearance • Wall hyperemia • Appendicolith	• Increased echogenicity of periappendiceal fat • Periappendiceal fluid and abscess • Enlargement of mesenteric nodes

17. USG in ectopic pregnancy. [10] [DNB June 22]

Definition of ectopic pregnancy: Implantation of the blastocyst anywhere other than the endometrial cavity.

- **Types of ectopic pregnancy**:
  - Tubal (most common)
  - Interstitial
  - Cornual

- Ovarian
- Cervical
- Scar
- Intraabdominal
- **Incidence**: 6–16%
- **Risk factors**:
  - Past history of ectopic pregnancy
  - Pelvic inflammatory disease
  - Past history of gynaecological surgery
  - Presence of IUCD
  - In vitro fertilization
  - Congenital anomalies of uterus

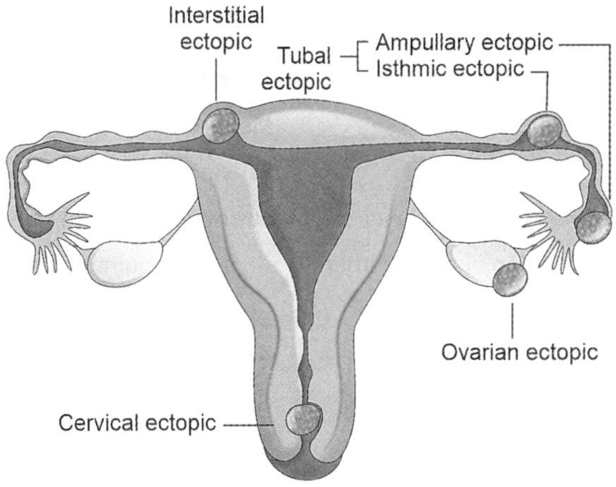

FIG. 44: Schematic diagram showing different locations of ectopic gestation.

USG Findings in Ectopic Pregnancy (Table 28 and Fig. 44)

Pregnancy of Unknown Location

- A transient stage when no definite intrauterine pregnancy (IUP) is detected on transvaginal ultrasound and no sign of ectopic pregnancy detected.
- **Beta human chorionic gonadotropin (hCG) level**: 1,000–2,000 mIU/mL without an IUP—suspicion of ectopic pregnancy.
- Serial beta HCG monitoring is needed.
- If rise of beta HCG >35% in the next 48 hours—highly suggestive of IUP
- <35% rise—indicates ectopic pregnancy.

18. Role of USG, CT and MRI in Endometrial Carcinoma. [10] [DNB Dec 21, DNB Dec 18]

Introduction

Carcinoma of the endometrium of the uterus is the most common gynaecological malignancy. Often develops from endometrial hyperplasia with atypia.

Epidemiology

More common in 6th–7th decade. Mean age 65 years.

Risk Factors

- Early menarche
- Late menopause
- Nulliparity
- Obesity
- Diabetes
- Hypertension
- **Drugs**: Hormone replacement therapy, Tamoxifen
- **Estrogen producing tumors**: Granulosa cell tumor, thecoma, endometroid carcinoma
- Lynch syndrome, polycystic ovarian syndrome
- Hereditary nonpolyposis colorectal cancer

Histological Types (Table 40)

Imaging Features

- **Ultrasound**:
  - Enlarged uterus
  - Thickened heterogenous poorly defined endometrium

TABLE 40: Histological types of endometrial carcinoma.		
Features	***Type 1***	***Type 2***
	More common (80%)	Rare (20%)
Prone population	Early postmenopausal women	Older patients
Relation with estrogen	Strong relation with estrogen excess and obesity	No relation
Condition of endometrium	Atypical endometrial hyperplasia	Small atrophic uterus
Prognosis	Good	Worse
Pattern	—	May have pattern of ovarian malignancy
Examples	Grade 1and 2 endometrioid carcinoma	• Grade 3 endometrioid carcinoma • Clear cell • Serous • Papillary • Mixed • Undifferentiated • Carcinosarcoma

- Large endometrial mass may look polypoidal expanding the endometrial cavity
- May be seen as well-defined homogeneously echogenic lesion within the endometrial cavity—difficult to differentiate from endometrial hyperplasia or polyp.
- Cystic changes within the lesion.
- Collection within the endometrial cavity due to obstruction
- Interruption of subendometrial halo indicates invasion of myometrium.
- Cannot assess involvement of cervix, parametrium and suspicious lymph nodes

- **Doppler**:
  - Low resistance flow in subendometrial, endometrial and uterine arteries
  - No definite vascular stalk (to differentiate from endometrial polyp)
- **CT**:
  - Can detect advanced disease (stage III and above)
  - Important for assessing pelvic lymph nodes and extension to pelvic side walls
  - Cannot accurately evaluate myometrial and cervical invasion and bladder and rectal wall invasion.
- **PET CT**:
  - Useful for assessment of pelvic recurrence and distant metastasis.
  - Metabolically active lesions seen as FDG avid.
- **MR**:
  - Oblique axial and coronal images taken perpendicular to the axis of the endometrium
  - On T1WI, the mass is isointense to normal endometrium and on T2WI the mass is hypointense as compared to normal endometrium but hypointense as compared to the junctional zone.
  - The mass shows less contrast enhancement as compared to myometrium but is more enhancing as compared to the endometrium.
  - Thickened poorly defined endometrium
  - Hematometra or pyometra
  - Enlarged uterus
- **Invasion of cervix**:
  - Tumor may prolapse into the cervix—intactness of the cervical mucosa rules out cervical invasion
  - Invasion of junctional zone and myometrium assessed on T2w images.
  - Extension to the cervix—endocervical mucosa may or may not be disrupted.
  - If myometrium above the cervix is involved, microscopic extension into the cervix cannot be ruled out.

- **Invasion of bladder or rectum**:
  - Interruption of the T2 hypointense muscular wall of bladder and rectum
  - Mass lesion involving the rectal and bladder mucosa
  - Postcontrast images and DWI images increase the diagnostic confidence.
- **Postcontrast study**:
  - Postcontrast images crucial to determine the degree of invasion
  - Endometrial tumors are hypoenhancing except sarcomas (intense enhancement)
    - Early postcontrast (30–60 second)—for superficial myometrial invasion
    - Equilibrium phase (120–180 second)—for for deep myometrial invasion
    - Delayed phase (4–5 minutes)—cervical stromal invasion
- **DWI**:
  - Helps in delineation of the tumor from adenomyosis, fibroids, cornual lesions
  - Useful when junctional zonal anatomy is distorted.
  - Can show vaginal drop metastasis and peritoneal deposits.
  - Invasion into the parametrium:
    - Parametrial soft tissue intensity mass
    - Parametrial fat stranding
    - Whickering of the mass into the surrounding parametrium
    - Assessed on T2W images.
  - Evaluation of lymph nodes:
    - Pelvic, paraaortic and common iliac nodes are the drainage sites.
  - Lymph nodes with suspicious features:
    - More than 10 mm in short axis
    - Round morphology
    - Irregular margin
    - Heterogenous appearance
- **Pitfalls**:
  - Overestimation of the depth of invasion due to the presence of leiomyoma, adenomyosis, cornual tumor.
  - Uterine cornua are thin so overestimation of myometrial invasion is possible.
  - Mimics of endometrial cancer:
    - Secretory or hyperplastic endometrium
    - Retained blood products
  - These are differentiated by T1 and postcontrast images.
  - Metastasis to ovary:
    - Bilateral
    - Morphologically similar to endometrial mass
    - Endometrial mass is larger than ovarian mass
- **Primary synchronous tumor of ovary**:
  - Unilateral
  - Presence of lesions like endometriosis
  - Low grade endometrial mass without invasion

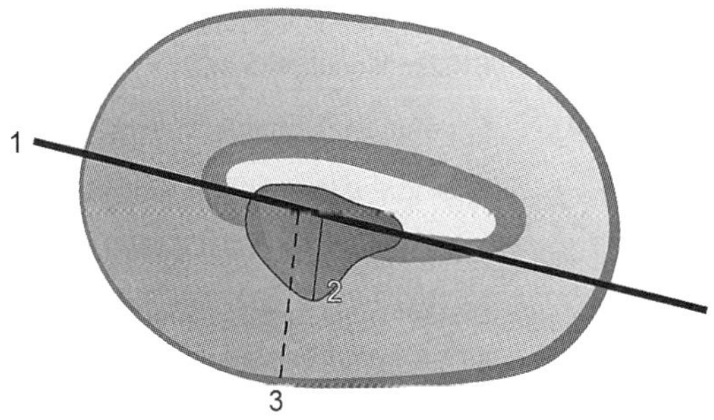

FIG. 45: Measurement of myometrial invasion.

Measurement of Myometrial Invasion (Gordon's Method) (Fig. 45)

- A Line is drawn over the expected inner edge of the myometrium
- Two lines are drawn perpendicular to the previous line
  - A line measuring the thickness of the tumor (2)
  - Another line measuring the thickness of the whole of the myometrium (3)
  - (2)/(3) gives percentage of myometrial invasion.
  - >50% means deep myometrial invasion upstaging the tumor to IB.

Staging of Endometrial Carcinoma (Table 41)

TABLE 41: FIGO staging of endometrial carcinoma.

Stage	*Description*
Stage I	Confined to the uterine corpus and ovary
IA	Disease limited to the endometrium OR nonaggressive histological type, i.e., low-grade endometrioid, with invasion of less than half of myometrium with no or focal lymphovascular space involvement (LVSI) OR good prognosis disease **IA1**: Nonaggressive histological type limited to an endometrial polyp OR confined to the endometrium **IA2**: Nonaggressive histological types involving less than half of the myometrium with no or focal LVSI **IA3**: Low-grade endometrioid carcinomas limited to the uterus and ovary
IB	Nonaggressive histological types with invasion of half or more of the myometrium, and with no or focal LVSI
IC	Aggressive histological types limited to a polyp or confined to the endometrium
Stage II	Invasion of cervical stroma with extrauterine extension OR with substantial LVSI OR aggressive histological types with myometrial invasion
IIA	Invasion of the cervical stroma of nonaggressive histological types
IIB	Substantial LVSI of nonaggressive histological types
IIC	Aggressive histological types with any myometrial involvement
Stage III	Local and/or regional spread of the tumor of any histological subtype
IIIA	Invasion of uterine serosa, adnexa, or both by direct extension or metastasis **IIIA1**: Spread to ovary or fallopian tube (except when meeting stage IA3 criteria) **IIIA2**: Involvement of uterine subserosa or spread through the uterine serosa
IIIB	Metastasis or direct spread to the vagina and/or to the parametria or pelvic peritoneum **IIIB1**: Metastasis or direct spread to the vagina and/or the parametria **IIIB2**: Metastatic to the pelvic peritoneum
IIIC	Metastasis to the pelvic or para-aortic lymph nodes or both **IIIC1**: Metastasis to the pelvic lymph nodes **IIIC1a**: Micrometastasis **IIIC1b**: Macrometastasis **IIIC2**: Metastasis to para-aortic lymph nodes up to the renal vessels, with or without metastasis to the pelvic lymph nodes **IIIC2a**: Micrometastasis **IIIC2b**: Macrometastasis
Stage IV	Spread to the bladder mucosa and/or intestinal mucosa and/or distant metastasis
IVA	Invasion of the bladder mucosa and/or the intestinal/bowel mucosa
IVB	Abdominal peritoneal metastasis beyond the pelvis
IVC	Distant metastasis, including metastasis to any extra- or intra-abdominal lymph nodes above the renal vessels, lungs, liver, brain, or bone

19. Role on USG and MRI in morbidly adherent placenta. [10] [DNB Dec 21, AIIMS May 23]

Introduction

Morbid adhesions of placenta also called Placenta accreta spectrum (PAS), is a term used to describe placenta accreta, increta and percreta. It results due to trophoblast invasion beyond decidua basalis.

Risk Factors

- Most commonly due to previous caesarean section and placenta previa.
- The risk factors for morbid adhesions of placenta (MAP) are presented as follows **(Table 27)**

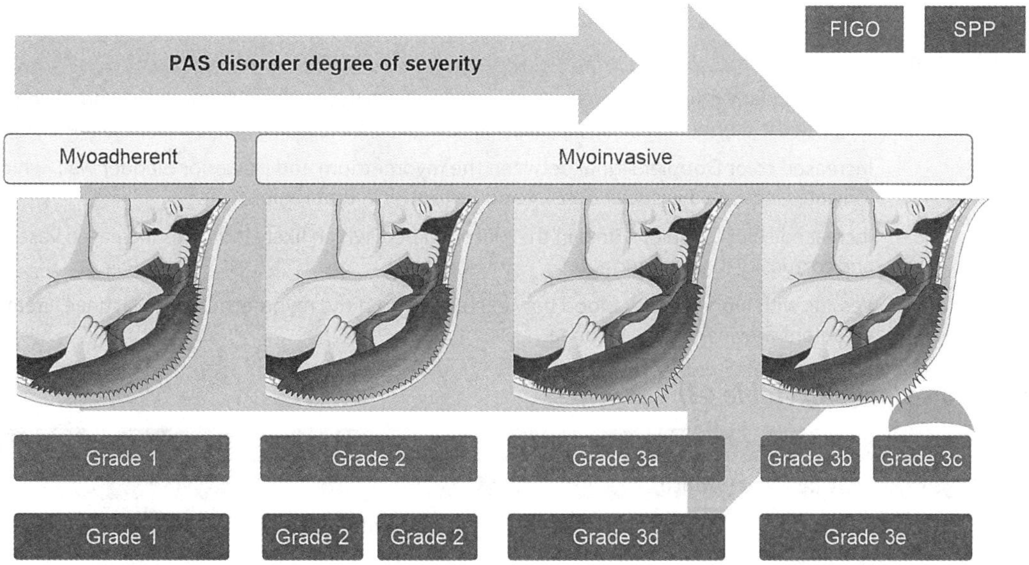

FIG. 46: Placenta accreta spectrum (PAS).

Pathophysiology

Occurs due to placental implantation at an area of abnormal decidualization allowing the chorionic villi to attach and invade into the myometrium.

Classification of Morbidly Adherent Placenta (Fig. 46)

- **Accreta**: Villi attach to the myometrium
- **Increta**: Villi penetrate into the myometrium
- **Percreta**: Villi penetrate through the myometrium to the uterine serosa or adjacent organs.

Imaging Features

Ultrasound with Color Doppler Findings (Table 42)

TABLE 42: US findings of PAS disorders.

US finding	*Description*
Gray-scale US features	
Abnormal placental lacunae	Presence of multiple lacunae, which are large irregularly shaped placental hypoechoic spaces that give the placenta a moth-eaten appearance. They can contain internal turbulent flow at gray-scale US Lacunae are usually centered within a lobule or cotyledon and are adjacent to the involved myometrium. These are not to be confused with placental lakes, which are features of a normal placenta and appear as a few small hypoechoic spaces with regular margins scattered throughout the placental tissue with slow flow (Movie 2).
Loss of retroplacental clear zone	Marked by obliteration or irregularity of the hypoechoic plane between the placenta and myometrium. This area can be falsely obscured by pressure from a distended urinary bladder and excess pressure from the ultrasound transducer.
Myometrial thinning	Asymmetric thinning of myometrium overlying the placenta relative to myometrium not covered by placenta. This can be focal or diffuse, with the myometrium measuring <1 mm or being nonvisible. It is associated with prior hysterotomy scars or placental invasion.
Placental bulge	Focal bulge of the placenta in an area of myometrial thinning, leading to deviation of the uterine serosa from its expected plane and uterine contour deformity.
Bladder wall interruption	Disruption of the normally smoothly echogenic bladder wall, located between the uterine serosa and urinary bladder lumen.
Focal exophytic mass	Focal extension of placental trophoblastic tissue beyond the uterine serosa, most commonly into the bladder.

Continued...

Continued...

Color Doppler US features	
Bridging vessels	Perpendicularly oriented vessels seen extending from the placenta through the underlying myometrium and into the uterine serosa or extrauterine structures, including but not limited to the bladder.
Uterovesical hypervascularity	Increased color Doppler signal between the myometrium and posterior bladder wall, which likely indicates increased vascular density and tortuosity in that region.
Subplacental hypervascularity	Increased color Doppler signal in the placental bed, which likely indicates increased vascular density and tortuosity in that region.
Placental lacunae feeder vessels	Vessels with high-velocity blood flow extending from the myometrium into lacunae, creating turbulent flow within the lacunae.

Magnetic Resonance Imaging (Table 43)

TABLE 43: MRI findings of PAS.			
Spectral MRI findings of PAS (inside out approach)			
		Placenta percreta	
Placenta accreta and placenta increta			
IN	⟶		***OUT***
Placenta	***Placenta-myometrial interface***	***Myometrium***	***Extrauterine invasion***
• Dark intraplacental band • Heterogeneous placenta • Placental bulge • Lumpy contour and rounded edge • Abnormal/disorganized placental vascularity	Thinning or loss of retroplacental T2 dark zone	• Myometrial thinning • Focal disruption of myometrium	• Bladder or adjacent structural invasion • Focal exophytic mass sign

- **Dark intraplacental bands**:
  - Random linear T2 hypointense bands, at maternal surface of placenta.
  - Caused by fibrin due to recurrent hemorrhage and infarction.
  - Irregular and thicker than placental septa
- **Heterogeneous placenta**:
  - Due to hemorrhage, intraplacental bands and flow voids
  - Different from heterogeneity due to aging in third trimester – because of calcifications, vascular lakes
  - Subjective indicator
- **Placental bulge**:
  - Implantation of placenta in lower uterine segment causes bulging of the uterus
  - Diffuse or focal
  - Snowman appearance of uterus (normally inverted pear shaped)
- **Lumpy contour, rounded edge**:
  - Smooth placental contour, angled edges
  - Due to tethering of placenta
- **Abnormal vascularity**:
  - Dilated tortuous signal voids or clump of placental vessels on T2
  - May extend into myometrium
  - Can cross uterine serosa
  - Extensive vascularity around uterus, cervix, bladder and vagina
  - Adjacent to areas of dark intraplacental bands
  - Stripped fetal vessel sign: Large caliber vessel between fetal and maternal placental surface with no change in vessel caliber

- **Loss of retroplacental dark zone**:
  - If present—interruption of placenta—myometrial interface
  - Associated with—focal myometrial defect or thinning
  - Extension of placental tissue into myometrium
- **Thinning of myometrium**:
  - Earliest MRI sign suggesting PAS
  - Can be <1 mm or imperceptible
- **Focal myometrial disruption**: Site of invasion

Complications

- Incomplete expulsion of the placenta at delivery
- Torrential hemorrhage when placenta is attempted to be taken out

Role of Interventional Radiology

Balloon occlusion of the internal iliac arteries or distal aorta till the time of delivery and hysterectomy.

20. Bleeding PV at 18 weeks. Causes and imaging findings. [5] [DNB Dec 21]

Bleeding PV at 18 Weeks

Causes

- Nonobstetric causes—cervicitis, vaginitis, polyp
- **Obstetric causes**:
  - Subchorionic hemorrhage
  - GTD
  - Spontaneous abortion
- USG features of causes of second-trimester bleeding **(Table 44)**:

Imaging Features of Spontaneous Abortion

Threatened Abortion

- **Definition**: Vaginal bleeding occurs, but the cervix remains closed, and the pregnancy may continue.
- **Ultrasound findings**:
  - Normal gestational SAC: A visible intrauterine gestational sac with an embryo and detectable fetal cardiac activity.
  - Subchorionic hemorrhage: This appears as a hypoechoic or anechoic crescent-shaped area adjacent to the gestational sac, indicating a subchorionic hematoma, a risk factor for miscarriage.

Inevitable Abortion

- **Definition**: Vaginal bleeding occurs with an open cervix, indicating that miscarriage is unavoidable.
- **Ultrasound findings**:
  - Cervical dilation: The internal cervical os appears open.
  - Gestational Sac in the lower uterine segment: The sac may be descending toward or through the cervix, which may indicate imminent expulsion.

TABLE 44: USG features of causes of second trimester bleeding.

Subchorionic hemorrhage	Hyperechoic collection elevating membranes, which becomes heterogeneous and heterogeneous and then hypoechoic (cystic) in 1–2 weeks
Gestational trophoblastic disease	• Complete mole—distended uterine cavity with multiple small cystic spaces, no embryonic tissue in utero • Partial mole—cystic spaces surrounding a distorted gestational sac; and • A fetal pole GTN—nonspecific focal masses within the endometrium and myometrium with marked vascularity due to arteriovenous shunting, cystic space representing focal necrosis or vascular spaces

Incomplete Abortion

- **Definition**: Partial expulsion of pregnancy tissue, with some retained products of conception (RPOC) in the uterus.
- **Ultrasound findings**:
  - Heterogeneous echogenic material in uterine cavity: Mixed echogenic material within the endometrium, indicating retained products.
  - Absence of intact gestational sac: The gestational sac is often disrupted or absent.
  - Thickened endometrial stripe: Endometrial thickness greater than 15 mm suggests retained tissue.

Complete Abortion

- **Definition**: All products of conception have been expelled, and the uterus is empty.
- **Ultrasound findings**:
  - Empty uterus: No gestational sac or significant echogenic material is seen in the endometrial cavity.
  - Thin endometrial stripe: The endometrium appears thin, typically <15 mm, indicating that no retained products are present.
  - Resolution of symptoms: The patient's clinical symptoms (e.g., cramping, bleeding) typically resolve.

Retained Products of Conception (RPOC)

- **Definition**: Residual pregnancy tissue remains in the uterus after a miscarriage.
- **Ultrasound findings**:
  - Heterogeneous echogenic material: Echogenic material in the endometrial cavity, sometimes with blood flow on color Doppler imaging, indicates retained tissue.
  - Thickened endometrial stripe: The endometrium may appear thickened (>15 mm).

Role of Doppler Ultrasound

Doppler imaging: Color Doppler may show increased blood flow in cases of retained products of conception (RPOC), distinguishing it from normal postpartum changes or clot.

Algorithm for Managing Second Trimester Bleeding (Table 45 and Flowchart 21)

The different types of spontaneous abortion and their characteristics are presented in the following table **(Table 45)**.

TABLE 45: Different types of spontaneous abortion and their characteristics.

Types of spontaneous abortion			
Abortion classification	***Characteristics***	***Cervical Os***	***Passage of fetal tissue***
Threatened	Abdominal pain or bleeding in the first 20 weeks of gestation	Closed	None
Inevitable	Abdominal pain or bleeding in the first 20 weeks of gestation	Open	None
Incomplete	Abdominal pain or bleeding in the first 20 weeks of gestation	Open	Yes (some products of conception still remain in uterus)
Complete	Abdominal pain or bleeding in the first 20 weeks of gestation	Closed	• Complete passage of fetal parts and placenta • Uterus contracted
Septic	Infection of uterus during miscarriage, fever and chills. Usually due to *Staph. aureus*	• Open with purulent cervical discharge • Uterine tenderness	None or may be incomplete

21. Oligohydramnios. [5] [DNB Dec 21]

Introduction

Oligohydramnios is defined as amniotic fluid volume less than expected for the gestational age.

Associated with

- Posterior urethral valve
- Urethral atresia
- Prune belly syndrome
- Bilateral ureteropelvic junction obstruction
- Cloacal abnormalities in female fetus
- Fetal growth restriction—due to redistribution of more blood to cerebral arteries and less amount of blood to kidney
- Meckel gruber syndrome
- Sacral agenesis
- Vacterl association

Causes of Oligohydramnios

A. **Maternal**:
- Uteroplacental insufficiency:
  - Hypertensive disorders such as preeclampsia
  - Chronic hypertension
  - Collagen vascular disease
  - Nephropathy
  - Thrombophilia
- Maternal exposure to medications:
  - Angiotensin-converting enzyme (ACE) inhibitors
  - Angiotensin receptor blockers (ARBs)
  - Nonsteroidal anti-inflammatory drugs
  - Calcium channel blockers

B. **Placental**:
- Abruption
- Insufficiency
- Thrombosis
- Infarction
- Twin polyhydramnios—oligohydramnios sequence

C. **Fetal**:
- Renal anomalies:
  - Bladder outlet obstruction
  - Bilateral renal agenesis
  - Bilateral multicystic dysplastic kidney
  - Autosomal recessive polycystic kidney
  - Posterior urethral valve
  - Congenital megalourethra
- Chromosomal anomalies:
  - Trisomy 18
  - Triploidy

FLOWCHART 21: Algorithm for managing second trimester bleeding.

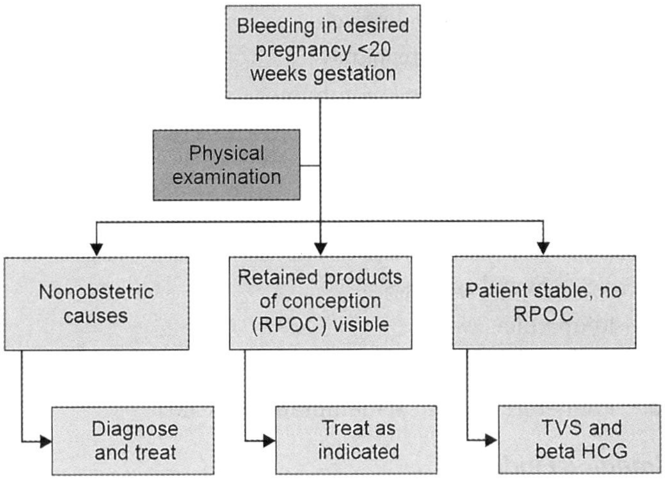

- Growth restriction
- Intrauterine demise
- Post-term pregnancy
- Ruptured fetal membranes
- TORCH and Parvovirus B19 infection

▪ Other anomalies:
- Meckel gruber syndrome
- VACERL
- Sacral agenesis

d. Idiopathic

c. Post-term pregnancy.

d. Premature rupture of membranes (PROM)

Imaging Findings

Diagnosed on transabdominal ultrasound.

- **Subjectively**:
  - Lack of fluid
  - Crowding of fetal parts
- **Criteria to diagnose oligohydramnios**:
  - Amniotic fluid index (AFI) <5 cm
  - AFI <5th centile for gestational age
  - Single deep vertical pocket (SDV) <2 cm
  - Borderline oligohydramnios- 5–8 cm
- **Grading oligohydramnios by SDP**:
  - <1cm—severe
  - 1–2 cm—mild
  - >2 cm—< 8 cm—normal

Complications of Oligohydramnios

1. **Pulmonary hypoplasia**:
   - Associated with long standing oligohydramnios.
   - There are five stages of lung development-
     - Embryonic
     - Pseudoglandular
     - Canalicular
     - Saccular
     - Alveolar

   In oligohydramnios, there is inadequate development of the acini and vascularization is restricted that occur during the **canalicular stage**.
2. Fetal growth restriction

Management

Depends on the etiology, severity and the gestational age at which oligohydramnios is discovered.

1. **Amnioinfusion**:
   - Can help detect fetal anomalies
   - Can prevent pulmonary hypoplasia in second trimester.
   - Can prevent cord compression in third trimester.

2. **Maternal hydration**: Drinking 1-2 liter of water can increase amniotic fluid volume in hypovolemic and idiopathic oligohydramnios patients.
3. **Left lateral decubitus**

22. MRI in Ca cervix. [5] [DNB Dec 21, AIIMS May 24]

Introduction

Cancer of the cervix is the third most common cancer after endometrial and ovarian cancers.

Epidemiology

- 35-50 years females
- Mean age 45 years

Risk Factors

- **Infection**: HPV 16 and 18
- **Sexual activity**: Multiple sexual partners, early age at first intercourse, high parity
- **Drugs**: Smoking oral contraceptives
- Low socioeconomic status

Pathophysiology

- Infection of the lower genital tract by HPV 16 and 18
- Precursor lesions develop in the **squamocolumnar junction** in a sequential manner
- Low grade dysplasia
- High grade dysplasia
- Cervical intraepithelial neoplasia
- Carcinoma in situ

Imaging Modality of Choice: MRI

- **Protocol**:
  - Magnet: 1.5T or 3T
  - Coil: pelvic phased array coil
  - Position: supine
  - Sequences taken:
    - T2W axial, coronal, sagittal images of pelvis
    - T1W axial images from kidneys to perineum
    - Oblique axial T2W—perpendicular to long axis of the cervix
    - Fat suppressed T2 axial
    - DWI with B value 800-1000 sec/mm^2
    - Dynamic postcontrast T1W (if required)
- **Patient preparation**:
  - 3-4 hours of fasting
  - Administration of Buscopan to reduce bowel movements

Imaging Features

- T2W images—cervix is normally hypointense due to dense fibrocollagenous stroma.
- Microscopic disease (stage IA) cannot be visualized.
- Macroscopic disease (stage IB and above) are well visualized on MRI.

Cervical Region

- Ulcerating, infiltrating or exophytic mass lesion
- Loss of normal hypointensity of the cervix on T2w images.
- Mass shows T1W isointense, T2W intermediate to hyperintense signal intensity
- Diffusion restriction in the mass lesion

- Early contrast enhancement
- Hydro/pyometra due to cervical obstruction.

Vaginal Extension

- Loss of normal T2 hypointensity of vaginal wall in case of invasion
- In case of extension, obliteration of the fornices without infiltration of the vaginal wall.

Invasion to Parametrium

- Spiculated extensions from the tumor to the parametrium
- Soft tissue intensity mass in parametrium
- Parametrial fat stranding
- Tumor infiltration into the surrounding vessels and ureter

Extension to Pelvic Wall

- Involvement of obturator internus, piriformis, or levator ani muscles by tumor
- Involvement of ureter may cause hydronephrosis
- Postcontrast enhancement of the mass and accurate delineation of the extension

Bladder and Rectal Invasion

- Nodular wall thickening
- Interruption of the normal T2 hypointense wall
- Postcontrast enhancement of the mass and accurate delineation of the extension

Lymph Node

- Pelvic and retroperitoneal lymph nodes measuring 10 mm or more in short axis.
- **Suspicious morphological characteristics**:
  - Round shape
  - Irregular margin
  - Central necrosis
  - Nodal group formation
- Assessed on T2W and DWI images—shows DWI restriction
- **Reporting checklist**:
  - Tumor size, extent
  - Involvement of bladder, rectum, ureter, vagina
  - Metastasis to bones, liver, peritoneum if any
  - Pelvic and para-aortic lymph nodes.

Staging

FIGO 2018 staging system for cervical cancer **(Box 7)**

BOX 7: FIGO 2018 staging system for cervical cancer.

Cervical cancer—FIGO stage

I Tumor confined to cervix (disregard extension to uterine corpus)

- IA Stromal invasion ≤5 mm (diagnosed by microscopy)
- IB Stromal invasion >5 mm
  Greatest tumor dimension ≤2 cm= IB1; 2-4 cm=1B2; >4 cm=1B3

II Invasion beyond uterus, but *not* to the lower 1/3 of vagina or pelvic sidewall

- IIA Invasion limited to upper 2/3 of vagina
- IIB With parametrial invasion

III Invasion of lower 1/3 of vagina, pelvic sidewall, or causing hydronephrosis

- IIIA Invasion of lower 1/3 of vagina
- IIIB Invasion of pelvic sidewall and/or hydronephrosis

IVA Invasion of bladder or rectal mucosa, or distant metastases

23. Antenatal MRI—indications, safety and protocols. [5] [DNB Dec 21]

Introduction

A novel technique in which the pregnant mother is put under MR scanner and fetal anatomic anomalies and placental abnormalities can be assessed.

Need of fetal MRI arises because of various limitations of ultrasound.[19]

Limitations of ultrasound leading to inadequate evaluation are:

- Due to oligohydramnios
- Due to fetal position obscuring some of the anatomical structures
- Maternal abdominal fat
- Inexperienced sonographer

Indications of fetal MRI (*refer* **Table 36**)

Patient Preparation

- The mother should not take anything peroral 4 hours before the examination to prevent artifacts from bowel peristalsis.
- Bladder should be emptied before the examination.

Protocol of Fetal MRI

- **Magnet**: 1.5T
- **Coil**: 4 or 8 element phased array surface coil, over the region of interest.
- **Position**: Supine or left decubitus to prevent compression of the inferior vena cava by the gravid uterus with feet entering the magnet.
- **H/O claustrophobia**: Sublingual BZD 1 hour prior to the examination.

Following the acquisition of a localizer sequence with respect to the mother using SSFSE T2 weighted sections (slice thickness 6-8 mm, gap 1-2 mm), images are graphically specified in fetal anatomic planes.

- For most studies, we capture single-shot rapid acquisition T2-weighted pictures with refocused echoes in the axial, coronal, and sagittal planes. T2-weighted images are useful to assess both anatomy and pathology.
- Certain sequences may need to be repeated because fetal mobility during acquisition distorts the image or causes images that are not in proper anatomic planes between sequences.
- Fetal landmarks may not be trustworthy due to transposition, hence fetal anatomy should be lateralized as either right or left based on an examination of the fetal position in relation to the mother.
- Although having a large matrix, thin sections and small field of view gives us high spatial resolution images, it shouldn't be overdone since gains might be negated by the "wrap" artifact and a lower signal-to-noise ratio.
- **Fetal brain**: 3 mm slice thickness in all planes.
- **Other fetal organs**: 4 mm slice thickness
- **Special techniques used in fetal MRI**:
  - Parallel imaging
  - Fast sequences to reduce motion artifacts
  - Free breathing sequences
  - Single slice acquisitions techniques used
- Usually done after 20 weeks
- After 26 weeks—all organs seen in detail.
- **Exposure limit according to FDA for maternal body**: 4 W/kg
- SAR of mother—2 W/kg
- SAR of fetus—1.24 W/kg in 1.5T and 1.14 W/kg in 3T

MRI Sequences

- T1-2D GRE
- T2-SSH-TSE/T2-SSFSE/HASTE
- b-FFE/FIESTA/true-FISP
- **Ultrafast GRE**: TFE/FMPSPGR/turbo-FLASH
- DWI (b: 0 and 700s/mm^2)

Advantages

1. Superior soft tissue contrast—in regions like brain and spine
2. Detailed brain imaging for detecting brain abnormalities such as ventriculomegaly, cortical malformations and hemorrhage that might not be clear on an ultrasound.
3. No ionizing radiation—unlike CT, MRI does not use ionizing radiation, making it safe for both the mother and the fetus.
4. Improved evaluation of complex anatomy: MRI offers a detailed view of the anatomy of vital organs, which is especially beneficial for diagnosing complex congenital malformations.
5. Complementary to ultrasound—fetal MRI is often used in conjunction with ultrasound when the latter's results are inconclusive, providing a more detailed follow-up investigation.
6. Better visualization in cases of maternal obesity or oligohydramnios
7. Detection of subtle anomalies—MRI can detect subtle fetal anomalies like small hemorrhages or white matter injuries that are difficult to visualize on an ultrasound.

Disadvantages of Fetal MRI

- High cost
- Limited availability
- Maternal pacemaker, ferromagnetic implants
- Claustrophobia
- Energy deposition (SAR)
- Acoustic noise reaching the fetal ears
- Fetal nerve stimulation
- Potential teratogenic effects due to heating by gradient changes and nonthermal interaction of fetal tissue with electromagnetic field

24. Different variety of gestational trophoblastic disease and role of imaging. [10] DNB June 21]

Introduction

Gestational trophoblastic disease (GTD)—a group of benign and malignant tumors which arise due to abnormal trophoblastic proliferation within the uterus.

Different Types of Gestational Trophoblastic Diseases

- Complete hydatidiform mole
- Partial mole or triploidy
- Invasive mole or chorioadenoma destruens
- Choriocarcinoma
- Placental site trophoblastic tumor
- Epithelioid trophoblastic tumor

Varieties of Gestational Trophoblastic Disease

1. **Hydatidiform mole (molar pregnancy)**:
   - Complete mole: Occurs when secondary oocyte with no genetic material is fertilized, leading to abnormal proliferation of trophoblastic tissue. No fetal tissue is present. It is benign but has malignant potential.

- Partial mole: Occurs when two sperm fertilize a normal egg, resulting in an abnormal fetus and trophoblastic proliferation. Fetal tissue may be present but is nonviable.

2. **Invasive mole**: This is a locally invasive tumor derived from a hydatidiform mole that invades the uterine wall. It is still composed of trophoblastic tissue but has the potential to spread to other organs.
3. **Choriocarcinoma**: A highly malignant form of GTD that arises from trophoblastic tissue. It can occur after a molar pregnancy, abortion, or normal pregnancy. It has a high propensity to metastasize to the lungs, liver, and brain.
4. **Placental site trophoblastic tumor (PSTT)**: A rare form of GTD that arises from the placental implantation site. It is slower-growing compared to choriocarcinoma but can still be malignant and metastasize.
5. **Epithelioid trophoblastic tumor (ETT)**: Another rare form of GTD that can mimic choriocarcinoma but is generally less aggressive. It arises from intermediate trophoblasts and may appear years after pregnancy.

Imaging Modalities

1. **Ultrasound (US)**: Primary modality for diagnosis:
   - Complete mole: Ultrasound typically shows a "snowstorm" or "cluster of grapes" appearance, where numerous cystic spaces replace the normal placental tissue. No identifiable fetus is present.
   - Partial mole: A fetus may be present with an abnormally large placenta containing cystic areas.
   - Invasive mole and choriocarcinoma: These may present as a heterogeneous uterine mass with areas of necrosis and hemorrhage on ultrasound, though definitive diagnosis may require further imaging.
   - Monitoring uterine involution and detecting persistent disease following evacuation of the mole.
   - Theca lutein cysts: Bilaterally enlarged ovaries with multiseptated cysts.
2. **Chest X-ray**: Since choriocarcinoma and other malignant forms of GTD often metastasize to the lungs, a chest X-ray is part of the initial workup. Multiple nodular lesions may be present in cases of lung metastases.
3. **CT scan (computed tomography) for staging and metastasis detection**:
   - Chest, abdomen, and pelvis CT: This is used to evaluate for metastatic disease in cases of malignant GTD, especially in choriocarcinoma. Common metastatic sites include the lungs, liver, brain, and pelvic lymph nodes.
   - Uterine invasion: In invasive moles and choriocarcinoma, CT can reveal the extent of the tumor's invasion into the uterine wall and surrounding structures.
4. **MRI (magnetic resonance imaging)**:
   - For evaluating local invasion of GTD into the myometrium and adjacent tissues
   - Superior soft-tissue contrast.
   - Differentiating GTD from other causes of abnormal uterine growth (e.g., fibroids or retained products of conception).
   - MRI findings: GTD typically shows heterogeneous signals with areas of hemorrhage. MRI is often used when there is concern about uterine or pelvic spread, particularly in invasive moles and placental site trophoblastic tumors (PSTT).
5. **PET-CT (positron emission tomography-computed tomography)**:
   - PET-CT is used in cases of suspected or confirmed metastatic choriocarcinoma.
   - For identifying distant metastatic disease
   - Monitoring response to chemotherapy.
   - Choriocarcinoma is highly metabolically active and shows increased uptake of radiotracers.

Imaging Findings by GTD Variety

1. **Complete mole**:
   - Ultrasound: No fetus, cystic or "snowstorm" appearance with diffuse trophoblastic tissue.
   - CT or MRI: May show an enlarged uterus filled with heterogeneous masses or cysts.

     MR findings

     i. Isointense to myometrium on T1. Hemorrhagic areas are hyperintense
     ii. Markedly hyperintense mass on T2
     iii. Post-contrast study: Avid enhancement
     iv. Modality of choice for evaluating myometrial invasion

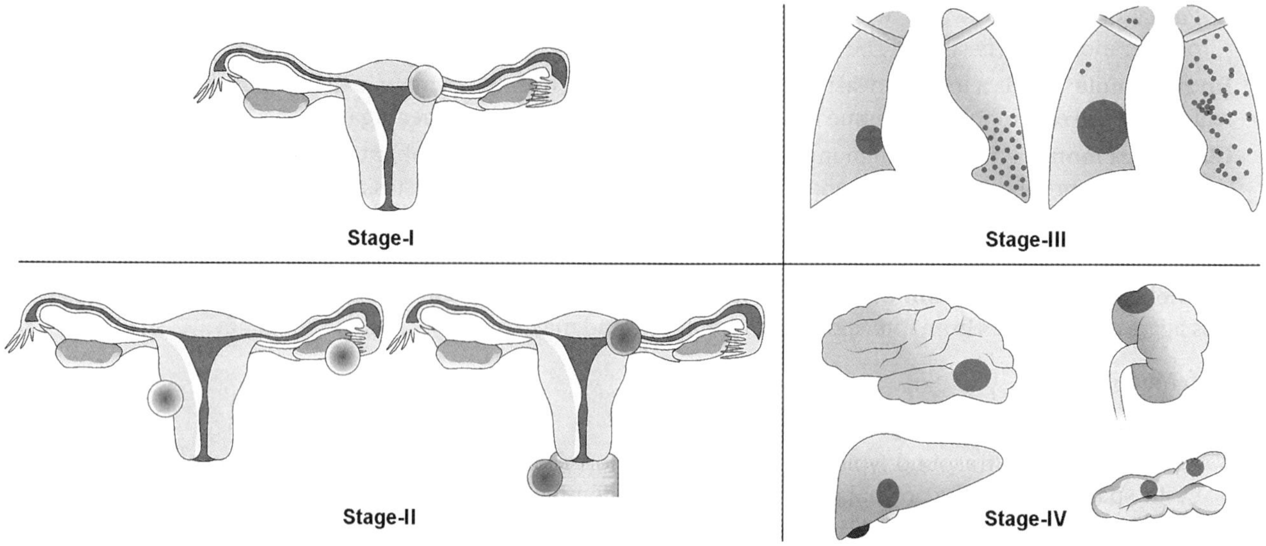

FIG. 47: The FIGO anatomic staging of GTD.

2. **Partial mole**: Ultrasound—fetus may be present, along with a thickened placenta with cystic spaces.
3. **Invasive mole**:
   - Ultrasound: Similar to molar pregnancy but with invasion into the myometrium.
   - CT/MRI: Shows myometrial invasion with uterine enlargement and heterogeneous mass.
4. **Choriocarcinoma**:
   - Ultrasound: Irregular masses within the uterus, possibly with hemorrhage.
   - CT/MRI: Uterine mass with potential invasion, hemorrhage, and necrosis. Metastasis can be seen in the lungs, liver, or brain.
   - PET-CT: High metabolic activity, useful for metastatic disease assessment.
5. **PSTT and ETT**:
   - MRI/CT: Localized uterine masses with myometrial invasion. These tumors have a more solid appearance compared to other forms of GTD.

The FIGO anatomic staging of GTD is presented as follows **(Fig. 47 and Table 46)**

TABLE 46: The FIGO anatomic staging of GTD.

Stage I	Disease confined to the uterus
Stage II	GTN extends outside of the uterus but is limited to genital structures (adnexa, vagina, broad ligament)
Stage III	GTN extends to the lungs, without genital tract involvement
Stage IV	All other metastatic sites

25. (a) Imaging evaluation of female presented with infertility, (b) MRI imaging feature of uterine adenomyosis. [10] [DNB June 21, AIIMS May 23]

Introduction

Infertility is failure of conception for 12 months or more by a couple having regular unprotected sexual intercourse after ruling out physiological causes such as lactational amenorrhea.

- Primary infertility—infertility in a couple who never had a child.
- Secondary infertility—failure of conception following a previous pregnancy.
- The causes of female infertility are listed (*refer* **Boxes 4 and 5**).
- Tubal occlusion is the most common cause of female infertility-assessed with hysterosalpingography first.

Imaging Evaluation of a Female Patient Presenting with Infertility

- **Modalities available**:
  - Hysterosalpingography (HSG)
  - Ultrasonography (USG)—color Doppler and 3D USG
  - Sonohysterosalpingography (SSG)
  - Hystero-salpingo-contrast sonography (HyCoSy)
- **Ultrasound of thyroid**: To look for causes of hypo/hyperparathyroidism
- **Transabdominal ultrasound**:
  - Position of kidneys
    - Presence or absence of uterus
    - Position of uterus: Ante/retroverted
    - Presence of intrauterine contraceptive or other devices
    - Endometrial thickness corresponding to the day of the cycle
    - Evaluation of fibroid, endometriosis, Müllerian anomalies (by using 3D ultrasound), hydrosalpinx
    - Volume of ovaries for polycystic ovarian syndrome (better evaluated on transvaginal scan)
- **Transvaginal ultrasound**: Evaluation of the same structures as transabdominal scan with better detail.

Hysterosalpingography—evaluation (Fig. 48):
- Fibroid, polyp
- Uterine synechiae
- Müllerian anomalies
- Infections like tuberculosis
- Cornual block

Fallopian tube abnormalities are better evaluated on HSG
MRI pelvis and hypothalamo-pituitary axis with dynamic contrast:

1. **MRI pelvis**:
   - Protocol:
     - 1.5–3T magnet
     - Pelvic phased array coil
     - Consent taken
     - Supine position of patient
     - Sequences taken:
       - Axial T1, T2, T2FS, DWI
       - Sagittal T2
       - Oblique coronal T2
   - Müllerian anomalies—septate, bicornuate uterus most commonly
   - The different congenital malformations of female genital tract (*refer* **Fig. 34**).

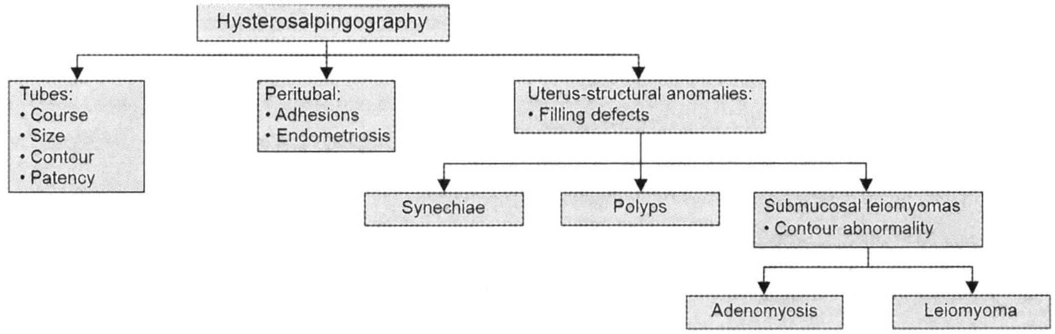

FIG. 48: Role of HSG in female infertility.

- The ESHRE-ESGE consensus on the classification of congenital malformations of the female genital tract (*refer* **Table 33**)
  - Pelvic masses—fibroid
  - Evaluation of endometriosis
2. MRI hypothalamo-pituitary axis with dynamic contrast: To look for pituitary micro or macroadenoma
   Process diagram showing systematic approach to diagnostic imaging for female infertility (*refer* **Flowchart 18**).

MRI Imaging Features of Uterine Adenomyosis

Introduction

- Benign pathological condition in which there is presence of ectopic endometrium within the myometrium
- Can be diffuse or focal
- Impaired uterine contractions lead to infertility
- Associated with endometriosis in <36 years of age

Hysterosalpingography

Diverticula filled with contrast protruding beyond endometrial cavity in a focal or diffuse manner.

Ultrasound

- Enlarged uterus with heterogenous myometrium
- Cysts within the myometrium
- Endomyometrial interface is indistinct
- Echogenic nodules in subendometrial location
- Linear striations
- Asymmetrical thickening of myometrium

Modality of choice: Pelvic MRI

Imaging features in MRI:

- Focal, diffuse or cystic variety
- Thickening of the junctional zone ≥12 mm.
- T1 foci of high signal—presence of hemorrhage
- Ill-defined or ovoid focal or diffuse thickening
- Features of endometriosis

Focal Adenomyosis or Adenomyoma (Figs. 49 and 50)

- Ill defined, noncapsulated
- T2 hypointense area with T2 hyperintense foci—suggestive of ectopic endometrial glands
- No diffusion restriction

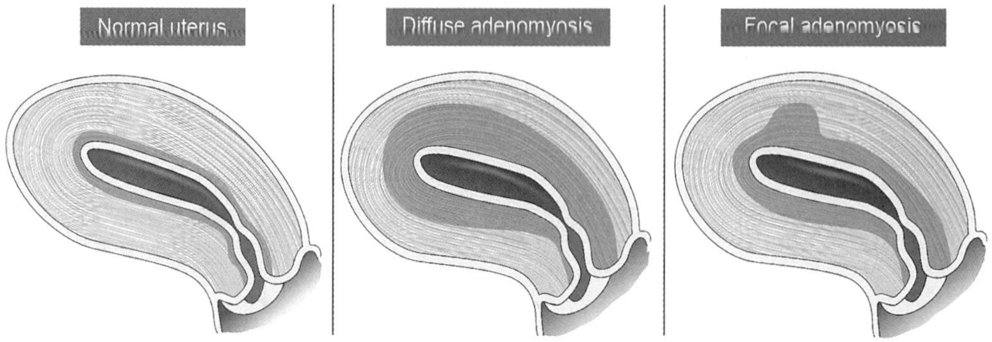

FIG. 49: Diffuse vs focal adenomyosis.

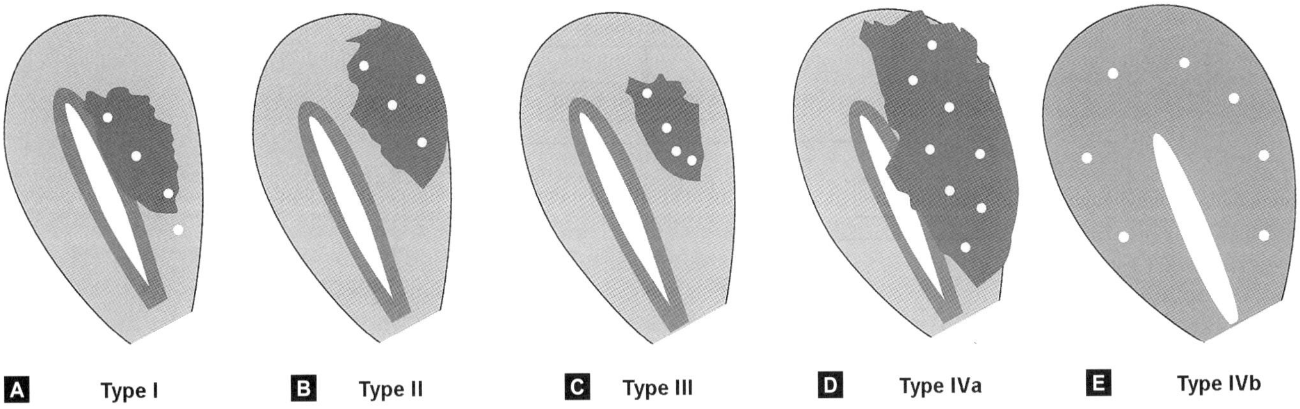

FIGS. 50A TO E: Schematic drawings of MRI classification of adenomyosis: (A) Type I—intrinsic focal adenomyosis; (B) Type II—extrinsic focal adenomyosis; (C) Type III—intramural focal adenomyosis; (D) Type IVa—diffuse adenomyosis with unilateral myometrium involved; (E) Type IVb—diffuse adenomyosis with bilateral myometrium involved.

26. (a) MRI evaluation method in ovarian mass, (b) differentiating features of benign and malignant ovarian mass on USG and MRI. [10] [DNB June 21]

The approach to incidental adnexal mass on CT or MR and MR evaluation of ovarian masses are presented **(Flowcharts 22–25)**.[20,21]

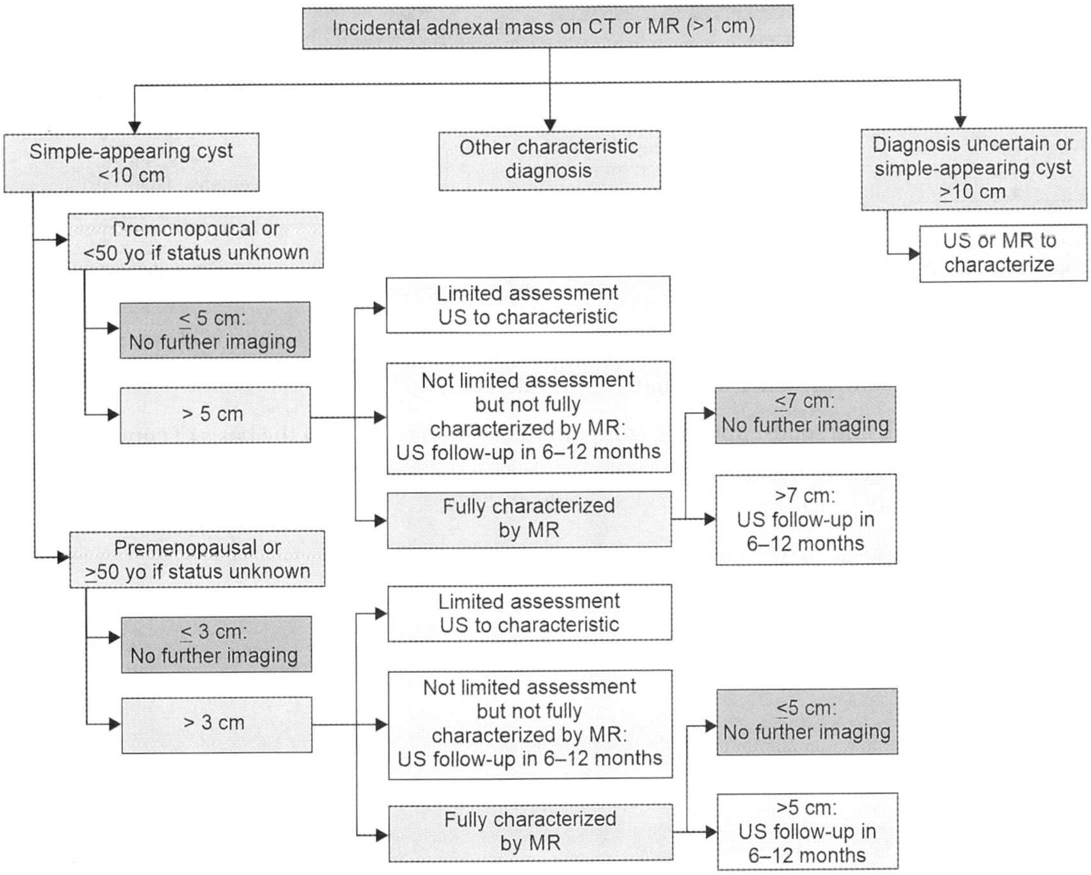

FLOWCHART 22: Algorithm for MRI evaluation of ovarian mass.

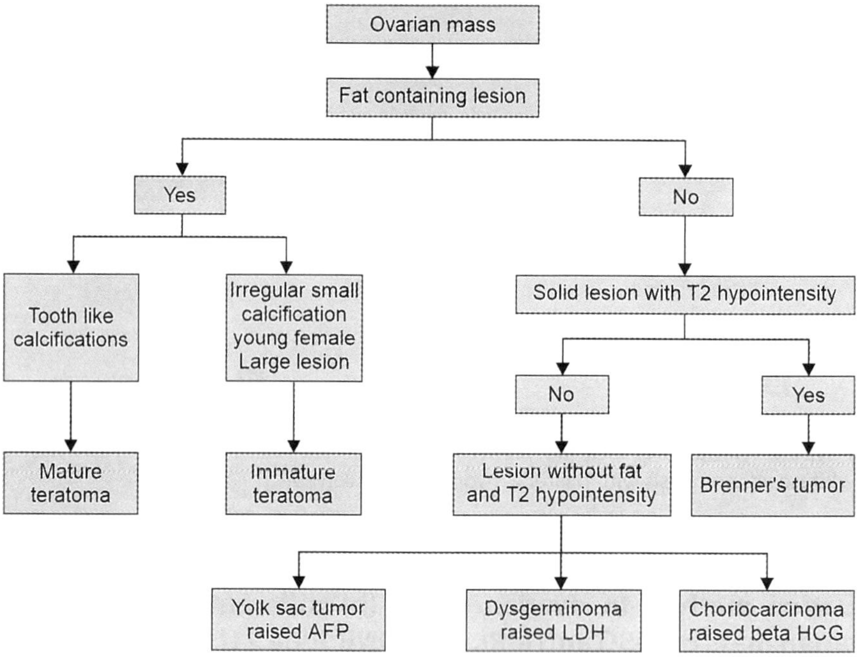

FLOWCHART 23: MR evaluation of ovarian masses.

Major sequences for evaluation of ovarian masses are T2W and T1FS.

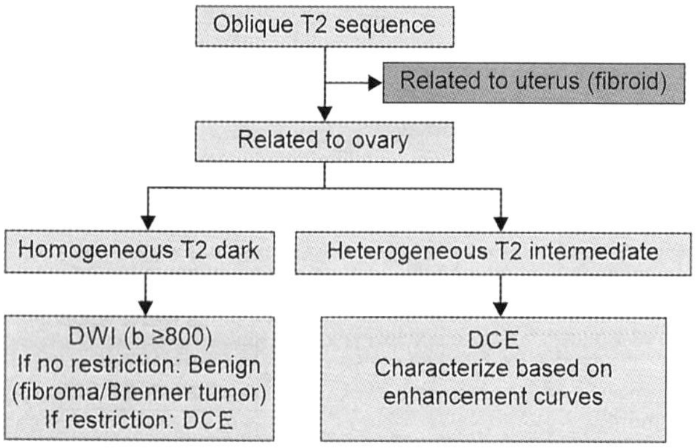

FLOWCHART 24: MR evaluation of ovarian masses–T2W.

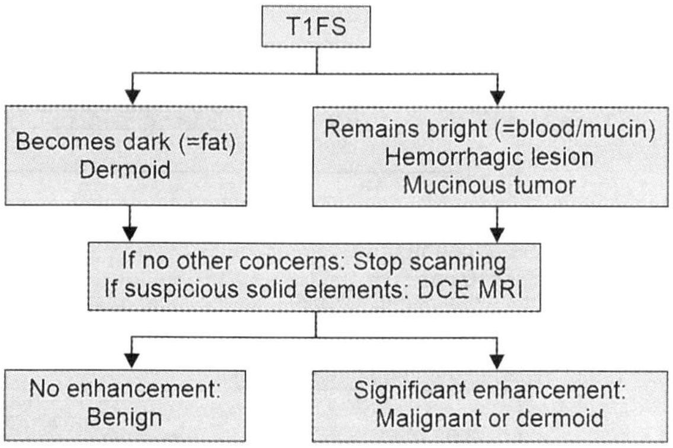

FLOWCHART 25: MR evaluation of ovarian masses–T1FS.

If no solid component is present, presence of malignancy is ruled out.

Differentiation between solid and solid-appearing component of lesion is done on the basis of contrast enhancement.

- **Solid enhancement on CE MRI**:
  - Mural nodule/Papillary projection
  - Irregular wall
  - Irregular septations
  - Large solid component
- **Solid-appearing component**:
  - Thin
  - Blood clot
  - Fat
  - Fibrin
  - Non-enhancing debris

Dynamic Contrast Enhancement Study (Figs. 51A to C)

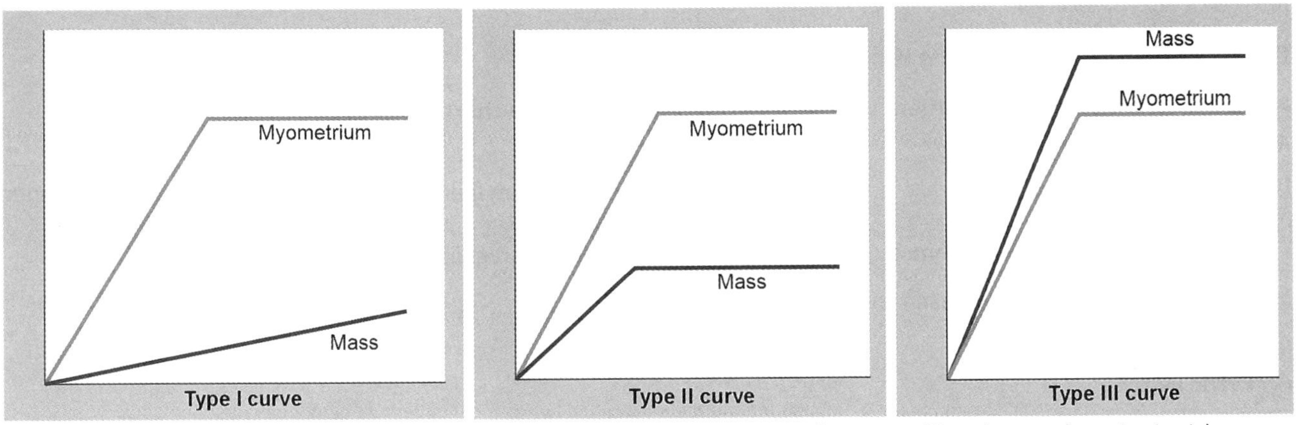

- Gradual increase in contrast uptake
- No plateau
- Most likely benign

- Moderate increase in contrast uptake
- Plateau present
- Indeterminate lesion

- Steep increase in contrast uptake
- Plateau at higher level than myometrium
- Most likely malignant

FIGS. 51A to C: (A) Type I curve on dynamic contrast enhanced study; (B) Type II curve on dynamic contrast enhanced study; (C) Type III curve on dynamic contrast enhanced study.

Differentiating Features of Benign and Malignant Ovarian Mass (Table 47)

TABLE 47: US and MRI features of benign and malignant adnexal masses.

	IOTA Simple Rules (US)	*A_{DNEX} MR Scoring System (MRI)*
Benign	B features: • Unilocular cyst • Solid components <7 mm in largest diameter • Presence of acoustic shadows • Smooth multilocular cystic mass <10 cm in largest diameter • No blood flow	A_{DNEX} MR Score 2: Benign mass • Purely cystic or fatty or endometriotic • No wall enhancement • + solid tissue with low signal on DWI and T2 sequences A_{DNEX} MR Score 3: Probably benign • Cystic + wall enhancement but no solid tissue, or • Solid tissue with a type 1 enhancement curve (gradual increase in signal intensity without a well-defined 'shoulder')
Malignant	M features: • Irregular solid tumor • Presence of ascites • >3 papillary structures • >3 mm in height • Irregular multilocular cystic-solid tumor 210 cm • Very strong blood flow	A_{DNEX} MR Score 5: Probably malignant mass • Peritoneal implants, or • Solid tissue with a type 3 enhancement curve (initial increase in signal intensity steeper than that of myometrium)
Comments	Rule 1: If one or more M features are present in the absence of B features, the mass is classified as *malignant* Rule 2: If one or more B features are present in the absence of M features, the mass is classified as *benign* Rule 3: If both M and B features are present, or if no M or B features are present, the result is *inconclusive* and a second stage test is recommended	NB: • A_{DNEX} MR Score 1: No adnexal mass • A_{DNEX} MR Score 4: Indeterminate • Solid tissue with a type 2 enhancement curve (moderate initial increase in signal intensity less steep than that of myometrium, followed by a plateau)

27. (a) Enumerate the causes of acute pelvic pain in a young female patient. (b) Role of imaging in ovarian torsion. [4+6]

Causes of Acute Pelvic Pain in a Young Female Patient (Box 8)

Approach to a Young Female Patient with Acute Pelvic Pain (*refer* Flowchart 20)

Role of imaging in ovarian torsion

Introduction: Twisting of the ovary along its vascular pedicle. Most often fallopian tube is also involved. So a broader term "adnexal torsion" is used.

Most commonly found on women of reproductive age especially in pregnancy.

Most common cause: Mature cystic teratoma

Clinical features

- Pelvic pain
- Tenderness
- Guarding
- Rigidity

Pathophysiology

- Twisting of vascular pedicle
- Blockage of venous flow and lymphatic drainage (walls are more collapsible as compared to muscular wall of arteries)
- Reduction of arterial flow
- Rapid engorgement
- Enlargement of the ovary
- Complete blockage of arterial flow
- Ovarian infarct

BOX 8: Causes of acute pelvic pain in a young female patient.

Gynecologic causes

- Complications of pregnancy
  - Abortion
  - Ectopic pregnancy
- Ovary
  - Rupture of a cyst
  - Torsion of a cyst
  - Bleeding of corpus luteum
  - Mittelschmerz
  - Ovarian hyperstimulation syndrome
- Fallopian tubes
  - Torsion
  - Infection
- Uterus
  - Degeneration of leiomyomas
  - Torsion of a fibroid
  - Pyometra
  - Endometritis
- Acute pelvic inflammatory disease

Nongynecologic causes

- Gastrointestinal tract
  - Appendicitis
  - Diverticulitis
  - Mesenteric lymphadenitis
  - Bowel obstruction
- Urinary tract
  - Cystitis
  - Pyelonephritis
  - Nephrolithiasis
- Vascular
  - Mesenteric vascular disease
  - Aortic aneurysm
- Musculoskeletal
- Metabolic
  - Porphyria
  - Sickle-cell crisis
- No evident organic abnormality

Modality of choice: Ultrasound with color Doppler

Imaging Features of Ovarian Torsion

B-mode ultrasound:

- Enlarged midline ovary
- Heterogenous echogenicity due to edema and hemorrhage
- May be hypoechoic or hyperechoic
- Follicles displaced towards periphery
- Central echogenic stroma
- Follicular ring sign—echogenicity around the follicles
- Adnexal mass identified as the cause of torsion
- Intraperitoneal free fluid in pelvis
- Probe tenderness

Doppler:

- Reduced or absent arterial flow
- High resistance flow
- **Whirlpool sign**: Twisted pedicle giving the appearance of whirlpool
- Blood flow may be normal if concomitant uterine artery supply is present.

Contrast enhanced CT or MR:

- Enlarged midline ovary
- May be deviated to one side
- Non enhancing - if infarcted.
- Presence of edema, hemorrhage and necrosis
- Tubal thickening may be present.

Management

- Surgical emergency
- Detorsion and adnexal preservation tried as soon as possible—in young.
- Salpingo-oophorectomy—if family is complete.

28. Enumerate various causes of post-menopausal bleeding in a 60-year-old female. Discuss the role of imaging in evaluation of endometrial carcinoma and its management based on staging. [2+(5+3)] [MD (WBUHS) 24]

Causes of Post-menopausal Bleeding in a 60-year-old Woman

- **Endometrium**:
  - Endometritis
  - Fibroid
  - Endometrial hyperplasia
  - Endometrial polyp
  - Endometrial carcinoma
  - Leiomyosarcoma of uterus
  - Infections: Pyometra
- **Cervix**:
  - Cervicitis
  - Cervical trauma

  - Cervical polyp
  - Cervical carcinoma
- **Vagina**:
  - Atrophic vaginitis
  - Vaginal malignancy
- **Ovary**:
  - Ovarian malignancy (estrogen producing)
- **Vulva**:
  - Trauma
  - Vulvar carcinoma
- **Drugs**:
  - Anticoagulant use
  - Hormone replacement therapy
- **Systemic disease**: Bleeding disorder (thrombocytopenia, leukemia, pancytopenia)
- No cause found

Imaging Features of Endometrial Carcinoma

- **Ultrasound**:
  - Enlarged uterus
  - Thickened heterogenous poorly defined endometrium
  - Large endometrial mass may look polypoidal expanding the endometrial cavity
  - May be seen as well-defined homogenously echogenic lesion within the endometrial cavity—difficult to differentiate from endometrial hyperplasia or polyp.
  - Cystic changes within the lesion.
  - Collection within the endometrial cavity due to obstruction
  - Interruption of subendometrial halo indicates invasion of myometrium.
  - Cannot assess involvement of cervix, parametrium and suspicious lymph nodes
- **Doppler**:
  - Low resistance flow in subendometrial, endometrial and uterine arteries
  - No definite vascular stalk (to differentiate from endometrial polyps)
- **CT**:
  - Can detect advanced disease (Stage III and above)
  - Important for assessing pelvic lymph nodes and extension to pelvic side walls
  - Cannot accurately evaluate myometrial and cervical invasion and bladder and rectal wall invasion.
- **PET CT**:
  - Useful for assessment of pelvic recurrence and distant metastasis.
  - Metabolically active lesions seen as FDG avid.
- **MR**:
  - Oblique axial and coronal images taken perpendicular to the axis of the endometrium
  - On T1WI, the mass is isointense to normal endometrium and on T2WI the mass is hypointense as compared to normal endometrium but hypointense as compared to the junctional zone.
  - The mass shows less contrast enhancement as compared to myometrium but is more enhancing as compared to the endometrium.
  - Thickened poorly defined endometrium
  - Hematometra or pyometra
  - Enlarged uterus

- **Invasion of cervix**:
  - Tumor may prolapse into the cervix—intactness of the cervical mucosa rules out cervical invasion
  - Invasion of junctional zone and myometrium assessed on T2W images.
  - Extension to the cervix—endocervical mucosa may or may not be disrupted.
  - If myometrium above the cervix is involved, microscopic extension into the cervix cannot be ruled out.
- **Invasion of bladder or rectum**:
  - Interruption of the T2 hypointense muscular wall of bladder and rectum
  - Mass lesion involving the rectal and bladder mucosa
  - Post contrast images and DWI images increase the diagnostic confidence.
- **Post-contrast study**:
  - Post-contrast images crucial to determine the degree of invasion
  - Endometrial tumors are hypoenhancing except sarcomas (intense enhancement)
  - Early postcontrast (30-60 sec)—for superficial myometrial invasion
  - Equilibrium phase (120-180 sec)—for deep myometrial invasion
  - Delayed phase (4-5 min)—cervical stromal invasion
- **DWI**:
  - Helps in delineation of the tumor from adenomyosis, fibroids, cornual lesions
  - Useful when junctional zonal anatomy is distorted.
  - Can show vaginal drop metastasis and peritoneal deposits.
  - Invasion into the parametrium:
    - Parametrial soft tissue intensity mass
    - Parametrial fat stranding
    - Whickering of the mass into the surrounding parametrium
    - Assessed on T2W images.
- **Evaluation of lymph nodes**: Pelvic, para-aortic and common iliac nodes are the drainage sites.
- **Lymph nodes with suspicious features**:
  - More than 10 mm in short axis
  - Round morphology
  - Irregular margin
  - Heterogenous appearance
- **Pitfalls**:
  - Overestimation of the depth of invasion due to the presence of leiomyoma, adenomyosis, cornual tumor.
  - Uterine cornu are thin so overestimation of myometrial invasion is possible.
  - Mimics of endometrial cancer:
    - Secretory or hyperplastic endometrium
    - Retained blood products
  - These are differentiated by T1 and postcontrast images.
- **Metastasis to ovary**:
  - Bilateral
  - Morphologically similar to endometrial mass
  - Endometrial mass is larger than ovarian mass
- **Primary synchronous tumor of ovary**:
  - Unilateral
  - Presence of lesions like endometriosis
  - Low grade endometrial mass without invasion

Measurement of Myometrial Invasion (Gordon's Method) (Fig. 52)

- 1 Line is drawn over the expected inner edge of the myometrium
- 2 lines are drawn perpendicular to the previous line
    - A line measuring the thickness of the tumor (2)
    - Another line measuring the thickness of the whole of the myometrium (3)
    - (2)/(3) gives percentage of myometrial invasion.
    - >50% means deep myometrial invasion upstaging the tumor to IB.

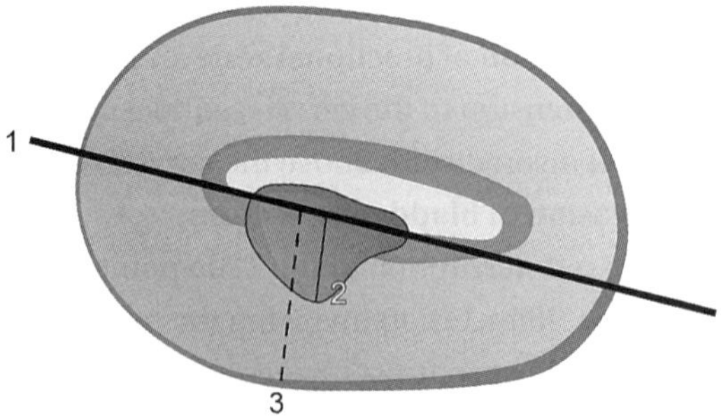

FIG. 52: Measurement of myometrial invasion.

Staging of Endometrial Carcinoma (refer Table 41)

Management

Based on lymph node status, staging, histological grade

- Stage 1A—total abdominal hysterectomy and bilateral salpingo-oophorectomy
- Stage 1B—total abdominal hysterectomy and bilateral salpingo-oophorectomy and **lymph node dissection**
- Stage 2—total abdominal hysterectomy and bilateral salpingo-oophorectomy and lymph node dissection ± **radiotherapy**
- Stages 3 and 4—debulking surgery with radiotherapy or brachytherapy ± chemotherapy

For type 2 endometrial carcinoma—total abdominal hysterectomy and bilateral salpingo-oophorectomy and lymph node dissection + **omentectomy and peritoneal biopsy**.

Recurrence or metastasis: Surgery or radiotherapy or chemotherapy or hormonotherapy or combination.
Absence of myometrial involvement is necessary for fertility sparing surgery **(Box 9)**.

BOX 9: Eligibility criteria for fertility preservation in patients with endometrial cancer.

All criteria to be met

- *Histopathology*
    - Histologic diagnosis with dilatation and curettage
    - Grade I (well differentiated) endometrioid adenocarcinoma

    Or
    - Premalignant conditions such as atypical hyperplasia or endometrial intraepithelial neoplasia
- MRI: Tumor confined to the endometrium (absence of myometrial invasion, cervical stromal invasion, ovarian metastases or synchronous primary ovarian cancer, and absence of lymphadenopathy)
- Clinical: Patient compliance for close follow-up during and after conservative treatment

29. Describe imaging algorithm in a suspected case ectopic pregnancy. Describe role of imaging in differentiating three common clinical mimics of ectopic pregnancy. [5+5] [MD (WBUHS) 24, DNB June 20]

The algorithm for diagnosis and management of suspected ectopic pregnancy is as follows **(Flowchart 26)**.

Clinical mimics of ectopic pregnancy:

1. Corpus luteum
2. Ovarian torsion
3. Early pregnancy loss
4. Incidental adnexal mass
5. Appendicitis
6. Ureteric calculi

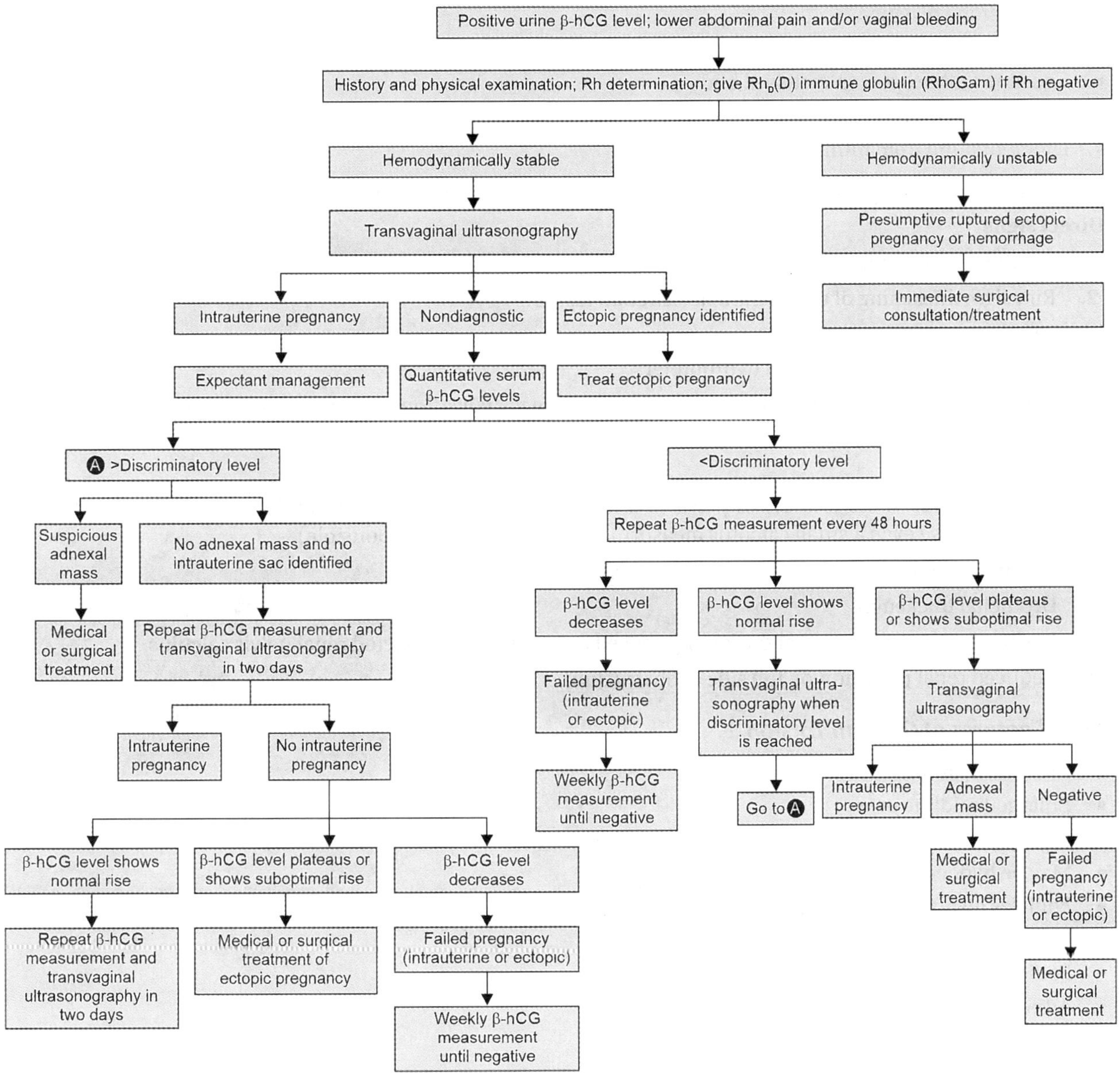

FLOWCHART 26: Algorithm for diagnosis and management of suspected ectopic pregnancy.

7. Subchorionic hemorrhage in viable intrauterine pregnancy
8. Pelvic inflammatory disease

Imaging Features of Ureteric Calculi

- **Ultrasound**:
  - Hyperechoic round to oval or curvilinear structure giving posterior acoustic shadowing
  - Most commonly found at vesicoureteric junction
  - Color Doppler—twinkling artifact
  - Proximal hydroureteronephrosis
- **CT**:
  - Location, size, HU value (for hardness on 120 kVp scan)
  - Stone heterogeneity index

- Skin to stone distance
- Distance from VUJ or PUJ
- Location with respect to vertebral body
- Stone characterization using dual energy CT scan
- Differentiation from mimics

Computed tomography signs of an obstructed system caused by ureteric calculus

- **Direct signs**
  1. Identification of stone
  2. Rim sign: thickening of urothelium in a circular fashion
- **Indirect signs**
  1. Hydronephrosis and proximal hydroureter
  2. Perinephric fat stranding, which is represented by the visualization of perirenal septa due to edema (perirenal cobwebs)
  3. Perinephric fluid
  4. Rupture of one of the fornices or pelvis in a high-pressure obstructed system. (This is unrelated to the size of stone because even a small calculus measuring 3 or 4 mm can be responsible).
  5. Periureteral edema
  6. Urothelial thickening
  7. Pyelitis: Inflammatory mural thickening caused by chronically impacted renal pelvis calculus
  8. Reduced renal perfusion on the side of obstruction.

Imaging Features of Ovarian Torsion

- **B-Mode ultrasound**:
  - Enlarged midline ovary
  - Heterogenous echogenicity due to edema and hemorrhage
  - May be hypoechoic or hyperechoic.
  - Follicles displaced towards periphery
  - Central echogenic stroma
  - Follicular ring sign-echogenicity around the follicles
  - Adnexal mass identified as the cause of torsion.
  - Intraperitoneal free fluid in pelvis.
  - Probe tenderness
- **Doppler**:
  - Reduced or absent arterial flow
  - High resistance flow
  - Whirlpool sign: Twisted pedicle giving the appearance of whirlpool
  - Blood flow may be normal if concomitant uterine artery supply is present.
- **Contrast enhanced CT or MR**:
  - Enlarged midline ovary
  - May be deviated to one side
  - Nonenhancing—if infarcted.
  - Presence of edema, hemorrhage and necrosis
  - Tubal thickening may be present.
- **Management**:
  - Surgical emergency
  - Detorsion and adnexal preservation tried as soon as possible – in young.
  - Salpingo-oophorectomy—if family is complete.

Imaging Features of Acute Appendicitis (Table 39)

CT

- Highly sensitive
- Radiation exposure
- Reserved for patients having
  - Equivocal ultrasound findings
  - Perforation
  - Complications like abscess, etc.
- Wall thickening, hyperenhancement
- Appendicolith may be present
- Periappendiceal fat stranding
- Mesenteric lymphadenopathy
- Upper limit of diameter of appendix 10 mm, 6–10 mm equivocal in the absence of other findings.
- Cecal wall thickening
- Arrowhead sign—administration of contrast gives a triangular configuration at the cecum due to wall thickening
- Cecal bar sign—bar like inflammatory tissue between cecum and appendix
- Features of perforation:
  - Extraluminal air or appendicolith
  - Phlegmon (enhancing inflammatory soft tissue)
  - Rim enhancing complex collections
  - Bowel obstruction

30. Describe various indications, protocol, advantages and disadvantages of fetal MRI. [2+3+3+2] [DNB June 20]

Introduction

A novel technique in which the pregnant mother is put under MR scanner and fetal anatomic anomalies and placental abnormalities can be assessed.

Need of fetal MRI arises because of various limitations of ultrasound.

Limitations of ultrasound leading to inadequate evaluation are:

- Due to oligohydramnios
- Due to fetal position obscuring some of the anatomical structures
- Maternal abdominal fat
- Inexperienced sonographer.

Indications of Fetal MRI (Table 36)

Patient Preparation

- The mother should not take anything peroral 4 hours before the examination to prevent artifacts from bowel peristalsis.
- Bladder should be emptied before the examination.

Protocol of Fetal MRI

- **Magnet**: 1.5T
- **Coil**: 4 or 8 element phased array surface coil, over the region of interest.
- **Position**: Supine or left decubitus to prevent compression of the inferior vena cava by the gravid uterus., with feet entering the magnet.

History of Claustrophobia—Sublingual BZD 1 hour prior to the examination.

Following the acquisition of a localizer sequence with respect to the mother using SSFSE T2 weighted sections (slice thickness—6–8 mm, gap 1–2 mm), images are graphically specified in fetal anatomic planes.

- For most studies, we capture single-shot rapid acquisition T2-weighted pictures with refocused echoes in the axial, coronal, and sagittal planes. T2-weighted images are useful to assess both anatomy and pathology. Certain sequences may need to be repeated because fetal mobility during acquisition distorts the image or causes images that are not in proper anatomic planes between sequences.
- Fetal landmarks may not be trustworthy due to transposition, hence fetal anatomy should be lateralized as either right or left based on an examination of the fetal position in relation to the mother.
- Although having a large matrix, thin sections and small field of view gives us high spatial resolution images, it should not be overdone since gains might be negated by the "wrap" artifact and a lower signal-to-noise ratio.
- Fetal brain—3 mm slice thickness in all planes.
- **Other fetal organs**: 4 mm slice thickness
- **Special techniques used in fetal MRI**:
  - Parallel imaging
  - Fast sequences to reduce motion artifacts
  - Free breathing sequences
  - Single slice acquisitions techniques used
- Usually done after 20 weeks
- After 26 weeks—all organs seen in detail.
- **Exposure limit according to FDA for maternal body**: 4W/kg
- SAR of mother—2W/kg
- SAR of fetus—1.24W/kg in 1.5T and 1.14W/kg in 3T

MRI Sequences

- T1-2D GRE
- T2-SSH-TSE/T2-SSFSE/HASTE
- b-FFE/FIESTA/true-FISP
- **Ultrafast GRE**: TFE/FMPSPGR/turbo-FLASH
- DWI (b: 0 and 700s/mm^2)

Advantages

1. Superior soft tissue contrast—in regions like brain and spine
2. Detailed brain imaging for detecting brain abnormalities such as ventriculomegaly, cortical malformations and hemorrhage that might not be clear on an ultrasound.
3. **No ionizing radiation**: Unlike CT, MRI does not use ionizing radiation, making it safe for both the mother and the fetus.
4. **Improved evaluation of complex anatomy**: MRI offers a detailed view of the anatomy of vital organs, which is especially beneficial for diagnosing complex congenital malformations.
5. **Complementary to ultrasound**: Fetal MRI is often used in conjunction with ultrasound when the latter's results are inconclusive, providing a more detailed follow-up investigation.
6. Better visualization in cases of maternal obesity or oligohydramnios
7. **Detection of subtle anomalies**: MRI can detect subtle fetal anomalies like small hemorrhages or white matter injuries that are difficult to visualize on an ultrasound.

Disadvantages of Fetal MRI

- High cost
- Limited availability
- Maternal pacemakers, ferromagnetic implants
- Claustrophobia
- Energy deposition (SAR)
- Acoustic noise reaching the fetal ears
- Fetal nerve stimulation
- Potential teratogenic effects—due to heating by gradient changes and due to nonthermal interaction of fetal tissue with electromagnetic field.

Prostate

1. Imaging of prostate cancer with regards to TRUS and MRI. [5+5] [MD (WBUHS) 23]

Prostate cancer can be imaged with the help of Transrectal ultrasound and MRI (modality of choice).[22]

Transrectal ultrasound is an examination in which transrectal probe is inserted into the rectum after optimal patient preparation and consent, giving a good field of view of the prostate, seminal vesicles, vas deferens and posterior urethra.

Role of Transrectal Ultrasound (TRUS) in Prostate Cancer

1. **Prostate cancer detection**:

   Guidance for prostate biopsy: The most common role of TRUS is to guide biopsy needles during a prostate biopsy. TRUS is used to image the prostate gland in real-time, allowing us to take tissue samples from areas of prostate, based on PSA levels or abnormalities found in a digital rectal exam (DRE).
2. **Prostate volume assessment**: For measurement of prostate volume and calculation of PSA density **(Fig. 53)**
3. **Cancer staging**:
   - Evaluation of extracapsular spread of prostate cancer
   - Involvement of seminal vesicles present or not
   - Local staging of prostate cancer
4. **Monitoring and follow-up**:
   - TRUS and TRUS guided biopsies can be repeated periodically for follow-up in case of low risk prostate cancer
   - For monitoring progression of disease or treatment response after radiotherapy or chemotherapy.
5. **Treatment guidance**:
   - Brachytherapy: TRUS is crucial in guiding the placement of radioactive seeds during prostate brachytherapy, a common treatment for localized prostate cancer. The real-time imaging provided by TRUS allows precise seed placement within the prostate.
   - Cryotherapy: In cryotherapy, TRUS helps monitor the placement of probes and the freezing of prostate tissue to ensure that the cancerous tissue is targeted while minimizing damage to surrounding structures.

PSA Density

$$\text{Prostate volume} = \text{Length} \times \text{Width} \times \text{Height} \times 0.52$$

$$\text{PSA density} = \frac{\text{PSA value}}{\text{Prosate Volume}}$$

FIG. 53: PSA density measurement.

Advantages of TRUS in Prostate Cancer

- Widely available
- Less expensive
- Real-time imaging procedures like biopsy and treatment placement is possible.
- Repeated imaging is possible.

TRUS Guided Biopsy

- Indicated after screening test (PSA or DRE) detects abnormality.
- Hypoechoic (most common)/isoechoic/hyperechoic (rarely) lesion in Peripheral zone close to capsule.
- Asymmetry or bulge along lateral aspect.
- Less reliable than DRE for predicting extracapsular extension and involvement of seminal vesicles.

Patient Preparation

- Adequate bowel preparation with laxatives for 2 days prior to the procedure.
- Oral antibiotic cover for 24 hrs prior to the procedure

Procedure

- 12 cores are taken from different areas (as described below) with the help of 18 gauze biopsy gun **(Fig. 54)**
- Transperineal approach can also be taken.

Postprocedure

Color of urine to be observed due to chances of urethral injury

Complications

- Urethral injury
- Rectal bleeding

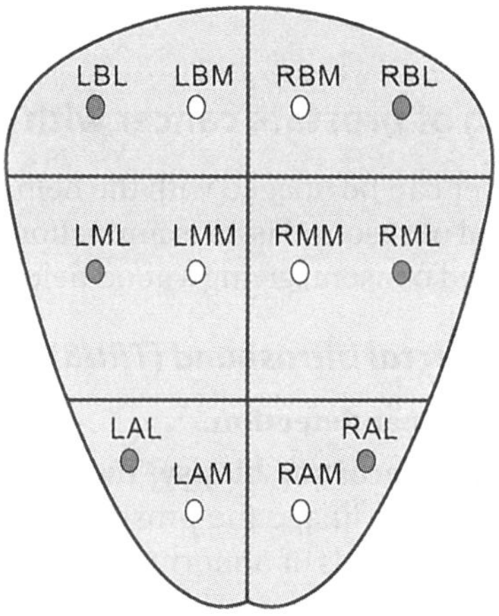

FIG. 54: Schematic representation of nontarget prostatic biopsy. LAL: left apex lateral; LAM: left apex medial; LBL: left base lateral; LBM: left basal medial; LML: left mid lateral; LMM: left mid medial; RAL: right apex lateral; RAM: right apex medial; RBl: right base lateral; RBM: right basal medial; RML: right mid lateral; RMM: right mid medial.

Role of MRI in Prostate Cancer

1. **Detection and diagnosis**:
   - **Multiparametric MRI (mpMRI)** is the most widely used MRI technique **(Table 48)** in prostate cancer. It combines several imaging sequences, including T2-weighted imaging, diffusion-weighted imaging (DWI), and dynamic contrast-enhanced imaging (DCE), providing detailed anatomical and functional information about the prostate.
   - Studies have demonstrated that mpMRI has high sensitivity and specificity in identifying clinically significant prostate cancer, improving detection compared to traditional methods like TRUS (transrectal ultrasound)-guided biopsy.
   - The **Prostate Imaging Reporting and Data System (PI-RADS)** scoring system, developed to standardize the interpretation of prostate mpMRI, helps stratify patients based on the likelihood of significant cancer. A higher PI-RADS score correlates with a higher probability of finding clinically significant cancer.
2. **MRI-guided biopsy**:
   - Targeted biopsy, particularly through **MRI/ultrasound fusion-guided biopsy**.
   - More precise sampling of suspicious areas identified on mpMRI
   - Improved detection rates of significant cancers while reducing over-diagnosis of indolent tumors.

TABLE 48: MRI findings in prostate cancer.

Imaging techniques	*Typical findings*	*Advantages*	*Limitations*
T1W	Iso signal	Detecting postbiopsy hemorrhage and LN metastasis	Low accuracy of tumor detection
T2W	Low signal	Differentiating zonal anatomy, assessing extracapsular extension, seminal vesicle invasion and adjacent structure invasion	False-positive (inflammation, hemorrhage, atrophy, scar, BPH, post-treatment changes), similar signal with central zone cancer and BPH nodule, LN staging
DCE	Early nodular enhancement and early washout	Evaluating vascular distribution of tumor, improved tumor localization and detection, improved staging accuracy, improved accuracy of recurred cancer detection	Low specificity for differentiation with prostatitis, transition zone cancer or BPH nodule, potential nephrogenic systemic fibrosis in renal insufficiency patients
DW	High signal on DW image and low signal on ADC map	Fast scan time, improved specificity of tumor detection, qualitative and quantitative evaluation of tumor, offering useful information before and after treatment, assessing tumor aggressiveness, improved staging accuracy	Differentiation with low Gleason score cancer, prostatitis or BPH nodule, low spatial resolution, susceptibility and motion artifacts
MRS	↑ Choline ↓ citrate	Providing metabolic information, improved specificity of tumor detection, assessing tumor aggressiveness, improved staging accuracy	Technical difficulty, wide variation related to postprocessing and shimming, differentiation with BPH nodule, long postprocessing time

- MRI-targeted biopsy has been shown to detect more high-grade cancers compared to systematic biopsy and can reduce the number of unnecessary biopsies in men with low-risk profiles.

3. **Staging of prostate cancer**:
   - Superior visualization of the prostate and surrounding structures compared to other imaging modalities.
   - T2-weighted MRI is used to assess the local extent of the tumor, including extracapsular extension, seminal vesicle invasion, and involvement of adjacent organs (e.g., bladder).
   - Accurate assessment of extracapsular extension (ECE) and seminal vesicle invasion (SVI).
4. **Active surveillance**:
   - Non-invasive monitoring of prostate tumors, reducing the need for repeated biopsies
   - Monitoring changes in tumor size or PI-RADS score.
5. **Treatment planning**:
   - Accurate mapping of the extent of the tumor
6. **Post-treatment monitoring**:
   - For the detection of recurrence after treatment

Protocol

- **Magnet**: 1.5–3T
- **Coil**: Pelvic phase array coil
- **Position**: Supine
- **Sequences taken**:
  A. Large FOV Axial T1
  B. Large FOV Axial T2
  C. Large FOV Sagittal T2
  D. Small FOV Axial T2
  E. Small FOV Coronal T2
  F. Small FOV Axial DWI and ADC
  G. Small FOV Axial T1 and T1 FS
  H. Small FOV Axial T1 FS with dynamic contrast

Imaging Features of Prostatic Carcinoma

- Ill-defined T2 hypointense nodules in peripheral zone
- T2 hypointense nodule in central gland is difficult to differentiate from BPH nodule
- Erased charcoal appearance
- Diffusion restriction present
- **Dynamic contrast enhanced images**: Early enhancement and rapid washout
  - Assignment of PIRADS according to zones
- PIRADS is prostate imaging and data system **(Tables 49 and 50 and Fig. 55)**

TABLE 49: Prostate imaging-reporting and data system (PI-RADS).

PI-RADS	
PI-RADS 1	Very low (clinically significant cancer highly unlikely)
PI-RADS 2	Low (clinically significant caner unlikely)
PI-RADS 3	Intermediate (clinically significant cancer equivocal)
PI-RADS 4	High (clinically significant cancer likely)
PI-RADS 5	Very high (clinically significant cancer highly likely)

TABLE 50: PI-RADS assessment on MRI.

PI-RADS assessment for T2W in peripheral zone	
Score	***Peripheral zone***
1	Uniform hyperintense signal intensity (normal)
2	Linear or wedge-shaped hypointensity or diffused mild hypointensity usually indistinct margin
3	Heterogeneous signal intensity or circumscribed, rounded moderate hypointensity Includes others that do not qualify as 2, 4 or 5
4.	Circumscribed homogeneous moderate hypointense focus/mass confined to prostate and <1.5 cm in greatest dimension
5	Same as 4 but 1.5 cm in greatest dimension or definite extra prostatic extension/invasive behavior
PI-RADS assessment for T2W in transition zone (TZ)	
Score	***Transition zone***
1	Normal appearing TZ (rare) or a round, completely encapsulated nodule ("typical nodule')
2	A mostly encapsulated nodule OR a homogeneous circumscribed nodule without encapsulation ('atypical nodule') OR a homogeneous mildly hypointense area between nodules
3	Heterogeneous signal intensity with obscured margins includes others that do not qualify as 2.4, or 5
4	Lenticular or noncircumscribed, homogeneous, moderately hypointense, and <1.5 cm in greatest dimension
5	Same as 4, but >1.5 cm in greatest dimension or definite extra prostatic extension invasive behavior
PI-RADS assessment of DM	
Score	***Peripheral zone or transition zone***
1.	No abnormality (i.e. normal) on ADC and high b-value DWI
2.	Linear or wedge-shaped hypointense on ADC and/or linear or wedge-shaped hyperintense on high b-value DWI
3.	Focal (discrete and different from the background) hypointense on ADC and/or focal hyperintense on high b-value DVA: may be markedly hypointense on ADC or markedly hyperintense on high b-value DWI. but not both
4.	Focal markedly hypointense on ADC and markedly hyperintense on high b-value DWI: <1.5 cm in greatest dimension
5.	Same as 4 but >1.5 cm in greatest dimension or definite extra prostatic extension/invasive behavior
PI-RADS Assessment for DCE	
Score	***Peripheral zone or transition zone***
(–)	No early or contemporaneous enhancement: or diffuse mutt local enhancement NOT corresponding to a focal finding on T2WI and /or DIM or focal enhancement corresponding to a lesion demonstrating features of BPH on T2WI (including features of extruded BPH in the PZ)
(+)	Focal and earlier than or contemporaneously with enhancement of adjacent normal prostatic tissues. and corresponds to suspicious fin ding on T 2W and/or DW

(T2W: T2-weighted; PI-RADS: prostate imaging-reporting and data system; DWI: diffusion-weighted imaging; ADC: apparent diffusion coefficient; DCE: dynamic contrast-enhanced: T2WI: T2-weighted image: DW: diffusion weighted imaging; BPH: benign prostatic hyperplasia: PZ: peripheral zone)

- Radiological estimation of likelihood of malignancy
- Dominant sequence score is to applied for final PIRADS score—DWI for PZ and T2 for TZ.
- **Artifacts encountered in multiparametric MRI of prostate**:
  - Chemical shift artifact
  - Wraparound
  - Motion
  - Susceptibility

2. Describe the protocols and MR imaging features in prostatic carcinoma. [3+7] [MD (WBUHS) 21]

mpMRI pelvis—modality of choice for imaging prostatic carcinoma

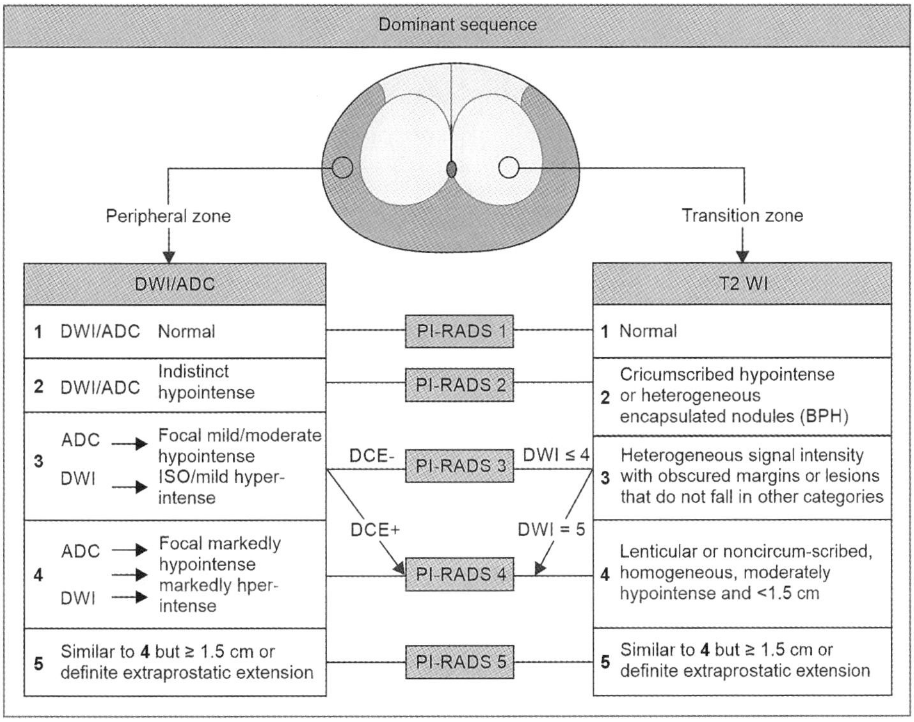

FIG. 55: PI-RADS assessment on MRI.

Protocol

- **Magnet**: 1.5- 3T
- **Coil**: Pelvic phase array coil
- **Position**: Supine
- **Sequences taken**:
  - A. Large FOV axial T1
  - B. Large FOV axial T2
  - C. Large FOV sagittal T2
  - D. Small FOV axial T2
  - E. Small FOV coronal T2
  - F. Small FOV axial DWI and ADC
  - G. Small FOV axial T1 and T1 FS
  - H. Small FOV axial T1 FS with dynamic contrast

Multiparametric MRI (mpMRI) is the most widely used MRI technique **(Table 48)** in prostate cancer.

Imaging Features of Prostatic Carcinoma

- Ill-defined T2 hypointense nodules in peripheral zone
- T2 hypointense nodule in central gland is difficult to differentiate from BPH nodule
- Erased charcoal appearance
- Diffusion restriction present
- **Dynamic contrast enhanced images**: Early enhancement and rapid washout
- **Assignment of PIRADS according to zones**:
  - PIRADS is prostate imaging and data system **(Tables 49 and 50 and Fig. 56)**
  - Radiological estimation of likelihood of malignancy
  - Dominant sequence score is to applied for final PIRADS score—DWI for PZ and T2 for TZ.

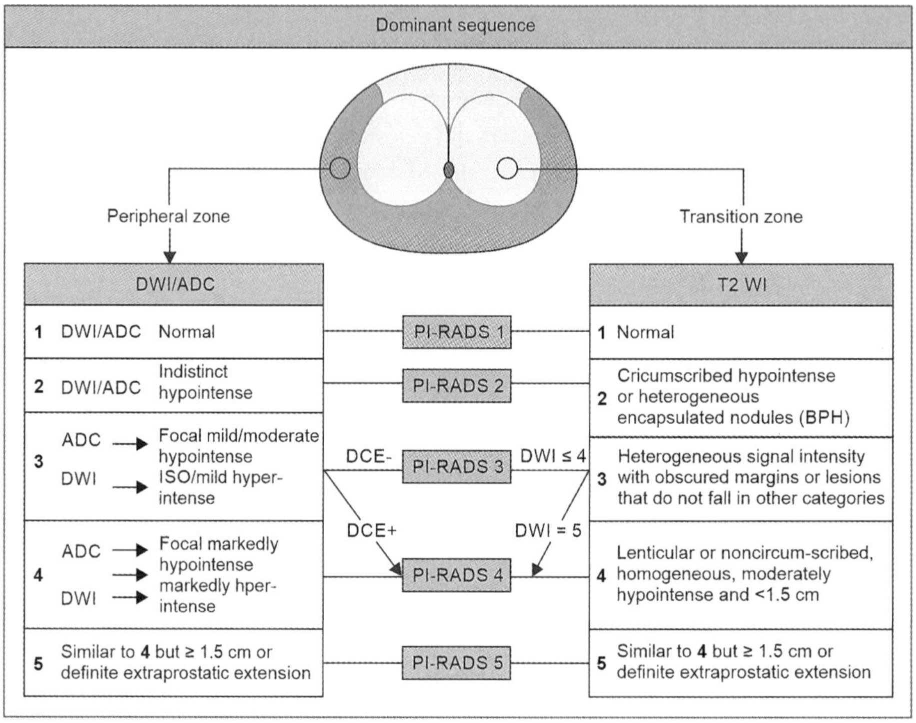

FIG. 56: PI-RADS assessment on MRI.

- **Artifacts encountered in multiparametric MRI of prostate**:
  - Chemical shift artifact
  - Wraparound
  - Motion
  - Susceptibility

3. Discuss Multiparametric MR imaging of the prostate. [10] [MD (WBUHS) 21]

Multiparametric MRI (mpMRI) refers to a sophisticated imaging technique that combines multiple MRI sequences to provide detailed anatomical and functional information about tissues, particularly in evaluating diseases such as cancer. Each "parameter" or sequence offers a different type of information about the tissue being imaged, allowing for a more comprehensive assessment.

It is used in:

- Prostate cancer
- Breast cancer
- mpMRI pelvis—modality of choice for imaging prostatic carcinoma

Protocol

- **Magnet**: 1.5–3T
- **Coil**: Pelvic phase array coil
- **Position**: Supine
- **Sequences taken**:
  A. Large FOV Axial T1
  B. Large FOV Axial T2
  C. Large FOV Sagittal T2
  D. Small FOV Axial T2
  E. Small FOV Coronal T2
  F. Small FOV Axial DWI and ADC

G. Small FOV Axial T1 and T1 FS
H. Small FOV Axial T1 FS with dynamic contrast

Multiparametric MRI (mpMRI) is the most widely used MRI technique **(Table 48)** in prostate cancer.

Imaging Features of Prostatic Carcinoma

- Ill-defined T2 hypointense nodules in peripheral zone
- **T2 hypointense nodule in central gland is difficult to differentiate from BPH nodule**
- **Erased charcoal appearance**
- **Diffusion restriction present**
- **Dynamic contrast enhanced images**: Early enhancement and rapid washout
- Assignment of PIRADS according to zones
- PIRADS is prostate imaging and data system **(Tables 49 and 50 and Fig. 57)**
- Radiological estimation of likelihood of malignancy
- Dominant sequence score is to applied for final PIRADS score—DWI for PZ and T2 for TZ.

Artifacts encountered in multiparametric MRI of prostate:

- Chemical shift artifact
- Wraparound
- Motion
- Susceptibility

3. Discuss in brief about Radiological Anatomy of prostrate with its radiological implications. [5+5] [MD (WBUHS) 22]

- Radiological anatomy of prostate **(Fig. 58)**:
- **Four glandular zones around the prostatic urethra**:
  - Peripheral zone
  - Transition zone
  - Central zone
  - Anterior fibromuscular stroma

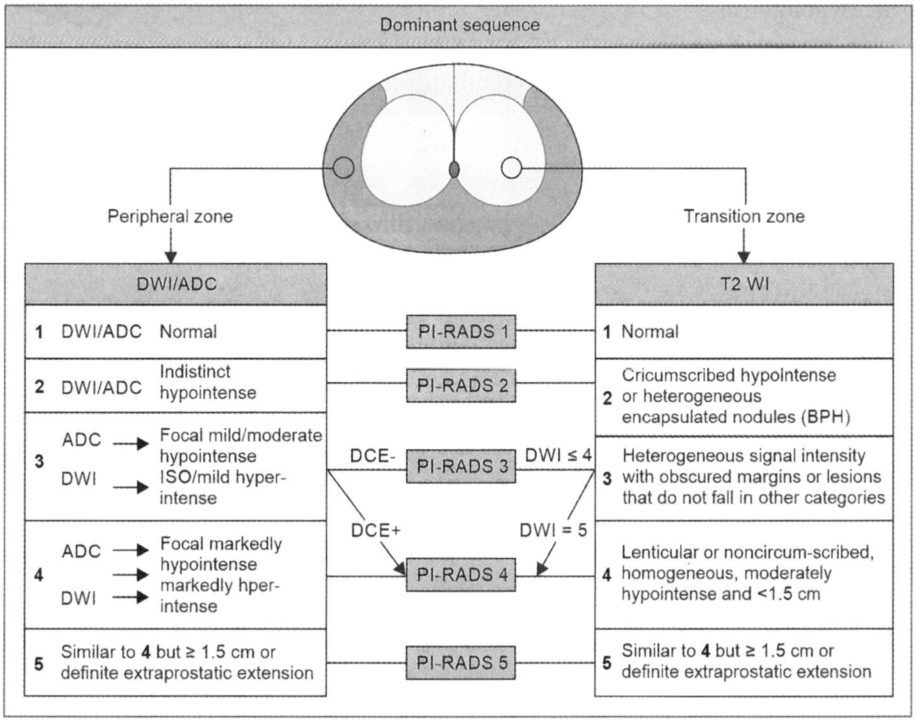

FIG. 57: PI-RADS assessment on MRI.

- **Surfaces**:
  - Anterior
  - Posterior
  - Inferior lateral surface
- **Regions**:
  - Apex (1/3rd)
  - Mid gland (1/3rd)
  - Base (1/3rd)
- **Blood supply**: Prostatic and vesical arteries—branch of internal iliac arteries
- **Lymphatic drainage**: Internal iliac nodes
- **Nerve supply**:
  - Prostatic plexus (parasympathetic nerves from S2-S4)
  - Sympathetic supply—hypogastric nerve
- **Capsule of prostate**:
  - Fibromuscular tissue made of smooth muscle
  - Covers the entire gland
- **Peripheral zone**:
  - Largest zone
  - 70% of prostate tissue
  - Separated from central and transition zones by a capsule
  - Composed of ductal and acinar elements, interwoven smooth muscles
  - High signal intensity on T2W
  - Prostatic carcinoma—75% in Central zone
- **Transition zone**:
  - 5% of prostatic tissue
  - Superior to verumontanum
- **Composed of two types of tissue**: Glandular and stromal tissue
  - Glandular tissue: Hyperintense
  - Stromal tissue: Hypointense
  - Benign prostatic hyperplasia arises here.
  - T2 hypointense cancer nodule—difficult to differentiate from normal tissue
- **Central zone**:
  - 25% of prostatic tissue
  - Between peripheral and central zone at base of prostate
  - Prostatic carcinoma—5% in Central zone
  - Low signal intensity on T2W
- **Anterior fibromuscular stroma**:
  - Nonglandular tissue
  - Continuous with detrusor muscle
  - Low signal on T2W
  - Not a region for prostatic carcinoma
  - Loss of symmetry indicates underlying prostatic nodule.

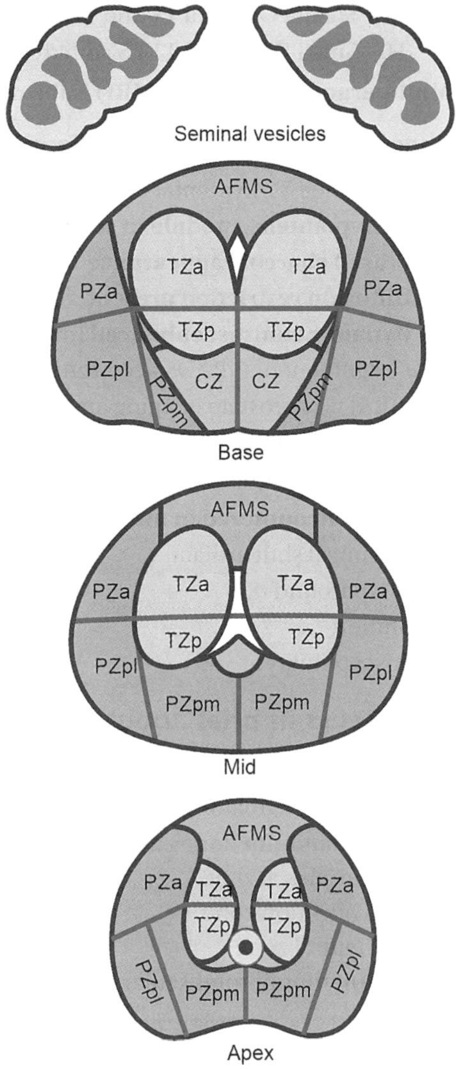

FIG. 58: Schematic diagram of prostatic anatomy

Radiological Implications

Multiparametric MRI (mpMRI) is the most widely used MRI technique in prostate cancer.

Imaging Features of Prostatic Carcinoma

- Ill-defined T2 hypointense nodules in peripheral zone

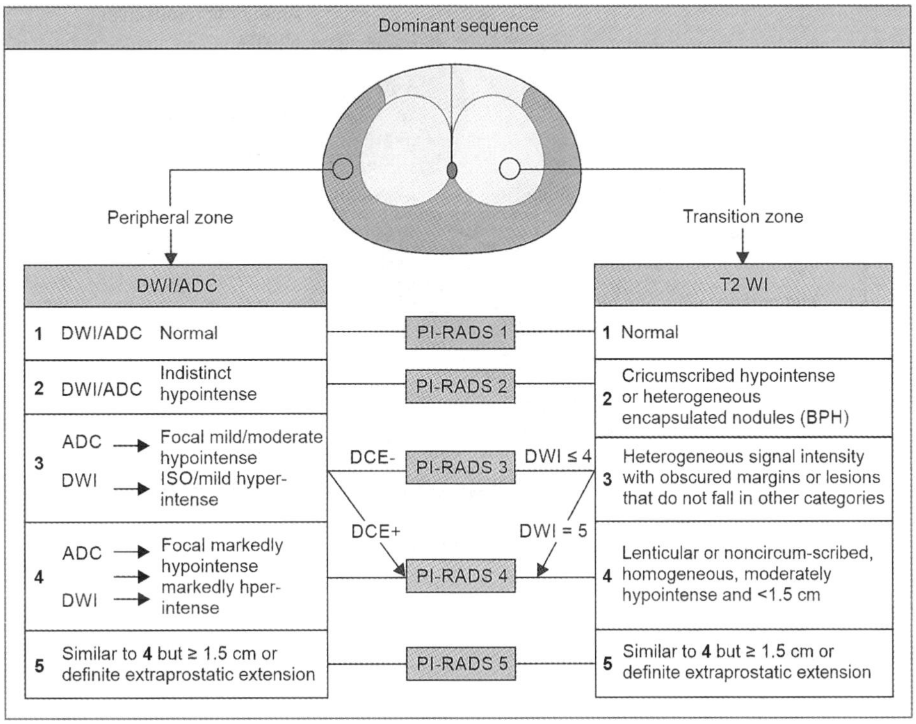

FIG. 59: PI-RADS assessment on MRI.

- **T2 hypointense nodule in central gland is difficult to differentiate from BPH nodule**
- **Erased charcoal appearance**
- **Diffusion restriction present**
- **Dynamic contrast enhanced images**: Early enhancement and rapid washout
- Assignment of PIRADS according to zones
- PIRADS is prostate imaging and data system **(Tables 49 and 50 and Fig. 59)**
- Radiological estimation of likelihood of malignancy
- Dominant sequence score is to applied for final PIRADS score DWI for PZ and T2 for TZ.

4. Draw cross-sectional anatomy of prostate. Discuss briefly the role of MRI in prostate pathologies. [2+5] Discuss PIRADS. [3] [MD (WBUHS) 24]

Cross-sectional Anatomy of Prostate (Figs. 60A and B)

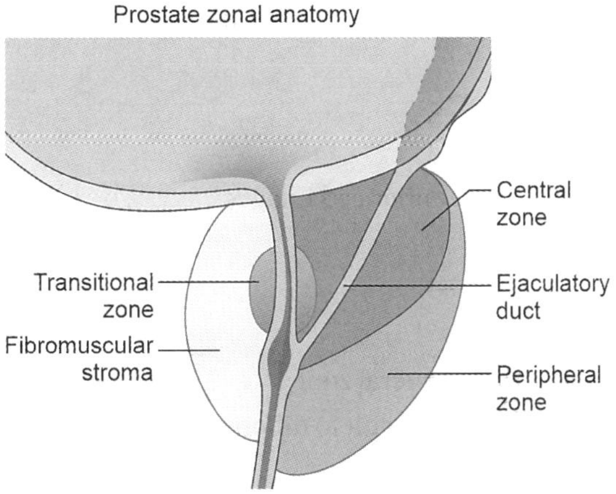

FIG. 60A: Sagittal anatomy of prostate.

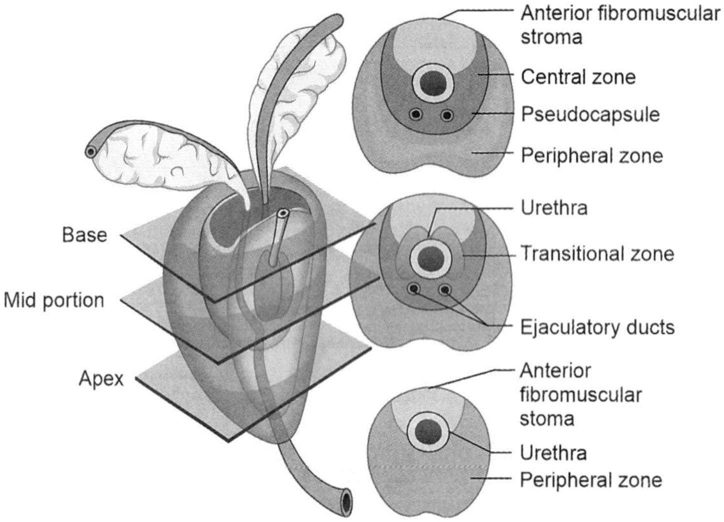

FIG. 60B: Cross-sectional anatomy of prostate.

MRI in Prostate Pathologies

- **Benign prostatic hyperplasia**:
  - Enlargement of TZ
  - Heterogenous TZ with multiple nodules.
  - Variable appearance due to varying proportion of glandular and stromal elements
  - Well defined smooth margins, round to oval shape
  - Glandular nodules—hyperintense on T2W (secretions present)
  - Stromal nodules: Hypointense on T2W, similar appearance as carcinoma
  - Diffusion restriction present in stromal nodules like carcinoma
  - Dynamic contrast enhanced images: Early enhancement and rapid washout.
- **Findings in bladder**:
  - Bladder base indented and thickened
  - Trabeculations
  - Diverticula and calculi

Prostatitis and Prostatic Abscess

- **Focal**: Band like or geographic area of hypointensity
- **Diffuse**: Peripheral zone is lower in signal than expected on T2W
- **Prostatitis**:
  - Hyperintense on DWI, low signal on ADC.
  - ADC value higher than prostatic carcinoma
  - Hyperenhancement on dynamic contrast enhanced images
  - Mass effect absent
  - Capsule preserved
- **Prostatic carcinoma**
  - Ill-defined T2 hypointense nodules in peripheral zone
  - T2 hypointense nodule in central gland is difficult to differentiate from BPH nodule
  - Erased charcoal appearance
  - Diffusion restriction present

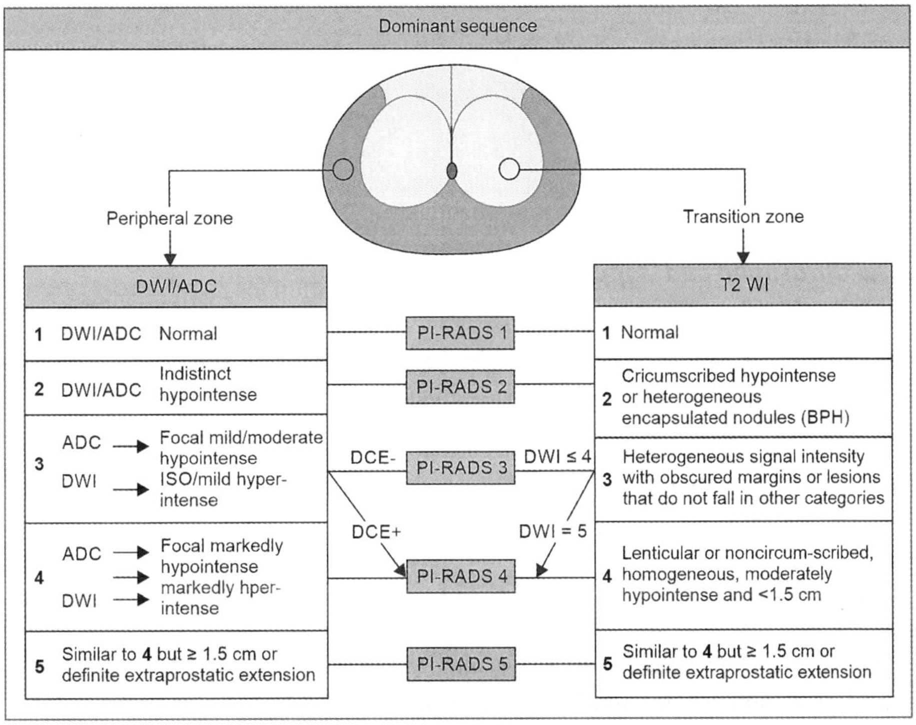

FIG. 61: PI-RADS assessment on MRI.

  - Dynamic contrast enhanced images: Early enhancement and rapid washout
  - Assignment of PIRADS according to zones
- PIRADS is prostate imaging and data system **(Tables 49 and 50 and Fig. 61)**
- Radiological estimation of likelihood of malignancy
- Dominant sequence score is to applied for final PIRADS score—DWI for PZ and T2 for TZ.

Scrotum and Male Sexual Dysfunction

1. Discuss the role of Sonogram in various scrotal pathologies. [10] [MD (WBUHS) 19]

Causes of Acute Unilateral Scrotal Pain in an Young Adult

- **Infection/inflammation**:
  - Epididymo-orchitis
  - Funiculitis
  - Pyocele
  - Fournier's gangrene
- **Vascular**:
  - Torsion of testis or appendix
  - Thrombosed varicocele
  - Vasculitis (Henoch-Schonlein purpura)
- **Trauma**:
  - Hematoma
  - Rupture
  - Fracture
  - Torsion

- **Tumor**:
  - Seminomatous or nonseminomatous germ cell tumor
  - Incarcerated inguinal hernia
- **Referred pain**:
  - Ureteric colic
  - Appendicitis.

Technique of Scrotal Ultrasound and Doppler

- High frequency probe (10–15MHz).
- Lower frequency probe or curvilinear probe in case of grossly thickened and edematous scrotal wall
- Comfortable room and warm gel to avoid cremasteric reflex.
- Penis positioned up on the pelvis.
- Towel used in case of enlarged scrotum
- Patient's thigh used for support.
- Ample amount of gel used to avoid contact artifacts due to rugae.
- **For Doppler**: High PRF, low wall filter, max color gain but avoid noise and color vs echo priority (70–90%) and high color persistence
- Power Doppler, B flow, microflow imaging, microvascular imaging.
- Standing up and Valsalva maneuver for hernia and varicocele.

Individual Scrotal Pathologies

Epididymitis or Epididymo-orchitis

- Sexually active age group—*Chlamydia, Neisseria*
- Older age group—UTI retrograde from vas—*E. coli*, Proteus
- Children—genitourinary anomalies, dysfunctional micturition
- Orchitis (involvement of testis) from epididymitis
- Isolated orchitis is uncommon—mumps
- Chronic epididymoorchitis—TB
- **Positive prehn's sign**: When the medial aspect of the thigh is scratched the scrotum is lifted-up.

Ultrasound Findings

- Thickened epididymis. Focal and diffuse
- Hypoechoic or heterogenous
- Increased echogenicity in chronic cases.
- Reactive hydrocele/pyocele and scrotal wall thickening.
- Hypoechoic, enlarged and striated testis in case of acute orchitis.
- Increased vascularity in epididymis, flow more than testis
- Increased vascularity in testis
- PSV of TA >or equal to 15 cm/sec or testis ratios > or equal to 1.9
- Epididymal PSV ratio > or equal to 1.7
- Normal PSV of epididymis < or equal to 5 cm/sec
- Low resistance wave pattern RI <0.5 in testis and <0.7 in epididymis

Hydro/Pyo/Hematocele

- Collection of fluid between the layers of tunica vaginalis
- Congenital or acquired
- Acquired due to infection, trauma, tumor or idiopathic.

- Snow fall sign—echogenic debris in pyocele have vertical motion (up to down) in the presence of ultrasound probe due to the ultrasound pulses
- Pyocele—parietal layer of tunica vaginalis is hyperemic

Types—partial (<360 degree), complete, intermittent

USG Findings

- Normal/swollen testis, rounded contour or shape
- Altered axis
- Echogenicity—normal, hypoechoic or heterogenous
- Segmental or global testicular infarct
- Extratesticular mass causing mass effect due to twisted spermatic cord (whirlpool sign)
- Associated hydrocele and scrotal wall thickening
- Whirlpool sign is the most specific sign of testicular torsion—twisted vascular pedicle on b mode and color Doppler.
- Other signs—snail sign (twisted spermatic cord giving the appearance of a spiral mass like snail), FIGURE OF EIGHT SIGN (two separate masses lying side by side - one due to the twisted cord and other one is the testis)

Doppler Findings

- Vascular whirlpool sign—twisted vascular pedicle on color Doppler giving the appearance of a whirlpool.
- No flow/reduced flow in intratesticular arteries
- High resistance to blood flow (RI >0.75)
- Low resistance increased flow in intratesticular arteries in case of partial torsion - detorsion.
- Normal flow can also be seen.
- **Infarction**: Increased RI values.

Testicular appendix can also undergo torsion.

Clinical Features

- Blue dot sign—acute scrotum with firm tender nodule in upper pole of scrotum
- cremasteric reflex—present.

USG Findings

- Round to oval echogenic or heterogenous supra testicular lesion measuring >5mm
- Hydrocele and scrotal wall thickening can be present.
- Rule out infection and testicular torsion.

Doppler

- No internal vascularity
- Perilesional hyperemia

Seminoma

- Most common germ cell tumor
- **Age group**: 35–45 yrs
- **Ultrasound features**: Homogenously hypoechoic lesion, may replace parenchyma completely
- No calcifications
- Cystic spaces rare
- <1.5 cm hypovascular
- >1.6 cm hypervascular
- Associated hydrocele
- Assessment of retroperitoneal lymphadenopathy.

Varicocele

- Abnormal dilatation of pampiniform plexus in spermatic cord
- Asymptomatic or symptomatic
- **Types**: Primary or secondary
- Primary—due to incompetent valves in the testicular vein
- Left> bilateral>right
- Left side predominant due to right angle insertion of left testicular vein into the left renal vein and long left testicular vein (8–10 cm longer).
- Secondary—due to compression of left renal vein due to nutcracker syndrome or obstruction due to thrombus.
- Normal—0.5–1.5 mm. >2 mm is abnormal.
- Ultrasound performed in supine, erect and Valsalva.

Ultrasound Findings

- Serpiginous structures superior and posterolateral to the testis.
- May show internal flow echoes (due to slow flow)
- >2mm diameter and >1mm increase with Valsalva
- May have testicular atrophy
- Reversal of flow or enhancement with Valsalva maneuver
- If no change with Valsalva then secondary.
- Screen the retroperitoneum, kidney and renal vein
- Reflux >2 sec with Valsalva
- Obstructive type—no change with respiration or position
- Reflux of 1 sec can be present without varicocele.

Sarteschi Grading of Varicocele (Table 51)

TABLE 51: Sarteschi grading of varicocele.

Grade	*Description*
1	Reflux in vessels in the inguinal channel is detected only during the Valsalva maneuver, while scrotal varicosity is not evident in the standard ultrasound study.
2	Small posterior varicosities that extend to the superior pole of the testis. Their diameters increase and venous reflux is seen in the supratesticular region only during the Valsalva maneuver.
3	Vessels appear enlarged at the inferior pole of the testis when the patient is evaluated in a standing position; no enlargement is detected if the patient is examined in a supine position. Reflux observed only under during the Valsalva maneuver.
4	Vessels appear enlarged even when the patient is studied in a supine position; the dilatation is more marked in the upright position and during the Valsalva maneuver. Testicular hypotrophy is common at this stage.
5	Venous ectasia is evident even in the prone decubitus and supine positions. Reflux is observed at rest and does not increase during the Valsalva maneuver.

Testicular trauma: Blunt trauma—most common

- **Hematoma**:
  - Types: Testicular or extratesticular
  - Testicular hematoma:
    - Hypoechoic avascular area in testicular parenchyma
    - Clot may appear echogenic
    - Tunica albuginea—intact
    - Chronic hematoma—hypo/anechoic

- **Extratesticular hematoma**:
  - Most common finding in blunt injury
  - Echogenic collection in tunica vaginalis
  - Large size-urgent surgical management
  - Scrotal wall hematoma-echogenic wall thickening or fluid collection
  - Testicular rupture
    - Irregularity or disruption of tunica albuginea
    - Heterogenous echogenicity
    - Focal bulge in contour
    - Absence of vascularity within the testes
    - Surgical management
  - Testicular fracture:
    - Linear or complex
    - Linear hypoechoic avascular area
    - Pseudoaneurysm can occur
  - Testicular torsion (discussed later)
  - Scrotal abscess:
    - Heterogenous collection in thickened scrotal wall
    - Increased vascularity in scrotal wall
  - Fournier gangrene—air pockets underneath the scrotal skin.

2. What are the common causes of a young adult presenting with acute unilateral scrotal pain and swelling? Discuss the Ultrasound/Doppler evaluation of such cases. [5+5] [MD (WBUHS) 22, MD (WBUHS) 17, AIIMS May 24]

Causes of Acute Unilateral Scrotal Pain in an Young Adult

- **Infection/inflammation**:
  - Epididymoorchitis
  - Funiculitis
  - Pyocele
  - Fournier's gangrene
- **Vascular**:
  - Torsion of testis or appendix
  - Thrombosed varicocele
  - Vasculitis (Henoch-schonlein purpura)
- **Trauma**:
  - Hematoma
  - Rupture
  - Fracture
  - Torsion
- **Tumor**: Seminomatous or non seminomatous germ cell tumor
  - Incarcerated inguinal hernia
- **Referred pain**:
  - Ureteric colic
  - Appendicitis

Technique of Scrotal Ultrasound and Doppler

- High frequency probe (10-15MHz).
- Lower frequency probe or curvilinear probe in case of grossly thickened and edematous scrotal wall

- Comfortable room and warm gel to avoid cremasteric reflex.
- Penis positioned up on the pelvis.
- Towel used in case of enlarged scrotum
- Patient's thigh used for support.
- Ample amount of gel used to avoid contact artifacts due to rugae.
- **For Doppler**: High PRF, low wall filter, max color gain but avoid noise and color vs echo priority (70-90%) and high color persistence
- Power Doppler, B flow, microflow imaging, microvascular imaging.
- Standing up and Valsalva maneuver for hernia and varicocele.

Individual Scrotal Pathologies

- **Epididymitis or Epididymoorchitis**:
  - Sexually active age group—*Chlamydia, Neisseria*
  - Older age group—UTI retrograde from vas—*E. coli*, Proteus
  - Children—genitourinary anomalies, dysfunctional micturition
  - Orchitis (involvement of testis) from epididymitis
  - Isolated orchitis is uncommon—mumps
  - Chronic epididymoorchitis—TB
  - Positive prehn's sign—when the medial aspect of the thigh is scratched the scrotum is lifted up.
- **Ultrasound findings**:
  - Thickened epididymis. Focal and diffuse
  - Hypoechoic or heterogenous
  - Increased echogenicity in chronic cases.
  - Reactive hydrocele/pyocele and scrotal wall thickening.
  - Hypoechoic, enlarged and striated testis in case of acute orchitis.
  - Increased vascularity in epididymis, flow more than testis
  - Increased vascularity in testis
  - PSV of TA >or equal to 15 cm/sec or testis ratios > or equal to 1.9
  - Epididymal PSV ratio > or equal to 1.7
  - Normal PSV of epididymis < or equal to 5 cm/sec
  - Low resistance wave pattern RI <0.5 in testis and <0.7 in epididymis
- **Hydro/pyo/heamatocele**:
  - Collection of fluid between the layers of tunica vaginalis
  - Congenital or acquired
  - Acquired due to infection, trauma, tumor or idiopathic.
  - Snow fall sign—echogenic debris in pyocele have vertical motion (up to down) in the presence of ultrasound probe due to the ultrasound pulses
  - Pyocele—parietal layer of tunica vaginalis is hyperemic
- **Types**: Partial (<360 degree), complete, intermittent
- **USG findings**:
  - Normal/swollen testis, rounded contour or shape altered axis
  - Echogenicity—normal, hypoechoic or heterogenous
  - Segmental or global testicular infarct
  - Extratesticular mass causing mass effect due to twisted spermatic cord (whirlpool sign)
  - Associated hydrocele and scrotal wall thickening
  - Whirlpool sign is the most specific sign of testicular torsion-twisted vascular pedicle on b mode and color Doppler.

- Other signs—snail sign (twisted spermatic cord giving the appearance of a spiral mass like snail), figure of eight sign (two separate masses lying side by side - one due to the twisted cord and other one is the testis)

- **Doppler findings**:
  - Vascular whirlpool sign—twisted vascular pedicle on color Doppler giving the appearance of a whirlpool.
  - No flow/reduced flow in intratesticular arteries
  - High resistance to blood flow (RI > 0.75)
  - Low resistance increased flow in intratesticular arteries in case of partial torsion—detorsion.
  - Normal flow can also be seen.
  - Infarction: Increased RI values

Testicular appendix can also undergo torsion.

- **Clinical feature**: Blue dot sign—acute scrotum with firm tender nodule in upper pole of scrotum cremasteric reflex-present
- **USG findings**:
  - Round to oval echogenic or heterogenous supra testicular lesion measuring >5mm
  - Hydrocele and scrotal wall thickening can be present.
  - Rule out infection and testicular torsion.
- **Doppler**:
  - No internal vascularity
  - Perilesional hyperemia
- **Seminoma**:
  - Most common germ cell tumor
  - Age group: 35-45 yrs
- **Ultrasound features**: Homogenously hypoechoic lesion, may replace parenchyma completely
  - No calcifications
  - Cystic spaces rare
  - <1.5 cm hypovascular
  - >1.6 cm hypervascular
  - Associated hydrocele
  - Assessment of retroperitoneal lymphadenopathy
- **Varicocele**:
  - Abnormal dilatation of pampiniform plexus in spermatic cord
  - Asymptomatic or symptomatic
  - Types: Primary or secondary
  - Primary—due to incompetent valves in the testicular vein
  - Left > bilateral > right
  - Left side predominant due to right angle insertion of left testicular vein into the left renal vein and long left testicular vein (8-10 cm longer).
  - Secondary—due to compression of left renal vein due to nutcracker syndrome or obstruction due to thrombus.
  - Normal—0.5-1.5mm. >2 mm is abnormal.
  - Ultrasound performed in supine, erect and valsalva.
- **Ultrasound findings**:
  - Serpiginous structures superior and posterolateral to the testis.
  - May show internal flow echoes (due to slow flow)
  - >2mm diameter and >1mm increase with Valsalva
  - May have testicular atrophy
  - Reversal of flow or enhancement with Valsalva maneuver
  - If no change with Valsalva then secondary

- Screen the retroperitoneum, kidney and renal vein
- Reflux >2 sec with Valsalva
- Obstructive type—no change with respiration or position
- Reflux of 1 sec can be present without varicocele.

Sarteschi Grading of Varicocele (Table 51)

Testicular trauma: Blunt trauma—most common

- **Hematoma**:
  - Types: Testicular or extratesticular
  - Testicular hematoma:
    - Hypoechoic avascular area in testicular parenchyma
    - Clot may appear echogenic
    - Tunica albuginea—intact
    - Chronic hematoma—hypo/anechoic
  - Extratesticular hematoma:
    - Most common finding in blunt injury
  - Echogenic collection in tunica vaginalis
  - Large size—urgent surgical management
  - Scrotal wall hematoma—echogenic wall thickening or fluid collection
  - Testicular rupture
    - Irregularity or disruption of tunica albuginea
    - Heterogenous echogenicity
    - Focal bulge in contour
    - Absence of vascularity within the testes
    - Surgical management
  - Testicular fracture:
    - Linear or complex
    - Linear hypoechoic avascular area
    - Pseudoaneurysm can occur
  - Testicular torsion (discussed later)

Scrotal Abscess

- Heterogenous collection in thickened scrotal wall
- Increased vascularity in scrotal wall
- Fournier gangrene-air pockets underneath the scrotal skin.

3. Color Doppler in testicular torsion. [5]

- Torsion of the testis due to twisting of the spermatic cord causing vascular compromise. It is a surgical emergency.
- Salvage rate is 100 % in <6 hrs, <10% in >24 hrs.
- Cause—bell clapper deformity
- Tunica vaginalis covering whole of the testis and high insertion of the tunica vaginalis.

Pathophysiology

- Twisting of the spermatic cord
- Venous occlusion
- Venous engorgement
- Arterial occlusion

- Ischemia
- Infarction

Clinical Feature

- Acute scrotum in children and young adults
- Cremasteric reflex absent
- High placed testis with altered axis
- Types—partial (<360°), complete, intermittent

USG Findings

- Normal/swollen testis, rounded contour or shape altered axis
- Echogenicity-normal, hypoechoic or heterogenous
- Segmental or global testicular infarct
- Extratesticular mass causing mass effect due to twisted spermatic cord (whirlpool sign)
- Associated hydrocele and scrotal wall thickening
- Whirlpool sign is the most specific sign of testicular torsion—twisted vascular pedicle on B mode and color Doppler.
- Other signs—snail sign (twisted spermatic cord giving the appearance of a spiral mass like snail), Figure of eight sign (two separate masses lying side by side—one due to the twisted cord and other one is the testis)

Doppler Findings

- Vascular whirlpool sign—twisted vascular pedicle on color Doppler giving the appearance of a whirlpool.
- No flow/reduced flow in intratesticular arteries
- High resistance to blood flow (RI >0.75)
- Low resistance increased flow in intratesticular arteries in case of partial torsion—detorsion.
- Normal flow can also be seen.

Testicular appendix can also undergo torsion.

Clinical Features

- Blue dot sign—acute scrotum with firm tender nodule in upper pole of scrotum
- Cremasteric reflex—present

USG Findings

- Round to oval echogenic or heterogenous supra testicular lesion measuring >5mm
- Hydrocele and scrotal wall thickening can be present.
- Rule out infection and testicular torsion.

Doppler

- No internal vascularity
- Perilesional hyperemia

4. Role of radiology in erectile dysfunction. [10] [DNB June 22]

Cross-sectional anatomy of penis **(Fig. 62)**

Etiologies of Erectile Dysfunction

- Psychogenic—most common cause
  - Performance anxiety
  - Depression
- Endocrinologic
  - Hypogonadism
  - Hyperprolactinemia

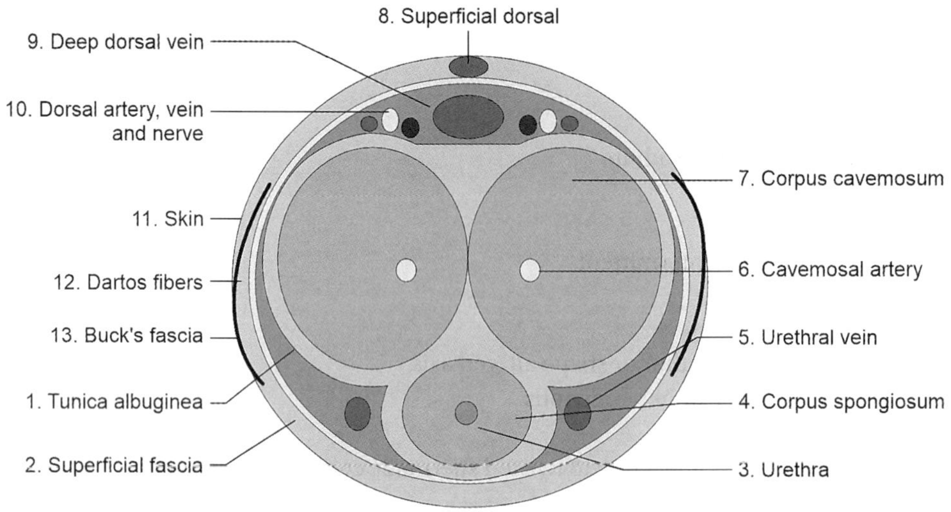

FIG. 62: Schematic diagram of cross-sectional anatomy of penis. Three distensible corpora chambers—corpora spongiosum enveloping the urethra. This does not play significant role in erection. Paired Corpora cavernosa—dorsal in position. Midline septum separates the two corpora cavernosa. Thick fascia (*Tunica albuginea*) encircles the corpora cavernosa. Buck's fascia covers corpora cavernosa and spongiosa together.

- Neurologic
  - Stroke
  - Spinal cord injury
  - Diabetic retinopathy
- Vascular—arterial and venous (more common)
  - Atherosclerosis
  - Hypertension
- Medication induced
  - Antihypertensives
  - Antidepressants
  - Alcohol
  - Smoking

Mechanism of Erection

Arrival of autonomic nerve impulse

⇓

Vasodilatation of cavernosal arteries

⇓

Blood fills in corpora cavernosa

⇓

Causes elongation

⇓

Veins get compressed against tunica albuginea

⇓

Subtunical veins get blocked

⇓

Complete venous occlusion causes tumescence

Role of Radiology

Penile Doppler is used to assess the vascular etiology.[23]

- **Procedure of penile Doppler**:
  - B mode ultrasound of scrotum and penis done with 7–15 MHz linear high frequency probe.
    - Assessment of calcification, plaques, tumor, hematoma.
    - Assessment of intact tunica albuginea, corpora cavernosa and the 2 cavernosal arteries within them identified by echogenic wall.
  - Injection of papaverine in the two corpora cavernosa
    - The penis is cleaned with alcohol swab.
    - Under USG guidance, Papaverine is injected at 10 and 2O'clock position by insulin syringe/26 G needle
    - Central artery is avoided.
    - Digital pressure is given at the area of injection.
    - Postinjection measurements are taken at 5, 10, 15, 20 minutes with color and spectral Doppler.

Observations on Color and Spectral Doppler

Arterial Insufficiency

- B mode—failure of cavernosal artery dilatation, i.e., <75% of the arterial dilatation from normal.
- PSV <25 cm/s (>30 - arterial competence, 25–30 not specific)
- Stenosis, occlusions of small arteries or systolic arterial flow reversal causing inadequate intracavernosal pressure.

Veno-occlusive Dysfunction

- Assessed by EDV and RI
- Normal cutoff—EDV <5 cm/sec, RI >0.8
- Should be considered only if PSV >25 cm/s
- **Causes**:
  - Venous leak
  - Inadequate intracavernosal pressure
- **Doppler findings**:
  - Presence of persistent and elevated diastolic flow
  - EDV >5cm/sec, RI <0.8
  - Persistent dorsal vein flow may reflect veno-occlusion failure.
- When Intracavernosal pressure < diastolic blood pressure—appearance of Diastolic notch
- When Intracavernosal pressure = diastolic blood pressure—diastolic cutoff
- When Intracavernosal pressure > diastolic blood pressure—reversal of diastolic flow

Correlation between erection phases and spectral Doppler **(Table 52)**:

TABLE 52: Correlation between erection phases and spectral Doppler.

Erection phases	*Spectral Doppler phases*	*Spectral Doppler waveform*
Flaccid	Phase 0: Monophasic with minimal diastolic flow	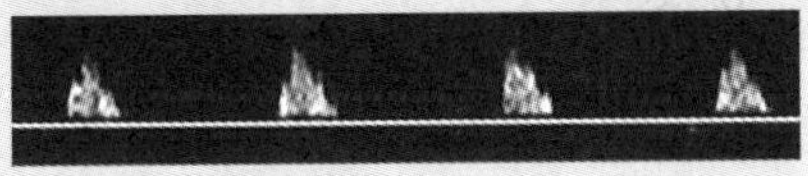
Filling	Phase 1: Increased peak systolic velocity and end-diastolic velocity	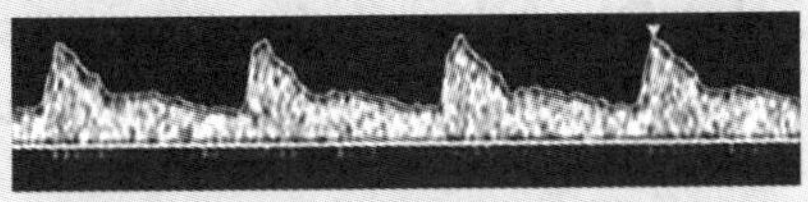
Tumescence	Phase 2: Decrease in diastolic flow with classic dicrotic notch	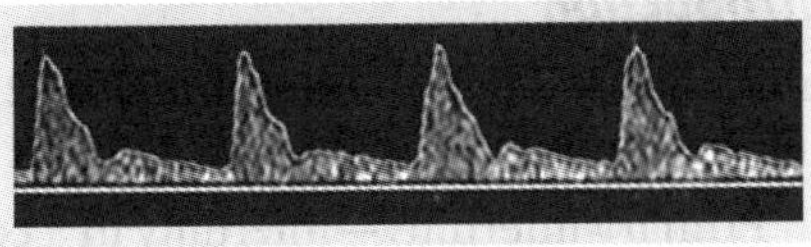

Continued...

Continued...

Erection phases	***Spectral Doppler phases***	***Spectral Doppler waveform***
	Phase 3: Decrease in diastolic flow approaching 0 cm/s	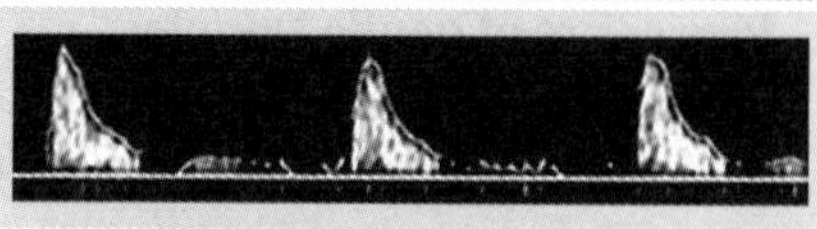
Full erection	Phase 4: Diastolic flow reversal	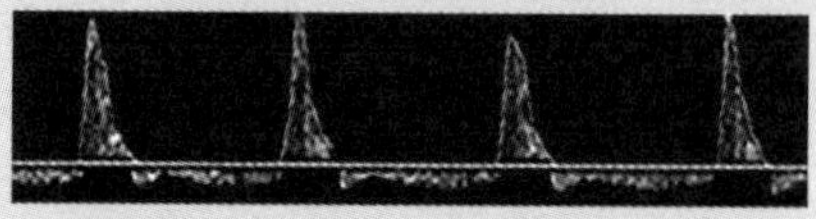
Rigidity	Phase 5: Decrease in peak systolic velocity and end-diastolic velocity	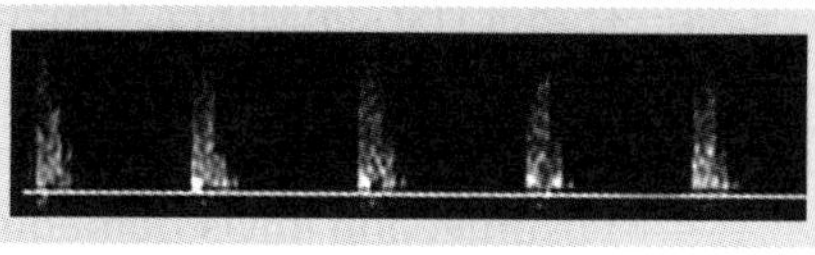

Golden Rule to Remember: Rule of 5/25

- EDV >5 cm/s—veno-occlusive dysfunction
- PSV <25cm/s—arterial insufficiency

Role of Intervention Radiology

- Cavernosography
- Arteriography
- In case arterial insufficiency is present, concurrent presence of venous insufficiency cannot be assessed by penile Doppler study.
- In these cases, cavernosography and arteriography is required.

Extra Points

- When there is discrepancy of >10 cm/sec between the 2 cavernosal arteries, it represents unilateral arterial disease.
- High velocity jets and dampened waveform indicates proximal artery stenosis.
- If there is flow reversal noted in systolic phase, it represents proximal penile artery occlusion.
- Alprostadil or phentolamine can be used. But papaverine is the safest drug.

Complications

1. Hypotension
2. Priapism (painful erection for >4 hrs)
   - Call urologist on call.
   - Administration of alpha-adrenergic agonist
   - Draining out some blood from the corpora cavernosa.
3. Pain
4. Hematoma

5. (a) Describe various causes and role of imaging modalities in male infertility. (b) Role of sonography in erectile dysfunction. [(3+3)+4] [AIIMS Dec 24, AIIMS Dec 23]

Introduction

Infertility is failure of conception for 12 months or more by a couple having regular unprotected sexual intercourse after ruling out physiological causes such as lactational amenorrhea.

- Primary infertility—infertility in a couple who never had a child.
- Secondary infertility—failure of conception following a previous pregnancy.

Common Causes of Male Infertility

A. **Pretesticular**:
   1. Endocrine:
      i. Gonadotrophin deficiency
      ii. Obesity
      iii. Thyroid dysfunction
      iv. Hyperprolactinemia
   2. Psychosexual:
      i. Erectile dysfunction
      ii. Impotence
   3. Drugs:
      i. Antihypertensives
      ii. Antipsychotics
   4. Genetics:
      i. 47 XXY
      ii. Y chromosome deletions
      iii. Single gene mutations

B. **Testicular**:
   1. Immotile cilia syndrome
   2. Cryptorchidism
   3. Infection (mumps orchitis)
   4. Toxins: Drugs, smoking, radiation
   5. Varicocele
   6. Immunologic
   7. Sertoli cell only syndrome
   8. Primary testicular failure
   9. Oligoasthenoteratozoospermia
   10. Neoplasms (primary/metastasis)

C. **Post-testicular**:
   - Obstruction of efferent duct:
     - Congenital
     - Absence of vas deferens (cystic fibrosis)
     - Young syndrome
     - Acquired: Infection (tuberculosis, gonorrhea)
     - Surgical
     - Herniorrhaphy
     - Vasectomy
   - Others:
     - Ejaculatory failure
     - Retrograde ejaculation
     - Hypospadias
     - Bladder neck surgery

- **Radiological investigations in male infertility**:
  - Micturating cystourethrogram (MCU)
  - Retrograde urethrography (RGU)

- Chest X-ray—to rule out Kartagener's syndrome
- Ultrasound: B-mode, color Doppler, transrectal ultrasound
- MRI brain and spine to look for tumors

- **Role of MCU**: Assessment of patency of posterior urethra, stricture, diverticula
- **Role of RGU**: Assessment of patency of anterior urethra, stricture, diverticula
- **Role of chest X-ray**: Dextrocardia with bronchiectasis may indicate Kartagener syndrome
- **Role of ultrasound in male infertility**:
  - Scrotal ultrasound
  - Transrectal ultrasound of vas deferens, seminal vesicles and ejaculatory duct
  - Color Doppler for erectile dysfunction, varicocele, torsion, infections
  - Transabdominal ultrasound for looking at the kidneys and cause of varicocele (if any)
- **Ultrasound of scrotum**:
  - Normal parameters of testis:
    - Ovoid shape
    - 3–5 cm in length
    - 2–3 cm in AP diameter
    - 2–3 cm in width
  - 16–20 cc in volume (reduces with age)
- **B mode ultrasound to look for**:
  - Small volume of testis
  - Undescended testis—in inguinal canal or intrabdominal
  - Testicular lithiasis—multiple tiny calculi in testis
  - Testicular tumor—seminomatous or nonseminomatous germ cell tumor, lymphoma
  - Testicular torsion—twisting of the spermatic cord along its axis
  - Testicular infarction—patchy hypoechoic areas in testis
  - Infections—abscess, tuberculosis
- **Doppler ultrasound to look for**:
  - Varicocele:
    - Erectile dysfunction:
      - EDV >5 cm/s—veno-occlusive dysfunction
      - PSV <25cm/s—arterial insufficiency
- **Role of transrectal ultrasound**:
  - For thorough evaluation of vas deferens, prostate, seminal vesicles, ejaculatory duct, prostatic and membranous urethra.
  - Infections, abscess, obstructing cyst can be seen.
- **Role of transabdominal ultrasound**:
  - To look for intra-abdominal mass causing varicocele, position of kidneys, any associated anomaly.
- **Role of magnetic resonance imaging**:
  - MRI BRAIN + HPA with dynamic contrast—To look for hypothalamo pituitary axis—in prolactinoma, pituitary adenoma may be seen.
  - MRI whole spine screening—spinal cord tumors or any space occupying lesion causing compression of the autonomic nerves.

Role of Sonography in Erectile Dysfunction

Penile Doppler is used to assess the vascular etiology.

- **Procedure of penile Doppler**:
  - B mode ultrasound of scrotum and penis done with 7–15 MHz linear high frequency probe.
    - Assessment of calcification, plaques, tumor, hematoma.

    - Assessment of intact tunica albuginea, corpora cavernosa and the 2 cavernosal arteries within them identified by echogenic wall.
  - **Injection of papaverine in the two corpora cavernosa**:
    - The penis is cleaned with alcohol swab.
    - Under USG guidance, Papaverine is injected at 10 and 2 O'clock position by insulin syringe/26 G needle
    - Central artery is avoided.
    - Digital pressure is given at the area of injection.
    - Postinjection—measurements are taken at 5, 10, 15, 20 minutes with color and spectral Doppler.
- **Observations on color and spectral Doppler**:
  - Arterial insufficiency
  - B mode-failure of cavernosal artery dilatation, i.e., <75% of the arterial dilatation from normal.
  - PSV <25 cm/s (>30—arterial competence, 25–30 not specific)
  - Stenosis, occlusions of small arteries or systolic arterial flow reversal causing inadequate intracavernosal pressure.
- **Veno-occlusive dysfunction**:
  - Assessed by EDV and RI
  - Normal cutoff—EDV <5 cm/sec, RI >0.8
  - Should be considered only if PSV >25 cm/s
  - Causes
    - Venous leak
    - Inadequate intracavernosal pressure
- **Doppler findings**:
  - Presence of persistent and elevated diastolic flow
  - EDV >5cm/sec, RI <0.8
  - Persistent dorsal vein flow may reflect veno-occlusion failure.
- When intracavernosal pressure < diastolic blood pressure—appearance of diastolic notch
- When intracavernosal pressure = diastolic blood pressure—diastolic cutoff
- When intracavernosal pressure > diastolic blood pressure—reversal of diastolic flow

Correlation between erection phases and spectral Doppler **(Table 52)**.

Golden Rule to Remember: Rule of 5/25

- EDV >5 cm/s—veno-occlusive dysfunction
- PSV <25cm/s—arterial insufficiency.

Vascular Diseases

1. What are the common types of renal artery Dysplasia with its clinical features? What are the Angiographic features of FMD? [10] [MD (WBUHS) 19]

Introduction

Fibromuscular dysplasia is a noninflammatory, nonatherosclerotic disease of small to medium sized arteries.

Clinical Features

- **Symptoms due to renal artery involvement**: Hypertension
- **Symptoms due to carotid or vertebral artery involvement**: Headache, pulsatile tinnitus, TIA, stroke, dissection
- **Symptoms due to coronary artery involvement**: Angina, sudden cardiac death, myocardial infarction
- **Symptoms due to mesenteric artery involvement**: Mesenteric ischemia

Types: Three types based on the vessel wall layer affected:

- **Media**: 90–95%: Medial fibromuscular dysplasia
- Medial fibroplasia (most common type)
- Perimedial fibroplasia
- Medial hyperplasia
- **Intima**: Intimal fibroplasia
- **Adventitia**: Adventitial fibroplasia (rare)

Angiographic Features of Fibromuscular Dysplasia

- Gold standard modality is **Digital Subtraction angiography**.
- Evaluation of small arteries and peripheral lesions.
- **Intimal and adventitial type of FMD**:
  - Focal/diffuse concentric stenosis
  - Diverticular outpouching
- **Other appearance**:
  - Renal ischemic changes when renal arteries are involved
  - Vascular loops
  - Fusiform ectasia
- Dissection
- Aneurysm
- Subarachnoid hemorrhage

Medial FMD

Histology: Alternating areas of collagen and loss of elastic membrane with preserved internal elastic lamina.

Angiographic appearance:

- String of beads pattern in medial type of FMD-alternating narrowing and dilatation in mid and distal renal arteries.
- Ostial part of renal artery is not affected (in contrast to atherosclerosis).

Intimal FMD

- **Histology**:
  - Circumferential deposition of collagen in intima
  - Fragmentation of internal elastic lamina
- **Angiographic appearance**: Concentric smooth stenosis.

Adventitial FMD

- **Histology**: Deposition of collage in adventitia
- **Angiographic appearance**: Concentric smooth stenosis
- **Angiographic variants of FMD**:
  - Multifocal: Multiple areas of stenosis with string of beads appearance
  - Tubular: Concentric stenosis >1 cm in length
  - Focal: Single area of stenosis <1 cm in length
  - Mixed type

2. Imaging in renal artery stenosis. [5] [DNB Dec 21, MD (WBUHS) 24]

Introduction

It refers to focal or diffuse narrowing of the renal arteries.

Causes

- Atherosclerosis
- Fibromuscular dysplasia
- Vasculitis—Takayasu arteritis, Polyarteritis nodosa
- Neurofibromatosis—1
- Post-traumatic sequalae
- Entrapment of renal artery in psoas muscle or crus of diaphragm in case of high origin of renal artery

Imaging Features

- **Ultrasound**:
  - Assessment of:
    - Renal size (length, width, and parenchymal thickness)
    - Renal cortical scars (due to ischemia or infarction)
    - Renal mass (pheochromocytoma or paraganglioma)
    - Features of end stage renal disease—small kidney with parenchymal thinning
  - Doppler study of abdominal aorta and renal arteries
  - Size of abdominal aorta
  - Atherosclerotic changes
  - PSV in prerenal segment of aorta
  - Doppler of both renal arteries at origin, mid and distal segment and se
- **Color Doppler**:
  - Direct signs (at stenosis site)
    - Aliasing at the site of stenosis (turbulent flow)
    - Peak systolic velocity >180 cm/sec
    - Turbulent flow distal to the stenosis with spectral broadening
    - Main renal artery to abdominal aorta peak systolic velocity ratio >3.5 **(Table 53)**
  - Indirect signs (distal to stenosis site)
    - Increased acceleration time >70ms
    - Decreased acceleration index <300 cm/s^2
    - Low velocity blood flow
  - Spectral doppler (distal to stenosis site):
    - Tardus parvus waveform within segmental arteries.
- **CT angiography**:
  - Modality of choice for evaluation of the abdominal aorta and its branches.
  - Calcifications, soft plaques, atherosclerotic changes in abdominal aorta and renal arteries
  - String of beads pattern in medial type of FMD—alternating narrowing and dilatation in mid and distal renal arteries.
  - **Kidneys**: Decreased in size and decreased enhancement
  - Highly sensitive and specific.

TABLE 53: Classification of renal artery stenosis.

Severity	*Renal artery diameter reduction*	*PSV (cm/s)*	*Renal artery— aorta PSV ratio*
Normal	Normal	<180	<3.5
Mild	<60%	>180	<3.5
Moderate	>60%	>180	>3.5
Occlusion	Complete occlusion	Absent signal	Absent signals

- **MR angiography**:
  - Used when CT angiography is contraindicated.
  - Patients with raised serum creatinine
  - Non contrast—evaluation of abdominal aorta and main branches
  - Contrast MRA—evaluation of smaller segmental and intrarenal arteries
  - High sensitivity and specificity but less than CT angiography.

3. Discuss Imaging features of renal artery stenosis on ultrasonography and MR angiography and briefly the role of interventions in its management. [3+3+4] [MD (WBUHS) 24, AIIMS Dec 24]

Introduction

It refers to focal or diffuse narrowing of the renal arteries.

Causes

- Atherosclerosis
- Fibromuscular dysplasia
- Vasculitis—Takayasu arteritis, Polyarteritis nodosa
- Neurofibromatosis—1
- Post-traumatic sequalae
- Entrapment of renal artery in psoas muscle or crus of diaphragm in case of high origin of renal artery.

Imaging Features

- **Ultrasound**:
  - Assessment of
    - Renal size (length, width and parenchymal thickness)
    - Renal cortical scars (due to ischemia or infarction)
    - Renal mass (pheochromocytoma or paraganglioma)
    - Features of end stage renal disease—small kidney with parenchymal thinning
  - Doppler study of abdominal aorta and renal arteries
  - Size of abdominal aorta
  - Atherosclerotic changes
  - PSV in prerenal segment of aorta
  - Doppler of both renal arteries at origin, mid and distal segment and se
- **Color Doppler**:
  - Direct signs (at stenosis site)
    - Aliasing at the site of stenosis (turbulent flow)
    - Peak systolic velocity >180 cm/sec
    - Turbulent flow distal to the stenosis with spectral broadening
    - Main renal artery to abdominal aorta peak systolic velocity ratio >3.5 **(Table 52)**
  - Indirect signs (distal to stenosis site)
    - Increased acceleration time >70ms
    - Decreased acceleration index <300 cm/s^2
    - Low velocity blood flow
  - Spectral Doppler (distal to stenosis site): Tardus parvus waveform within segmental arteries.
- **MR angiography**:
  - Used when CT angiography is contraindicated.

- Patients with raised serum creatinine
- Noncontrast—evaluation of abdominal aorta and main branches
- Contrast MRA—evaluation of smaller segmental and intrarenal arteries
- High sensitivity and specificity but less than CT angiography
- Gadolinium contrast agent—0.2 mmol/kg injected at the rate of 1.5–2 mL/s.

Imaging Methods

1. Time of flight (TOF)—high velocity jet of blood at stenosed part—signal void
2. Phase contrast technique
3. Gadolinium enhanced MR angiography:
   - Breath hold—3D spoiled gradient echo imaging
   - T1—shortening effect—intravenous administration of paramagnetic contrast agent
   - Blood—bright
   - Stationary tissues—dark
   - Subtracted images—removal of signal and improvement of vessel to background signal.
   - Stenosis in proximal 3–3.5 cm of renal arteries can be diagnosed
   - Limited visualization of stenosis of distal renal arteries and segmental renal arteries
   - Limited visualization in the presence of metallic stent

Patients with Renal Impairment: TOF Imaging

- **Interventions in renal artery stenosis**:
  - Endoluminal stent placement (preferred)
  - Balloon angioplasty
  - Percutaneous angioplasty in FMD
- If renal function is normal, revascularization is recommended if the following criteria are fulfilled:
  - Degree of RAS >80–85%
  - Degree of RAS -50–80% and captopril scintigraphy shows intrarenal RAS
- If renal function is abnormal, the following criteria has to fulfilled:
  - Serum creatinine <4mg/dl
  - Serum creatinine >4mg/dl with renal artery thrombosis
  - Degree of RAS >80%
  - Degree of RAS - 50–80% and scintigraphy positive for RAS
  - Increase of serum creatinine with ACE inhibitors.

Recent Advances

1. Discuss radiological evaluation of renal transplant donor. [10] [MD (WBUHS) 20]

Modality of Choice for Evaluation of Potential Renal Donor

MDCT angiography of renal vessels and abdominal vessels **(Table 54)**

- **Postprocessing methods**:
  - Multiplanar reconstruction (MPR)
  - Curved MPR
  - Maximum intensity projection (MIP)
  - 3D volume rendered images
- Arterial anatomy and the variants **(Table 55)**
- Venous anatomy and the variants **(Table 56)**:

TABLE 54: CT Protocol for assessment of donor renal system.

Computed tomography protocol for assessment of the donor renal system		
Phase	***Timing of image acquisition***	***Utility***
Precontrast	Before intravenous contrast administration	For detection of renal calculi and calcifications
Arterial	Through bolus tracking	Assessment of arterial anatomy
Nephrogenic	100 sec postcontrast injection	Renal parenchymal assessment and venous anatomy assessment
Excretory	5–10 minutes postcontrast injection	Assessment of collecting system and urothelial pathologies

TABLE 55: Renal arterial anatomy and the variants.

Variants	***Description***	***Implications***	
Extra-renal arteries	Accessory arteries	• They extend to the kidney through the hilum with the main renal artery • Mostly arise from the aorta	• The presence of accessory arteries increases the risk of thrombosis and intra-operative time • The presence of more than two arteries within a kidney is a contraindication for donation
	Aberrant arteries	• They can be capsular arteries or polar arteries • Capsular arteries are thin vessels that course along the renal capsule tangentially • Polar arteries enter the kidneys through the superior or inferior pole	• Small upper polar and intracapsular arteries of caliber <2 mm can be sacrificed because the renal infarct produced is very small • Lower polar arteries should be preserved because their excision can lead to ureteral complications because they may supply the ureter
Early branching of renal artery		• The first branch at <10–15 mm of its origin in the case of left renal artery • Branching behind the IVC or within 1 cm of the right IVC margin in the case of the right renal artery	• Expert surgeons require at least 1 cm of the main renal artery to properly anastomose the artery in the recipient • Working posterior to the IVC is difficult because of the possibility of injuring a large vessel

TABLE 56: Renal venous anatomy and the variants.

Variant	***Description***	***Implications***
Multiple renal veins	This is the most common variant. These supernumerary double or triple renal veins are more common on the right side	• In case of multiple renal veins inserting into the IVC, the insertion should be evaluated for circumferential and craniocaudal separation • Circumferential separation without craniocaudal separation creates difficulty for the surgeon in IVC repair
Circumaortic and retroaortic renal veins	• These are common on the left side. • Whereas circumaortic vein embraces the dorsal and ventral aorta and is more common retroaortic veins are present posterior to the aorta	In the case of a circumaortic vein, if there is a significant discrepancy between the calibers of anterior and posterior veins or if one of the veins is significantly small, then the surgeon may completely ligate the smaller vein

Pretransplant Workup in Donor

A. **Kidneys**:

- Size, shape, echogenicity, location
- Presence of calculi-single calculi ≥5 mm or multiple renal calculi—contraindication to donation
- Perirenal fat-more fat—more time taken for surgery, difficulty to dissect the hilum

B. Renal arteries—main and accessory renal arteries, multiple renal arteries.[24]
- Interarterial distance between accessory renal artery and main renal artery
- In the presence of multiple renal arteries, the artery with the largest diameter is considered the main renal artery.
- Diameter of main renal artery is measured in orthogonal plane and should be 3 mm.
- Calcification, if present can hinder clamping and cause incomplete occlusion and laceration
- Significant atherosclerotic changes—endarterectomy
- Fibromuscular dysplasia of B/L renal arteries—contraindication to donation
- Main renal artery:
  - Diameter
  - Length (origin to bifurcation)
  - Early segmentation—Present or absent
  - Right renal artery—arterial branching 1 cm or less from right margin of IVC
  - Left renal artery—arterial branching 1.5 cm or less from LRA origin
- Accessory renal artery:
  - Present or absent
  - Diameter
  - Arising from aorta above/below main renal artery—distance in mm/cm
  - Distance between main and accessory renal artery
- Aberrant renal artery: Polar, capsular
  - Number—single, double, triple
  - Length

C. **Renal veins**:
- Number
- Late confluence—joining of venous tributaries within 1.5 cm of the left lateral margin of the aorta on the left side and 1.5 cm from confluence of the renal vein with IVC on the right side.
- Length of right renal vein
- Length of left renal vein
- Distance between the confluence of the left renal vein and lumbar vein and confluence of left renal vein and IVC
- Left gonadal vein
- Left circumaortic, retroaortic veins

D. Urinary bladder

E. IVC

F. Other solid organs and bowel

2. How would you evaluate donor kidney for renal transplant. Discuss role of ultrasonography and scintigraphy in various types of renal graft dysfunction. [4+3+3] [MD (WBUHS) 21]

Modality of Choice for Evaluation of Potential Renal Donor

MDCT angiography of renal vessels and abdominal vessels **(Table 54)**

- **Postprocessing methods**:
  - Multiplanar reconstruction (MPR)
  - Curved MPR
  - Maximum intensity projection (MIP)
  - 3D volume rendered images
- Arterial anatomy and the variants **(Table 55)**
- Venous anatomy and the variants **(Table 56)**:

Pretransplant Workup in Donor

A. **Kidneys**:
   - Size, shape, echogenicity, location
   - Presence of calculi-single calculi ≥5 mm or multiple renal calculi—contraindication to donation
   - Perirenal fat-more fat—more time taken for surgery, difficulty to dissect the hilum

B. Renal arteries—main and accessory renal arteries, multiple renal arteries
   - Interarterial distance between accessory renal artery and main renal artery
   - In the presence of multiple renal arteries, the artery with the largest diameter is considered the main renal artery.
   - Diameter of main renal artery is measured in orthogonal plane and should be 3 mm.
   - Calcification, if present can hinder clamping and cause incomplete occlusion and laceration
   - Significant atherosclerotic changes—endarterectomy
   - Fibromuscular dysplasia of B/L renal arteries-contraindication to donation
   - Main renal artery:
     - Diameter
     - Length (origin to bifurcation)
     - Early segmentation—present or absent
     - Right renal artery—arterial branching 1 cm or less from right margin of IVC
     - Left renal artery—arterial branching 1.5 cm or less from LRA origin
   - Accessory renal artery:
     - Present or absent
     - Diameter
     - Arising from aorta above/below main renal artery—distance in mm/cm
     - Distance between main and accessory renal artery
   - Aberrant renal artery: Polar, Capsular
     - Number—Single, double, triple
     - Length

C. **Renal veins**:
   - Number
   - Late confluence—joining of venous tributaries within 1.5 cm of the left lateral margin of the aorta on the left side and 1.5 cm from confluence of the renal vein with IVC on the right side.
   - Length of right renal vein
   - Length of left renal vein
   - Distance between the confluence of the left renal vein and lumbar vein and confluence of left renal vein and IVC
   - Left gonadal vein
   - Left circumaortic, retroaortic veins

D. Urinary bladder

E. IVC

F. Other solid organs and bowel.

Role of Ultrasonography in Renal Graft Dysfunction

It is the first investigation of choice post-transplant.

- Done within 24 hours.
- Transplant kidney is superficially located—provides good acoustic window

Imaging Features

- **B-mode**:
  - Size and shape of graft kidney
  - Echogenicity of parenchyma
  - Corticomedullary differentiation lost and Cortical echogenicity increased—graft dysfunction
  - Renal sinus fat less echogenic
  - Collecting system
  - Dilatation due to obstruction
  - Grading of hydronephrosis
  - Cortical thinning
  - Ureteric stricture and thickening
  - Ureterovesical junction
  - Bladder
  - Presence of calculi
  - Perirenal collection—abscess, hematoma, urinoma, lymphocele
  - Stents and tubes: Location, migration, kinking, patency
- **Color Doppler**:
  - Patency of vessels
  - Flow direction
  - Vascular stenosis or thrombosis
  - Anomalies of aorta
  - Aorta, internal iliac artery, external iliac artery, transplanted vessels
  - Examination of the carrel's patch—in case of cadaveric donor, part of the iliac vessels is grafted along with the kidney.
- Spectral Doppler of segmental and interlobar arteries **(Table 57)**:
  - Fast upstroke with slow decay and forward flow
  - Resistivity index (RI), pulsatility index (PI) and systolic to diastolic ratio—for quantification of flow.

Ultrasound Guided Procedures

Biopsy and drainage of collection easy to perform with lower incidence of complications because of its superficial location.

- **Contrast enhanced ultrasound**:
  - Not FDA approved
  - Contrast media is not nephrotoxic.
  - For assessment of graft perfusion and infarcts
  - Confirmation of renal artery stenosis and estimation of degree
  - Confirmation of renal abscess, masses
  - Graft nephropathy—reduced blood flow

TABLE 57: Color Doppler and spectral analysis in transplanted kidneys.

	Where to measure	*Application*	*Values*
Resistivity Index	Renal segmental or interlobar artery measured by duplex Doppler USG	Differentiate a normal from abnormal allograft function	>0.8 associated with allograft dysfunction
Peak systolic velocity	In the renal artery	RAS	>200–300 cm/sec highly suggestive of RAS

(RAS: renal artery stenosis; USG: ultrasonography)

- **Ultrasound elastography**:
  - Parenchymal fibrosis assessed by measuring stiffness
  - Higher values indicates diseased kidney

Role of Scintigraphy in Renal Graft Dysfunction

- Noninvasive assessment of transplant kidney
- Serial images for assessing renal function
- Independent of serum creatinine.

Agents used: Technetium-99m DTPA, technetium-99m MAG3 (mercapto-acetyl-triglycine) (preferred)

Useful for assessment of:
- The graft and native kidney separately
- Baseline investigation for assessing renal function post-transplant, return of function post-ATN (acute tubular necrosis) or rejection
- Assessment of urinary leakage—leakage of agent in abnormal location
- Renal artery stenosis or obstruction—ACE inhibitors or diuretics used.

Interpretation: Reduced or absence of perfusion of the graft on time intensity curve in case of renal artery thrombosis, renal artery stenosis.

3. Briefly discuss USG features of renal transplant. [10] [MD (WBUHS) 19]

USG Features of Renal Transplant

- It is the first investigation of choice post-transplant.
- Done within 24 hrs.
- Transplant kidney is superficially located - provides good acoustic window

Imaging Features

- **B-mode**:
  - Size and shape of graft kidney
  - Echogenicity of parenchyma
  - Corticomedullary differentiation lost and cortical echogenicity increased—graft dysfunction
  - Renal sinus fat less echogenic
  - Collecting system
  - Dilatation due to obstruction
  - Grading of hydronephrosis
  - Cortical thinning
  - Ureteric stricture and thickening
  - Ureterovesical junction
  - Bladder
  - Presence of calculi
  - Perirenal collection—abscess, hematoma, urinoma, lymphocele
  - Stents and tubes: Location, migration, kinking, patency
- **Color Doppler**:
  - Patency of vessels
  - Flow direction
  - Vascular stenosis or thrombosis
  - Anomalies of aorta

  - Aorta, internal iliac artery, external iliac artery, transplanted vessels
  - Examination of the CARREL'S PATCH - in case of cadaveric donor, part of the iliac vessels is grafted along with the kidney.
- **Spectral Doppler of segmental and interlobar arteries (Table 57)**:
  - Fast upstroke with slow decay and forward flow
  - Resistivity index, pulsatility index, and systolic to diastolic ratio—for quantification of flow
- **Ultrasound guided procedures**:
  - Biopsy and drainage of collection easy to perform with lower incidence of complications because of its superficial location
- **Contrast enhanced ultrasound**:
  - Not FDA approved
  - Contrast media is not nephrotoxic
  - For assessment of graft perfusion and infarcts
  - Confirmation of renal artery stenosis and estimation of degree
  - Confirmation of renal abscess, masses
  - Graft nephropathy reduced blood flow
- **Ultrasound elastography**:
  - Parenchymal fibrosis assessed by measuring stiffness
  - Higher values indicates diseased kidney

4. Briefly discuss the role of ultrasound Doppler in postoperative evaluation of AV fistula for dialysis. [5]

Introduction

Ultrasound Doppler evaluation is the modality of choice for pre and post operative AVF. The various complications and functionality can be assessed and measures for intervention can be taken.[25]

Indications

- **Preoperative indications for USG and CD Imaging**:
  - To detect suitable vein
  - To determine surgical technique
  - In patients with previous AVF failure
  - In patients with history of CVC placement
- **Postoperative indications for USG and CD Imaging**:
  - Abnormal functioning fistula
  - Loss of thrill
  - Distal limb ischemia
  - Difficult cannulation
  - Obvious limb swelling
  - Elevated venous pressure >200 mm Hg
  - Elevated recirculation time (≥15%)

The different types of AVF are as follows **(Figs. 63A to C)**:

- **Procedure of post operative evaluation of AVF**:
  - Doppler evaluation in postoperative day 1 or 2—counted as first scan
  - Done again in 2nd and 6th week
  - Tourniquet is not used.

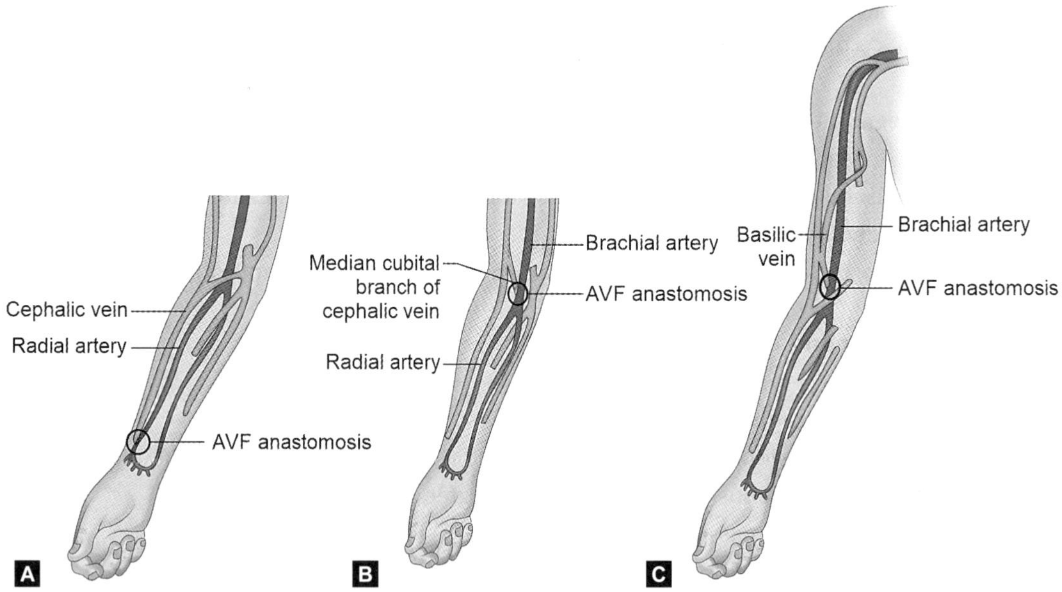

FIGS. 63A to C: Various types of AVF.

- Optimum amount of gel and minimal pressure
- Maximum gate in the middle of the vessel with an angle of insonation <60 degrees
- Feeding artery, draining vein and AVF assessed—show aliasing flow
- Puncture site evaluated for thrombosis
- Patency, narrowing assessed.
- Blood flow in mid part of AVF and continuous draining vein approximately 10 away from anastomosis is measured.
- Evaluation of deep veins of upper limb for ruling out DVT
- Neck veins evaluated for steal syndrome, thrombosis and obstruction
- Branches of large veins within 10 cm of draining vein are assessed because of possibility of decreased blood flow to the fistula and causing immaturity.

- **Evaluation of maturation of AVF**:
  - Ultrasound is the ideal modality
  - Size, diameter, length, depth of outflow vein
  - Flow pattern and volume
  - Obstruction—site, nature (valve hypertrophy, valve dysfunction)
  - Collateral vessels—in case of stenosis collaterals open up
  - Accessory veins: Normal, duplicated or variant veins competing against the flow in cannulation segment
  - Decision whether fistulogram or venoplasty required or not
  - Subcutaneous edema
  - Hematoma
  - Lymphocele
  - Interventions to reduce the collections
- **Features of a mature fistula**:
  - Rule of 6:
    - Flow velocity >600 mL/min
    - >6 mm diameter
    - <6 mm below skin
    - Examination done <6 weeks post op

- Causes of AVF immaturity:
    - Inflow blockage
    - Outflow blockage

Inflow Blockage

Can occur anywhere from heart to needle cannulation segment

- Arterial stenosis (subclavian, axillary, brachial, radial)
- Venous juxta anastomotic stenosis

Juxta anastomotic stenosis or swing point venous stenosis
1-4 cm beyond AV anastomosis

Etiology

- Trauma during surgery-twisting or kinking of vein during maneuvering causing adventitial ischemia
- Altered flow dynamics in case of end to side anastomosis.

AVF Stenosis

- **Anywhere in the circuit**:
    - Inflow artery
    - AV anastomosis
    - Juxta-anastomotic 1-3 cm
    - Cannulation zone
    - Outflow veins
    - Cephalic arch
- **Complications**:
    - Thrombosis
    - Aneurysm
    - Infection
    - Stenosis
    - Heart failure
    - Steal syndrome
- **Highest risk of stenosis in radiocephalic fistula**: At the anastomotic site
- **Highest risk of stenosis in brachiocephalic fistula**: Cephalic arch
- Recurrence of stenosis is common
- In case of failed or difficult dialysis, reevaluation is done.

5. Role of imaging in management of renal transplant patient. [10] [DNB June 22]

USG Features of Renal Transplant

- It is the first investigation of choice post-transplant.
- Done within 24 hrs.
- Transplant kidney is superficially located-provides good acoustic window

Imaging Features

- **B-mode**:
    - Size and shape of graft kidney
    - Echogenicity of parenchyma
    - Corticomedullary differentiation lost and cortical echogenicity increased—graft dysfunction

- Renal sinus fat less echogenic
- Collecting system
- Dilatation due to obstruction
- Grading of hydronephrosis
- Cortical thinning
- Ureteric stricture and thickening
- Ureterovesical junction
- Bladder
- Presence of calculi
- Perirenal collection—abscess, hematoma, urinoma, lymphocele
- Stents and tubes: Location, migration, kinking, patency

- **Color Doppler**:
  - Patency of vessels
  - Flow direction
  - Vascular stenosis or thrombosis
  - Anomalies of aorta
  - Aorta, internal iliac artery, external iliac artery, transplanted vessels
  - Examination of the carrel's patch—in case of cadaveric donor, part of the iliac vessels is grafted along with the kidney.
- Spectral Doppler of segmental and interlobar arteries **(Table 57)**:
  - Fast upstroke with slow decay and forward flow
  - Resistivity index, pulsatility index, and systolic to diastolic ratio - for quantification of flow
- **Ultrasound guided procedures**: Biopsy and drainage of collection easy to perform with lower incidence of complications because of its superficial location.
- **Contrast enhanced ultrasound**
  - Not FDA approved
  - Contrast media is not nephrotoxic.
  - For assessment of graft perfusion and infarcts
  - Confirmation of renal artery stenosis and estimation of degree
  - Confirmation of renal abscess, masses
  - Graft nephropathy—reduced blood flow
- **Ultrasound elastography**
  - Parenchymal fibrosis assessed by measuring stiffness
  - Higher values indicates diseased kidney

Assessment of Renal Transplant Complications

Transplant kidney is at the risk of perioperative and iatrogenic complications

Classified as:

1. **Vascular complications**:
   - Renal artery thrombosis
   - Rean vein thrombosis
   - Arteriovenous malformation
   - Pseudoaneurysm
   - Renal artery stenosis
2. **Nonvascular complications (Table 58)**:
   - Acute tubular necrosis (ATN)
   - Acute rejection

TABLE 58: Describing nonvascular complications post renal transplant.

Acute event	*Timeline*	*USG or Doppler features*	*Remarks*
ATN	Within 24–48 hours	• Enlarged kidneys with a loss of corticomedullary differentiation • Diminished cortical flow and increased intraparenchymal arterial RIs on Doppler	• BOLD MRI can distinguish acute rejection from ATN • Ultrasound-guided biopsy is recommended for final diagnosis
Acute infection	Within 1 week	Normal appearance to bulky and hypoechoic kidney	Contrast-enhanced computed tomography in complications such as abscess or emphysematous pyelonephritis
Acute rejection	A few days to weeks	• Edematous thickened cortex • Diminished diastolic blood flow and resultant elevated RIs	• Contrast-enhanced USG evaluates microvascular renal perfusion, predicts graft viability and an impending loss of renal function • Newer functional MRI may be helpful

- Hydronephrosis
- Infections: Pyonephrosis, Pyelonephritis, Emphysematous pyelonephritis
- Herniation of transplant kidney
- Stone formation (struvite and calcium phosphate) is more common post-transplant than in nontransplant patients
- Neoplasm: Post-transplant lymphoproliferative disorders, renal cell carcinoma
- Perirenal collections: Hematoma, urinoma, abscess, lymphocele **(Table 59)**

TABLE 59: Complications comprising fluid collections in post renal transplant.

Fluid collection	*Timeframe*	*Imaging features*	*Fluid analysis*
Hematoma	Immediate postoperative —5 days	• Complex, heterogeneous fluid collection with septations, retracting clot • Hyperdense components at unenhanced CT	Not usually aspirated due to risk of superinfection
Abscess	5 days, but variable according to infectious etiology	• Peripheral enhancement at CECT • Increased peripheral color Doppler flow at US • Thickened wall	Purulent material, numerous polymorphonucleocytes (PMNs)
Urinoma	10 days	• Simple fluid-attenuation collection • Contrast extravasation at delayed CECT • Extra-urinary tracer excretion at renal scintigraphy (e.g., 99mTc-MAG3 or 99mTc-DTPA)	• Fluid creatinine > serum creatinine • Fluid K > serum K
Lymphocele	10 days–2 months	Fluid-attenuation collection lacking epithelial lining ± thin septations, often adjacent to the allograft or along pelvic sidewall	• Fluid creatinine serum creatinine • Fluid K serum creatinine

Vascular Complications of Transplant Kidney

Renal Artery Thrombosis

- Within minutes to hours
- Fatal, rare complication
- Hyperacute rejection, occlusion at anastomotic site, kinking of renal artery, dissection-lead to renal artery thrombosis.
- **Imaging features**:
  - Ultrasound: Hypoechoic region with indistinct or well-defined echogenic margins
  - Color Doppler: Global absence of color flow (also seen in hyperacute rejection or renal vein thrombosis)

  - CT or MR angiography: Decreased or absent flow
  - Renal scintigraphy: Reduced or absence of perfusion of the graft on time intensity curve.
- **Management**: Transplant nephrectomy

Renal Vein Thrombosis

- After postoperative day 5
- More common in children <6yrs and adults > 50 yrs
- **Higher risk**:
  1. Patients having atherosclerotic, hypercoagulable states, or undergoing peritoneal dialysis, diabetic patients
  2. Left iliac fossa transplant kidney—due to compression of left iliac vein by aorta or overlying artery.
- **Clinical features**: Pain, oliguria, anuria
- **Imaging features**:
  - Ultrasound:
    - Edematous, enlarged transplant kidney, corticomedullary differentiation is lost, perinephric fluid
    - Dilated renal vein with thrombus
  - Color Doppler:
    - Absence of color flow
    - Reversal of color flow in renal artery (also seen in torsion of vascular pedicle, allograft rejection, ATN)
- **Management**: Surgical thrombectomy
- Late renal vein thrombosis—endovascular thrombolysis

Renal Artery Stenosis

- Most common vascular complication
- May be focal or diffuse
- Classified as preanastomotic, anastomotic and postanastomotic depending on the site of stenosis.
- **Duration**: 3 months to 2 years
- **Clinical features**: Refractory hypertension
- **Risk factors**:
  - Donor—recipient related: Atherosclerosis, infection, old age of recipient or donor, immunological causes
- **Recipient factors**:
  - Rejection
  - Delayed graft function
  - Ischemic heart disease
  - Extrinsic compression due to polycystic kidney or pseudoaneurysm
  - Iatrogenic trauma
- **Imaging features**:
  - Ultrasound with color Doppler
  - Stenotic site—aliasing
  - Elevated PSV>200-300 cm/s
  - Tardus parvus waveform—small amplitude peak with delayed upstroke
  - Acceleration time—0.1 sec
  - Renal artery—external iliac artery ratio—cutoff 1.8
  - Elevated PSV >250cm/s
- **CT and MR angiography**:
  - For confirmation
  - Done before endovascular intervention

Perirenal Hematoma

- Postoperative 0–5 days
- Due to inadequate surgical anastomosis
- Anticoagulation
- Postbiopsy
- **Imaging features**:
  - Ultrasound:
    - Acute—anechoic, echogenic debris
    - Subacute—heterogeneously hyperechoic
    - Chronic—centrally hypoechoic or cystic, thin internal septations—indicates clot lysis
  - NCCT:
    - Acute—hyperdense (>30–40 HU)
    - Subacute—iso to hyperdense
    - Chronic—hypodense
  - MRI:
    - Blooming on gradient sequences
    - Hyperintense on T1
    - Depending on the age, T1 and T2 appearances vary

Renal Arteriovenous Malformation

Laceration of vessel wall leads to communication of artery with adjacent vein

- **Clinical features**:
  - Gross hematuria
  - Hypertension
  - High output cardiac failure (AV fistula)
- **Ultrasound**: Simple or complex cystic structure
- **Color Doppler**:
  - Mosaic appearance
  - Feeding artery—high velocity, low resistance waveform
  - Draining vein—pulsatile waveform
- **Management**: Catheter embolization

Pseudoaneurysm of Renal Artery

- Postbiopsy
- During transplant surgery
- **Ultrasound**:
  - B-mode: Simple or complex cystic structure
  - Color Doppler: Yin-Yang sign to-and-fro pattern in the aneurysm sac
- **CT angiography**:
  - Identification of Feeding vessel, draining vein
  - Determination of size and extension
  - Done before endovascular intervention
- **Management**: Endovascular intervention (coiling) when pseudoaneurysm >2 cm in size
- Ultrasound guided percutaneous thrombin injection also done.

6. (a) Imaging workup of a potential renal donor. (b) Imaging evaluation of vascular complications of a transplant kidney. [5+5] [DNB June 20]

Modality of Choice for Evaluation of Potential Renal Donor

MDCT angiography of renal vessels and abdominal vessels **(Table 54)**

- Postprocessing methods:
  - Multiplanar reconstruction (MPR)
  - Curved MPR
  - Maximum intensity projection (MIP)
  - 3D volume rendered images
- Arterial anatomy and the variants **(Table 55)**
- Venous anatomy and the variants **(Table 56)**:

Pretransplant Workup In Donor

A. **Kidneys**:
  - Size, shape, echogenicity, location
  - Presence of calculi-single calculi ≥ 5 mm or multiple renal calculi - contraindication to donation
  - Perirenal fat-more fat—more time taken for surgery, difficulty to dissect the hilum

B. Renal arteries—main and accessory renal arteries, multiple renal arteries
  - Interarterial distance between accessory renal artery and main renal artery
  - In the presence of multiple renal arteries, the artery with the largest diameter is considered the main renal artery.
  - Diameter of main renal artery is measured in orthogonal plane and should be 3 mm.
  - Calcification, if present can hinder clamping and cause incomplete occlusion and laceration
  - Significant atherosclerotic changes-endarterectomy
  - Fibromuscular dysplasia of B/L renal arteries-contraindication to donation
  - Main renal artery:
    - Diameter
    - Length (origin to bifurcation)
    - Early segmentation—Present or absent
    - Right renal artery—arterial branching 1 cm or less from right margin of IVC
    - Left renal artery—arterial branching 1.5 cm or less from LRA origin
  - Accessory renal artery:
    - Present or absent
    - Diameter
    - Arising from aorta above/below main renal artery—distance in mm/cm
    - Distance between main and accessory renal artery.
  - Aberrant renal artery—polar, capsular
    - Number—single, double, triple
    - Length

C. **Renal veins**:
  - Number
  - Late confluence-joining of venous tributaries within 1.5 cm of the left lateral margin of the aorta on the left side and 1.5 cm from confluence of the renal vein with IVC on the right side.
  - Length of right renal vein
  - Length of left renal vein
  - Distance between the confluence of the left renal vein and lumbar vein and confluence of left renal vein and IVC
  - Left gonadal vein
  - Left circumaortic, retroaortic veins

D. Urinary bladder
E. IVC
F. Other solid organs and bowel

Vascular Complications of Transplant Kidney

Renal Artery Thrombosis

- Within minutes to hours
- Fatal, rare complication
- Hyperacute rejection, occlusion at anastomotic site, kinking of renal artery, dissection- lead to renal artery thrombosis.
- **Imaging features**:
  - **Ultrasound**:
    - Hypoechoic region with indistinct or well defined echogenic margins
    - Color Doppler: Global absence of color flow (also seen in hyperacute rejection or renal vein thrombosis)
    - CT or MR angiography: Decreased or absent flow
- **Renal scintigraphy**: Reduced or absence of perfusion of the graft on time intensity curve.
- **Management**: Transplant nephrectomy

Renal Vein Thrombosis

- After postoperative day 5
- More common in children <6 years and adults > 50 years
- **Higher risk**:
  1. Patients having atherosclerotic, hypercoagulable states, or undergoing peritoneal dialysis, diabetic patients
  2. Left iliac fossa transplant kidney-due to compression of left iliac vein by aorta or overlying artery.
- **Clinical features**: Pain, oliguria, anuria
- **Imaging features**:
  - **Ultrasound**:
    - Edematous, enlarged transplant kidney, corticomedullary differentiation is lost, perinephric fluid
    - Dilated renal vein with thrombus
  - **Color Doppler**:
    - Absence of color flow
    - Reversal of color flow in renal artery (also seen in torsion of vascular pedicle, allograft rejection, ATN)
- **Management**: Surgical thrombectomy
- Late renal vein thrombosis—endovascular thrombolysis

Renal Artery Stenosis

- Most common vascular complication
- May be focal or diffuse
- Classified as preanastomotic, anastomotic and postanastomotic depending on the site of stenosis.
- Duration: 3 months to 2 years
- **Clinical features**: Refractory hypertension.
- **Risk factors**:
  - Donor—recipient related: Atherosclerosis, infection, old age of recipient or donor, immunological causes
- **Recipient factors**:
  - Rejection
  - Delayed graft function
  - Ischemic heart disease
  - Extrinsic compression due to polycystic kidney or pseudoaneurysm
  - Iatrogenic trauma

- **Imaging features**:
  - Ultrasound with color Doppler
  - Stenotic site—aliasing
  - Elevated PSV>200–300 cm/s
  - Tardus parvus waveform—small amplitude peak with delayed upstroke
  - Acceleration time—0.1 sec
  - Renal artery—external iliac artery ratio-cutoff 1.8
  - Elevated PSV >250cm/s
- **CT and MR angiography**:
  - For confirmation
  - Done before endovascular intervention

Perirenal Hematoma

- Postoperative 0–5 days
- Due to inadequate surgical anastomosis
- Anticoagulation
- Postbiopsy
- **Imaging features**:
  - Ultrasound:
    - Acute—anechoic, echogenic debris
    - Subacute—heterogeneously hyperechoic
    - Chronic—centrally hypoechoic or cystic, thin internal septations—indicates clot lysis
  - NCCT:
    - Acute—hyperdense (>30–40 HU)
    - Subacute—iso to hyperdense
    - Chronic—hypodense
  - MRI:
    - Blooming on gradient sequences
    - Hyperintense on T1
    - Depending on the age, T1 and T2 appearances vary

Renal Arteriovenous Malformation

Laceration of vessel wall leads to communication of artery with adjacent vein

- **Clinical features**:
  - Gross hematuria
  - Hypertension
  - High output cardiac failure (AV fistula)
- **Ultrasound**: Simple or complex cystic structure
- **Color Doppler**:
  - Mosaic appearance
  - Feeding artery—high velocity, low resistance waveform
  - Draining vein—pulsatile waveform
- **Management**: Catheter embolization

Pseudoaneurysm of Renal Artery

- Postbiopsy
- During transplant surgery
- **Ultrasound**:
  - B mode: Simple or complex cystic structure
  - Color Doppler: YIN-YANG sign- to and fro pattern in the aneurysm sac

- **CT Angiography**:
  - Identification of feeding vessel, draining vein
  - Determination of size and extension
  - Done before endovascular intervention
- **Management**: Endovascular intervention (coiling) when pseudoaneurysm >2 cm in size
- Ultrasound guided percutaneous thrombin injection also done.

REFERENCES

1. Kawashima A, Vrtiska TJ, LeRoy AJ, Hartman RP, McCollough CH, King Jr BF. CT urography. Radiographics. 2004;24(suppl_1):S35-54.
2. Gulati P, Chidambaranathan N, Ahuja A, Anbarasu A, Mahajan A. Comprehensive Textbook of Clinical Radiology. Principles of Clinical Radiology. Philadelphia: Elsevier Health Sciences; 2023.
3. Sutton D. A textbook of Radiology and Imaging, 8th edition. Mosby, Churchill: Elsevier; 2023.
4. Adam A, Dixon AK, Gillard JH, Schaefer-Prokop C. Grainger & Allison's diagnostic radiology. Philadelphia: Elsevier Health Sciences; 2020.
5. Khandelwal N, Gupta AK, Chowdhury V. AIIMS-MAMC-PGI's Comprehensive Textbook of Diagnostic Radiology. New Delhi: Jaypee Brothers Medical Publishers; 2016.
6. Verma S, Rajesh A, Prasad SR, Gaitonde K, Lall CG, Mouraviev V, Aeron G, et al. Urinary bladder cancer: role of MR imaging. Radiographics. 2012;32(2):371-87.
7. Woo KT. Clinical nephrology. Singapore: World Scientific; 2011.
8. Dixe de Oliveira Santo I, Sailer A, Solomon N, Borse R, Cavallo J, Teitelbaum J, et al. Grading abdominal trauma: changes in and implications of the revised 2018 AAST-OIS for the spleen, liver, and Kidney. Radiographics. 2023;43(9):e230040.
9. Bhargavi DV, Avantsa R, Kala P. (2015). MDCT signs differentiating retroperitoneal and intraperitoneal lesions-diagnostic pearls. [online] Available from https://www.semanticscholar.org/paper/MDCT-signs-differentiating-retroperitoneal-and-Bhargavi-Avantsa/54dd8e25665180f0d7944b9fcac3247387fd5e33 [Last accessed January, 2025].
10. Chorney E, Rosen A, Lewis S, Wilck E, Simpson W. Radiologic Differentiation of Adrenal Lesions and Its Impact on Patient Management. Contemp Diagn Radiol. 2016;39(3):1-5.
11. Wagner-Bartak NA, Baiomy A, Habra MA, Mukhi SV, Morani AC, Korivi BR, et al. Cushing syndrome: diagnostic workup and imaging features, with clinical and pathologic correlation. Am J Roentgenol. 2017;209(1):19-32.
12. Singh A, Kumar A, Kumar P, Kumar S, Gamanagatti S. "Beyond saving lives": current perspectives of interventional radiology in trauma. World J Radiol. 2017;9(4):155.
13. Dworkin LD, Cooper CJ. Renal-artery stenosis. N Engl J Med. 2009;361(20):1972-8.
14. Patel-Lippmann KK, Planz VB, Phillips CH, Ohlendorf JM, Zuckerwise LC, Moshiri M. Placenta accreta spectrum disorders: update and pictorial review of the SAR-ESUR joint consensus statement for MRI. RadioGraphics. 2023;43(5):e220090.
15. Melamed N, Baschat A, Yinon Y, Athanasiadis A, Mecacci F, Figueras F, et al. FIGO (international Federation of Gynecology and obstetrics) initiative on fetal growth: best practice advice for screening, diagnosis, and management of fetal growth restriction. *Int J Gynaecol Obstet*. 2021;*152*(Suppl 1):3.
16. Histed SN, Deshmukh M, Masamed R, Jude CM, Mohammad S, Patel MK. Ectopic pregnancy: a trainee's guide to making the right call: women's imaging. Radiographics. 2016;36(7):2236-7.
17. Jaising I. Pre-conception & Pre-natal Diagnostic Techniques Act: A Users Guide to the Law. New Delhi: Universal Law Publishing; 2004.
18. Maheshwari E, Nougaret S, Stein EB, Rauch GM, Hwang KP, Stafford RJ, et al. Update on MRI in evaluation and treatment of endometrial cancer. Radiographics. 2022;42(7):2112-30.
19. Coakley FV, Glenn OA, Qayyum A, Barkovich AJ, Goldstein R, Filly RA. Fetal MRI: a developing technique for the developing patient. American Journal of Roentgenology. 2004;182(1):243-52.
20. Patel MD, Ascher SM, Horrow MM, Pickhardt PJ, Poder L, Goldman M, et al. Management of incidental adnexal findings on CT and MRI: a white paper of the ACR Incidental Findings Committee. J Am Coll Radiol. 2020;17(2):248-54.
21. Sadowski EA, Thomassin-Naggara I, Rockall A, Maturen KE, Forstner R, Jha P, et al. O-RADS MRI risk stratification system: Guide for assessing adnexal lesions from the ACR O-RADS committee. Radiology. 2022;303(1):35-47.
22. Moses KA, Sprenkle PC, Bahler C, Box G, Carlsson SV, Catalona WJ, et al. NCCN Guidelines® Insights: Prostate cancer early detection, version 1.2023: featured updates to the NCCN guidelines. J Natl Compr Canc Netw. 2023;21(3):236-46.
23. Varela CG, Yeguas LA, Rodríguez IC, Vila MD. Penile Doppler ultrasound for erectile dysfunction: technique and interpretation. Am J Roentgenol. 2020;214(5):1112-21.
24. Leckie A, Tao MJ, Narayanasamy S, Khalili K, Schieda N, Krishna S. The renal vasculature: What the radiologist needs to know. RadioGraphics. 2021;41(5):1531-48.
25. Patel VA. (2021). Hemodialysis AV Fistula: What a Radiologist Should Know? [online] Available from https://www.intechopen.com/chapters/78986 [Last accessed January, 2025].

CHAPTER

6 Musculoskeletal and Breast Imaging

Soumik Das, Manideepa Maiti, Sayeka Khatun, Himadri Shee, Anisha Sharma, Rohan Dey, Omkar Oraon, Arghya Chattopadhyay, Azhar Molla, Hasibur Rahaman

QUESTIONS

Imaging Modalities

1. Discuss the radiological anatomy of the shoulder joint. [10] [DNB Dec 19, MD (WBUHS) 21]
2. Define osteoporosis. Mention the different imaging modalities to assess bone mineral density. [10] [MD (WBUHS) 21]
3. Imaging techniques for cartilage imaging. Common sites for osteochondral defects and their imaging appearances. [10] [DNB Dec 21]
4. (a) Discuss the radiological anatomy of ankle ligaments. (b) Briefly state various MR sequences and planes used to evaluate ankle joints on magnetic resonance imaging. [3+(3+4)] [DNB Dec 20]

Congenital Diseases

1. Classify skeletal dysplasia. Briefly describe the radiological features of different types of osteogenesis imperfecta. [10] [MD (WBUHS) 21]

Infections/Inflammations

1. Discuss the pathophysiology and radiographic features of rheumatoid arthritis. [4+6] [MD (WBUHS) 23]
2. Discuss the differential diagnosis of the radiological appearance of absorption of terminal phalanges. [10] [MD (WBUHS) 23, MD (WBUHS) 21]
3. Enumerate the causes and imaging features in hypertrophic osteoarthropathy. [10] [MD (WBUHS) 20]
4. Ultrasound and MRI findings of rheumatoid arthritis. [10] [MD (WBUHS) 17, DNB June 21]

Metabolic Bone Diseases

1. Mention the causes of a generalized increase in bone density. Write the radiographic features of Paget's disease of bone. [4+6] [MD (WBUHS) 23, MD (WBUHS) 18]
2. Write short notes on radiological features of hyperparathyroidism. [5] [MD (WBUHS) 23]
3. What are metabolic and endocrine disorders affecting bones? Describe the radiological findings of hyperparathyroidism. [5+5=10] [MD (WBUHS) 19]
4. Discuss about the metabolic disorders of bone and the role of imaging to arrive at the diagnosis. [5+5] [MD (WBUHS) 24, MD (WBUHS) 22, RG 18]
5. What are the causes of increased bone density? Briefly describe the radiological features of pyknodysostosis. [4+6] [MD (WBUHS) 22]
6. Discuss various radiographic findings in rickets and osteomalacia. [5+5] [MD (WBUHS) 24]

7. Write a short note on: Rickets. [5] [DNB Dec 21, MD (WBUHS) 18]
8. Renal osteodystrophy—imaging findings. Approach to imaging in hyperparathyroidism. [10] [DNB June 21]
9. Discuss in brief, various types of hyperparathyroidism. Describe imaging features of various types of hyperparathyroidism. [5+5] [MD (WBUHS) 17, DNB June 20, DNB Dec 19]

Bone Tumors

1. Enumerate the bone-forming tumors. Discuss the imaging features of osteosarcoma. [2+8] [AIIMS Dec 23]
2. Write a short note on: Ewing sarcoma. [5] [DNB Dec 21]

Musculoskeletal MRI

1. Describe the radiographic and MRI findings in avascular necrosis of the hip. [4+6] [MD (WBUHS) 23, MD (WBUHS) 20, RG 18]
2. Write a short note on MRI features of anterior cruciate ligament injury of knee. [5] [MD (WBUHS) 23]
3. CT and MRI finding of recurrent dislocation of shoulder joint. [10] [MD (WBUHS) 19]
4. MRI findings of anterior and posterior cruciate ligament tear. [10] [MD (WBUHS) 19]
5. Write a short note on: SLAP. [5] [MD (WBUHS) 22]
6. Meniscal tear MRI and MR arthrogram role. [5] [DNB June 22]
7. Latest nomenclature of disc herniation. Osteoporotic vertebral collapse vs. metastatic vertebral collapse. [10] [DNB June 21, MD (WBUHS) 18]
8. Imaging features of recurrent shoulder dislocation. Role MR arthrography in shoulder displacement. [10] [DNB June 21]
9. Radiological anatomy of ligaments of the knee joint. MR evaluation of cartilages of the knee joint. [10] [DNB June 21]
10. What is lipoma arborescens? Enumerate imaging findings on US and MRI. Discuss any two differential diagnosis. [2+4+4] [DNB Dec 20]
11. Discuss the etiology of femoroacetabular impingement and imaging findings on plain radiographs and MRI. [10] [DNB Dec 20]

Trauma and Soft Tissues

1. Enumerate various causes of paravertebral masses and their imaging features. [3+7] [MD (WBUHS) 23, MD (WBUHS) 21]
2. MRI in soft tissue tumors—discuss. [10] [MD (WBUHS) 20]
3. What is a growth plate? Discuss imaging of growth plate disorders and Salter-Harris classification of fractures. [2+4+4] [MD (WBUHS) 24, MD (WBUHS) 21]
4. Write a short note on: Types of meniscus injury of the knee with MRI features. [5] [MD (WBUHS) 24, MD (WBUHS) 22]
5. Write a short note on: Rotator cuff injury. [5] [MD (WBUHS) 22]
6. Internal derangement of knee causes. MRI knee protocol. ACL tear findings. [10] [MD (WBUHS) 17, DNB Dec 21]
7. Pelvic fractures—classification and Imaging approach. Osseous and soft tissue injury patterns of pelvic fractures. [10] [DNB June 21]

Miscellaneous

1. Write a short note on: Single dense vertebra. [5] [MD (WBUHS) 19]
2. Discuss the differential diagnosis of radiological appearance of metaphyseal lucent bands in child. [10] [MD (WBUHS) 24, MD (WBUHS) 22]
3. Radiological evaluation of a child with limping. [10] [MD (WBUHS) 20]
4. Briefly describe the radiological features of various paragangliomas. [10] [MD (WBUHS) 21]

5. 1-year-old boy with limping since 1 month: (a) Radiological role (b) Causes and imaging. [10] [DNB June 22]
6. Skeletal finding in leukemia and hemolytic anemia. [10] [DNB June 22, DNB Dec 19]
7. Diffuse hyperostosis of the skull: Imaging. [10] [DNB Dec 21]
8. Write a short note on: Perthe's disease. [5] [DNB Dec 21]
9. Write a short note on: Cleidocranial dysplasia. [5] [DNB Dec 21]
10. Enumerate various causes for unilateral painful hips in a 10-year-old child. Discuss the role of imaging in any two pathologies. [2+8] [DNB June 20]
11. A 14-year-old male presented with fever, pain, and swelling of the right proximal arm. (a) What are the various differential diagnoses? (b) Discuss in brief, the role of imaging in the evaluation of such a case. [3+7] [DNB June 20]

Breast Imaging

1. USG findings in solid breast lesions. [10] [MD (WBUHS) 20]
2. Discuss the role of MR in breast diseases. [10] [MD (WBUHS) 21]
3. Describe the anatomy of the breast with a diagram. Discuss the basic physics with the instrumentation of a mammography unit. What are the different mammographic projections? [4+4+2] [MD (WBUHS) 22, AIIMS May 24]
4. Ultrasound lexicon of BI-RADS. [5] [MD (WBUHS) 22, AIIMS Dec 23]
5. BI-RADS classification system. [5] [DNB Dec 19]
6. Describe the role of sonography in the evaluation of breast lumps. [5] [MD (WBUHS) 17]
7. 60 year female breast masses d/d: Benign vs. malignant on USG and MRI. [10] [DNB Dec 21]
8. Indications of MRI breast. Technique of MRI breast. Nonenhancing mass in MRI breast. [10] [DNB June 21]
9. Indications, technique, advantages, and limitations of MRI in imaging of breast cancer. [2+3+3+2] [DNB Dec 20, DNB June 20, MD (WBUHS) 17]

Vascular Diseases and Interventions

1. Doppler evaluation of acute lower limb ischemia. [5]
2. Role of interventional radiology in intra-arterial management of various neoplasms including paragangliomas. [DNB June 20, MD (WBUHS) 20]

ANSWERS

Imaging Modalities

1. Discuss the radiological anatomy of the shoulder joint. [10] [DNB Dec 19, MD (WBUHS) 21]

The shoulder joint or the glenohumeral joint is primarily a ball and socket joint with articulation involving the humeral head and the glenoid cavity of the scapula. The small size of the glenoid fossa and the relatively larger head size of the humerus and the laxity of the joint capsule render the joint relatively unstable and prone to subluxation and dislocation. The labral cartilage, joint capsule, and surrounding soft tissues provide stability by deepening the glenoid fossa.[1]

I. **Bony anatomy**:

a. **Humerus**: The articular surface of the humeral head is covered with hyaline cartilage. Bony landmarks of the proximal humerus are the greater tuberosity, lesser tuberosity, and bicipital groove, where rotator cuff (RC) tendons are attached.

b. **Scapula**: Flat bone that glides over the thoracic surface to facilitate rotating arm movement. The osseous glenoid fossa is markedly smaller than the humeral head.

There are three bony projections of the scapula—anteriorly coracoid process, scapular spine posteriorly, and acromion process superiorly.

The shape of the acromion can contribute to impingement. There are four acromial types **(Fig. 1)** as per Bigliani classification. These are:

Type 1-flat or slightly convex undersurface.

Type 2-concave undersurface.

Type 3-hooked undersurface.

Type 4-convex undersurface.

Os acromiale: The four ossification centers of the acromion fuse at varying ages up to 25 years. Failure of fusion of these ossification centers results in os acromiale.

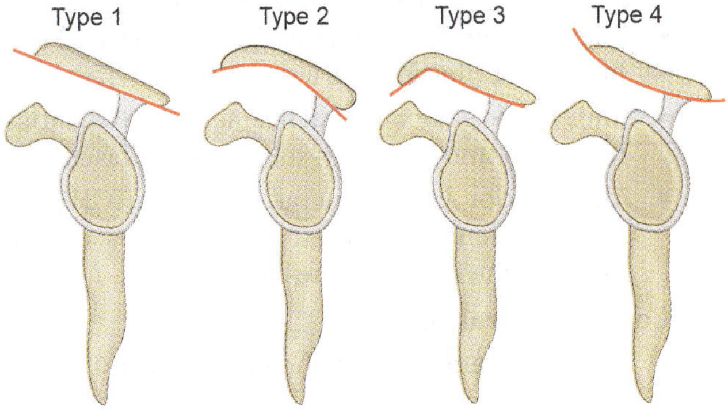

FIG. 1: Shows types of acromion.

c. **Clavicle**: Medially articulates with the sternum at the sternoclavicular (SC) joint. Laterally it connects to the scapula with the AC joint.

II. **Rotator cuff anatomy**:

The shoulder joint is reinforced by the rotator cuff muscles/tendons. The RC is also referred to as the SITS muscle, (Supraspinatus, Infraspinatus, Teres minor, and Subscapularis, respectively). The muscles arise from the scapula and connect to the head of the humerus, forming a cuff around the glenohumeral (GH) joint **(Table 1)**.

III. **Labral anatomy**:

- Is a tough triangular fibrocartilaginous tissue that is attached along the bony margins of the glenoid fossa. This increases the surface area and the depth of the glenoid fossa, resulting in GH joint stability.
- For imaging purposes, the glenoid is divided into four quadrants or described as a clock face with 12'o clock located superiorly and 3'o clock anteriorly.

TABLE 1: Rotator cuff muscles—origin, insertion, and action.

Muscles	*Origin*	*Insertion*	*Action*
Supraspinatus	Supraspinous fossa	The superior facet of the greater tuberosity	Initiation of abduction of arm
Infraspinatus	Infraspinous fossa	Middle facet on the greater tubercle	External rotation of the arm
Subscapularis	Subscapularis fossa	Inferior facet on the greater tubercle	Internal rotation of the arm
Teres minor	The lateral border of the scapula	Lesser tubercle	Internal rotation of the arm

- Three types of superior labral attachments have been described at the 12 o'clock position with respect to biceps tendon insertion.
  - Type 1: There is no recess between the labrum and glenoid cartilage
  - Type 2: There is a small recess
  - Type 3: There is a large sublabral recess between the 11 and 1 o'clock positions

IV. **Capsule**:
- GH joint stability is provided by the joint capsule and the labrum.
- The insertion of the anterior joint capsule can be variable.
- Insertion from the base of the glenoid labrum and more medially into the scapula.
- According to Moseley and Övergaard there are three capsular insertions **(Fig. 2)** that can be differentiated in the axial plane:
  - Type I: Insertion at the tip or basis of the anterior labrum
  - Type II: Insertion of the capsule not >1 cm medial to the labrum.
  - Type III: Insertion of the capsule >1 cm medial to the labrum.

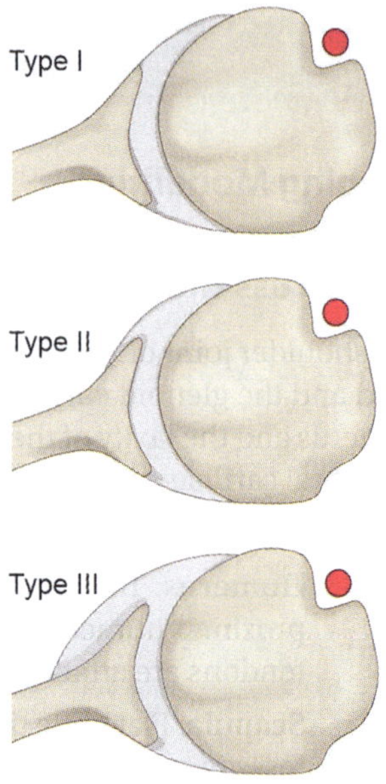

FIG. 2: The types of capsular insertion.

V. **Glenohumeral ligaments**:
- These are the capsular ligaments that fuse with RC muscles or attach to the glenoid labrum.
- The superior glenohumeral ligament (SGHL) arises from the supraglenoid tubercle and merges with the CHL before inserting into the lesser tuberosity.
- The middle glenohumeral ligament (MGHL) arises most commonly from the labrum and inserts into the lesser tuberosity and fuses with subscapularis fascia.
- The inferior glenohumeral ligament (IGHL) is the largest and most important component of the GH labroligamentous complex and is composed of the anterior band, posterior band, and axillary pouch. It extends between the labrum to the humeral neck.

VI. **Coracohumeral ligament**:
- A strong ligament of the shoulder joint and is a part of the RC interval.
- It originates from the lateral aspect of the base of the coracoid process, runs laterally, and envelops the LHBT tendon superiorly.
- It attaches to the margin of the greater and lesser tubercles of the humerus.

VII. **Rotator interval**:
- Is a triangular space between the tendons of the subscapularis and supraspinatus and the base of the coracoid process.
- The LHBT and SGHL are the content of the RI.
- The CHL and SGHL act as stabilizers, preventing subluxation and anterior dislocation of the LHBT.
- The RI may show abnormal soft tissue on USG or MRI, which may suggest a frozen shoulder.

Arterial Supply

From the branches of the axillary artery:
- Suprascapular artery.
- Circumflex scapular artery.
- Anterior and posterior circumflex humeral arteries.

Venous Drainage

Veins with corresponding names, accompany the arteries and drain the shoulder via a periscapular venous plexus.

Innervation:
By the nerves of:
- Suprascapular nerve

- Lateral pectoral nerve
- Axillary nerve

The bones, tendons, and ligaments around the shoulder joint are represented schematically in the following figures **(Figs. 3 to 5)**.[2]

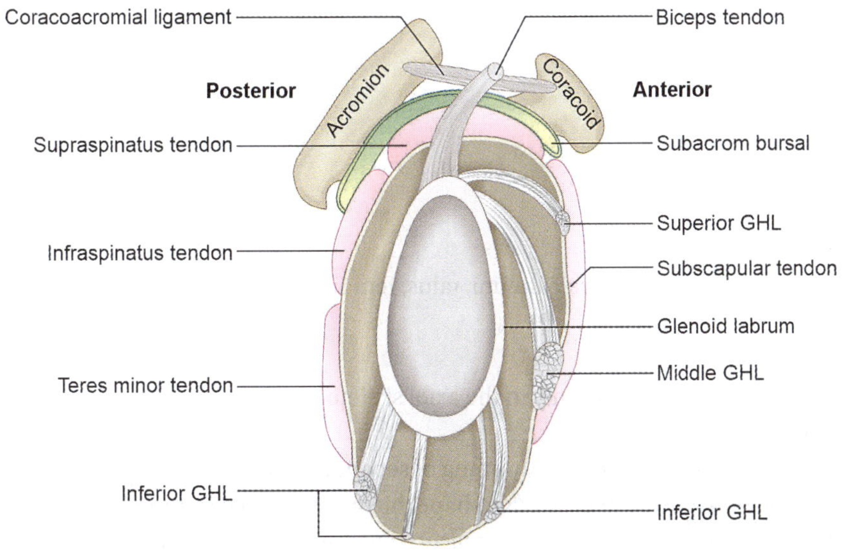

FIG. 3: Illustrated images of tendons and ligaments around the shoulder joint.

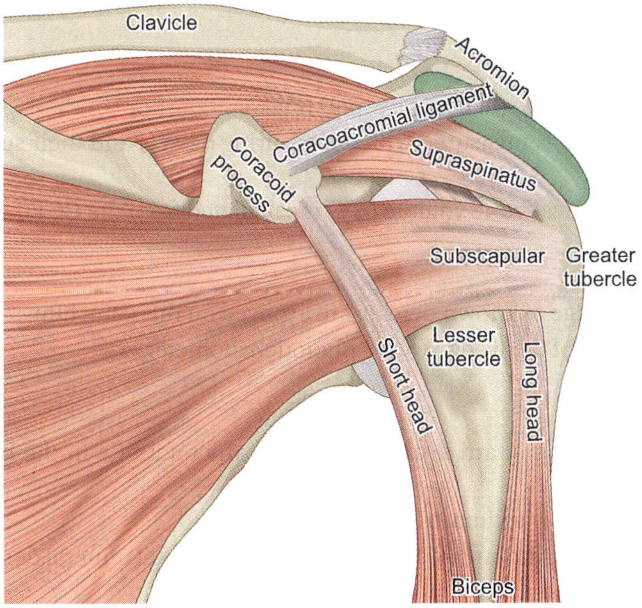

FIG. 4: Anterior view of the shoulder joint.

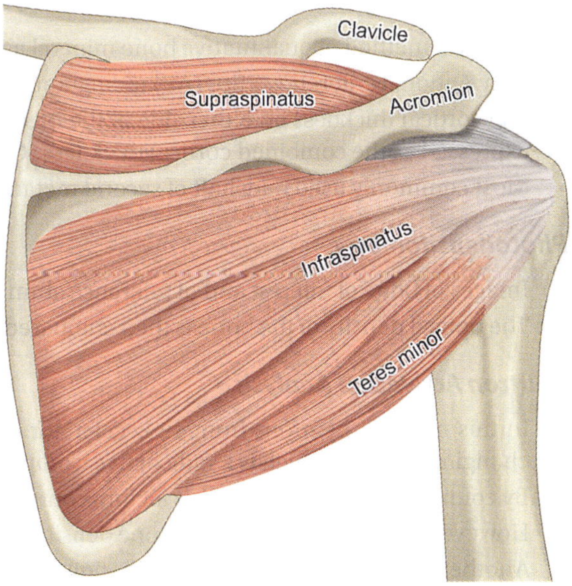

FIG. 5: Posterior view of the shoulder joint.

2. Define osteoporosis. Mention the different imaging modalities to assess bone mineral density. [10] [MD (WBUHS) 21]

Osteoporosis: It is defined by the World Health Organization (WHO) as "a skeletal disease, characterized by low bone mass and microarchitectural deterioration of bone tissue, with a consequent increase in bone fragility and susceptibility to fracture." The strength of the bone depends upon two features, its quality and density (mass/volume). Bone quality is a composite of bone architecture, turnover, mineralization, and damage incurred. The bone mineral density (BMD) can be subject to measurement and has been used in the quantitative WHO definition of osteoporosis, with bone density <2.5 standard deviations (SD) for the diagnosis of osteoporosis.[3]

The various modalities which may be utilized are as follows:

- Standard radiography
- Radiogrammetry
- Photodensitometry
- Compton scattering
- Neutron activation analysis
- Single and dual photon absorptiometry
- Dual-energy X-ray absorptiometry
- Quantitative computed tomography
- Quantitative ultrasound

Standard Radiography

a. Assessment is done on the metacarpal, calcaneum, talus, femoral neck, and vertebral bodies.
b. Mainly based on subjective criteria.
c. The findings are:
   - Generalized osteopenia, most commonly in the axial skeleton.
   - Reduced thickness of cortex.
   - Accentuation of primary trabeculae with thinning of secondary trabeculae.
   - Changes in vertebral body shape like—wedge shape, biconcave, and compression.
   - Insufficiency fractures seen in the sacrum, supraacetabular regions, os pubis, etc., are common sites. The fracture may be difficult to find radiographically and may be detected by computed tomography (CT).

Radiogrammetry

- Simplest method of quantitative bone mineral assessment.
- Conventional anteroposterior (AP) radiograph of a tubular bone (like metacarpal) is taken.
- The cortical thickness on either side of the medullary space is measured with a measuring device, and their sum is expressed as the combined cortical thickness (CCT).
- Most commonly used midshaft of second metacarpal. Cortical bone volume (BV) is calculated from the CCT.

Photodensitometry

- Images of bone of interest and of reference aluminum wedge of known density are exposed on the same film.
- The optical density of the bone is then compared with that of the wedge with a photodensitometer.

Neutron Activation Analysis

- In this method, neutrons from an accelerator or a reactor bombard a small fraction of the total ^{48}Ca in the body, changing it to ^{49}Ca which is a radioactive isotope.
- By counting its activity, the total calcium content of the body is estimated.
- However, it does not quantify the bone density of trabecular bone and does not correlate with spinal mineral density.
- Another disadvantage is the large radiation dose (200–300 mrem).

Compton Scattering

- Measures the absolute density of a volume of tissue based on its electron density.
- Can measure purely trabecular bone.
- It is based on the measurement of scattered radiation from a source of 100–700 keV gamma rays.
- Used for calcaneum, spine, and radius.

Single-energy Photon Absorptiometry

- This technique uses a gamma ray source (^{125}I), a detector, and intervening electronics that measure the beam attenuation through bone and express the result in bone mineral per cm^2 scanned.

- Generally, radius is measured at two sites, the mid-diaphysis consists of nearly 100% cortical bone, and the distal radial metaphysis contains about 75% cortical bone and 25% trabecular bone.
- A major clinical limitation of this technique is that it quantifies the status of peripheral long bone and measures primarily the cortex.

Dual-energy Photon Absorptiometry

- Dual-energy photon absorptiometry (DPA) technique utilizes a radioisotope that emits photons at two different energy levels.
- The chief advantage is that the gamma-ray energy of the source is higher (^{153}Gd with photons of 42 and 100 keV) and it has a uniform path length.
- The lumbar spine from L1 to L4 is usually scanned.
- This technique yields integral of all minerals within the scan path including the vertebral bodies, endplates, and posterior elements.
- Used to determine the total body mineral content.

Dual-energy X-ray Absorptiometry

Dual-energy X-ray absorptiometry (DXA) is the **gold standard** for assessing bone mineral density. It is widely used due to its accuracy, low radiation exposure, and ability to assess BMD in various anatomical sites (such as the **lumbar spine**, **hip**, and **forearm**).

- **Mechanism**: DXA uses two X-ray beams of different energies to measure bone mineral content and bone mass. The amount of X-ray absorbed by the bone is used to calculate the **BMD**.
- **Indications**: DXA is commonly used for diagnosing **osteoporosis**, monitoring **fracture risk**, and assessing **treatment efficacy** (e.g., for patients receiving **bisphosphonates**, **hormone replacement therapy**, etc.).
- **Common Sites Measured**:
  - **Lumbar spine** (L1-L4)
  - **Femoral neck**
  - **Total hip**
  - **Radius** (for peripheral DXA, in patients with contraindications for spine/hip assessment)
- **Advantages**:
  - Quick and non-invasive.
  - Low radiation exposure.
  - High accuracy and precision.
- **Disadvantages**:
  - Cannot assess bone quality (only bone quantity).
  - Sensitivity to **vertebral deformities** (which may affect lumbar spine readings).
  - Not suitable for assessing **children** or **pregnant women**.
- BMD is expressed in terms of SD as a T-score and a Z-score.
- The T-score compares the BMD of the interrogated subject/patient with the mean BMD of a standard young adult individual (between 20 and 30 years of age).
- The Z-score reflects the difference between the examined BMD of the patient and the mean BMD of age and gender-matched controls.
- The WHO classifies BMD based on the T-score **(Table 2)**.
- This definition is applied to DXA measurements made in the lumbar spine, proximal femur, and forearm.

TABLE 2: WHO definitions of osteoporosis and osteopenia.

The World Health Organization (WHO) definitions of osteoporosis and osteopenia.

Terminology	*T-score definition*
Normal	$T \geq -1.0$
Osteopenia	$-2.5 < T < -1.0$
Osteoporosis	$T \leq -2.5$
Severe osteoporosis	$T \leq -2.5$ in the presence of one or more fragility fractures

Quantitative Computed Tomography (QCT)

Quantitative computed tomography (QCT) is another imaging modality used to measure BMD. It involves the use of a **CT scanner** to obtain high-resolution images of the bone.

- **Mechanism**: QCT uses **CT scans** to directly assess the **volume** of trabecular bone (in contrast to DXA, which measures areal BMD). It provides a **three-dimensional** analysis of bone density and can differentiate between **trabecular** and **cortical bone**.
- **Indications**: QCT is sometimes used for patients with **vertebral deformities** that may affect DXA results, or in situations where the patient is at high risk for **vertebral fractures**.
- **Common Sites Measured**:
  - **Spine** (lumbar vertebrae)
  - **Peripheral sites** (e.g., forearm)
- **Advantages**:
  - It is more sensitive than DXA for **trabecular bone**.
  - Can assess **volumetric bone density**, which is less affected by **bone size**.
- **Disadvantages**:
  - **Higher radiation dose** compared to DXA.
  - Less widely available than DXA.
  - Higher cost.

Peripheral Quantitative Computed Tomography (pQCT)

Peripheral quantitative computed tomography (pQCT) is similar to QCT but focuses on measuring BMD at peripheral sites, such as the **forearm**, using lower radiation than conventional CT.

- **Mechanism**: pQCT provides a **three-dimensional** image of the bone and measures both **cortical and trabecular bone** separately.
- **Indications**: Used for assessing **cortical and trabecular bone** density in the **distal radius** or other peripheral sites, often in research settings or for **athletes** with bone stress.
- **Common Sites Measured**:
  - **Distal radius** (most commonly).
  - **Tibia** and other peripheral bones.
- **Advantages**:
  - Ability to differentiate **cortical and trabecular bone**.
  - Provides **volumetric BMD** (in contrast to the areal BMD of DXA).
- **Disadvantages**:
  - Limited availability.
  - Higher radiation exposure compared to DXA.
  - Less commonly used in clinical practice.

Quantitative Ultrasound (QUS)

Quantitative ultrasound (QUS) measures BMD using **high-frequency sound waves**. It is a noninvasive, radiation-free technique, often used for **screening** or in settings where access to DXA is limited.

- **Mechanism**: QUS measures the **speed of sound** (SOS) and **broadband ultrasound attenuation** (BUA) in bone. These measurements can then be used to calculate an **estimated bone density**.
- **Indications**: QUS is commonly used for **osteoporosis screening**, especially for patients who cannot undergo DXA, or in areas where DXA is not available.
- **Common Sites Measured**:
  - **Calcaneus (heel bone)**.
  - **Tibia** (less commonly).
- **Advantages**:
  - **No radiation** exposure.

- Portable and can be done at the point of care.
- Lower cost compared to DXA.

- **Disadvantages**:
  - Less accurate than DXA in quantifying exact BMD.
  - Cannot be used to directly diagnose **osteoporosis** or **fracture risk**.
  - Limited ability to assess bone quality compared to DXA.

Magnetic Resonance Imaging (MRI)

While MRI is not primarily used for BMD measurement, it can provide important **indirect information** about bone quality and **bone marrow changes**, which can be relevant for assessing bone health.

- **Mechanism**: MRI detects differences in **bone marrow composition** (e.g., fatty marrow, edema) and can visualize **trabecular bone structure**.
- **Indications**: MRI is useful in assessing **bone marrow diseases** (such as **osteonecrosis** or **metastatic disease**), **bone stress injuries**, or **osteoporosis complications** like **vertebral fractures**.
- **Advantages**:
  - **No radiation** exposure.
  - High-resolution imaging of **bone marrow** and **trabecular structure**.
- **Disadvantages**:
  - Not suitable for routine BMD assessment.
  - Expensive and less widely available than DXA.
  - Not standardized for bone density measurement.

X-ray Absorptiometry (XA)

X-ray absorptiometry (XA) is similar to DXA but typically used for **assessing bone mineral content** in specific bones such as the **heel** or **wrist**.

- **Mechanism**: Measures the **attenuation of X-rays** as they pass through the bone to estimate its mineral density.
- **Indications**: Used in screening for **osteoporosis** in patients who cannot undergo DXA or when more localized measurements are needed.
- **Advantages**:
  - Noninvasive and relatively easy.
  - **Portable** devices available.
- **Disadvantages**:
  - Less accurate than DXA.
  - Limited to certain anatomical sites.

3. Imaging techniques for cartilage imaging. Common sites for osteochondral defects and their imaging appearances. [10] [DNB Dec 21]

Imaging of cartilage is crucial for diagnosing and monitoring conditions like osteoarthritis, cartilage defects, and joint degeneration. These are the imaging techniques are used to visualize cartilage, each with its own advantages and limitations.[4]

Magnetic Resonance Imaging (MRI)

MRI is considered one of the most effective methods for cartilage imaging due to its ability to provide detailed soft tissue contrast without the need for radiation. Several specialized MRI techniques are used to assess cartilage structure and composition:

- **Standard MRI**: Provides excellent visualization of the articular cartilage and subchondral bone. High-resolution MRI sequences, such as T1-weighted (T1W) and T2-weighted (T2W) images, are often used to evaluate cartilage morphology and joint space narrowing.
- **T2 Mapping**: T2 mapping is a quantitative MRI technique that measures the relaxation time of water molecules in tissues. Changes in T2 values are associated with cartilage degeneration, such as collagen loss or increased water content in the cartilage.

- **T1ρ Mapping**: T1ρ imaging assesses proteoglycan content and cartilage integrity. It is especially useful for early-stage cartilage degeneration before visible morphological changes occur.
- **Delayed Gadolinium-Enhanced MRI of Cartilage (dGEMRIC)**: This technique uses a contrast agent (gadolinium) to assess the biochemical composition of cartilage. The gadolinium binds to glycosaminoglycans (GAGs) in the cartilage, and the imaging highlights areas of reduced GAG content, which is an early sign of cartilage degeneration.
- **MR Arthrography**: This technique involves injecting a contrast agent into the joint space to provide enhanced visualization of the cartilage, labrum, and other intra-articular structures. It is especially useful for detecting cartilage defects in the knee, shoulder, and hip.

X-ray Imaging

X-ray is commonly used for detecting joint space narrowing and osteophyte formation, which are signs of cartilage degradation in conditions like osteoarthritis. While it does not provide direct visualization of cartilage itself, it can be used to monitor the progression of joint disease over time.

- **Conventional Radiography**: This is the standard X-ray approach for observing bone changes that indirectly reflect cartilage loss.
- **Quantitative Radiography (e.g., X-ray Cartilage Thickness Measurement)**: More advanced techniques, such as high-resolution X-rays, can be used to estimate cartilage thickness, though they are not as precise as MRI for cartilage assessment.

Ultrasound Imaging

Ultrasound is a noninvasive and relatively inexpensive imaging technique that can be used for assessing cartilage, especially in the knee and other peripheral joints. However, it is more commonly used to evaluate synovial tissue and joint effusion rather than cartilage directly. That said, it can provide useful information for:

- Assessing cartilage surface integrity and thickness.
- Guiding injections or aspirations in the joint space.

Limitations: Ultrasound lacks the spatial resolution of MRI and does not provide detailed information about cartilage composition.

Computed Tomography (CT) and CT Arthrography

CT imaging can be useful for evaluating bony structures and joint alignment, particularly when combined with contrast agents (CT arthrography) for better visualization of soft tissue structures, including cartilage. However, CT is not commonly used for direct cartilage assessment because of its limited ability to visualize soft tissue compared to MRI.

High-resolution CT: This may be used for assessing subchondral bone and joint architecture, but it provides little direct information about cartilage quality or integrity.

Arthroscopy

While not a traditional imaging technique, **arthroscopy** allows direct visualization of the cartilage surface via a small camera inserted into the joint. This is particularly useful for assessing cartilage defects, grading their severity, and guiding surgical decisions. Arthroscopy can also be combined with other imaging methods to provide a comprehensive view of cartilage pathology.

Integrated PET–MRI

- Integrating Positron Emission Tomography (PET) with MRI is used to understand the disease process at a molecular level before structural or compositional changes occur.
- Can assess cartilage metabolism and inflammation using tracers like 18F-FDG.

Optical Coherence Tomography (OCT)

- Provides microscopic imaging of cartilage layers.
- Useful for assessing cartilage repair and early degeneration.

Single Photon Emission Computed Tomography (SPECT)

Evaluate joint activity and cartilage degeneration.

Common Sites for Osteochondral Defects and Their Imaging Appearances

Below are the **common sites** for osteochondral defects and their typical **imaging appearances.**[5,6]

Knee Joint (Most Common Site)

Femoral Condyles (Medial > Lateral)

The **femoral condyles**, especially the **medial femoral condyle**, are the most common sites for osteochondral defects in the knee. These defects typically result from acute trauma (e.g., fractures or dislocations) or from **degenerative changes**.

- **Imaging Modality**:
  - **X-ray**:
    - **Plain X-rays** may show **subchondral sclerosis**, **joint space narrowing**, or **osteophytes. Loose bodies** within the joint may also be visible if the cartilage has been damaged severely.
    - **Osteochondral fractures** may appear as **bone fragments** detached from the underlying subchondral bone.
  - **MRI**:
    - **MRI** is the gold standard for detecting osteochondral defects.
    - **T2-weighted images** typically show **cartilage thinning**, **subchondral bone edema**, and **osteochondral lesions** with hyperintensity in the bone (indicating edema).
    - **T1-weighted images** can show **defects in the cartilage** and **subchondral bone**, with low signal intensity corresponding to bone and high signal intensity corresponding to fluid or cartilage.
    - **Gadolinium-enhanced MRI** may help evaluate the cartilage surface integrity and underlying bone.
  - **CT**:
    - **CT scans** are used to assess **osseous involvement** and the **depth of the defect**.
    - It is useful for evaluating **fractures** of the subchondral bone or for preoperative planning (e.g., for **osteochondral autograft transplantation**).

Patella

Osteochondral defects of the **patella** often result from trauma, patellar instability, or repetitive overload (e.g., in athletes).

- **Imaging Modality**:
  - **X-ray**:
    - Plain radiographs may show **subchondral sclerosis**, **joint effusion**, or **patellar malalignment** (which predisposes to OCD).
  - **MRI**:
    - **MRI** typically demonstrates **cartilage defects**, **subchondral bone changes**, and **joint effusion**. High signal intensity on **T2-weighted** sequences can indicate **cartilage damage** or **bone marrow edema**.
    - A **high-grade osteochondral defect** may show a well-defined area of **cartilage loss** with underlying **subchondral bone changes**.

Ankle Joint

Talus (most common)

The **talus** is the most common site for osteochondral defects in the **ankle joint**, especially in the **medial talar dome** (often associated with ankle sprains or fractures).

- **Imaging Modality**:
  - **X-ray**:
    - **Plain radiographs** may show **joint effusion**, **osteophytes**, or **subchondral bone changes**.
    - **Loose bodies** in the joint can sometimes be seen in cases where the osteochondral defect involves fragmentation of the talus.
  - **MRI**:
    - **MRI** is highly sensitive for detecting **osteochondral lesions** in the talus.
    - **T1-weighted** images show **low signal intensity** for the subchondral bone and **cartilage**.

    - **T2-weighted** or **Proton Density (PD)** images show **high signal intensity** in the areas of **edema** in the bone and **cartilage defects**.
    - Gadolinium contrast enhancement can further highlight the defects and assess **cartilage integrity**.
  - **CT**:
    - **CT scans** can provide detailed imaging of **osseous lesions** and are useful for evaluating the **extent** and **depth** of the osteochondral defect.

Shoulder Joint

Humeral Head

The **humeral head** is a less common but significant site for osteochondral defects, particularly in cases of **repetitive overhead motion** (e.g., in athletes or heavy lifting) or after **trauma** (such as a **shoulder dislocation**).

- **Imaging Modality**:
  - **X-ray**:
    - **Plain X-rays** can reveal **osteochondral fractures**, **joint effusion**, and **subchondral sclerosis. Loose bodies** may be visible in cases of **traumatic lesions.**
  - **MRI**:
    - **MRI** is the best imaging modality for assessing the **extent** and **location** of osteochondral defects in the humeral head.
    - **T2-weighted images** may show **bone marrow edema** and **cartilage thinning**.
    - **T1-weighted** images typically highlight **defects in cartilage and subchondral bone** and **fluid-filled cystic changes**.
  - **CT**:
    - **CT** is used to assess the **degree of bone involvement** in **osteochondral fractures**, particularly in complex cases.

Elbow Joint

Capitellum

The **capitellum** of the elbow joint is another common site for osteochondral defects, particularly in **adolescents** (as in **Panner's disease**) or following **trauma**.

- **Imaging Modality**:
  - **X-ray**:
    - **Plain radiographs** may show **osteochondral fractures**, **subchondral cysts**, and **joint effusion.** Early lesions may appear as areas of **cartilage loss** with associated subchondral sclerosis.
  - **MRI**:
    - **MRI** is sensitive in detecting **early cartilage defects**, **bone marrow edema**, and **joint effusion.**
    - **T2-weighted** MRI images show **high signal intensity** in areas of **cartilage loss** and underlying **bone edema.**
    - **Gadolinium-enhanced MRI** can help delineate the cartilage defect more clearly.

Hip Joint

Femoral Head

Osteochondral defects in the **femoral head** (often secondary to conditions like **avascular necrosis (AVN)** or **trauma**) can lead to **arthritis** and functional disability.

- **Imaging Modality**:
  - **X-ray**:
    - **Plain X-rays** may show **joint space narrowing**, **subchondral cysts**, and **osteophytes**. In cases of **avascular necrosis**, radiographs may reveal **collapsed femoral head.**
  - **MRI**:
    - **MRI** is the most sensitive modality for detecting early **avascular necrosis** and associated **osteochondral defects** in the femoral head.

    - **T1-weighted** images show **low signal intensity** in the affected bone, and **T2-weighted** images show **high signal intensity** from **bone edema** and **cartilage damage**.
  - **CT**:
    - **CT** is helpful in assessing **osseous defects** and **bone collapse** in the femoral head.

Osteochondral injury staging system for MRI attempts to grade the stability and severity of osteochondral injury and is used to plan management.

Classification

- **Stage I**:
  - Injury limited to articular cartilage
  - MRI findings: Subchondral edema
  - X-ray findings: None
- **Stage II**:
  - Cartilage injury with associated subchondral fracture but without detachment
  - Thin sclerotic margin
  - X-ray findings: Usually none; may see fracture as sclerotic or osteopenic area
  - Two subtypes
    - **Type A**: Cystic on CT and/or edema on MRI
    - **Type B**: Nondisplaced and incompletely undercut by fluid (MR) or lucency (CT), with an open connection to the articular cartilage
- **Stage III**:
  - Detached, nondisplaced fragment
  - MRI findings: High signal around osteochondral fracture (rim sign) but not displaced
  - X-ray findings: Slight lucency between osteochondral fragment and remainder of the bone
- **Stage IV**:
  - Osteochondral fragment displaced
  - Usually joint effusion present, surrounding fragment and filling donor site
  - X-ray findings: Increased lucency between osteochondral fragment and remainder of the bone, or loose body with donor site irregularity
- **Stage V**:
  - Subchondral cyst formation
  - Secondary degenerative change
  - X-ray findings: Secondary osteoarthritis

4. (a) Discuss the radiological anatomy of ankle ligaments. (b) Briefly state various MR sequences and planes used to evaluate ankle joint on magnetic resonance imaging. [3+(3+4)] [DNB Dec 20]

The ankle joint is stabilized by a network of ligaments that help control motion and maintain the integrity of the joint. These ligaments can be visualized through various imaging modalities such as X-ray, ultrasound, MRI, and CT. Each imaging modality offers different insights into the ankle's ligamentous structure, with MRI being the gold standard for soft tissue evaluation.[7]

Lateral Ligament Complex (Lateral Collateral Ligaments)

The lateral ligament complex of the ankle consists of three primary ligaments:

- **Anterior Talofibular Ligament (ATFL)**:
  - **Radiological Appearance**: This ligament is most commonly injured in inversion sprains. On MRI, it appears as a low signal intensity structure on T1-weighted images and a high signal on T2-weighted images when injured.

  - **Position**: The ATFL runs from the anterior aspect of the fibula to the talus.
  - **Function**: It stabilizes the ankle against inversion and plantar flexion forces.
- **Calcaneofibular Ligament (CFL)**:
  - **Radiological Appearance**: On MRI, the CFL can be seen as a band-like structure between the fibula and the calcaneus, with low signal intensity on T1 and high signal intensity on T2 images if injured.
  - **Position**: The CFL runs from the distal fibula to the lateral surface of the calcaneus.
  - **Function**: It prevents excessive inversion of the foot and limits dorsiflexion.
- **Posterior Talofibular Ligament (PTFL)**:
  - **Radiological Appearance**: The PTFL is often seen as a low-signal band in T1-weighted MRI images.
  - **Position**: It runs from the fibula to the talus on the posterior aspect of the ankle.
  - **Function**: It stabilizes the posterior aspect of the ankle, limiting excessive dorsiflexion and inversion.

Medial Ligament Complex (Deltoid Ligament)

The deltoid ligament is a strong and broad ligament complex that provides stability to the medial side of the ankle.

- **Radiological Appearance**: On MRI, the deltoid ligament appears as a fan-shaped, low-signal structure on T1-weighted images.
- **Components**: It consists of several parts, including:
  - **Tibionavicular Ligament**: Runs from the tibia to the navicular.
  - **Tibiocalcaneal Ligament**: Runs from the tibia to the calcaneus.
  - **Posterior Tibiotalar Ligament**: Connects the tibia to the talus posteriorly.
  - **Anterior Tibiotalar Ligament**: Connects the tibia to the talus anteriorly.
- **Function**: The deltoid ligament primarily prevents eversion and provides medial stability to the ankle.

Syndesmotic Ligaments (Distal Tibiofibular Ligament)

The syndesmosis is a fibrous joint that holds the tibia and fibula together at the distal end of the leg.

- **Radiological Appearance**: MRI is the preferred modality to assess syndesmotic injury, which may show widening of the syndesmosis and disruption of the ligamentous structures. On X-rays, a positive "mortise view" may indicate syndesmotic disruption.
- **Components**:
  - **Anterior Inferior Tibiofibular Ligament (AITFL)**
  - **Posterior Inferior Tibiofibular Ligament (PITFL)**
- **Function**: These ligaments prevent separation of the tibia and fibula and stabilize the distal ankle during weight-bearing.

Posterior Ankle Ligaments

- **Radiological Appearance**: MRI can visualize the posterior ligaments, but they are less frequently injured compared to the anterior and lateral ligaments. The posterior ankle ligaments include:
  - **Posterior Talofibular Ligament (PTFL)**: As mentioned earlier, this ligament stabilizes the posterior part of the ankle.
  - **Ligamentum Flavum**: In the posterior aspect of the ankle, this ligament contributes to stabilizing the ankle and is seen on MRI as a low-signal structure.

MR Sequences and Planes Used to Evaluate Ankle Joint

Common MR Sequences for Ankle Imaging

MRI sequences are generally categorized into **T1-weighted**, **T2-weighted**, and **Special Sequences**. The choice of sequence depends on the clinical indication (e.g., detecting ligament tears, bone marrow edema, or soft tissue pathology).[8]

a. **T1-Weighted Imaging (T1WI)**:
  - **Appearance**: On T1-weighted images, **fat** appears bright (hyperintense), while **water** and **edematous tissue** appear dark (hypointense).

- **Clinical Use**: T1 sequences are useful for evaluating the **anatomical detail** of normal structures like ligaments, tendons, and bone marrow. They are also helpful for detecting **chronic tears** or **atrophy** and for assessing bone marrow abnormalities.
- **Advantages**: Provides excellent anatomical resolution, particularly for visualizing normal anatomical structures and for detecting bone marrow changes.

b. **T2-Weighted Imaging (T2WI)**:

- **Appearance**: On T2-weighted images, **water** or **fluid** (such as in edema or inflammation) appears bright (hyperintense), while **fat** appears darker.
- **Clinical Use**: T2 sequences are ideal for assessing **soft tissue injuries** such as **ligament tears**, **tendinitis**, and **joint effusion**. They are also used to detect **acute inflammation**, **bone marrow edema**, and **swelling**.
- **Advantages**: Excellent for detecting **acute injuries** and inflammation, including ligament and tendon tears, and soft tissue edema.

c. **Proton Density (PD) Weighted Imaging**:

- **Appearance**: PD-weighted images can show intermediate signal intensity for **muscle** and **tendons** and low signal intensity for **bone**. Fluid appears hyperintense (bright).
- **Clinical Use**: This sequence is used for evaluating **soft tissue structures** like **tendons** and **ligaments** with relatively good contrast resolution between different soft tissues.
- **Advantages**: Good for visualizing **muscle**, **tendons**, and **ligaments**, with a higher signal-to-noise ratio than T2WI for structures of similar composition.

d. **Short-Tau Inversion Recovery (STIR)**:

- **Appearance**: This is a fat-suppressed sequence that reduces the signal from fat, allowing **fluid** and **edema** to appear hyperintense.
- **Clinical Use**: STIR is useful for detecting **inflammatory conditions**, **bone marrow edema**, **acute ligament tears**, or **soft tissue edema** around the ankle joint.
- **Advantages**: Best for detecting **inflammation** and **edema** in the soft tissues and bone marrow without interference from fat.

e. **Gradient Echo (GRE) Sequences**:

- **Appearance**: GRE sequences offer a good balance of **high spatial resolution** and **sensitivity** for detecting **bone marrow lesions** and **cartilage** defects.
- **Clinical Use**: GRE is often used to evaluate **bone marrow edema**, **cartilage** integrity, and **bone lesions** (e.g., stress fractures).
- **Advantages**: Provides detailed imaging of the **bone marrow** and **cartilage**.

Special MRI Sequences

a. **Contrast-Enhanced Imaging (Gadolinium Contrast)**:

- **Clinical Use**: Contrast enhanced MRI can help identify **areas of active inflammation** or **infection** in the joint or soft tissues.
- **Advantages**: Used for assessing **vascular abnormalities**, **joint effusion**, and **inflammatory conditions** that might not be apparent on non-contrast images.

b. **Diffusion-Weighted Imaging (DWI)**:

- **Clinical Use**: DWI is particularly useful for detecting **acute tissue injury** or **infection** (e.g., osteomyelitis or abscess formation).
- **Advantages**: Allows for the early detection of **acute ischemia** or **infection**, though less commonly used for standard ankle evaluations.

MRI Planes for Ankle Imaging

The MRI ankle examination typically involves three orthogonal planes to provide comprehensive visualization of the ankle joint and its surrounding structures. The most common planes are:

a. **Sagittal Plane**:

- **Description**: The sagittal plane cuts the body from front to back (dividing it into left and right halves).

- **Clinical Use**: The sagittal view is critical for evaluating the **anterior and posterior structures** of the ankle, such as:
  - **Anterior talofibular ligament (ATFL)**
  - **Posterior talofibular ligament (PTFL)**
  - **Tendon and muscle structures** (e.g., Achilles tendon, peroneal tendons)
  - **Cartilage** and **joint space** in the **talocrural joint**.
- **Advantages**: Provides a detailed view of the **joint space** and **ligamentous structures** in a weight-bearing position.

b. **Coronal Plane**:
- **Description**: The coronal plane divides the body into front (anterior) and back (posterior) halves.
- **Clinical Use**: The coronal view is useful for evaluating:
  - **Deltoid ligament** (medial ligament complex)
  - **Calcaneofibular ligament (CFL)**
  - **Tibiofibular syndesmosis**
  - **Tendon sheaths** and **muscles** (e.g., peroneal muscles and tendons).
- **Advantages**: Offers a good view of the **medial and lateral ligament complexes** and **soft tissues** of the ankle.

c. **Axial Plane**:
- **Description**: The axial plane cuts the body horizontally from top to bottom (dividing it into superior and inferior halves).
- **Clinical Use**: The axial view is important for evaluating:
  - **Joint spaces** and **osteochondral lesions**
  - **Tendons** (e.g., flexor tendons, Achilles tendon)
  - **Bone fractures** or **bone contusions**.
- **Advantages**: Provides a **cross-sectional view** of the **bone** and **joint** from below, helpful for assessing **osteochondral lesions**, **fractures**, and the relationship of bones and soft tissues.

Combined Views

- To ensure accurate assessment of the **ligaments**, **tendons**, **joint structures**, and **bones** of the ankle, **multiple plane views** are often combined. This may include:
  - **Sagittal** and **coronal** views to assess **ligamentous injuries** and **joint alignment**.
  - **Axial** and **sagittal** views for detailed assessment of **bone marrow** and **soft tissue injuries**

Congenital Diseases

1. Classify skeletal dysplasia. Briefly describe the radiological features of different types of osteogeneses imperfecta. [10] [MD (WBUHS) 21]

Classification of Skeletal Dysplasia

1. **Disorders of Bone Growth (Chondrodysplasias)**: These conditions primarily affect **cartilage** and **bone growth**, leading to abnormalities in the length of long bones,[9] resulting in **short stature** or **dwarfism**. Examples include:
   - **Achondroplasia**
   - **Hypochondroplasia**
   - **Thanatophoric dysplasia**
   - **Metatropic dysplasia**
2. **Disorders of Bone Remodeling**: These disorders involve defects in **bone remodeling** and are often associated with **fragile bones**, increased bone density, or bone deformities. Examples include:
   - **Osteogenesis imperfecta**
   - **Osteopetrosis**
   - **Paget's disease of bone**

3. **Disorders of Bone Mineralization**: These conditions lead to **defective bone mineralization** and can result in **soft bones**, fractures, or other skeletal abnormalities. Examples include:
   - **Rickets** (due to vitamin D deficiency)
   - **Hypophosphatasia**
4. **Metabolic Bone Disorders**: These involve abnormalities in bone metabolism, including mineralization and resorption. Examples include:
   - **Osteoporosis**
   - **Renal osteodystrophy**
   - **Fibrous dysplasia**
5. **Disorders of Collagen or Connective Tissue**: These disorders affect the **collagen** and other connective tissues, leading to brittle bones, abnormal joint flexibility, and other skeletal features. Examples include:
   - **Ehlers-Danlos syndrome**
   - **Marfan syndrome**
6. **Disorders of the Skeletal System with Other Organ Involvement**: These conditions affect not just the skeleton but also other systems such as the **eyes**, **skin**, or **cardiovascular system**. Examples include:
   - **Pachyonychia congenita**
   - **Osteogenesis imperfecta (OI)**, which also has a connective tissue component.

Radiological Features of Osteogenesis Imperfecta (OI)

Osteogenesis Imperfecta (OI) is a genetic disorder characterized by **brittle bones** that are prone to fractures. OI is caused by mutations in the genes responsible for collagen type I synthesis, resulting in weak, fragile bones. It has a variable clinical spectrum, with fractures occurring from birth or childhood and continuing throughout life. Radiologically, different types of OI can be distinguished based on the severity of bone involvement and other associated features.

OI is classified into **4 main types** (I-IV), with **additional subtypes** identified based on genetic and clinical features.

1. **Type I OI (Classic Mild)**:
   - **Genetic Basis**: Autosomal dominant, most common type (mutation in COL1A1).
   - **Radiological Features**:
     - **Normal birth length**, but **short stature** develops later.
     - **Fractures** are common in childhood, but decrease in frequency with age.
     - **Bowing of long bones** (e.g., femurs and tibias), especially in the lower extremities.
     - **Cortical thinning** and **moderate bone fragility**, leading to **fragility fractures**.
     - **Dentinogenesis imperfecta** (DI) may be present, seen as abnormal dental pulp calcification.
     - **Fractures in early childhood** may result in **deformities**.
     - **Normal or mildly reduced bone density**.
2. **Type II OI (Perinatal Lethal)**:
   - **Genetic Basis**: Autosomal dominant, caused by mutations in **COL1A1** or **COL1A2**.
   - **Radiological Features**:
     - **Severe bone fragility**, leading to **multiple fractures** even in utero or shortly after birth.
     - **Cranial deformities** (e.g., **soft skull** due to multiple fractures).
     - **Extremely fragile bones** with **shortened limbs** and **severe skeletal deformities**.
     - **Severe rib fractures**, leading to **respiratory insufficiency**.
     - **Underdeveloped lung tissue**, contributing to **perinatal death** due to respiratory failure.
     - **Intracranial hemorrhages** may also be present.
     - **Newborns** may present with **severe deformities**, and **fractures** may be seen in the **long bones** and **ribs**.
3. **Type III OI (Progressive Deformity)**:
   - **Genetic Basis**: Autosomal dominant, mutations in **COL1A1** or **COL1A2**.

- **Radiological Features**:
  - **Severe bone fragility** and **short stature.**
  - **Multiple fractures** starting in infancy, leading to **deformities.**
  - **Bowing of the limbs** due to recurrent fractures and insufficient bone healing.
  - **Vertebral compression fractures** result in **kyphosis** and **scoliosis.**
  - **Wormian bones** (extra bones in the sutures of the skull) can be seen on X-ray.
  - **Thinned cortices**, especially in the long bones.
  - **Dentinogenesis imperfecta** is also common.
  - **Joint laxity** and **muscle weakness.**
  - **Radiographic findings** include **fractures**, **shortened bones**, and **deformities** from early childhood.

4. **Type IV OI (Normal to Mildly Severe)**:
   - **Genetic Basis**: Autosomal dominant, mutations in **COL1A1** or **COL1A2.**
   - **Radiological Features**:
     - **Milder bone fragility** than Type III but still prone to fractures, particularly in childhood.
     - **Normal birth length** and **growth** but **short stature** in adulthood.
     - **Bowing of the long bones** and **fractures** in childhood and adolescence.
     - **Fractures** may heal with some deformity but are less severe than in Type III.
     - **Normal bone mineralization**, but **thinned cortical bone.**
     - **Skeletal deformities**, including **osteopenia**, **curvature of the spine**, and **joint contractures.**

Other Radiological Features Across Types of OI

- **General Features**: The radiographic hallmark of all types of OI is **bone fragility**, which leads to frequent fractures. In some cases, fractures may heal with deformities.
- **Bowing of Long Bones**: Characteristic in many forms of OI, especially in **Type III and IV.**
- **Wormian Bones**: Extra bones in the sutures of the skull, often seen in more severe forms (Type III and IV).
- **Bone Density**: In some forms, particularly in Type I, bone density may appear **normal** or mildly **reduced.** In more severe forms, such as Type II, the bones are **extremely fragile** and may show **severe cortical thinning.**
- **Dentinogenesis Imperfecta**: Present in most individuals with OI, leading to **discolored teeth**, often with a **bluish-grey or yellowish hue**, and increased risk of dental fractures.

Infections/Inflammations

1. Discuss the pathophysiology and radiographic features of rheumatoid arthritis. [4+6] [MD (WBUHS) 23]

Rheumatoid arthritis (RA) is a **chronic, systemic autoimmune disease** characterized primarily by **inflammation of the synovial joints**, leading to progressive joint damage and deformity. It typically affects multiple joints, particularly in the hands, wrists, and knees, and can have extra-articular manifestations. The exact cause of RA is unknown, but it is believed to result from a combination of **genetic**, **environmental**, and **immunological factors.**

1. **Immunological Mechanisms**:
   - **Autoimmune Attack on Synovium**: RA is thought to begin with an autoimmune response where the body's immune system attacks the synovium (the lining of the joints). This leads to **synovial inflammation (synovitis)** and an abnormal immune response involving **T cells**, **B cells**, and **macrophages.** These immune cells infiltrate the synovium and produce various pro-inflammatory cytokines (e.g., **TNF-alpha, IL-1, IL-6**) and **autoantibodies.**
   - **Rheumatoid Factor (RF) and Anti-Citrullinated Protein Antibodies (ACPA)**: These are key autoantibodies often present in RA. Rheumatoid factor (RF) is an antibody against **IgG** antibodies, and **ACPA (anti-CCP antibodies)** target citrullinated proteins and are highly specific for RA. Their presence can aid in diagnosis and can also be used to predict disease severity.

- **Cytokine Involvement**: **TNF-alpha** and **IL-1** are major cytokines involved in the pathogenesis of RA. They activate synovial fibroblasts and chondrocytes, leading to the production of enzymes such as **matrix metalloproteinases (MMPs)** and **cathepsins**, which degrade cartilage and bone. **IL-6** plays a key role in systemic manifestations, contributing to fever, malaise, and acute-phase reactant production (e.g., C-reactive protein or CRP).
- **Formation of Pannus**: As a result of synovial inflammation, **pannus** (an abnormal layer of fibrovascular tissue) forms over the articular cartilage. Pannus contains immune cells, inflammatory mediators, and enzymes that promote **cartilage degradation** and **bone erosion**.

2. **Joint Destruction**:
   - The prolonged inflammation leads to the destruction of the **cartilage**, **bone**, and **ligaments** of the affected joints. This manifests in **joint deformities**, **loss of joint function**, and **pain**.
   - **Bone Erosion**: As inflammation persists, **osteoclast activation** results in the resorption of bone in the joints. This is most evident at the **joint margins**, where the bone is gradually eroded. **Erosions** are a hallmark feature of RA and typically appear at the **bare areas** of the joint (i.e., areas without articular cartilage) such as the **metacarpophalangeal joints (MCP)** and **proximal interphalangeal joints (PIP)**.
   - **Joint Deformities**: As the disease progresses, **ligamentous and tendinous structures** become involved. This leads to **joint instability**, subluxation (partial dislocation), and deformities, including **ulnar deviation** and **swan-neck deformities** in the fingers.
3. **Systemic Involvement**:

   RA is a **systemic disease**, meaning it affects the body beyond just the joints. Extra-articular manifestations include:
   - **Rheumatoid nodules**: Firm, subcutaneous nodules that form over pressure points (e.g., elbows).
   - **Vasculitis**: Inflammation of blood vessels that can lead to organ damage.
   - **Lung involvement**: Interstitial lung disease and pleuritis are common in RA.
   - **Cardiovascular risk**: Increased risk of heart disease due to chronic inflammation.

Radiographic Features of Rheumatoid Arthritis

Radiographic imaging plays a critical role in the diagnosis and monitoring of RA, as well as assessing the extent of joint damage. The following are the key radiographic features:

1. **Early Stage (Initial Changes)**:
   - **Soft Tissue Swelling**: One of the earliest signs is **soft tissue swelling** around the affected joints due to synovial inflammation and fluid accumulation.
   - **Periarticular Osteopenia**: Decreased bone density around the affected joint due to **increased blood flow** and **osteoclastic activity**. This is seen as **juxta-articular bone loss** (bone loss next to the joint) on radiographs.
   - **No Erosions**: In the very early stages of RA, radiographs may show **soft tissue swelling** and **periarticular osteopenia** but no joint erosions.
2. **Mid Stage (Progressive Disease)**:
   - **Joint Erosions**: These are **focal defects** in the bone at the joint margin, most commonly seen in the **proximal interphalangeal (PIP)** and **metacarpophalangeal (MCP)** joints in the hands. Erosions are typically located at the **bare areas** of bone (areas without cartilage), where inflammation is most intense.
   - **Joint Space Narrowing**: As cartilage is destroyed, there is **progressive narrowing of the joint space**, particularly in weight-bearing joints like the knees and hips.
   - **Subchondral Cysts**: Small cyst-like areas of bone that develop within the subchondral bone, adjacent to the articular surface, as a result of inflammation and bone resorption.
   - **Bone Deformities**: As the disease progresses, deformities such as **subluxation**, **ulnar deviation** (especially in the hands), and **swelling of the joints** become more apparent. The **"pencil-in-cup" deformity** can be seen in advanced stages, particularly in the fingers.
   - **Joint Subluxation**: Partial dislocation due to progressive ligament damage and synovial swelling, particularly in the small joints (e.g., wrists, MCP joints).

3. **Late Stage (Severe Disease):**
   - **Severe Joint Deformities**: This may include **fibrous ankylosis** (loss of joint movement due to fibrosis), **bony ankylosis** (fusion of bones), and severe joint destruction.
   - **Marginal Erosions**: These become more extensive, leading to significant **joint instability** and **deformities**, especially in the **hands** and **feet**.
   - **Deformities**: Characteristic deformities in the hands include **swan-neck deformities**, **boutonnière deformities**, and **ulnar deviation.**
   - **Bone Destruction**: Loss of the normal joint architecture with severe destruction of both cartilage and bone. **Joint ankylosis** can occur, and the **joint space** may be obliterated.
   - **Bony Ankylosis**: In severe cases, the joints can become completely fused due to the inflammatory process leading to bony union.
4. **Extra-Articular Findings**:
   - **Rheumatoid Nodules**: These can be visible on radiographs as soft-tissue masses, commonly seen over pressure points such as the elbows and forearms.
   - **Pericardial Effusion or Cardiovascular Abnormalities**: These may be noted incidentally, as RA can have systemic effects that are seen in imaging studies beyond the joints.

2. Discuss the differential diagnosis of the radiological appearance of absorption of terminal phalanges. [10] [MD (WBUHS) 23, MD (WBUHS) 21]

Following are the main differential diagnoses for the **absorption of the terminal phalanges**:[10]

1. **Psoriatic Arthritis (PsA):**
   - **Radiological Features**: Psoriatic arthritis can involve the **distal interphalangeal joints (DIPs)**, leading to **distal phalanx resorption**. This is typically characterized by **"pencil-in-cup" deformity** in more advanced stages, where the distal phalanx is tapered and eroded. **Absorption of the terminal phalanges** is often seen early and can be asymmetric.
   - **Associated Features**:
     - **Joint erosion** at the DIPs.
     - **Soft tissue swelling**.
     - **Nail changes** (onycholysis, pitting).
     - **Skin psoriasis** (may be present or history of it).
2. **Rheumatoid Arthritis (RA):**
   - **Radiological Features**: In **Rheumatoid arthritis**, resorption of the **distal phalanx** can occur due to chronic inflammation and **joint destruction**. The **distal interphalangeal joints** can show **peripheral erosions** and **bone resorption** as a part of the inflammatory process.
   - **Associated Features**:
     - **Symmetrical joint involvement**.
     - **Proximal interphalangeal (PIP) joint involvement**.
     - **Periarticular osteoporosis** and **joint space narrowing**.
     - **Ulnar deviation** and **swan-neck deformity** in later stages.
3. **Acroosteolysis**:
   - **Radiological Features**: Acroosteolysis refers to **atrophy or resorption of the distal phalanges** without significant joint destruction. It can be seen as a **loss of bone at the distal tips** of the fingers or toes, leading to a **blunted or tapered appearance** of the affected phalanges.
   - **Associated Features**:
     - **Symmetrical** or **asymmetrical** involvement.
     - **Progressive loss of bone mass**.
     - Can be isolated or part of a broader systemic condition.

- **Causes**: Acroosteolysis can occur in various conditions, including:
  - **Systemic sclerosis** (scleroderma).
  - **Hyperparathyroidism**.
  - **Chronic renal failure**.
  - **Increased calcium metabolism** or **low vitamin D** levels.

4. **Systemic Sclerosis (Scleroderma)**:
   - **Radiological Features**: In **systemic sclerosis**, a specific form of **acroosteolysis** may develop, often involving **distal phalanges**. This leads to the characteristic **resorption** and **atrophy** of the distal tips of the fingers, creating a **"tuft-like" appearance**.
   - **Associated Features**:
     - **Skin thickening** and **tightening**, particularly on the hands.
     - **Raynaud's phenomenon**.
     - **Digital ulcers** and **vascular abnormalities** (e.g., dilated capillaries, arteriovenous shunting).
     - **Pulmonary fibrosis** (in more advanced stages).
5. **Hyperparathyroidism**:
   - **Radiological Features**: **Hyperparathyroidism** can cause **"osteitis fibrosa cystica"**, leading to **resorption of the terminal phalanges** and **subperiosteal bone resorption**. This is often seen as a **loss of bone in the distal phalanges** and can lead to a **"salt-and-pepper" skull** or **osteopenia** in the hands.
   - **Associated Features**:
     - **Brown tumors** (osteolytic lesions).
     - **Subperiosteal resorption** of bone, often noted at the **proximal phalanges** and **metacarpals**.
     - **Increased serum calcium** and **parathyroid hormone levels**.
     - **Cystic bone lesions** on radiographs.
6. **Diabetic Cheiroarthropathy (Diabetic Scleroderma)**:
   - **Radiological Features**: Diabetic cheiroarthropathy is a complication of long-term diabetes, and it can cause **soft tissue calcification** and **joint contractures**. Though it is not primarily characterized by phalangeal resorption, some patients may exhibit **distal phalanx involvement** with **mild osteopenia** or **resorption**.
   - **Associated Features**:
     - **Limited joint mobility**.
     - **"Praying hands"** sign (inability to flatten hands).
     - **Flexion contractures of fingers**.
7. **Chronic Renal Failure and Secondary Hyperparathyroidism**:
   - **Radiological Features**: In **chronic renal failure**, **secondary hyperparathyroidism** often causes **resorption of the terminal phalanges**. This leads to **distal phalanx resorption** and **soft tissue calcification**. On radiographs, there may be **peripheral osteopenia**, **osteosclerosis**, and **subperiosteal bone resorption**.
   - **Associated Features**:
     - **Metabolic bone disease** due to disturbances in calcium and phosphate metabolism.
     - **Calciphylaxis** (calcium deposition in soft tissues).
     - **Erosion of bone** at the phalanges and other sites.
8. **Langerhans Cell Histiocytosis (Histiocytosis X)**:
   - **Radiological Features**: Langerhans cell histiocytosis can cause **osteolytic lesions** in various bones, including the **distal phalanges**, leading to **absorption** or **resorption** of the terminal phalanges. This is more commonly seen in children or young adults.
   - **Associated Features**:
     - **Lytic bone lesions** elsewhere (skull, ribs, etc.).
     - **Soft tissue masses** or swelling around the joints.
     - **Systemic symptoms** (e.g., fever, weight loss, and organ involvement).

9. **Sickle Cell Disease**:
   - **Radiological Features: Sickle cell disease** can cause **osteonecrosis** and **bone infarcts**. While not primarily causing terminal phalanx absorption, it can lead to **distal phalanx changes**, particularly if there are associated bone infarcts and changes in bone density.
   - **Associated Features**:
     - **Bone infarcts** and **osteonecrosis** (especially in the **hands** and **hips**).
     - **Radiological evidence** of **bone marrow changes**.
     - **Painful episodes (crisis)** and **splenomegaly**.
10. **Infectious Causes (Osteomyelitis)**:
    - **Radiological Features**: **Osteomyelitis** of the distal phalanx (often due to **direct trauma**, **puncture wounds**, or **hematogenous spread**) can cause **localized bone destruction** or resorption. **Absorption** of the terminal phalanges can occur with **chronic infection**.
    - **Associated Features**:
      - **Soft tissue swelling**.
      - **Bone destruction** and **periosteal reaction**.
      - **Fistula formation** and **abscesses**.

3. Enumerate the causes and imaging features in hypertrophic osteoarthropathy. [10] [MD (WBUHS) 20]

Causes of Hypertrophic Osteoarthropathy (HOA)

HOA can be classified into two types: **primary** (idiopathic) and **secondary** (associated with systemic diseases).[11]

1. **Primary (Idiopathic) Hypertrophic Osteoarthropathy**:
   - Rare, and the cause is unknown.
   - No associated systemic condition is identified.
2. **Secondary Hypertrophic Osteoarthropathy**:

   Secondary HOA is more common and is usually linked to systemic diseases, especially those affecting the chest or heart. The most frequent causes include:

   1. **Lung Diseases (Most Common Cause)**:
      - **Chronic Pulmonary Diseases**:
        - **Lung cancer** (especially **bronchogenic carcinoma**, including **small-cell lung cancer**).
        - **Pulmonary tuberculosis**.
        - **Chronic obstructive pulmonary disease (COPD)**.
        - **Cystic fibrosis**.
        - **Pulmonary fibrosis**.
        - **Bronchiectasis**.
      - **Hypoxia** due to chronic lung diseases is thought to be a contributing factor in the development of HOA.
   2. **Cardiac Diseases**:
      - **Congenital cyanotic heart disease** (e.g., **tetralogy of Fallot**).
      - **Chronic heart failure**, especially with **right-sided heart failure** or **chronic cor pulmonale**, leading to secondary pulmonary hypertension.
   3. **Malignancies**:
      - **Nonlung cancers** can also cause secondary HOA, including:
        - **Breast cancer**.
        - **Ovarian cancer**.
        - **Esophageal cancer**.
        - **Gastrointestinal cancer**.
      - **Nonsmall cell lung carcinoma** is the most frequent malignancy linked to HOA.

4. **Infectious Causes**:
   - **Endocarditis** (infective endocarditis).
   - **Tuberculosis.**
   - **Abscess formation** (often pulmonary).
5. **Endocrine Disorders**:
   - **Hyperthyroidism** (Graves' disease).
   - **Acromegaly** (growth hormone excess).
6. **Vascular Diseases**:
   - **Arteriovenous malformations** or **vascular shunts** can lead to altered blood flow and contribute to HOA.
7. **Other Conditions**:
   - **Crohn's disease.**
   - **Ulcerative colitis.**
   - **Cirrhosis of the liver.**
   - **Chronic kidney disease.**
   - **Familial HOA** (rare genetic form).

Imaging Features of Hypertrophic Osteoarthropathy

The hallmark of HOA is **periosteal bone formation**, which can be seen on radiographs, as well as **joint changes** typical of osteoarthritis. The imaging features may vary depending on the severity of the condition and the underlying cause.

1. **Digital Clubbing (Most Prominent Clinical Feature)**:
   - **Radiographic Features**: Not typically visible on X-ray, but **digital clubbing** can be seen clinically as **thickening of the nail beds** and **curvature of the nails**, along with **swelling** of the distal phalanges.
2. **Periosteal Bone Formation**:
   - **Radiographic Findings**:
     - **Periosteal new bone formation** at the **metaphyseal** and **diaphyseal** regions of the long bones, especially the **distal limbs** (hands, feet).
     - **"Onion-skin" appearance**: This refers to concentric layers of new bone formation around the shaft of long bones, especially in the **distal phalanges**.
     - **Cortical thickening** and **new bone formation** can be seen on **X-rays**.
     - **Symmetrical involvement** of the limbs, particularly the **distal ends** of the long bones.
3. **Joint Changes**:
   - **Radiographic Features**:
     - **Osteoarthritis**-like changes in the affected joints, including:
       - **Joint space narrowing.**
       - **Osteophyte formation** (bone spurs).
       - **Subchondral sclerosis.**
     - These changes are typically more prominent in the **fingers**, **toes**, **wrists**, and **elbows**, but **weight-bearing joints** like the knees and hips can also be involved.
4. **Soft Tissue Changes**:
   - **Soft Tissue Swelling**: Soft tissue swelling due to inflammation around the joints and periosteal reaction can be seen on **X-rays** or **MRI**.
   - **Synovial Proliferation**: This can occur with joint involvement, resulting in **joint effusions** or **synovitis**, which can be seen on MRI.
5. **Bone Resorption**:
   - In severe cases, **osteolytic lesions** or **resorption** of the terminal phalanges can be observed. This is more common in advanced stages and when HOA is associated with other systemic conditions like **malignancy** or **chronic pulmonary diseases**.

- **Acroosteolysis**: This is the resorption of the distal phalanx, typically seen in diseases like **hyperthyroidism** and **chronic renal failure** but can also occur in HOA, especially with **lung cancer** or **chronic infections**.

6. **Radiographic Locations**:
   - **Hands and Feet**: Periosteal bone formation, **subperiosteal bone resorption**, and **joint changes** are most prominent in the **distal phalanges, metacarpals, phalanges of the feet**, and **distal parts of long bones**.
   - **Lower Extremities**: The **tibias** and **fibulas** may also show **periosteal thickening** and **new bone formation**, although less commonly than in the upper extremities.

4. Ultrasound and MRI findings of rheumatoid arthritis. [10] [MD (WBUHS) 17, DNB June 21]

Ultrasound Findings in Rheumatoid Arthritis

Ultrasound is a highly sensitive imaging modality for detecting **synovitis** (inflammation of the synovial membrane) and **early joint damage** in RA. It can also be used to monitor disease activity, guide joint injections or aspirations, and assess treatment efficacy.

Key Ultrasound Findings in RA

1. **Synovitis**:
   - **Synovial Hypertrophy**: Ultrasound can detect **thickening of the synovial membrane**, which is one of the earliest signs of RA. The increased thickness is often seen as a **hypoechoic (dark) area** surrounding the joint, which indicates fluid accumulation or thickening of the synovium.
   - **Power Doppler**: Doppler ultrasound is particularly useful in detecting **increased blood flow** in the synovial vessels, a hallmark of active inflammation in RA. **Power Doppler signal** can quantify the level of vascularization in the synovium, indicating the presence of **active synovitis**.
2. **Effusion**:
   - **Joint Effusion**: Fluid accumulation in the joint space is common in active RA. Ultrasound can detect **fluid accumulation** in the synovial cavity, often appearing as **anechoic (black)** or **hypoechoic** areas in the joint. Effusions may be seen in the wrist, knee, and MCP joints, among others.
   - **Bursitis**: Ultrasound can also identify inflammation in periarticular structures like **bursae**, which may be involved in RA (e.g., **olecranon bursitis**).
3. **Tenosynovitis**:
   - **Tendon Sheath Inflammation**: RA can involve **tendon sheaths**, leading to **tenosynovitis**. Ultrasound can identify **thickening of the tendon sheath** and **fluid within the tendon sheath** (hypoechoic areas).
   - Commonly seen in the **flexor tendons** of the hands and wrists and **extensor tendons** in the feet.
4. **Bone Erosions**:
   - **Early Erosions**: While ultrasound is not typically used for detecting bone erosions in RA (MRI is more sensitive for this), it can sometimes detect **superficial cortical erosions**. These appear as **irregularities** or **breaks** in the bone cortex, often located near the joint margins.
   - **Subchondral Bone Erosion**: When present, erosions may show a **hypoechoic defect** in the bone surface.
5. **Cartilage Loss**:
   - **Cartilage Thinning**: In advanced stages of RA, ultrasound can detect **joint space narrowing** due to **cartilage loss**, although this is more accurately assessed on X-ray and MRI.
6. **Vascular Involvement**:
   - **Vascularity**: Ultrasound can evaluate the vascularity of inflamed joints and tendons using **Power Doppler**. Increased vascularity in the synovium correlates with **active inflammation** in RA.

MRI Findings in Rheumatoid Arthritis

MRI is a highly sensitive imaging modality for assessing **soft tissue involvement**, including synovitis, **cartilage damage**, **bone erosions**, and **bone marrow edema**, making it ideal for evaluating the full spectrum of RA.

Key MRI Findings in RA

1. **Synovitis**:
   - **Synovial Thickening**: MRI shows **synovial hypertrophy** as **increased signal intensity** on **T2-weighted images** and **short tau inversion recovery (STIR)** images. Inflammation and synovial fluid accumulate in the synovium, which appears hyperintense.
   - **Synovial Enhancement**: After contrast administration (gadolinium), inflamed synovium enhances, providing a clear indication of **active synovitis**.
2. **Bone Erosions**:
   - **Subchondral Erosions**: **Bone erosions** are one of the most important MRI findings in RA. They appear as **areas of bone loss** with irregular margins on **T1-weighted images**, with surrounding **bone marrow edema** or **osteitis** visible on **T2-weighted** or **STIR images**.
   - **Early Erosions**: MRI is more sensitive than X-ray in detecting **early bone erosions** (before they are visible on plain radiographs), making it a valuable tool for **early RA detection**.
3. **Bone Marrow Edema (BME)**:
   - **Bone Marrow Edema**: One of the earliest and most sensitive findings in RA. BME appears as **hyperintense areas** on **STIR** or **T2-weighted MRI** sequences, indicating **inflammation** and **bone stress**. This finding is associated with **active disease** and may precede visible erosions.
4. **Cartilage Damage**:
   - **Cartilage Loss**: MRI is excellent for detecting **cartilage thinning** and **joint space narrowing**, which are indicative of cartilage damage. **T2-weighted images** may show **increased signal** in the cartilage, indicating damage or **degeneration**.
   - **Focal Cartilage Defects**: MRI is particularly useful in assessing **focal cartilage defects** in weight-bearing joints like the **knee** and **hip** in RA patients.
5. **Tendon and Ligament Involvement**:
   - **Tenosynovitis**: Similar to ultrasound, MRI can show **inflammation of the tendon sheaths**. **T2-weighted images** highlight the **increased signal** in tendons affected by **tenosynovitis**.
   - **Tendon Ruptures**: MRI can detect tendon ruptures or **degenerative changes** resulting from chronic inflammation.
6. **Joint Deformities**:
   - **Joint Subluxation/Dislocation**: Advanced RA may result in **joint instability** and deformities, which can be evaluated on MRI. **Subluxation** (partial dislocation) is especially common in the **wrist**, **MCP joints**, and **PIP joints**.
   - **Deformities** such as **ulnar deviation** in the fingers and **bony ankylosis** (fusion of joints) can also be seen in later stages of the disease.
7. **Vascular Involvement**:
   - **Vascular Changes**: MRI can also demonstrate **vascular changes**, such as increased blood flow to inflamed synovium, which may correlate with active disease.

Metabolic Bone Diseases

1. Mention the causes of a generalized increase in bone density. Write the radiographic features of Paget's disease of bone. [4+6] [MD (WBUHS) 23, MD (WBUHS) 18]

A generalized increase in bone density, also known as **osteosclerosis**, can result from a variety of systemic conditions, metabolic disorders, and certain pathologies. These conditions are associated with increased **bone formation** or **decreased bone resorption**, leading to the thickening of bones. Some of the key causes include:

1. **Osteopetrosis (Marble Bone Disease)**:
   - **Description**: Osteopetrosis is a rare hereditary disorder characterized by **abnormal bone resorption** due to dysfunctional osteoclasts, leading to the accumulation of dense bone.

- **Radiographic Features**: The bones appear **uniformly dense**, with a **"bone within bone" appearance**, and may show **long bone cortical thickening** and **narrowed medullary cavities**.

2. **Paget's Disease of Bone**:
   - **Description**: Paget's disease is a **chronic bone disorder** characterized by abnormal bone remodeling, with **excessive bone resorption** followed by **disorganized bone formation**. This results in structurally weakened but dense bones.
   - **Radiographic Features**: Paget's disease exhibits a **"cotton wool" appearance** of the skull, **broadening of long bones**, and **trabecular thickening** with **areas of sclerosis and lytic lesions**.
3. **Hyperparathyroidism (Secondary)**:
   - **Description**: In **secondary hyperparathyroidism**, typically due to **renal failure** or **vitamin D deficiency**, there is compensatory **parathyroid hormone (PTH) overproduction**, leading to **osteoclast activation** and abnormal bone remodeling, which can result in increased bone density in some areas.
   - **Radiographic Features**: Often **bone sclerosis** in certain areas, like the **pelvis**, **wrists**, and **knees**, with **subperiosteal resorption** being more prominent in other regions.
4. **Fluoride Poisoning**:
   - **Description**: Chronic exposure to high levels of fluoride can lead to **fluorosis**, where **excessive fluoride deposition** causes increased bone mineralization.
   - **Radiographic Features**: **Dense, sclerotic bones**, with **cortical thickening**, **calcification of ligaments** and tendons, and **joint space narrowing**.
5. **Osteoblastic Metastases**:
   - **Description**: **Osteoblastic metastases** from cancers such as **prostate cancer**, **breast cancer**, or **carcinoid tumors** can lead to areas of increased bone density.
   - **Radiographic Features**: **Diffuse or localized sclerotic lesions**, especially in the **spine**, **pelvis**, and **long bones**.
6. **Hemochromatosis**:
   - **Description**: **Hemochromatosis** is a disorder of iron overload that can result in **increased bone density** due to **iron deposition** in bone tissues.
   - **Radiographic Features**: **Increased bone density** with **sclerosis of joints** and sometimes **generalized osteosclerosis**.
7. **Acromegaly**:
   - **Description**: Acromegaly, caused by excessive **growth hormone** secretion, leads to **bone thickening**, especially in the **hands**, **feet**, and **face**, resulting in generalized **increased bone density**.
   - **Radiographic Features**: **Enlarged bones**, particularly **hands**, **feet**, and **facial bones**; **sclerosis of the skull** and **mandible**.
8. **Osteopoikilosis (Spotty Bone Disease)**:
   - **Description**: This is a rare, benign genetic condition that leads to **multiple small, round, or oval bone sclerosis** in the **epiphyses**, **metaphyses**, and **diaphyses** of long bones, often with no associated symptoms.
   - **Radiographic Features**: **Multiple small, round, or oval areas of increased bone density** scattered throughout the bones, resembling "spots" on X-ray.
9. **Lead Poisoning**:
   - **Description**: Chronic lead poisoning can result in **bone lead deposition**, which leads to increased bone density in some areas.
   - **Radiographic Features**: **Lead lines** in the **metaphysis** of long bones and generalized sclerosis in severe cases.

Radiographic Features of Paget's Disease of Bone

Paget's disease of bone is a chronic condition of abnormal bone remodeling, characterized by a **combination of excessive bone resorption** followed by **disorganized and excessive bone formation**. It typically affects the **pelvis**, **spine**, **skull**, and **long bones**. The radiographic findings of Paget's disease are distinct and can evolve over time, depending on the stage of the disease (lytic, mixed, or sclerotic phases).

1. **Lytic Phase**:
   - **Radiographic Features**:
     - **Bone resorption**: In the early stages, **areas of bone destruction** are evident, especially in the **skull**, **pelvis**, **spine**, and **long bones**. The affected bones may appear **lucent** with **sharp-bordered lytic lesions**.
     - **"Blade of Grass" Sign**: This is a characteristic feature in the long bones, especially the **femur** and **tibia**, where the **cortex** appears **splayed** and **expanded** in a **widening flare**, resembling the blade of a grass.
2. **Mixed Phase (Lytic and Sclerotic)**:
   - **Radiographic Features**:
     - **Cotton Wool Appearance**: In the skull, Paget's disease often shows a **cotton wool appearance** due to **irregular bone sclerosis** with areas of **trabecular thickening** and **coarse bone patterns**.
     - **Cortical Thickening**: The cortex of long bones may become **thickened**, resulting in **bowing of the bones**, which is particularly noticeable in the **femur** and **tibia**.
     - **Bone Enlargement**: The affected bones may **enlarge**, leading to deformities. This is particularly evident in the **skull**, where the bones become **enlarged**, giving rise to a **"hat size increase"**.
     - **Trabecular Pattern Changes**: The trabecular bone pattern becomes **coarse** and **irregular**, and the overall **bone density** increases.
3. **Sclerotic Phase**:
   - **Radiographic Features**:
     - **Dense Sclerotic Bone**: In the later stages of Paget's disease, the bone becomes **dense** and **sclerotic**, often appearing as **bone sclerosis** on X-ray. The bone architecture may become **homogeneous** or show **marked cortical thickening**.
     - **"Osteoporosis circumscripta"**: In the skull, this appears as **localized, sharply demarcated areas of sclerosis** with a **reversal of the normal cortical-trabecular bone architecture**.
4. **Bowing Deformities**:
   - **Radiographic Features**: Paget's disease can lead to **bone deformities** due to **excessive bone formation** and **softening of bone structure**. Common deformities include **bowing of the long bones**, such as the **tibia** (known as **tibial bowing** or **"shepherd's crook deformity"**), and in the **femur**.
5. **Fractures**:
   - **Radiographic Features**: Due to the **abnormal bone remodeling** and **weakened bone structure**, Paget's disease is associated with **pathological fractures**. These fractures are particularly common in the **long bones** and **pelvis**.
6. **Increased Bone Density**:
   - **Radiographic Features**: In the later stages of Paget's disease, **increased bone density** is evident, particularly in the **pelvis**, **vertebrae**, and **long bones**. The bone density is often **heterogeneous** with areas of **high sclerosis** and **irregular trabeculae**.
7. **Vertebral Involvement**:
   - **Radiographic Features**: In the spine, Paget's disease can cause **vertebral body enlargement**, **increased bone density**, and **flattening of the vertebral bodies**. This may lead to **vertebral fractures** or **kyphosis**.

2. Write short notes on radiological features of hyperparathyroidism. [5] [MD (WBUHS) 23]

Hyperparathyroidism is a condition characterized by excessive secretion of **parathyroid hormone (PTH)**, which leads to abnormalities in calcium, phosphate, and bone metabolism. There are two types of hyperparathyroidism:

- **Primary hyperparathyroidism**: Due to an abnormality in the parathyroid glands themselves (e.g., adenoma, hyperplasia).
- **Secondary hyperparathyroidism**: Often associated with chronic renal disease, where there is an impaired calcium-phosphate balance.
- **Tertiary hyperparathyroidism**: Resulting from long-standing secondary hyperparathyroidism, often seen in patients with chronic kidney disease.

Radiologically, hyperparathyroidism leads to characteristic changes in the bones and soft tissues, most notably in the **bones** due to the effects of increased PTH on bone resorption.

Key Radiological Features of Hyperparathyroidism

1. **Subperiosteal Bone Resorption**:
   - **Description**: One of the hallmark radiographic findings in **primary hyperparathyroidism** is **subperiosteal resorption**, particularly in the **phalanges**, **metacarpals**, **radius**, and **tibia**.
   - **Appearance**: The resorption is most pronounced along the **distal phalanges** (in the fingers) and **distal radius** (in the forearm), where the periosteum is more active. This leads to **lucent areas** along the bone surface, giving a **"sharp" or "pointed" appearance** to the tips of the fingers (also called **"rat bite" lesions**).
2. **Osteitis Fibrosa Cystica** (also known as **Brown Tumor**):
   - **Description**: A late manifestation of **primary hyperparathyroidism**, where there is **localized bone resorption** and **fibrosis**, leading to the formation of cyst-like spaces in bones. This is caused by the excessive release of calcium from bone.
   - **Appearance**: It results in **lytic lesions** (areas of bone destruction), which are often **multilocular** and filled with **fibrous tissue**. These are most commonly seen in the **jaw**, **ribs**, **pelvis**, and **long bones**.
   - **"Brown tumor"**: These cystic lesions are sometimes referred to as **brown tumors** because of the presence of hemosiderin from **hemorrhage** within the cysts, which gives them a **brownish color**.
3. **Osteopenia/Osteoporosis**:
   - **Description**: The chronic effects of elevated PTH lead to **increased bone resorption**, which results in **generalized bone loss**.
   - **Appearance**: X-rays can show **decreased bone density** throughout the skeleton, particularly affecting **trabecular bone**. The **vertebrae** may show **vertebral body collapse** (wedge-shaped) due to the loss of the trabecular network.
   - **"Salt and Pepper" Skull**: A characteristic finding on skull radiographs is a **"salt-and-pepper" appearance** due to the combination of **bone resorption** and **trabecular pattern** changes in the skull, creating a mottled appearance.
4. **Metacarpal and Metatarsal Enlargement**:
   - **Description**: In severe hyperparathyroidism, there may be **soft tissue swelling** and **enlargement of the metacarpals** and **metatarsals** due to **subperiosteal bone resorption** and **fibrous tissue formation**.
   - **Appearance**: This results in a **"thickened" or "widened" appearance** of the bones at the ends of the fingers or toes.
5. **Calcifications in Soft Tissues**:
   - **Description**: **Ectopic calcifications** are common in both **primary** and **secondary hyperparathyroidism**. These are often due to the **elevated calcium levels** in the blood.
   - **Appearance**: The most common sites of calcification include the **skin**, **kidneys** (nephrocalcinosis), and **blood vessels**. In the kidneys, the radiograph may show **calcified renal stones** or **renal parenchymal calcifications**.
6. **Rugger-Jersey Spine**:
   - **Description**: This is a characteristic finding in **secondary hyperparathyroidism** (more commonly associated with chronic kidney disease).
   - **Appearance**: The **spine** shows a **"rugger-jersey" appearance**, where the **endplates of the vertebral bodies** are sclerotic (dense), while the **central part** of the vertebral body shows **osteopenia** (loss of bone density). This results in a **band-like appearance** on lateral radiographs.
7. **Fractures**:
   - **Description**: Due to the bone weakening caused by hyperparathyroidism, **pathological fractures** are more common, especially in the **vertebrae**, **ribs**, and **long bones**.
   - **Appearance**: The fractures are often **compression fractures** of the spine or **fractures of weakened long bones** that may show **evidence of chronic osteopenia**.
8. **Chondrocalcinosis** (in secondary hyperparathyroidism):
   - **Description**: In secondary hyperparathyroidism, there may be **calcium deposition in the cartilage** (chondrocalcinosis), particularly in the **knees**, **wrist**, and **shoulders**.
   - **Appearance**: X-rays may show **calcifications within joint cartilage**, which appear as fine **linear or stippled calcifications**.

3. What are metabolic and endocrine disorders affecting bones? Describe the radiological findings of hyperparathyroidism. [5+5=10] [MD (WBUHS) 19]

Metabolic and Endocrine Disorders Affecting Bones

Metabolic and endocrine disorders significantly influence bone metabolism, either by altering bone formation or increasing bone resorption. Several conditions are associated with abnormal bone density, shape, and structural integrity. These disorders often manifest in radiographic findings that help in diagnosis.

1. **Osteoporosis**:
   - **Cause**: Imbalance between bone resorption and formation, leading to reduced bone mass.
   - **Radiological Features**:
     - **Generalized bone thinning**.
     - **Decreased bone density**.
     - **Fractures**: Particularly **vertebral compression fractures** (wedge-shaped vertebrae), **colles fractures** (distal radius), and hip fractures.
     - **Trabecular thinning** with **loss of vertical trabeculae**.
2. **Osteomalacia and Rickets**:
   - **Cause**: **Vitamin D deficiency** leading to impaired mineralization of the bone matrix.
   - **Radiological Features**:
     - **Looser zones (pseudofractures)**: Bilateral, symmetrical, radiolucent areas near joints, particularly in the **pelvis**, **proximal femora**, and **scapulae**.
     - **Cupping and fraying of metaphyses** in **children** (Rickets).
     - **Widening of epiphyseal plates** in children.
3. **Paget's Disease of Bone**:
   - **Cause**: Abnormal bone remodeling, with increased resorption followed by chaotic bone formation.
   - **Radiological Features**:
     - **Cotton wool appearance** (skull).
     - **Bone expansion** with cortical thickening (long bones).
     - **Mixed lytic and sclerotic lesions** (classic stage).
     - **Bow-shaped deformities** (long bones).
     - **"Osteoporosis circumscripta"** (localized skull sclerosis).
4. **Hyperparathyroidism**:
   - **Cause**: Excess **parathyroid hormone (PTH)** leads to increased bone resorption and abnormal calcium metabolism.
   - **Radiological Features**: (See below)
5. **Acromegaly**:
   - **Cause**: Excess growth hormone, leading to abnormal bone growth.
   - **Radiological Features**:
     - **Enlargement of hands, feet**, and **facial bones**.
     - **Thickening of cortical bone** and **enlarged sella turcica**.
     - **Spinal changes**: Widening of intervertebral disc spaces, bony overgrowth.
6. **Cushing's Syndrome**:
   - **Cause**: Chronic excess of **cortisol** (often due to prolonged corticosteroid therapy or Cushing's disease).
   - **Radiological Features**:
     - **Osteopenia** or **osteoporosis**.
     - **Compression fractures** of the vertebrae.
     - **Cortical thinning**.

7. **Hypoparathyroidism**:
   - **Cause**: Low levels of parathyroid hormone (PTH), leading to hypocalcemia and decreased bone resorption.
   - **Radiological Features**:
     - **Increased bone density** in some areas.
     - **Basal ganglia calcifications** (rare).
     - **Dental changes**: Delayed eruption of teeth, malformed teeth.
8. **Osteogenesis Imperfecta (OI)**:
   - **Cause**: Genetic disorder causing **collagen type I defects**, leading to fragile bones.
   - **Radiological Features**:
     - **Multiple fractures** (with varying stages of healing).
     - **Wormian bones** (extra bones in sutures of the skull).
     - **Bow-shaped long bones**.
     - **Decreased bone density** (increased fragility).

Radiological Findings of Hyperparathyroidism

Hyperparathyroidism is a condition characterized by excessive secretion of **parathyroid hormone (PTH)**, which leads to abnormalities in calcium, phosphate, and bone metabolism. There are two types of hyperparathyroidism:

- **Primary hyperparathyroidism**: Due to an abnormality in the parathyroid glands themselves (e.g., adenoma, hyperplasia).
- **Secondary hyperparathyroidism**: Often associated with chronic renal disease, where there is an impaired calcium-phosphate balance.
- **Tertiary hyperparathyroidism**: Resulting from long-standing secondary hyperparathyroidism, often seen in patients with chronic kidney disease.

Radiologically, hyperparathyroidism leads to characteristic changes in the bones and soft tissues, most notably in the **bones** due to the effects of increased PTH on bone resorption.

Key Radiological Features of Hyperparathyroidism

1. **Subperiosteal Bone Resorption**:
   - **Description**: One of the hallmark radiographic findings in **primary hyperparathyroidism** is **subperiosteal resorption**, particularly in the **phalanges**, **metacarpals**, **radius**, and **tibia**.
   - **Appearance**: The resorption is most pronounced along the **distal phalanges** (in the fingers) and **distal radius** (in the forearm), where the periosteum is more active. This leads to **lucent areas** along the bone surface, giving a **"sharp" or "pointed" appearance** to the tips of the fingers (also called **"rat bite" lesions**).
2. **Osteitis Fibrosa Cystica** (also known as **Brown Tumor**):
   - **Description**: A late manifestation of **primary hyperparathyroidism**, where there is **localized bone resorption** and **fibrosis**, leading to the formation of cyst-like spaces in bones. This is caused by the excessive release of calcium from bone.
   - **Appearance**: It results in **lytic lesions** (areas of bone destruction), which are often **multilocular** and filled with **fibrous tissue**. These are most commonly seen in the **jaw**, **ribs**, **pelvis**, and **long bones**.
   - **"Brown tumor"**: These cystic lesions are sometimes referred to as **brown tumors** because of the presence of hemosiderin from **hemorrhage** within the cysts, which gives them a **brownish color**.
3. **Osteopenia/Osteoporosis**:
   - **Description**: The chronic effects of elevated PTH lead to **increased bone resorption**, which results in **generalized bone loss**.
   - **Appearance**: X-rays can show **decreased bone density** throughout the skeleton, particularly affecting **trabecular bone**. The **vertebrae** may show **vertebral body collapse** (wedge-shaped) due to the loss of the trabecular network.
   - **"Salt and Pepper" Skull**: A characteristic finding on skull radiographs is a **"salt-and-pepper" appearance** due to the combination of **bone resorption** and **trabecular pattern** changes in the skull, creating a mottled appearance.

4. **Metacarpal and Metatarsal Enlargement**:
   - **Description**: In severe hyperparathyroidism, there may be **soft tissue swelling** and **enlargement of the metacarpals** and **metatarsals** due to **subperiosteal bone resorption** and **fibrous tissue formation**.
   - **Appearance**: This results in a **"thickened" or "widened" appearance** of the bones at the ends of the fingers or toes.
5. **Calcifications in Soft Tissues**:
   - **Description**: **Ectopic calcifications** are common in both **primary** and **secondary hyperparathyroidism**. These are often due to the **elevated calcium levels** in the blood.
   - **Appearance**: The most common sites of calcification include the **skin**, **kidneys** (nephrocalcinosis), and **blood vessels**. In the kidneys, the radiograph may show **calcified renal stones** or **renal parenchymal calcifications**.
6. **Rugger-Jersey Spine**:
   - **Description**: This is a characteristic finding in **secondary hyperparathyroidism** (more commonly associated with chronic kidney disease).
   - **Appearance**: The **spine** shows a **"rugger-jersey" appearance**, where the **endplates of the vertebral bodies** are sclerotic (dense), while the **central part** of the vertebral body shows **osteopenia** (loss of bone density). This results in a **band-like appearance** on lateral radiographs.
7. **Fractures**:
   - **Description**: Due to the bone weakening caused by hyperparathyroidism, **pathological fractures** are more common, especially in the **vertebrae**, **ribs**, and **long bones**.
   - **Appearance**: The fractures are often **compression fractures** of the spine or **fractures of weakened long bones** that may show **evidence of chronic osteopenia**.
8. **Chondrocalcinosis** (in secondary hyperparathyroidism):
   - **Description**: In secondary hyperparathyroidism, there may be **calcium deposition in the cartilage** (chondrocalcinosis), particularly in the **knees**, **wrist**, and **shoulders**.
   - **Appearance**: X-rays may show **calcifications within joint cartilage**, which appear as fine **linear or stippled calcifications**.

4. Discuss about the metabolic disorders of bone and the role of imaging to arrive at the diagnosis. [5+5] [MD (WBUHS) 24, MD (WBUHS) 22, RG 18]

Metabolic bone disorders are a group of diseases that affect bone metabolism, either by increasing bone resorption or decreasing bone formation. These disorders can result in changes in bone density, structure, and function, and their recognition often requires a combination of **clinical evaluation**, **laboratory tests**, and **imaging studies** to establish a diagnosis and assess disease severity.

Imaging plays a critical role in diagnosing and monitoring metabolic bone disorders. Common imaging modalities include **X-ray**, **CT**, **MRI**, and **bone scintigraphy**. The choice of imaging depends on the specific condition being assessed, the clinical scenario, and the desired level of detail.

Here is an overview of the most important metabolic bone disorders, their radiological features, and the role of imaging in diagnosis:

1. **Osteoporosis**:

   Pathophysiology:
   - Osteoporosis is characterized by **decreased bone mass** and **deterioration of bone microarchitecture**, which results in increased bone fragility and susceptibility to fractures.
   - Common causes include **age-related bone loss**, **postmenopausal changes**, **chronic corticosteroid use**, and **nutritional deficiencies** (e.g., calcium or vitamin D deficiency).

   Radiological Features:
   - **X-ray**: Early stages show **decreased bone mineral density** (BMD), especially in **trabecular bone** (e.g., spine, wrist). **Compression fractures** of the vertebrae and **fractures** of the long bones may also be visible in advanced cases.
   - **Bone Density Measurement (DXA)**: **Dual-energy X-ray absorptiometry (DXA)** is the gold standard for diagnosing osteoporosis, providing a quantitative measure of BMD at critical sites (spine, hip, wrist). A **T-score** of –2.5 or lower is diagnostic of osteoporosis.

- **CT**: **Quantitative CT** can assess **vertebral trabecular bone density**, offering additional detail in cases of osteoporosis, especially for evaluating vertebral fractures.
- **MRI**: Used in cases of vertebral fractures to assess for **bone marrow edema**, which can suggest acute fractures or **osteonecrosis**.

Role of Imaging:

- **X-rays** are typically the first imaging modality to evaluate suspected fractures in osteoporotic patients.
- **DXA** is essential for confirming the diagnosis and monitoring disease progression.
- **CT and MRI** may be used to evaluate fractures and complications like **osteonecrosis** or **vertebral deformities**.

2. **Osteomalacia and Rickets**:

Pathophysiology:

- **Osteomalacia** (in adults) and **rickets** (in children) are caused by **vitamin D deficiency** or impaired calcium metabolism, leading to defective **bone mineralization**.
- In osteomalacia, the bones become soft and prone to deformities and fractures.

Radiological Features:

- **X-ray**:
  - **Looser zones** (pseudofractures): Radiolucent bands across the **pelvis**, **proximal femora**, and **scapulae**. These are stress fractures at sites of weakened bone.
  - **Widened metaphyses** (rickets): In children, **metaphyseal widening**, **cupping**, and **fraying** of the distal femur and tibia.
  - **Rachitic rosary**: Enlargement of the **costochondral junctions** in children.
- **Bone Scintigraphy** (bone scan): Can help identify areas of **increased bone turnover** and **microfractures** (useful in detecting pseudofractures).
- **MRI**: Can detect bone marrow changes and **bone deformities** in severe cases.

Role of Imaging:

- **X-ray** is essential for identifying characteristic skeletal changes in osteomalacia and rickets, including **fractures**, **deformities**, and **widening of the metaphyses**.
- **Bone scintigraphy** can help identify regions of increased activity, especially in children with rickets.

3. **Paget's Disease of Bone**:

Pathophysiology:

- Paget's disease is a **chronic disorder** of bone remodeling characterized by **excessive bone resorption** followed by **disorganized new bone formation**, leading to abnormal bone architecture.
- It most commonly affects the **pelvis**, **spine**, **skull**, and **long bones**.

Radiological Features:

- **X-ray**:
  - **Lytic lesions** in the early stages.
  - **Cotton wool appearance** in the skull, due to **mixed sclerotic and lytic** bone changes.
  - **Bone expansion** with **cortical thickening**, particularly in long bones (e.g., **femur**, **tibia**).
  - **Bow-shaped deformities** (especially in the **tibia**), due to abnormal bone growth.
- **Bone Scintigraphy**: **Increased uptake** in the affected bones, reflecting areas of **active bone remodeling**.
- **MRI**: Shows areas of **trabecular bone thickening**, **bone marrow changes**, and **bony deformities**.

Role of Imaging:

- **X-ray** is the primary modality for diagnosing Paget's disease, revealing classic findings such as **cotton wool appearance** and **bone expansion**.
- **Bone scintigraphy** can assess **disease activity** and involvement of multiple skeletal sites.
- **MRI** is useful for detecting **bone marrow involvement** and **complications** such as **fractures** or **osteosarcoma**.

4. **Hyperparathyroidism**:

Pathophysiology:

- **Primary hyperparathyroidism** results from **overproduction of parathyroid hormone (PTH)**, which leads to **excessive bone resorption**, **elevated calcium levels**, and **bone weakening**.
- **Secondary hyperparathyroidism** typically occurs due to **renal disease** and **vitamin D deficiency**, with compensatory **PTH overproduction**.

Radiological Features:

- **X-ray**:
  - **Subperiosteal resorption**: Especially in the **phalanges**, **distal radius**, and **tibia**, giving a **rat-bite** appearance.
  - **Osteitis fibrosa cystica (brown tumors)**: Lytic lesions with **fibrous tissue** in bones like the **jaw**, **pelvis**, and **ribs**.
  - **Generalized osteopenia** or **osteoporosis** in advanced disease.
- **MRI**: Useful to assess bone marrow changes in cases of **brown tumors** or fractures.
- **Bone Scintigraphy**: May show increased **uptake** in areas of bone resorption.

Role of Imaging:

- **X-ray** is used to identify characteristic findings such as **subperiosteal resorption** and **brown tumors**.
- **MRI** may be used to assess the extent of **bone involvement**, especially in cases of **brown tumors**.
- **Bone scintigraphy** can be used to assess **disease activity** and monitor skeletal involvement.

5. **Osteogenesis Imperfecta (OI)**:

Pathophysiology: Osteogenesis imperfecta is a genetic disorder characterized by defects in **collagen type I**, resulting in **brittle bones** and a propensity for **fractures**.

Radiological Features:

- **X-ray**:
  - **Multiple fractures** at varying stages of healing.
  - **Decreased bone density**, with **thin cortices** and **trabecular bone loss**.
  - **Wormian bones** (extra bones in cranial sutures).
  - **Bow-shaped long bones**, particularly the **femur** and **tibia**.
- **Bone Scintigraphy**: Can help in assessing **bone turnover** and identifying fractures.

Role of Imaging:

- **X-ray** is crucial for detecting **fractures** and **deformities** in OI patients.
- **Bone scintigraphy** may be used to assess **bone turnover** or evaluate **fractures**.

6. **Hypercalcemia of Malignancy**:

Pathophysiology: **Osteolytic bone metastases** (e.g., from **breast**, **prostate**, **lung** cancer) and **parathyroid hormone-related peptide (PTHrP)** secretion by tumors can lead to **hypercalcemia**.

Radiological Features:

- **X-ray**:
  - **Lytic lesions** in bones such as the **vertebrae**, **ribs**, and **pelvis**.
  - **Pathological fractures** due to weakened bones.
- **Bone Scintigraphy**: Can help detect **osteoblastic** or **osteolytic** metastases.
- **CT/MRI**: Best for identifying **bone metastases** and assessing the extent of disease.

Role of Imaging:

- **X-ray** is often the first modality for detecting **lytic lesions** or **fractures**.
- **CT and MRI** are more sensitive for evaluating **soft tissue involvement** and **bone metastases**.
- **Bone scintigraphy** is helpful in detecting **metastatic bone disease** and assessing **skeletal involvement**.

5. What are the causes of increased bone density? Briefly describe the radiological features of pyknodysostosis. [4+6] [MD (WBUHS) 22]

Causes of Increased Bone Density (Osteosclerosis)

Increased bone density (osteosclerosis) refers to an abnormal increase in bone mass and mineralization, which can result from several metabolic, genetic, or pathological conditions. These conditions may lead to **abnormal bone formation, decreased bone resorption**, or both, causing bones to become abnormally dense.

Causes of Increased Bone Density

1. **Hereditary and Genetic Disorders**:
   - **Pyknodysostosis**: A genetic disorder characterized by increased bone density and short stature.
   - **Osteopetrosis (Marble Bone Disease)**: A group of inherited disorders where bone resorption is impaired due to dysfunctional osteoclasts, leading to dense, brittle bones.
   - **Albers-Schönberg disease**: A form of osteopetrosis with more moderate findings compared to other types.
   - **Craniometaphyseal Dysplasia**: A rare inherited condition that leads to sclerosis of the skull and metaphyses of long bones.
2. **Metabolic Bone Diseases**:
   - **Hyperparathyroidism** (early or compensated): In some cases, mild hyperparathyroidism can lead to sclerosis or dense bone areas, particularly if associated with other conditions.
   - **Lead Poisoning**: Chronic lead exposure can cause dense metaphyseal lines, often referred to as **"lead lines"** visible on radiographs, especially in children.
   - **Vitamin D Deficiency** (in certain cases): Can lead to osteosclerosis or bone thickening, especially in cases of rickets or osteomalacia.
3. **Chronic Osteomyelitis**: Chronic infection can lead to sclerosis of the bone as part of the body's response to infection.
4. **Metastatic Disease**: Certain cancers, such as **prostate cancer** or **breast cancer**, can cause **osteoblastic metastasis**, leading to areas of increased bone density.
5. **Paget's Disease of Bone**: Early stages may show areas of **osteosclerosis** as the bone remodels and becomes overly thickened and dense before progressing to a more mixed phase with both sclerotic and lytic areas.
6. **Fibrous Dysplasia**: Although this typically causes the **ground-glass** appearance of the bones, some forms may lead to areas of increased density.
7. **Bone Islands (enostosis)**: These are small, benign areas of increased bone density, often found incidentally on radiographs.

Radiological Features of Pyknodysostosis

Pyknodysostosis is a rare, autosomal recessive genetic disorder characterized by **increased bone density** (osteosclerosis), short stature, **brittle bones**, and **delayed bone maturation**. It results from mutations in the **cathepsin K gene** (CTSK), leading to impaired osteoclast function and abnormal bone resorption. This results in excessively dense bones that are fragile and prone to fractures.

Radiological Features of Pyknodysostosis

1. **Generalized Increased Bone Density**:
   - **Bone sclerosis** is most prominent in the **skull**, **vertebrae**, **pelvis**, and **long bones**.
   - **The skull**: The most characteristic feature is **thickening of the calvarium**, leading to a **"generalized sclerosis"** of the skull bones. The **skull vault** may appear **uniformly dense** or have **thickened trabeculae**.
   - **Frontal bossing** (prominent forehead) may be seen due to skull changes.
2. **Short Stature** and **Disproportionate Limb Length**:
   - The bones are often **shortened**, particularly in the **long bones**, leading to **dwarfism** and **disproportionately short limbs**.
   - **Radiographs of long bones** show **abnormal thickening of cortical bone** and **narrowing of the medullary canal**.

3. **Delayed Bone Age**:
   - On **X-rays**, there may be **delayed closure of the epiphyses**, indicating a delay in bone maturation compared to chronological age.
   - **Ossification centers** may appear **delayed or absent** in early childhood.
4. **Fractures**:
   - Bones are **brittle** and prone to fractures, which are often noted in patients with pyknodysostosis. These fractures may appear on **radiographs** as **bone breaks** with **minimal displacement** due to the high bone density and brittle nature.
5. **Facial Abnormalities**:
   - **Mandibular sclerosis**: The mandible is thickened, and the **coronoid process** may be prominent. This sclerosis often leads to a **"ground-glass" appearance** of the mandible.
   - **Maxillary hypoplasia**: The maxilla may be underdeveloped, leading to **facial disproportion**.
6. **Osteoporosis with High Bone Density**:
   - The bones in pyknodysostosis are not only **dense** but are also more prone to fractures, leading to findings of **microfractures** and **thin cortices** in radiographic studies.

6. Discuss various radiographic findings in rickets and osteomalacia. [5+5] [MD (WBUHS) 24]

Rickets (in Children)

Radiographic findings are crucial for diagnosing rickets, and they often reveal characteristic changes in the **growth plates** (epiphyseal cartilage) and **metaphyses** (bone growth zones) of long bones.

1. **Widened Growth Plates**: The **metaphyses** of long bones, such as the **distal femur**, **proximal tibia**, and **radius**, become **widened** and **flared** due to defective mineralization. This is often referred to as **metaphyseal widening**.
2. **Cupping and Fraying of Metaphyses**: The **edges of the growth plates** appear **cupped** (concave), and **fraying** of the metaphyseal region is seen. This occurs due to the accumulation of **unmineralized cartilage** at the growth plate.
3. **Rachitic Rosary**: **Enlargement** of the **costochondral junctions** (where the ribs meet the cartilage) causes a **beaded appearance** along the **anterior chest wall**, termed **rachitic rosary**. This is one of the classic radiographic findings.
4. **Bowlegs (Genu Varum)**: The **tibia** and **femur** may show **bowing** due to insufficient mineralization, resulting in a **genu varum** deformity (outward angulation of the lower legs).
5. **Knock knees (Genu Valgum)**: In some cases, especially if there is **severe rickets**, **genu valgum** (inward angulation of the lower legs) may occur as the weight-bearing bones are affected.
6. **Widening of the Wrist and Ankle Joints**: The **wrist** and **ankle** joints may appear **widened**, and the **distal radius** and **ulna** may show **swelling** due to the growth plate involvement.
7. **Fractures and Deformities**: **Stress fractures** or **compression fractures** can occur, particularly in the **spine** and **long bones**, which may be detected radiographically.
8. **Scoliosis or Spinal Deformities**: Due to bone weakness, spinal **deformities** like **scoliosis** or **kyphosis** (hunched back) may develop.

Osteomalacia (in Adults)

Osteomalacia refers to the **softening of bones** in adults due to inadequate mineralization of the **bone matrix**, often due to a **vitamin D deficiency** or **phosphate deficiency**. Unlike rickets, osteomalacia does not affect the growth plates (as the bones have already matured), but it does result in the weakening of the **cortical bone** and **trabecular bone**.

Radiographic Features of Osteomalacia

1. **Generalized Osteopenia**:
   - There is **decreased bone density** or **osteopenia**, which is often visible on **X-ray** as a **generalized thinning** of the **cortex** of the bones.
   - The **trabecular bone** pattern becomes less distinct, especially in areas like the **pelvis**, **spine**, **femoral neck**, and **ribs**.

2. **Looser Zones (pseudofractures)**: **Looser zones** (also called **pseudofractures**) are characteristic radiographic findings. These are **bilateral, symmetric radiolucent lines** that appear perpendicular to the bone cortex, often seen in the **pelvis**, **proximal femur**, **scapula**, **ribs**, and **tibia**. These are stress fractures with a surrounding area of **unmineralized bone** and are a hallmark of osteomalacia.
3. **Widening of the metaphyses**: Similar to rickets, **widening of the metaphyses** can occur, but it is usually less pronounced because the bones have already finished growing.
4. **Bowing of Long Bones**: In **chronic osteomalacia**, there may be **bowing deformities** of weight-bearing bones, particularly the **femur** and **tibia**, due to the weakened bone structure.
5. **Fractures**: **Pathological fractures** are common in osteomalacia due to bone weakness. These fractures may occur with minimal trauma, and they often appear on radiographs as **incomplete fractures** or **microfractures**.
6. **Rugger-Jersey Spine**: In cases of **secondary hyperparathyroidism** (often due to **vitamin D deficiency**), a characteristic finding is **"rugger-jersey spine"**, where the **vertebral endplates** become **sclerotic**, giving the appearance of **striped patterns** (alternating dense and lucent bands) in the spine, resembling a rugby shirt.
7. **Frontal Bossing**: **Frontal bossing** (prominent forehead) may be seen in severe cases of osteomalacia due to the effect of **bone softening** on the skull.
8. **Pelvic and Pelvic Girdle Changes**: In some cases, the **pelvic bones** show **increased lucency** and deformity due to the softening of the bone.

7. Write a short note on: Rickets. [5] [DNB Dec 21, MD (WBUHS) 18]

Rickets is a childhood bone disorder caused by **defective mineralization** of the growing bone, leading to weakened bones, skeletal deformities, and impaired growth. The condition typically results from a deficiency in **vitamin D**, **calcium**, or **phosphate**, which are essential for proper bone mineralization. Inadequate levels of these nutrients cause the bone matrix to become soft, resulting in skeletal abnormalities.

Etiology of Rickets

The primary causes of rickets include:

1. **Vitamin D Deficiency**:
   - The most common cause of rickets worldwide, often due to **insufficient sunlight exposure** (especially in regions with limited sunlight), **dietary deficiencies**, or **malabsorption syndromes**.
   - **Vitamin D** is necessary for the absorption of **calcium** and **phosphate** in the gut.
2. **Calcium Deficiency**: Insufficient intake of **calcium** or impaired calcium metabolism can also lead to rickets. This can be secondary to **poor dietary intake** or **malabsorption** due to conditions like **celiac disease**.
3. **Phosphate Deficiency**: Rare, but can occur in conditions like **X-linked hypophosphatemia**, where there is **renal phosphate wasting** or genetic defects that reduce phosphate reabsorption.
4. **Renal Disorders**: Chronic kidney diseases can impair phosphate handling and **vitamin D activation**, leading to **secondary rickets**.
5. **Genetic Disorders**: In rare cases, **genetic mutations** affecting the **vitamin D receptor** or **enzymes** involved in **phosphate metabolism** can result in inherited forms of rickets (e.g., **hypophosphatemic rickets**).

Clinical Features of Rickets

- **Growth Retardation**: Children with rickets may show **delayed growth** and short stature.
- **Deformities**:
  - **Bowing of legs** (genu varum) is the most common skeletal deformity, particularly in **weight-bearing bones** like the **tibia** and **femur**.
  - **Knock-knees** (genu valgum) may develop as the disease progresses.
- **Frontal Bossing**: The forehead may become prominent due to **softening of the skull bones**.
- **Rachitic Rosary**: Enlargement of the **costochondral junctions** (where the ribs meet the cartilage) results in a beaded appearance along the **anterior chest wall**.

- **Pigeon Chest**: The breastbone (sternum) protrudes forward.
- **Widening of Wrist and Ankle Joints**: The **growth plates** in these areas may become widened and deformed.
- **Muscle Weakness**: Children with rickets may experience **muscle weakness**, difficulty walking, and **delayed motor milestones**.
- **Fractures**: The bones are fragile and prone to **stress fractures** due to softening.

Radiological Features of Rickets

- **Widened and Cupped Growth Plates**: The most characteristic radiological finding in rickets is the **widening** and **cupping** (concavity) of the **metaphyses** at the distal femur, proximal tibia, and radius.
- **Fraying of the Metaphysis**: The edges of the metaphyses appear irregular and frayed due to defective mineralization of the growing bone.
- **Rachitic Rosary**: Radiographs of the chest will show **enlargement** at the **costochondral junctions**.
- **Bowing Deformities**: **Genu varum** (bowing of the legs) or **genu valgum** (knock knees) are visible on **X-rays** of the lower limbs.
- **Widening of Wrist and Ankle Joints**: **Widened radiolucent zones** are visible at the wrist and ankle, where the cartilage growth plate is abnormally developed.
- **Fractures**: Pathological fractures, especially in weight-bearing bones, may be seen.

Diagnosis

- **Clinical Evaluation**: Diagnosis is based on clinical signs such as **skeletal deformities** (bow legs, frontal bossing, etc.), **growth delay**, and **muscle weakness**.
- **Laboratory Tests**:
  - **Serum calcium** and **phosphate** levels are often low.
  - **Alkaline phosphatase (ALP)** levels are elevated, reflecting increased bone turnover.
  - **Vitamin D levels**: Low levels of **25-hydroxyvitamin D** (the active form of vitamin D) confirm vitamin D deficiency.
  - **PTH levels**: Parathyroid hormone (PTH) levels may be elevated in secondary rickets due to low calcium levels.
- **X-rays**: The characteristic findings of **widened growth plates**, **cupping**, **fraying**, and **rachitic rosary** help confirm the diagnosis.

Treatment of Rickets

The treatment of rickets aims to correct the underlying deficiency or disorder and to promote normal bone growth and development:

1. **Vitamin D Supplementation**: The primary treatment for **vitamin D deficiency rickets**. This may be given orally in high doses or through **sunlight exposure**.
2. **Calcium and Phosphate Supplements**: These may be necessary, especially in cases of **hypocalcemia** or **phosphate deficiency**.
3. **Dietary Modifications**: Ensure an adequate intake of **vitamin D**, **calcium**, and **phosphate** through diet or supplements.

Management of Underlying Conditions: If rickets is secondary to another condition (such as **chronic kidney disease** or **genetic disorders**), specific treatment for that condition is essential.

8. Renal osteodystrophy—imaging findings. Approach to imaging in hyperparathyroidism. [10] [DNB June 21]

Renal osteodystrophy refers to a group of bone disorders associated with **chronic kidney disease (CKD)**, where abnormalities in **calcium**, **phosphate**, and **vitamin D** metabolism lead to disturbances in bone formation and mineralization. These disturbances may result in a range of skeletal changes, including **osteopenia**, **osteosclerosis**, and **bone deformities**. The underlying pathophysiology often involves **secondary hyperparathyroidism**, **mineralization defects**, and **impaired bone turnover**.

Osteitis Fibrosa Cystica (Secondary Hyperparathyroidism)

Osteitis fibrosa cystica is caused by **secondary hyperparathyroidism**, which is often due to impaired kidney function and **hyperphosphatemia**, leading to excessive **parathyroid hormone (PTH)** secretion. This results in increased bone resorption.

Radiographic Findings

- **Subperiosteal Resorption**:
  - This is the hallmark finding in osteitis fibrosa cystica. **Resorption of the cortical bone** at the **phalanx**, **radius**, **ulna**, and **proximal femur** may be seen.
  - **Subperiosteal resorption** is most evident in the **distal phalanges** of the fingers and toes.
- **Cystic Lesions**:
  - **Brown tumors**: These are **osteolytic lesions** that can be seen in the **bones** (particularly in the hands, ribs, and skull) due to excessive osteoclast activity.
  - These cyst-like areas often appear **radiolucent** on X-rays and are associated with **fibrous tissue**.
- **Hyperostosis and Sclerosis**:
  - In some cases, there may be **peripheral cortical sclerosis** in response to high PTH levels, leading to increased bone density.
  - **Rugger-jersey spine**: This is a characteristic finding where the **vertebral endplates** become **sclerotic** (dense) and **lucent** in the center, giving the spine a "striped" appearance.
- **Fractures**: Weakened bones are prone to **fractures**, which can be seen on X-ray, often with **bony deformities** in long bones and vertebrae.

Osteomalacia (Renal Rickets)

Osteomalacia in renal osteodystrophy is typically caused by **impaired vitamin D activation** (due to kidney dysfunction) and **phosphate deficiency**. This results in **impaired bone mineralization**, leading to soft bones.

Radiographic Findings

- **Widening of Growth Plates** (in children): If the patient is a child, **widened growth plates** with **cupping** and **fraying** of the metaphyses may be seen, similar to rickets.
- **Osteopenia**: There is often **generalized decreased bone density** on X-rays, which can make the bones appear **more lucent** than usual.
- **Looser Zones** (pseudofractures):
  - These are **radiolucent bands** that appear perpendicular to the bone cortex, often found in the **pelvis**, **proximal femur**, **scapula**, and **ribs**.
  - **Looser zones** represent incomplete fractures or stress fractures that occur due to weak, inadequately mineralized bone.
- **Fractures**: Due to the softening of bones, **stress fractures** or **pathological fractures** can occur. These are common in weight-bearing bones such as the **spine** and **long bones**.

Adynamic Bone Disease (Low Bone Turnover)

In **adynamic bone disease**, which is seen in some patients with **chronic kidney disease (CKD)**, there is **decreased osteoclastic activity** and **low bone turnover**. This condition often occurs when patients are treated with **high-dose calcium** or **calcimimetics** (which suppress PTH secretion).

Radiographic Findings

- **Normal or Mild Osteopenia**: The X-rays may show little change or mild **osteopenia** (loss of bone mineral density).
- **Absence of Significant Bone Resorption**: Unlike osteitis fibrosa cystica, there is no obvious **subperiosteal resorption** or **bone cysts**.
- **Fractures**: **Fractures** due to bone fragility are less common than in osteitis fibrosa cystica but may occur due to **low bone turnover**.

Mixed Renal Osteodystrophy

Mixed renal osteodystrophy occurs when a patient has features of both **osteitis fibrosa cystica** (secondary hyperparathyroidism) and **osteomalacia** (impaired mineralization), often as a result of chronic kidney disease progression. In this case, the radiographic findings may show a combination of bone resorption, sclerosis, and poor mineralization.

Radiographic Findings

- **Features of Osteitis Fibrosa**: Such as **subperiosteal resorption** and **brown tumors**.
- **Features of Osteomalacia**: Such as **Looser zones**, **widening of growth plates**, and **osteopenia**.

Other Radiographic Features in Renal Osteodystrophy

1. **Renal Osteosclerosis**:
   - In some cases, there may be increased **bone density** (osteosclerosis) due to **vascular calcifications** or **hyperphosphatemia**. This is more common in patients with **long-standing kidney disease**.
   - **X-rays** of the **skull** and **long bones** may show areas of increased bone density.
2. **Cystic Changes in the Skull**: In advanced cases, **cystic bone lesions** can be seen in the skull, particularly in the **calvarium**, which can be associated with **brown tumors** and **osteitis fibrosa cystica**.
3. **Soft Tissue Calcifications**: **Soft tissue calcifications** (such as in the **skin**, **blood vessels**, and **muscles**) may also be seen, typically related to **hyperphosphatemia** and **secondary hyperparathyroidism**. These calcifications can appear as **radiopaque** areas on X-ray or CT scans.

9. Discuss in brief, various types of hyperparathyroidism. Describe imaging features of various types of hyperparathyroidism. [5+5] [MD (WBUHS) 17, DNB June 20, DNB Dec 19]

Types of Hyperparathyroidism and Their Imaging Features

Hyperparathyroidism is a condition characterized by excessive secretion of **parathyroid hormone (PTH)** from the parathyroid glands, leading to disturbances in calcium and phosphate metabolism. There are three main types of hyperparathyroidism, each with distinct causes, clinical presentations, and imaging findings:

1. **Primary Hyperparathyroidism**
2. **Secondary Hyperparathyroidism**
3. **Tertiary Hyperparathyroidism**

Primary Hyperparathyroidism (PHPT)

Primary hyperparathyroidism occurs when there is an abnormality in the parathyroid glands themselves, leading to the overproduction of PTH. This is most often due to a **parathyroid adenoma**, but can also be caused by **hyperplasia** or rarely, **parathyroid carcinoma**.

Etiology:

- **Parathyroid adenoma** (most common cause)
- **Parathyroid hyperplasia**
- **Parathyroid carcinoma** (rare)

Pathophysiology: Excessive PTH increases calcium levels in the blood by promoting calcium release from bones, increasing renal calcium reabsorption, and enhancing intestinal calcium absorption. This results in **hypercalcemia** and **hypophosphatemia**.

Imaging Features:

1. **X-ray**:
   - **Osteitis fibrosa cystica** (OFC): This is a classic finding, especially in advanced cases, with **subperiosteal resorption** (most often at the distal phalanges, radial side of the hand) and **cystic lesions** in the bones (brown tumors).
   - **Osteopenia**: Generalized reduction in bone density.

- **Cystic lesions** (brown tumors): These are lytic areas seen in bones like the **hands**, **ribs**, **skull**, and **pelvis** due to excessive bone resorption from high PTH levels.

2. **Ultrasound**: **Parathyroid adenoma**: On neck ultrasound, a **well-defined hypoechoic mass** is typically seen, usually located **posterior to the thyroid gland**. The adenoma may have **vascularity** on Doppler imaging.
3. **Sestamibi Scan (Parathyroid Scintigraphy)**:
   - **99mTc-sestamibi** is the imaging modality of choice for localizing **parathyroid adenomas**.
   - The adenoma appears as a **hot spot** that is **hyperfunctional** (due to increased blood flow and PTH production), usually localized in the **lower neck** near the thyroid gland.
4. **CT/MRI**: In more complex cases or when the parathyroid adenoma is located ectopically (e.g., in the **mediastinum**), **CT** or **MRI** may help locate the abnormal parathyroid tissue. On CT, the adenoma may appear as a **soft tissue mass** that enhances after contrast injection.

Secondary Hyperparathyroidism

Secondary hyperparathyroidism is a compensatory response to chronic hypocalcemia, most often due to **chronic kidney disease (CKD)** or **vitamin D deficiency**. The parathyroid glands overproduce PTH in an attempt to normalize calcium levels, but the underlying cause (e.g., kidney failure or low vitamin D) prevents effective calcium regulation.

Etiology:

- **Chronic kidney disease (CKD)**: Leads to reduced phosphate excretion and impaired vitamin D activation, both of which cause hypocalcemia and stimulate PTH secretion.
- **Vitamin D deficiency**: Leads to decreased calcium absorption, which stimulates PTH release.
- **Malabsorption syndromes** or **chronic liver disease** can also result in secondary hyperparathyroidism.

Pathophysiology: Secondary hyperparathyroidism is marked by **elevated PTH** levels in response to **low calcium** or **phosphate imbalance**, resulting in the **hypertrophy** or **hyperplasia** of parathyroid glands.

Imaging Features:

1. **X-ray**:
   - **Osteomalacia**: The bones may appear soft and poorly mineralized. **Looser zones** (pseudofractures) may be seen as radiolucent bands at sites of stress, particularly in the **pelvis**, **femoral neck**, and **scapula**.
   - **Osteopenia**: Decreased bone density, particularly in the **cortical bone** (e.g., **ribs**, **vertebrae**, **proximal femur**).
   - **Rugger-Jersey Spine**: A characteristic finding where the **vertebral endplates** show **sclerosis**, leading to a striped appearance (dense bands at the top and bottom of vertebrae, with lucent areas in the middle).
2. **Ultrasound**: Parathyroid glands may be **enlarged** due to **hyperplasia** in secondary hyperparathyroidism, which is visible on neck ultrasound. However, **specific localization** of abnormal parathyroid tissue may be less distinct compared to primary hyperparathyroidism.
3. **Sestamibi Scan**:
   - **Sestamibi scans** can show **bilateral parathyroid hyperplasia** but may be less specific than in primary hyperparathyroidism, where a single adenoma is usually the cause.
   - In **tertiary hyperparathyroidism** (a sequel of secondary hyperparathyroidism), **multiple parathyroid glands** may show increased uptake due to hyperplasia.
4. **Bone Scintigraphy**: Increased bone turnover may be detected, with **increased uptake** in areas of bone resorption.

Tertiary Hyperparathyroidism

Tertiary hyperparathyroidism occurs when **secondary hyperparathyroidism** (usually due to CKD) becomes **autonomous**, meaning the parathyroid glands continue to overproduce PTH despite correction of the original calcium imbalance (e.g., after kidney transplant or treatment of vitamin D deficiency). This condition results in **parathyroid hyperplasia** and hypercalcemia.

Etiology:

- **Chronic kidney disease**: Prolonged secondary hyperparathyroidism that leads to irreversible **parathyroid hyperplasia**.

- **Kidney transplant**: After kidney transplantation, the parathyroid glands may become unresponsive to the normalization of calcium and phosphate levels.

Pathophysiology: The parathyroid glands become **hyperplastic** due to long-term overstimulation by elevated PTH levels, and they continue to secrete excessive PTH even when the calcium and phosphate levels normalize. This results in **hypercalcemia** and increased bone resorption.

Imaging Features:

1. **X-ray**:
   - **Osteitis fibrosa cystica** (similar to primary hyperparathyroidism) can be seen with **subperiosteal resorption**, especially in the distal phalanges, and **brown tumors**.
   - **Osteopenia** and **generalized bone loss** may also be observed due to prolonged high PTH levels.
2. **Ultrasound**: Ultrasound may show **bilateral parathyroid hyperplasia**. In some cases, **multiple enlarged parathyroid glands** can be identified.
3. **Sestamibi scan**: A **sestamibi scan** may show **multiple areas of increased uptake** due to **bilateral parathyroid hyperplasia**. This is different from primary hyperparathyroidism, where a single adenoma is usually seen.
4. **CT/MRI**: In advanced tertiary hyperparathyroidism, **parathyroid adenomas** or **hyperplasia** may become large enough to be visualized on **CT** or **MRI**. The imaging may also show **calcifications** in the **parathyroid glands** due to prolonged disease.

Bone Tumors

1. Enumerate the bone-forming tumors. Discuss the imaging features of osteosarcoma. [2+8] [AIIMS Dec 23]

Bone Forming Tumors

- **Benign**:
  - Osteoid Osteoma
  - Osteoblastoma
  - Ossifying Fibroma
- **Intermediate (Locally Aggressive or Rarely Metastatic)**:
  - Osteofibrous dysplasia
  - Fibrous Dysplasia (may exhibit bone formation, though not a true neoplasm)
- **Malignant**: Osteosarcoma—
  - Conventional (osteoblastic, chondroblastic, and fibroblastic)
  - Telangiectatic
  - Parosteal
  - Periosteal
  - High-grade surface
  - Small-ccll ostcosarcoma
  - Secondary osteosarcoma (e.g., post-Paget's disease, post-radiation)

Imaging Features of Osteosarcoma

Osteosarcoma is the most common primary malignant bone tumor of adolescence, characterized by the production of osteoid matrix by malignant cells. The imaging features depend on the subtype of osteosarcoma and vary between conventional and rare variants.

Below is a detailed discussion:

- **General Imaging Features (Common to Most Types)**: **Plain Radiograph**:
- **Location**: Typically involves the metaphysis of long bones (distal femur, proximal tibia, proximal humerus).

- **Appearance**:
  - Mixed lytic and sclerotic lesions (classic presentation).
  - Wide zone of transition with poorly defined margins.
- **Periosteal reactions**:
  - Codman triangle (periosteal elevation).
  - Sunburst or spiculated pattern (radiating bone spicules).
  - Cortical destruction and extension into soft tissues.
- **CT**:
  - **Superior for detecting**:
    - Mineralized osteoid matrix within the lesion.
    - Cortical destruction.
    - Intramedullary and soft tissue extension.
    - Often used for surgical planning and evaluation of chest metastases.
- **MRI**:
  - **Modality of choice for local staging and determining tumor extent**:
  - **T1**: Hypointense to isointense signal relative to muscle.
  - **T2**: Hyperintense signal with areas of heterogeneous signal due to necrosis, hemorrhage, and mineralization.
  - **T1 C+ (Gd)**: Marked heterogeneous enhancement.
  - **Soft tissue extension**: Seen as lobulated soft tissue with low signal striations (representing mineralized osteoid).
  - **Skip lesions**: Can be visualized as distant tumor foci within the same bone or across a joint.
- **Nuclear Medicine**:
  - Technetium-99m Bone Scan: Increased uptake in the primary lesion and potential skip metastases.
  - **FDG-PET/CT**: High sensitivity for metastasis, skip lesions, and treatment response evaluation.

Subtypes of Osteosarcoma

1. **Conventional Osteosarcoma**:
   - Most common subtype (80–90%).
   - **Radiographic features as described above**: Mixed lytic-sclerotic pattern, aggressive periosteal reaction, and soft tissue mass.
   - Often presents with a large destructive lesion with prominent osteoid matrix.
2. **Telangiectatic Osteosarcoma**:
   - Rare (4% of cases).
   - **Radiograph/CT**:
     - Purely lytic lesion resembling an aneurysmal bone cyst (ABC).
     - Minimal or no periosteal reaction.
   - **MRI**:
     - Multiloculated cystic appearance with fluid-fluid levels.
     - Enhancing nodular components representing viable tumor cells.
3. **Parosteal Osteosarcoma**:
   - Low-grade surface osteosarcoma.
   - **Radiograph/CT**:
     - Dense, heavily ossified mass arising from the cortical surface, typically posterior distal femur.
     - Broad base with minimal soft tissue involvement.
   - **MRI**: Shows marrow invasion in advanced cases.

4. **Periosteal Osteosarcoma**:
   - Intermediate-grade surface osteosarcoma.
   - **Radiograph/CT**:
     - Lobulated mass arising from the cortical surface, usually along the diaphysis.
     - Sunburst-type periosteal reaction.
   - **MRI**: Confirms periosteal origin and shows soft tissue involvement.
5. **High-grade Surface Osteosarcoma**:
   - Rare, highly aggressive surface variant.
   - **Radiograph/CT**:
     - Osteolytic lesion with minimal ossification.
     - Extensive soft tissue component.
6. **Small-cell Osteosarcoma**:
   - Resembles Ewing sarcoma histologically.
   - **Radiograph**: Moth-eaten, permeative lesion without prominent osteoid formation.
   - **MRI**: Similar to Ewing sarcoma but with intratumoral matrix mineralization.
7. **Secondary Osteosarcoma**:
   - Occurs in pre-existing bone conditions (e.g., Paget's disease, chronic osteomyelitis, prior radiation).
   - **Radiograph/CT**: Mineralized osteoid within areas of previously abnormal bone.

2. Write a short note on: Ewing sarcoma. [5] [DNB Dec 21]

Epidemiology

- **Age**: Children and adolescents (10–20 years; 95% between 4–25 years).
- **Sex**: Male predominance (M:F = 1.5:1).
- **Ethnicity**: Primarily in White patients; lower incidence in Black and Asian/Pacific Islander populations.

Clinical Presentation

- Localized pain (most common symptom).
- Soft tissue mass (occasionally palpable).
- Systemic symptoms: Fever, elevated ESR, and serum LDH.
- Pathological fractures may occur.

Pathology

- **Histology**: Small round blue cell tumor.
- **Genetics**: t(11;22)(q24;q12) chromosome rearrangement.
- **Related Tumors**: pPNET, Askin tumor, neuroepithelioma (collectively ESFT).

Common Locations

- **Lower Limb**: 45% (femur most common).
- **Pelvis**: 20%.
- **Upper Limb**: 13%.
- **Spine and Ribs**: 13% (thoracic).
- **Skull/Face**: 2%.
- **Long Bones**: 50–60% (metadiaphysis or diaphysis most common).

Radiographic Features

- **Plain Radiograph/CT**:
  - Permeative lesion (76%).
  - Lamellated (onion skin) periosteal reaction (57%).

  - Sclerosis (40%).
  - May show Codman triangles, spiculated (sunburst) reaction, bone expansion, or cystic components.
  - Rare soft tissue calcification (<10%).
- **MRI**:
  - **T1**: Low to intermediate signal.
  - **T1 C+ (Gd)**: Heterogeneous but prominent enhancement.
  - **T2**: High signal with possible hair-on-end striations.
- **Nuclear Medicine**: Increased uptake on Gallium-67 and Technetium-99m bone scans.

Treatment and Prognosis

- **Primary Treatment**: Systemic chemotherapy.
- **Adjuvant Options**: Surgery and/or radiotherapy based on size and location.

Musculoskeletal MRI

1. Describe the radiographic and MRI findings in avascular necrosis of the hip. [4+6] [MD (WBUHS) 23, MD (WBUHS) 20, RG 18]

Avascular necrosis (AVN) of the hip is the most common site for osteonecrosis, presumably due to a combination of precarious blood supply and high loading when standing.[12]

Epidemiology

Usually affects adults below 50 years of age.

Clinical Presentation

The commonest presenting feature is pain in the region of the affected hip, groin, thigh, and buttock.

Pathology

Classically, it affects the superior articular surface (between 10 and 2 o'clock) and begins in the most anterior part of the hip.

Etiology

It can be traumatic (secondary to neck of femur fractures) or nontraumatic. Traumatic osteonecrosis is mostly unilateral. In nontraumatic cases, it is usually bilateral in 70–80%.

- Traumatic
- Alcoholism
- Chronic corticosteroid therapy
- Sickle cell disease
- Systemic lupus erythematosus (SLE)
- Smoking
- Hyperlipidemias
- Gaucher disease
- HIV
- Chronic renal failure
- Pregnancy-related
- Diabetes mellitus
- Pancreatitis

Radiographic Features

Following are necessary details to be included in the report as they affect the treatment and prognosis:

- Position
- Coexisting osteoarthritis

- Estimating percentage volume of the head involved (axial) and percentage weight-bearing surface involved (coronal)
- Joint effusion
- Subchondral fractures
- Presence of a potentially unstable osteochondral fragment: Rim sign

CT

CT is more sensitive in depicting subchondral fractures than plain film.

MRI

MRI is the most sensitive imaging modality for avascular necrosis.

- **T1**: Usually the initial specific findings are areas of low signal intensity representing edema, which can be bordered by a hyperintense line that represents blood products.
- **T2**: May show a second hyperintense inner line between normal marrow and ischemic marrow; this appearance is highly specific for osteonecrosis of the hip and is known as the "double-line sign".

Staging

The Association Research Circulation Osseous classification (ARCO classification) is one of the staging systems used to assess **femoral head osteonecrosis** and includes radiographic and MRI findings.[13]

Classification

- **Stage 0**:
  - Clinically: No symptoms
  - Plain radiograph: Normal
  - MRI: Normal
- **Stage I**:
  - Clinically: No symptoms or presence symptoms
  - Plain radiograph: Normal
  - MRI or bone scan: Abnormal
- **Stage II**:
  - Clinically: Symptoms present
  - Plain radiograph: Trabecular bone changes without changes in subchondral bone; preserved joint space
  - MRI: Abnormal, diagnostic appearance
- **Stage III**:
  - Clinically: Symptoms present
  - Presence of trabecular bone changes and subchondral fracture (crescent sign or subchondral bone collapse); preserved joint space
  - Further subdivided with regard to the depth of femoral head depression: IIIA—depression ≤2 mm, IIIB—depression >2 mm
- **Stage IV**:
  - Clinically: Symptoms present
  - Features of osteoarthritis, with distorted femoral head shape, acetabular changes and narrowed joint space

Differential Diagnosis

- Idiopathic transient osteoporosis of the hip (ITOH): Hyperemia with diffuse increased uptake of radiotracer by the femoral head, neck, and intertrochanteric region
- Infection:
  - Pain and fever
  - Usually involves both sides of the joint
- Fracture

- Chondroblastoma
- Metastases

2. Write a short note on MRI features of anterior cruciate ligament injury of knee. [5] [MD (WBUHS) 23]

The MRI findings for Anterior Cruciate Ligament (ACL) tear are as follows:

ACL Tear MRI Findings

1. **Primary Signs**:
   - Absence or disruption of the ACL fibers: The ACL appears torn, frayed, or absent.
   - ACL fiber discontinuity: The ACL fibers are disrupted, and the ligament is no longer intact.
   - Increased signal on T2 or fat-saturated PD
   - ACL angle [angle between the intercondylar line (Blumensaat line) and ACL] >15° with the apex of the angle located anteriorly, indicating a less steep ACL line—this indicates a ruptured and collapsed ligament
   - Empty notch sign: A fluid signal at the site of femoral attachment at the intercondylar notch, denotes avulsion at the femoral attachment
2. **Secondary Signs**:
   - Anterior tibial translation: The tibia is displaced anteriorly relative to the femur by >7 mm.
   - Kissing contusion: Bone bruises on the lateral femoral condyle and the posterior tibial plateau.
   - Meniscal injuries: Tears or displacement of the menisci, particularly the lateral meniscus. Uncovered posterior horn of the lateral meniscus: Posterior displacement >3.5 mm
   - Bony avulsion: A fragment of bone is avulsed from the tibial spine or the femoral condyle.
   - Bowing of PCL: Reduced PCL angle <107° or bowing ratio >0.39
   - Lateral femoral sulcus deeper than 1.5 mm

It is essential to note that MRI findings should be correlated with clinical examination and other diagnostic tests to confirm the diagnosis of ACL tear.

3. CT and MRI finding of recurrent dislocation of shoulder joint. [10] [MD (WBUHS) 19]

Imaging Features of Recurrent Shoulder Dislocation

Recurrent shoulder dislocation, commonly due to anterior instability, often results from underlying structural abnormalities. Imaging plays a critical role in identifying the features contributing to instability and planning appropriate management. Key imaging findings include:

1. **Bone Lesions**:
   - Hill-Sachs lesion: A compression fracture of the posterolateral humeral head caused by impaction against the glenoid during dislocation. Best visualized on axial MRI or MR arthrography.
   - Bony Bankart lesion: Fracture or erosion of the anteroinferior glenoid rim. CT is particularly sensitive for detecting bony defects, but MRI can also demonstrate associated soft tissue injuries.
2. **Soft Tissue Lesions**:
   - Bankart lesion: Detachment of the anteroinferior glenoid labrum with possible capsulolabral avulsion. Visualized on MR arthrography, especially in the abduction and external rotation (ABER) position.
   - Anterior labroligamentous periosteal sleeve avulsion (ALPSA) lesion: Labrum displacement medially along the glenoid rim while remaining attached to the periosteum.
   - Humeral avulsion of the glenohumeral ligament (HAGL) lesion: Disruption of the anterior band of the inferior glenohumeral ligament from the humeral attachment. Best seen on MR arthrography.
   - Capsular Laxity: Stretching or thinning of the joint capsule, often due to repetitive trauma or hypermobility.
3. **Associated Findings**:
   - Rotator Cuff Tears: May occur in older patients or after significant trauma.

- Glenoid Bone Loss: Chronic instability can lead to significant anterior glenoid bone loss, which predisposes to further dislocations.

Role of MR Arthrography in Shoulder Dislocation

MR arthrography (MRA) is the gold standard imaging modality for assessing recurrent shoulder dislocations. Its advantages include superior visualization of soft tissue injuries and dynamic evaluation of joint stability.

Key roles of MR arthrography include:

1. **Evaluation of Labral Pathology**:
   - Provides detailed visualization of labral tears (e.g., Bankart, ALPSA) and their extent.
   - Identifies subtle labral detachment or degenerative changes.
2. **Assessment of Ligamentous and Capsular Integrity**:
   - Identifies capsular tears, laxity, or thinning.
   - Detects HAGL lesions and abnormalities in the glenohumeral ligament complex.
3. **Dynamic Imaging**: The ABER position improves visualization of anterior labral and ligamentous injuries.
4. **Differentiating Chronic from Acute Changes**: Distinguishes acute labral or ligament tears from chronic scarring or degenerative changes.
5. **Quantification of Glenoid Bone Loss**: While CT is better for detailed bony analysis, MRA can provide estimates of bone loss and its effect on stability.

In conclusion, MR arthrography is invaluable in evaluating recurrent shoulder dislocation, especially for soft tissue injuries and capsulolabral pathology. Combining MRA with CT for complex cases (e.g., significant bone loss) allows comprehensive preoperative assessment and improved surgical planning.

4. MRI findings of anterior and posterior cruciate ligament tear. [10] [MD (WBUHS) 19]

The MRI findings for Anterior Cruciate Ligament (ACL) and Posterior Cruciate Ligament (PCL) tears are as follows:

ACL Tear MRI Findings

1. **Primary Signs**:
   - Absence or disruption of the ACL fibers: The ACL appears torn, frayed, or absent.
   - ACL fiber discontinuity: The ACL fibers are disrupted, and the ligament is no longer intact.
   - Increased signal on T2 or fat-saturated PD
   - ACL angle [angle between the intercondylar line (Blumensaat line) and ACL] >15° with the apex of the angle located anteriorly, indicating a less steep ACL line—this indicates a ruptured and collapsed ligament
   - Empty notch sign: A fluid signal at the site of femoral attachment at the intercondylar notch, denotes avulsion at the femoral attachment
2. **Secondary Signs**:
   - Anterior tibial translation: The tibia is displaced anteriorly relative to the femur by >7 mm.
   - Kissing contusion: Bone bruises on the lateral femoral condyle and the posterior tibial plateau.
   - Meniscal injuries: Tears or displacement of the menisci, particularly the lateral meniscus. Uncovered posterior horn of the lateral meniscus: Posterior displacement >3.5 mm
   - Bony avulsion: A fragment of bone is avulsed from the tibial spine or the femoral condyle.
   - Bowing of PCL: Reduced PCL angle <107° or bowing ratio >0.39
   - Lateral femoral sulcus deeper than 1.5 mm

PCL Tear MRI Findings

1. **Primary Signs**:
   - Absence or disruption of the PCL fibers: The PCL appears torn, frayed, or absent.
   - PCL fiber discontinuity: The PCL fibers are disrupted, and the ligament is no longer intact.

- Enlarged and swollen PCL: >7 mm AP diameter of the vertical portion on sagittal imaging is indicative of a tear

2. **Secondary Signs**:
   - Posterior tibial translation: The tibia is displaced posteriorly relative to the femur by >2-3 mm.
   - Kissing contusion: Bone bruises on the medial femoral condyle and the anterior tibial plateau.
   - Meniscal injuries: Tears or displacement of the menisci, particularly the medial meniscus.
   - Bony avulsion: A fragment of bone is avulsed from the tibial spine or the femoral condyle.

It is essential to note that MRI findings should be correlated with clinical examination and other diagnostic tests to confirm the diagnosis of ACL or PCL tears.

5. Write a short note on: SLAP. [5] [MD (WBUHS) 22]

Superior labral anterior posterior (SLAP) tears are injuries of the glenoid labrum, and can often be confused with a sublabral sulcus on MRI.

Pathology

SLAP tears involve the superior glenoid labrum, where the long head of biceps tendon inserts. They can extend into the tendon, involve the glenohumeral ligaments or extend into other quadrants of the labrum. Unlike Bankart lesions and ALPSA lesions, they are uncommonly (20%) associated with shoulder instability.

Classification

The most widely used system for classifying SLAP tears was initially described by Snyder, who on the basis of arthroscopic findings, described four patterns of labral injury:

- **Type I**: Fraying of the superior labrum free margin
  - Commonly asymptomatic
  - Often due to degeneration
- **Type II**: Detachment of the superior labrum and biceps anchor from the underlying superior glenoid at the chondrolabral junction (undercuts the anchor)
  - In younger patients (<40 years of age) these are associated with Bankart lesions
  - In older patients (>40 years of age) they are associated with rotator cuff tears
  - Seen in overhead athletes
- **Type III**: Bucket handle tear of the superior labrum without extension into the long head of biceps tendon
- **Type IV**: Bucket handle tear of the superior labrum with extension into the long head of biceps tendon

Beyond these four original types, multiple additional types have been described, although their clinical relevance is controversial.

MRI

The investigation of choice is an MR arthrogram, which is variably reported as having accuracies of 75–90%, although distinguishing between subtypes can be difficult.

High signal (fluid on T2WI or arthrographic contrast on T1WI) is seen extending into the superior labrum, and tracking into the labrum, and sometimes into the biceps tendon is the characteristic finding.

Treatment and Prognosis

- **Type I**: Usually asymptomatic and do not require treatment
- **Type II**: Require surgical reattachment
- **Type III**: Usually require resection of the bucket handle tear

6. Meniscal tear MRI and MR arthrogram role. [5] [DNB June 22]

MRI is the modality of choice when a meniscal tear is suspected, with sagittal images being the most sensitive.

There are three basic MRI characteristics/criteria of meniscal tears:
- High intrameniscal signal extending to at least one articular surface, which should be seen in at least two slices: Two-slice touch rule (do not have to be contiguous, e.g., sagittal and coronal slices)
- Distortion of the normal meniscal morphology if no prior surgery

Each type of meniscal tear has its own characteristics on MRI, but in most cases, the following can be seen:
- **T1**: A hyperintense line in the meniscus can be seen, but it is difficult to differentiate between degeneration and meniscal tear on this sequence; in the case of a bucket-handle tear an empty groove can sometimes be seen
- **T2**: A hyperintense line in the meniscus, which indicates synovial fluid in the meniscus
  - The high T2 signal in mid-substance of the meniscus without extension to the surface is not necessarily a tear and can be:
    - In adults: Secondary to degeneration
    - In children: High vascularity of meniscus

MR Arthrogram Findings for Meniscal Tears

1. **Contrast extravasation**: Contrast material can leak into the tear, confirming the diagnosis.
2. **Meniscal surface irregularity**: The contrast material can outline the irregular meniscal surface, indicating a tear.
3. **Meniscosynovial communication**: Contrast material can flow between the meniscus and synovium, indicating a tear.

Associated features that are suggestive of a meniscal tear include:
- Tibial subchondral bone edema
- Parameniscal cyst
- Meniscal extrusion

There are several signs associated with meniscal tears:
- Absent bow tie sign
- Truncated triangle sign
- Double posterior cruciate ligament sign
- Double anterior cruciate ligament sign
- Marching cleft sign
- Fragment-in-notch sign
- Flipped meniscus sign
- Ghost meniscus sign
- Jack and Jill lesion
- Quadruple sign

7. Latest nomenclature of disc herniation. Osteoporotic vertebral collapse vs. metastatic vertebral collapse. [10] [DNB June 21, MD (WBUHS) 18]

Latest Nomenclature for Disc Herniation

Disc herniation refers to the displacement of intervertebral disc material beyond the normal confines of the disc but involving less than 25% of the circumference (to distinguish it from a disc bulge). A herniation may contain nucleus pulposus, vertebral endplate cartilage, apophyseal bone/osteophyte and annulus fibrosus.

The combined task forces of the North American Spine Society (NASS), the American Society of Spine Radiology (ASSR), and the American Society of Neuroradiology (ASNR) have proposed a new nomenclature for disc herniation:

1. **Disc Protrusion**:
   - A disc herniation where the greatest dimension of the herniated material is less than the diameter of the disc space.
   - Base wider than herniation
   - Confined to disc level
   - Outer annular fibers intact

2. **Disc Extrusion**:
   - A disc herniation where the greatest dimension of the herniated material is greater than the diameter of the disc space.
   - Base narrower than herniation 'dome'
   - May extend above or below endplates or adjacent vertebrae
   - Complete annular tear with passage of nuclear material beyond disc annulus
3. **Disc Sequestration**: A type of disc extrusion where the herniated material has separated from the parent disc.
4. **Disc Migration**: A type of disc extrusion where the herniated material has moved away from the parent disc.

Herniations can further be classified as:
- **Contained**:
  - With intact outer fibers of annulus fibrosus and posterior longitudinal ligament, or
  - With intact posterior longitudinal ligament alone
- **Not contained**: Tear of outer fibers of annulus fibrosus and posterior longitudinal ligament.

Osteoporotic Vertebral Collapse vs. Metastatic Vertebral Collapse

Osteoporotic collapse is common in the elderly and in postmenopausal women. In the acute setting it may be difficult to distinguish it from malignant collapse, as the presence of edema gives rise to hypointense signal on T1W images and hyperintense signal on T2W and STIR sequences.

However, the following points may help us significantly in differentiating between these 2 conditions **(Table 3)**.

Accurate diagnosis and differentiation between these two conditions are crucial for guiding treatment and management decisions.

TABLE 3: Main differences between osteoporotic and metastatic vertebral collapse.

Osteoporotic collapse	*Metastatic collapse*
Anterior wedging, height relatively maintained posteriorly	Uniform collapse
Posterior margin flat	Posterior margin convex
Patchy abnormal signal, some fatty marrow present	Uniform replacement of fatty marrow by tumor giving uniform abnormal signal
Fracture line present	Fracture line absent
Absence of extraosseous soft tissue	Presence of extraosseous soft tissue

8. Imaging features of recurrent shoulder dislocation. Role MR arthrography in shoulder displacement. [10] [DNB June 21]

Imaging Features of Recurrent Shoulder Dislocation

Recurrent shoulder dislocation, commonly due to anterior instability, often results from underlying structural abnormalities. Imaging plays a critical role in identifying the features contributing to instability and planning appropriate management. Key imaging findings include:

1. **Bone Lesions**:
   - Hill-Sachs Lesion: A compression fracture of the posterolateral humeral head caused by impaction against the glenoid during dislocation. Best visualized on axial MRI or MR arthrography.
   - Bony Bankart Lesion: Fracture or erosion of the anteroinferior glenoid rim. CT is particularly sensitive for detecting bony defects, but MRI can also demonstrate associated soft tissue injuries.
2. **Soft Tissue Lesions**:
   - Bankart Lesion: Detachment of the anteroinferior glenoid labrum with possible capsulolabral avulsion. Visualized on MR arthrography, especially in the abduction and external rotation (ABER) position.
   - Anterior labroligamentous periosteal sleeve avulsion (ALPSA) lesion: Labrum displacement medially along the glenoid rim while remaining attached to the periosteum.

- Humeral avulsion of the glenohumeral ligament (HAGL) lesion: Disruption of the anterior band of the inferior glenohumeral ligament from the humeral attachment. Best seen on MR arthrography.
- Capsular Laxity: Stretching or thinning of the joint capsule, often due to repetitive trauma or hypermobility.

3. **Associated Findings**:
   - Rotator Cuff Tears: May occur in older patients or after significant trauma.
   - Glenoid Bone Loss: Chronic instability can lead to significant anterior glenoid bone loss, which predisposes to further dislocations.

Role of MR Arthrography in Shoulder Dislocation

MR arthrography (MRA) is the gold standard imaging modality for assessing recurrent shoulder dislocations. Its advantages include superior visualization of soft tissue injuries and dynamic evaluation of joint stability.

Key roles of MR arthrography include:

1. **Evaluation of Labral Pathology**:
   - Provides detailed visualization of labral tears (e.g., Bankart and ALPSA) and their extent.
   - Identifies subtle labral detachment or degenerative changes.
2. **Assessment of Ligamentous and Capsular Integrity**:
   - Identifies capsular tears, laxity, or thinning.
   - Detects HAGL lesions and abnormalities in the glenohumeral ligament complex.
3. **Dynamic Imaging**: The ABER position improves visualization of anterior labral and ligamentous injuries.
4. **Differentiating Chronic from Acute Changes**: Distinguishes acute labral or ligament tears from chronic scarring or degenerative changes.
5. **Quantification of Glenoid Bone Loss**: While CT is better for detailed bony analysis, MRA can provide estimates of bone loss and its effect on stability.

In conclusion, MR arthrography is invaluable in evaluating recurrent shoulder dislocation, especially for soft tissue injuries and capsulolabral pathology. Combining MRA with CT for complex cases (e.g., significant bone loss) allows comprehensive preoperative assessment and improved surgical planning.

9. Radiological anatomy of ligaments of the knee joint. MR evaluation of cartilages of the knee joint. [10] [DNB June 21]

Radiological Anatomy of Knee Ligaments

The knee joint has multiple ligaments that provide stability, which can be divided into intra-articular and extra-articular groups. Their detailed imaging evaluation, particularly on MRI, is essential for diagnosing ligamentous injuries.

Intra-articular Ligaments

- **Anterior Cruciate Ligament (ACL)**:
  - Originates from the anterior intercondylar area of the tibia and attaches to the lateral femoral condyle.
  - Best evaluated on sagittal T2-weighted or proton density (PD) fat-saturated MRI sequences.
  - Normal ACL appears as a hypointense band; disruptions indicate tears.
- **Posterior Cruciate Ligament (PCL)**:
  - Originates from the posterior intercondylar area of the tibia and attaches to the medial femoral condyle.
  - Thicker and stronger than the ACL; also seen as hypointense on MRI.
  - Partial or complete tears may present with abnormal thickening or discontinuity.

Extra-articular Ligaments

- **Medial Collateral Ligament (MCL)**:
  - Superficial and deep layers run along the medial aspect of the knee.
  - Seen as a hypointense band on coronal MRI sequences.
  - Injuries are graded (I to III) based on thickening, disruption, and fiber alignment.

- **Lateral Collateral Ligament (LCL)**:
  - Extends from the lateral femoral condyle to the fibular head.
  - Best evaluated on coronal and axial MRI, appearing as a thin hypointense band.
- **Patellar Ligament (Tendon)**: Connects the patella to the tibial tuberosity; appears hypointense on sagittal MRI.
- **Posterolateral Corner (PLC)**:
  - Includes the arcuate ligament, popliteus tendon, and lateral capsule.
  - Injuries to this region are challenging but well-visualized on MRI.

MRI Evaluation of Knee Cartilages

MRI is the most sensitive modality for evaluating knee cartilage, particularly for detecting early degenerative changes and focal defects. Cartilage is best visualized on sequences that highlight the joint spaces.

Normal Cartilage Anatomy

- The knee joint cartilage covers the femoral condyles, tibial plateaus, and patellar surfaces.
- Appears as a smooth, homogenous, intermediate-to-low signal layer on T1-weighted images and a hyperintense layer on T2 or PD-weighted sequences.

Sequences for Cartilage Evaluation

- **Proton Density (PD) Fat-Suppressed Imaging**: Commonly used for assessing cartilage thickness and defects.
- **T2-Weighted Imaging**: Evaluates cartilage hydration and matrix integrity. Fissures or edema appear as signal changes.
- **3D Gradient Echo (GRE) or SPGR Sequences**: High-resolution sequences for quantitative cartilage evaluation and detecting subtle defects.
- **T2 Mapping and dGEMRIC**: Quantitative techniques to assess cartilage composition and glycosaminoglycan content.

Common Pathologies

- **Chondral Defects**: Focal defects appear as thinning, irregularity, or signal changes in cartilage layers.
- **Osteochondritis Dissecans**: Associated with subchondral bone abnormalities, with overlying cartilage disruption.
- **Osteoarthritis**: Features include cartilage thinning, delamination, and bone marrow edema.
- **Patellar Chondromalacia**: Softening or degeneration of patellar cartilage, often graded on MRI (Grades I-IV).

MRI allows for the noninvasive assessment of cartilage quality, early detection of degenerative changes, and precise localization of injuries, which is crucial for treatment planning.

10. What is lipoma arborescens? Enumerate imaging findings on US and MRI. Discuss any two differential diagnosis. [2+4+4] [DNB Dec 20]

Lipoma arborescens (LA) is a rare, benign intra-articular condition characterized by diffuse villous proliferation of synovium, which is replaced by mature adipose tissue. It typically affects large joints like the knee, although other joints can be involved.

Etiology: Often associated with chronic joint inflammation, trauma, or degenerative joint disease, though idiopathic cases also occur.

Clinical Presentation:

- Chronic, painless joint swelling.
- Reduced range of motion.
- Symptoms of joint effusion or mechanical obstruction.

Imaging Findings in Lipoma Arborescens

1. **Ultrasound (US)**:
   - Appearance:
     - Hyperechoic frond-like structures within the joint, corresponding to fat.

 - Moves freely with joint motion.
 - Associated joint effusion or synovial thickening.
- Doppler Imaging: Usually shows no vascularity, helping differentiate it from synovial proliferative disorders (e.g., rheumatoid synovitis).

2. **Magnetic Resonance Imaging (MRI)**:
   - MRI is the modality of choice for diagnosing lipoma arborescens.
   - T1-Weighted Images:
     - Fat signal intensity (hyperintense), similar to subcutaneous fat.
     - Frond-like or villous synovial proliferation.
   - T2-Weighted and PD Fat-Saturated Images:
     - Fat suppression reveals hypointense villous structures.
     - Joint effusion appears hyperintense on T2.
   - Postcontrast T1 with Gadolinium:
     - Minimal or no enhancement of the lipomatous tissue.
     - Synovial enhancement if associated with inflammation.
   - Associated Findings:
     - Joint effusion.
     - Degenerative changes, including osteophytes and cartilage thinning.

Differential Diagnosis

1. **Synovial Chondromatosis**
   - **Pathophysiology**: Benign proliferation of synovium with metaplastic formation of cartilaginous nodules, which may calcify.
   - **Imaging Features**:
     - MRI: Multiple intra-articular loose bodies with variable signal intensity (low signal on T1 and T2 if calcified).
     - May show synovial thickening and joint effusion.
     - Calcified nodules are hypointense on all MRI sequences.
     - Radiographs often show visible calcifications.
     - Key Differentiator: Presence of calcified or ossified loose bodies, absent in lipoma arborescens.
2. **Pigmented Villonodular Synovitis (PVNS)**
   - **Pathophysiology**: Synovial proliferation with hemosiderin deposition due to recurrent hemorrhage.
   - **Imaging Features**:
     - MRI: Low signal intensity on both T1 and T2 sequences due to hemosiderin.
     - Postcontrast: Significant synovial enhancement.
     - May demonstrate erosions of adjacent bone.
     - Key Differentiator: Hemosiderin deposition causing low signal on all MRI sequences and erosive bone changes, absent in lipoma arborescens.

Conclusion: Lipoma arborescens has characteristic imaging findings, particularly on MRI, that differentiate it from other intra-articular disorders. Recognizing its features is crucial for diagnosis and guiding appropriate treatment.

11. Discuss the etiology of femoroacetabular impingement and imaging findings on plain radiographs and MRI. [10] [DNB Dec 20]

Etiology of Femoroacetabular Impingement (FAI)

Femoroacetabular impingement (FAI) is a pathological condition resulting from abnormal contact between the femoral head-neck junction and the acetabular rim during hip motion, particularly flexion and rotation. This abnormality can lead to labral damage, cartilage degeneration, and early osteoarthritis.

Types of FAI

1. **Cam Type**:
   - Due to an aspherical femoral head or head-neck offset deformity.
   - The abnormal morphology causes the femoral head to impact the acetabular rim during hip flexion and rotation.
   - Associated with conditions like slipped capital femoral epiphysis (SCFE) and Legg-Calvé–Perthes disease.
2. **Pincer Type**:
   - Caused by excessive acetabular coverage, resulting in impingement between the acetabular rim and the femoral head-neck junction.
   - Seen in cases of acetabular retroversion, coxa profunda, or acetabular protrusion.
3. **Mixed Type**: Combines features of both cam and pincer types.

Risk Factors

- Congenital or developmental hip deformities.
- Prior trauma to the hip.
- Overuse injuries in athletes, especially those involving repetitive hip flexion.

Imaging Findings

1. **Plain Radiographs**: Plain radiographs are the initial imaging modality for assessing bony abnormalities in FAI. Key views include an anteroposterior (AP) pelvis view, frog-leg lateral view, and Dunn view.
   - **Cam Impingement**:
     - Alpha Angle:
       - Measured on cross-table lateral or Dunn views.
       - Increased alpha angle (>50°) indicates abnormal femoral head-neck offset.
     - Pistol-Grip Deformity: Flattening of the femoral head-neck junction.
     - Anterior Offset Ratio: Reduced ratio due to loss of the concave contour of the femoral neck.
   - **Pincer Impingement**:
     - Coxa Profunda: Deep acetabulum with the medial acetabular wall crossing the ilioischial line.
     - Acetabular Retroversion: Posterior wall sign or crossover sign (anterior acetabular rim crosses posterior rim on AP view).
     - Os acetabuli: Small ossicle at the acetabular rim indicating chronic impingement.
   - **Other Findings**:
     - Joint space narrowing in advanced cases (early osteoarthritis).
     - Subchondral sclerosis or cyst formation.
2. **Magnetic Resonance Imaging (MRI)**: MRI, especially MR arthrography (MRA), is superior in detecting soft tissue injuries, cartilage damage, and labral tears associated with FAI.
   - **Cam Impingement**:
     - Femoral Head-Neck Offset: Loss of the normal concavity at the femoral head-neck junction.
     - Labral Tears: High signal intensity at the labral base on fluid-sensitive sequences (e.g., T2-weighted or PD fat-saturated sequences).
     - Chondral Damage: Cartilage thinning or delamination at the anterosuperior acetabulum.
   - **Pincer Impingement**:
     - Labral Degeneration: Labrum appears hypertrophied or ossified.
     - Cartilage Damage: Posterior cartilage wear due to leverage effect from anterior overcoverage.
   - **Common Findings in Both Types**:
     - Bone Marrow Edema: Reactive edema in the femoral head, neck, or acetabulum due to chronic impingement.

- Subchondral Cysts: Fluid-filled defects in the subchondral bone.
- Synovitis or Joint Effusion.

Conclusion: FAI is caused by structural abnormalities in the femoral head-neck junction and/or acetabulum, leading to impingement and joint damage. Plain radiographs help identify bony abnormalities, while MRI, especially MR arthrography, is critical for evaluating associated labral and cartilage injuries. Early diagnosis and intervention.

Trauma and Soft Tissues

1. Enumerate various causes of paravertebral masses and their imaging features. [3+7] [MD (WBUHS) 23, MD (WBUHS) 21]

Paravertebral masses are abnormal growths located adjacent to the vertebral column, and they can arise from a variety of causes. Below is a list of the main causes of paravertebral masses, along with their common imaging features.

1. **Neurogenic Tumors**:
   - **Types**:
     - Schwannomas
     - Neurofibromas
     - Ganglioneuromas
   - **Imaging Features**:
     - CT/MRI: Well-circumscribed masses, often iso- to hyperdense on CT and iso- to hypointense on T1 MRI, with variable enhancement on T2 depending on the tumor type.
     - Schwannomas often have a "target sign" on MRI (hypointense center and hyperintense peripheral zone).
     - Neurofibromas may show a "spaghetti" appearance due to multiple, irregular strands of tissue.
2. **Spinal Infections**:
   - **Types**:
     - Tuberculosis (Pott's disease)
     - Epidural abscess
     - Osteomyelitis
   - **Imaging Features**:
     - CT/MRI: Bone destruction and soft tissue mass in the epidural or paravertebral space.
     - MRI shows low signal intensity on T1-weighted images and high signal on T2-weighted images for abscesses or granulation tissue.
     - The abscess appears as a ring-enhancing lesion with surrounding edema.
     - Epidural abscesses may cause compression of the spinal cord, visible on MRI.
     - Paravertebral abscesses can cause significant bony destruction in the case of infections like tuberculosis.
3. **Lymphadenopathy**:
   - **Types**:
     - Lymphoma
     - Metastatic involvement from other cancers (e.g., lung, breast)
   - **Imaging Features**:
     - CT/MRI: Enlarged lymph nodes with irregular borders, often with central necrosis and peripheral enhancement. Lymphoma can present with bulky, asymmetrical masses.
     - Lymph node enlargement is typically seen in the paravertebral region, especially in mediastinal or retroperitoneal lymphoma.
4. **Metastatic Disease**:
   - **Types**:
     - Lung cancer

  - Breast cancer
  - Renal cell carcinoma
- **Imaging Features**:
  - CT/MRI: Metastatic lesions often present as poorly defined or lobulated masses with contrast enhancement.
  - MRI typically shows mixed signal intensity depending on the nature of the mass. Bone involvement may be noted on CT.

5. **Vertebral Tumors**:
   - **Types**:
     - Multiple myeloma
     - Osteosarcoma
     - Chondrosarcoma
   - **Imaging Features**:
     - CT/MRI: Bony destruction is often seen with irregular mass formation in the paravertebral space.
     - Myeloma often presents with lytic lesions of the vertebrae, while sarcomas may have soft tissue extension into the paravertebral space.
6. **Hemangiomas**:
   - **Types**: Vertebral hemangiomas
   - **Imaging Features**:
     - CT/MRI: Vertebral hemangiomas are typically well-circumscribed, with a "honeycomb" or "polka-dot" appearance on CT.
     - MRI may show a hyperintense mass on T2-weighted images due to the vascular content.
7. **Muscle or Soft Tissue Masses**:
   - **Types**:
     - Lipomas
     - Fibromas
   - **Imaging Features**: CT/MRI: Lipomas appear as well-defined, homogeneous masses with low attenuation on CT and high signal intensity on T1 and T2 MRI. Fibromas typically appear as well-defined, fibrous masses with low signal intensity on T2 MRI.
8. **Congenital Lesions**:
   - **Types**:
     - Dermoid cysts
     - Neuroenteric cysts
   - **Imaging Features**: CT/MRI: Cysts appear as well-circumscribed, fluid-filled structures with low density or low signal intensity on T1 MRI, and high signal intensity on T2 MRI. Some may have peripheral enhancement or contain fat, leading to mixed signal intensities.
9. **Pediatric Tumors**:
   - **Types**: Neuroblastomas (typically in children)
   - **Imaging Features**: CT/MRI: Often show large, heterogeneous masses with areas of necrosis and hemorrhage. Calcifications may be present, particularly in neuroblastomas.
10. **Fibrosarcoma**:
    - **Imaging Features**: CT/MRI: A large, infiltrating soft tissue mass with irregular borders, possible calcifications, and enhancement after contrast. MRI reveals heterogeneous signal intensity.
11. **Aneurysmal Bone Cyst**:
    - **Imaging Features**: CT/MRI: A well-defined cystic lesion with bony destruction and fluid-fluid levels in the mass (due to blood or serous fluid collection), often presenting as an expansile lesion.

Summary of Imaging Techniques

- **CT**: Excellent for bone involvement and detailed soft tissue contrast. Often used in trauma or to evaluate for bony lesions.

- **MRI**: Superior for evaluating soft tissue masses, especially in the paravertebral region. It provides detailed information on the extent of soft tissue involvement, tumor characteristics, and the presence of edema or necrosis. T1 and T2 imaging is essential for characterizing masses.

Each type of paravertebral mass has distinct imaging features that help differentiate between them, and often, a combination of imaging modalities is necessary to arrive at the correct diagnosis.

2. MRI in soft tissue tumors—discuss. [10] [MD (WBUHS) 20]

MRI is the imaging modality of choice for evaluating soft tissue tumors due to its superior soft tissue contrast, multiplanar imaging capability, and ability to characterize tumor components. Below is a detailed discussion of its role in diagnosing and evaluating soft tissue tumors:

1. **Indications for MRI in Soft Tissue Tumors**
   - Detection and localization of the tumor.
   - Characterization of the tumor (benign vs malignant).
   - Assessment of tumor extent, including size, depth, and relationship to surrounding structures. Presurgical planning and biopsy guidance.
   - Monitoring treatment response and post-treatment follow-up.
2. **MRI Sequences in Soft Tissue Tumor Evaluation**
   - **T1-Weighted Imaging (T1WI)**:
     - Provides excellent anatomical detail.
     - Tumors are usually isointense to slightly hypointense compared to muscle. Detects fat content in lipomatous tumors (high signal intensity).
   - **T2-Weighted Imaging (T2WI)**:
     - Highlights water content, edema, or cystic/necrotic areas. Tumors typically appear hyperintense.
     - Helps differentiate cystic and solid components.
   - **Fat-Suppressed Sequences (STIR or Fat-Sat T2)**:
     - Improves the detection of high-signal intensity tumors by suppressing fat signals.
     - Useful for identifying edema, inflammation, or subtle tumor margins.
   - **Contrast-Enhanced T1-Weighted Imaging**:
     - Uses gadolinium-based contrast agents.
     - Helps evaluate vascularity and enhancement patterns, crucial for characterizing malignancy. Differentiates viable tumor tissue from necrosis or fibrosis.
   - **Diffusion-Weighted Imaging (DWI)**:
     - Evaluates cellular density by measuring the diffusion of water molecules.
     - Restricted diffusion (low ADC values) suggests high cellularity, seen in many malignant tumors.
3. **Key MRI Features of Soft Tissue Tumors**

   A. **Benign Tumors**:

      1. **Lipomas**:
         - T1: High signal intensity (fat signal).
         - T2: High signal intensity, suppressed on fat-suppressed sequences. No significant enhancement after contrast.
      2. **Hemangiomas**:
         - T2: High signal due to vascular components.
         - T1: May contain fat or thrombi, appearing as mixed signals. Post-contrast: Intense enhancement of vascular channels.
      3. **Schwannomas/Neurofibromas**:
         - T1: Iso- to hypointense.
         - T2: Hyperintense with a "target sign" (central low signal surrounded by high signal). Postcontrast: Uniform or peripheral enhancement.

B. **Malignant Tumors**:
   1. **Soft Tissue Sarcomas**:
      - T1: Iso- to hypointense to muscle.
      - T2: Heterogeneous hyperintensity with necrotic or cystic areas.
      - Postcontrast: Heterogeneous enhancement, with central necrosis often seen.
   2. **Rhabdomyosarcoma**:
      - T2: Hyperintense.
      - Postcontrast: Strong enhancement due to vascularity.
   3. **Synovial Sarcoma**: T2: Mixed hyperintensity with areas of calcification. Postcontrast: Heterogeneous enhancement.
   4. **Malignant Peripheral Nerve Sheath Tumors (MPNSTs)**:
      - T2: Heterogeneous with no clear "target sign."
      - Postcontrast: Irregular enhancement.

C. **Cystic Lesions**:
   1. **Ganglion Cysts**:
      - T1: Hypointense.
      - T2: Hyperintense, with well-defined margins. No significant postcontrast enhancement.
   2. **Abscesses**:
      - T2: High signal intensity.
      - Postcontrast: Peripheral ring enhancement with central nonenhancing area.

4. **Role of MRI in Differentiating Benign and Malignant Tumors**:
   - **Margins**: Benign: Well-defined margins. Malignant: Ill-defined, infiltrative margins.
   - **Signal Intensity**: Malignant tumors often show heterogeneous signals on T2 due to necrosis and hemorrhage.
   - **Enhancement Patterns**: Benign: Minimal or uniform enhancement. Malignant: Heterogeneous enhancement.
   - **Peritumoral Edema**: More common in malignant tumors, appearing as hyperintensity on T2/STIR.
   - **Infiltration**: Malignant tumors may invade adjacent muscles, vessels, or bone.
5. **Advantages of MRI in Soft Tissue Tumors**:
   - Superior soft tissue contrast for detailed tumor characterization.
   - Multiplanar capability for precise localization and surgical planning.
   - Differentiates between solid, cystic, necrotic, and fatty components.
   - Assesses involvement of neurovascular structures.
   - Nonionizing, making it safer for long-term monitoring.
6. **Limitations of MRI**:
   - Cannot reliably distinguish all benign from malignant tumors.
   - Gadolinium use is contraindicated in renal impairment.
   - Less effective in detecting calcifications (CT is better).
   - May not be suitable for patients with contraindications to MRI (e.g., metallic implants, claustrophobia).

Conclusion: MRI plays a pivotal role in the evaluation of soft tissue tumors by providing critical information about the tumor's size, extent, composition, and relationship to surrounding structures. By integrating anatomical, signal intensity, and enhancement characteristics, MRI aids in differentiating benign from malignant lesions and assists in guiding biopsy, treatment planning, and follow-up.

3. What is a growth plate? Discuss imaging of growth plate disorders and Salter-Harris classification of fractures. [2+4+4] [MD (WBUHS) 24, MD (WBUHS) 21]

The growth plate, also known as the epiphyseal plate or physis, is a layer of cartilage located at the ends of long bones in children and adolescents. It is where bone growth occurs, allowing bones to lengthen and the skeleton to mature.

Key Features

1. **Location**: Found at the ends of bones like the femur, tibia, and humerus.
2. **Composition**: Made up of cartilage, which is less dense and more flexible than bone tissue.
3. **Function**:
   - Cells in the growth plate multiply and gradually ossify (turn into bone), contributing to the elongation of the bone.
   - The growth plate is responsible for most of the bone's lengthening during childhood and adolescence.

Closure

As a child reaches the end of puberty, the growth plates harden and close, turning into solid bone. Once this occurs, bones stop growing in length.

Imaging of growth plate disorders is crucial for diagnosing, monitoring, and planning treatment for conditions affecting the growth plate (epiphyseal plate). Various imaging modalities are used, depending on the suspected disorder or injury.

1. **X-rays**
   - Advantages: Widely available, inexpensive, and fast.
   - Uses:
     - Growth Plate Injuries (Salter-Harris Fractures): X-rays are the first-line imaging to assess fractures involving the growth plate. These are classified into types I–V using the Salter-Harris system.
     - Growth Arrest: X-rays may show bony bridges or disruptions in the growth plate.
     - Bone Age Assessment: By comparing the appearance of growth plates to standardized charts (e.g., Greulich-Pyle Atlas).
   - Limitations: May not detect subtle cartilage injuries or early abnormalities.
2. **Magnetic Resonance Imaging (MRI)**
   - Advantages: Superior soft tissue contrast and detailed visualization of cartilage.
   - Uses:
     - Cartilage Damage: Detects early changes in the growth plate cartilage that are invisible on X-rays.
     - Physeal Bar Formation: Identifies small areas of premature bone bridging within the growth plate.
     - Infections and Tumors: Helps assess soft tissue and surrounding structures for conditions like osteomyelitis or neoplasms.
   - Limitations: Expensive and not always readily available.
3. **Computed Tomography (CT)**
   - Advantages: High-resolution imaging for detailed bone structure.
   - Uses:
     - Complex Fractures: Provides precise anatomical detail for surgical planning.
     - Physeal Bars: Used in 3D reconstructions to map the extent of bony bridging.
   - Limitations: Higher radiation exposure compared to X-rays.
4. **Ultrasound**:
   - Advantages: Noninvasive, radiation-free, and cost-effective.
   - Uses:
     - Early Growth Plate Injury: Can detect fluid or damage in the growth plate.
     - Dynamic Assessment: Useful for real-time evaluation of joint and growth plate movement.
   - Limitations: Operator-dependent and less detailed than MRI or CT.
5. **Nuclear Medicine (Bone Scans)**:
   - Advantages: Sensitive for detecting increased metabolic activity.
   - Uses:
     - Growth Plate Activity: Helps assess whether growth plates are still active.
     - Infections or Tumors: Identifies areas of high bone turnover.
   - Limitations: Low spatial resolution and involves radioactive tracers.

Common Growth Plate Disorders Evaluated by Imaging

1. Salter-Harris Fractures: Graded from I to V based on growth plate involvement and visible on X-rays or MRI.
2. Growth Arrest/Physeal Bar Formation: Diagnosed with MRI or CT for surgical planning.
3. Infections (e.g., Osteomyelitis): MRI is preferred for assessing inflammation around the growth plate.
4. Endocrine Disorders (e.g., Hypothyroidism): X-rays may show delayed bone age.
5. Bone Dysplasias (e.g., Achondroplasia): X-rays reveal characteristic changes in growth plate morphology.

By choosing the appropriate imaging modality, clinicians can ensure accurate diagnosis and management of growth plate disorders.

Salter-Harris Classification of Fractures

The classification has five primary types (I–V), based on the relationship of the fracture line to the growth plate, epiphysis, and metaphysis:

1. **Type I**:
   - Description: The fracture occurs through the growth plate only.
   - Imaging: The physis appears widened; no bone involvement.
   - Prognosis: Excellent; minimal risk of growth disturbance.
   - Example: Slipped capital femoral epiphysis (SCFE).
2. **Type II**:
   - Description: The fracture involves the growth plate and metaphysis but not the epiphysis.
   - Imaging: A triangular metaphyseal fragment (Thurston-Holland sign) is seen.
   - Prognosis: Good; usually heals without significant growth issues.
   - Prevalence: Most common type (~75% of cases).
3. **Type III**:
   - Description: The fracture involves the growth plate and epiphysis, sparing the metaphysis.
   - Imaging: A vertical fracture extending into the joint space is visible.
   - Prognosis: Guarded; potential for growth disturbances and joint issues if not properly aligned.
4. **Type IV**:
   - Description: The fracture crosses the epiphysis, growth plate, and metaphysis.
   - Imaging: A vertical fracture through all three zones.
   - Prognosis: Poor; high risk of growth plate damage and deformities if not treated correctly.
5. **Type V**:
   - Description: Crush injury of the growth plate with no visible fracture line.
   - Imaging: Subtle or no changes acutely; later, growth arrest or deformity may develop. Prognosis: Worst; almost always leads to growth disturbances.

Management and Prognosis

- **Early Diagnosis**: Accurate imaging (X-ray, MRI) is essential.
- **Treatment**:
  - Nonsurgical (e.g., casting) for stable fractures (Type I–II).
  - Surgical intervention for complex cases (Type III–V) to realign the growth plate.
- **Long-term Monitoring**: Follow-up is critical to detect growth arrest or deformities.

Proper classification helps predict complications and tailor treatment to prevent growth and functional impairments.

4. Write a short note on: Types of meniscus injury of the knee with MRI features. [5] [MD (WBUHS) 24, MD (WBUHS) 22]

Types of Meniscus Injury of Knee with MRI Features

Meniscus injuries of the knee are common and can be classified into several types based on their morphology and location. MRI is the imaging modality of choice for detecting and characterizing meniscal injuries because it provides high-resolution images of soft tissue and cartilage.

Types of Meniscal Injuries and Their MRI Features

1. **Vertical Longitudinal Tear**:
   - **Description**: A tear running parallel to the long axis of the meniscus.
   - **MRI Features**:
     - Linear high signal intensity within the meniscus extending to the articular surface on at least one side.
     - Often associated with bucket-handle tears if displaced.
2. **Radial Tear**:
   - **Description**: A tear perpendicular to the long axis of the meniscus, disrupting its circumferential fibers.
   - **MRI Features**:
     - High signal intensity extending from the inner edge radially toward the periphery.
     - Truncation or absence of the meniscus on coronal or sagittal images ("ghost meniscus" sign).
3. **Horizontal Tear**:
   - **Description**: A tear parallel to the tibial plateau, splitting the meniscus into upper and lower leaflets.
   - **MRI Features**: Horizontal high signal intensity on T2-weighted images reaching the articular surface. May appear as a "cleavage tear."
4. **Oblique Tear**:
   - **Description**: A combination of horizontal and vertical components at an angle to the meniscal planes.
   - **MRI Features**: Irregular high signal intensity at the posterior horn or body of the meniscus, extending obliquely.
5. **Bucket-Handle Tear**:
   - **Description**: A displaced longitudinal tear where a fragment of the meniscus is displaced into the intercondylar notch.
   - **MRI Features**:
     - "Double PCL sign": The displaced meniscal fragment mimics the posterior cruciate ligament.
     - Absence of meniscus in its normal location on sagittal images.
6. **Flap Tear**:
   - **Description**: A tear creating a mobile fragment (flap) of the meniscus.
   - **MRI Features**:
     - Irregular high signal extending to the meniscal surface with a displaced fragment.
     - Seen on sagittal or coronal images as an abnormal contour.
7. **Complex Tear**:
   - **Description**: A combination of two or more tear patterns (e.g., horizontal, radial, or oblique).
   - **MRI Features**: Multiple intersecting high-signal lines on various planes. Irregular morphology with possible fraying.
8. **Meniscal Root Tear**:
   - **Description**: A tear at the meniscal root attachment to the tibial plateau, leading to extrusion.
   - **MRI Features**:
     - High signal intensity at the root insertion.
     - Meniscal extrusion >3 mm beyond the tibial edge.
     - Associated with subchondral bone edema in the adjacent tibial plateau.
9. **Degenerative Tear**:
   - **Description**: Chronic fraying and tearing associated with wear and tear, not discrete.
   - **MRI Features**:
     - Inhomogeneous high signal intensity within the meniscus.
     - No discrete tear lines extending to the articular surface.

Classification by Meniscus Location

- **Medial Meniscus**: More common for longitudinal and degenerative tears.
- **Lateral Meniscus**: More common for radial and complex tears due to its increased mobility.

Grading on MRI

Meniscal signal changes on MRI are often graded to evaluate tears:

- **Grade 1**: Small focal increased signal within the meniscus not extending to the surface.
- **Grade 2**: Linear increased signal not extending to the surface.
- **Grade 3**: Increased signal intensity extending to at least one articular surface, indicating a tear.

MRI plays a pivotal role in determining the type, extent, and location of meniscal injuries, which is critical for guiding treatment decisions such as conservative management or surgical repair.

5. Write a short note on: Rotator cuff injury. [5] [MD (WBUHS) 22]

Four muscles (supraspinatus, infraspinatus, teres minor, subscapularis), together with their tendons, form the rotator cuff. Of these muscles, the supraspinatus is most prone to injury.

Rotator cuff injury can occur due to acute causes such as trauma, sudden heavy lifting or sports injuries where there is direct impact on or sudden stretch of rotator cuff muscles. Chronic wear and tear and degenerative changes can also lead to injury.[14]

Rotator cuff injury can be of two types: Partial-thickness tears or full-thickness tears.

Imaging Findings

Partial-thickness Tears:

- Focal areas of increased signal intensity on short echo time (TE) images; these areas increase in relative signal intensity on long-TE images but need not match the signal intensity of joint fluid. The abnormal focus does not extend through the entire thickness of the tendon.
- If the partial tear is on the articular side, there may be increased fluid in the glenohumeral joint; and if the partial tear lies on the bursal side of the tendon, then fluid may be seen in the subacromial-subdeltoid bursa.
- The depth of tendon fiber involvement is also used as a criterion for grading of partial tears:
  1. Less than 3 mm deep
  2. 3 to 6 mm deep and less than 50% of the cuff thickness involved
  3. High-grade partial-thickness tear more than 6 mm deep with more than 50% of the rotator cuff thickness involved
- **Full-thickness tears**:
  - The tendon is interrupted by an abnormal focus of increased T2-weighted signal intensity extending across its complete superior-to-inferior extent on at least one image.
  - Fluid in the subacromial-subdeltoid bursa is a common association.
  - Tendon retraction (more obvious when the size of the tear is bigger).
  - Atrophy of the involved muscles with associated fatty infiltration.
  - Cephalad migration of the humeral head maybe the only sign when there is little joint fluid to communicate with the tear.
  - Occasional accompanying sign is irregularity of the bony elements of the glenohumeral joint as a result of rotator cuff arthropathy.

6. Internal derangement of knee causes. MRI knee protocol. ACL tear findings. [10] [MD (WBUHS) 17, DNB Dec 21]

Internal derangement of the knee (IDK) is injury to one or more internal stabilizing elements of the knee (ligaments, cartilages or menisci) resulting in ongoing or intermittent signs and symptoms such as pain, instability, or abnormal mobility of that knee.[14,15]

It is a chronic disorder of the knee which can be due to:

- Torn, ruptured or deranged meniscus of the knee, or
- Partial or complete cruciate rupture with or without injury to the capsular ligament of the knee.

The **essential features** of IDK are as follows:

1. The appearance of locking and/or recurrent locking of the knee causing the knee to buckle during weight-bearing, i.e., sometimes in locking, a person's knee may give way because both the extensors and flexors of the knee have failed.
2. Sudden loss of motion, usually of full extension.
3. Sudden loss of function of the knee, often associated with a minor injury.
4. Possible restoration of the knee to normal function by manipulation.
5. Subjective complaint of "something moving around in the knee."

The **causes** of IDK are as follows:

1. **Traumatic Injuries**:
   - Sports injuries: Activities involving sudden stops, twists, or impacts (e.g., football, basketball, skiing) often result in ligament or meniscal damage.
   - Direct blows to the knee: A fall, collision, or car accident can cause tears, fractures, or joint instability.
   - Hyperextension or over-rotation: Overstretching or twisting the knee beyond its normal range can damage internal structures.
2. **Overuse and Repetitive Stress**:
   - Repetitive movements: Activities like running, jumping, or squatting may cause gradual wear on cartilage or ligaments.
   - Chronic strain: Over time, repeated stress without adequate rest can lead to microtears in the menisci or ligaments.
3. **Degenerative Changes**: Osteoarthritis or age-related degeneration can lead to wear and tear of the cartilages and weakening of the ligaments.
4. **Congenital or Developmental Abnormalities**:
   - Alignment Issues: Conditions like bowlegs or knock knees may put uneven stress on the joint, increasing the risk of derangement.
   - Weak Supporting Muscles: Weakness in the quadriceps or hamstrings may lead to instability and subsequent injury.
5. **Other Contributing Factors**:
   - Obesity: Excess weight puts additional stress on the knee joint, contributing to wear and potential damage.
   - Poor Technique: Incorrect techniques in sports or heavy lifting can lead to injuries.

MRI Knee Protocol

- **Patient position**: Supine with the knee positioned centrally in the coil, slightly flexed (10–15 degrees) to relax the joint.
- **Coil**: Knee coil or a dedicated extremity coil for high-resolution imaging.
- **Slice Thickness**: 3–4 mm
- **Sequences**:
  1. 3 plane LOC
  2. T1 Sagittal
  3. PD Sagittal
  4. PDFS Sagittal: Sagittal, Coronal, Axial
  5. T2FS Coronal
  6. Volumetric sequence: MENSA
  7. GRE Sagittal

Advantages of individual sequences:

- **T1**: To detect any bony lesion or marrow changes.

- **PD**: Detailed anatomy of ligaments, fat helps to identify structures.
- **PDFS**: Fat saturation helps detect fluids.
- **T2FS Coronal**: Best coronal sequence for meniscal root tear detection.
- **GRE**: For articular cartilage
- **MENSA**: Can be reformatted for 3D visualization of meniscal body.

ACL Tear Findings

Direct Signs

Complete interstitial tear:

- Fairly ill-defined mass of reactive edema and hemorrhage.
- Complete discontinuity of the ACL fibers, often with increased T2 signal traversing buckled indistinct ligament fibers
- The absence of these low-signal fibers at the expected site of attachment is occasionally the most definitive sign of proximal ACL tear in subtle cases (*empty notch sign*)
- Avulsion fractures at the tibial eminence or (less commonly) the femoral attachment may occur

Partial tear:

- Increased T2 signal with contour irregularity.
- Obscuration of the fasciculi within the ligament.

Indirect or Secondary Signs of ACL Tear

- Anterior translation of the tibia relative to the femur of >7mm (the *anterior tibial translocation sign*)
- Buckling of the PCL
- Posterior displacement of the lateral meniscus from the tibial plateau (the *uncovered lateral meniscus sign*),
- Indentation of the anterior margin of the medial femoral condyle,
- Avulsion fracture of the lateral tibial plateau (the *Segond fracture*)
- Fairly specific combinations of bone contusions that depend on the mechanism of trauma—in lateral femoral condyle and posterolateral tibial plateau

Injury to other supporting structures of the knee is also commonly seen along with ACL injury:

- Peripheral vertical tears of the posterior horn of the medial meniscus are characteristically encountered in the setting of clip injuries.
- Medial or lateral collateral ligaments injuries.

7. Pelvic fractures—classification and imaging approach. Osseous and soft tissue injury patterns of pelvic fractures. [10] [DNB June 21]

Tile Classification of Pelvic Fractures

It takes into account the stability, force direction, and pathoanatomy. Stability is defined as the 'ability of the pelvis to withstand physiologic force without deformation.[16,17]

Three basic stability descriptions are used, each with degrees of severity.

Classification

Type A: Stable (posterior arch intact)

- **A1**: Avulsion injury
- **A2**: Iliac-wing or anterior-arch fracture due to a direct blow
- **A3**: Transverse sacrococcygeal fracture

Type B: Partially stable (incomplete disruption of the posterior arch)—unstable to rotation but vertically stable.

- **B1**: Open-book injury (external rotation)

- **B2**: Lateral-compression injury (internal rotation)
  - B2-1: Ipsilateral anterior and posterior injuries
  - B2-2: Contralateral (bucket-handle) injuries
- **B3**: Bilateral

Type C: Unstable (complete disruption of the posterior arch)—unstable to both rotation and vertical displacement.

- **C1**: Unilateral
  - C1-1: Iliac fracture
  - C1-2: Sacroiliac fracture-dislocation
  - C1-3: Sacral fracture
- **C2**: Bilateral, with one side type B, one side type C
- **C3**: Bilateral

Young and Burgess Classification

It is a modification of the Tile classification. It is the recommended and most widely used classification system for pelvic ring fractures. It takes into account force type, severity, and direction, as well as injury instability. Three basic mechanistic descriptions are used, each with degrees of severity.

Classification

Lateral compression: Transverse overlapping obturator ring fractures (Most common type)

- **LC I**: Stable
  - Oblique fracture of pubic rami
  - Ipsilateral anterior compression fracture of the sacral ala
  - Intact ligaments
- **LC II**: Rotationally unstable, vertically stable
  - Fracture of pubic rami
  - Iliac crescent fracture (posterior fracture with dislocation of the ipsilateral iliac wing)
- **LC III**: Globally unstable
  - Ipsilateral type 1 or 2 lateral compression and contralateral anteroposterior compression injury.

Anteroposterior compression: Diastasis of pubic symphysis without anterior fracture

- **APC I**: Stable
  - Pubic diastasis <2.5 cm
- **APC II**: Rotationally unstable, vertically stable
  - Pubic diastasis >2.5 cm
  - Disruption and diastasis of the anterior part of the sacroiliac joint, with intact posterior sacroiliac joint ligaments
- **APC III**: Globally unstable; equates to a complete hemipelvis separation (but without vertical displacement)
  - Pubic diastasis >2.5 cm (often more than 5 cm)
  - Disruption-diastasis of both anterior and posterior sacroiliac joint ligaments with dislocation

Vertical shear: Most severe and unstable type with a high association of visceral injuries.

- Vertical displacement of hemipelvis, pubic and sacroiliac joint fractures

Combined: Stability depends on the individual components of this injury.

- Complex fracture, including a combination of anteroposterior compression, lateral compression, and/or vertical shear

Approach

The osseous and ligamentous components of the pelvis cause it to biomechanically function as a ring, and disruption of one portion of the pelvic ring must raise suspicion for disruption in a second location. Further, the complex anatomy of the pelvis and its often-subtle imaging findings may be challenging to the radiologist. Thus, it is critical to adhere to a systematic and rigorous approach in evaluating pelvic images.

Radiographs:

- Initial radiographic evaluation of the pelvic ring—standard AP view as part of the initial trauma series.
  - Anterior ring fractures are most often evident on AP radiographs.
  - Posterior ring injuries, such as sacral fractures, are often occult and require careful scrutiny of the sacral arcs and, often, further imaging

Additional projections to the pelvic trauma series include:

- Pelvic outlet (Ferguson) view—AP view obtained with the X-ray tube angled 25–45° cephalad.
  - It best depicts the SI joints,
  - Vertical fractures of the sacrum,
  - Extension of fractures into the neural foramina, and
  - Cranial or caudad displacement of fracture fragments or hemipelvis.
- Pelvic inlet view—AP view obtained with X-ray tube angled 30–60° caudad.
  - For evaluation of the sacral arcuate lines
  - AP displacement or internal rotation of fracture fragments, and
  - Alignment of the pubic symphysis.
- Judet views—comprises of two projections: Iliac oblique and obturator oblique.
  - Obtained to better depict associated acetabular fractures.

CT: Provides better depiction and characterization of radiographically occult posterior ring fractures.

MRI: Impractical in acute setting due to longer acquisition time, however have shown value in depicting acute pelvic ring disruptions and additional information on ligamentous injuries.

Osseous and Soft Tissue Injury Patterns of Various Pelvic Fractures

Lateral compression fracture **(Table 4)**:

TABLE 4: Types of lateral compression pelvic fracture.

Type	*Osseous pattern*
LC 1	• Impaction fracture of the anterior sacrum on the side of the compression • Small buckle fracture in the sacral ala • Disruption or angulation of the sacral arcuate line • Superior and inferior rami fractures
LC 2	• Crescent shaped fracture of the posterior iliac blade • Superior and inferior rami fractures
LC 3	• Ipsilateral pattern of LC1 or LC2 • Contralateral pubic diastasis and disruption of SI joint • Disruption of the sacrospinous, sacrotuberous, and anterior and posterior SI ligaments

Soft tissue injuries.

1. Internal rotation of the hemipelvis drives the osseous spike of the fractured pubic rami into a branch of the internal iliac artery or the urinary bladder, resulting in
   - Hemorrhage, or
   - Extraperitoneal bladder rupture.
2. Increased intrapelvic pressure may lead to intraperitoneal bladder rupture
3. Posteriorly, a compression injury of the sacrum through the foramina may compress the sacral nerve roots
4. Iliac crescent fractures may also extend to the greater sciatic foramen, with injury to the sciatic or superior gluteal nerve

Anteroposterior compression fracture **(Table 5)**:

TABLE 5: Types of anteroposterior compression pelvic fracture.

Type	*Osseous pattern*
APC 1	• Disruption of pubic symphysis (diastasis <2.5 cm) • Vertical fracture through one or both pairs of pubic rami
APC 2	• Pubic symphysis diastasis >2.5 cm • Asymmetry of SI joint (due to anterior SI joint widening) • Occult L5 transverse process fracture
APC 3	• Same as APC 2 with instability • Broader than normal iliac wing (due to external rotation at SI joint)

Soft tissue injuries: Substantial hemorrhage and arterial bleeding are most common with AP injuries. Most commonly severed arteries are the superior gluteal (in posterior pelvic injuries) and the internal pudendal (in anterior pelvic arch injuries) arteries.

Vertical shear injury:
Osseous pattern:
- Pubic symphysis and SI joint disruptions.
- Vertically oriented pubic rami fractures anteriorly
- Sacral fractures posteriorly—characteristically extend from the sacral notch obliquely to the midportion of the body of the first sacral segment.
- Cephalad displacement of the iliac crest of the injured hemipelvis relative to the opposite side.
- Severe SI joint widening with pubic symphysis diastasis of less than 2.5 cm.

Soft tissue injuries: Associated with other visceral injuries:
1. **Extraperitoneal bladder rupture**
2. **Urethral injury**: Typically, urethral rupture occurs at the apex of the prostate at the junction of the prostatic and membranous urethra, above the urogenital diaphragm

Combined mechanism injury: The most common type of combined mechanism injury is a lateral compression and vertical shear injury. They demonstrate elements of more than one pattern.

Miscellaneous

1. Write a short note on: Single dense vertebra. [5] [MD (WBUHS) 19]

A single dense vertebra refers to a vertebral body that appears abnormally dense on radiological imaging compared to adjacent vertebral bodies. It is often an incidental finding during imaging studies.

The sclerosis can be of two patters:
i. Diffuse giving rise to what is known as ivory vertebra, where the spongiosa is entirely replaced by an amorphous homogenous bony mass.
ii. Coarsened trabeculae, where the spongiosa is otherwise atrophic.

Single dense vertebra can result from various causes which depends on the age of the patient:
- **Pediatric causes**:
    1. Lymphoma (usually Hodgkin's): Most common cause.
    2. Primary bone tumors: Osteosarcoma/osteoblastoma.
    3. Osteoblastic metastases: From medulloblastoma or neuroblastoma.
- **Adult causes**:
    1. Osteoblastic metastases: From prostate or breast cancer.
    2. Lymphoma (usually Hodgkin's)

3. Infection: Tuberculous spondylitis
4. Paget disease of the bone
5. Hemangioma
6. Chordoma

Imaging Features

Radiograph or CT:

- A single vertebra stands out with increased density compared to adjacent vertebrae.
- Generally, the shape, size and contour of the vertebral body is maintained.
- In Paget's disease, there will be expansion of the vertebral body with coarsened trabeculae. Double contour of the vertebral body may be seen due to subcortical sclerosis.
- Diffuse homogenous sclerosis is seen in lymphomatous involvement.
- Osteoblastic metastasis shows punctate and confluent, dense, irregular spotting of bone.

MRI: Hypointense signal seen within the corresponding vertebra.

The finding of a single dense vertebra warrants investigation to rule out serious underlying conditions like metastasis or systemic bone disease. Clinical history, laboratory studies, and additional imaging are critical for diagnosis.

2. Discuss the differential diagnosis of radiological appearance of metaphyseal lucent bands in child. [10] [MD (WBUHS) 24, MD (WBUHS) 22]

Radiological Appearance of Metaphyseal Lucent Bands in Children

Metaphyseal lucent bands are radiolucent (darker) lines seen in the metaphysis of long bones on radiographs. These bands are typically 2–15 mm wide and can be caused by various conditions that interfere with normal bone growth and development.

Characteristics

- **Appearance**: Radiolucent bands that appear as dark lines within the metaphysis of long bones.
- **Width**: Typically, 2–15 mm wide.
- **Location**: Seen in the metaphysis, which is the growing part of the bone adjacent to the growth plate (physis).

Differential Diagnosis of Metaphyseal Lucent Bands in Children

1. **Normal Growth Variants**:
   - **Rapid Bone Growth**: In rapidly growing children, especially during growth spurts, metaphyseal lucent bands can sometimes be observed. These bands are generally physiological and not associated with any pathology.
2. **Infections**:
   - **Congenital Infections (TORCH)**:
     - **Toxoplasmosis, Rubella, Cytomegalovirus, Herpes, Syphilis**: These infections can lead to metaphyseal lucent bands due to congenital bone abnormalities.
     - **Radiological Features**: Typically, these bands are seen in multiple bones and may be associated with other signs of congenital infection like hepatosplenomegaly or intracranial calcifications.
   - **Osteomyelitis**:
     - **Acute or Chronic Bone Infection**: Osteomyelitis can cause localized metaphyseal lucent bands due to bone destruction and reactive changes.
     - **Radiological Features**: Ill-defined lucent areas in the metaphysis, sometimes with periosteal reaction or soft tissue swelling.
3. **Hematologic Conditions**:
   - **Leukemia**:
     - **Bone Marrow Infiltration**: Leukemia can present with metaphyseal lucent bands due to marrow infiltration by malignant cells.

  - **Radiological Features**: Diffuse, bilateral metaphyseal bands, often accompanied by generalized osteopenia and other skeletal changes.
- **Anemia**:
  - **Severe chronic anemia**: Conditions like thalassemia and sickle cell anemia can lead to changes in the bone marrow and subsequently metaphyseal lucent bands.
  - **Radiological Features**: Expansion of marrow spaces, cortical thinning, and lucent bands in the metaphysis.

4. **Nutritional Deficiencies**:
   - **Rickets**:
     - **Vitamin D Deficiency**: Leads to defective mineralization of growing bones, resulting in metaphyseal lucent bands.
     - **Radiological Features**: Widened and irregular growth plates, metaphyseal cupping, and fraying. Lucent bands are due to unmineralized osteoid.
   - **Malnutrition**:
     - **General Malnutrition**: Can affect overall bone growth and development, leading to lucent bands.
     - **Radiological Features**: Diffuse osteopenia and possible metaphyseal lucent bands.
5. **Metabolic Disorders**:
   - **Hypophosphatasia**:
     - **Genetic Disorder**: Affecting alkaline phosphatase activity, leading to defective mineralization.
     - **Radiological Features**: Metaphyseal lucent bands, along with premature loss of teeth and generalized bone abnormalities.
   - **Hyperparathyroidism**:
     - **Parathyroid Hormone Excess**: Causes increased bone resorption, leading to lucent bands.
     - **Radiological Features**: Subperiosteal bone resorption, particularly along the radial aspects of the middle phalanges, and metaphyseal lucent bands.
6. **Neoplastic Conditions**:
   - **Bone Tumors**:
     - **Primary Malignancies (e.g., Osteosarcoma, Ewing Sarcoma)**: These can cause metaphyseal changes, including lucent bands.
     - **Radiological Features**: Irregular metaphyseal lucent areas, sometimes with periosteal reaction or a soft tissue mass.
   - **Metastatic Neuroblastoma**:
     - **Pediatric Malignancy**: Can metastasize to bones, causing lucent bands.
     - **Radiological Features**: Multiple, ill-defined metaphyseal lucent bands, often associated with cortical bone destruction.
7. **Trauma**
   - **Fractures**:
     - **Healing Fractures**: Metaphyseal lucent bands can be seen during the healing process of fractures.
     - **Radiological Features**: Lucent lines at the metaphysis, sometimes associated with callus formation.
8. **Genetic Disorders**:
   - **Osteogenesis Imperfecta**:
     - **Brittle Bone Disease**: A genetic disorder causing fragile bones.
     - **Radiological Features**: Multiple fractures at various stages of healing, metaphyseal lucent bands, and generalized osteopenia.

Clinical Relevance

The presence of metaphyseal lucent bands in children necessitates a thorough clinical and radiological evaluation to determine the underlying cause. The specific radiological features, along with the clinical presentation and patient history, can help narrow down the differential diagnosis and guide appropriate management and treatment strategies.

3. Radiological evaluation of a child with limping. [10] [MD (WBUHS) 20]

Radiological Evaluation of a Child with Limping

Limping in children can be caused by a variety of conditions, ranging from mild injuries to serious systemic diseases. A systematic approach to radiological evaluation is essential to accurately diagnose the underlying cause. Here is a detailed overview:

Initial Assessment

History and Physical Examination

- **History**: Focus on the onset, duration, and progression of limping, any history of trauma, pain, fever, weight loss, or other systemic symptoms.
- **Physical Examination**: Assess the gait, check for tenderness, range of motion, and any visible deformities or masses.

Radiological Imaging Modalities

1. **Plain Radiographs (X-rays)**:
   - **Indications**: First-line imaging for initial assessment of musculoskeletal complaints.
   - **Techniques**: Anteroposterior (AP) and lateral views of the affected limb, sometimes including the contralateral limb for comparison.
   - **Findings**:
     - **Fractures**: Displacement, angulation, and healing stages of fractures.
     - **Bone Tumors**: Lytic or sclerotic lesions, periosteal reaction.
     - **Infections**: Osteomyelitis presents as bone destruction, and periosteal reaction.
     - **Developmental Disorders**: Legg–Calvé–Perthes disease shows fragmentation and sclerosis of the femoral head; slipped capital femoral epiphysis (SCFE) shows displacement of the femoral head.
2. **Ultrasound**:
   - **Indications**: Useful for soft tissue evaluation and detecting joint effusions.
   - **Techniques**: Real-time imaging with the possibility of dynamic assessment.
   - **Findings**:
     - **Hip Effusion**: Fluid collection in the joint capsule.
     - **Soft Tissue Masses**: Characterization of cystic vs. solid masses.
     - **Tendon Injuries**: Tendon thickening, tears, or inflammation.
3. **Magnetic Resonance Imaging (MRI)**:
   - **Indications**: Detailed evaluation of soft tissues, bone marrow, and joint structures.
   - **Techniques**: T1-weighted, T2-weighted, and contrast-enhanced sequences; sometimes includes fat suppression.
   - **Findings**:
     - **Osteomyelitis**: Bone marrow edema, abscess formation.
     - **Bone Tumors**: Extent of the tumor, involvement of adjacent structures.
     - **Soft Tissue Injuries**: Muscle tears, ligament injuries.
     - **Inflammatory Conditions**: Juvenile idiopathic arthritis shows synovial thickening, joint effusion.
4. **Computed Tomography (CT) Scan**:
   - **Indications**: Detailed evaluation of bone architecture and complex fractures.
   - **Techniques**: High-resolution axial images with multiplanar reconstructions.
   - **Findings**:
     - **Complex Fractures**: Detailed assessment of fracture lines, bone fragments.
     - **Bone Lesions**: Characterization of cortical involvement, mineralization patterns.
     - **Intra-articular Pathology**: Joint surface irregularities, loose bodies.

5. **Bone Scintigraphy (Bone Scan)**:
   - **Indications**: Highly sensitive for detecting bone abnormalities, especially when the source of pain is unclear.
   - **Techniques**: Involves intravenous injection of a radiotracer followed by imaging.
   - **Findings**:
     - **Infections**: Increased radiotracer uptake in areas of osteomyelitis.
     - **Tumors**: Increased uptake in malignant bone lesions.
     - **Fractures**: Stress fractures show focal areas of increased uptake.

Diagnostic Considerations

1. **Infectious Etiologies**:
   - **Radiographs**: May show soft tissue swelling, periosteal reaction, or lytic lesions.
   - **MRI**: Superior for detecting early osteomyelitis and abscess formation.
   - **Bone Scan**: High sensitivity for early detection of osteomyelitis.
2. **Traumatic Injuries**:
   - **Radiographs**: First-line for detecting fractures and dislocations.
   - **CT**: Detailed assessment of complex fractures and joint involvement.
   - **Ultrasound**: Useful for evaluating soft tissue injuries and effusions.
3. **Neoplastic Conditions**:
   - **Radiographs**: Initial identification of suspicious lesions.
   - **MRI**: Detailed assessment of the extent of the lesion and soft tissue involvement.
   - **CT**: Characterization of bone lesions and surgical planning.
4. **Inflammatory and Developmental Disorders**:
   - **Radiographs**: Initial assessment of bone and joint morphology.
   - **MRI**: Detailed evaluation of joint structures, bone marrow, and inflammation.
   - **Ultrasound**: Useful for detecting joint effusions and guiding aspirations.

Summary

Radiological imaging plays a vital role in the evaluation of a child with limping. The choice of imaging modality depends on the clinical presentation, suspected underlying condition, and the need for detailed anatomical assessment. Combining different modalities often provides a comprehensive understanding of the pathology and guides appropriate management.

4. Briefly describe the radiological features of various paragangliomas. [10] [MD (WBUHS) 21]

Paragangliomas are rare neuroendocrine tumors that arise from paraganglionic cells. They can occur anywhere along the sympathetic and parasympathetic paraganglia.

Here are the main types of paragangliomas, along with their detailed radiological features:

1. **Carotid Body Paraganglioma**:
   - **Location**: Arises from the carotid body, located at the bifurcation of the common carotid artery.
   - **Radiological Features**:
     - **CT**: Homogeneous or slightly heterogeneous mass with intense enhancement post-contrast.
     - **MRI**: Hyperintense on T2-weighted images, with a characteristic "salt and pepper" appearance on T1-weighted images due to numerous small blood vessels.
     - **Ultrasound**: Hypoechoic mass with increased vascularity on Doppler imaging.
     - **MIBG Scintigraphy**: Positive uptake indicating catecholamine secretion.
2. **Jugulotympanic Paraganglioma (Glomus Jugulare)**:
   - **Location**: Arises from the jugular foramen, involving the temporal bone.

  - **Radiological Features**:
    - **CT**: Mass with bone erosion and intense contrast enhancement.
    - **MRI**: Hyperintense on T2-weighted images, with a "salt and pepper" appearance on T1-weighted images.
    - **Ultrasound**: Hypoechoic mass with increased vascularity.
    - **MIBG Scintigraphy**: Positive uptake indicating catecholamine secretion.
3. **Vagal Paraganglioma (Glomus Vagale)**:
  - **Location**: Arises from the vagal body, located in the neck.
  - **Radiological Features**:
    - **CT**: Homogeneous mass with intense enhancement.
    - **MRI**: Hyperintense on T2-weighted images, with a "salt and pepper" appearance on T1-weighted images.
    - **Ultrasound**: Hypoechoic mass with increased vascularity.
    - **MIBG Scintigraphy**: Positive uptake indicating catecholamine secretion.
4. **Tympanic Paraganglioma (Glomus Tympanicum)**:
  - **Location**: Arises from the middle ear.
  - **Radiological Features**:
    - **CT**: Mass with bone erosion and intense enhancement.
    - **MRI**: Hyperintense on T2-weighted images, with a "salt and pepper" appearance on T1-weighted images.
    - **Ultrasound**: Hypoechoic mass with increased vascularity.
    - **MIBG Scintigraphy**: Positive uptake indicating catecholamine secretion.
5. **Aorticopulmonary Paraganglioma (Pulmonary Paraganglioma)**:
  - **Location**: Arises from the aorticopulmonary region.
  - **Radiological Features**:
    - **CT**: Homogeneous mass with intense enhancement.
    - **MRI**: Hyperintense on T2-weighted images, with a "salt and pepper" appearance on T1-weighted images.
    - **Ultrasound**: Hypoechoic mass with increased vascularity.
    - **MIBG Scintigraphy**: Positive uptake indicating catecholamine secretion.
6. **Abdominal Paraganglioma (Organ of Zuckerkandl)**:
  - **Location**: Arises from the organ of Zuckerkandl, located near the aorta.
  - **Radiological Features**:
    - **CT**: Homogeneous mass with intense enhancement.
    - **MRI**: Hyperintense on T2-weighted images, with a "salt and pepper" appearance on T1-weighted images.
    - **Ultrasound**: Hypoechoic mass with increased vascularity.
    - **MIBG Scintigraphy**: Positive uptake indicating catecholamine secretion.
7. **Mediastinal Paraganglioma**:
  - **Location**: Arises in the mediastinum.
  - **Radiological Features**:
    - **CT**: Homogeneous mass with intense enhancement.
    - **MRI**: Hyperintense on T2-weighted images, with a "salt and pepper" appearance on T1-weighted images.
    - **Ultrasound**: Hypoechoic mass with increased vascularity.
    - **MIBG Scintigraphy**: Positive uptake indicating catecholamine secretion.
8. **Pheochromocytoma**:
  - **Location**: Arises from the adrenal medulla.

    Pheochromocytomas are rare catecholamine-secreting tumors that arise from chromaffin cells in the adrenal medulla or extra-adrenal paraganglia. Here are the detailed radiological features of pheochromocytomas across various imaging modalities:

- **Computed Tomography (CT)**:
  - **Non-contrast**: The tumor appears as a well-defined mass with variable attenuation.
  - **Contrast Enhanced**: Shows heterogeneous enhancement due to areas of necrosis or cystic degeneration. Pheochromocytomas often enhance more during the portovenous phase compared to the arterial phase.
  - **Findings**: Large size at presentation (usually >3 cm), presence of calcifications, and possible local invasion to adjacent structures.
- **Magnetic Resonance Imaging (MRI)**:
  - **T1-Weighted**: The tumor may appear isointense or slightly hyperintense compared to muscle.
  - **T2-Weighted**: Typically shows a hyperintense signal.
  - **Postcontrast**: Exhibits intense enhancement with a characteristic "salt and pepper" appearance due to the presence of numerous small blood vessels.
  - **Fat Suppression**: Helps in better delineation of the tumor from surrounding fat.
  - **Findings**: High T2 signal intensity in approximately one-third of solid tumors.
- **Ultrasound**:
  - **Echogenicity**: Pheochromocytomas can appear as hypoechoic or isoechoic masses.
  - **Vascular Flow**: Demonstrates prominent vascular flow within the tumor on Doppler imaging.
  - **Findings**: Presence of cystic areas and calcifications.
- **Nuclear Medicine (MIBG Scintigraphy)**:
  - **Metaiodobenzylguanidine (MIBG) Scintigraphy**: Useful for detecting extra-adrenal pheochromocytomas, especially those that are catecholamine-secreting.
  - **Uptake**: Pheochromocytomas typically show increased uptake of MIBG.
  - **Findings**: Helps in identifying the extent of the disease and detecting metastatic lesions.

Clinical Relevance

Identifying the radiological features of paragangliomas is crucial for accurate diagnosis and management. The imaging characteristics help differentiate paragangliomas from other tumors and guide treatment planning, including surgical intervention and monitoring for recurrence.

5. 1-year-old boy with limping since 1 month—(a) Radiological role (b) Causes and imaging. [10] [DNB June 22]

Radiological Role

When a 1-year-old boy presents with limping for a month, radiological imaging plays a crucial role in diagnosing the underlying cause.

Here is a detailed overview of the radiological evaluation process:

Initial Clinical Assessment

1. **History and Physical Examination**:
   - **History**: Detailed history including onset, duration, progression, associated symptoms (pain, fever, weight loss), and any history of trauma.
   - **Physical Examination**: Assess gait, check for tenderness, range of motion, and any visible deformities or masses.

Radiological Imaging Modalities

1. **Plain Radiographs (X-rays)**:
   - **Indications**: First-line imaging for initial assessment of musculoskeletal complaints.
   - **Techniques**: Anteroposterior (AP) and lateral views of the involved limb, sometimes including the contralateral limb for comparison.
   - **Findings**:
     - **Fractures**: Displacement, angulation, and healing stages of fractures.

    - **Bone Tumors**: Lytic or sclerotic lesions, periosteal reaction.
    - **Infections**: Osteomyelitis presents as bone destruction and periosteal reaction.
    - **Developmental Disorders**: Legg–Calvé–Perthes disease shows fragmentation and sclerosis of the femoral head; slipped capital femoral epiphysis (SCFE) shows displacement of the femoral head.
2. **Ultrasound**:
    - **Indications**: Useful for soft tissue evaluation and detecting joint effusions.
    - **Techniques**: Real-time imaging with the possibility of dynamic assessment.
    - **Findings**:
        - **Hip Effusion**: Fluid collection in the joint capsule.
        - **Soft Tissue Masses**: Characterization of cystic vs. solid masses.
        - **Tendon Injuries**: Tendon thickening, tears, or inflammation.
3. **Magnetic Resonance Imaging (MRI)**:
    - **Indications**: Detailed evaluation of soft tissues, bone marrow, and joint structures.
    - **Techniques**: T1-weighted, T2-weighted, and contrast-enhanced sequences; sometimes includes fat suppression.
    - **Findings**:
        - **Osteomyelitis**: Bone marrow edema, abscess formation.
        - **Bone Tumors**: Extent of the tumor, involvement of adjacent structures.
        - **Soft Tissue Injuries**: Muscle tears, ligament injuries.
        - **Inflammatory Conditions**: Juvenile idiopathic arthritis shows synovial thickening, joint effusion.
4. **Computed Tomography (CT) Scan**:
    - **Indications**: Detailed evaluation of bone architecture and complex fractures.
    - **Techniques**: High-resolution axial images with multiplanar reconstructions.
    - **Findings**:
        - **Complex Fractures**: Detailed assessment of fracture lines, bone fragments.
        - **Bone Lesions**: Characterization of cortical involvement, mineralization patterns.
        - **Intra-articular Pathology**: Joint surface irregularities, loose bodies.
5. **Bone Scintigraphy (Bone Scan)**:
    - **Indications**: Highly sensitive for detecting bone abnormalities, especially when the source of pain is unclear.
    - **Techniques**: Involves intravenous injection of a radiotracer followed by imaging.
    - **Findings**:
        - **Infections**: Increased radiotracer uptake in areas of osteomyelitis.
        - **Tumors**: Increased uptake in malignant bone lesions.
        - **Fractures**: Stress fractures show focal areas of increased uptake.

Laboratory Tests

1. **Blood Tests**:
    - **Inflammatory Markers**: Erythrocyte sedimentation rate (ESR), C-reactive protein (CRP), and white blood cell count (WBC) to assess for infection or inflammation.
    - **Specific Tests**: Blood cultures, serological tests for infections, and tumor markers if malignancy is suspected.
2. **Joint Aspiration**:
    - **Septic Arthritis**: Aspiration of joint fluid for culture and analysis, especially in cases of suspected septic arthritis.

Interpretation of Findings

- **Fractures**: Look for signs of acute or healing fractures, including displacement and alignment.
- **Bone Tumors**: Assess for lytic lesions, periosteal reactions, and soft tissue involvement.
- **Infections**: Identify signs of osteomyelitis or septic arthritis, such as bone destruction, periosteal reaction, and joint effusion.

- **Neuromuscular Disorders**: Evaluate for muscle atrophy, fatty infiltration, and other signs of neuromuscular conditions.

Causes and Imaging

Limping in a 1-year-old boy can be due to various causes, each with distinct radiological features.

Here are some detailed potential causes along with their imaging features:

1. **Physical Injury**:
   - **Cause**: Minor trauma, falls, or bumps.
   - **Imaging Features**:
     - **Plain Radiographs (X-rays)**: Fractures may show displacement, angulation, and healing stages.
     - **Ultrasound**: Soft tissue injuries, such as sprains or strains, may show fluid collection or tendon injuries.
2. **Transient Synovitis (Irritable Hip)**
   - **Cause**: Inflammation of the hip joint lining, often following a viral infection.
   - **Imaging Features**:
     - **Ultrasound**: Joint effusion (fluid collection) in the hip.
     - **MRI**: Increased signal intensity in the synovium and joint fluid.
3. **Infections**:
   - **Cause**: Septic arthritis (bacterial infection in the joint) or osteomyelitis (bone infection).
   - **Imaging Features**:
     - **Plain Radiographs (X-rays)**: Bone destruction, periosteal reaction.
     - **MRI**: Bone marrow edema, abscess formation.
     - **Bone Scintigraphy (Bone Scan)**: Increased radiotracer uptake in areas of infection.
4. **Juvenile Idiopathic Arthritis (JIA)**
   - **Cause**: Chronic arthritis affecting children.
   - **Imaging Features**:
     - **Plain Radiographs (X-rays)**: Joint space narrowing, erosions.
     - **MRI**: Synovial thickening, joint effusion, bone marrow edema.
5. **Legg–Calvé–Perthes Disease**:
   - **Cause**: Reduced blood flow to the femoral head, leading to bone death.
   - **Imaging Features**:
     - **Plain Radiographs (X-rays)**: Fragmentation and sclerosis of the femoral head.
     - **MRI**: Bone marrow edema, subchondral fractures.
6. **Slipped Capital Femoral Epiphysis (SCFE)**:
   - **Cause**: Slipping of the femoral head due to a weakened growth plate.
   - **Imaging Features**:
     - **Plain Radiographs (X-rays)**: Displacement of the femoral head.
     - **MRI**: Detailed assessment of the epiphyseal slip and any associated complications.
7. **Congenital Hip Dislocation**:
   - **Cause**: Developmental issue present from birth.
   - **Imaging Features**:
     - **Plain Radiographs (X-rays)**: Dislocation of the hip joint.
     - **Ultrasound**: Assessment of hip joint stability and alignment.
8. **Tumors**:
   - **Cause**: Rare bone tumors causing pain and limping.
   - **Imaging Features**:
     - **Plain Radiographs (X-rays)**: Lytic or sclerotic lesions, periosteal reaction.

    - **MRI**: Extent of the tumor, involvement of adjacent structures.
    - **Bone Scintigraphy (Bone Scan)**: Increased radiotracer uptake in malignant lesions.
9. **Neuromuscular Disorders**:
    - **Cause**: Conditions affecting muscle strength and coordination.
    - **Imaging Features**:
        - **MRI**: Muscle atrophy, fatty infiltration, and other signs of neuromuscular conditions.
10. **Leg Length Discrepancy**:
    - **Cause**: Structural difference in leg lengths.
    - **Imaging Features**:
        - **Plain Radiographs (X-rays)**: Measurement of leg lengths and assessment of alignment.
11. **Other Causes**:
    - **Cause**: Inflammatory diseases, serious bone diseases.
    - **Imaging Features**:
        - **MRI**: Detection of inflammation, bone marrow change.

A thorough clinical evaluation, including history, physical examination, and appropriate radiological imaging, is essential for diagnosing the cause of limping in children. Early and accurate diagnosis ensures appropriate management and treatment, preventing potential complications and improving outcomes.

6. Skeletal finding in leukemia and hemolytic anemia. [10] [DNB June 22, DNB Dec 19]

Skeletal Finding in Leukemia and Hemolytic Anemia

Leukemia

Introduction: Leukemia is a hematological neoplasm characterized by the overproduction of immature (blasts) or abnormally differentiated cells of the hematopoietic system in the bone marrow that often, but not always, extends into the peripheral blood and, therefore, may involve multiple organs, including also the muscles and soft tissues.

Radiological findings: Skeletal leukemia (leukemic involvement of the bones) can present with various radiological findings, depending on the type of leukemia (acute or chronic) and the extent of bone involvement. These findings are typically observed on X-rays, CT scans, and MRI.

Below are the common radiological features of skeletal leukemia:

1. **Bone Marrow Infiltration (Bone Marrow Edema)**:
    - **MRI**: One of the most sensitive imaging modalities to detect bone marrow involvement. It shows bone marrow edema, which appears as a hyperintense signal on T2-weighted images and hypointense on T1-weighted images.
    - **CT**: May show diffuse or patchy low-density areas in the bones due to marrow replacement by leukemic cells.
2. **Osteolytic Lesions**:
    - **X-ray/CT**: Osteolytic lesions are the most common skeletal manifestation, presenting as ill-defined, punched-out areas of bone destruction. These can occur in any part of the skeleton, but are especially common in the pelvis, spine, ribs, and long bones.
    - The lesions may be unilateral or bilateral and may range from small, well-circumscribed to large, more diffuse areas of bone loss.
    - **"Moth-eaten" appearance**: This is characterized by multiple small, irregular lytic areas, resembling a moth-eaten pattern, which can be seen in both acute and chronic leukemias.
3. **Periosteal Reaction**:
    - **X-ray**: A periosteal reaction is often seen in acute leukemia (especially in the context of infiltration and inflammation), appearing as new bone formation on the surface of the affected bones.
    - This may manifest as a laminated or spiculated appearance, indicative of reactive bone changes, which are also seen in other malignant conditions.

4. **Fractures**:
    - **X-ray/CT/MRI**: Due to the loss of bone density from leukemic infiltration, pathologic fractures are common, particularly in the long bones, pelvis, and spine. These fractures often occur without significant trauma.
5. **Joint Involvement**:
    - **X-ray/MRI**: Leukemic involvement may extend into the joints, causing synovial thickening or even joint effusions. This can result in joint deformities or limited range of motion.
    - In the case of chronic leukemia, there may be chronic osteoarthritis-like changes with joint space narrowing and sclerosis.
6. **Skeletal Deformities and Bone Shape Changes**:
    - **X-ray**: In chronic cases of leukemia, particularly chronic myelogenous leukemia (CML), skeletal deformities can develop, including subluxation, bone erosion, or bony sclerosis.
    - In children with acute lymphoblastic leukemia (ALL), growth disturbances may result in abnormal bone shape and length.
7. **Sclerosis**:
    - **X-ray/CT**: In chronic leukemias like CML, bone sclerosis may occur as a reactive change. This can be seen as increased bone density in the form of patchy or generalized sclerosis, particularly in the metaphyseal regions of the long bones.
8. **Leukemic Infiltration in the Spine**:
    - **MRI**: Spinal involvement in leukemia can present as vertebral body collapse, bone marrow infiltration, and in severe cases, spinal cord compression.
    - **X-ray**: Involvement of the spine may appear as vertebral lysis or deformity due to bone destruction.
9. **Soft Tissue Swelling**:
    - **X-ray/CT/MRI**: Soft tissue masses or swelling, due to leukemic infiltration, may be observed. This is often seen around joints or at the site of bone destruction, and the masses can be heterogeneous in appearance.
10. **Leukemic Infiltration of the Skull**:
    - **X-ray/CT**: Leukemic infiltration can cause diffuse thinning of the calvarial bones or perforation of the skull with lumpy, bumpy lesions, particularly in the orbital and paranasal sinuses.
11. **Changes in Bone Density**:
    - **X-ray/CT**: Due to marrow infiltration by leukemic cells, the bone density may be reduced, leading to osteopenia or osteoporosis. This is a common feature in acute leukemias.

Summary of Common Imaging Modalities in Skeletal Leukemia:

- **X-ray**: Best for detecting bone lesions, fractures, periosteal reaction, and bone deformities.
- **CT Scan**: Provides detailed imaging of bone destruction, osteolytic lesions, and fractures.
- **MRI**: Most sensitive for detecting bone marrow infiltration, soft tissue involvement, and spinal cord compression.
- **Bone Scintigraphy**: Sometimes used to assess bone involvement, particularly in chronic leukemias.

Hemolytic Anemia

Skeletal changes in hemolytic anemia are primarily seen in chronic forms, especially in sickle cell anemia, thalassemia, and other hereditary hemolytic anemias. The bone changes are due to chronic bone marrow hyperactivity, secondary complications (like osteonecrosis or bone infarcts), and the effects of chronic hemolysis. Radiological findings may vary depending on the specific type of hemolytic anemia and the presence of associated complications.

Below are some key radiological findings related to skeletal involvement in hemolytic anemia:

1. **Bone Marrow Expansion**:
    - **X-ray**: In chronic hemolytic anemia (e.g., thalassemia and sickle cell anemia), the body attempts to compensate for the excessive RBC destruction by increasing bone marrow production. This leads to medullary expansion and a resultant thinning of the cortical bone, often seen on X-ray.
    - **"Hair-on-end" Appearance**: A classic radiological feature, especially in thalassemia, is the hair-on-end appearance of the skull on X-ray, due to expanded bone marrow in the flat bones of the skull. This results from trabecular bone formation in response to increased hematopoiesis.

- **MRI**: MRI is more sensitive and can show bone marrow hyperplasia, with an increased signal on T2-weighted images, reflecting increased marrow activity and expansion.

2. **Osteoporosis and Osteopenia**:
   - **X-ray/CT**: Chronic hemolysis and increased bone marrow activity can lead to osteopenia or osteoporosis, particularly in individuals with sickle cell disease and thalassemia. Radiographs may show generalized bone thinning and decreased bone density, making the bones more prone to fractures.
   - **MRI**: MRI can show bone marrow changes and areas of marrow fat replacement in cases of chronic anemia and marrow expansion.
3. **Osteonecrosis (Avascular Necrosis)**:
   - **X-ray/CT/MRI**: One of the more serious skeletal complications, especially in sickle cell disease, is osteonecrosis or avascular necrosis (AVN), typically involving the hip, shoulders, knees, and spine. This occurs due to vascular occlusion by sickled red blood cells, leading to decreased blood flow and bone death.
   - **X-ray**: Early osteonecrosis may appear as subtle subchondral lucency or flattening of the joint surfaces, particularly in the femoral head.
   - **MRI**: MRI is the gold standard for detecting osteonecrosis in sickle cell disease. It shows subchondral bone lesions, bone marrow edema, and joint space narrowing. In later stages, the bone may appear collapsed, and changes in the articular surface are visible.
4. **Bone Infarcts**:
   - **X-ray/CT/MRI**: In sickle cell disease and thalassemia, bone infarcts can occur due to impaired blood flow, leading to local ischemia and death of bone tissue. These infarcts can affect the long bones, spine, ribs, and pelvis. On X-ray, bone infarcts may appear as ill-defined, patchy, lytic areas.
   - **MRI**: MRI is the most sensitive imaging modality for detecting bone infarcts. It typically shows areas of low signal on T1-weighted images and high signal on T2-weighted images, indicating bone marrow edema and ischemia. In chronic infarcts, bone sclerosis or cystic changes may be seen.
5. **Joint Deformities and Changes**:
   - **X-ray/MRI**: Chronic hemolytic anemia can lead to joint deformities, especially in sickle cell anemia, due to the effects of osteonecrosis, bone infarcts, and vascular compromise. Commonly affected joints include the hips, knees, shoulders, and spine. X-rays may show joint space narrowing, degenerative changes, and subchondral sclerosis.
   - In sickle cell disease, degenerative joint disease can develop as a result of avascular necrosis or chronic infarction.
   - **MRI**: In cases of osteonecrosis or bone infarction, MRI can detect the involvement of the joint space and soft tissues, such as joint effusions or synovial thickening.
6. **Sickle Cell Disease Specific Findings**:
   - **"Crew-Cut" Skull**: In sickle cell anemia and thalassemia, expansion of the bone marrow in the skull can cause a characteristic "crew-cut" appearance on X-ray, which is caused by increased trabecular bone formation in the calvarium. This is also associated with bone marrow hyperplasia.
   - **Spinal Changes**: In sickle cell anemia, there can be vertebral collapse due to infarction and ischemia, leading to kyphosis or scoliosis. These changes can be seen on X-ray as vertebral body flattening or wedge-shaped deformities.
   - **MRI**: MRI of the spine can show spinal infarcts and bone marrow changes, such as decreased signal intensity on T1-weighted images and increased signal intensity on T2-weighted images, indicating ischemia or infarction of the vertebrae.
7. **Fractures**:
   - **X-ray**: Due to bone weakness from marrow expansion, osteopenia, and osteonecrosis, individuals with chronic hemolytic anemia are at an increased risk of pathologic fractures. These fractures may be subtle or occur in areas of previously healthy bone.
   - **MRI**: In case of fracture, MRI may help assess soft tissue involvement and the extent of any associated damage (e.g., joint or muscle injury).

8. **Skeletal Changes Due to Iron Overload (Thalassemia)**:
   - **X-ray/CT**: Thalassemia patients may develop skeletal changes related to iron overload, especially in the liver and heart. Although these changes are more often seen on MRI, X-ray and CT can sometimes show cardiomegaly, sclerosis, and deposits in the liver.
   - **MRI**: MRI is sensitive in detecting iron deposition in organs, which can indirectly affect bone health due to altered hematopoiesis and organ function.
9. **Chronic Osteomyelitis**:
   - **X-ray/CT/MRI**: Sickle cell disease can increase the risk of osteomyelitis (bone infection) due to impaired blood flow and the increased susceptibility to bacterial infections. Radiographs may show bone lysis, periosteal reaction, or sequestra (dead bone) in affected bones.
   - **MRI**: MRI is highly sensitive for detecting osteomyelitis, showing bone marrow edema, periosteal reaction, and abscess formation.

Summary of Radiological Findings in Skeletal Hemolytic Anemia:

- Splenomegaly and Hepatomegaly (Ultrasound/CT)
- Bone Marrow Expansion (X-ray: "Hair-on-end" appearance, MRI: Bone marrow hyperplasia)
- Osteopenia/Osteoporosis (X-ray, CT, MRI)
- Osteonecrosis and Bone Infarcts (X-ray, MRI, CT)
- Joint Changes (X-ray, MRI)
- "Crew-Cut" Skull (X-ray)
- Spinal Deformities (X-ray, MRI)
- Fractures (X-ray, MRI)
- Iron Overload (MRI)
- Osteomyelitis (X-ray, CT, MRI)

7. Diffuse hyperostosis of the skull: Imaging. [10] [DNB Dec 21]

Diffuse hyperostosis of the skull refers to a condition where there is widespread abnormal bone formation or thickening of the bones of the skull. It can be associated with several conditions, and the radiological findings depend on the underlying cause of the hyperostosis. Below are some key radiological features seen in diffuse hyperostosis of the skull:

General Radiological Features of Diffuse Hyperostosis of the Skull

1. **Increased Bone Density (Sclerosis)**:
   - The most notable feature is the generalized **increased bone density** or sclerosis of the skull. This means that the bone appears denser than normal on X-rays or CT scans.
   - The cortical bone (outer layer) and sometimes the trabecular bone (inner layer) show thickening and sclerosis.
2. **Diffuse Skull Thickening**:
   - The calvarium (the dome of the skull) appears uniformly thickened. This can involve the frontal, parietal, and occipital bones, or in some cases, the entire skull.
   - The thickness is often more pronounced in the diploic space (the inner cancellous bone between the inner and outer tables of the skull), leading to a "trabecular pattern" on imaging.
3. **Cortical Thickening**: The **outer cortical bone** may appear especially thickened. This is often seen as a smooth, expanded outer table of the skull, while the inner table may remain relatively unaffected.
4. **Loss of Normal Cranial Landmarks**: Due to thickening and sclerosis, **normal cranial landmarks**, such as sutures, foramina (openings for blood vessels or nerves), and venous sinuses, may be obscured or diminished.
5. **Sutural Changes**: In some cases, **sutures** may be obliterated or appear prematurely closed, especially if the hyperostosis extends along the sutural lines. However, this is not always the case, and some sutures may remain patent even in the presence of significant hyperostosis.

6. **Hyperostosis May Involve Other Craniofacial Structures**:
   - In certain conditions, other parts of the craniofacial skeleton (such as the jaw, orbits, or facial bones) may also show signs of hyperostosis, though this is less common.
   - **Mandibular hyperostosis** or abnormal bone growth in the jaw may be seen in some syndromes, for example.
7. **Potential for Soft Tissue Involvement**: There may be evidence of soft tissue changes in some conditions associated with diffuse hyperostosis, such as abnormal calcifications or periosteal reactions in severe cases.

Specific Conditions Associated with Diffuse Hyperostosis of the Skull

1. **Hyperostosis Corticalis Generalisata (HCG)**: Also known as **van Buchem disease**, this rare condition involves generalized thickening of the cortical bone, particularly in the skull. The radiographic findings include:
   - Widespread **cortical thickening** of the skull, leading to a "heavy skull" appearance.
   - Obliteration of the **frontal and parietal sutures**.
   - The diploic space may be narrow or obliterated, and the inner cortical bone is often unaffected.
2. **Paget's Disease of Bone**:
   - Paget's disease can involve the skull, leading to **enlargement and deformity** of the affected bones.
   - Radiological findings include **increased bone density**, along with **coarsened trabeculae** and **increased bone turnover**, leading to thickened, enlarged bones that may have a "cotton-wool" appearance.
   - Paget's disease may cause **skull deformities**, including a **wide and thickened calvarium**.
3. **Osteopetrosis (Albers-Schönberg Disease)**:
   - This genetic disorder causes **increased bone density** due to impaired bone resorption, leading to **diffuse sclerosis** of the skull.
   - Radiological findings may include the **"bone within a bone" appearance**, which is the result of thickened trabeculae, and the **"sandwich vertebra"** appearance in the spine.
   - The skull shows **uniform thickening**, particularly of the calvarial bones.
4. **Fibrous Dysplasia**:
   - Although not typically diffuse, **fibrous dysplasia** can cause localized hyperostosis of the skull, often leading to **ground-glass opacity** or a **"blade of grass" appearance** on imaging.
   - This condition can result in asymmetric thickening of bones but may involve the entire skull in more severe cases.
5. **Diffuse Idiopathic Skeletal Hyperostosis (DISH)**:
   - DISH is a condition characterized by **calcification of ligaments and tendons**, particularly the anterior longitudinal ligament of the spine, and may occasionally affect the skull.
   - Radiographs may show **flowing ossification** along the spine, but skull involvement is less frequent.
6. **Chronic Renal Failure and Uremic Osteodystrophy**:
   - Chronic kidney disease can lead to **metabolic bone disease**, where diffuse **hyperostosis** of the skull is sometimes seen due to **secondary hyperparathyroidism**.
   - Imaging may show **generalized bone sclerosis** or **thickening** in the skull and other skeletal structures.
7. **Cranial Calcifications in Infectious or Inflammatory Diseases**:
   - Some chronic infections (e.g., **tuberculosis**) or conditions that cause **chronic inflammation** may lead to **hyperostosis** or calcification of the skull bones.
   - Radiological features may include areas of **calcification** or **hyperostosis** in the skull, though this is usually localized and not diffuse.

Imaging Modalities for Evaluation

- **X-ray**: The most common and initial imaging technique, especially to assess the density and thickness of the skull bones.
- **CT Scan**: Provides more detailed images of the bone, allowing assessment of cortical and trabecular involvement. It is particularly useful when the skull deformities are subtle or complex.

- **MRI**: While not typically used to evaluate bone sclerosis, MRI may be helpful to assess soft tissue involvement, including brain or dural changes if there is suspicion of associated conditions (e.g., tumors, infections).

8. Write a short note on: Perthe's disease. [5] [DNB Dec 21]

Perthe's disease, also known as Legg-Calvé-Perthes disease, is a condition where there is avascular necrosis (loss of blood supply) to the femoral head in children, typically between the ages of 4 and 8. This leads to degeneration, collapse, and potential deformity of the femoral head and the hip joint. The disease is divided into different stages based on the progression of the condition, and radiological findings are critical in assessing the extent of involvement.

Stages of Perthe's Disease

Perthes disease is divided into five stages, based on the progression of the disease and the changes in the femoral head. These stages include:

1. **Initial Stage (Stage I)**: **Avascular Necrosis Phase**:
   - The first phase occurs when the blood supply to the femoral head is disrupted. This leads to bone death (necrosis) and a decrease in the size and density of the femoral head.
   - **Radiological Findings**:
     - **X-ray**: Initial softening of the femoral head may be seen, with a loss of bone density.
     - The femoral head may appear rounder and less well-defined, as the bone begins to lose its structural integrity.
     - A radiolucent area (area that appears darker on the X-ray) may be seen in the femoral head, indicating the loss of bone density due to necrosis.
2. **Fragmentation Stage (Stage II)**: **Resorption and Fragmentation Phase**:
   - During this stage, the femoral head begins to fragment, and the bone undergoes resorption. The bone starts to break apart and collapse. This stage is characterized by the loss of bone structure and the development of joint space narrowing.
   - **Radiological Findings**:
     - **X-ray**: Fragmentation of the femoral head can be seen, with parts of the femoral head appearing fragmented and irregular.
     - There may be increased radiolucency (more dark areas) due to the breakdown of the femoral bone.
     - The joint space may appear narrowed as the femoral head loses its spherical shape and begins to collapse.
     - Subchondral cysts or osteophytes (bone spurs) may begin to develop.
3. **Re-ossification Stage (Stage III)**: **Rebuilding and Healing Phase**:
   - In the re-ossification phase, new bone starts to replace the resorbed bone. The femoral head begins to heal, and new bone begins to form in the area of necrosis.
   - **Radiological Findings**:
     - **X-ray**: Regeneration of the femoral head can be seen as it starts to regain its density.
     - The femoral head may start to become rounder and more defined, though it may still have some deformity.
     - New bone formation can appear as increased radiopacity (lighter areas on the X-ray) as the femoral head revascularizes and reforms.
4. **Residual Stage (Stage IV)**: **Healing and Remodeling Phase**:
   - During this stage, the femoral head continues to heal and remodel. However, the femoral head may still have some residual deformity, which can affect the overall shape and function of the hip joint.
   - **Radiological Findings**:
     - **X-ray**: The femoral head may still appear flattened, with signs of residual deformity or irregularities.
     - Joint space narrowing may persist, and secondary osteoarthritis changes may be evident in the acetabulum (the socket of the hip joint).
     - Some sclerosis (hardening of the bone) may occur in the femoral head and neck.

5. **Healing and Remodeling Stage (Stage V): Final Stage**:
   - In the final stage, the femoral head is healed, but the shape may be permanently altered. The hip joint may develop secondary arthritis or changes due to the deformity of the femoral head.
   - **Radiological Findings**:
     - **X-ray**: The femoral head may appear deformed or flattened due to the changes that occurred during the disease process.
     - Osteoarthritis changes, such as joint space narrowing, acetabular changes, and osteophyte formation, may be visible.
     - The hip joint may show signs of degenerative changes due to the abnormal femoral head shape and the altered mechanics of the joint.

Radiological Findings at Each Stage of Perthes Disease

1. **Initial Stage (Avascular Necrosis)**:
   - **X-ray**:
     - Loss of bone density in the femoral head (radiolucency).
     - Slight flattening of the femoral head.
     - Possible soft tissue swelling around the hip joint.
2. **Fragmentation Stage (Resorption and Fragmentation)**:
   - **X-ray**:
     - Fragmentation of the femoral head with irregularities.
     - Increased radiolucency due to bone loss.
     - Joint space narrowing and changes in the acetabulum.
     - Possible presence of subchondral cysts and osteophytes.
3. **Re-ossification Stage (Rebuilding)**:
   - **X-ray**:
     - Early re-ossification with the femoral head beginning to regain bone density.
     - Femoral head may begin to regain a more rounded shape.
     - Some residual deformity may persist, such as flattening or irregularities.
4. **Residual Stage (Healing and Remodeling)**:
   - **X-ray**:
     - Femoral head may still appear flattened or misshapen.
     - Continued joint space narrowing.
     - Possible signs of secondary degenerative joint disease (DJD) or osteoarthritis in the hip joint.
     - Presence of sclerosis (bone hardening) in the femoral head.
5. **Final Stage (Healing and Remodeling)**:
   - **X-ray**:
     - The femoral head may show flattening, deformity, or irregularity due to permanent changes.
     - Arthritic changes such as joint space narrowing, osteophyte formation, and acetabular changes may be evident.
     - Secondary osteoarthritis can be seen in the hip joint.

Additional Imaging Modalities

- **MRI**: MRI is sometimes used to provide more detailed images of the soft tissue, bone marrow, and cartilage. It is particularly useful in detecting early changes in the femoral head, bone edema, and early stages of necrosis, especially when X-rays are inconclusive.
- **CT Scan**: CT can be used in more advanced stages to assess bone deformity or to evaluate the extent of joint destruction, especially if surgery is being considered.

9. Write a short note on: Cleidocranial dysplasia. [5] [DNB Dec 21]

Cleidocranial dysplasia (CCD) is a rare autosomal dominant disorder that affects the development of bones and teeth. The radiological findings associated with CCD primarily involve the skeleton, particularly the clavicles, skull, spine, and pelvis.

Here are the key radiological features of cleidocranial dysplasia:

1. **Clavicle Abnormalities**:
   - **Hypoplasia or Aplasia of the Clavicles**: The most characteristic feature of CCD is the underdevelopment or complete absence of the clavicles (collarbones). This results in shoulder deformities and an increased range of motion of the shoulders.
   - **Bilateral Absence or Hypoplasia**: In many cases, both clavicles are affected, although unilateral involvement is also possible.
2. **Skull and Facial Features**:
   - **Delayed Closure of Sutures**: The skull may show delayed closure of the sutures, leading to a relatively large, "open" skull in some individuals.
   - **Fontanelles**: The fontanelles (soft spots on the skull) may remain open for longer periods.
   - **Frontal and Parietal Bossing**: Prominent foreheads and parietal bulging can be seen, giving the skull a "dome-shaped" appearance.
   - **Midface Hypoplasia**: Underdevelopment of the middle face (especially the maxilla) is common, leading to a flattened facial profile.
   - **Absent or Underdeveloped Nasal Bones**: This may result in a flattened nasal bridge.
3. **Teeth and Jaw**:
   - **Supernumerary Teeth**: Radiographs often show multiple extra (supernumerary) teeth, especially in the upper jaw.
   - **Delayed Eruption of Teeth**: Tooth eruption is usually delayed, and permanent teeth may fail to erupt or erupt in an irregular pattern.
   - **Impacted Teeth**: Many teeth may be impacted or fail to emerge from the gums.
4. **Spine**:
   - **Spinal Abnormalities**: There may be anomalies in the vertebrae, such as scoliosis (lateral curvature of the spine), kyphosis (forward curvature), or other deformities.
   - **Rugger-Jersey Spine**: In some cases, a "rugger-jersey" spine appearance may be seen on X-rays, characterized by sclerosis of the vertebral endplates (appearance of a striped pattern on radiographs).
5. **Pelvis and Limbs**:
   - **Abnormal Pelvic Bones**: Radiographic findings may show broadening of the iliac wings (the top parts of the pelvis).
   - **Abnormalities of Long Bones**: The long bones of the limbs, including the femur and humerus, may show variations in shape or size, but they are typically less affected than other skeletal regions.
6. **Other Skeletal Findings**:
   - **Short Stature**: While not directly visible on X-ray, short stature is often present and may be associated with other skeletal anomalies.
   - **Bony Lesions**: Some individuals with CCD may have other bony abnormalities, such as an abnormal density or shape of bones.

Imaging Modalities

- X-rays are the most common imaging technique for identifying the skeletal features of CCD, particularly for clavicle hypoplasia or aplasia, skull abnormalities, and dental findings.
- CT scans can provide more detailed views of the craniofacial structures, particularly for assessing the skull and clavicles.
- MRI may be used in cases of spinal involvement or to assess the presence of any other soft tissue abnormalities.

10. Enumerate various causes for unilateral painful hips in a 10-year-old child. Discuss the role of imaging in any two pathologies. [2+8] [DNB June 20]

Unilateral Painful Limp in a Child <10 Years of Age

1. **Transient Synovitis**:
   - Common in this age group often self-limiting inflammation of the hip joint.
   - **Etiology**: Often follows a viral infection or minor trauma.
   - **Symptoms**: Sudden onset of hip pain and limping, often without fever.
   - **Diagnosis**: Clinical diagnosis supported by ultrasound showing joint effusion.
2. **Legg Calvé-Perthes Disease**:
   - **Description**: Avascular necrosis of the femoral head.
   - **Etiology**: Unknown, possibly related to vascular interruption.
   - **Symptoms**: Gradual onset of limp and hip pain, sometimes referred to the knee, with limited hip movement.
   - **Diagnosis**: X-ray shows increased density of the femoral head followed by fragmentation and reossification.
3. **Slipped Capital Femoral Epiphysis (SCFE)**:
   - **Description**: Displacement of the femoral head relative to the neck at the growth plate. Etiology: Often occurs during rapid growth spurts, associated with obesity or hormonal imbalances.
   - **Symptoms**: Gradual onset of hip, thigh, or knee pain, with a limp and restricted hip movement.
   - **Diagnosis**: X-ray showing the femoral head displaced posteriorly and inferiorly relative to the femoral neck.
4. **Septic Arthritis**:
   - **Description**: Infection of the hip joints
   - **Etiology**: Bacterial infection, commonly *Staphylococcus aureus*.
   - **Symptoms**: Acute onset of severe hip pain, fever, and inability to bear weight.
   - **Diagnosis**: Elevated white blood cell count, ESR, CRP, and ultrasound showing joint effusion. Joint aspiration confirms the diagnosis.
5. **Osteomyelitis**:
   - **Description**: Infection of the bone, commonly affecting the proximal femur.
   - **Etiology**: Bacterial infection, often hematogenous spread.
   - **Symptoms**: Gradual onset of localized bone pain, fever, and swelling.
   - **Diagnosis**: Elevated inflammatory markers, MRI showing bone marrow oedema, and possible bone biopsy.
6. **Juvenile Idiopathic Arthritis (JLA)**:
   - **Description**: Chronic arthritis in children under 16, affecting one or more joints.
   - **Etiology**: Autoimmune disease.
   - **Symptoms**: Chronic joint pain and swelling, morning stiffness, and decreased range of motion.
   - **Diagnosis**: Clinical diagnosis supported by elevated inflammatory markers and imaging showing joint effusion or synovitis.
7. **Trauma**:
   - **Description**: Fractures or soft tissue injuries to the hip or proximal femur.
   - **Etiology**: Falls, sports injuries, or accidents.
   - **Symptoms**: Acute onset of pain, inability to bear weight, and localized tenderness,
   - **Diagnosis**: X-rays to detect fractures or dislocations; MRI may be needed for soft tissue injuries.
8. **Developmental Dysplasia of the Hip (DDH)**:
   - **Description**: Abnormal development of the hip joint.
   - **Etiology**: Congenital or developmental factors.
   - **Symptoms**: Limping, pain, or decreased hip movement.
   - **Diagnosis**: Clinical examination with Ortolani and Barlow tests, confirmed by ultrasound or X-ray.

Role of Imaging

Slipped Capital Femoral Epiphysis (SCFE)

Imaging Modalities

1. **X-ray**:
   - **Role**: Primary diagnostic tool for SCFE.
   - **Views**: Anteroposterior (AP) and frog-leg lateral views are typically obtained.
   - **Findings**:
     - Frog-Leg Lateral View: Best for visualizing the degree of slippage. The "ice cream slipping off the cone" sign is characteristic.
     - AP View: Widening and irregularity of the growth plate, decreased height of the epiphysis, and alignment changes.
2. **MRI**:
   - **Role**: Used when X-rays are inconclusive or to assess early, pre-slip SCFE, and complications.
   - **Findings**:
     - Edema: Increased signal in the metaphysis and growth plate on T2-weighted images, indicating early slip before it becomes apparent on X-ray.
     - Physeal Abnormalities: Detailed view of the growth plate showing irregularity and widening.
     - Associated Changes: Assessment of surrounding soft tissues and detection of concurrent conditions like synovitis.
3. **CT Scan**:
   - **Role**: Less commonly used but can be helpful for preoperative planning and in complex cases where 3D reconstruction of the hip is beneficial.
   - **Findings**: Precise delineation of the extent of slippage and any associated deformities of the femoral head and neck.
4. **Ultrasound**:
   - **Role**: Rarely used for diagnosis but can be helpful in very early cases or in patients who cannot undergo MRI.
   - **Findings**: May show joint effusion and subtle changes in the epiphyseal plate.

Clinical Utility:

- **Diagnosis**: X-rays are crucial for initial diagnosis and classification of the slip severity (mild, moderate, or severe).
- **Monitoring**: Serial imaging is important to monitor the progression of the slip and the response to treatment.
- **Preoperative Planning**: Detailed assessment of the slip and femoral head position to guide surgical intervention.
- **Postoperative Follow-Up**: Imaging, particularly X-ray and sometimes MRI, is used to assess the success of surgical treatment and detect complications such as avascular necrosis.

Developmental Dysplasia of Hip (DDH)

Imaging Modalities

1. **Ultrasound (US)**:
   - **Role**: Primary imaging modality for newborns and infants under 6 months of age.
   - **Techniques**:
     - Static Ultrasound: Measures key angles and assesses the position of the femoral head within the acetabulum.
     - Dynamic Ultrasound: Evaluates the stability of the hip using stress maneuvers (e.g., Barlow and Ortolani tests).
   - **Findings**:
     - Graf Classification: Uses measurements like the alpha and beta angles to classify hip maturity and dysplasia.
     - Hip Subluxation or Dislocation
     - Acetabular Development
2. **X-ray**:
   - **Role**: Preferred imaging modality for children over 6 months when the femoral head begins to ossify.

- **Views**:
  - Anteroposterior (AP) Pelvis: Standard view for assessing hip development.
  - Frog-Leg Lateral View: Sometimes used to provide additional information about hip positioning.
- **Findings**:
  - Acetabular Index: Angle measurement to assess acetabular slope and depth.
  - Hilgenreiner's Line: A horizontal line through the triradiate cartilages; used as a reference for other measurements.
  - Perkin's Line: A vertical line from the lateral aspect of the acetabulum; used to assess femoral head positioning.
  - Shenton's Line: A continuous curve formed by the superior margin of the obturator foramen and the inferior border of the femoral neck; interruption suggests dislocation.
  - Delayed Ossification: Indicates developmental delays in the femoral head ossification.

3. **Magnetic Resonance Imaging (MRI)**:
   - **Role**: Used in complex cases, preoperative planning, and postoperative follow-up.
   - **Findings**:
     - Cartilage Anatomy: Detailed view of the acetabular cartilage, labrum, and the femoral head.
     - Reduction Assessment: Useful in evaluating the success of closed or open reduction procedures.
     - Associated Pathologies: Identifies concurrent abnormalities like labral tears or synovitis.
4. **Computed Tomography (CT)**:
   - **Role**: Less commonly used due to radiation exposure but valuable in specific scenarios.
   - **Applications**:
     - Preoperative Planning: Detailed bony anatomy and alignment, particularly in complex or recurrent cases.
     - Postoperative Assessment: Evaluates the position of the femoral head and the quality of the reduction.
   - **Findings**:
     - 3D Reconstructions: Provides detailed anatomical views of the hip joint, aiding in surgical planning.
     - Bony Alignment: Accurate assessment of the acetabulum and femoral head relationship.

Clinical Utility

- **Diagnosis**
  - **Screening**: Ultrasound is the preferred method for early screening in at-risk infants (e.g., breech presentation, family history of DDH).
  - **Confirmation**: Ultrasound can confirm instability or dysplasia seen in physical examination using dynamic techniques.

11. A 14-year-old male presented with fever, pain and swelling of the right proximal arm. (a) What are the various differential diagnosis? (b) Discuss in brief, the role of imaging in the evaluation of such a case. [3+7] [DNB June 20]

Differential diagnoses in a case of 14-year-old male presented with fever, pain and swelling of right proximal arm:

1. **Osteomyelitis**:
   - **Description**: An infection and inflammation of the bone.
   - **Clinical Features**: Fever, localized pain, swelling, warmth, and sometimes redness over the affected area.
   - **Diagnosis**: Elevated white blood cell count, ESR, CRP, blood cultures, and imaging (X-ray, MRI, or bone scan).
2. **Septic Arthritis**:
   - **Description**: Infection within a joint, commonly bacterial.
   - **Clinical Features**: Severe pain, fever, swelling, and limited range of motion in the affected joint.
   - **Diagnosis**: Joint aspiration and analysis, blood cultures, elevated inflammatory markers, and imaging.
3. **Cellulitis**:
   - **Description**: A bacterial skin infection that can extend to deeper tissues.

- **Clinical Features**: Red, swollen, warm, and tender skin. Fever and lymphangitis (red streaks) may also be present.
- **Diagnosis**: Clinical examination, blood cultures, and possibly ultrasound to check for abscess formation.

4. **Pyomyositis**:
   - **Description**: A bacterial infection of the skeletal muscles, often caused by *Staphylococcus aureus.*
   - **Clinical Features**: Localized muscle pain, swelling, tenderness, and fever.
   - **Diagnosis**: MRI, ultrasound, blood cultures, and elevated inflammatory markers.
5. **Ewing's Sarcoma**:
   - **Description**: A malignant bone tumor commonly affecting adolescents.
   - **Clinical Features**: Pain and swelling at the site of the tumor, fever, and sometimes a palpable mass.
   - **Diagnosis**: Imaging (X-ray showing a characteristic "onion-skin" appearance, MRI, CT), biopsy, and bone scan.
6. **Osteosarcoma**:
   - **Description**: A primary malignant bone tumor typically occurring in children and adolescents.
   - **Clinical Features**: Progressive pain, swelling, and sometimes a palpable mass. Fever is less common but may occur.
   - **Diagnosis**: X-ray (showing a "sunburst" pattern), MRI, CT, biopsy, and bone scan.
7. **Rhabdomyosarcoma**:
   - **Description**: A malignant tumor of skeletal muscle origin, more common in children.
   - **Clinical Features**: Pain, swelling, and sometimes fever, depending on the location.
   - **Diagnosis**: Imaging (MRI or CT), biopsy, and possibly PET scan.
8. **Leukemia**:
   - **Description**: A malignancy of the blood and bone marrow.
   - **Clinical Features**: Bone pain, fever, fatigue, pallor, and other signs of bone marrow suppression (anemia, thrombocytopenia).
   - **Diagnosis**: Complete blood count (CBC), bone marrow biopsy, and imaging if localized pain is present.
9. **Trauma/Fractures**:
   - **Description**: Injury to the bone or surrounding tissues.
   - **Clinical Features**: History of trauma, localized pain, swelling, and sometimes deformity.
   - **Diagnosis**: X-ray, CT scan for complex fractures.
10. **Juvenile Idiopathic Arthritis (JIA)**:
    - **Description**: An autoimmune disorder causing inflammation of the joints.
    - **Clinical Features**: Joint pain, swelling, stiffness, fever, and fatigue.
    - **Diagnosis**: Clinical examination, blood tests (RF, ANA), and imaging (ultrasound, MRI).
11. **Bursitis**:
    - **Description**: Inflammation of a bursa (a small fluid-filled sac near joints).
    - **Clinical Features**: Localized swelling, pain, and reduced movement in the affected area.
    - **Diagnosis**: Clinical examination, ultrasound, and MRI if needed.
12. **Reactive Arthritis**:
    - **Description**: Arthritis that develops in response to an infection elsewhere in the body.
    - **Clinical Features**: Joint pain and swelling, often accompanied by other systemic symptoms such as fever.
    - **Diagnosis**: Clinical examination, blood tests, and imaging if necessary.

Role of Imaging

1. **X-ray**:
   - **Purpose**: The first-line imaging tool used to assess bone structure and integrity. X-rays can quickly identify fractures, bone lesions, or abnormal growths.
   - **Utility**: Helps rule out or confirm fractures, detect bone tumors (like osteosarcoma and Ewing's sarcoma), or show signs of osteomyelitis (such as periosteal reactions and bone destruction).

2. **Ultrasound**:
   - **Purpose**: Utilized to evaluate soft tissues, muscles, and smaller structures not well visualized on X-rays.
   - **Utility**: Useful for detecting soft tissue abnormalities such as cellulitis, abscesses, pyomyositis, can also guide diagnostic procedures like aspiration or biopsy.
3. **Magnetic Resonance Imaging (MRI)**:
   - **Purpose**: Provides detailed images of bone and soft tissue, including marrow.
   - **Utility**: Excellent for diagnosing osteomyelitis, which might show bone marrow oedema before changes are visible on X-rays. MRI is invaluable for evaluating bone tumors, soft tissue tumors (like rhabdomyosarcoma), and differentiating between benign and malignant lesions. It also helps in assessing joint diseases such as septic arthritis or juvenile idiopathic arthritis.
4. **Computed Tomography (CT) Scan**:
   - **Purpose**: Offers detailed images of bone and can provide finer details than an X-ray.
   - **Utility**: Particularly useful when complex bone structures are involved or when precise details about bone destruction or tumor extension are needed. CT can be superior for evaluating complex fractures or in surgical planning.
5. **Bone Scan**:
   - **Purpose**: A nuclear imaging method that helps detect bone metabolism and blood flow.
   - **Utility**: Useful in detecting osteomyelitis, metastatic bone disease, or primary bone tumors over the whole body, indicating active bone processes that might not yet be visible on X-rays.
6. **Positron Emission Tomography (PET)**:
   - **Purpose**: Combined with CT (PET/CT), this provides metabolic and anatomical details.
   - **Utility**: Useful for identifying malignant tumors and their metastases, differentiating between benign and malignant lesions, and sometimes for infection.

Breast Imaging

1. USG findings in solid breast lesions. [10] [MD (WBUHS) 20]

Introduction: Ultrasound (USG) is a key modality in breast imaging, particularly for characterizing solid lesions. It complements mammography and is particularly useful in evaluating dense breasts, guiding biopsies, and distinguishing cystic from solid masses. Using the Breast imaging reporting and data system (BI-RADS) guidelines, ultrasound findings help stratify the risk of malignancy and plan management accordingly.

1. **Shape**:
   - **Benign**:
     - Round or oval shape with smooth contours, suggesting a noninfiltrative process.
     - Example: Fibroadenoma, which often presents as an oval, well-marginated mass.
   - **Malignant**: Irregular shapes with angulated or spiculated borders suggest malignancy due to infiltrative growth.
2. **Margins**:
   - **Benign**: Circumscribed and well-defined margins without invasion into surrounding tissue.
   - **Malignant**: Noncircumscribed margins with features like microlobulation, indistinct or angular edges, or spiculation. These suggest invasion or desmoplastic reaction.
3. **Orientation**:
   - **Benign**: Lesions with a "wider-than-tall" orientation are generally benign, as they grow parallel to tissue planes.
   - **Malignant**: A "taller-than-wide" orientation is a strong predictor of malignancy, indicating the lesion's tendency to invade deeper tissue planes.
4. **Echogenicity**:
   - **Benign**: Isoechoic or mildly hypoechoic. Homogeneous texture is typical of benign masses like fibroadenomas.

- **Malignant**: Markedly hypoechoic lesions with heterogeneous internal texture, indicating malignant transformation or necrosis.

5. **Posterior Acoustic Features**:
   - **Benign**: Posterior acoustic enhancement, particularly in cystic or fibroadenomatous lesions.
   - **Malignant**: Posterior acoustic shadowing caused by desmoplastic reaction or stromal fibrosis.
6. **Internal Characteristics**:
   - **Benign**: Homogeneous internal texture. Examples include fibroadenomas and lipomas.
   - **Malignant**: Heterogeneous internal architecture with necrosis, calcifications, or debris. Microcalcifications are particularly suspicious.
7. **Calcifications**: Calcifications can be identified on high-resolution ultrasound, although mammography remains superior for their detection. The appearance and distribution of calcifications are important in differentiating benign from malignant processes.
   - **Benign Calcifications**:
     - Coarse, macrocalcifications, or "popcorn-like" calcifications, often associated with fibroadenomas or involuting lesions.
     - Echogenic foci without posterior shadowing.
     - Often scattered and not clustered.
   - **Malignant Calcifications**:
     - Microcalcifications appear as punctate echogenic foci, sometimes forming clusters.
     - Associated with posterior shadowing if embedded in a hypoechoic lesion.
     - Often indicative of ductal carcinoma in situ (DCIS) or invasive malignancy.
   - **Significance of Calcifications on USG**
     - Calcifications in fibroadenomas: "Popcorn-like" macrocalcifications are diagnostic of older fibroadenomas undergoing involution.
     - Malignant calcifications: Microcalcifications in a hypoechoic mass or ductal distribution are highly suspicious for malignancy.

   The combination of calcifications and other features (e.g., spiculated margins, taller-than-wide orientation) significantly increases the likelihood of malignancy.
8. **Doppler Findings**:
   - **Benign**: Minimal or peripheral vascularity.
   - **Malignant**: Increased central vascularity with chaotic flow patterns. High resistive index (>0.7) is suggestive of malignancy.
9. **Additional Features**:
   - **Elastography**: Malignant lesions show increased stiffness compared to benign ones, with strain ratios above thresholds (e.g., >4.5).
   - **Axillary Lymph Nodes**: Enlarged nodes with cortical thickening (>3 mm) and loss of the fatty hilum suggest malignancy.

Role of Ultrasound in Common Solid Breast Lesions

- **Benign Lesions**:
  - **Fibroadenoma**:
    - Oval, wider-than-tall, well-defined, homogeneous hypoechoic with posterior enhancement.
    - Common in younger women.
  - **Abscess**: Complex cystic lesion with peripheral hyperemia on Doppler.
- **Malignant Lesions**:
  - **Invasive Ductal Carcinoma (IDC)**: Irregular, taller-than-wide, spiculated, hypoechoic, posterior shadowing.
  - **Invasive Lobular Carcinoma (ILC)**: Subtle, ill-defined masses with architectural distortion.

2. Discuss the role of MR in breast diseases. [10] [MD (WBUHS) 21]

1. **Indications for Breast MRI**: MRI is used in specific clinical scenarios where mammography and ultrasound may have limitations. Key indications include:
   - **Screening in High-Risk Patients**:
     - Recommended annually for women with a ≥20–25% lifetime risk of breast cancer (e.g., BRCA mutation carriers).
     - Detects cancers missed on mammography, especially in dense breasts.
   - **Diagnosis and Characterization**:
     - Differentiating benign from malignant lesions.
     - Identifying multifocal, multicentric, or contralateral disease in newly diagnosed breast cancer.
   - **Preoperative Planning**:
     - To assess tumor size, extent, and chest wall invasion in locally advanced cancers.
     - Detecting satellite lesions for breast-conserving surgery planning.
   - **Assessment of Treatment Response**:
     - Monitoring response to neoadjuvant chemotherapy (NAC).
     - Evaluating residual tumor post-treatment.
   - **Evaluation of Breast Implants**: Best modality for assessing implant integrity and detecting complications like rupture or silicone leakage.
   - **Problem-Solving Tool**: Clarifying inconclusive findings on mammography or ultrasound.
2. **MRI Techniques for Breast Imaging**:
   - **Dynamic Contrast-Enhanced MRI (DCE-MRI)**:
     - Most commonly used technique.
     - Involves rapid acquisition of sequences before and after intravenous gadolinium injection.
     - Kinetic curves (Type I, II, III) help differentiate benign from malignant lesions. Malignancies often show rapid enhancement with washout (Type III).
   - **Diffusion-Weighted Imaging (DWI)**:
     - Measures tissue cellularity via apparent diffusion coefficient (ADC).
     - Malignant lesions: Low ADC values due to restricted diffusion.
     - Benign lesions: Higher ADC values.
   - **MR Spectroscopy**:
     - Detects choline peaks in malignant lesions.
     - Useful in differentiating benign from malignant lesions.
   - **Fat-Suppressed Imaging**: Enhances lesion conspicuity, particularly in dense breasts.
   - **T2-Weighted Imaging**: Highlights cystic or necrotic components within lesions.
3. **MRI Features of Breast Diseases**:
   - **Enhancing lesions are divided into three main categories**: Characterize as focus/foci, masses, and areas of nonmass enhancement.
   - **Focus (or when multiple, foci)**: It is defined as an area of enhancement measuring less than 5 mm in diameter which is too small to characterize.
   - **A mass**:
     - It is a three-dimensional lesion that occupies a space within the breast.
     - Just as in mammography and ultrasound, we look at its shape, its margins and its internal characteristics: This includes its T1- and T2-characteristics as well its enhancement pattern.
   - **Nonmass like enhancement**:
     - There are areas of enhancement without a detectable three-dimensional mass.
     - Features of nonmass enhancement include its distribution, its internal enhancement pattern, and whether the enhancement is symmetric or asymmetric.

- **Benign Diseases**:
  - **Fibroadenomas**:
    - Well-defined, oval, hypointense on T1, hyperintense on T2.
    - Slow, persistent contrast enhancement (Type I curve).
  - **Breast Abscesses**: T2 hyperintense lesions with peripheral rim enhancement and restricted diffusion.
  - **Cystic Lesions**: High signal intensity on T2 with no enhancement post-contrast.
- **Malignant Diseases**:
  - **Invasive Ductal Carcinoma (IDC)**:
    - Irregular, spiculated mass with rapid enhancement and washout.
    - Associated with surrounding edema or skin thickening.
  - **Ductal Carcinoma in Situ (DCIS)**:
    - Nonmass enhancement in ductal distribution.
    - "Clumped" or "linear" enhancement pattern.
  - **Lobular Carcinoma**: Ill-defined lesions with diffuse enhancement, often multifocal or multicentric.
  - **Breast Metastases**: Multiple, well-circumscribed masses with peripheral enhancement.

4. **Advantages of MRI in Breast Imaging**:
   - **High Sensitivity**: Sensitivity of >90% for breast cancer detection, especially in dense breasts and high-risk populations.
   - **Multiplanar Imaging Capability**: Allows precise localization and characterization of lesions.
   - **Nonionizing Radiation**: Safe for younger patients and those requiring frequent imaging.
   - **Superior Soft Tissue Contrast**: Differentiates between fat, glandular tissue, and abnormal lesions.
5. **Limitations of MRI**:
   - **High Cost**: Limits availability and use in resource-constrained settings.
   - **Lower Specificity**: High false-positive rates lead to unnecessary biopsies.
   - **Contrast Agent Use**: Risk of nephrogenic systemic fibrosis in renal dysfunction patients.
   - **Longer Examination Time**: Requires patient cooperation, especially in claustrophobic individuals.
6. **Clinical Importance**:
   - **Post-Treatment Evaluation**: Differentiates scar tissue (no enhancement) from residual/recurrent tumor (enhancement).
   - **Male Breast Diseases**: Useful in gynecomastia versus male breast cancer differentiation.
   - **Breast Implants**: MRI is the gold standard for evaluating implant rupture.
   - **Intracapsular rupture**: "Linguine sign."
   - **Extracapsular rupture**: Free silicone in surrounding tissues.

3. Describe the anatomy of the breast with a diagram. Discuss the basic physics with the instrumentation of a mammography unit. What are the different mammographic projections? [4+4+2] [MD (WBUHS) 22, AIIMS May 24]

Anatomy of the Breast

1. **Type and Function**:
   - **Type**: Apocrine gland in both males and females.
   - **Function (Females)**: Milk production for neonatal nutrition and immune support.
2. **Gross Anatomy (Fig. 6)**:
   - **Structure**: Inhomogeneous, composed of:
     - Adipose tissue
     - Glandular tissue (parenchyma: acini and ducts)
     - Fibrous tissue (stroma: Cooper's ligaments and connective tissue)

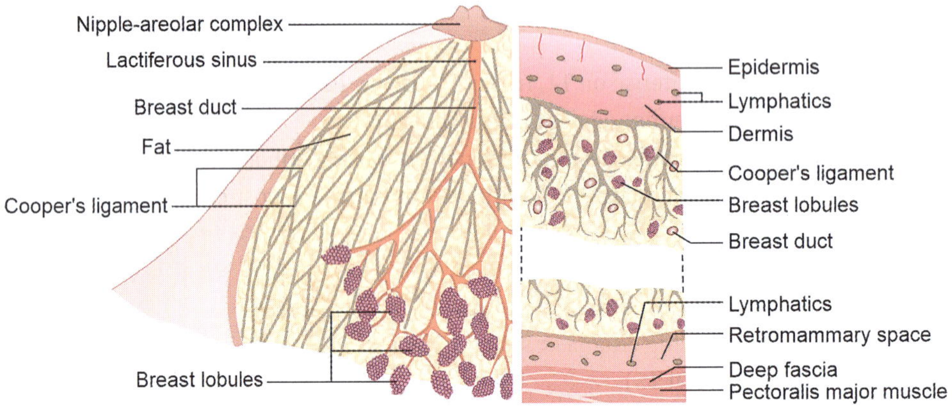

FIG. 6: Normal breast anatomy.

- **Lobes**: 14–18 lactiferous lobes, each with several lobules and acini.
- **Ducts**: Each lobe drains via a lactiferous duct to the nipple-areola complex.

3. **Hormonal Influence**:
   - **Estrogen-Dependent Growth**:
     - Increases glandular tissue during adolescence.
     - Further proliferation during pregnancy and lactation.
     - Atrophies postlactation and accelerates after menopause.
4. **Relations**:
   - **Superior**: Clavicle.
   - **Inferior**: 6th rib and middle sternum.
   - **Lateral**: Midaxillary line.
   - **Medial**: Sternum.
   - **Axillary Tail**: Extension of breast tissue into the axilla.
5. **Blood Supply**:
   - **Arteries**:
     - Internal thoracic artery perforators (2nd–5th).
     - Thoracoacromial artery.
     - Lateral thoracic artery.
     - Intercostal perforators (3rd–8th).
   - **Veins**: Axillary vein, internal thoracic vein, and posterior intercostal vein.
6. **Lymphatic Drainage**: Major route for the spread of malignancy. Includes axillary, internal mammary, and supraclavicular nodes.
7. **Innervation**:
   - **Thoracic intercostal nerves**: T3–T5.
   - **Supraclavicular nerves**: From cervical plexus

Basic Physics of Mammography

- **Principles of X-Ray Generation**:
  - Mammography utilizes low-energy X-rays (17–24 keV) to achieve high contrast between soft tissues.
  - The primary interaction in mammography is the photoelectric effect, enhancing contrast between glandular and fatty tissues.
- **Breast Compression**: Compression spreads tissue evenly, reduces radiation dose, minimizes motion, and improves image sharpness.

- **Key Physical Concepts**:
  - **Contrast**: Achieved by optimizing the X-ray beam's energy to differentiate between tissues.
  - **Spatial Resolution**: Essential for detecting small microcalcifications or masses.

Instrumentation of a Mammography Unit

- **X-Ray Tube**:
  - Molybdenum or rhodium targets produce low-energy X-rays ideal for soft tissue imaging.
  - Operates at 25–35 kVp for optimal contrast.
- **Compression Paddle**: Reduces breast thickness for uniform imaging, improving sharpness and lowering dose.
- **Detector System**:
  - **Film-Screen Mammography**: Combines film with a fluorescent screen for image capture.
  - **Digital Mammography**: Uses flat-panel detectors to directly capture and store images.
- **Anti-Scatter Grid**: Reduces scatter radiation, improving image contrast. Grid ratio is ~4:1 to 5:1.
- **Automatic Exposure Control (AEC)**: Adjusts exposure based on breast density and size.
- **Magnification View**: A smaller focal spot (0.1–0.3 mm) enhances resolution for evaluating microcalcifications.

Mammographic Projections

1. **Standard Views**:
   - **Craniocaudal (CC)**:
     - Vertical X-ray beam
     - Nipple seen in profile.
     - Demonstrates subareolar, medial and lateral portions.
   - **Adequacy**:
     - Difference between PNL measurement on MLO and CC view is <1 cm.
     - On 30% of CC: Pectoralis major muscle visible, medial tissue should be included.
     - If lesion seen in only CC view-rolled cc view.
   - **Mediolateral Oblique (MLO)**:
     - Tube angled at 45 degree to the horizontal.
     - Angle depends on orientation of pectoralis muscle (45–60).
     - Breast pulled upward and out.
     - Maximum breast tissue is demonstrated.
   - **Adequacy**:
     - Pectoralis major visible till level of axis of nipple.
     - Open inframammary fold.
     - No motion blur (exception oedema).
     - No artifact: Dust, scratches, bad pixel.
   - **Lesion seen on only MLO**:
     - Obscured on CC view or located far lateral.
     - Exaggerated CC view or true lateral view.
2. **Additional Views**:
   - **Lateral (Mediolateral—ML)**: Useful for lesion localization.
   - **Spot Compression View**: Isolates and compresses a specific area to clarify findings.
   - **Magnification View**: Used to assess microcalcifications.
   - **Cleavage View**: Evaluates medial portions of both breasts.
   - **Axillary tail view**: Cleopatra view.

4. Ultrasound lexicon of BI-RADS. [5] [MD (WBUHS) 22, AIIMS Dec 23]

The Breast imaging-reporting and data system (BI-RADS) ultrasound lexicon provides standardized terminology to describe ultrasound findings in breast imaging. It ensures uniform communication among radiologists, clinicians, and surgeons. Below are the key components of the BI-RADS 5th edition ultrasound lexicon **(Table 6)**:[18]

TABLE 6: Key components of the BI-RADS 5th edition ultrasound lexicon.

Ultrasound		
Tissue composition (screening only)	a. Homogeneous background echotexture—fat b. Homogeneous background echotexture—fibroglandular c. Heterogeneous background echotexture	
Masses	**Shape**	• Oval • Round • Irregular
	Orientation	• Parallel • Not parallel
	Margin	• Circumscribed • Not circumscribed – Indistinct – Angular – Microlobulated – Spiculated
	Echo pattern	• Anechoic • Hyperechoic • Complex cystic and solid • Hypoechoic • Isoechoic • Heterogeneous
	Posterior features	• No posterior features • Enhancement • Shadowing • Combined pattern
Calcifications	Calcifications in a mass	
	Calcifications outside of a mass	
	Intraductal calcifications	
Associated features	Architectural distortion	
	Duct changes	
	Skin changes	• Skin thickening • Skin retraction
	Edema	
	Vascularity	• Absent • Internal vascularity • Vessels in rim
	Elasticity assessment	• Soft • Intermediate • Hard

Continued...

Continued...

Ultrasound		
Special cases	Simple cyst	
	Clustered microcysts	
	Complicated cyst	
	Mass in or on skin	
	Foreign body including implants	
	Lymph nodes—intramammary	
	Lymph nodes—axillary	
	Vascular abnormalities	• Ateriovenous malformations/pseudoaneurysms (VMs) • Mondor disease
	Postsurgical fluid collection	
	Fat necrosis	

5. BI-RADS classification system. [5] [DNB Dec 19]

The breast imaging-reporting and data system (BI-RADS) classification system is a standardized system developed by the American College of Radiology (ACR) for reporting breast imaging findings. It includes categories for mammography, ultrasound, and MRI to provide a structured approach to describing findings, assessing malignancy risk, and guiding management.

Here is the BI-RADS 5th edition classification system **(Table 7)**:

TABLE 7: BI-RADS 5th edition: Final assessment categories.

Final assessment categories			
Category		***Management***	***Likelihood of cancer***
0	Need additional imaging or prior examinations	Recall for additional imaging and/or await prior examinations	n/a
1	Negative	Routine screening	Essentially 0%
2	Benign	Routine screening	Essentially 0%
3	Probably benign	Short interval-follow-up (6 months) or continued	>0% but <2%
4	Suspicious	Tissue diagnosis	4a. Low suspicion for malignancy (>2% to ≤10%) 4b. Moderate suspicion for malignancy (>10% to ≤50%) 4c. High suspicion for malignancy (>50% to ≤95%)
5	Highly suggestive of malignancy	Tissue diagnosis	≥95%
6	Known biopsy-proven	Surgical excision when clinically appropriate	n/a

Application Across Modalities

The BI-RADS classification can be applied to findings in:

- **Mammography**: Focuses on mass, asymmetry, calcifications, and architectural distortion.
- **Ultrasound**: Uses features like shape, orientation, margins, echo pattern, and posterior acoustic features.
- **MRI**: Includes dynamic contrast enhancement patterns, lesion morphology, and kinetic curves.
- **Utility of BI-RADS**:
  - Standardizes communication between radiologists and clinicians.

- Facilitates comparison of results across institutions.
- Helps guide management decisions based on risk stratification.
- Aids in patient education about breast imaging findings.

6. Describe the role of sonography in the evaluation of breast lumps. [5] [MD (WBUHS) 17]

Sonography (ultrasound) plays a crucial role in evaluating breast lumps, particularly as an adjunct to mammography. It is a real-time, noninvasive imaging modality that provides high-resolution images, especially for dense breast tissue. The following points summarize its role:

1. **Differentiation of Cystic vs. Solid Lesions**:
   - **Simple Cysts**:
     - Anechoic with posterior acoustic enhancement.
     - Thin-walled and well-circumscribed.
   - **Solid Lesions**:
     - Evaluates echotexture, margins, and vascularity (via Doppler imaging).
     - Helps determine if a palpable lump is benign or requires further evaluation.
2. **Characterization of Solid Masses**:
   - **Benign Features**:
     - Oval shape, parallel orientation (wider than tall).
     - Circumscribed margins and uniform internal echoes (e.g., fibroadenomas).
   - **Suspicious Features**:
     - Irregular shape, nonparallel orientation (taller than wide).
     - Spiculated or microlobulated margins.
     - Heterogeneous echotexture and posterior shadowing.
3. **Assessment of Elastography**:
   - **Elastography adds functional information by assessing tissue stiffness**:
   - **Shear-Wave Elastography (SWE)**: Measures quantitative stiffness values (kPa). Malignant lesions are typically stiffer (>80–100 kPa).
   - **Strain Elastography**:
     - Qualitative comparison of lesion deformability under compression.
     - Malignant lesions appear darker and less compressible than benign ones.

   Elastography increases specificity in distinguishing benign vs. malignant lesions when used with B-mode imaging.
4. **Evaluation of Vascularity (Doppler Imaging)**:
   - **Doppler ultrasound is essential for assessing lesion vascularity**:
   - **Benign Lesions**:
     - Minimal or peripheral vascularity (e.g., fibroadenomas).
   - **Malignant Lesions**:
     - Increased central vascularity with penetrating vessels.
     - Chaotic or tortuous vessel architecture.

   Doppler findings correlate with tumor angiogenesis and are often combined with elastography and morphology to improve diagnostic accuracy.
5. **Characterization of Calcifications**: Although mammography remains the gold standard for evaluating calcifications, sonography can detect and characterize specific types:
   - **Benign Calcifications**: Large, coarse, and associated with fibroadenomas or fat necrosis.
   - **Malignant Calcifications**:
     - Microcalcifications in soft tissue masses or ductal distributions (e.g., DCIS).
     - Use of high-frequency transducers improves detection.

6. **Evaluation of Axillary Lymph Nodes**: Ultrasound assesses axillary nodes for metastatic involvement:
   - **Benign Nodes**: Oval with a preserved fatty hilum and thin cortex (<3 mm).
   - **Suspicious Nodes**: Enlarged, round, with cortical thickening (>3 mm) or loss of hilum.

   Doppler imaging evaluates vascularity patterns (displaced or absent hilar vessels suggest malignancy).
7. **Guidance for Interventions**:
   - **Biopsy**: Core needle biopsy or fine-needle aspiration of suspicious masses or lymph nodes.
   - **Cyst Aspiration**: For symptomatic relief or to confirm diagnosis in atypical cysts.
   - **Localization**: Presurgical placement of wire markers for excision of non-palpable lesions.

Advantages of Sonography

- **Real-Time Imaging**: Excellent for assessing mobility and compressibility of masses.
- **No Radiation Exposure**: Ideal for young, pregnant, or lactating patients.
- **Adjunct in Dense Breasts**: Complements mammography by improving lesion detection.
- **Multifunctional Assessment**: Morphology, vascularity, stiffness, and calcifications evaluated in one modality.

Limitations of Sonography

- **Operator Dependence**: Image quality and interpretation vary with expertise.
- **Limited Sensitivity for Microcalcifications**: Mammography remains superior.
- **Reduced Specificity**: Benign lesions may appear suspicious, leading to unnecessary biopsies.

7. 60 year female breast masses d/d: Benign vs. malignant on USG and MRI. [10] [DNB Dec 21]

Breast masses in postmenopausal women, such as a 60-year-old female, require thorough evaluation because the risk of malignancy increases with age. The differentiation between benign and malignant masses relies on imaging modalities like ultrasound (USG) and MRI, which provide complementary information.

Benign Breast Masses

Common Benign Lesions in a 60-Year-Old Female

- Fibroadenomas (may calcify postmenopause).
- Cysts (simple, complex, or infected).
- Lipomas.
- Sclerosing Adenosis.
- Post-Surgical Changes/Scar Tissue.

Ultrasound Features of Benign Masses

- **Shape and Orientation**: Oval or round; parallel orientation (wider than tall).
- **Margins**: Smooth, circumscribed, and well-defined.
- **Echotexture**:
  - Homogeneous; simple cysts appear anechoic.
  - Lipomas show hyperechoic fat lobules.
- **Posterior Acoustic Features**: Posterior enhancement in cysts; shadowing uncommon unless calcified.
- **Vascularity**: Minimal or absent internal vascularity on Doppler imaging.

MRI Features of Benign Masses

- **Morphology**:
  - **Shape**: Round, oval, or lobulated.
  - **Margins**: Smooth and well-defined.

- **Internal Features**:
  - Nonenhancing dark internal septations typical of fibroadenomas.
  - Fat-containing lesions such as lipomas, hamartomas, or fat necrosis.
- **T1 and T2 Signal Characteristics**:
  - **T1**: High signal intensity indicates fat-containing lesions like hamartomas or fat necrosis.
  - **T2**: High signal on T2-weighted images typically indicates cysts, fibroadenomas, or benign lymph nodes.

  Most benign lesions are bright on T2 except for colloid carcinoma, which is malignant but also hyperintense on T2.
- **Enhancement Pattern**:
  - **Homogeneous enhancement**: Uniform enhancement throughout the lesion.
  - **Persistent kinetic curve (Type 1)**: Slow and continuous enhancement over time.
  - Punctate or faint, scattered nonmass enhancement often symmetric and diffuse.
- **Calcifications**: Nonenhancing punctate calcifications may be seen in fibroadenomas or fat necrosis.
- **Benign NME**:
  - **Distribution**: Focal or patchy.
  - **Pattern**: Homogeneous or stippled.

  Associated with benign conditions like fibrocystic changes, sclerosing adenosis, or hormonal effects.
- **Associated Findings**: Absence of skin thickening, nipple retraction, or axillary lymphadenopathy.

Malignant Breast Lesions

- Common Malignant Lesions
- Invasive Ductal Carcinoma (IDC)
- Invasive Lobular Carcinoma (ILC)
- Ductal Carcinoma in Situ (DCIS)
- Metastases or Secondary Tumors

Ultrasound Features of Malignant Lesions

- **Shape and Orientation**: Irregular, taller-than-wide (nonparallel orientation).
- **Margins**: Spiculated, microlobulated, or indistinct.
- **Echotexture**: Heterogeneous or hypoechoic; necrosis may appear as complex cystic areas.
- **Posterior Features**: Posterior acoustic shadowing, associated with desmoplastic reaction.
- **Vascularity (Doppler Imaging)**: Increased vascularity with central tortuous vessels.

MRI Features of Malignant Lesions

A. **Morphology**:
  - **Shape**: Irregular.
  - **Margins**: Irregular or spiculated (80% likelihood of malignancy).

B. **Internal Features**:
  - Enhancing internal septations or central enhancement often indicate high grade malignancy.
  - Rim enhancement, especially in invasive ductal carcinoma, indicates necrosis or aggressive tumor.

C. **T1 and T2 Signal Characteristics**:
  - **T1**: Low-to-intermediate signal intensity is typical of solid tumors.
  - **T2**: Intermediate to low signal intensity. Exception: Colloid carcinoma, which is bright on T2.

D. **Enhancement Pattern**:
  - Heterogeneous or rim enhancement patterns.
  - **Washout kinetic curve (Type 3)**: Rapid initial rise with subsequent drop in enhancement.
  - **Segmental or linear enhancement** is often indicative of ductal carcinoma in situ (DCIS).

E. **Non-Mass Enhancement (NME)**: Clumped or heterogeneous enhancement.

F. **Distribution**:
- **Ductal (60% malignant)**: Enhancement confined to a single duct.
- **Segmental (78% malignant)**: Multiple ducts involved.
- **Linear (31% malignant)**: Linear or branching pattern without a ductal orientation.

G. **Associated Findings**:
- Skin or nipple thickening or retraction.
- Chest wall invasion.
- Axillary or internal mammary lymphadenopathy.

8. Indications of MRI breast. Technique of MRI breast. Nonenhancing mass in MRI breast. [10] [DNB June 21]

Indications of MRI Breast

Breast MRI is a highly sensitive imaging modality used for various diagnostic and screening purposes. Its indications include:

1. **Screening**:
   a. **High-risk patients**:
      - BRCA1/BRCA2 mutation carriers.
      - First-degree relatives of BRCA mutation carriers.
      - Lifetime risk >20–25% based on risk models.

   b. **History of chest radiation therapy (e.g., for Hodgkin's lymphoma).**

   c. **Dense breasts on mammography in high-risk individuals.**
2. **Diagnosis**:
   - Problem-solving for inconclusive findings on mammography or ultrasound.
   - Evaluation of lesions with suspicious or malignant features on other imaging.
3. **Preoperative Staging**:
   - Assessing extent of disease in newly diagnosed breast cancer.
   - Detecting multifocal, multicentric, or contralateral lesions.
   - Evaluating tumor size and invasion (e.g., into chest wall or pectoral muscles).
4. **Evaluation of Response to Therapy**: Neoadjuvant Chemotherapy: Monitoring tumor response to treatment.
5. **Assessment of Silicone Breast Implants**: Detection of implant rupture (intracapsular or extracapsular).
6. **Recurrence Detection**: Differentiating between postsurgical changes or scarring and tumor recurrence.
7. **Problem-Solving**:
   - Nipple discharge with negative mammography and ultrasound.
   - Screening in individuals with lobular carcinoma in situ (LCIS) or atypical ductal/lobular hyperplasia

Technique of Breast MRI

- **Patient Preparation**:
  - **Scheduling**:
    - Premenopausal women: Perform in the mid-menstrual cycle (days 7–14) to reduce hormonal influence.
    - Postmenopausal women: No specific timing required.
  - **Contrast**: Gadolinium-based contrast agent is typically used.
  - **Fasting**: 4–6 hours prior to minimize motion artifacts due to bowel activity.
  - **Positioning**: Patient lies prone with breasts suspended in a dedicated breast coil to reduce motion and provide uniform fat suppression.

- **MRI Sequences**:
  - **Precontrast Sequences**:
    - **T1-weighted**: For anatomical detail.
    - **T2-weighted**: For edema, cystic lesions, and assessing tissue characteristics.
    - **Fat-suppressed T2-weighted**: Differentiates fat-containing lesions.
  - **Dynamic Contrast-Enhanced (DCE) MRI**:
    - Series of T1-weighted images postgadolinium injection.
    - Acquired at multiple time points for kinetic analysis.
  - **Types of Curves**: Persistent, plateau, or washout (suspicious).
  - **Diffusion-Weighted Imaging (DWI)**: Assesses cellularity and diffusion restriction (malignant lesions show restriction with low ADC values).
  - **Postprocessing**:
  - **Subtraction Images**: Highlight enhancement.
  - **Maximum Intensity Projection (MIP)**: 3D visualization of enhancement patterns.

Nonenhancing Mass in MRI Breast

A nonenhancing breast mass refers to a lesion that does not exhibit significant uptake of gadolinium contrast during dynamic contrast-enhanced (DCE) MRI. While most malignant breast lesions demonstrate enhancement due to increased vascularity and permeability, some lesions may not enhance or only minimally enhance. Understanding non-enhancing masses requires careful evaluation of their imaging characteristics and clinical context.

1. **Typical Causes of Nonenhancing Masses**:
   - **Benign Lesions**:
     - **Simple Cysts**:
       - High signal intensity on T2-weighted images.
       - No internal enhancement on postcontrast sequences.
       - Well-defined, thin-walled, and anechoic on ultrasound.
     - **Fibroadenomas (Nonhyalinized)**:
       - May show minimal or absent enhancement, particularly in older fibroadenomas with stromal hyalinization.
       - Often oval, well-circumscribed, and homogeneous on T2.
     - **Lipomas**:
       - High signal intensity on T1, suppresses on fat-saturated sequences.
       - No internal enhancement.
     - **Fat Necrosis**:
       - T1 hyperintense (liquefied fat) or T2 hyperintense with no enhancement.
       - Irregular morphology may mimic malignancy, requiring correlation with clinical history.
     - **Hematomas**:
       - T1 hyperintense (acute hemorrhage) and no contrast enhancement.
       - Gradual signal changes over time.
   - **Malignant Lesions (Rare)**:
     - **Necrotic Tumors**:
       - Central nonenhancement due to necrosis surrounded by an enhancing viable tumor rim.
       - Typical in large, aggressive malignancies or poorly vascularized regions.
     - **Sclerotic or Desmoplastic Tumors**: May not enhance due to fibrotic stroma.
     - **Post-Treatment Changes**:
       - **Radiation Fibrosis or Scarring**: Nonenhancing, low T2 signal, and may distort architecture.
       - **Postsurgical Scars**: Linear or irregular, often non-enhancing with time.

2. **MRI Findings of Nonenhancing Masses**:
   - **MRI Sequences**:
     - **T1-Weighted Imaging**:
       - High signal intensity in fat-containing lesions (e.g., lipomas, fat necrosis).
       - Useful for detecting hemorrhage in hematomas.
     - **T2-Weighted Imaging**:
       - High signal intensity in fluid-filled lesions (e.g., cysts).
       - Low signal in fibrotic masses or sclerotic areas.
     - **Fat-Suppressed Sequences**: Suppression of signal in fat-containing lesions (e.g., lipomas, fat necrosis).
     - **Diffusion-Weighted Imaging (DWI)**:
       - Low signal with high ADC values in benign masses (e.g., cysts, fibroadenomas).
       - Restricted diffusion with low ADC in necrotic areas of some malignancies.
3. **Diagnostic Approach**:
   - **Evaluate Signal Characteristics**:
     - **T1**: High (fat necrosis, hematoma), Low (fibrous lesions).
     - **T2**: High (cyst, necrosis), Low (sclerotic tumors).
   - **Check Morphology**:
     - Well-circumscribed masses are more likely benign (e.g., fibroadenomas).
     - Irregular or spiculated lesions with non-enhancing components warrant concern.
   - **Assess with DCE MRI**: Persistent lack of enhancement after contrast excludes most malignancies.
   - **Use Ancillary Techniques**:
     - DWI: Evaluate for restricted diffusion in necrotic or cellular components.
     - Compare with mammography/ultrasound for correlation.
4. **Nonenhancing vs. Minimal Enhancing Masses**:
   - **Nonenhancing Masses**: Suggest benignity, though necrotic tumors are exceptions.
   - **Minimal Enhancement**: Seen in low-grade malignancies, some fibrotic tumors, and certain DCIS.
5. **Clinical Considerations**:
   - Patient history (e.g., prior surgery, trauma).
   - Symptoms (e.g., pain, nipple discharge).
   - Risk factors (e.g., age, family history, genetics).

9. Indications, technique, advantages, and limitations of MRI in imaging of breast cancer. [2+3+3+2] [DNB Dec 20, DNB June 20, MD (WBUHS) 17]

Indications of MRI Breast

Breast MRI is a highly sensitive imaging modality used for various diagnostic and screening purposes. Its indications include:

1. **Screening**:
   a. **High-risk patients**:
      - BRCA1/BRCA2 mutation carriers.
      - First-degree relatives of BRCA mutation carriers.
      - Lifetime risk >20–25% based on risk models.

   b. **History of chest radiation therapy (e.g., for Hodgkin's lymphoma).**

   c. **Dense breasts on mammography in high-risk individuals.**
2. **Diagnosis**:
   - Problem-solving for inconclusive findings on mammography or ultrasound.
   - Evaluation of lesions with suspicious or malignant features on other imaging.

3. **Preoperative Staging**:
   - Assessing extent of disease in newly diagnosed breast cancer.
   - Detecting multifocal, multicentric, or contralateral lesions.
   - Evaluating tumor size and invasion (e.g., into chest wall or pectoral muscles).
4. **Evaluation of Response to Therapy**: Neoadjuvant chemotherapy: Monitoring tumor response to treatment.
5. **Assessment of Silicone Breast Implants**: Detection of implant rupture (intracapsular or extracapsular).
6. **Recurrence Detection**: Differentiating between postsurgical changes or scarring and tumor recurrence.
7. **Problem-Solving**:
   - Nipple discharge with negative mammography and ultrasound.
   - Screening in individuals with lobular carcinoma in situ (LCIS) or atypical ductal/lobular hyperplasia.

Technique of Breast MRI

- **Patient Preparation**:
  - **Scheduling**:
    - Premenopausal women: Perform in the mid-menstrual cycle (days 7–14) to reduce hormonal influence.
    - Postmenopausal women: No specific timing required.
  - **Contrast**: Gadolinium-based contrast agent is typically used.
  - **Fasting**: 4–6 hours prior to minimize motion artifacts due to bowel activity.
  - **Positioning**: Patient lies prone with breasts suspended in a dedicated breast coil to reduce motion and provide uniform fat suppression.
- **MRI Sequences**:
  - **Precontrast Sequences**:
    - **T1-weighted**: For anatomical detail.
    - **T2-weighted**: For edema, cystic lesions, and assessing tissue characteristics.
  - **Fat-suppressed T2-weighted**: Differentiates fat-containing lesions.
  - **Dynamic Contrast-Enhanced (DCE) MRI**:
    - Series of T1-weighted images postgadolinium injection.
    - Acquired at multiple time points for kinetic analysis.
  - **Types of curves**: Persistent, plateau, or washout (suspicious).
  - **Diffusion-Weighted Imaging (DWI)**: Assesses cellularity and diffusion restriction (malignant lesions show restriction with low ADC values).
  - **Postprocessing**:
    - **Subtraction images**: Highlight enhancement.
    - **Maximum intensity projection (MIP)**: 3D visualization of enhancement patterns.

Advantages of Breast MRI

- **High Sensitivity for Breast Cancer Detection**: **Sensitivity for invasive cancers approaches 93–100%.**
- **Especially effective in**:
  - Dense breasts where mammography sensitivity is reduced.
  - Detecting small, multifocal, or multicentric cancers.
  - Identifying cancer in patients with silicone implants.
- **Preoperative Staging and Assessment of Tumor Extent**:
  - **Superior to mammography and ultrasound for assessing**:
    - Multifocal disease (additional lesions in the same quadrant).
    - Multicentric disease (lesions in different quadrants).
    - Contralateral cancer (5–10% detected in newly diagnosed cases).

- **Functional Imaging Capabilities**:
  - Dynamic Contrast-Enhanced (DCE) MRI: Characterizes lesions based on vascularity and kinetic enhancement patterns.
  - Diffusion-Weighted Imaging (DWI): Adds specificity by evaluating diffusion restriction (malignant lesions typically show low ADC values).
  - Differentiates scar tissue from recurrence, assesses treatment response during neoadjuvant chemotherapy, and identifies tumor residuals post-treatment.
- **No Radiation Exposure**: Safe for repeated imaging, making it ideal for high-risk screening and follow-up in younger patients.

Limitations of Breast MRI

1. **High False Positive Rate**:
   - While MRI is highly sensitive, its specificity is lower (72–88%), leading to unnecessary biopsies.
   - Benign lesions such as fibroadenomas, papillomas, and adenosis can enhance, mimicking malignancy.
2. **Cost and Limited Availability**:
   - Breast MRI is significantly more expensive than mammography or ultrasound, limiting its widespread use.
   - Requires specialized equipment (dedicated breast coil) and trained radiologists for interpretation.
3. **Not Suitable for All Patients**:
   - **Contraindications**:
     - Gadolinium: Risk of nephrogenic systemic fibrosis (NSF) in patients with severe renal dysfunction.
     - Claustrophobia or inability to lie prone.
     - Metal implants incompatible with MRI
4. **Overdiagnosis and Over-staging**: MRI may identify clinically insignificant lesions, leading to overtreatment or unnecessary surgical interventions.
5. **Timing and Hormonal Influence**: Premenopausal women require precise scheduling (mid-menstrual cycle) to avoid hormone-induced enhancement, which can reduce specificity

Vascular Diseases and Interventions

1. Doppler evaluation of acute lower limb ischemia. [5]

Doppler ultrasound is a key imaging modality for evaluating acute lower limb ischemia (ALLI). It is noninvasive, readily available, and provides real-time information about blood flow dynamics.

1. **Background and Indications**: Acute limb ischemia is defined as a sudden decrease in limb perfusion threatening tissue viability, usually within 14 days of symptom onset.
   - **Etiology**:
     - Embolism: Abrupt occlusion, often at bifurcations (e.g., common femoral artery).
     - Thrombosis: Typically superimposed on pre-existing atherosclerosis.
     - Trauma, dissection, or iatrogenic causes.
2. **Doppler Ultrasound Techniques**:
   - **Gray-Scale Imaging**:
     - Visualizes thrombus (echogenic or hypoechoic filling defect).
     - Detects vessel wall thickening or plaques in chronic disease.
   - **Color Doppler**:
     - Detects absent or reduced color flow in the occluded segment.
     - Presence of "aliasing" proximal to the stenosis.
     - Identification of collaterals.

- **Spectral Doppler**:
  - Evaluates velocity and waveform morphology at various levels.
  - Assesses the severity of occlusion or stenosis.

3. **Spectral Doppler Findings in ALLI**:
   - **Proximal to Occlusion**:
     - High-resistance waveform with decreased diastolic flow or reversal of diastolic flow.
     - Indicative of downstream resistance due to complete occlusion.
   - **At the Site of Occlusion**:
     - No flow signal in complete occlusion.
     - High-velocity "jet" in partial occlusion with turbulence (aliasing).
     - Peak systolic velocity (PSV) ratio >2: suggests >50% stenosis.
   - **Distal to Occlusion**:
     - Dampened, monophasic waveforms.
     - Reduced PSV.
     - Loss of triphasic or biphasic pattern due to low perfusion.
   - **Collaterals**: Low-velocity monophasic flow, often irregular in waveform.
4. **Systematic Approach**:
   - **Examine the entire arterial tree**: Starting from the iliac arteries to distal vessels (popliteal, tibial).
   - **Identify collateral flow**: Seen as low-velocity signals bypassing the occlusion site.
   - **Evaluate venous patency**: Rule out concurrent deep vein thrombosis (DVT), which may influence management.
5. **Findings in Acute Ischemia**:
   - **Complete Occlusion**: No detectable flow in the affected segment.
   - **Thrombotic vs. Embolic Occlusion**:
     - Thrombotic: Usually in the setting of pre-existing atherosclerosis; chronic plaques may be visible.
     - Embolic: Abrupt occlusion without underlying plaque; distal branches are often spared.
   - **Reduced Pulsatility**: Monophasic flow distal to the occlusion.
6. **Clinical Applications**:
   - **Acute vs. Chronic Ischemia**: Differentiated by Doppler findings: Chronic conditions show more collateral flow and vessel wall thickening.
   - **Postintervention Monitoring**: Evaluate success of revascularization or thrombolysis.
   - **Dynamic Studies**: Assess positional changes or exercise-induced flow alterations if relevant.
   - **Advantages of Doppler in ALLI**:
     - Immediate Diagnosis: Noninvasive, quick bedside evaluation.
     - Functional Assessment: Offers real-time information on hemodynamics.
     - Collateral Assessment: Critical for surgical planning.
   - **Limitations**:
     - Inability to visualize proximal aortoiliac segments.
     - Reduced accuracy in calcified vessels.
     - Operator dependency.

2. Role of interventional radiology in intra-arterial management of various neoplasms including paragangliomas. [DNB June 20, MD (WBUHS) 20]

Intra-arterial management of neoplasms involves delivering therapeutic agents directly into the blood supply of a tumor, which can enhance treatment efficacy while minimizing systemic side effects. This approach is particularly useful for highly vascular tumors.

One of the tumors where intraarterial chemotherapy was most successful is retinoblastoma.

Below is a detailed overview of various intra-arterial techniques and their applications in the management of different neoplasms:

1. **Transarterial Chemoembolization (TACE)**:
   - **Indications**: Primarily used for hepatocellular carcinoma (HCC) and metastatic liver tumors.
   - **Procedure**:
     - **Catheterization**: A catheter is inserted into the femoral artery and advanced to the hepatic artery.
     - **Chemotherapy Delivery**: A chemotherapeutic agent (e.g., doxorubicin) is infused directly into the tumor's blood supply.
     - **Embolization**: After chemotherapy, embolic agents (e.g., gelatin sponge, polyvinyl alcohol particles) are injected to occlude the blood vessels feeding the tumor, leading to ischemia and tumor necrosis.
   - **Benefits**: Reduces systemic toxicity, delivers high local drug concentrations, and can shrink tumors before surgery.
2. **Transarterial Radioembolization (TARE)**:
   - **Indications**: Commonly used for liver tumors, particularly in cases where TACE is ineffective or not feasible.
   - **Procedure**:
     - **Catheterization**: Similar to TACE, a catheter is placed into the hepatic artery.
     - **Radioactive Beads**: Small radioactive microspheres (e.g., Yttrium-90) are injected directly into the tumor's arterial supply.
     - **Mechanism**: The radiation emitted by the beads targets tumor cells while sparing normal liver tissue.
   - **Benefits**: Provides localized radiation therapy, potentially longer-lasting effects compared to traditional radiotherapy.
3. **Selective Internal Radiation Therapy (SIRT)**:
   - **Indications**: Used for patients with unresectable liver tumors or those who are not candidates for surgery.
   - **Procedure**:
     - **Microsphere Injection**: Similar to TARE, SIRT involves injecting microspheres that emit radiation directly into the tumor's blood supply.
   - **Benefits**: Minimally invasive, can be repeated if needed, and maintains the integrity of surrounding healthy tissue.
4. **Intra-Arterial Chemotherapy for Other Tumors**:
   - **Indications**: Used for a variety of tumors, including soft tissue sarcomas, pancreatic cancer, and neuroendocrine tumors.
   - **Procedure**:
     - **Direct Delivery**: Chemotherapy agents are delivered via a catheter into the artery supplying the tumor.
     - **Embolization**: Sometimes combined with embolization to enhance drug uptake and effectiveness.
   - **Benefits**: Higher local concentrations of chemotherapy and reduced systemic side effects.
5. **Transarterial Ablation Techniques**:
   - **Radiofrequency Ablation (RFA)**:
     - **Indications**: Suitable for small, localized tumors (e.g., liver, kidney).
     - **Procedure**: A needle electrode is inserted into the tumor through imaging guidance, and radiofrequency energy generates heat to destroy tumor cells.
   - **Microwave Ablation (MWA)**:
     - **Indications**: Similar to RFA, used for various tumors.
     - **Procedure**: Utilizes microwave energy to heat and destroy tumor tissue effectively.
6. **Embolization Techniques**:
   - **Indications**: Used for various tumors, including renal cell carcinoma, hepatocellular carcinoma, and uterine fibroids.
   - **Procedure**:
     - **Selective Embolization**: Catheter is placed in the artery supplying the tumor, and embolic agents (e.g., coils, particles) are deployed to occlude the vessel.
   - **Benefits**: Can lead to tumor necrosis, control bleeding, and alleviate symptoms.

7. **Management of Specific Neoplasms**:
   - **Neuroendocrine Tumors**: Selective arterial chemoembolization or TARE may be used, especially for liver metastases.
   - **Pancreatic Cancer**: Intra-arterial chemotherapy can be considered, particularly in advanced cases.
   - **Soft Tissue Sarcomas**: Intra-arterial chemotherapy may help in reducing tumor burden before surgical intervention.
   - **Paragangliomas**: Selective embolization may be performed to reduce vascularity and facilitate surgical excision.
   - **Brain tumor**: Intra-arterial (IA) chemotherapy is a form of regional delivery to brain tumors, designed to enhance the intra-tumoral concentrations of a given drug, in comparison with the intravenous route. Drugs that are likely to benefit from IA delivery have a rapid systemic clearance and include carmustine and other nitrosoureas, cisplatin, carboplatin, etoposide, and methotrexate. Recent studies suggest that toxicity can be reduced by the use of carboplatin- and methotrexate-based regimens.
   - **Retinoblastoma**: The three principal chemotherapeutics used intra-arterially are melphalan, topotecan and carboplatin. The alkylating agent melphalan (trade name Alkeran®) has been the most extensively used intra-arterial chemotherapeutic agent for the treatment of intraocular retinoblastoma.
   - **Hepatocellular carcinoma**: Intra-arterial (IA) therapies are a type of catheter-based treatment for hepatocellular carcinoma (HCC) that deliver therapeutic agents directly to the tumor. These therapies are considered palliative and are used to treat intermediate-stage HCC in patients with sufficient liver reserve.

Some types of IA therapies for HCC include:

- **Transarterial Chemoembolization (TACE)**: Involves injecting drug-eluting beads (DEBs) into the liver arteries to slowly release chemotherapy drugs.
- **Transarterial Radioembolization (TARE)**: Involves delivering a compound linked to radio-emitter particles to the tumor or hepatic end-arterioles.
- **Yttrium-90 Radioembolization (Y-90 RE)**:
  - Involves delivering yttrium-90 microspheres to deliver homogeneous irradiation to large tumors.
  - Other IA therapies include transarterial embolization (TAE) and hepatic artery infusion (HAI).

Paraganglioma

The cellular polymorphism of head and neck paragangliomas confers these tumors with their characteristics hyper-vascularization (angioarchitecture) with characteristic arteriographic signs and hemorrhage that justify presurgical embolization.

Intra-arterial management of paraganglioma depends on the type of paraganglioma and the extent of the tumor:

Cardiac Paraganglioma

Surgical resection is the primary treatment for cardiac paragangliomas. The surgical approach depends on the location and size of the tumor, and may involve:

- **Aortic Cannulation**: Usually performed in the distal ascending aorta
- **Venous Cannulation**: Typically, bicaval, with cannulation into the superior vena cava and the inferior vena cava
- **Cardiopulmonary Bypass**: Used to perform en-bloc excision and complex reconstruction
- **Cardiac Autotransplantation**: May be necessary for large, complex left atrial paragangliomas

Carotid and Vagal Paraganglioma

The extent of the tumor and the surgeon's experience determine the type of resection required. For example, simple arteriography has a lower stroke rate than reconstruction or ligation.

Conclusion: Intra-arterial management of neoplasms is a powerful tool in the oncologist's arsenal, allowing for targeted therapy that can improve outcomes while reducing systemic toxicity.

REFERENCES

1. Luijkx T, Wong K, Walizai T. Shoulder. [Online] Available from https://doi.org/10.53347/rID-33453 [Last accessed January, 2025].
2. Sutton D (Ed). A Textbook of Radiology and Imaging. 8th edition. New Delhi: Elsevier; 2023.
3. Khandelwal N, Gupta AK, Chowdhury V (Eds). AIIMS-MAMC-PGI's Comprehensive Textbook of Diagnostic Radiology. New Delhi: Jaypee Brothers Medical Publishers Pvt Ltd; 2016.
4. Nischal N, Iyengar KP, Herlekar D, Botchu R. Imaging of cartilage and chondral defects: an overview. Life (Basel). 2023;13(2):363.
5. Gaillard F, Knipe H, Yap J. Osteochondral defect. [Online] Available from: https://doi.org/10.53347/rID-1795 [Last accessed January 2025].
6. Gaillard F, Knipe H, Jones J. Osteochondral injury staging. [Online]. Available from: https://doi.org/10.53347/rID-1796 [Last accessed January 2025].
7. Pau GA. Anatomy of the ankle ligaments: a pictorial essay. Knee Surg Sports Traumatol Arthrosc. 2010;18(5):557-69.
8. Sawant YN, Sanghvi D. Magnetic resonance imaging of ankle ligaments: a pictorial essay. Indian J Radiol Imaging. 2018;28(4):419-26.
9. Weerakkody Y, Campos A, Ranchod A. Skeletal dysplasia. [Online]. Available from: https://doi.org/10.53347/rID-8804 [Last accessed January 2025].
10. Weerakkody Y, Kearns C, Odedeyi A. Acro-osteolysis. [Online] Available: https://doi.org/10.53347/rID-8610. [Last accessed January 2025].
11. Gaillard F, Ranchod A, Sharma R. Hypertrophic osteoarthropathy. [Online]. Available from: https://doi.org/10.53347/rID-1479 [Last accessed January 2025].
12. Gaillard F, Walizai T, Le L. Osteonecrosis of the femoral head. [Online] Available from: https://doi.org/10.53347/rID-7577 [Last accessed January 2025].
13. Chmiel-Nowak M, Campos A, Knipe H. ARCO classification of femoral head osteonecrosis. [Online]. Available from: https://doi.org/10.53347/rID-79781. [Last accessed January 2025].
14. Haaga JR, Boll D, editors. Computed Tomography & Magnetic Resonance Imaging of the Whole Body e-book. Amsterdam: Elsevier Health Sciences; 2008.
15. World Health Organization. Entitlement Eligibility Guideline Posttraumatic Stress Disorder. [Online] Available from: https://public.cdn.cloud.veterans.gc.ca/pdf/dispen/eeg/internal_derangement_knee. pdf [Last accessed January 2025].
16. Harvey H, Walizai T, Collins E. Pelvic fractures. [Online] Available from: https://doi.org/10.53347/rID-15002 [Last accessed January 2025].
17. Khurana B, Sheehan SE, Sodickson AD, Weaver MJ. Pelvic ring fractures: what the orthopedic surgeon wants to know. Radiographics. 2014;34(5):1317-33.
18. Mendelson EB, Böhm-Vélez M, Berg WA, Whitman GJ, Feldman MI, Madjar H. ACR BI-RADS® Ultrasound. ACR BI-RADS® Atlas, Breast Imaging Reporting and Data System. Reston, VA: American College of Radiology; 2013. p. 149.

CHAPTER

7 Interventional Radiology

Soumik Das, Suparna Sahu

QUESTIONS

1. Describe briefly various embolizing agents used in interventional procedures. [10] [DNB Dec 24, DNB Dec 18, MD (WBUHS) 24, AIIMS May 24]
2. Classify the commonly used embolizing agents. Discuss their advantages, disadvantages, and clinical applications. [3+(2+2+3)] [DNB June 20]

ANSWERS

1. Describe briefly various embolizing agents used in interventional procedures. [10] [DNB Dec 24, DNB Dec 18, MD (WBUHS) 24, AIIMS May 24]

Embolizing Agents

Embolizing agents are materials used to acutely stop blood flow in a vessel by mechanical occlusion. The clinical uses are to stop hemoptysis, hematuria, hematochezia, internal bleed or a pseudoaneurysm. Embolization may also be done as an adjunct to surgery or for palliation of malignant tumors. The embolizing agents can be temporary or permanent. The embolization can be done in proximal vessel or in distal bed. Further, the embolization may or may not lead to organ/cellular death.[1]

Based on these requirements, the embolizing agents are divided into four main categories:

Permanent Proximal Occluders

- **Coils**: These are made of steel or platinum. They commonly have constituent thrombogenic polyester fibers. They are introduced within the vessel in straightened condition but form a spring shape when ejected out of the distal end of delivery catheter. They form a scaffolding upon which thrombus forms leading to permanent occlusion of the vessel. The coils come in various sizes depending upon the size of the wire used, the length of the coil and the diameter of the unconstrained coil. A typical example is 35-3-4. The 35 represents the diameter of the wire used to make the coil in inches which in turn determines the catheter lumen through which it will pass through. The 3 represents the length of straightened coil in cm which is chosen based on length of vessel available for deployment of coil and the 4 represents the diameter of the unconstrained coil loop in mm which is chosen based on diameter of the vessel in which the coil is to be deployed. Coils measuring 0.018 inches or less are termed microcoils and require microcatheters for their deployment. Nester coils are special fibered coils on a platinum strut which are soft and pliable. They conform to the target vessel anatomy when deployed and mainly used for filling up space in large vessels or aneurysms as they bunch up within the lumen. The coils are of two types based on method of deployment:
    1. **Pushable**—can be pushed out of the catheter by a guidewire or coil pushers
    2. **Detachable**—are detached from the catheter tip in vivo by either mechanical pressure or electrolytically.
- **Amplatzer vascular plug**: It is a nitinol mesh device which is self-expandable occlusive agent. It is deployed by mechanical detachment and is used to occlude vessels ranging from 4 to 16 mm diameter. The other less commonly used materials in this category are detachable balloons made of latex or silicon (used for treatment of carotid-cavernous fistulas), small intestinal submucosa, suture material and bare angiographic wires.

Permanent Distal Occluders

Polyvinyl alcohol (PVA) particles: This is an inert plastic particle which comes in varying sizes from 100 to 1100 μm. It is available in small vials with each vial having particles of a range of sizes e.g., 300–500 μm, 500–700 μm, etc. It is in fine dry coarse powder form which needs to be suspended in saline or contrast before it is injected through the catheter. The size of the particles to be injected is chosen based on the size of the distal vessel bed to be embolized. The particles go and form clumps within the vessels to permanently occlude it. If larger size particles are chosen, they may cause clumping within the catheter or proximal vessel itself to lead to their occlusion. These are most commonly used in tumor bed embolizations (often preoperatively to decrease the vascularity), bronchial artery embolizations, uterine fibroid embolizations, etc. The endpoint is distal occlusion of the small arterioles without proximal vessel occlusion thereby keeping the option of future repeat embolization of the same vascular territory. PVA is also available in the form of spherical PVA which makes it more compressible and therefore facilitates the delivery. The typical examples are bead block made of hydrogel PVA or embospheres constituted from tris-acryl gelatin spherical hydrophilic spheres.

- **Sclerosants**: These are liquid agents which produce vascular occlusion by causing inflammation and thrombosis. Absolute alcohol and sodium tetradecyl sulfate (STS) are the two most commonly used sclerosants. Absolute alcohol, besides causing permanent vessel occlusion, also leads to cell death and tissue ablation. It is therefore reserved for use where the end organ cell death is acceptable, e.g., in renal cell carcinomas. It is a very painful procedure and thus is best performed under general anesthesia or liberal analgesia at least. The use of protective devices like proximal balloons is often required with the use of alcohol to prevent non-target embolization. Sodium tetradecyl sulphate (STS) is a relatively milder sclerosant which does not lead to cell death. A 3% concentration solution is used. It is not used intra-arterially but is mainly used for spermatic vein ablations, pelvic congestion syndrome and for venous vascular malformations. Bleomycin and polidocanol are other sclerosants which are used for same indications as above. They are comparatively of lesser efficacy but have an advantage of causing lesser inflammation and hence have lesser side effects.

- **Cyanoacrylates**: These are tissue adhesives. The most common used product is N-butyl cyanoacrylate (NBCA) or glue. These are in the form of clear liquids at room temperature which get instantly polymerized when they come in contact with an ionic environment. Thus, even a small amount of saline or blood leads to initiation of polymerization reaction of cyanoacrylates. For this reason, when they are to be injected via the delivery catheter, the catheter should be flushed completely with a non-ionic solution (most commonly used 20% dextrose) before and after each injection to prevent polymerization of the agent within the catheter. As soon as the agent ejects out of the distal catheter tip within the vessel, it comes in contact of blood (ionic) and gets polymerized to form a cast. Also, since the cyanoacrylates are radiolucent, they are delivered by mixing them with a radiopaque substance to make them visible under fluoroscopy. Ethiodol (brand name Lipiodol by Guerbet) is the most commonly used non-ionic substance for the same. It is usually mixed in ratio of 1:1 to 5:1 to make 50–20% concentration of glue respectively. The higher concentration of glue (lesser the amount of ethiodol added), the more proximal and earlier is the cast formation of glue when it comes in contact with blood at the distal end of catheter within the body. A lesser concentration leads to farther delivery of the embolic agent with a slightly delayed cast formation. The embolus which ultimately forms is larger than anticipated with the amount of cyanoacrylate as the substance draws blood elements within it. It is of reasonably lower cost compared to coils.
- **Onyx**: It is a liquid embolic agent formed by combination of ethylene-vinyl alcohol copolymer, dimethyl sulfoxide and tantalum powder. It comes in the form of two vials, one containing the copolymer mixed with tantalum powder and the other containing dimethyl sulfoxide. These need to mixed and placed in a shaker for 20 minutes immediately prior to injection for the agent to become ready for use. The onyx forms a cast as soon as it gets in contact with ionic material (like glue). The cast formation starts from outer surface to inner region. The major advantage of using onyx is much better control over the injection than glue but the deterrent is the significantly higher cost compared with other agents of this category.
- **Thrombin**: It is an enzyme which participates in the coagulation pathway and converts fibrinogen to fibrin. It is mainly used for hemostasis on surgically cut surfaces in the operation theatre. Intravascularly it has been used to induce thrombosis of pseudoaneurysms. Care is required to prevent its propagation into main vessel so as to prevent its occlusion.
- **Ethiodol**: Manufactured under the brand name Lipiodol. It is an inert oil-based contrast agent which is also used as embolizing agent. The radiopaque properties of Lipiodol help to make it visible during embolization procedure. Once injected into the vessel, the fat droplets get released and travel distally into smaller vessels till they cannot cross due to their size and then occlude the vessel. This level of distal embolization is at the level of small arterioles. It is commonly used mixed with glue for embolization. The radiopacity of Lipiodol adds contrast to glue while the oil-based structure does not allow glue to solidify within the syringe/catheter till it comes in contact with ionic blood. Lipiodol is also used for embolization of hepatocellular carcinoma in combination with chemotherapeutic agents. It has affinity for the lesion and gets deposited in it even when injected non-selectively besides providing radio-opacity to the mixture.

Temporary Proximal Occluders

- **Gelatin sponge**: It is most commonly used in the form of gelfoam. It is available as a block which is cut into small pledgets and is made as a slurry mixed with contrast agent for intravascular injection. It leads to temporary mechanical occlusion of proximal vessels for a period of one week to few months. It is used in situations where preservation of blood flow is required in the long-term, e.g., to control bleeding from liver, spleen and in immediate preoperative embolization of tumors. Being inexpensive and easy to use, it is often used as a scaffold for combined embolization with coils.
- **Autologous clot**: Used for very short-term temporary embolization as it gets lysed within few hours. May be used in coagulopathic patients to control bleeding.
- **Nondetachable occlusion balloon**: Used in specific situations like before surgery to reduce intraoperative blood loss, for precise placement of embolic material or to reduce reflux of embolizing material into parent vessel.

Temporary Distal Occluders

- **Starch microspheres**: These are produced from vegetable sources like corn and potato. They are used for very short duration (few minutes) occlusion of distal small vessels, e.g., in procedures like intra-arterial chemotherapy.
- **Gelatin-sponge powder**: It is also available in powder form. When delivered it reaches distal circulation to block it temporarily.

2. Classify the commonly used embolizing agents. Discuss their advantages, disadvantages, and clinical applications. [3+(2+2+3)] [DNB June 20]

The idea behind catheter-directed embolization is to use a temporary or permanent agent to mechanically obstruct a blood artery or vascular region, therefore abruptly stopping flow.

In the history of interventional radiology, embolization has been a distinctive defining procedure, along with angioplasty.

The technique's beauty highlights the benefits of less invasive treatment.

Since the first autologous clot instances were documented in 1972, embolization procedures have advanced with the use of numerous agents and tools to produce genuinely remarkable outcomes.

Embolizing agents can be broadly divided into four main categories:

- Permanent proximal occluders
- Permanent distal occluders
- Temporary proximal occluders
- Temporary distal occluders

Permanent Proximal Occluders

- **Coils**: Made of steel or platinum, commonly have constituent thrombogenic polyester fibers.
  - Upon delivery to the target vessel, coils form a scaffolding helping in thrombus formation. They are introduced in a straight shape but become spring at the time of deployment.
  - Nester coils are special fiber coils which are soft and pliable.
  - Coils are offered in a range of diameters from 0.010 to 0.052 inch.
  - Coils may be pushable or detachable.
  - Coils mostly used to permanently occlude relatively large vessel.
- **Amplatzer vascular plug**: Self-expandable agent made of nitinol mesh.
  - Used to occlude vessel ranging from 4 to 16 mm diameter.

Permanent Distal Occluders

- **PVA particles**: Made of inert plastic particles:
  - Comes in various sizes ranging from 100 to 1100 μm.
  - They come in a dry powder form, before use they need to be suspended in normal saline or contrast.
  - Very effective in embolization of tumor bed, reduction of tumor vascularity.
  - Used in bronchial artery, uterine artery embolization.
  - **Disadvantage**: If larger sizes are used, chance of clumping in the vessel or within the catheter is there.
  - **Advantage**: There is always a chance of second embolization.
- **Sclerosants**: These are liquid agents which causes vessel thrombosis by inflammation.
  - Absolute alcohol—permanent occlusion with cell death
    - Used where permanent damage is desirable, like-renal cell carcinoma
    - Disadvantage—painful condition, requiting anesthesia.
  - Sodium tetradecyl sulfate—3% used
    - Used in venous malformation, pelvic congestion, etc.
    - Milder sclerosant than absolute alcohol.

- **Cyanoacrylates**:
  - Most commonly used—N-butyl cyanoacrylates
  - Tissue adhesive
  - In presence of ionic environment, it gets polymerized
  - Delivered by catheter with non-ionic fluid flash before and after
  - Used with radio-opaque substance—Lipiodol
  - **Advantages**:
    - Amount of thrombus is higher than expected
    - Relatively cheaper than coils
- **Onyx**:
  - Combination of ethylene-vinyl alcohol, dimethyl sulfoxide and tantalum powder.
  - Comes in two vials which needs to be mixed and shaken well 20 minutes before the use.
  - Better control than glue but high cost.
- **Thrombin**: Component of coagulation, mainly used for hemostasis
- **Ethiodiol**: Brand name—Lipiodol
  - Radio-opaque
  - Oil based, often used with glue
  - Once released, fat droplets deposited into the distal small arterioles
  - **Use**—in HCC with chemotherapeutic agent [by Trans-arterial chemo embolization (TACE)]
  - **Advantage**—radio-opaque, traceable post intervention
  - Has affinity to lesion, even in case of non-selective embolization it gets deposited in lesion.

Temporary Proximal Occluders

- **Gelatin sponge**:
  - Most commonly known as gelfoam.
  - Useful for temporarily occluding the vascular supply.
  - Comes in block which are cut into small pieces and mixed with contrast to apply.
  - Used for pre-operative tumor embolization, stop bleeding from liver, spleen, etc.
- **Autologous clot**: Short-term treatment, gets dissolved in hours.

Temporary Distal Occluders

- **Starch microsphere**:
  - Made of vegetable sources
  - Can stop bleeding for few minutes
  - Used in TACE.
- **Gelatin sponge powder**

REFERENCE

1. Khandelwal N, Gupta AK, Chowdhury V, editors. AIIMS-MAMC-PGI's Comprehensive Textbook of Diagnostic Radiology. New Delhi: Jaypee Brothers Medical Publishers (P) Ltd.; 2016.

CHAPTER

8 Biomedical Research

Soumik Das, Suparna Sahu

QUESTIONS

1. What is plagiarism in scientific writing? What are the various common types of plagiarism? Describe, how plagiarism can be detected in scientific writings. Briefly mention a few measures to avoid plagiarism. [1+4+2+3] [DNB June 20, MD (WBUHS) 24]
2. (a) Predatory journals and publishing. (b) Techniques of randomization of samples in a research study. [5+5] [DNB June 20]

ANSWERS

1. What is plagiarism in scientific writing? What are the various common types of plagiarism? Describe, how plagiarism can be detected in scientific writings. Briefly mention a few measures to avoid plagiarism. [1+4+2+3] [DNB June 20, MD (WBUHS) 24]

Plagiarism in Scientific Writing

Plagiarism is the act of representing someone else's ideas, language, or work as your own:[1,2]

- Using another person's ideas, language, or original knowledge without acknowledging the source
- Passing off another person's work as your own
- Presenting an existing idea as original or new:
  - Most common form of plagiarism is copying text word-for-word
  - Considered as serious publication misconduct

Types

- **Self-plagiarism**: Duplication of own work or publishing separately
- **Salami slicing**: Publishing parts of work in different journals, not publishing the paper as a total unit
- **Paraphrasing plagiarism**: Changing a few phrases or even the entire text from a source with maintenance of the key thing
- **Direct plagiarism**: Intentionally copying other's work or manuscript and publish by own name
- **Mosaic plagiarism**: Content taken from multiple sources without proper citation
- **Source based plagiarism**: When person uses information from a source but during citation mention it differently
- **Complete plagiarism**: Stealing someone else's work and presenting it as your own
- **Accidental plagiarism**: Occurrence is more than expectation; unintentionally one author using other's writing. It is because huge amount of data is available for a single topic.

Four-stage Plagiarism Detection Process

Text-based plagiarism: This is the detection of similarities between documents.

- It includes identification of redundancy or similarity of wards, tables, charts, images, etc., in case of partially plagiarized document, chance of detection is low.
- Following are the stages of detection of plagiarism on the basis of text:
  - **Stage one**: Collection of information
  - **Stage two**: Analysis—check for similarity.
  - **Stage three**: Confirmation
  - **Stage four**: Investigation—it relies on human intelligence; someone has to check the information depicted is true or false.

Different Techniques for Detection of Textual Plagiarism

- **Grammar-based method**: Focuses on the grammar of the documents, and measure similarity between the documents. This method is suitable for detection of exact replica devoid of any modification.
- **External plagiarism detection method**: Checking the citations, from which a specific portion or para may have been taken.
- **Citation-based method**: Proper citation at proper places done or not.

Software-based tools for plagiarism detection: Some software systems are commercially available that can determine reliably if a submitted document or an online text is plagiarized or not. These software can only compare the syntax, at the level of a word or character, and try to determine if any similarity exists between the texts. Experimental work is currently ongoing in the domain of semantic recognition. However, this seems successful only in case of a highly structured text, e.g., program language code.

- PlagAware
- PlagScan
- CheckForPlagiarism.net
- iThenticate
- PlagiarismDetection.org
- Viper

Ways to avoid plagiarism in your writing:

- **Proper citation**: Actual and serial wise citation is a key to avoid plagiarism.
- **Include quotations**: If a source's words are inserted into the writing, verbatim, then one of the simplest ways to avoid plagiarism is to use quotation marks around the said text. The source should always be cited in a direct quote.
- **Paraphrase**: Paraphrasing is rewriting an idea or information in your own language, without altering its meaning. Successful paraphrasing without plagiarizing requires a bit of effort. The writing needs to be formatted in original way avoiding too many similar phrases or words from the source. Even then, the source should be cited because another person's idea is being used.
- **Present your own idea**: Always present your own idea of the matter. Contribute a unique perspective on the topic in your writing.
    - If the same topic is being written for multiple assignments, some of the author's previous words may be used—this is named "self-plagiarism". However, this is illegal unless permission has been obtained from publisher regarding reuse of one's own work.
- **Use a plagiarism checker**: Using a plagiarism checking tool can help the author to catch any inadvertent use of phrases before submitting his work.

These tools also show the source from which the text or phrases have been copied.

2. (a) Predatory journals and publishing. (b) Techniques of randomization of samples in a research study. [5+5] [DNB June 20]

(a) **Predatory journals and publishing**: Predatory journals are publishers that encourages unethical publication by seeking money from the authors. They can exploit the authors either by taking money without publishing the paper or can publish the paper without proper peer review or checking.

Characteristics:

- The primary aim is to make money
- Minimal checking or editing
- Quick response
- False demand about impact factor or indexing
- Using ISSN incorrectly
- Very less information about editorial board and peer review system
- Hidden fees
- Poor website link
- Republishing published paper
- Unauthorized use of images
    - One must be very careful about the indexing—PUBMED, DOAJ, Google scholar; these are some authentic indices.
- One must be very aware of this publisher as many times academic and career achievement depends upon paper publication.

Cabell's Blacklist: A New Way to Tackle Predatory Journals:

- Jeffrey Beall, Librarian at the University of Colorado in Denver, coined the term "predatory publishers."
- It was launched on June 15.
- It would publish both "Black List" and "White List".
- Approximately 4,000 journals were included in the list.

- Both subscription-based and open access—journals are included.
- The whitelist database includes 18 academic disciplines from more than 13,000 international scholarly publications as per the website.

Importance of peer-review: It is the scrutiny of someone's work by other expert in the same field to validate the authenticity and check the quality. Ethical aspect of the paper was also taken care of.

Solutions: Some software tools are there to check the authenticity of journals.

- **Endnote manuscript matcher**: After login, it can suggest journal by checking the keywords, title and abstract. At the same time, it also denotes impact factor of journals.
- **Journal/author name estimator (JANE)**: Tags journal indexed in MEDLINE OR DOAJ.
- **IEEE publication recommender**: It matches periodicals, submission to publication time to suggest best journal for publishing.

(b) **Techniques of randomization of samples in a research study**: Randomization is a research strategy that randomly assigns participants to different groups in a clinical trial or study.[3]

Purpose: Randomization prevents bias and ensures that the results are trustworthy:

- **Bias**: Bias occurs when factors other than the treatment being tested affect the results. For example, a doctor might assign healthier patients to the new treatment group, making it seem more effective.
- **Validity**: Randomization increases the validity of clinical trials by producing comparable study groups.

How it works: Participants are randomly assigned to groups using a method that ensures each participant has an equal chance of being assigned to any group. Neither the researcher nor the participant chooses which treatment the participant will receive.

Methods: Randomization can be done using:

- **Simple randomization**: Randomization based on a single sequence of random assignments is known as simple randomization.
- **Block randomization**: The block randomization method is designed to randomize participants into groups that result in equal sample sizes. This method is used to ensure a balance in sample size across groups over time. Blocks are small and balanced with predetermined group assignments, which keeps the numbers of participants in each group similar at all times.
- **Stratified randomization**: The stratified randomization method addresses the need to control and balance the influence of covariates. This method can be used to achieve balance among groups in terms of participants' baseline characteristics (covariates).
    - Specific covariates must be identified by the researcher who understands the potential influence each covariate has on the dependent variable. Stratified randomization is achieved by generating a separate block for each combination of covariates, and participants are assigned to the appropriate block of covariates. After all participants have been identified and assigned into blocks, simple randomization occurs within each block to assign participants to one of the groups.
    - The stratified randomization method controls for the possible influence of covariates that would jeopardize the conclusions of the clinical trial.
- **Covariate adaptive randomization**: Covariate adaptive randomization has been recommended by many researchers as a valid alternative randomization method for clinical trials. In covariate adaptive randomization, a new participant is sequentially assigned to a particular treatment group by taking into account the specific covariates and previous assignments of participants. Covariate adaptive randomization uses the method of minimization by assessing the imbalance of sample size among several covariates.

The salient features of different techniques of randomization are outlined in **Table 1**.[3]

TABLE 1: Salient features of different techniques of randomization.

Simple randomization	• Single sequence of random assignment • Simple and easy method • Computer can generate random numbers to allocate people if groups • Difficult for small number of participants

Continued...

Continued...

Block randomization	• The purpose is to randomize subjects into groups so as to maintain the sample size equal • Useful for small sample size to maintain balance • Small blocks are made • Once the block size has been established, all possible combinations of assignments within the block must be determined
Stratified randomization	• Stratified randomization is done by generating separate blocks for each and every combination of covariates, and the participants are allocated to the specified block of covariates. After that, simple randomization within each block is done to assign the participants to one of these groups. • The stratified randomization method controls for the possible influence of covariates that would jeopardize the conclusions of the clinical trial.
Covariate adaptive randomization	In this method of randomization, new participant is assigned sequentially to a particular group after taking into account all the specific covariates and the previous assignments of the participants.

Flowchart 1 depicts selecting appropriate randomization technique.[3]

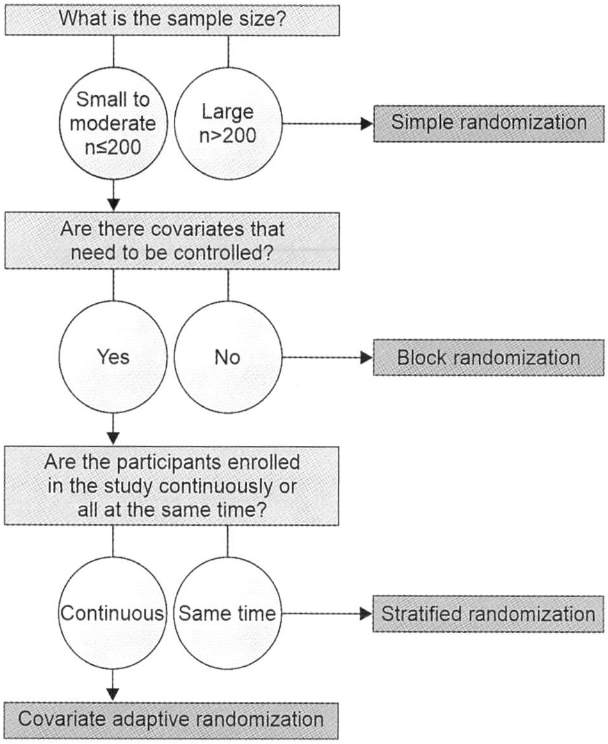

FLOWCHART 1: Selecting appropriate randomization technique. The gray boxes represent appropriate techniques.

Randomization is important because it:

- Ensures that the effects of the treatment can be compared fairly
- Prevents false results due to bias
- Produces comparable study groups in terms of baseline risk factors
- Eliminates or minimizes systematic error
- Ensures uniform distribution of confounders between groups.

REFERENCES

1. Sengupta S, Honavar SG. Publication ethics. Indian J Ophthalmol. 2017;65(6):429-32.
2. Sheikh A. Publication ethics and the research assessment exercise: Reflections on the troubled question of authorship. J Med Ethics. 2000;26(6):422-6.
3. Kang M, Ragan BG, Park JH. Issues in outcomes research: An overview of randomization techniques for clinical trials. J Athl Training. 2008;43(2):215-21.